T0179227

Alcohol, Drugs, and Impaired Driving

Alcohol, Drugs, and Impaired Driving

Forensic Science and Law Enforcement Issues

Edited by
A. Wayne Jones
Jørg G. Mørland
Ray H. Liu

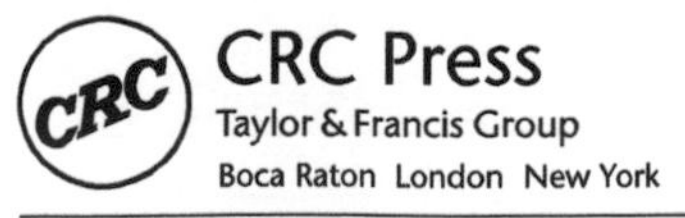

CRC Press is an imprint of the
Taylor & Francis Group, an **informa** business

First edition published 2020
by CRC Press
6000 Broken Sound Parkway NW, Suite 300, Boca Raton, FL 33487-2742

and by CRC Press
2 Park Square, Milton Park, Abingdon, Oxon, OX14 4RN

ISBN: 978-0-367-25162-8 (hbk)
ISBN: 978-1-003-03079-9 (ebk)

Typeset in Minion
by Lumina Datamatics Limited

In Fond Remembrance of Two Inspirational Leaders
in Traffic Safety and Police Science on Two Continents

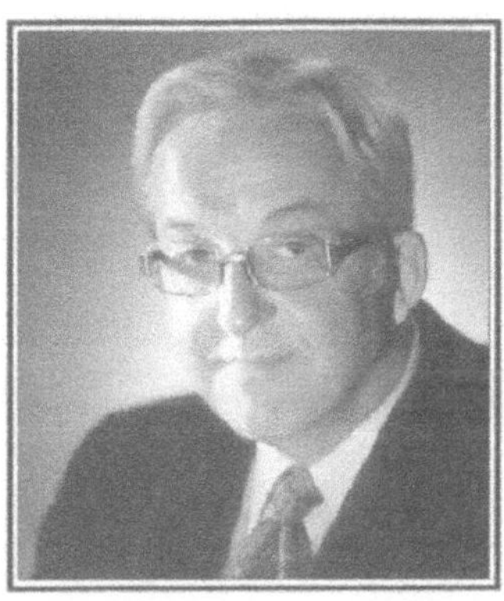

Robert F. Borkenstein, AB, HonScD, HonLLD
(August 31, 1912–August 10, 2002)
Indiana University
Bloomington, Indiana
United States of America

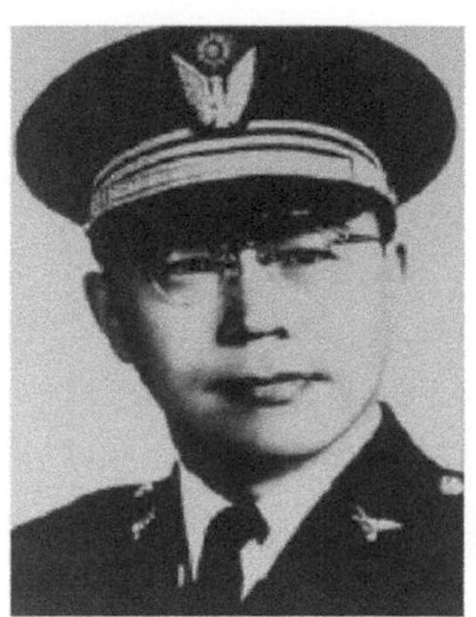

Ko-wang Mei, BA, MA, PhD
(March 16, 1918–April 1, 2016)
Central Police University
Taipei
Taiwan

Contents

Section V

EPIDEMIOLOGY, ENFORCEMENT, AND COUNTERMEASURES

Foreword

I am delighted to have been invited by three of my esteemed colleagues—the editors of this book—to write a foreword. The book represents a comprehensive and timely review of the multidisciplinary field of alcohol, drugs, and traffic safety—science, research, public policy, and litigation. The editors have assembled an outstanding roster of contributors, representing an international "who's who" of academics, researchers, and thought leaders in the field. The various chapters give a broad perspective of the past, present, and future of the science of alcohol, drugs, and impaired driving.

The field has reached a level of maturity, reflected by the many international efforts towards science-based laws and countermeasures, including widespread adoption of zero-tolerance and concentration *per se* laws for both illicit and selected licit psychoactive drugs in a driver's blood; use of emerging technologies, such as roadside analysis of drugs in oral fluid; and collection of more reliable information about the negative influence of drugs on human performance and traffic safety. New problems requiring scientific solutions will, however, always emerge, as exemplified by the current trend in the United States and elsewhere towards legalization of marijuana use and the negative impact this might have on public health and traffic safety.

My own involvement in the field of alcohol, drugs, and impaired driving began in 1990, as the newly appointed Washington State program director with responsibility for blood-/breath-alcohol testing and postmortem toxicology. I found myself working alongside Sergeant Rod Gullberg (author of two chapters in this book), who supervised the Washington State Patrol breath-test program. Not knowing what to expect from a police sergeant, but assuming that my task was to add scientific credentials to the program, I quickly realized that Rod was an expert on quality assurance aspects of breath-alcohol analysis and reliability of the results when these are used as evidence for prosecution of traffic offenders. Through Rod I was introduced to many of the world's leading experts, including Professor Robert (Bob) Borkenstein (1912–2002), Professor Alan Wayne Jones, and Professor Kurt M. Dubowski (1921–2017), all of whom were members of the faculty of the legendary Borkenstein Course on Alcohol and Highway Safety, held biannually at Indiana University (Bloomington campus).

In 1991 Dr. Jones nominated me as a member of the National Safety Council Committee on Alcohol and Other Drugs (NSC-CAOD) as well as the International Council on Alcohol, Drugs and Traffic Safety (ICADTS). By attending ICADTS meetings I met Professor Jørg G. Mørland—then head of the Division of Forensic Toxicology, the Norwegian Institute of Public Health, a leading international research group actively engaged in the emerging field of drug impaired driving.

In the United States in the 1960s through the 1990s, Professor Borkenstein was a leading voice and inspiration for research and policy in promoting traffic safety. Professor Borkenstein was also a driving force in developing interest in alcohol, drugs, and traffic safety worldwide as a long-serving president of ICADTS (1969–1983). During his tenure at Indiana University (where the Borkenstein Alcohol Course continues to this day, recently celebrating its 60th anniversary), Dr. Borkenstein influenced the lives of many of the major contributors to the field of traffic safety. Among others, Dr. Doug Lucas, an internationally renowned Canadian forensic scientist and director emeritus of the Centre of Forensic Sciences in Toronto, spearheaded introduction of the Borkenstein Breathalyzer® instrument in his home province and throughout the country. Indeed, Breathalyzer results served as the primary evidence for prosecuting drunken drivers throughout the United States, Canada, and Australia.

Dr. Ray Liu, who has been the editor-in-chief of the influential journal *Forensic Science Review* (FSR) for over 30 years, was a graduate student of Borkenstein and did an internship under Dr. Lucas in Toronto. Later, Dr. Liu was appointed professor and head of the Forensic Science Program at the University of Alabama, Birmingham, where he is currently professor emeritus. Dr. Liu has been continuously working with his mentor Dr. Ko-wang Mei (1918–2016), retired president of the Taiwanese Central Police University, and younger colleagues in further development of forensic science in his native Taiwan.

The network of influential scientists and policy makers contributing chapters to this book devoted to the subject of alcohol, drugs, and impaired driving will help to raise the profile of this important public health and safety issue. These individuals have already made significant contributions through their writings and research and have encouraged, trained, and/or mentored many of today's leaders in the field.

This book is a compilation of peer-reviewed articles previously published in FSR, most of which have been updated to include recent developments and current status of the subject matter. In addition, several new articles are included from the July 2019 and January 2020 issues of the journal. The readers of this book owe a debt of gratitude to the authors of the various chapters for their career-long contributions to the field of alcohol, drugs, and traffic safety. Others can trace their introduction to the subject of impaired driving to attending various ICADTS meetings and also as participants at the Borkenstein Alcohol and Drug Courses.

Most of the advances in road-traffic safety made in the United States, especially in the 1960s to 1980s, have a direct link to Dr. Borkenstein and the Center for Studies of Law in Action, which he founded at Indiana University. I attended the Borkenstein Alcohol Course as a student and novice researcher in 1990, and today I am proud to serve as its executive director.

The many and sustained contributions made by Dr. Borkenstein have had a major impact on the field of traffic safety, both in the United States and internationally, which is reflected in the narrative of various chapters in this book. First and foremost, he invented the Breathalyzer® instrument in 1954, which became the principal means of enforcing drunk-driving laws throughout North America when traffic offenders were prosecuted. In 1963–1964 Dr. Borkenstein led a team of researchers that produced the landmark "Grand Rapids Study," an epidemiological survey of crash risk in relation to a drivers' blood- and breath-alcohol concentration. There is no doubt that Dr. Borkenstein's efforts helped to change public opinion about drinking alcohol before driving, and his legacy continues to inspire new research initiatives in the on-going fight to improve traffic safety.

Barry K. Logan, PhD, F-ABFT
Executive Director, Center for Studies of Law in Action, Indiana University
Executive Director, Center for Forensic Science Research and Education
Chief Scientist, NMS Labs
ICADTS Widmark Award Laureate 2013

Preface

The contents of this book were derived from articles previously published in *Forensic Science Review* (FSR), an international peer-reviewed journal established in 1989 to publish invited review articles covering all aspects of the forensic sciences. To commemorate FSR's over 30 years of continuous publication, the July 2019 issue was devoted to the subject of *"Alcohol, Drugs, and Impaired Driving."* Three of the articles from this special edition of FSR are included in the book. Other chapters are updated versions of selected articles previously published in FSR on the subject of alcohol, drugs, and driving. Some authors made extensive revisions and opted to modify the titles of the articles published as book chapters.

Forensic science is a multidisciplinary subject dealing with the application of a wide range of scientific methods and techniques for the investigation of criminal offenses by examination of physical and biological evidence. This interaction between science and law makes the discipline of *impaired driving and the use of chemical evidence for prosecution of traffic offenders* an important sub-domain of the forensic sciences. The main key words for the chapters included in this book are:

> Alcohol, Analysis, Biomarkers of Alcohol Abuse, Blood, Breath, Crash-Risk, Drugged Driving, Drugs, Drunk-Driving, Epidemiology, Ethanol, Forensics, Impairment, Interlocks, Law Enforcement, Psychoactive Substances, Substance Abuse, Toxicology, Traffic Safety.

****

Sir Winston Churchill (1874–1965) is claimed to have said "*Those who fail to learn from history are doomed to repeat it.*" Others have added that in order to understand any scientific discipline you need to know its history. With this sound advice, we are keen to acknowledge the individuals who were instrumental in advancing knowledge about impaired driving and improving the way that traffic offenders are prosecuted. One man in particular deserves special mention and that is Professor Robert Frank Borkenstein (1912–2002), Department of Criminal Justice, Indiana University (Bloomington, IN, US). Dr. Borkenstein served as president of the International Council on Alcohol, Drugs, and Traffic Safety (ICADTS) between 1969 and 1983. On the occasion of the 6th ICADTS meeting held in Toronto in 1974 Dr. Borkenstein became the third recipient of the prestigious Widmark award.

When Dr. Borkenstein died, obituaries appeared in several scientific journals as well as national and international newspapers, exemplified by the *New York Times*, *The Washington Post*, *The Times of London*, *The Independent* (UK), *The Guardian* (UK), *The Economist*, and even *Time Magazine*. A summary of the life and work of Dr. Borkenstein, with focus on the man and his impact was written by his friend and colleague from Toronto, Dr. Douglas Lucas, whose tribute is included as Chapter 2 in this book.

Dr. Borkenstein made two fundamental contributions to the field of alcohol and traffic safety. The first was the development of the Breathalyzer instrument in 1954, the availability of which simplified and strengthened the scientific evidence necessary for successful prosecution of drunken drivers. The Breathalyzer was approved for use by police forces in Australia, Canada, and throughout the US. The wide acceptance and approval of the Breathalyzer prompted police authorities to allocate more resources in the fight against drunken driving and intensify their efforts to remove drunken drivers from the roads and highways.

The second major contribution made by Dr. Borkenstein was to the design and execution of a large-scale epidemiological study to determine the risk of involvement in a traffic crash in relation to a driver's blood-alcohol concentration (BAC). This became known as the "Grand Rapids Study" named after the city in Michigan where a roadside survey of drivers was conducted in 1963 and 1964. In this case-controlled study, the Breathalyzer instrument was used to test drivers involved in crashes and compare results with a control group of motorists not involved in crashes. The latter group was matched in various ways in terms of demographics and other variables with the drivers involved in crashes.

****

This first part of the book (Section I) consists of a single chapter (Chapter 1) that looks back at historical developments in drunk and drugged driving legislation worldwide. Although driving under the influence of alcohol is as old as motor-driven transportation dating to the start of the twentieth century, the impairment caused by other drugs did not attract much attention until the 1950s. Driving under the influence of non-alcohol drugs then became a separate criminal offence and proof of impairment depended on the results of clinical tests of impairment done by a physician or police surgeon. More recently, the concept of establishing concentration *per se* limits in blood, as done with BAC, has been extended to cover other psychoactive substances, both prescription medications and illicit recreational drugs of abuse.

The second part of the book (Section II) comprises three chapters of historical interest and important events, including a tribute to the life and work of Professor Borkenstein (Chapter 2) and a chapter by Patricia Waller, PhD (Chapter 3) dealing with the Grand Rapids Study. She emphasizes that driving with BAC above 0.04% is definitely associated with an increased crash risk. The probability of a crash increases rapidly as BACs reach 0.08%, and is extremely high at 0.15%. Single vehicle crashes were more common in drivers with higher BAC as was the severity of their injuries and material damage was also more extensive.

Dr. Waller was an authority on the subject of injury prevention in connection with traffic safety research. She was among a group of experts invited to attend a symposium held in Taipei, Taiwan on December 1–2, 1999 to honor the many contributions made by Dr. Borkenstein to traffic safety research. In honor of Dr. Waller (1932–2003) and her contributions to the field of traffic safety research, we include an unabridged version of her article in this book.

Chapter 4 presents a historical survey of the evolution of qualitative and quantitative methods for the determination of ethanol in blood and breath for legal purposes.

The third part of the book (Section III) focuses primarily on driving impairment caused by excessive drinking and the enforcement of BAC *per se* laws. The first chapter Chapter 5 discusses the pros and cons of BAC as evidence for prosecuting traffic offenders compared with methods of breath-alcohol analysis for evidential testing. The latter are more convenient and non-invasive; they provide on-the-spot results and permit making decisions about whether a driving permit should be revoked or a vehicle impounded.

The technology available for breath-alcohol analysis has improved considerably since the days of the Breathalyzer, and the use of micro-processors allows automated sampling of breath, detection of mouth alcohol, and calibration control of the accuracy of results, etc. The performance of modern instruments for breath-alcohol analysis matches the accuracy and precision of BAC determinations by gas-liquid chromatography. Nevertheless, results of forensic breath-alcohol analysis are more often challenged in a legal context, probably because of the weight given to this type of chemistry-based evidence in drunken-driving litigation.

Chapter 6 reviews the merits of common defense arguments and court decisions reached when scientific evidence in drunken driving cases is challenged. Because of the importance attached to the results of blood- and breath-alcohol testing, the analytical methods used require careful validation using rigorous quality assurance (QA) procedures to ensure that the methodology is fit for its intended purpose. The background and statistical methods applied in QA of forensic breath-alcohol testing are included in this section as Chapter 7.

Chapter 8 is a forensic primer on the subject of ethanol pharmacokinetics. Aspects of absorption, distribution, metabolism, and excretion of alcohol often arise in a typical drunken-driving prosecution. For example, this might entail comparing BAC with the quantity of alcohol a person admits drinking before driving. Another common request is to perform a back calculation of BAC from time of sampling blood to an earlier time, such as the time of driving, which is often several hours earlier. The practice of back-calculating a person's BAC is a mandatory requirement in some jurisdictions, and this requires knowledge of the many factors influencing the clinical pharmacokinetics of ethanol.

The final chapter (Chapter 9) in Section III deals with the increasing use of biomarkers to detect heavy drinking and the use of this information in forensic casework. Use of biomarkers is particularly important when dealing with repeat offenders because many suffer from an alcohol-use disorder and might clinically be diagnosed as being alcohol dependent. Before these individuals are sentenced, and when they apply for relicensing, objective evidence of their current drinking habits is obviously important. This can be achieved by the determination of various biomarkers, including liver enzymes (AST, ALT, and GGT), and other markers, such as MCV, CDT, EtG, and Peth.

The fourth part of the book (Section IV) shifts the focus toward the role played by drugs other than alcohol in causing driver impairment. Although drunken driving is the more serious problem for road-traffic safety, the prevalence of drivers impaired by non-alcohol drugs is rapidly increasing. Inappropriate use of prescription medications (such as sleep aids, anti-anxiety agents, and pain medications), as well as other drugs active in the central nervous system are hazardous for traffic safety. Added to this is the problem of taking psychoactive recreational drugs for pleasure and excitement, such as central stimulants (amphetamines and cocaine) and cannabis/marijuana. The latter represents a serious challenge for traffic safety because of the emphasis on legalizing/decriminalizing its use in some jurisdictions. Chapter 10 gives a broad overview of driving under the influence of non-alcohol drugs and the state of knowledge until the end of the twentieth century. Chapters 11 and 12 update this knowledge to the twenty-first century and delve deeper into experimental and epidemiological studies of impairment caused by certain classes of psychoactive drugs, which are over-represented in crash statistics. The quantitative relationships and the strength of the evidence relating impairment of body functions and the concentrations of active substances in blood are reviewed in depth. The final chapter

(Chapter 13) in Section IV looks at international trends in alcohol and drug use among motor vehicle drivers, the prevalence of road traffic crashes (RTC) involving impaired drivers, and the importance of study design, law enforcement strategies, and the toxicological methods used to confirm intake of impairing substances.

The final part of the book (Section V) is concerned with the epidemiology of impaired driving and the choice of enforcement strategies to deter traffic offenders and reduce their involvement in road traffic crashes. Revocation of driving permits is not always effective, because many drivers—especially hardcore offenders—continue to drive even without a valid license. Chapter 14 attempts to place alcohol-impaired driving in a public health perspective and underscores the importance of enforcing concentration *per se* alcohol limits for driving and paying more attention to improving the detection and prosecution of traffic offenders.

The relationship between alcohol/drug use and impairment can be assessed in various ways and with different types of methodological approaches. This is the subject of Chapter 15, which explores the relevance of controlled laboratory studies of drug influence, the use of computer software and driving simulators, as well as on-the-road driving tests under real-world conditions. These different methodologies have certain advantages and limitations. For safety and ethical reasons, human dosing studies are limited to therapeutic amounts of the medication, often a single acute dose, which is unlike many apprehended drivers who overdose and also combine multiple psychoactive substances. The authors present unequivocal evidence of the impairment effects of various classes of drugs on skills necessary for safe driving, and they reiterate the importance of toxicological analysis of blood samples from all victims of road traffic crashes, thus furnishing real-world case studies.

The final two chapters in Section V take a closer look at the effectiveness of various sanctions to deter and diminish driving under the influence of alcohol and/or drugs. Foremost among these, in the case of alcohol, is the fitting of ignition interlock devices to vehicles owned by a convicted drunken driver (Chapter 16). This necessitates that a person must pass a breath-alcohol test before being able to start and drive their vehicle. This approach has proven particularly effective in reducing recidivism among hard-core traffic delinquents. The final chapter (Chapter 17) looks at various approaches for reducing impaired driving, such as evidence-based legislation, more effective law enforcement deterrence strategies, and options for different ways of sentencing, including drug or DUI courts and mandatory treatment and rehabilitation programs in lieu of jail for a DUI or DUID conviction.

A. Wayne Jones, Jørg G. Mørland, and Ray H. Liu

Editors

Professor **A. Wayne Jones** earned a BSc degree (1969) and a PhD degree (1974) in chemistry from the University of Wales (Cardiff, UK). In 2013 Dr. Jones retired from his appointment as senior scientist at Sweden's National Laboratory of Forensic Medicine, Division of Forensic Genetics and Forensic Toxicology (Linköping, Sweden). He currently serves as a guest professor at the Department of Clinical Pharmacology, Division of Drug Research at University of Linköping, Sweden.

Prof. Jones's doctoral thesis was entitled "Equilibrium Partition Studies of Alcohol in Biological Fluids" which dealt with analytical and physiological aspects of ethanol analysis in blood and exhaled breath. Since 1973, his research activities have involved studies of the pharmacology and toxicology of ethanol and other drugs of abuse. He has been particularly interested in the determination of ethanol and drugs in biological specimens from living and deceased persons, as well as the disposition and fate of psychoactive substances in the body and their detrimental effects on performance and behavior. Dr. Jones received a senior doctorate degree (DSc) from the University of Wales in 1993 for his body of published work entitled: "Methods of Analysis, Distribution and Metabolism in the Body and Biological Effects of Alcohol and Narcotics."

Since his first publication in 1974, Dr. Jones's name now appears as author or co-author on more than 400 journal articles, reviews, and book chapters, most of which were published in peer-reviewed journals. His publications are widely cited in scientific articles, and also in court cases involving driving under the influence of alcohol and/or other drugs.

In recognition of his career-long contributions to the field of forensic science and toxicology, Dr. Jones has received numerous awards including the Widmark Award from the International Council on Alcohol, Drugs and Traffic Safety (ICADTS) in 1997.

Professor **Jørg G. Mørland** earned an MD degree from the University of Oslo in 1967 and a PhD degree in pharmacology from the same university in 1975. Dr. Mørland is now a senior scientist at the Division of Health Data and Digitalization of the Norwegian Institute of Public Health and a professor emeritus at the University of Oslo.

Throughout his professional career, Dr. Mørland has served as professor of pharmacology at the University of Oslo and the University of Tromsø (Tromsø, Norway), director of the former Norwegian National Institute of Forensic Toxicology, and was director of the Division of Forensic Medicine and Drug Abuse Research of the Norwegian Institute of Public Health (Oslo, Norway) until 2012.

He is a medical specialist in clinical pharmacology. His main research field is biomedical effects of alcohol and drugs of abuse, their metabolites and metabolism. He has been the principal supervisor for approximately 30 PhD students, as well as the scientific project manager for several projects supported by the Research Council of Norway.

Dr. Mørland has published more than 400 articles in peer-reviewed journals on pharmacology, toxicology, forensic medicine, neuroscience, alcoholism, epidemiology, drug analysis, and road-traffic safety. He has also written more than 8,000 expert-witness statements for the police and courts in Norway and has appeared hundreds of times as an expert witness in courts at all levels in Norway as well as in some Swedish courts.

He was the recipient of a Widmark Award from the International Council on Alcohol, Drugs and Traffic Safety (ICADTS) in 2004.

Professor **Ray H. Liu** began his career with a degree in law (1965) from the police academy (now Central Police University) in Taiwan before earning a PhD (1976) in chemistry from Southern Illinois University (Carbondale, IL). Before his doctoral thesis, Dr. Liu studied forensic science under the guidance of Professor Robert F. Borkenstein at Indiana University (Bloomington, IN) and received internship training at the Centre of Forensic Sciences in Toronto, Canada, headed by Dr. Doug Lucas.

Dr. Liu has held positions at the University of Illinois at Chicago (Chicago, IL), the US Environmental Protection Agency's Central Regional Laboratory (Chicago, IL), and the US Department of Agriculture's Eastern Regional Research Center (Philadelphia, PA) and Southern Regional Research Center (New Orleans, LA). He was a faculty member at the University of Alabama at Birmingham (UAB) for 20 years (serving as the director of the University's graduate program in forensic science for the last 10 years) before his retirement in 2004; he was granted professor emeritus status in 2005. Following his retirement from UAB, Dr. Liu taught at Fooyin University (Kaohsiung, Taiwan) for 8 years (2004–2012).

Dr. Liu's scientific works have been mainly in the field of analytical and toxicological chemistry of drugs of abuse (criminalistics and forensic toxicology), with a significant number of publications in each of the following areas: enantiomeric analysis, quantitative determination using isotopic analogs as internal standards, correlation of immunoassay and GC-MS test results, specimen source differentiation, and analytical method development. He has authored/edited (or coauthored/coedited) approximately 150 journal articles, book chapters, and 5 books. Dr. Liu has long served as editor-in-chief of *Forensic Science Review* and is a member of the editorial boards for several international journals.

Contributors

Federica Bortolotti
Department of Diagnostics and Public Health
University of Verona
Verona, Italy

Dennis V. Canfield
Civil Aerospace Medical Institute
Federal Aviation Administration
Oklahoma City, Oklahoma

Asbjørg S. Christophersen
Department of International Public Health
Norwegian Institute of Public Health
Oslo, Norway

Mack Cowan
Texas Department of Public Safety
Austin, Texas

Kurt M. Dubowski (1921–2017)
Oklahoma University Health Sciences Center
Oklahoma City, Oklahoma

James C. Fell
Department of Economics, Justice, and Society
National Opinion Research Center (NORC) at the University of Chicago
Bethesda, Maryland

Hallvard Gjerde
Department of Forensic Sciences
Oslo University Hospital
Oslo, Norway

Rod G. Gullberg
Clearview Statistical Consulting
Snohomish, Washington

Patrick M. Harding
Toxicology Section (Retired)
Wisconsin State Laboratory of Hygiene
Madison, Wisconsin

A. Wayne Jones
Department of Clinical Pharmacology
University of Linköping
Linköping, Sweden

Jørg G. Mørland
Division of Health and Digitalization
Norwegian Institute of Public Health
and
Institute of Clinical Medicine
University of Oslo
Oslo, Norway

Ray H. Liu
Department of Criminal Justice
University of Alabama at Birmingham
Birmingham, Alabama

Douglas M. Lucas
Centre of Forensic Sciences
Toronto, Ontario, Canada

Johannes G. Ramaekers
Department of Neuropsychology and Psychopharmacology
University of Maastricht
Maastricht, the Netherlands

Kathryn Stewart
Prevention Research Center
Safety and Policy Analysis International
Oakland, California

Maren C. Strand
Department of Forensic Sciences
Oslo University Hospital
Oslo, Norway

Franco Tagliaro
Department of Diagnostics and Public Health
University of Verona
Verona, Italy

Robert B. Voas
Pacific Institute for Research and Evaluation
Beltsville, Maryland

Patricia F. Waller (1932–2003)
Department of Psychology
University of Michigan
Ann Arbor, Michigan

History of Driving Under the Influence

I

Driving Under the Influence of Psychoactive Substances

A Historical Review*

1

A. WAYNE JONES, JØRG G. MØRLAND, AND RAY H. LIU

Contents

* This chapter is an updated version of a review article previously published in *Forensic Science Review*: Jones AW, Mørland JG, Liu RH: Driving under the influence of psychoactive substances—A historical review; *Forensic Sci Rev* 31:103; 2019.

1.1 Introduction

Compared with drunken driving, which is as old as motor-driven transportation, driving under the influence of psychoactive substances other than alcohol is a relatively new problem for road-traffic safety. According to a 2018 report from the World Health Organization (WHO), approximately 1.3–1.4 million people die each year as a result of road-traffic accidents (WHO 2018). Among these fatalities many drivers are impaired by excessive drinking or taking other psychoactive substances before driving, thereby increasing the risk of involvement in a traffic crash. Drug-impaired driving represents a global problem for public health and longevity and more effective ways of dealing with traffic delinquents and high-risk offenders should be made a top priority for government action.

1.1.1 Early Development

When the first "motor-wagons" appeared on the roads, driving under the influence of alcohol was not considered a criminal offense. The UK Licensing Act of 1872 had made it an offense to be "drunk while in charge on any highway or other public place of any carriage, horse, cattle or steam engine" (UK Government 1872). It was not until the UK Criminal Justice Act of 1925 that this requirement was extended to cover "any mechanically propelled vehicle." In 1930 it became illegal to drive, attempt to drive, or be in charge of a vehicle on a road or other public place while "under the influence of drink or drugs to such an extent as to be incapable of having proper control of the vehicle" (UK Government 1930).

The proof necessary to convict a person for drunken driving was elusive, because of the difficulty in convincing a judge or jury that a person was drunk to the extent of not being able to drive safely. The crux of the problem was that opinions among ordinary people differed as to what constituted being drunk and incapable (British Medical Association 1965). Meanwhile, a person might be charged with an offense based on their own admission of excessive drinking before driving and on eyewitness or police reports about the traffic incident (Lerner 2011). The person's general appearance and behavior and the smell of alcohol on the breath were taken as indications that alcohol was the culprit (Moskowitz et al. 1999).

The prosecution of impaired drivers was strengthened in the 1930s when medical evidence was presented to the court as proof that a driver was impaired by alcohol or drugs. A physician or police surgeon was charged with examining suspects, asking them about their alcohol consumption and also administering simple clinical tests of drunkenness to arrive at a diagnosis (Alha 1963). An important reason for the medical examination was to distinguish impairment caused by alcohol or other drugs from a medical condition mimicking the signs and symptoms of drunkenness (British Medical Association 1965).

The evaluation of clinical signs and symptoms of drunkenness is rather subjective, and different physicians could reach different conclusions when people with the same blood-alcohol concentration (BAC) were examined. This was well illustrated in a study from

Sweden in 1940 (Liljestrand 1940). Seven physicians each examined 100 apprehended drivers and reached a conclusion about alcohol impairment and their fitness to drive. Large discrepancies were noted in percentage of individuals judged as under the influence of alcohol within the same range of BAC. For example, in the 0.10–0.15 g% range, one of the doctors considered that 43% of suspects were "under the influence" whereas another concluded that 91% were similarly impaired at this same BAC.

The protocol used to examine traffic offenders gradually became more standardized for its intended purpose and the conclusions were less dependent on the experience and training of the examining physicians (Penttila and Tenhu 1976). It was also widely recognized that people reacted differently to the effects of alcohol and some impairment tests were more sensitive than others in detecting alcohol influence (British Medical Association 1927). Moreover, some people were able to "pull themselves together" in a critical situation, such as when threatened with criminal prosecution.

The results from clinical tests of drunkenness were, to some extent, influenced by the suspect's age, gender, drinking pattern (type of beverage consumed), time after end of drinking when the examination was made, and the individual's previous experience with alcohol consumption (habituation), etc. Other human factors that warranted consideration when traffic crashes were investigated included the driver's personality, mental health status, passengers and other distractions (such as children in the vehicle), aspects of the vehicle itself (brakes, steering, speed), the motoring environment, day or night-time driving, weather conditions, and so on (Petridou and Moustaki 2000).

1.1.2 First Conviction for Impaired Driving

According to a British newspaper report, the first conviction for a drunk-driving offense occurred in London, England, in 1897 (Editorial 1897). The suspect, Mr. George Smith (25 years old), drove his electric motor cab erratically, swerving from one side of the road to the other, crossed a footway (side-walk) and crashed into a building on New Bond Street. When helped from the wreckage by passersby, Mr. Smith appeared to be drunk, and when questioned by police he admitted drinking three glasses of beer before driving. He was later charged with being "unfit to drive through drink" and pleaded guilty, but said he was very sorry. He was fined 20 shillings or 1 GBP (roughly 150 GBP in today's money). The presiding magistrate warned him to be more careful in the future and remarked that "the police have a very happy knack of stopping a runaway horse, but to stop a motor is a very different thing."

The prosecution evidence in this case rested on Mr. Smith's own admission of drinking beer before driving, the fact he crashed his cab, and the testimony of the police and eyewitnesses to the crash. Accordingly, there was no medical or scientific evidence that Mr. Smith was under the influence of alcohol at the time of the crash.

The first prosecution for driving under the influence of drugs (DUID) has been more difficult to trace. Psychoactive drugs other than alcohol were not widely available at the start of the twentieth century; however, opiates and cocaine were recognized as drugs of abuse in some quarters and were used for recreational purposes (Musto 1991). Furthermore, until the 1960s the analytical methods needed to identify drugs other than alcohol in blood and urine were rudimentary and gave only qualitative results for a few selected substances, such as barbiturates and chloral hydrate (Sharma 1976). Barbiturate-type drugs were widely prescribed during the first half of the twentieth century to treat insomnia; therefore, it is reasonable to assume that inappropriate use of this medication represented a hazard for traffic safety.

If a driver showed signs and symptoms of impairment but there was no smell of alcohol on the breath, this raised a warning flag that other drugs might be involved. One of the tasks of the physician was to rule out a medical condition "simulating" drunkenness, such as mental instability, a nervous disorder, or metabolic disturbance, such as low blood sugar (diabetes) or epilepsy, all of which warranted consideration.

1.2 Alcohol, Drugs, and Crash Risk

At the turn of the twentieth century, ownership of motor-driven vehicles by ordinary people was uncommon. This soon changed and by the 1920–1930s automobiles were the main form of transportation in some nations, especially in the United States (Lerner 2011). However, impaired driving was not a major issue of concern; regulations, such as having a valid driving permit, basic rules of the road (e.g., a speed limit), and a highway code, were considered as elements requiring more attention from policymakers.

The prevalence of alcohol and drug use by drivers is usually determined through a close collaboration with the police authorities and in some nations they are allowed to make random checks of driver sobriety by requesting samples of blood, breath, or oral fluids for analysis of alcohol and other drugs (Walsh et al. 2008). A review article from 1993 found large differences between countries in the prevalence of alcohol-positive drivers in the traffic flow and among those fatally injured in crashes (Ross 1993).

A 12-month study (2016–2017) of alcohol and drug use by drivers in Norway (Furuhaugen et al. 2018), involving checks made on drivers of all types of vehicle, found:

- Only 0.2% were alcohol positive (BAC > 0.02 g%);
- Medicinal drugs were identified in 3% of drivers and the most prevalent of these was zopiclone, a prescription sleep-aid medication; and
- Illicit drugs were positive in 1.7% of samples, mostly cannabis as verified by finding THC in blood or saliva.

The low prevalence of alcohol-positive cases (0.2%) above the legal limit of 0.02 g% confirmed the findings from an earlier study done in 2008–2009 (Gjerde et al. 2008).

Detection rates of alcohol-positive drivers depended to some extent on day of week and time of day when traffic stops were made. The highest prevalence was found in drivers tested on weekend nights. Other roadside surveys, including mandatory testing of oral fluid specimens, have identified the prevalence of drivers using drugs other than alcohol (Alcaniz et al. 2018). Depending on the country concerned, between 5% and 10% of drivers test positive for one or more psychoactive substance other than alcohol, in part dependent on weekday and the time of day (Alcaniz et al. 2018; Gjerde et al. 2013, 2008). Worldwide trends in alcohol and drug use by drivers were the subject of a 2016 review article, which drew attention to the need for better standardization of the material collected in different countries and the need for more research on the role of alcohol and drugs in crashes utilizing a comprehensive program of toxicological analysis of biological samples (Christophersen et al. 2016).

The prevalence of alcohol use by drivers in the United States decreased from 1973 to 2014, whereas use of other drugs, both on prescription and illicit substances, increased over the same time period (Berning et al. 2015). The results from a 2014 national roadside survey, done on weekdays during daytime, found 1.1% of drivers tested positive for alcohol use

(BAC > 0.005 g%) and 0.4% were above the 0.08 g% statutory limit. The alcohol-positive rates for a similar roadside survey done on weekend nights were appreciably higher: 8.3% positives and 1.5% above the statutory BAC limit (Berning et al. 2015).

In the same US study, the drivers testing positive for non-alcohol drugs (both licit and illicit) rose to 22.4% in midweek daytime tests and 22.5% positives on weekend nights, suggesting no statistical difference (Berning et al. 2015). Of the drug-positive cases, roughly 12%–15% involved illegal drugs and 7%–10% of drivers had used prescribed medicines. The dominant illicit drug was cannabis with a prevalence of 15.2%, followed by prescription drugs in 7.3% of the drivers tested on weekend nights. These positive results were ratified by toxicological analysis of drugs in blood and/or saliva specimens, although the concentrations of pharmacologically active substances present were not reported.

Further convincing evidence that driving under the influence of alcohol and/or other drugs is a danger for traffic safety comes from postmortem toxicology results in drivers killed in crashes. However, making such comparisons between countries is problematic because different procedures and practices are adopted in selecting crash victims for forensic autopsy and conducting toxicological analysis (Berning and Smither 2014). For example, in Norway 58% of the drivers killed in crashes included information from drug analysis (Gjerde et al. 2011), while the corresponding rate was >95% in Sweden (Jones et al. 2009).

Reliable information about drug use by drivers killed in crashes in the United States is difficult to obtain because there is no consistent policy or procedures about who is actually tested. Much seems to depend on age and/or gender of the deceased and the jurisdiction where the crash occurred. Some medical examiners are content with toxicological testing for ethanol, whereas others require a broad drug-screening analysis. If only 50% of drivers killed are autopsied, there is nothing known about alcohol and drug use by the remaining 50%. Furthermore, information is lacking on the scope of the analytical toxicology, such as the number of drugs tested, the body fluids analyzed, and the analytical cutoff concentrations for reporting positive results (Berning and Smither 2014). In this connection, it is important to appreciate that a positive drug finding does not necessarily mean the driver was impaired by that substance or that the driver was to blame for the road traffic crash (Berghaus et al. 2007).

1.2.1 Role of Alcohol

An early reminder that consumption of alcohol before driving was a dangerous activity appeared in *Quarterly Journal of Inebriety* in 1904 (Crothers 1904). This editorial mentions an investigation of 25 accidents involving “motor wagons” in which 20 drivers were killed or fatally injured, and 19 of the victims had used spirits within an hour or more of the disaster. This editorial probably represents the first epidemiological data linking risk of a crash with drinking alcohol before driving. The editorial ended with the warning: “With the increasing popularity of these wagons, accidents of this kind will rapidly multiply, and we invite our readers to make notes of disasters of this kind.”

During the following decades, information was accumulating from different sources that between 20% and 50% of drivers killed in crashes had been drinking alcohol and that their BAC at autopsy exceeded the legal limit for driving in that particular country. In Norway and Sweden, where the statutory limit is 0.02 g%, statistics showed that 20%–25% of crash victims had a punishable BAC (Gjerde et al. 2011; Jones et al. 2009), whereas in many US states, 30%–40% of drivers killed were above the 0.08 g% limit (Voas et al. 2012). Alcohol-positive drivers were overrepresented in single-vehicle crashes, which supports the notion that alcohol impairment was a causative factor in the crash. Moreover, the mean autopsy BAC in drivers killed in traffic crashes is often in the 0.15–0.19 g% range, which is a level associated with gross impairment of driving skills.

The relationship between BAC and diminished performance has been verified in hundreds of experiments using different types of methodology. One approach is the use of controlled drinking experiments—with healthy volunteers under laboratory conditions, which usually involve moderate doses of ethanol (Drew et al. 1959). Subjects are required to perform a battery of cognitive and psychomotor tests before they drink alcohol, to establish baseline values, and the same tests are administered again at various times post-dosing (Goldberg 1943). The behavioral test scores are then compared with BAC or breath-alcohol concentration (BrAC) at the time of testing. Many such laboratory studies find a strong association between performance decrement (error rates) and BAC, but a lot also depends on complexity of the task, the time after drinking, and whether testing was done on the absorptive or postabsorptive limb of the BAC curve (Jongen et al. 2016; Martin et al. 2013).

Controlled drinking studies in a laboratory environment are unlike real-world conditions, because the volunteer subjects almost always consume a bolus dose of ethanol in 15–30 minutes after an overnight fast (Jones and Neri 1994). Under these conditions, absorption of ethanol into the blood is fast and initial impairment tends to be more pronounced. Thereafter a subject's performance in the behavioral tests rapidly improves and, by 90–120 minutes post dosing, their test scores are often not significantly different from baseline measurements before drinking. The general finding from many such studies is that both subjective feelings of intoxication and objective measures of impairment are more pronounced on the rising limb of the BAC curve and close to the peak (Jones and Neri 1985, 1994). On reaching the postabsorptive phase, the volunteer subjects feel tired and sleepy and might perform worse in behavioral tests for these reasons. Acute tolerance develops to impairment effect during a single exposure to ethanol; results of cognitive and psychomotor tests 2–3 hours after drinking are not significantly different from pre-drinking scores, despite BAC still being elevated and above 0.05–0.08 g% (Jones and Neri 1994; Mellanby 1920).

Another methodological approach to establish a relationship between BAC and impairment of driving skills makes use of closed track driving courses. This approach allows for evaluating complex maneuvers at speed, avoiding traffic cones, and other tasks that require divided attention, and braking in emergency situations (Bjerver and Goldberg 1950; Laurell 1977). Fairly sophisticated computer-aided tests are available to investigate other skills and traits associated with driving, such as tracking, divided attention, and simple and choice reaction times, all of which are relevant for traffic safety (Strand et al. 2016).

In the Netherlands, investigators have developed on-the-road driving tests to measure impairment from alcohol or other drugs, using specially designed dual-controlled vehicles with electronic recording of various aspects of the driving. The test subject is expected to drive on the normal highway in the traffic flow and is required to hold a steady lateral position and maintain a constant speed (O'Hanlon 1984; Ramaekers 2017; Verster and Roth 2011). The measure of impairment caused by psychoactive substances is the standard deviation of lateral position (SDLP), which is a quantitative indication of the amount of weaving during the driving task. Studies have shown that SDLP is a reliable and stable index of driving performance and provides an easily understood quantitative measure of weaving with high test-retest reproducibility. The SDLP shows a significant dose–response relationship to increasing levels of BAC, which can be used to compare with the effects of taking other drugs—using alcohol impairment as a calibrator to judge the dangerousness of other psychoactive substances (Jongen et al. 2017).

Also available are driving simulators of various complexity, which can be programmed to mimic real-world conditions, including weather (such as rain, snow, and icy roads), urban vs rural traffic, and surprise situations requiring emergency braking (Kenntner-Mabiala et al. 2015). All these different methodologies; laboratory studies, on-the-road driving tasks, driving simulators, computer software, cognitive and psychomotor performance tests, etc., confirm a dose–response relationship between impairment and BAC, albeit with large intersubject variations (Hadland et al. 2017; Jongen et al. 2016).

A review of 112 published articles, mainly involving laboratory experiments aimed at evaluating the effects of alcohol on skills considered relevant for driving, was funded by US Department of Transportation (Moskowitz and Fiorentino 2000). The authors concluded that some driving skills were impaired after any significant departure from zero BAC. Most of the articles reviewed found that, on reaching a BAC of 0.05 g% there was some degree of impairment in cognitive and psychomotor performance. At BAC of 0.08 g%, the results from the vast majority (~94%) of these studies indicated that subjects performed worse and that their driving-related skills were impaired. A more recent (2010) meta-analysis of a large number of published studies, dealing with the effects of alcohol on skills necessary for safe driving, came to the same conclusion, namely that BACs >0.04 g% cause performance decrements in most subjects (Schnabel et al. 2010).

In retrospect, it is unfortunate that more attention was not given to the pharmacokinetic profile of ethanol and whether testing was done on the absorptive or postabsorptive limbs of the BAC curve (Amlung et al. 2014). It has been known since the 1920s that impairment is more pronounced on the absorption phase of the BAC curve compared with the same BAC in the postabsorptive period (Mellanby 1920). However, a more recent laboratory study of alcohol impairment did not find much difference in relation to time after drinking and whether BAC was rising or declining (Gustavsen et al. 2012).

Perhaps the most convincing epidemiological evidence of an increased crash risk after drinking alcohol before driving comes from case-controlled studies of drivers involved in crashes compared with a control group not involved in crashes. The BAC or BrAC of drivers involved in crashes is then compared with a control group of drivers matched for day of week, time of day, location of the crash, and other variables, such as age, gender, years of driving experience, and ethnicity. This type of study is very demanding in resources, but is considered highly relevant furnishing a relative risk curve linking probability of involvement in a crash to the driver's BAC (or BrAC) (Gjerd et al. 2018).

The best-known case-control study was done in Grand Rapids, MI, in 1962–1963 and lasted for about 12 months—generally known as the Grand Rapids Study (Borkenstein et al. 1974). The BACs of 5,895 drivers involved in crashes were determined by breath analysis and compared with 7,590 matched control drivers. This allowed calculating odds ratios for involvement in a crash as a function of the driver's BAC. As the BAC increased above 0.04 g%, the probability of a crash increased compared with the control group of drivers not involved in crashes. The risk of being involved in a crash increased appreciably when BAC exceeded 0.08 g%, especially for single-vehicle crashes, when the outcome in terms of property damage and injury severity was greater.

The overall results from the Grand Rapids Study were later verified in more recent case-control studies of risk of involvement in a crash after drinking alcohol

(Blomberg et al. 2009). These newer studies used more modern technology for breath-alcohol analysis and efforts were made to track down and test hit-and-run drivers (Lacey et al. 2015). The design of case-control studies has some common weaknesses as does all types of epidemiological research and these have been discussed elsewhere (Gjerde et al. 2018b; Kim and Mooney 2016).

Studies done in Sweden over a 12-year period found that 20%–22% of drivers killed in crashes had been drinking and their postmortem BACs were above the statutory limit for driving (0.02 g%), actually eight times higher; mean 0.15–0.17 g% (Ahlner et al. 2014). These findings are noteworthy because the material consisted of traffic deaths occurring throughout the whole country and >95% of the victims were subjected to a forensic autopsy and toxicological analysis of blood and urine. In other countries, the autopsy rate is considerably less—probably under 40% in some US regions and reportedly 70% in Norway (Mørland et al. 2011).

The most recent case-controlled study of a driver's BAC and the risk of involvement in a crash was done in Virginia Beach, VA, during 2013–2014 (Lacey et al. 2016). This epidemiological survey involved testing 3,000 crash-involved drivers and 6,000 control drivers (not involved in crashes). Breath-alcohol was determined in 10,221 drivers, and other drugs were analyzed in 9,285 specimens of oral fluid as well as in 1,764 blood samples. Research teams worked 24 × 7 and responded to crashes over a 20-month period. Attempts were made to match control drivers to crash-involved drivers for weekday, time of day, vicinity of the crash, and direction of travel (Lacey et al. 2016). The results showed that drivers with a BAC of 0.05 g% were roughly twice as likely to be involved in a crash, while the odds ratio indicated a four times higher risk at 0.08 g%. When BAC passed 0.15 g%, the crash risk was increased by a factor of 12 compared with sober drivers (Berning et al. 2015).

1.2.2 Role of Other Drugs

A research project (2006–2011) funded by the European Union—referred to as DRUID (Driving Under the Influence of Drugs, Alcohol and Medicines)—was designed to investigate the prevalence of drug use by drivers and the role of drug-related impairment in traffic crashes. This project involved combined resources from 13 countries, each with its own traditions, including traffic safety legislation and enforcement strategies as well as statutory BAC limits and laboratory procedures for the analysis of non-alcohol drugs in body fluids (Houwing et al. 2011; Schulze et al. 2012). The police procedures and priorities for dealing with the problem of impaired driving differs between countries, including use of random testing of motorists in some but not all nations. Moreover, the panorama of drugs analyzed in blood and/or saliva, as well as the methodology and analytical cutoffs for reporting positive drug use, are also country-specific. All in all, scores of behavioral scientists, toxicologists, and traffic safety researchers participated in the DRUID project and many useful scientific articles, including a recent comprehensive update were published (Schulze et al. 2012).

The most prevalent impairing substance used by the general driving population, as might be expected, was alcohol and roadside breath-alcohol tests were positive in ~3.5% of drivers stopped in the normal traffic flow (Marillier and Verstraete 2019). Illicit drugs, mainly cannabis, were found in 1.9% of drivers based on analyzing saliva or blood samples. Potentially impairing medicinal drugs were detected in ~1.4% of drivers stopped by the police (Houwing et al. 2011). In an evaluation of alcohol and drug use by drivers injured in traffic crashes in six EU countries, an elevated BAC was reported in 18%–43%

of the victims and this was mostly above 0.13 g% (Legrand et al. 2013). The second-most prevalent drug in this study was cannabis (0.5%–7.6%) followed by benzodiazepines (0%–10%).

Evaluation of medical examiner reports from drivers killed in crashes provides useful information about the dangers of alcohol and drug use by drivers (Gjerde et al. 2018b; Legrand et al. 2014; Robertson and Drummer 1994). The results from such studies show a high prevalence of drunken driving, between 20% and 50% depending on the country, and particularly single-vehicle crashes (Mørland et al. 2011). The most prevalent non-alcohol drugs were amphetamines, followed by opioids, cocaine, benzodiazepines, and similar medicinal drugs, were identified in fatally injured drivers (Legrand et al. 2014). Even in drivers surviving the crash but seriously injured, the evidence is clear-cut that the use of alcohol and other psychoactive substances is a danger for traffic safety (Legrand et al. 2013). Drivers who combined different impairing substances (poly-drug users) are particularly vulnerable and run a greater risk of being involved in a traffic crash (Hels et al. 2013; Legrand et al. 2012). The most prevalent prescription medications in killed and injured drivers were various benzodiazepines (1.8%–3.3%), which are used to treat anxiety and panic attacks and also as sleep-aids and often subject to overdosing and abuse. The central stimulant amphetamine was highly prevalent in blood of drivers killed in traffic crashes in Sweden, a country where amphetamine abuse has been a problem since the 1950s (Jones et al. 2015).

The DRUID project indicated that illicit drugs represented a more serious risk for involvement in a road traffic crash, compared with drivers taking psychoactive prescription medicines (Verstraete and Legrand 2014). These results corroborate investigations done on weekend nights in the United States, where illicit drugs, such as cannabis, methamphetamine, and/or cocaine were overrepresented (Gjerde et al. 2011; Jones et al. 2015).

In the previously mentioned Virginia Beach study, the investigators reported statistically significant unadjusted odds ratios ($p < 0.01$) for drivers using illicit drugs (1.21 times) and those using cannabis (1.25 times). However, when the results were adjusted for background variables, such as a driver's age, gender, ethnicity, and alcohol use, the resulting odds ratios were no longer statistically significant compared with control drivers (Lacey et al. 2016).

Cannabis was the most prevalent non-alcohol drug detected in 234 drivers involved in crashes. Least prevalent were prescription medications, such as antidepressants ($n = 44$ cases), and sedatives ($n = 90$ cases). Elevated BAC (>0.08 g%) was highly correlated with the risk of having a crash, which verified earlier case-controlled studies (Kuypers et al. 2012).

The numbers of drivers testing positive for non-alcohol drugs in the Virginia Beach study were relatively low, which might have given insufficient statistical power to find elevated odds ratios. Another complicating factor was that some drivers ingested multiple drugs, making it difficult to attribute risk of a crash to a single substance. Furthermore, the concentrations of the various non-alcohol drugs detected in oral fluid and/or blood were not reported, simply if drugs were present or not. For many prescription drugs it is important to know the concentrations in blood and whether therapeutic levels were present. Many antidepressants, such as SSRI or SNRI, are not considered a traffic safety hazard—if these are used as prescribed by a physician. The situation can be very different when prescription drugs are taken in overdose or abused.

Poly-drug use is common in traffic offenders and consumption of alcohol and taking an illicit or prescription drug is the norm, rather than the exception, among impaired drivers arrested in most countries (Holmgren et al. 2007). Many drivers drink alcohol and take one or more other psychoactive substance, which poses a greater threat to traffic safety owing to more severe impairment and increased risk of a crash (Berning et al. 2015). Especially common in many countries is the consumption of alcohol and the smoking of marijuana, the potency of which has increased appreciably over the last decade and some products now contain up to 10% THC on average (Ramaekers et al. 2006a). The more potent the cannabis product, the higher is the THC concentration in blood, resulting in more pronounced effects on cognition and executive functions.

An Australian study of fatally injured drivers ($n = 3398$) calculated odds ratios for involvement in a fatal crash in relation to previous alcohol and drug use by the deceased (Drummer et al. 2004). The investigators also made efforts to address culpability on the part of the driver by use of a previously published responsibility analysis (Robertson and Drummer 1994). Drivers testing positive for psychotropic drugs in autopsy blood were more likely to be culpable for the crash than drug-free drivers. The odds ratios were statistically significant for drivers with increasing concentrations of THC in blood and >5 ng/mL was more dangerous than having a BAC in the range 0.1–0.15 g%. A statistically significant positive association with culpability was reported for cannabis/marijuana users and having a BAC >0.05 g%.

The design and execution of case-control studies requires special efforts to minimize selection bias, information bias, and other confounding factors such as poly-drug use, the choice of biological specimen analyzed (blood, saliva, or urine), and the cutoff concentrations for reporting positive drug findings (Gjerde et al. 2018b). Nevertheless, the take-home message from many epidemiological surveys of alcohol- and drug-impaired driving is that drunken drivers with high BAC (> 0.08 g%) pose the biggest threat to traffic safety, although the prevalence of non-alcohol drugs is definitely increasing.

1.3 Impaired Driving Legislation

1.3.1 Alcohol

When prohibition of alcohol was abrogated in 1933, the US federal government became concerned about the consequence this might have for traffic safety, because in the intervening years (1919–1933) motor transportation had proliferated on roads and highways (Ellerbrook and VanGaasbeek 1943). Furthermore, the evidence was mounting that many victims of road-traffic accidents had consumed alcohol before their deaths, especially those involved in single-vehicle crashes (Heise 1934). An early (1938) investigation of alcohol use and crash risk done in Evanston, IL, found that 46.6% of the crash-involved drivers (n = 270) were alcohol-positive compared with 12.1% of the control group (n = 1,750), which strongly implicates elevated BAC as a hazard for traffic safety (Holcomb 1938).

The first impaired driving laws in US states (Lerner 2011) made it illegal "to operate a motor vehicle when under the influence of alcohol or any other intoxicating substance or the combination of alcohol and other intoxicating substances." The definition of being "under the influence" was formulated in a judgment handed down by the Supreme Court of Arizona (Steffani *vs* State of Arizona 42 P.2d 615, 1935), which stated:

> The expression 'under the influence of intoxicating liquor' covers not only all the well-known and easily recognized conditions and degrees of intoxication, but any abnormal mental and physical condition which is the result of indulging in any degree in intoxicating liquors, and which tends to deprive him of that clearness of intellect to control himself which he would otherwise possess. If the ability of the driver of an automobile has been lessened in the

> slightest degree by the use of intoxicating liquors, then the driver is deemed to be under the influence of intoxicating liquor. The mere fact that the driver has taken a drink does not place him under the ban of the statute unless such drink has some influence upon him lessening in some degree his ability to handle said automobile.

In 1936 US National Safety Council's Committee on Alcohol and Other Drugs (NSC-CAOD) was formed. Thereafter, this organization played a leading role in research and teaching about impaired driving, particularly the scientific evidence necessary for prosecution. The committee was proactive in supporting use of chemical evidence based on the concentration of ethanol determined in specimens of blood or breath.

Until the 1950s, drunken driving was the major concern for state legislators and the need for countermeasures. Statistics about the part played by drugs other than alcohol in traffic crashes and driver fatalities were mostly lacking. This can be gleaned by browsing through published proceedings from conferences held under the auspices of the International Council on Alcohol, Drugs and Traffic Safety (ICADTS), which is searchable via http://www.icadtsinternational.com. The first such meeting was held in Stockholm in 1950 and was entitled "Alcohol and Road Traffic." The importance of "other drugs" did not become apparent until the sixth meeting, which was held in 1974 in Toronto, when the theme was expanded to cover "Alcohol, Drugs and Traffic Safety." The twenty-second meeting of ICADTS was held in Edmonton, Canada, in 2019 and a major topic for discussion was *per se* limits for drugs other than alcohol, especially cannabis, which has been legalized in Canada and several US states.

In the United States it appears that the first state to criminalize drunken driving was New Jersey in 1906, closely followed by New York in 1910 (Lerner 2011). However, the requisite proof of "intoxication" or "drunkenness" at the wheel was a major stumbling block for the prosecution (Thornton 1928). In 1939, Indiana and Maine were the first states to adopt a punishable BAC limit for driving, which was set at 0.15 g%, considered by many as being unusually high. The NSC-CAOD (National Safety Council 2019) assisted government officials in developing this legislation as to how a person's BAC should be interpreted as evidence of intoxication:

> Evidence that there was, at the time, five hundredths percent, or less, by weight of alcohol in his blood, is prima facie evidence that the defendant was not under the influence of intoxicating liquor sufficiently to lessen his driving ability within the meaning of the statutory definitions of the offense. Evidence that there was, at the time, from five hundredths percent to fifteen hundredths percent by weight of alcohol in his blood, is relevant evidence but is not to be given prima facie effect in indicating whether or not the defendant was under the influence of intoxicating liquor within the meaning of this act. Evidence that there was, at the time fifteen hundredths percent, or more, by weight of alcohol in his blood, is prima facie evidence that the defendant was under the influence of intoxicating liquor sufficiently to lessen his driving ability within the meaning of statutory definitions of the offenses.

Accordingly, a BAC below 0.05 g% meant the driver was not impaired by alcohol, whereas 0.05–0.15 g% pointed toward impairment, but did not constitute prima facie evidence. A BAC above 0.15 g% was interpreted by the courts as prima facie evidence that the driver was impaired and in breach of the law.

Reliable information about the prevalence of alcohol and other drugs in road-traffic fatalities was difficult to obtain because many pathologists and medical examiners were reluctant to submit autopsy specimens for toxicological analysis (Selesnick 1938). Much seemed to depend on the victim's age and gender, as well as local policies and practices in communities where the crash occurred. Furthermore, even when blood and/or urine specimens were available, they were not always subjected to toxicological analysis for ethanol and other impairing drugs.

When concentration *per se* statutes were introduced in the United States, many suspects refused to provide the biological specimens necessary for analysis (Bavis 1940). Obtaining blood by force was problematic because this was considered an invasive procedure, and a search in breach of the US Constitution (the Fourth Amendment). Sampling breath or urine was less invasive and efforts were made to develop instruments for breath-alcohol analysis, already in the 1940s (Harger et al. 1938). However, a person could not be forced to blow into such an instrument, which required making a continuous exhalation for about 6–12 seconds. Some type of legislation was needed to ensure that a drunken driver would not refuse to provide blood or breath for analysis, which led to the creation of implied-consent laws (Voas et al. 2009).

All 50 states have adopted implied consent laws, which essentially meant that on being granted a driving license, the individual agrees to provide a specimen of blood or breath if there is probable cause to suspect impairment. Being allowed to drive a motor vehicle on the public roads and highways is considered a privilege as opposed to a right, and one of the conditions is consenting to provide body fluids for toxicological analysis. This type of legislation helped initially to eliminate refusals, but a 2005 nationwide survey found that an average of 22.4% (median 17.4%) of suspects refused to comply with sampling (Zwicker et al. 2005). Refusal rates varied among states, from a low of 4.4% to a high of 81%, despite serious consequences, such as monetary fines and revocation of the driver's license for 6–12 months.

The UK Road Traffic Act of 1930 (UK Government 1930) made it an indictable offense to be "under the influence of drink or a drug to such an extent as to be incapable of having proper control of a vehicle." The prosecution no longer needed to prove that a driver was "drunk" when in charge of the vehicle, but that the driver was "incapable of having proper control." This change in wording proved equally troublesome to interpret; in addition to driver impairment, other factors (such as road conditions, weather, passenger distractions, and medical health) might account for loss of control of the vehicle.

In 1967 a paradigm shift occurred in British drunk-driving law when the government introduced a statutory concentration *per se* BAC limit of 80 mg/100 mL (0.08 g%), which remains the same to this day. This particular limit was chosen on the basis of the results presented in the Grand Rapids Study of crash risk, which was published in 1964–1965 (see Section 1.2.1 for further detail). Because some suspects might refuse to provide the required blood sample, a separate offense was created, known as "failure to provide without reasonable cause," which carried the same penalty as if the BAC was above the prescribed limit for driving (UK Government 1967).

In many EU nations, refusal to provide a specimen for toxicological analysis is virtually nonexistent, because if this happens the police have powers to obtain the required specimen by force, whenever serious crimes, such as impaired driving, are being investigated.

1.3.1.1 Clinical Tests of Drunkenness

The prosecution of traffic offenders was strengthened considerably when medical evidence was included as part of the prosecution case. A physician or police surgeon was charged with examining arrested drivers, noting their general appearance and asking questions about state of health. It was important to rule out that a medical condition, such as diabetes or epilepsy, which might mimic the signs and symptoms of drunkenness was absent. The smell of alcohol on the breath was the first indication of overconsumption and a person's orientation in time and space were noted along with simple cognitive and psychomotor tests of alcohol influence. This might include a Romberg test of balance, finger-to-nose test, picking up small objects (like coins, from the floor), and errors incurred when counting backward starting at 107 (Kataja et al. 1975). At the end of the examination, the physician signed a form certifying whether or not the suspect was under the influence of alcohol or other drugs (Penttila and Tenhu 1976).

The medical examination was usually done at a police station about 60–90 minutes after a driver had been arrested by the police. The responsible physician could be summoned to appear in court and explain to the jury the basis for the conclusion reached, which meant of course that the expert opinion was open to cross-examination by defense counsel.

In the 1930s, developments in analytical chemistry made it possible to determine a person's BAC in a quantitative way and suspects were encouraged to provide the required samples for analysis in drunk-driving cases. However, the results were used as supporting evidence because the main thrust of the prosecution case rested on unfitness to drive based on the results of the clinical examination.

1.3.1.2 Alcohol Concentration per se *Limits*

The Swedish physiological chemist Erik Widmark developed a reliable method of blood-alcohol analysis in 1922 (Widmark 1922), the so-called micro-diffusion method, which required only a drop of capillary blood (~100 mg). Starting in 1934, the Swedish government approved this analytical method for legal purposes and BAC was presented to the court along with the results of clinical tests. Case law was gradually changing toward giving more weight to BAC results, which are considered more objective evidence of overconsumption of alcohol than a clinical or medical examination of traffic offenders.

The results of clinical tests of drunkenness showed that the percentage of suspects judged to be impaired increased with increasing BAC (Liljestrand 1940), but there were also many discrepancies. Some apprehended drivers with high BAC were declared as not under the influence of alcohol. This probably depends, at least in part, on the training and experience of the examining physician, the age and gender of the suspect, and the degree of tolerance to behavioral effects of the drug (Andreasson and Bonnichsen 1965).

In 1934, the physiological laws governing absorption, distribution, metabolism, and excretion of alcohol in the body were formulated, mainly as a result of research done in Sweden (Widmark 1981). He showed that BAC could be converted into the amount of alcohol absorbed and distributed in all body fluids and tissues, which was often easier for the judge and jury to understand. Furthermore, if the time drinking started was known, then an estimate could be made of the total consumption of alcohol before driving.

The availability of a reliable analytical method for blood alcohol analysis was a prerequisite when countries like Norway adopted a statutory *per se* BAC limit of 0.50 g/kg (50 mg% or 0.05 g% w/w) in 1936. Sweden followed this lead and adopted a BAC *per se* limit of 0.80 g/kg in 1941. The statutory BAC limit in Sweden was subsequently lowered from 0.80 g/kg (1941) to 0.50 g/kg (1956) and 0.20 g/kg (1990 to this day) for all drivers, regardless of their age and driving experience. There is also a more serious offense referred to as aggravated drunken driving if the BAC exceeds 1.0 g/kg (0.1 g%).

Statutory BAC limits differ between countries, ranging from 0.20 g/kg (0.02 g%) in Norway, Poland, and Sweden to 80 mg% (0.08 g%) in the UK, Canada, and the United

States. This fourfold difference in punishable BAC probably reflects political forces and the actions of public pressure groups rather than results of traffic-safety research and studies of crash risk. Most EU nations enforce a BAC limit of 0.05 g%, although more serious charges can be brought for those with very high BAC, such as 0.10 or 0.12 g%.

Scotland lowered its illegal *per se* BAC limit for driving in December 2014 from 80 to 50 mg% (0.08 to 0.05 g%), whereas the limit in England and Wales remains at 80 mg%. An investigation into the effects of lowering the BAC limit on road traffic accidents in Scotland failed to find any improvements compared with statistics from England, which were used as a control material (Haghpanahan et al. 2019). The investigators concluded that lowering the BAC limit should not be done in isolation; other measures are needed such as media coverage, public information campaigns, and increased traffic surveillance by the police, such as more frequent controls of driver sobriety and the possibility to stop and test drivers at random.

Many researchers in the United States strongly support lowering the statutory BAC limit from 0.08 to 0.05 g%, which they believe will improve road-traffic safety and save lives lost in alcohol-related crashes (Fell and Voas 2006b). But whether lowering the drink-drive limit will act as a general deterrent is an open question; many traffic offenders suffer from a substance-use disorder and drink compulsively with little regard to whether they intend to drive afterward (Brinkmann et al. 2002; Snenghi et al. 2015).

Beginning January 2019, one US state (Utah) enacted a statutory *per se* BAC limit for driving of 0.05 g%; other states are likely to follow this lead. This will give a good opportunity to evaluate the effects on traffic safety, including number of arrests, sales of alcohol in society, prevalence of alcohol-related crashes before and after lowering the statutory limit, and also making comparisons with states with a BAC limit of 0.08 g% (Fell and Voas 2006b).

1.3.2 Non-alcohol Drugs

In recent years, the use of psychoactive drugs, especially medicines for treatment of anxiety and sleep disorder as well as prescription pain medication, has increased appreciably in all age groups. This suggests that prevalence of drivers taking such drugs will also increase as verified by several roadside surveys (Legrand et al. 2013, 2014). Sleep-aid medication makes people drowsy and should be used before bedtime and not at other times of the day, when a need to drive might arise. Until the 1950s, most countries did not have any specific legislation prohibiting driving under the influence of drugs other than alcohol.

The road-traffic acts contained wording such as impairment caused by "drink or drugs," but the nature of the other drugs was not further elaborated upon. Attempts were made to define impairment as any process (e.g., drug use) that adversely influenced a person's reasoning and judgment, mental performance (as reflected in clarity and acuity), and/or physical performance, such as ability to concentrate, dexterity, and reaction time.

The protocol used by physicians to examine arrested drivers was originally designed with alcohol impairment in mind and some of the tests might not be appropriate for measuring the type of impairment caused by drugs other than alcohol. Modifications, including more attention given to appearance of the eyes, such as pupil size, color of conjunctiva, whether bloodshot, watery, etc., are important. The examining physician needed to consider pathological conditions, such as hypoglycemia, epilepsy, or a nervous disorder, in the person arrested for DUID. The prosecution case also needed to identify which drug (or drugs) was causing the impairment, and this required analysis of blood or urine samples, which was not feasible in the 1950s. The analytical chemistry for drug analysis in biofluids did not advance sufficiently until the 1960s–1970s when gas chromatography (GC) and mass spectrometry (MS) methods came into routine use in clinical and forensic toxicology laboratories (Maurer 1992).

Driver impairment caused by drugs other than alcohol was first mentioned in the Swedish Road Traffic Act of 1951, although no particular drugs were specified. If a driver was arrested by the police and a roadside breath-alcohol test was negative, this raised a suspicion that other drugs might be involved. The first studies of non-alcohol drugs used by drivers in Sweden were done in 1967–1970 and published in four articles under the rubric "Arzneimittel und Fahrtüchtigkeit" or in English "Medicines and Driving." In this early study, the main classes of drugs determined in the blood of drivers were barbiturates (Bonnichsen et al. 1969a), central stimulants and aromatic hydrocarbons (Bonnichsen et al. 1969b), benzodiazepine derivatives (Bonnichsen et al. 1970), and other pharmaceutical substances, mainly sedative-hypnotics (Bonnichsen et al. 1972).

As stated earlier, the results of toxicological analysis did not always agree with results of the clinical examination, which might have to do with sensitivity of the tests and the driver's individual tolerance to effects of certain drugs. The correlation between concentrations of drugs in blood and signs and symptoms of impairment was much better in a population of arrested drivers compared with controlled laboratory experiments in which much lower doses of alcohol and/or other drugs are administered for safety reasons (Hoiseth et al. 2017b). Some physicians preferred to attribute a person's unusual behavior to a medical condition rather than drug-induced impairment from psychoactive substances.

Until the 1960s, barbiturates were widely used and abused and were highly prevalent in apprehended drivers and in overdose deaths—both accidental and with suicidal intent (McBay 1965). Thereafter, a plethora of other central nervous system (CNS) depressants, including Valium and Librium, appeared on the market. These prototype benzodiazepines were much less toxic in overdose than barbiturates, but they were nevertheless subject to abuse and could be habit-forming (Greenblatt and Shader 1978; Lader 2011). The 1960s–1970s also saw a marked increase in abuse of central stimulants, such as amphetamine derivatives, which were often detected in blood samples from apprehended drivers (Bonnichsen et al. 1970).

Knowledge about driving under the influence of non-alcohol drugs was deficient in the 1960s–1970s because the main focus was on drunken driving. For example, if the BAC was above the legal limit for driving, the police usually weren't interested in searching for other drugs, because the penalty was the same regardless of whether the driver had taken multiple drugs. Even when psychoactive drugs other than alcohol were identified in blood, if the results of the physician's clinical examination were inconclusive, the charges were usually dropped.

In Finland, Norway, and Sweden, the toxicological analysis of blood and urine samples from people arrested by the police for impaired driving is centralized to one national laboratory in each country. Scientists in Norway took an early interest in the role of drugs other than alcohol in road-traffic safety as causative factors in crashes (Bjorneboe et al. 1987; Gjerde et al. 1993). They embarked on systematic studies of the prevalence of non-alcohol drugs in blood of apprehended drivers regardless of whether alcohol had been detected (Gjerde et al. 1990). This was in contrast to the practice in Sweden, where other drugs were analyzed in blood only if BAC was below the legal limit for driving. The Norwegian police were much more proactive in arranging for DUID suspects to be examined by a physician to obtain evidence of impairment based on clinical tests (Christophersen and Mørland 1997). The results from the medical examination along with the toxicology report and an expert assessment done by a clinical pharmacologist, who looked at all available information in the case, proved highly effective in the prosecution case.

In the early 1990s, the news media in Sweden reacted to court decisions in which people were acquitted from the charge of impaired driving despite toxicology reports showing high concentrations of illicit drugs in blood, such as central stimulant amines (e.g., amphetamine). This prompted the Swedish government to commission a review of the current practices and to make suggestions for tightening the DUID laws to make prosecution easier. The members of the expert committee agreed that a zero-tolerance law was appropriate for driving after the use of illicit drugs, but psychoactive prescription drugs were exempted, provided these were being used in accordance with a physician's ordination.

A summary of the current legislation in Denmark, Finland, Norway, Sweden, and the UK for drunk and drugged driving offenses is given in Table 1.1.

Table 1.1 Summary of Legislation Pertaining to Driving Under the Influence of Alcohol and/or Other Drugs in Some Selected European Countries

Country	Statutory BAC[a] Limits	Considerations for Other Psychoactive Substances
Denmark	0.50 g/kg[b]	• Threshold concentration limits in blood were established for a large number of illicit and prescription drugs with psychoactive properties • Expert group: decided on the drugs to be included and the punishable limits—based on pharmacological properties and available analytical technology
Finland	0.50 and 1.20 g/kg	• For controlled substance it is prohibited to drive if these are present in a sample of blood • No threshold concentration limits for illicit drugs (zero tolerance) • Psychoactive prescription drugs: the arrested drivers were examined by a physician for signs and symptoms of impairment
Norway	0.20, 0.50, and 1.2 g/kg	• Threshold concentration limits in blood were established for commonly abused psychoactive substances (both illicit and prescription medications) • Prescription drugs in blood: all relevant medical and pharmacological information in the case are considered • Enhanced sanctions: parallel to existing punishable BAC limits (see Tables 1.4 and 1.5)
Sweden	0.20 and 1.0 g/kg	• For controlled substance: prohibited to drive when these are present in blood • No threshold concentration limits for illicit drugs (zero tolerance) • Psychoactive prescription drugs: exempted if used in accordance with a physician's ordination
England and Wales[c]	80 mg% (0.08 g%)[d]	• Threshold concentration limits in blood: established for 17 psychoactive substances (8 illicit and 9 prescription drugs)

[a] BAC = blood alcohol concentration.

[b] Only a single BAC limit is mentioned in the law, but enhanced penalties are possible at higher BAC, such as 1.2 g/kg or 2.0 g/kg, depending on the circumstances.

[c] Scotland introduced a statutory BAC limit of 50 mg% (0.05 g%) in December 2014.

[d] BAC mass/volume is not exactly the same as BAC mass/mass, because the density of blood is 1.055 g/mL. This means that a statutory BAC limit of 0.50 g/kg is equal to limit of 0.53 g/L or 53 mg%.

Legislation pertaining to the enforcement of DUID laws in the United States differs among states as does the evidence necessary for prosecution and the penalties imposed for those convicted of this traffic crime (Walsh 2007). Most laws require that a person took the drug voluntarily and that the pharmacologically active substance was identified in samples of blood or urine. The drugs of major interest for traffic-safety legislation are those classified as controlled substances (Schedules I through V) for which a valid prescription is necessary.

Although an increasing number of states have enacted concentration *per se* laws, which puts more focus on the toxicology report, it is by no means certain whether the courts interpret the legislation that way and many still require evidence of driver impairment (Voas et al. 2013).

1.3.2.1 Clinical Tests and Impairment Laws

For much of the twentieth century, the main evidence necessary for a successful impaired driving prosecution was a signed statement by a physician that the driver was impaired by drugs other than alcohol. The protocol used to examine drugged drivers was the same as that used for drunken drivers, which was problematic, because the signs and symptoms of drunkenness are not necessarily applicable to impairing effects of other drugs (Kataja et al. 1975). The clinical examination was modified in various ways to include more information about the subject's eyes, including conjunctiva, pupil size, reaction to light, and any horizontal gaze nystagmus (HGN). There was also an option to conclude that an arrested driver was suffering from a medical condition, such as a psychiatric disorder, which was causing strange and erratic behavior (Bramness et al. 2003).

1.3.2.2 Drug Recognition Experts

In many US states, drivers arrested for DUID are examined by police officers with special training, known as "Drug-Recognition Expert" (DRE). This method originated in California, where suitably adept officers were trained in pharmacology and toxicology of psychoactive drugs and ways to recognize signs and symptoms of impairment caused by these substances (Page 2002). Use of DRE officers spread to other US states and now constitutes an important part of the prosecution evidence when a person is suspected of impaired driving by non-alcohol drugs.

In practice, a vehicle is usually stopped by the police because of a moving traffic offense, or after involvement in a crash. If the driver seemed impaired by alcohol or drugs because of appearance and/or behavior, or refuses to answer questions about alcohol and/or drug use, this was considered sufficient to motivate a more detailed assessment. In some communities, a driver might be known to the police as a user of illicit drugs, or lacking a valid driving license, or has previously been arrested for impaired driving. Some motorists admit that they had consumed alcohol or smoked a joint some time before driving.

The next step in the procedure is to perform field sobriety tests, which are done at the roadside close to where the vehicle was stopped. Based on an overall assessment of the evidence, the driver is arrested and transported to a police station, where a DRE is called to make a more thorough examination according to a standard protocol, which commonly consists of the following 12 steps:

1. The result of a handheld breath-alcohol test;
2. Interview with the arresting police officer;
3. Preliminary assessment of the suspect;
4. Evaluation of the suspect's eyes (e.g., pupil size, nystagmus, etc.);

5. Results of simple cognitive and psychomotor tests;
6. Presence of vital signs and orientation in time and space;
7. Examination of the suspect in a dark room;
8. Test of muscle tone;
9. Location and identification of any injection marks on the skin;
10. Interrogation of the suspect with respect to their use of drugs and medicines;
11. Conclusions about impairment by drugs and the type of drug concerned; and
12. Review of the results of toxicological analysis of blood and urine.

DRE officers are trained to recognize seven categories of drugs as defined in the Drug Evaluation and Classification Program (Smith et al. 2002). These include cannabis, central stimulants, depressants, hallucinogens, dissociative anesthetics, narcotic analgesics, and inhalants. The DRE examination was intended to establish impairment and to identify the class of drug or drugs involved. This was not so easy because many DUID suspects ingested multiple drugs, including stimulants, depressants, narcotic analgesics, cannabis, and/or alcohol (Beirness 2009).

The use of alcohol could usually be ruled out by a negative breath alcohol test (point 1 above). Some suspects tell the DRE officer which drugs they had taken at the material time, which is another confounding factor. Accordingly, the opinion of the DRE officer is not always in unison with the toxicological results of analyzing blood or urine specimens (point 12 above). When this happens, the results of the toxicology should trump the conclusions made by the DRE officer (Kane 2013).

When concentration *per se* DUID laws were introduced in Sweden (since July 1, 1999), the police were permitted to examine a suspect's eyes with a flashlight and measure the size of the pupils using a pupilometer device. The premise for examining the eyes was that use of drugs such as opiates/opioids causes pinpoint pupils and use of stimulants (cocaine/amphetamine) dilates the pupils. The police officer also paid attention to (a) existence of gaze nystagmus; (b) reaction of the pupils to light; and (c) other indications of recent drug use, such as slurred or slow speech, bloodshot eyes, drug paraphernalia in the vehicle, needle marks on arms, etc.

1.3.2.3 Zero-Tolerance Laws

The term "zero tolerance" implies an immediate sanction when a given rule or regulation is violated, with the aim of eliminating dangerous or antisocial behavior, such as drug-impaired driving. However, the same terminology conjures up the notion of low (zero) tolerance to the effects of drugs, which is not the case. Although the term zero tolerance is in common usage, it is not an accurate description of how the law actually works. For example, many American states and Canada enforce zero-tolerance drink-driving laws for people aged under 21 (Chamberlain and Solomon 2008; Voas et al. 2003), because this is also the age limit for legal purchase and consumption of alcohol. But in practice a threshold BAC of 0.02 g% is enforced for these individuals, which happens to be the statutory limit for all drivers in Norway, Sweden, and Poland (0.20 g/kg).

A zero-tolerance law for driving under the influence of non-alcohol drugs was introduced in Sweden in 1999 and similar legislation has now been adopted elsewhere (Table 1.1). However, there was no consensus or agreement reached about the requirements for prosecuting traffic offenders having non-alcohol psychoactive drugs in blood. In some countries, any detectable amount of an illicit drug in blood was breaking the law, whereas special regulations applied to psychoactive prescription drugs. The threshold concentration in blood for illicit drugs was equal to the lower limit of quantitation (LLOQ) by the analytical method used, usually by GC-MS or LC-MS technology. A result below LLOQ was reported to the police as "not detected" and when above LLOQ, a drug concentration was included on the toxicology report.

Driving after use of psychoactive prescription drugs is not an offense provided the driver holds a valid prescription and was using the medication in accordance with a physician's ordination (Jones 2005). The detection of a scheduled medicinal drug without a valid prescription meant a driver would be charged with impaired driving. Such a charge can also be brought if the concentration of active chemical substance in blood is higher than expected for accepted therapeutic usage, even if the driver has a prescription for the medication (Schulz and Schmoldt 2003). In such cases, an expert medical report is required from a forensic toxicologist (or a clinical pharmacologist) as additional evidence for prosecution. Finding a drug concentration above the upper point of the therapeutic interval indicates lack of patient compliance, overdosing, or abuse of the medication (Flanagan et al. 2008; Schulz and Schmoldt 2003).

By definition, a therapeutic drug concentration in serum or plasma is that which produces the desired effects without causing adverse reactions or toxicity for the patient. Dosing to reach a concentration in excess of the therapeutic interval can lead to adverse clinical effects including toxicity and death. A concentration in plasma lower than the accepted therapeutic level might fail to benefit the patient. Even therapeutic doses of some drugs can cause impairment, which is relevant to consider, especially when a medication is taken for the first time and before a tolerance develops or when the dose is increased to reach a higher steady-state level in plasma. Many prescription drugs are subject to abuse, such as sedative-hypnotics and opioid pain medication; hence, these substances are commonly encountered in overdose deaths and impaired drivers (Lader 1991; Volkow et al. 2018).

The types of drugs identified in blood samples from impaired drivers apprehended in four Scandinavian countries (Denmark, Finland, Norway, and Sweden) are listed in Table 1.2. There is clearly close agreement between the four countries with regard to the types and classes of drugs used and abused by traffic offenders, both illicit substances and psychoactive prescription medications (mainly benzodiazepines). In Denmark there was a high prevalence of ketamine, which is used clinically as an anesthetic agent and is also a recreational drug of abuse, but this substance was less of a problem in neighboring countries (Simonsen et al. 2018).

1.3.2.4 Drug Concentration per se *Limits*

In 1999 the Swedish Parliament approved a zero-tolerance law for driving under the influence of scheduled drugs and controlled substances (Jones 2005). The members of the expert government committee were unanimous that zero tolerance was appropriate for illicit drugs of abuse but not psychoactive prescription drugs. However, the evidence is overwhelming that misuse of prescription drugs, especially sedative-hypnotics and opiates/opioid analgesics, is a danger for traffic safety. These substances are also subject to abuse and lead to dependence (Lader 2011; Volkow et al. 2018). Experts on the committee recognized that psychoactive prescription drugs were a greater danger for traffic safety when taken for the first time. After compliance with the prescribed treatment regimen, an appreciable tolerance develops to the impairing effects of sedative-hypnotics and opioids (Neutel 1995).

Table 1.2 Examples of the Psychoactive Drugs Other Than Alcohol Most Frequently Identified in Blood Samples from Drivers Arrested in Four Nordic Countries—The Drugs Are Listed in Descending Order of Prevalence over the Past Few Years (the Actual Rank Order Is Not Static)

Rank	Sweden	Norway	Finland	Denmark
1	Amphetamine[a]	THC[b]	Amphetamine[a]	THC[b]
2	THC[b]	Amphetamine[a]	Diazepam	Cocaine/BZE[c]
3	Diazepam	Clonazepam	Alprazolam	Amphetamine[a]
4	Alprazolam	Methamphetamine	Clonazepam	Clonazepam
5	Clonazepam	Diazepam	Buprenorphine	Morphine/heroin
6	Morphine/heroin	Alprazolam	Oxazepam	GHB[d]
7	Cocaine/BZE[c]	Alprazolam	THC[b]	Methadone
8	Oxazepam	MDMA[e]	Temazepam	MDMA[e]
9	MDMA[e]	Buprenorphine	Pregabalin	Ketamine
10	Buprenorphine	Cocaine/BZE[c]	MDMA[e]	Diazepam
11	Tramadol	Pregabalin	Tramadol	Alprazolam
12	Zopiclone	Tramadol	Methamphetamine	Bromazepam

[a] Mainly an illicit drug of abuse although the *d*-isomer of amphetamine has some legitimate medical indications.
[b] THC = tetrahydrocannabinol, the active constituent of cannabis.
[c] BZE = benzoylecognine, a major metabolite of cocaine.
[d] GHB = γ-hydroxybutyrate
[e] MDMA = 3,4-methylenedioxymethamphetamine.

Creating a total ban on use of psychoactive medications when driving was obviously not an option, because many people need drug treatment to function normally in society. Furthermore, when psychoactive prescription drugs are used in accordance with a physician's ordination the dangers for traffic safety are minimal.

One basic requirement to avoid prosecution is possession of a valid prescription for the medication in question. Furthermore, the concentration of the active substance in blood should be within the limits observed after normal therapeutic usage (Schulz and Schmoldt 2003). Without a prescription or a supratherapeutic concentration of the pharmacologically active substance in blood motivates a prosecution for DUID. In such cases, an expert witness, usually a toxicologist or clinical pharmacologist, is instructed to review all evidence in the case including aspects of the driving, the clinical evidence of impairment if any, and the toxicological results and drug concentrations (Jones et al. 2007).

Finland adopted a similar approach including a zero-tolerance law for illicit drugs; any measurable amount in blood was a punishable offense (Lillsunde and Gunnar 2005). If the driver had a valid prescription for a scheduled prescription drug present in blood, then impairment evidence was necessary before a prosecution for DUID was made (Blencowe et al. 2011).

Denmark introduced threshold concentrations in blood for a large number of licit and illicit substances as recommended by a committee of experts (Steentoft et al. 2010). Their task was to review and evaluate the pharmacological literature including capabilities of the analytical methods and the relationship between concentration of drugs in blood and impairment of cognitive and psychomotor functioning. The most hazardous therapeutic drugs for traffic safety are sedative-hypnotics of the benzodiazepine class and sleep-aid medications or so-called z-hypnotics (zolpidem, zopiclone, and zaleplon) (Brandt and Leong 2017).

In 2015, the British government introduced threshold concentration limits in blood for 17 drugs comprising common recreational drugs of abuse (illegal drugs) and widely

Table 1.3 Statutory Concentration Limits of Certain Prescription and/or Illicit Substances in Blood of Drivers Apprehended in England and Wales Applicable Since 2015

	Blood Concentration			Blood Concentration	
Illicit Drugs	ng/mL[a]	mg/L	Prescription Drugs	ng/mL[a]	mg/L
Methamphetamine	10	0.01	Amphetamine[b]	250	0.25
Cocaine	10	0.01	Clonazepam	50	0.05
BZE[c]	50	0.05	Diazepam	550	0.55
THC[d]	2.0	0.002	Flunitrazepam	300	0.30
Ketamine	20	0.02	Lorazepam	100	0.10
LSD[e]	1.0	0.001	Temazepam	1,000	1.00
MDMA[f]	10	0.01	Methadone	500	0.50
6-Acetylmorphine[g]	5.0	0.005	Morphine	80	0.08
			Oxazepam	300	0.30

[a] The drug concentration unit in British law is ng/mL in blood, which is the same as µg/L. The threshold concentrations are also shown as mg/L, the unit used in many other countries.
[b] The *d*-isomer of amphetamine has some legitimate medical indications.
[c] BZE = benzoylecgonine, a major metabolite of cocaine.
[d] THC = tetrahydrocannabinol is the active constituent of cannabis/marijuana.
[e] LSD = lysergic acid diethylamide.
[f] MDMA = 3,4-methylenedioxymethamphetamine.
[g] 6-Acetylmorphine is the primary metabolite of heroin.

prescribed psychoactive prescription drugs (Wolff et al. 2013). Shown in Table 1.3 are the prohibited concentration limits (in blood) for eight illicit drugs and nine prescription drugs.

In England and Wales, the use of alcohol and drugs by drivers is regulated in the Road Traffic Act of 1988. Section 5 of this act pertains to alcohol and Section 5A concerns other intoxicating substances. The Road Traffic Act prohibits driving, attempting to drive, or being in charge of a motor vehicle with one of the 17 drugs in blood at concentrations listed in Table 1.3. If toxicology results show drug concentrations above these limits, then a driver is in breach of the law and is charged and prosecuted for impaired driving, even if there is no behavioral evidence of drug impairment.

In connection with the introduction of this new law in March 2015, the UK government provided the following further information for the benefit of the public:

- If you are taking medicines as directed by your physician and your driving is not impaired, then you are not breaking the law.
- Keep using your medicines as prescribed.
- Check the leaflet that comes with your medicines for information on whether they are likely to impair your driving ability.
- Do not drive after taking your medicines until you know how they affect you.
- Do not drive if you feel drowsy, dizzy, unable to concentrate or make decisions, or if you experience blurred or double vision.
- If your driving is impaired, then you are guilty of breaking the law.

Since July 1, 2017, The Netherlands enforces statutory concentration *per se* limits in blood mainly for illicit drugs, such as amphetamine, methamphetamine, cocaine, MDMA, MDEA, MDA, THC, heroin, morphine, and GHB. The statutory concentration limit for THC in blood is 3 ng/mL or 1 ng/mL if combined with other drugs, such as elevated BAC.

1.3.2.5 Graded or Enhanced Penalties

Norway was the first country to adopt graded or enhanced penalties depending on the concentration of psychoactive non-alcohol drugs in a driver's blood (Vindenes et al. 2012). Enhanced penalties are widely used in many countries depending on a suspect's BAC to represent a minor or more serious traffic offense. In Norway, three punishable BAC limits are enforced: 0.20‰ (0.02 g%), 0.50‰ (0.05 g%), and 1.2‰ (0.12 g%). The courts are accustomed to graded penalties when sentencing drunken drivers. A similar approach was suggested for driving under the influence of non-alcohol psychoactive substances (Vindenes et al. 2014). However, arriving at the appropriate limits for non-alcohol drugs was not easy because ethanol-induced impairment is not a good model for other CNS-active drugs, which have various mechanisms of action. Researchers in Norway argued that most individuals were impaired when BAC was above 0.10 g%, whereas the lower alcohol limit for prosecution in that country was already set at 0.02 g%, which is one-fifth of 0.10 g%. Accordingly, the concentration of a non-alcohol drug in blood that caused impairment in most subjects was divided by a factor of five to give the statutory concentration in blood corresponding to 0.02 g% BAC (Vindenes et al. 2012).

Specialists in clinical pharmacology attempted to ascertain the concentrations of psychoactive drugs in blood associated with impairment of body functions, based on various laboratory experiments and psychomotor and cognitive tests. Review of pharmacological evidence and data obtained from new experimental studies established a relationship between drug concentration in blood and impairment. Such a study was reported for the sleep-aid medication zopiclone in comparison with ethanol; a similar approach was used for other substances (Gustavsen et al. 2012). Other examples of medicinal drugs used by drivers that cause impairment of their ability to drive safely are benzodiazepine derivatives and opiate-opioid analgesics (Gustavsen et al. 2009; Strand et al. 2018). Other published studies were reviewed in which impairment from drinking alcohol and elevated BAC was compared with impairment from other psychoactive substances. The resulting threshold concentrations in blood obtained in this way were subsequently used to define statutory limits roughly equivalent to the BAC limits of 0.05 g% and 0.12 g% (Vindenes et al. 2012). However, this approach was not applicable to all drugs, especially those for which development of tolerance was more pronounced and the concentration-effect relationship was weak or not established (Blanke et al. 1985).

Nevertheless, concentration *per se* limits for graded penalties were established for many illicit and prescription drugs, whereas amphetamine and methamphetamine were excluded. People regularly taking opiates or opioid-like drugs, such as cancer patients, rapidly develop CNS tolerance and initial impairing effects on performance are less marked and subside after regular usage (Chihuri and Li 2017). Accordingly, people taking this type of medication and don't intentionally increase the dosage are unlikely to pose a problem for traffic safety (Vainio et al. 1995; Wilhelmi and Cohen 2012). Therefore, the Norwegian *per se* concentration limits for non-alcohol drugs don't apply to patients who are compliant with their medication as ordered by a physician (Vindenes et al. 2012). However, if the police have other tangible evidence that a driver was impaired, this triggers a thorough evaluation including a clinical examination of the suspect and a review of all toxicology evidence and an expert assessment by a clinical pharmacologist.

Tables 1.4 and 1.5 contain the threshold concentration *per se* limits in blood established in Norway for illicit drugs (Table 1.4) and various prescription medicines (Table 1.5).

Table 1.4 Concentration *per se* Limits in Blood for Driving after Use of Various Illicit Drugs in Norway—The Penalties for a Conviction Are Interpreted by the Courts in the Same Way as the Statutory Blood-alcohol Concentration (BAC) Limits of 0.20‰, 0.50‰, and 1.2‰ (g/kg)

Drugs in Blood	Concentration (mg/L)[a] Equal to 0.20‰ BAC	Concentration (mg/L)[a] Equal to 0.50‰ BAC	Concentration (mg/L)[a] Equal to 1.2‰ BAC
Amphetamine	0.041	Not set[b]	Not set[b]
Cocaine	0.024	Not set[b]	Not set[b]
MDMA[c]	0.097	Not set[b]	Not set[b]
Methamphetamine	0.045	Not set[b]	Not set[b]
GHB[d]	10.3	30.9	123.6
Ketamine	0.055	0.137	0.329
LSD[e]	0.001	Not set[b]	Not set[b]
THC[f]	0.0013	0.003	0.009

[a] The mg/L concentration units were calculated from the μmol/L concentration units written into the Norwegian legislation.
[b] No higher limits or graded penalties were set for these drugs.
[c] MDMA = 3,4-methylenedioxymethamphetamine.
[d] GHB = γ-hydroxybutyrate.
[e] LSD = lysergic acid diethylamide.
[f] THC = tetrahydrocannabinol active constituent of cannabis.

Table 1.5 Concentration *per se* Limits in Blood for Psychoactive Prescription Drugs in Norway When Used without a Prescription or When Higher Than the Prescribed Dosages Were Taken—The Courts Interpreted These Concentrations in the Same Way as Statutory Blood-alcohol Concentration (BAC) Limits of 0.20‰, 0.50‰, and 1.2‰ (g/kg)

Drugs in Blood	Concentration (mg/L)[a] Equal to 0.20‰ BAC	Concentration (mg/L)[a] Equal to 0.50‰ BAC	Concentration (mg/L)[a] Equal to 1.2‰ BAC
Alprazolam	0.003	0.006	0.015
Bromazepam	0.032	0.079	0.190
Clobazam	0.18	0.45	1.08
Clonazepam	0.0013	0.003	0.008
Desmethyldiazepam	0.108	0.270	0.650
Diazepam	0.057	0.143	0.342
Etizolam	0.014	0.034	0.082
Flunitrazepam	0.0016	0.003	0.008
Lorazepam	0.0096	0.024	0.058
Nitrazepam	0.017	0.042	0.098
Oxazepam	0.172	0.430	0.860
Phenazepam	0.0018	0.005	0.010
Triazolam	0.00034	0.00086	0.0021
Zolpidem	0.031	0.077	0.184
Zopiclone	0.012	0.023	0.058
Buprenorphine	0.0004	0.0009	0.0022
Methadone	0.025	0.062	0.148
Morphine	0.009	0.024	0.061
Oxycodone	0.016	0.038	0.095
Methylphenidate	0.0035	Not set[b]	Not set[b]

[a] The mg/L concentration units were calculated from the μmol/L concentration units written into the Norwegian legislation.
[b] No higher limits or graded penalties were set for methylphenidate.

The DUID laws operating in the United States depend on the particular state and some are more draconian than others (Walsh 2007). In some states, drivers are prosecuted with any detectable amount of a banned substance in a sample of blood, whereas other states bring a charge if inactive drug metabolites are identified in blood or urine. Most US states require that a controlled substance is identified in a sample of the driver's blood, because the blood transports the drug to the brain where impairment effects are elicited.

The recreational use of cannabis is currently legal in ten states (e.g., Colorado, Oregon, Nevada, and Michigan) and throughout Canada. This will undoubtedly have consequences for prevalence of positive THC findings in blood of arrested drivers. What THC concentration in blood should be equated with impairment (and decreased ability to drive safely) lacks any international consensus (Hartman and Huestis 2013; Wolff and Johnston 2014). In the state of Colorado, which was one of the first to legalize cannabis for recreational purposes, a threshold THC concentration in blood of 5 ng/mL (0.005 mg/L) is enforced. Other states have opted to enforce a 2 ng/mL (0.002 mg/L) limit, because THC concentration in blood decreases rapidly after smoking a joint (Grotenhermen et al. 2007). However, when interpreting analytical results, one needs to consider the possibility that THC might accumulate in lipid compartments of the body after a period of heavy usage. Several studies observed that THC was measurable in the blood from heavy users several days or longer after a period of abstinence (Schwope et al. 2012; Skopp and Potsch 2008). From a single determination of the THC concentration in blood, it is not possible to predict when cannabis was last used with any degree of certainty.

1.4 Synthetic Drugs and Pharmaceuticals

1.4.1 Development of Synthetic Drugs

Until the second half of the nineteenth century, treatment of human suffering and disease involved the use of drugs derived from natural sources. Foremost among "nature's pharmaceuticals" was opium or laudanum (a mixture of opium and alcohol). Advances in organic and physiological chemistry, mainly in German-speaking countries, led to the development of the first synthetic drugs, such as the barbiturates during the first decade of the twentieth century (Lopez-Munoz et al. 2005).

1.4.1.1 A Plethora of Pharmaceuticals

The pharmaceutical industry prospered after World War II; many new synthetic drugs appeared on the market, including a host of psychoactive medications for the treatment of anxiety and mental health problems. Understandably, some people attempted to drive after taking their medication; for example, taking a sleep-aid at the wrong time of the day obviously creates a danger for traffic safety. By the 1950s, road traffic acts in many countries were updated to include provisions for prosecuting people for driving under the influence of non-alcohol drugs.

During the 1950s and 1960s, a plethora of new psychoactive substances were registered to treat conditions such as anxiety and depression, including antipsychotics such as chlorpromazine, antidepressant (imipramine), and a range of sedative-hypnotics such as ethchlorvynol, chlormethiazole, meprobamate, methaqualone, and glutethimide. All these substances were subject to abuse and caused impairment of driving ability if taken in higher than normal doses. The benzodiazepines (Librium and Valium) appeared in the early 1960s; although less toxic in overdose, they were dependence-producing and represent a danger for traffic safety (Papoutsis et al. 2016; Thomas 1998).

Like barbiturates, the benzodiazepines function as agonists at the $GABA_A$ inhibitory receptors, thereby slowing down GABAergic neurotransmission, making people less anxious and worried (Sigel and Steinmann 2012). However, benzodiazepines and other $GABA_A$ agonists are subject to abuse, and increasing the dose causes more pronounced impairment of body functions (Barbone et al. 1998; Tan et al. 2011). As pharmaceutical agents, the benzodiazepines are highly prevalent in apprehended drugged drivers in most nations, which is probably a rough indication of their abuse potential (Bramness et al. 2002; Strand et al. 2017).

1.4.1.2 Scheduled Drugs and Controlled Substances

The US Controlled Substance Act (CSA) lists the pharmaceutical substances that are regulated under US federal law, subdividing these into Schedules I through V (US Drug Enforcement 2019). The scheduling for a particular drug rests on perceived dangerousness to the patient and the potential for abuse, and whether there are well-proven medical indications. According to US Federal Drug Administration (FDA), drugs included in Schedule I are those with highest potential for abuse and are expected to cause addiction and dependence after repeated usage. The potential for addiction decreases as the schedule numbering increases from Schedules I to V.

Table 1.6 explains in more detail the grounds for placing certain drugs in one of the five classes, along with some examples and generic names of the controlled substances.

Controlled substances in the UK are those listed in the Misuse of Drugs Act, which has three classes, A, B, and C, depending on potential of the drug to harm the user (UK Government 1971). Class A drugs are those with high potential for abuse and Class C are the least dangerous. Like the FDA listing, the UK Misuse of Drugs Act is intended to regulate distribution, possession, and sale of dangerous drugs, exemplified by sedative-hypnotics (benzodiazepines) and opioid/opiate pain medication (morphine, fentanyl, pethidine, methadone, etc.). The manufacture, distribution, transport, and sale of controlled substances are restricted to prevent them being obtained and sold illegally as drugs of abuse.

1.4.1.3 Public Awareness and Information

When patients are prescribed a psychoactive medicine for the first time, their physician is expected to inform them of any adverse drug-drug interactions and also whether it is safe to operate machinery or drive a motor vehicle after taking medication. Drug-induced

Table 1.6 Classification and Scheduling of Drugs as Controlled Substances by the US Federal Drug Administration (FDA) on the Basis of Legitimate Medical Indications and Dependence Liability—The Generic Drug Names Are Used in the Table Because Trade Names Differ between Countries and Some Medications Have Several Different Proprietary Names

Classification	Brief Explanation-Motivation	Examples of the Types of Drugs in Class
Schedule I	• High potential for abuse and dependence • Lack of any well-accepted clinical or medical benefits • Lack of information about appropriate safety margins when used under medical supervision	Heroin, lysergic acid diethylamide (LSD), marijuana/cannabis (THC), peyote, methaqualone, 3,4-methylenedioxymethamphetamine (MDMA)
Schedule II	• High potential for abuse • Psychological or physical dependence can develop after repeated usage • Have legitimate medical uses in treatment of certain conditions, especially centrally acting analgesics	Opioid pain medications: hydromorphone, methadone, meperidine, oxycodone, fentanyl Narcotic analgesics: morphine, opium, codeine, and hydrocodone Stimulants: amphetamine, methamphetamine, methylphenidate Others: amobarbital, glutethimide, pentobarbital
Schedule III	• Carry a risk for abuse and dependence, but less so than drugs in schedule I & II • Care is needed when prescribed to patients (risk of developing a physical and/or psychological dependence after repeated use)	Products containing less than 90 mg codeine per dosage unit, buprenorphine, benzphetamine, phendimetrazine, ketamine, anabolic steroids
Schedule IV	• Many are sedative-hypnotics and CNS depressants with a potential for abuse and dependence, but less so than for drugs in Schedules I–III • Can cause impairment of body functions, especially when used for the first time or in overdose	• Many benzodiazepine sedative-hypnotics: alprazolam, clonazepam, clorazepate, diazepam, lorazepam, oxazepam midazolam, temazepam, triazolam • Hypnotics zopiclone, zolpidem, zaleplone
Schedule V	• Have the lowest potential for abuse • Medications with low doses of certain narcotics	Formulations containing not more than 200 mg of codeine per dose, phenergan, ezogabine.

impairment is usually more pronounced when a patient takes the prescribed medication for the first time before reaching a steady-state concentration in blood or plasma, which might take several days or weeks, depending on the drug's half-life and frequency of intake. However, the development of tolerance to a drug's effects, such as morphine, can take a lot longer than the time needed to reach steady-state concentrations in blood—as exemplified by use of strong analgesics for cancer pain (Fishbain et al. 2003; Vainio et al. 1995).

Warnings about risk of impairment are first and foremost a responsibility for the prescribing physician, but should be reiterated by the dispensing pharmacist when a patient fills or refills their prescription. Package inserts contain detailed information about possible side effects and other untoward reactions, including dangers when driving, but few people bother to read these instructions.

Drugs listed in the Swedish pharmacopeia considered dangerous to use while driving were stamped with a red warning triangle on the packaging. This warning was easy to recognize, but was unfortunately removed by the pharmaceutical agencies for dubious reasons. In some countries, medicines considered dangerous to use before driving contain a "traffic light" warning system (RED, AMBER, and GREEN) to alert patients to the dangers if and when skilled tasks (like driving) are performed (Orriols et al. 2010; Orriols et al. 2016).

1.4.2 Upsurge of Recreational Drugs

1.4.2.1 Historical Background

According to historical records, raw opium has been used by mankind for thousands of years to relieve pain and suffering and for treatment of battle wounds (Macht 1915). During the sixteenth century, laudanum (from the Latin meaning "to praise") was heralded as a universal cure for man's ailments, but this medication was also habit-forming and addictive. Morphine was isolated from raw opium in 1806, and the hypodermic needle and glass syringe were invented in 1844, thus making parenteral administration of drugs possible. Heroin was synthesized from morphine in 1874 and marketed by the Bayer Pharmaceutical Company in 1898 as an effective antitussive agent, but was later withdrawn, owing to the high risk for abuse and dependence (Sneader 2005).

Cocaine was isolated from coca leaves in 1860 and first used in medicine as a local anesthetic for eye surgery (Jones 2013). The drug's stimulant effects were also discovered and cocaine was touted as substitution therapy for people addicted to opium or alcohol, although they later became addicted to cocaine (Musto 1992).

Amphetamine was first synthesized in Germany in 1897 and methamphetamine in 1893, but pharmacological testing did not occur until the 1930s. Amphetamine was first marketed to treat nasal decongestion and was inhaled, leading to discovery of the drug's stimulant properties. This led to off-label use of amphetamine as a general pick-me-up to make people feel happier, boost their energy, and as an appetite suppressant (slimming aid). Some people looked to amphetamine as a cure for depression, but the drug was also habit-forming and many became addicted to the medication (Rasmussen 2006).

Before World War II, recreational drugs were often referred to as "uppers" and "downers"—slang expressions referring to stimulants (amphetamine-like drugs) and depressants (barbiturate derivatives), respectively. Tranquilizers was another term used to describe drugs that calmed people down, making them drowsy, sedated, and able to relax and fall asleep.

The troops in the battlefield were supplied with central stimulants, to help them stay awake longer and be more alert during combat. Other stimulant drugs were later used as pick-me-ups to relieve fatigue, as exemplified by phenmetrazine (Preludin) and methylphenidate (Ritalin). However, potential for abuse of amphetamine and methamphetamine became a major problem in some countries when the intravenous route of administration became popular. Amphetamine and methamphetamine are still high on the list of abused drugs in Finland and Sweden, especially among impaired drivers (Jones and Holmgren 2013). Stimulant drugs have some legitimate indications. For example, methylphenidate (Concerta) is used for treating attention deficit hyperactivity disorder (ADHD; the *d*-isomer of amphetamine (Adderall) is used for the same condition and also less often for narcolepsy patients.

1.4.2.2 Abuse of Illicit Drugs

In the mid-1950s, Western society was changing: a more affluent middle class had more free time on their hands and money to spend. Home entertainment was changing from listening to radio broadcasts to watching television programs and young people purchased gramophones and vinyl records. They enjoyed listening to popular music, such as jazz, blues, and rock-and-roll, which was imported to Europe from the United States and along with it came an interest in recreational drug use. Smoking a joint (cannabis) or taking stimulants to lower their inhibitions and make them more daring and liberated was a common practice among people attending pop-music festivals.

According to a 1971 report by the Department of Defense, during the Vietnam War 51% of the armed forces had smoked cannabis; 31% had used psychedelics, such as LSD, mescaline, and psilocybin mushrooms; and an additional 28% had taken cocaine and/or heroin (Stanton 1976). When soldiers returned home from active service, many were addicted to heroin and had difficulties in adjusting to a normal way of life. This led to the development of various drug-abuse treatment programs including methadone maintenance for opiate addiction (Dole 1971).

Poly-drug use, including various combinations of illicit and licit substances and consumption of alcohol, is a common finding in blood samples from apprehended drivers (Jones and Holmgren 2012). Driving under the influence of multiple drugs is generally considered a bigger danger for traffic safety than a single psychoactive substance, which in some countries (e.g., Norway) is reflected in more severe penalties when sentencing offenders. However, in other countries, punishment for having one banned substance in blood is no different from a driver taking multiple drugs.

Furthermore, there is increasing evidence that many repeat offenders have a substance abuse problem and this often coexists with sensation-seeking behavior and mental health issues (Karjalainen et al. 2011, 2013). This suggests it might be beneficial to sentence this group of traffic delinquents in specialist drug courts with options for medical intervention and treatment rather than conventional penalties for traffic crimes (Impinen et al. 2009). The notion of sentencing repeat offenders to a drug-abuse treatment program is attractive, but this strategy incurs large costs for the health care system. In some jurisdictions specialist "drug-courts" are available to deal with repeat offenders with substance-use disorder (Fell et al. 2011). Early intervention including appropriate psychological or psychiatric counseling, rehabilitation, and substitution therapy (such as methadone maintenance for heroin users), might be more beneficial for the individual and society.

There is increasing interest in sentencing repeat offenders to treatment programs designed to educate them about the dangers of excessive drinking and use of recreational drugs. Furthermore, before re-licensing they are required to undergo a thorough medical examination, including use of alcohol biomarkers in body fluids and hair strands, to evaluate ongoing drinking problems (Bortolotti et al. 2018).

Mind-altering drugs have powerful reinforcing properties and are habit-forming. Many people resort to taking these substances to help them relax and lessen the burdens of everyday life, whereas others seek pleasurable effects, euphoria, and excitement to make them appear more friendly and sociable and willing to take risks—things that are not compatible with safe driving (Karjalainen et al. 2013).

1.5 Analytical Methods

The concentrations of ethanol in blood of drivers are roughly 1,000–10,000 times higher than the concentrations of other psychoactive substances used by motorists. This makes it obvious that more sophisticated analytical methods are needed when these non-alcohol drugs are determined in blood or urine samples. Ethanol is also easily separated from the biological matrix by its volatility, whereas other drugs must be extracted using organic solvents and/or other cleanup procedures, such as solid-phase extraction, prior to analysis.

Table 1.7 compares mean, median, and highest concentrations of ethanol and other psychotropic drugs determined in blood samples from impaired drivers arrested in Sweden over many years. The concentrations of ethanol are appreciably higher than for other impairing drugs listed, the lowest being for THC (1–2 ng/mL or 0.001–0.002 mg/L) from the intake of cannabis.

Table 1.7 The Mean, Median, and Highest Concentrations of Ethanol and Other Drugs Identified in Blood Samples from Motorists Apprehended in Sweden—The Results Represent Data Accumulated over Several Years during the Period 2000–2012

Drug Determined in Blood	*n*	Mean, mg/L	Median, mg/L	Highest, mg/L
Ethanol	32,814	1740	1780	5180
Amphetamine	9,162	0.77	0.60	22.3
Methamphetamine	644	0.34	0.20	3.7
MDMA[a]	493	0.23	0.10	3.5
THC[b]	7,750	0.0019	0.001	0.036
GHB[c]	548	89	82	340
Cocaine	160	0.069	0.05	0.31
BZE[d]	160	0.80	0.60	3.0
Morphine[e,f]	2,029	0.046	0.03	1.13
6-Acetylmorphine[e]	52	0.016	0.01	0.10
Codeine[f]	1,391	0.047	0.01	2.4
Diazepam[f]	1,950	0.36	0.20	6.2

[a] MDMA = 3,4-methylenedioxymethamphetamine.
[b] THC = tetrahydrocannabinol, the active constituent of cannabis.
[c] GHB = γ-hydroxybutyrate.
[d] BZE = benzoylecognine, a major metabolite of cocaine.
[e] Metabolites of heroin.
[f] Prescription drugs.

1.5.1 Roadside Screening Tests

The police forces in most countries are equipped with handheld instruments to control driver sobriety by means of a preliminary breath test (PBT). Several versions of the PBT are available, either fitted with a pass, warn, and fail indication (with fail being set at the statutory BAC or BrAC limits for driving) or with a digital readout of the alcohol level (Poon et al. 1987). In most countries, PBTs can be administered without any prior suspicion of driver impairment, although in the United States probable cause is needed before a roadside breath test is permissible. After a presumptive positive PBT, a driver is arrested and taken for further testing, either an evidential breath alcohol test or blood sampling for laboratory analysis (Kriikku et al. 2014). If the PBT test is negative and there are outward signs and/or symptoms of impairment, this suggests other psychoactive drugs were responsible or some medical condition had altered the driver's behavior. False-positive rates of PBTs are relatively low because the electrochemical oxidation method of analysis is highly selective for identification and quantification of ethanol (Zuba 2008).

Testing for use of drugs other than alcohol at the roadside is possible by the analysis of oral fluid, which is swabbed from the mouth or tongue onto an absorbent material sometimes referred to as a DrugWipe (Drummer 2006). Many drugs enter oral fluid from the blood supplying the salivary glands and are detectable by immunochemical methods targeted toward certain classes of abused substances (such as cocaine, cannabis, PCP, and amphetamine) but not prescription drugs or new psychoactive substances (NPS) purchased over the Internet (Drummer et al. 2007). The results from analysis of drugs in oral fluid must be confirmed by use of more sophisticated methods of analysis, such as LC-MS-MS or equivalent methodology, on blood samples to motivate a prosecution (Gjerde et al. 2018a; Krotulski et al. 2018).

1.5.1.1 Standardized Field Sobriety Tests

The police in the United States require reasonable suspicion that a driver is impaired by alcohol and/or other drugs before an arrest can be made (Burns 2003). Obtaining samples of blood or breath for toxicological analysis without probably cause is forbidden according to the article of the US Constitution that regulates unwarranted searches and seizures (Voas and Fell 2013). The police in many jurisdictions are not even allowed to administer a preliminary roadside breath test without reasonable suspicion that a driver is impaired by alcohol. This problem has—to some extent—been sidestepped by use of "passive alcohol sensors" (PAS) (Fell et al. 2008). These devices are fitted with electrochemical sensors and often look like a police flashlight; they are held in close proximity to the driver's mouth while he or she is engaged in conversation. The PAS aspirates a specimen of breath and any alcohol present is detected, indicating whether the driver was above or below a statutory limit for driving (Foss et al. 1993). The PAS device tends to underestimate the alcohol content of a deep-lung breath sample, but nevertheless give the police sufficient grounds to proceed with further testing. Passive sensors for drugs other than alcohol (e.g., cannabis) are highly desirable but are not yet available.

In the 1970s, the police in the United States made use of standardized field sobriety tests (SFSTs) to produce evidence that a driver was impaired by alcohol or drugs. SFSTs are administered at the roadside after a traffic stop and comprise: (a) one-leg stand;

(b) walk and turn; and (c) horizontal gaze nystagmus (HGN). The first suspicion might be aroused by: (a) a driver's way of responding to questioning, suspicious behavior, or exhibiting outward signs and symptoms; (b) slurred speech; (c) the smell of cannabis in the vehicle; and (d) finding drug paraphernalia (Rubenzer 2011). The original SFSTs were designed to detect impairment caused by overconsumption of alcohol and have not been fully evaluated for detecting impairment caused by other drugs (Brown et al. 2013). Nevertheless, the preliminary results are promising that SFSTs are able to detect if a driver is impaired by non-alcohol drugs (Porath-Waller and Beirness 2014).

Of the three types of test, the HGN test is probably the most sensitive. This measures involuntary jerking of the eyeball when a stimulus (small pen) is moved from side to side in front of the eyes. The walk-and-turn and one-leg stand test are "divided attention" tasks requiring a person to listen and follow instructions while performing simple physical movements (Burns 2003). According to several studies, divided-attention tasks are highly sensitive to the effects of alcohol (Jongen et al. 2016).

The reliability of SFSTs for the purpose of identifying drivers impaired by non-alcohol drugs (e.g., cannabis) will depend on several factors, such as time of last usage of the drug, the dose and concentration present in blood, and development of tolerance to drug-related effects (Hartman et al. 2016). The police are allowed to make a video recording of the driver to document his or her attitude and behavior when being questioned and subjected to field sobriety tests, which can later be introduced in evidence to support other evidence of impairment.

SFSTs are administered under different lighting and weather conditions at the roadside with other traffic in motion. Some individuals might experience difficulty in passing the test sober. In such cases, an option to administer a PBT would be worthwhile. Elderly people (>65 years) in poor health, suffering from hyper- or hypotension, or age-related disturbances in balance, might have difficulty standing on one leg for 30 seconds and follow orders even without drinking any alcohol.

The use of SFSTs has been thoroughly evaluated around the BAC limit of 0.08 g%, but less is known about their reliability at lower BAC, such as 0.05 g% (Stuster 2006). This question needs to be addressed if other US states follow the lead of Utah, where the BAC *per se* limit was lowered from 0.08 to 0.05 g% starting January 2019 (McKnight et al. 2002). Lowering the statutory alcohol limit for driving will hopefully prompt police authorities to make more use of PBTs as a noninvasive way to test driver sobriety. These handheld devices are highly reliable and are widely used in countries where the threshold BAC limit for driving is set at 0.02 g%.

Starting December 18, 2018, the police in Canada no longer need probable cause of impairment to administer a PBT. Changes in the Criminal Code of Canada removed the requirement for establishing impairment prior to arrest and administering a PBT. There is now a mandatory requirement that motorists submit to a PBT when asked to do so by a police officer in uniform (Canadian Centre on Substance Use and Addiction: 2019).

Since the late twentieth century, the police in most European countries (Dunbar et al. 1987) and in Australia (Homel 1993) and New Zealand have been allowed to stop any vehicle and demand a roadside breath-alcohol test, which is commonly referred to as random breath testing (RBT). This approach has proven a highly effective way to control driver sobriety, allowing immediate arrest and further evidential testing if necessary. Indeed, allowing the police to undertake RBTs is almost a prerequisite for effective enforcement of low BAC limits of 0.02 or 0.05 g%.

1.5.1.2 Breath Tests for Non-alcohol Drugs

Methods have been developed that permit collecting breath samples at the roadside for later analysis of drugs other than alcohol at a forensic laboratory. A driver is asked to exhale through a handheld device containing a chemical reagent that absorbs drugs and volatiles in the form of a breath aerosol. The tubes are then shipped to a laboratory for analysis by LC-MS/MS (Beck et al. 2013, 2016; Ullah et al. 2018). Human breath is saturated with water vapor at body temperature and during a forced exhalation drug molecules enter the breath as an aerosol of microparticles (Seferaj et al. 2018). Both illicit drugs, such as amphetamine, cocaine, and THC, as well as a range of therapeutic drugs, have been detected in breath after extraction from the absorbent material (Ullah et al. 2018). However, interpretation of the results from such tests in relation to impairment is difficult; correlations of drug concentrations in blood and oral fluid (let alone breath) are low and not significant, so the usefulness of sampling breath for analysis of non-alcohol drugs in traffic law enforcement is questionable (Beck and Olin 2016).

However, there is considerable commercial interest in developing a handheld device for analysis of THC in breath for use at the roadside to screen drivers, thus providing the police with more objective evidence of cannabis use before driving. Studies from several sources show that prevalence of driving under the influence of cannabis is increasing owing to its acceptance for medical purposes (such as treatment of multiple sclerosis, glaucoma, or idiopathic pain) and recreational use. Because use of cannabis for recreational purposes has been decriminalized in ten US states and throughout Canada, this paradigm shift will undoubtedly lead to more arrests for driving under the influence of THC (US National Highway Traffic Safety Administration 2017).

1.5.1.3 Oral Fluid Tests

The analysis of oral fluid for drugs is widely used by the police as a roadside screening test. One such oral fluid test is referred to as DrugWipe (Beirness and Smith 2017). A person wipes his or her tongue on a small absorbent material and within about 5 min the device indicates whether the person has drugs in saliva, with the primary focus on testing for cannabis and cocaine (Drummer et al. 2007). More sophisticated on-site oral fluid tests are also available from some manufacturers (e.g., Draeger DrugTest 5000), which responds to cocaine, cannabis, and methamphetamine. All positive results from roadside oral fluid tests need confirmation by more reliable analytical methods, such as GC-MS or LC-MS/MS (Gjerde et al. 2018a; Pehrsson et al. 2011). The false-positive and false-negative rates from analysis of oral fluid are fairly high, requiring more sensitive and specific methods for verification (Gjerde et al. 2010, 2015).

The correlation between concentrations of drugs in saliva and in blood (or plasma) taken at the same time is rather poor, which precludes the use of saliva-test results to estimate concentrations in plasma or blood (Busardo et al. 2018; Langel et al. 2014). Nevertheless, sampling of saliva is a non-invasive procedure, which can be done at the roadside and a decision made to arrest the driver and proceed with confirmatory oral fluid testing at a police station. If this second test is also positive, then the suspect is either sanctioned or asked to provide a sample of blood for laboratory analysis using GC-MS-MS to bring a more serious charge of impaired driving. The methods available for the analysis of drugs in oral-fluid have been much improved with regard to obtaining the required volume of specimen. Police authorities in many countries use this equipment, especially to screen drivers, for cocaine and/or cannabis use (Huestis et al. 2011).

1.5.2 Quantitative Analysis of Ethanol and Other Drugs

Handheld instruments for the determination of ethanol in breath have been used by the police to control sobriety since the early 1970s (Poon et al. 1987). Likewise, instruments suitable for evidential purposes have gone through six generations since the Breathalyzer was invented in 1954 (Wigmore and Langille 2009). The analytical principles for quantitative analysis of ethanol in breath either involve electrochemical oxidation with a fuel-cell sensor or infrared spectrometry; some devices incorporate both technologies (EC and IR) to enhance selectivity for identifying ethanol (Jones 2000). The accuracy and precision of modern breath-alcohol instruments matches that of GC analysis of ethanol in blood.

The gold standard method of blood-alcohol analysis involves the use of headspace gas chromatography with flame ionization detector (HS-GC-FID) or, more recently, a mass detector (HS-GC-MS) (Tiscione et al. 2011). This type of methodology has been used for legal purposes since the 1960s and gives accurate, precise, and specific results fit for its intended purpose (Jones 1996).

Table 1.8 summarizes major historical developments in the analytical methods used for determination of ethanol and other drugs in biological specimens for clinical and forensic purposes.

The quantitative analysis of drugs other than ethanol is a more challenging task for analytical toxicologists for several reasons. First, as stated earlier, the concentrations of non-alcohol drugs in blood and other biological fluids (see Table 1.7) are 1,000–10,000 times lower than concentrations of ethanol. Second, ethanol is easily separated from the biological matrix by its volatility, whereas other drugs need to be extracted with organic solvents or solid-phase cartridges, which is more troublesome and costly (Maurer 2018).

Table 1.8 Historical Landmarks in the Development of Methods for Analysis of Alcohol and Other Drugs in Biological Specimens for Legal Purposes

Time Period	Analytical Methods Used for Analysis of Abused Drugs in Body Fluids
1850–1950	• Analytical methods utilize chemical reactions to observe color changes after adding certain reagents or mixing with solvents, even formation of precipitates or oxidation-reduction reactions • Volumetric titration and gravimetric analysis was the basis for quantitative analysis of ethanol in blood • Making chemical derivatives of substances isolated from tissues and measuring melting points was the way that other drugs were identified (yielding only qualitative results) • Visible and other photometric methods, as well as polarography, became available after 1940
1950–1960	• After WWII, radioactive and stable isotopes were made commercially available and were incorporated in methods of analysis in biological chemistry • The isotopes of carbon, hydrogen, phosphorous and iodine were labeled and inserted into various organic compounds • Spectrometric methods including visible, ultraviolet and infrared more advanced including the highly sensitive technique of spectrophotofluorimetry, which was applied to the analysis of endogenous substances and therapeutic drugs • After certain enzymes were purified from animal tissues they were adopted for in-vitro diagnostic testing in clinical laboratories. Procedures were available for enzymatic analysis of glucose, ethanol, and many other substances

(*Continued*)

Table 1.8 (*Continued*) Historical Landmarks in the Development of Methods for Analysis of Alcohol and Other Drugs in Biological Specimens for Legal Purposes

Time Period	Analytical Methods Used for Analysis of Abused Drugs in Body Fluids
1960s–1970s	• Chromatographic separation methods dominated laboratory procedures: after solvent extraction and clean-up, drugs were separated and identified by paper and thin-layer chromatography and later gas-liquid chromatography (GLC) • The first GLC methods describing the quantitative analysis of ethanol and barbiturates in blood appeared at about this time
1970s–1980s	• Combination of GC separation technique for analysis of volatiles (headspace sampling) with flame ionization detector (FID), electron capture (EC) as well as a mass spectrometric (MS) detector • Widely applied and highly sensitive and specific hyphenated technique of GC-MS, revolutionizing the work done in forensic toxicology laboratories • Enzyme immunoassay became routine methods for drug screening analysis of urine, especially EMIT and CEDIA, ideally suited for mass screening of samples thus eliminating drug negatives (Positive screening results led to use of more specific and sensitive analysis being done)
1980s–1990s	• GC methods of analysis underwent further development, especially the use of capillary columns, which gradually replaced the traditional packed columns • More compact instruments became available thanks to development of microchip technology and integrated circuit boards • Laboratory computerization: the once bulky GC-MS instruments computerized and miniaturized leading to development of a range of benchtop models and GC-MS workstations • Deuterium labeled analogues of many drugs became available for use as internal standards
1990s–2000s	• Combination of liquid chromatograph (LC) for drug separation (and clean-up) with an MS detector began to replace/complement GC-MS methods of analysis (with LC methods, chemical derivatives prior to analysis often not required) • Basic LC-MS methodology was further advanced with tandem and high-resolution MS technologies
2000–present	• Methods based on LC-MS or LC-MS/MS continue to improve, and have gradually replaced GC-MS methods for the analysis of most drugs and toxins • Accurate mass identification of drug fragmentation patterns are widely used in toxicology laboratories worldwide • Time-of-flight (TOF) MS analysis, which allows making a simultaneous screening analysis of a wide range of drugs and metabolites in a single analytical run • Small quantities of drugs, in the ng or pg range, can be determined in blood and the same methodology also applied to alternative biological specimen, such as saliva and hair strands

The pharmacologically active substance is first extracted from blood or tissue by adjusting the pH so that drug molecules are in their unionized form and therefore more lipophilic. The buffered mixture is then shaken with organic solvents or added to specially designed solid-phase columns. In this way, the active drug is separated from interfering substance and/or any drug metabolites prior to analysis by GC or LC using various detector systems, such as flame ionization detector, electron capture detector, nitrogen-phosphorous detector, or a mass detector (MS) with selected ion monitoring (Maurer 1999).

An important advance occurred when capillary column GC methods appeared in the 1980s, which improved sensitivity and specificity of the assay considerably. The time elapsed after injecting the sample onto the GC column to the time of appearance of a peak is known as the retention time (RT) and serves to identify the analyte (qualitative analysis) by comparing RT with known authentic substances. Alternatively, relative retention time (RRT) is another way of identification, whereby the time for elution of the GC peak is compared with RT of an internal standard added to the biological specimen before analysis (Mbughuni et al. 2016). When GC-MS or LC-MS methods of analysis are used, it is customary to make use of deuterium-labeled internal standards and both RT and mass fragmentation patterns help to identify the drugs and/or metabolites in the sample (Maurer 1992).

Today's analytical methodology for the determination of drugs in biological specimens is highly sophisticated, fully automated, and controlled by computer systems and workstations. Separation methods based on GC or LC are first and foremost coupled with mass-selective detectors, often high-resolution instruments—so-called tandem detectors GC-MS-MS or LC-MS-MS (Maurer and Meyer 2016; Meyer et al. 2016). The positive identification of hundreds of psychoactive substance and their metabolites is no longer a difficult task for analytical toxicologists. However, the correct interpretation of the analytical results is more challenging, especially when compliance with some threshold concentration limit is an issue in criminal prosecutions. In this connection, making an allowance for uncertainty by subtracting a certain amount from the analytical result is highly recommended when concentration *per se* statutes are enforced (Kristoffersen et al. 2016) as is commonly done with forensic BAC determinations (Gullberg 2012). Neither should one forget pre-analytical factors, such as those associated with sampling, transport, storage, and chain-of-custody issues as well as stability of the target drug during storage (Kouri et al. 2005).

1.5.3 Interpretation of Analytical Results

After absorption into the bloodstream, drugs are transported to the brain and interact or bind with certain receptor sites and proteins causing impairment of thought processes, and altered performance and behavior, etc. The degree of impairment associated with drug use depends on the type of drug, the mechanism of action, the dose taken, and the time after intake when driving occurs. Drugs are eliminated from the body by metabolism and excretion at widely different rates, varying from a few hours to several days, depending on the drug's elimination half-life.

When toxicology results are interpreted in DUID cases, it is important to consider the entire case scenario. This includes observations about the driving, results of field sobriety tests if any, clinical signs and symptoms, and the DRE examination results along with the toxicology report. The totality of information available allows reaching an evidence-based opinion about impairment caused by drug use and whether the concentrations in blood are consistent with therapeutic usage or overdosing with medication (Launiainen and Ojanpera 2014). The question of whether a patient was compliant (or not) with their medication can be gleaned by comparison with therapeutic drug-monitoring programs and concentrations of the same drugs in plasma or serum (Jones et al. 2007).

Based on knowledge of the main pharmacokinetic parameters of the drug (such as distribution volume, elimination-rate constant, and half-life), tentative conclusions can be drawn about the amount of drug in the body and sometimes when it was taken in relation to driving (Huestis et al 2005). The concentrations of drugs in blood, plasma, or serum are more closely related to amounts reaching the brain and the pharmacologic response, including impairment of body functions (Nedahl et al 2019).

Urine is an excellent specimen for a preliminary screening analysis and also provides a wider window of detection compared with blood or plasma; but urinary concentrations cannot be used to draw inferences about concentrations existing in blood nor any drug-related effects on impairment (Liu 1992). Positive results from the analysis of urine verifies prior usage; however, calculating the dose administered or the time of last intake is not possible with any degree of scientific certainty.

In the field of forensic toxicology, drugs are almost always determined in blood, whereas clinical laboratories (dealing with therapeutic drug monitoring) analyze the concentrations in plasma or serum. The concentrations of drugs in these biological media are not necessarily the same, depending on lipid- to water-solubility and the amount of binding to plasma proteins and other biomolecules (Jantos et al. 2011). In general, drug concentrations in plasma/serum are higher than in an equal volume of blood. These distribution ratios should be considered when analytical results from forensic laboratories are interpreted and compared with therapeutic concentration in clinical pharmacology. Some examples of serum/blood distribution ratios for drugs determined in blood of drivers are 1.7–2.0 for THC (Gronewold and Skopp 2011), 1.6–1.8 for diazepam (Jones and Larsson 2004), and 1.01–1.15 for various alcohols, such as ethanol (Skopp et al. 2005).

1.6 Common Defense Arguments in DUID Cases

Defending impaired drivers has become a specialty area for many law firms, especially those operating in the US or the UK, where the adversarial system of justice operates as opposed to the inquisitorial system in continental Europe (Beran 2009; McBay 1965). Many defense lawyers are knowledgeable about the scientific issues involved including the analytical methods and physiological effects of drug intake (Fitzgerald 2001). As legal professionals, they are schooled in raising a reasonable doubt and are well versed in the pros and cons of rebuttable presumptions. Organizations such as "The National College of DUI Defense" (https://ncdd.com/) regularly hold seminars and symposia to discuss ways of challenging the admissibility of toxicology evidence in DUI and DUID cases. A library of books dealing with the science and law of impaired driving legislation is available—often coauthored by a lawyer and a scientist combining expertise in jurisprudence with analytical and toxicological chemistry.

Defense lawyers have a tendency to speculate about likely sources of laboratory error, including obtaining the requisite samples of blood, saliva, or urine; the chain of custody and deviations from good laboratory practice, and magnitude of analytical uncertainty. Many defense arguments lack merit and are simply a way to create a reasonable doubt in the eyes of the jury (Jones 1991) by finding flaws and technicalities in the prosecution case—legitimate trial tactics under the adversarial system (Williams 2018). In countries like Finland, Germany, and Sweden a very common defense argument in drunken-driving cases is the consumption of alcohol after being involved in a crash, to calm the nerves and reduce anxiety (Jones 1991). This same argument is increasingly observed among drugged drivers who claim they took certain drugs after driving. Defense lawyers tend to focus on the subjective nature of SFSTs and the qualifications, training, and possible bias on the part of the arresting police officer (Rubenzer 2008).

As of 2019, the use of cannabis for medical purposes in the USA is legal in 33 states and recreational use is permitted in 10 states. This change in attitude and liberalization of a hitherto controlled substance will have long-term consequences for public health and traffic safety. An obvious concern is drug-impaired driving, because cannabis use is almost as common as alcohol among some communities in the US (Compton 2017). The notion of introducing a threshold THC concentration in blood corresponding to the 0.05 or 0.08 g% BAC limits has been much discussed. The potency of THC as a pharmacologically active substance is several thousand times higher than ethanol. The threshold limits of THC in blood in most jurisdictions (ranging from 1 to 5 ng/mL) are probably appropriate for occasional users of cannabis (Ramaekers et al. 2006b). However, after chronic daily usage, the THC concentration tends to accumulate in fatty tissues and gets washed out over weeks or months during a period of abstinence (Skopp and Potsch 2008). There is increasing evidence that 1–2 ng/mL of THC might be measurable in blood or plasma for days or weeks after the person last took the drug and this needs consideration when punishable limits of THC are enforced (Bergamaschi et al. 2013). Some specialists in THC research have suggested setting a *per se* THC limit in blood of 5 ng/mL to avoid the problem of residual THC in heavy users (Grotenhermen et al. 2007). The median THC concentration in blood of drivers arrested in Sweden was 1–2 ng/mL, which means that many would evade prosecution if the statutory limit was 5 ng/mL, and much will depend on elapsed time between last use of the drug, the time of arrest, and any delay before sampling blood for toxicology (Jones et al. 2008).

Prior to the introduction of *per se* laws for drugs, the results and conclusions from clinical tests were often challenged, claiming a medical condition or complaint was mimicking the signs and symptoms of drug impairment. Examples include diabetes (hypoglycemia), epilepsy, and various psychiatric disorders or even failure to medicate with antidepressants or antipsychotics as prescribed by a physician. Understandably, problems arose when results of the medical examination stood in conflict with the toxicological report and the concentrations of drugs in blood.

Table 1.9 gives examples of excuses or arguments encountered during prosecution of DUID offenders in Sweden after a zero-tolerance law for illicit drugs was enacted and special requirements for use of psychoactive prescription drugs (in connection with driving) was enforced.

In a typical DUID investigation, it might take several hours after the time of driving (or involvement in a traffic crash) before blood samples are taken for toxicological analysis. Such delays have consequences for positive identification of certain drugs in blood, especially those with relatively short elimination half-lives. In many US states, the administration of SFSTs takes time, as does transporting the suspect to a police station or medical center for further evaluation and examination. If a driver was injured in a crash and needed emergency medical treatment, the time elapsed after driving before blood was taken for toxicology is often considerably longer.

Drugs such as GHB, cocaine, THC, zopiclone, and zolpidem are rapidly eliminated from the blood and even if present at time of driving might have dropped below the method's LLOQ (and thus reported as not detected) by the time blood was taken for toxicological analysis. The analysis of drugs in urine extends the window of detection by several hours, although urinary concentrations are not correlated with impairment effects.

Table 1.9 Examples of Some Defense Arguments (Challenges) Raised when Impaired Drivers Were Arrested in Sweden for Driving Under the Influence of Non-alcohol Drugs when Zero-Tolerance or Concentration *per se* Limits Were Enforced

1	I took my wife's medication by mistake, her bottle of pills stood next to mine in the bathroom cabinet and I inadvertently used her medication.
2	The prescribing physician failed to warn me about the dangers of taking the medication before driving and I had neglected to read the package insert that came with the medication.
3	The suspect claims to have been taking the same psychoactive medication for many years and had unintentionally increased the dose, but did not feel ability to drive safely had deteriorated.
4	Suffered from an acute anxiety episode when on vacation abroad and purchased medication at a local pharmacy store without the need for a prescription. The person continued using the medication on return home and had no idea it could cause driving impairment.
5	Smoked cannabis/marijuana intensively last weekend on a visit to Amsterdam, Canada, or a US state where recreational use of this drug is legal. The suspect claims to have been unaware that the active substance (THC) and/or its main metabolite (carboxy-THC) would be identified in body fluids for such a long time after last usage.
6	The suspect took an antianxiety or analgesic drug after being involved in a traffic crash to calm the nerves or to relieve pain from injuries sustained in the crash.
7	Drugs were taken by mistake when visiting a hospital clinic for substance use disorder.
8	When attending a nightclub someone must have spiked the person's drink while he or she was on the dance floor or away visiting the restroom (bathroom).
9	The positive test results for cannabis/marijuana must have arisen from unintentional exposure, such as when guests at a private party were smoking a joint. Close proximity or contact with these individuals resulted in passive inhalation of the smoke, hence causing the positive result of the analysis for THC or carboxy-THC.

Because some drugs are cleared rapidly from the bloodstream after intake, there is discussion in some circles about back-extrapolating the concentration determined at the time of sampling blood to the time of driving, sometimes a few hours earlier (Huestis et al. 2005). Such retrograde extrapolations are routine in some jurisdictions for drunk-driving cases and it is probably only a matter of time before similar procedures are generally adopted for other drugs, as they already are in Norway (Montgomery and Reasor 1992). However, knowledge about the human pharmacokinetics of ethanol is much more extensive and well documented than it is for other psychoactive substances.

Some of the things to consider when toxicological results for non-alcohol drugs are interpreted in DUID cases are listed below:

- Are the drugs identified in the driver's blood classified as controlled substances?
- If yes, does the driver have a valid prescription for the medication? Without such a prescription for a psychoactive medication the person can be charged with DUID. If supratherapeutic concentrations are detected in blood, this motivates prosecution for DUID, regardless of whether the driver has a prescription.
- What is the accepted therapeutic concentration range in blood, plasma, or serum for the active chemical substance in the medication?
- Are there any pharmacologically active metabolites of the drug present in blood?
- Some metabolites of illicit drugs, such as carboxy-THC or benzoylecgonine (the major breakdown product of cocaine) are not pharmacologically active. Finding these substances verifies prior use of cannabis or cocaine, but drawing conclusions about impairment are not possible.

- The concentrations of drugs determined in plasma/serum are not necessarily the same as in whole blood, owing to plasma protein binding and differences in lipid solubility.
- Differences in plasma/blood concentration need to be considered when analytical results for blood samples are compared with therapeutic concentrations determined in serum or plasma.
- What is known about the stability of drugs in blood during transport and storage of the specimens prior to analysis? Was there a sodium fluoride preservative in the evacuated tubes? The concentrations of some drugs and metabolites, such as cocaine, 6-acetyl morphine, and zopiclone, are stabilized in fluorinated tubes.
- What does the peer-reviewed literature say about the quantitative relationship between dose of the drug, the concentration measured in blood, and the impairment of cognitive and psychomotor functioning relevant for safe driving?

1.7 Age, Gender, and Drugs Detected

The demographics of people arrested for driving under the influence of alcohol and/or other drugs show a predominance of male traffic offenders (Skurtveit et al. 1995). Table 1.10 contains information about DUID suspects arrested in Sweden indicating a male-to-female ratio of 85% to 15% regardless of the drug used. These cases were selected from a national toxicology database if only a single psychoactive substance was verified present in the driver's blood, hence mono-drug intoxication. The number of cases, apart from ethanol, amphetamine, and THC, is therefore limited for the other psychoactive substances, because most DUID suspects take multiple drugs, combining prescription medication with alcohol and/or an illicit drug (Jones and Holmgren 2012).

When impaired driving cases in Norway were investigated over a 25-year period (1990–2015), the proportion of male traffic offenders remained fairly constant at 87% and these individuals were also more likely to have used illicit drugs (Valen et al. 2017).

Table 1.10 Demographics of People Arrested in Sweden for Driving Under the Influence of Alcohol and/or Other Psychoactive Drugs—The Results Represent Information Accumulated Over Several Years During the Period 2000–2012 When Only a Single Psychoactive Substance Was Identified in Blood

Drug in Blood Samples	*n*	Men (%)	Women (%)	Suspect's Age, y (mean ± SD)
Ethanol	32,814	90%	10%	40.0 ± 8.7
Amphetamine	9,162	85%	15%	36.5 ± 9.0
THC[a]	7,750	94%	6%	32.6 ± 8.4
MDMA[b]	493	92%	8%	26.4 ± 7.2
GHB[c]	548	96%	4%	26.0 ± 6.8
6-Acetylmorphine[d]	52	89%	11%	33.2 ± 8.7
Cocaine and/or BZE[e]	160	96%	4%	28.6 ± 7.0

[a] THC = tetrahydrocannabinol, the active substance in cannabis.
[b] MDMA = 3,4-methylenedioximethamphetamine.
[c] GHB = γ-hydroxybutyrate.
[d] Metabolite of heroin.
[e] BZE = benzoylecgonine, the major metabolite of cocaine.

The prevalence of amphetamine use by drivers in Norway increased after 2000, especially in male offenders aged >40. By contrast, the prevalence of drivers taking benzodiazepines decreased over the same time period studied; although diazepam remained highly prevalent, clonazepam seems to have replaced flunitrazepam, after the latter hypnotic became more difficult to obtain legally (Hoiseth et al. 2015). In the past decade, prevalence of THC-positive drivers has increased in the Nordic countries, indicating the popularity of cannabis as a recreational drug. However, decriminalization of cannabis is not on the Nordic horizon.

In a study of 410 drivers arrested in Norway aged over 65, toxicology results verified at least one impairing substance in blood in 92% of cases and ethanol was above the legal limit (0.02 g%) in 81% of cases (Hoiseth et al. 2017). Illegal drugs and amphetamine were rarely detected in blood in this elderly age group of traffic offenders; the dominant drugs were various benzodiazepine derivatives (15%) and certain hypnotics (13%). The drugs most frequently used as monotherapy by elderly drivers (>65) was zopiclone (9.8%) and diazepam (9.3%).

The ages of drunk and/or drugged drivers span from about 15 to 90, and the choice of drug seems to vary with their age. Alcohol-impaired drivers and abusers of amphetamine are generally older (late 30s to early 40s) than people taking other psychoactive substances. Users of cocaine or GHB were in their late 20s or early 30s. The drugs of choice by drivers probably reflects availability (and popularity) of psychoactive substances in the society as a whole, as reflected in prescribing practices for legal drugs and proximity to smuggling routes, such as from Eastern European nations for obtaining illicit drugs.

Driving under the influence of central stimulant amines has a long history in Sweden, whereas GHB appeared on the drug scene in the late 1990s. Results from toxicological analysis of blood samples from drivers apprehended in Norway over a 25-year period (n = 112,348) found that 63% were positive for at least one drug and 43% had used both alcohol and another impairing substance before driving (Valen et al. 2017).

The demographic profile of people arrested for drunk driving in Norway and Sweden is probably similar to other nations, being predominantly male offenders in their late 30s to early 40s, and binge drinkers with high BAC (mean 0.15–0.18 g%) when apprehended (Gjerde 1987). Furthermore, recidivism rates are high among impaired drivers, many of whom don't have a valid driving license, presumably because it was withdrawn for earlier convictions (Hubicka et al. 2007, 2008). By contrast, the typical DUID offender is about 5–10 years younger than drunk drivers and is more likely to have taken multiple impairing substances before driving; poly-drug use is rampant among some traffic offenders (Holmgren et al. 2007). Indeed, there is a strong association between early-onset drunken driving, violent criminality, mental health disorder, and premature death (Karjalainen et al. 2014; Rasanen et al. 1999).

Based on 10 years of DUID arrests, in three Nordic countries, the toxicology findings show a predominance of illicit drugs in blood and poly-drug use is normal (Holmgren et al. 2007; Lillsunde and Gunnar 2005; Valen et al. 2017). In Sweden the most prevalent illicit drug was amphetamine, closely followed by cannabis, morphine from heroin abuse, and cocaine; whereas for prescription drugs, benzodiazepine anxiolytics and opiate/opioid pain medication were highly prevalent (Ahlner et al. 2014).

Repeat offending is common among DUI and DUID offenders and deserves special attention from traffic-safety organizations and more effective legislation from the government (Christophersen et al. 1996; Jones et al. 2015). For this group of offenders, the conventional penalties are seemingly ineffective as a deterrent, because many suffer from a substance-use disorder and are arrested multiple times in the same calendar year (Marques et al. 2003). Much can be said for introducing special sanctions, such as drug or DUI courts with options for treatment and rehabilitation of repeat offenders and mandatory fitting of ignition interlock devices for drunk-driving recidivists (Fell et al. 2011; Voas et al. 2016).

1.8 Discussion and Conclusions

1.8.1 Discussion

This review has highlighted many of the similarities and differences in traffic-safety laws pertaining to drunk and drugged driving in various nations. The prosecution evidence was initially based on a driver's own admission of alcohol consumption or taking drugs before driving and supported by testimony from the arresting police officer or other witnesses. Later, the main evidence for charging a person with impaired driving came from a medical examination of the suspect by a physician or police surgeon or DRE officer. The current trend in most nations is toward enforcement of zero-tolerance laws for illicit drugs, which means that a prosecution is not dependent on impairment evidence; the evidence needed is the presence of any measurable amount of the banned substance in a sample of the driver's blood. In the case of taking psychoactive prescription drugs before driving, a valid prescription is necessary and the medication should not have been taken in overdose or abused.

There is a general agreement that zero-tolerance laws are acceptable for drivers taking illicit drugs, because use of these substances for nonmedical purposes is already a criminal offense. The situation is more complex for legitimate medicines, which are used by many in society to live a normal life. If a driver is judged to be impaired from use of a prescription drug, then he or she can be arrested and charged with impaired driving regardless of whether a valid prescription is presented. If the concentration of a prescription drug in blood is higher than expected for normal therapeutic usage, this suggests the person was noncompliant or had overdosed with the medication, which is not uncommon in the case of pain medication, such as opiate/opioid analgesics—often subject to abuse (Impinen et al. 2011; Volkow et al. 2018).

This historical review of impaired driving legislation would not be complete without mentioning the impact of an organization called Mothers Against Drunk Driving (MADD; https://www.madd.org). MADD was founded in 1980 in the US and functions as a victims' advocate group drawing attention to the dangers of drunken driving as a public health problem (Fell and Voas 2006a). MADD focuses its attention on the trauma and suffering caused to families who have lost loved ones in road traffic crashes involving a drunk or drugged driver. Among other things, MADD advocates lowering BAC limits for driving, increasing traffic surveillance, use of random breath testing, and more immediate sanctions, such as revocation of the driving permit, short periods of incarceration, and mandatory fitting of ignition interlock devices to vehicles owned by repeat offenders (Voas et al. 2016).

Taken together, the evidence is clear that zero-tolerance and *per se* laws are a pragmatic way to deal with the problem of impaired driving, because it simplifies the evidence necessary for prosecution and produces higher rates of conviction. The results from clinical tests of impairment are more subjective than chemistry-based evidence of drug intake and the latter evidence is more difficult to challenge in litigation.

Unfortunately, there does not exist any international agreement about what *per se* limits in blood should be enforced for non-alcohol psychoactive substances; these differ from jurisdiction to jurisdiction (Busardo et al. 2017). This situation is not unique as evidenced by statutory BAC limits, which vary fourfold between countries. Experimental work on drug-related impairment is hampered by ethical and safety considerations, because giving supratherapeutic doses of drugs to healthy volunteers is not feasible. Furthermore, the effect of an acute dose on one occasion will not necessarily be the same after repeated intake of the medication, such as when steady-state concentrations are reached in blood and when tolerance develops to some drug effects.

After a zero-tolerance DUID law was introduced in Sweden and Finland, the number of drivers arrested by the police increased appreciably (Jones et al. 2015; Karjalainen et al. 2015). For example, in Sweden, before a zero-tolerance law ~1,000 drivers/year were arrested for DUID, whereas 10 years later the number had increased to 13,000 and this has since remained fairly constant, corresponding to a 13-fold increase. Furthermore, in 85%–90% of the blood samples analyzed, one or more banned substances were identified. Similar increases in DUID arrest rates have been observed in Denmark (Simonsen et al. 2018), Norway (Valen et al. 2017), and Finland (Karjalainen et al. 2015). This apparent increased prevalence of DUID, despite a stricter legislation (zero tolerance and/or *per se* law), probably reflects increased activity and enthusiasm on the part of police authorities with the knowledge that now it is much more likely that a prosecution will be successful.

Many traffic delinquents are addicted to drugs and they combine illicit substances with psychoactive prescription drugs as well as consume alcohol. They invariably lack a valid prescription for the medications, especially in the case of sedative-hypnotics and centrally acting analgesics (Tjaderborn et al. 2016). The source of these medications is an open question, although several possibilities exist including drug-trafficking, theft, smuggling, black-market purchases, and via the Internet, especial the "Darknet," where almost anything can be obtained.

In an increasing number of US states, the use of cannabis preparations for medical purposes is legitimate and widely accepted. Ten US states also allow its purchase and use for recreational purposes, even though according to federal law cannabis is still a controlled substance. This decriminalization of cannabis will undoubtedly have negative consequences for traffic safety and more people will be arrested by the police for driving under the influence of THC. Legislation to control driving under the influence of cannabis is modeled on the crime of drunken driving, including the use of science-based jurisprudence and concentration *per se* limits of the active substance THC in a driver's blood (Roth 2015).

But ethanol is very different from THC in its properties and pharmacological effects. The question of establishing science-based limits for THC has been much debated and until now no legal or scientific consensus exists (Grotenhermen et al. 2007). Statutory *per se* limits of THC in blood are already implemented in EU nations, where cannabis is an illegal Class A drug. Punishable THC concentrations in blood range from a low of 0.3 ng/mL in Sweden (method LLOQ), 1.0 ng/mL in Denmark, 1.3 ng/mL in Norway (equivalent to 0.02 g% BAC), 2.0 ng/mL in the UK, and 3 ng/mL in The Netherlands. The suggested blood THC concentration limit for DUID offenders in US states (where this drug is decriminalized) is set at 5 ng/mL—e.g., in Colorado and Oregon.

The Canadian government decriminalized the cultivation, purchase, possession, and consumption of cannabis products for recreational purposes on October 17, 2018. Making a hitherto banned substance a legal commodity, albeit with some government restriction and control, will have negative consequences for traffic safety, because consumption of cannabis alters behavior and impairs driving skills. The government envisaged this problem and introduced statutory concentration limits in blood for the pharmacologically active constituent THC. Two types of offense are defined, one when the driver has a THC concentration in blood between 2.0–5.0 ng/mL and a more serious offense when THC in blood is >5 ng/mL. Because consumption of alcohol and cannabis together exacerbates the degree of impairment, 2.5 ng/mL THC in blood together with 0.05 g% ethanol is a punishable offense, even though the BAC limit for driving in Canada is 0.08 g% (European Monitoring Center for Drugs and Drug Addiction 2018). The enforcement of a threshold THC concentration in blood is analogous to the statutory BAC limits for drunken driving, because both ethanol and cannabis are now popular recreational drugs in some nations.

1.8.2 Conclusions

In this chapter we have reviewed key historical events related to driving under the influence of alcohol and/or other psychoactive substances, with the main focus on legislation and research from North America, the United Kingdom, some EU nations, and particularly in the Nordic countries. These latter nations were proactive in trying to improve traffic safety by enforcing concentration *per se* limits for alcohol in blood—Norway in 1936, Sweden in 1941. More recently *per se* limits or zero-tolerance legislation was introduced for other psychoactive substances—Sweden in 1999, Norway in 2012, Finland in 2003, Denmark in 2007, and The Netherlands in 2017.

Statistics from postmortem examination of drivers killed in crashes (and from roadside surveys of seriously injured) support the contention that drunken driving is more of a problem for traffic safety than impairment caused by other psychoactive substances. Indeed, many traffic offenders combine alcohol with other drugs, which makes them more of a danger on the roads. The impairment-BAC relationship is well established and more reproducible than the corresponding relationship for non-alcohol drugs, both licit and illicit. The odds ratios for being involved in a crash after use of non-alcohol psychoactive drugs by drivers, especially when background variables are adjusted for, are less significant compared with elevated BAC (Berning et al. 2015). Another consideration is severity of a crash, such as whether this manifested in material damage to the vehicle, minor injuries to the driver or passenger, or life-threatening injuries requiring emergency hospital treatment. When a multiple-vehicle crash occurs, it is obviously important to investigate culpability on the part of the drivers and who was responsible, which is not always easy (Drummer and Yap 2016).

Taking a psychoactive medication in accordance with a physician's ordination should not pose a threat to traffic safety. Unfortunately, many centrally active drugs are often habit-forming and are subject to abuse, resulting in some people increasing the dosage to obtain pleasurable effects, and consequently diminished performance. Taking drugs to treat insomnia is obviously a hazard for traffic safety, because people become drowsy and risk falling asleep at the wheel. Accordingly, when toxicological results are interpreted, it is crucial to consider the therapeutic indication and whether the concentrations in blood are higher than expected for normal usage of that particular medication.

The prescription drugs most often encountered in blood and urine from apprehended drivers are sedative-hypnotics (Bramness et al. 2002) and pain medication, such as methadone, oxycodone, morphine, hydrocodone, and fentanyl. Anxiolytics, especially benzodiazepines (such as alprazolam, clonazepam, diazepam, and lorazepam) are also overrepresented (Christophersen et al. 1999). A recent study showed that many arrested drivers lacked a valid prescription for the psychoactive medication identified in their blood, and in some cases 50% of those apprehended seemingly obtained the medication illegally (Tjaderborn et al. 2016). Many psychoactive medicinal drugs are available on the "black market" in many countries, being smuggled across borders or purchased anonymously over the Internet. The so-called Dark Net is a particularly active place for marketing and sales of illicit drugs, prescription medications, and NPS.

The use of non-alcohol drugs by drivers has increased in prevalence according to the results from oral-fluid analysis, especially when drivers are stopped and tested on weekend nights (Alcaniz et al. 2018). However, positive results from oral-fluid testing confirms intake, but not whether the driver was impaired. Salivary drug concentrations are poorly correlated with coexisting blood concentrations and the latter are needed to draw conclusions about impairment effects. Particularly troublesome for traffic safety are sedative-hypnotics and opiate/opioid pain medications, because both classes of drugs are habit-forming and often abused (Jones et al. 2007).

Drunken driving remains the biggest problem for road-traffic safety in most nations, despite the upsurge of other psychoactive substances. The traditional illegal drugs of abuse (such as cannabis, heroin, cocaine, and amphetamines) are still highly prevalent in DUID cases globally, despite the emergence in recent years of newer psychoactive substances (Hoiseth et al. 2016; Karinen et al. 2017). There is strong evidence that over the last 10–15 years the proportion of alcohol-related fatal road traffic crashes is decreasing in many countries, whereas the proportion of crashes involving non-alcohol drugs is increasing particularly after use of cannabis and stimulants, such as amphetamines and cocaine (Christophersen et al. 2016).

The existence of zero-tolerance or concentration *per se* laws does not seem to deter hardcore offenders, for whom re-arrest rates are high (Holmgren et al. 2008). There is abundant evidence that many traffic delinquents suffer from a substance-use disorder, which often coexists with a mental health problem (Holmgren et al. 2007). For this group of repeat offenders, many of whom are bipolar with a personality disorder and exhibit sensation-seeking behavior, mortality rates are higher than in the general population (Karjalainen et al. 2010). Early intervention and sentencing to a treatment program after a first or second impaired driving offense might be a better strategy to rehabilitate this troublesome group of traffic offenders.

References

Ahlner J, Holmgren A, Jones AW. Prevalence of alcohol and other drugs and the concentrations in blood of drivers killed in road traffic crashes in Sweden. *Scand J Public Health* 42:177, 2014.

Alcaniz M, Guillen M, Santolino M. Prevalence of drug use among drivers based on mandatory, random tests in a roadside survey. *PLoS One* 13:e0199302, 2018.

Alha A. The forensic medical demonstration of the presence of alcohol and clinical intoxication in Finland. In Havard DJ (Ed): *Alcohol and Traffic Safety*. British Medical Association: London, UK, p. 293, 1963.

Amlung MT, Morris DH, McCarthy DM. Effects of acute alcohol tolerance on perceptions of danger and willingness to drive after drinking. *Psychopharmacology* (Berl) 231:4271, 2014.

Andreasson R, Bonnichsen R. Results of a clinical study of different concentrations of alcohol in the blood. In Harger RN (Ed): *Proceedings—4th International Conference on Alcohol, Drugs and Traffic Safety*. Indiana University: Indianapolis, IN, p. 118, 1965.

Barbone F, McMahon AD, Davey PG, Morris AD, Reid IC, McDevitt DG, MacDonald TM. Association of road-traffic accidents with benzodiazepine use. *Lancet* 352:1331, 1998.

Bavis DF. Tests for concentration of alcohol in blood. *JAMA* 115:73, 1940.

Beck O, Olin AC, Mirgorodskaya E. Potential of mass spectrometry in developing clinical laboratory biomarkers of nonvolatiles in exhaled breath. *Clin Chem* 62:84, 2016.

Beck O, Stephanson N, Sandqvist S, Franck J. Detection of drugs of abuse in exhaled breath using a device for rapid collection: Comparison with plasma, urine and self-reporting in 47 drug users. *J Breath Res* 7:026006, 2013.

Beirness DJ, Beasley E, Lecavalier J. The accuracy of evaluations by drug recognition experts in Canada. *Can Soc Forensic Sci J* 42:75, 2009.

Beirness DJ, Smith DR. An assessment of oral fluid drug screening devices. *Can Soc Forensic Sci J* 50:55, 2017.

Beran RG. The role of the expert witness in the adversarial legal system. *J Law Med* 17:133, 2009.

Bergamaschi MM, Karschner EL, Goodwin RS, Scheidweiler KB, Hirvonen J, Queiroz RH, Huestis MA. Impact of prolonged cannabinoid excretion in chronic daily cannabis smokers' blood on per se drugged driving laws. *Clin Chem* 59:519, 2013.

Berghaus G, Ramaekers JG, Drummer OH. Demands on scientific studies in different fields of forensic medicine and forensic sciences: Traffic medicine, impaired driver, alcohol, drugs, diseases. *Forensic Sci Int* 165:233, 2007.

Berning A, Smither DD. *Understanding the Limitations of Drug Test Information, Reporting, and Tetsing Practices in Fatal Crashes* (DOT HS 812 072). US National Highway Traffic Safety Administration: Washington, DC, 2014.

Berning A, Compton RP, Wochinger K. *Results of the 2013–2014 National Roadside Survey of Alcohol and Drug Use by Drivers* (DOT HS 812 118). US National Highway Traffic Safety Administration: Washington, DC, 2015.

Bjerver K, Goldberg L. Effects of alcohol ingestion on driving ability: Results of practical road tests and laboratory experiments. *Quart J Stud Alc* 11:1, 1950.

Bjorneboe A, Bjorneboe GE, Gjerde H, Bugge A, Drevon CA, Mørland J. A retrospective study of drugged driving in Norway. *Forensic Sci Int* 33:243, 1987.

Blanke RV, Caplan YH, Chaimberlain RT, Dubowski KM, Finkle BS. Consensus report. Drug concentrations and driving impairment. *JAMA* 254:2618, 1985.

Blencowe T, Raaska K, Lillsunde P. Drug concentrations and impaired drivers—Consensus report. *Ther Drug Monit* 33:64, 2011.

Blomberg RD, Peck RC, Moskowitz H, Burns M, Fiorentino D. The Long Beach/Fort Lauderdale relative risk study. *J Safety Res* 40:285, 2009.

Bonnichsen R, Maehly AC, Åqvist S. Arzneimittel und fahrtüchtigkeit 1. Mitteilung: Barbiturate. *Blutalkohol* 6:165, 1969a.

Bonnichsen R, Maehly AC, Åqvist S. Arzneimittel und fahrtüchtigkeit II. Mitteilung—Zentralstimulierende Amine und aromatische Kohlenwasserstoffe. *Blutalkohol* 6:245, 1969b.

Bonnichsen R, Maehly AC, Åqvist S. Arzneimittel und fahrtüchtigkeit III. Mitteilung—Benzodiazepinderivate. *Blutalkohol* 7:1, 1970.

Bonnichsen R, Maehly AC, Marde Y, Ryhage R, Schubert B. Determination and identification of sympathomimetic amines in blood samples from drivers by a combination of gas chromatography and mass spectrometry. *Z Rechtsmed* 67:19, 1970.

Bonnichsen R, Maehly AC, Åqvist S. Arzneimittel und Fahrtüchtigkeit IV. Mitteilung—Übriga Pharmaca und Zusammenfassung der Resultate der I-IV Mitteilung. *Blutalkohol* 9:8, 1972.

Borkenstein RF, Crowther RF, Shumate RP, Ziel WB, Zylman R. The role of the drinking driver in traffic accidents (the Grand Rapids Study). *Blutalkohol* 11 (suppl 1):1, 1974.

Bortolotti F, Sorio D, Bertaso A, Tagliaro F. Analytical and diagnostic aspects of carbohydrate deficient transferrin (CDT): A critical review over years 2007–2017. *J Pharm Biomed Anal* 147:2, 2018.

Bramness JG, Skurtveit S, Mørland J. Clinical impairment of benzodiazepines—Relation between benzodiazepine concentrations and impairment in apprehended drivers. *Drug Alcohol Depend* 68:131, 2002.

Bramness JG, Skurtveit S, Mørland J. Testing for benzodiazepine inebriation—Relationship between benzodiazepine concentration and simple clinical tests for impairment in a sample of drugged drivers. *Eur J Clin Pharmacol* 59:593, 2003.

Brandt J, Leong C. Benzodiazepines and Z-drugs: An updated review of major adverse outcomes reported on in epidemiologic research. *Drugs R D* 17:493, 2017.

Brinkmann B, Beike J, Kohler H, Heinecke A, Bajanowski T. Incidence of alcohol dependence among drunken drivers. *Drug Alcohol Depend* 66:7, 2002.

British Medical Association. Test for drunkenness. *Br Med J* 1:53, 1927.

British Medical Association. *The Drinking Driver* (Report of a Special Committee). British Medical Association: London, UK, 1965.

Brown T, Milavetz G, Murry DJ. Alcohol, drugs and driving: Implications for evaluating driver impairment. *Ann Adv Automot Med* 57:23, 2013.

Burns M. An overview of field sobriety test research. *Percept Mot Skills* 97:1187, 2003

Busardo FP, Pichini S, Pacifici R. Driving under the influence of drugs: Looking for reasonable blood cutoffs and realistic analytical values. *Clin Chem* 63:781, 2017.

Busardo FP, Pichini S, Pellegrini M, Montana A, Lo Faro AF, Zaami S, Graziano S. Correlation between blood and oral fluid psychoactive drug concentrations and cognitive impairment in driving under the influence of drugs. *Curr Neuropharmacol* 16:84, 2018.

Canadian Centre on Substance Use and Addiction. *Mandatory Alcohol Screening Policy*. https://madd.ca/pages/impaired-driving/public-policy-initiatives/random-breath-testing/ (Accessed March 23, 2019).

Chamberlain E, Solomon R. Zero blood alcohol concentration limits for drivers under 21: Lessons from Canada. *Inj Prev* 14:123, 2008.

Chihuri S, Li G. Use of prescription opioids and motor vehicle crashes: A meta analysis. *Accid Anal Prev* 109:123, 2017.

Christophersen AS, Mørland J. Drugged driving, a review based on the experience in Norway. *Drug Alcohol Depend* 47:125, 1997.

Christophersen AS, Beylich KM, Bjornboe A, Skurtveit S, Mørland J. Recidivism among drunken and drugged drivers in Norway. *Alcohol Alcohol* 31:609, 1996.

Christophersen AS, Ceder G, Kristinsson J, Lillsunde P, Steentoft A. Drugged driving in the Nordic countries—A comparative study between five countries. *Forensic Sci Int* 106:173, 1999.

Christophersen AS, Mørland J, Stewart K, Gjerde H. International trends in alcohol and drug use among vehicle drivers. *Forensic Sci Rev* 28:37, 2016.

Compton C. *Marijuana-Impaired Driving—A Report to Congress* (DOT HS 812 440). US National Highway Traffic Safety Administration: Washington, DC, 2017.

Crothers TD. Editorial. *Q J Inebriety* XXV1:308, 1904.

Dole VP. Methadone maintenance treatment for 25,000 heroin addicts. *JAMA* 215:1131, 1971.

Drew GC, Colquhoun WP, Long HA. *Effect of Small Doses of Alcohol on a Skill Resembling Driving*. Her Majesty's Stationery Office: London, UK, p. 108, 1959.

Drummer OH. Drug testing in oral fluid. *Clin Biochem Rev* 27:147, 2006.

Drummer OH, Yap S. The involvement of prescribed drugs in road trauma. *Forensic Sci Int* 265:17, 2016.

Drummer OH, Gerostamoulos J, Batziris H, Chu M, Caplehorn J, Robertson MD, Swann P. The involvement of drugs in drivers of motor vehicles killed in Australian road traffic crashes. *Accid Anal Prev* 36:239, 2004.

Drummer OH, Gerostamoulos D, Chu M, Swann P, Boorman M, Cairns I. Drugs in oral fluid in randomly selected drivers. *Forensic Sci Int* 170:105, 2007.

Dunbar JA, Penttila A, Pikkarainen J. Drinking and driving: Success of random breath testing in Finland. *Br Med J (Clin Res Ed)* 295.101, 1987.

Editorial: Drunken motor car driver. *The Morning Post* September 11, 1897.

Ellerbrook LD, VanGaasbeek CB. The reliability of chemical tests for alcoholic intoxication the importance of the selection of proper material for analysis. *JAMA* 122:966, 1943.

European Monitoring Center for Drugs and Drug Addiction. *Cannabis and Driving—Questions and Answers for Policy Makers*. European Monitoring Center for Drugs and Drug Addiction: Lisbon, Portugal, 2018.

Fell JC, Voas RB. Mothers Against Drunk Driving (MADD): The first 25 years. *Traffic Inj Prev* 7:195, 2006a.

Fell JC, Voas RB. The effectiveness of reducing illegal blood alcohol concentration (BAC) limits for driving: Evidence for lowering the limit to .05 BAC. *J Safety Res* 37:233, 2006b.

Fell JC, Compton C, Voas RB. A note on the use of passive alcohol sensors during routine traffic stops. *Traffic Inj Prev* 9:534, 2008.

Fell JC, Tippetts AS, Ciccel JD. An evaluation of three driving-under-the-influence courts in Georgia. *Ann Adv Automot Med* 55:301, 2011.

Fishbain DA, Cutler RB, Rosomoff HL, Rosomoff RS. Are opioid-dependent/tolerant patients impaired in driving-related skills? A structured evidence-based review. *J Pain Symptom Manage* 25:559, 2003.

Fitzgerald EF. *Intoxicating Test Evidence*, 2nd ed. West Group: St Paul, MN, 2001.

Flanagan RJ, Brown NW, Whelpton R. Therapeutic drug monitoring (TDM). *CPD Clin Biohem* 9:3, 2008.

Foss RD, Voas RB, Beirness DJ. Using a passive alcohol sensor to detect legally intoxicated drivers. *Am J Public Health* 83:556, 1993.

Furuhaugen H, Jamt REG, Nilsson G, Vindenes V, Gjerde H. Roadside survey of alcohol and drug use among Norwegian drivers in 2016–2017: A follow-up of the 2008–2009 survey. *Traffic Inj Prev* 19:555, 2018.

Gjerde H. Daily drinking and drunken driving. *Scand J Soc Med* 15:73, 1987.

Gjerde H, Christophersen AS, Bjorneboe A, Sakshaug J, Mørland J. Driving under the influence of other drugs than alcohol in Norway. *Acta Med Leg Soc* (Liege) 40:71, 1990.

Gjerde H, Beylich KM, Mørland J. Incidence of alcohol and drugs in fatally injured car drivers in Norway. *Accid Anal Prev* 25:479, 1993.

Gjerde H, Normann PT, Pettersen BS, Assum T, Aldrin M, Johansen U, Kristoffersen L, Oiestad EL, Christophersen AS, Mørland J. Prevalence of alcohol and drugs among Norwegian motor vehicle drivers: A roadside survey. *Accid Anal Prev* 40:1765, 2008.

Gjerde H, Normann PT, Christophersen AS. The prevalence of alcohol and drugs in sampled oral fluid is related to sample volume. *J Anal Toxicol* 34:416, 2010.

Gjerde H, Christophersen AS, Normann PT, Mørland J. Toxicological investigations of drivers killed in road traffic accidents in Norway during 2006–2008. *Forensic Sci Int* 212:102, 2011.

Gjerde H, Christophersen AS, Normann PT, Assum T, Oiestad EL, Mørland J. Norwegian roadside survey of alcohol and drug use by drivers (2008–2009). *Traffic Inj Prev* 14:443, 2013.

Gjerde H, Langel K, Favretto D, Verstraete AG. Detection of illicit drugs in oral fluid from drivers as biomarker for drugs in blood. *Forensic Sci Int* 256:42, 2015.

Gjerde H, Clausen GB, Andreassen E, Furuhaugen H. Evaluation of drager DrugTest 5000 in a naturalistic setting. *J Anal Toxicol* 42:248, 2018a.

Gjerde H, Romeo G, Mørland J. Challenges and common weaknesses in case-control studies on drug use and road traffic injury based on drug testing of biological samples. *Ann Epidemiol* 28:812, 2018b.

Goldberg L. Quantitative studies on alcohol tolerance in man. *Acta Physiol Scand* 5(Supp 16):1, 1943.

Greenblatt DJ, Shader RI. Dependence, tolerance, and addiction to benzodiazepines: Clinical and pharmacokinetic considerations. *Drug Metab Rev* 8:13, 1978.

Gronewold A, Skopp G. A preliminary investigation on the distribution of cannabinoids in man. *Forensic Sci Int* 210:e7, 2011.

Grotenhermen F, Leson G, Berghaus G, Drummer OH, Kruger HP, Longo M, Moskowitz H, Perrine B, Ramaekers JG, Smiley A, et al. Developing limits for driving under cannabis. *Addiction* 102:1910, 2007.

Gullberg RG. Estimating the measurement uncertainty in forensic blood alcohol analysis. *J Anal Toxicol* 36:153, 2012.

Gustavsen I, Al-Sammurraie M, Mørland J, Bramness JG. Impairment related to blood drug concentrations of zopiclone and zolpidem compared to alcohol in apprehended drivers. *Accid Anal Prev* 41:462, 2009.

Gustavsen I, Hjelmeland K, Bernard JP, Mørland J. Individual psychomotor impairment in relation to zopiclone and ethanol concentrations in blood—A randomized controlled double-blinded trial. *Addiction* 107:925, 2012.

Hadland SE, Xuan Z, Sarda V, Blanchette J, Swahn MH, Heeren TC, Voas RB, Naimi TS. Alcohol policies and alcohol-related motor vehicle crash fatalities among young people in the US. *Pediatrics* 139, 2017.

Haghpanahan H, Lewsey J, Mackay DF, McIntosh E, Pell J, Jones A, Fitzgerald N, Robinson M. An evaluation of the effects of lowering blood alcohol concentration limits for drivers on the rates of road traffic accidents and alcohol consumption: A natural experiment. *Lancet* 393:321, 2019.

Harger RN, Lamb EB, Hulpieu HR. A rapid chemical test for intoxication employing breath a new reagent for alcohol and a procedure for estimating the concentration of alcohol in the body from the ratio of alcohol to carbon dioxide in the breath. *JAMA* 110:779, 1938.

Hartman RL, Huestis MA. Cannabis effects on driving skills. *Clin Chem* 59:478, 2013.

Hartman RL, Richman JE, Hayes CE, Huestis MA. Drug Recognition Expert (DRE) examination characteristics of cannabis impairment. *Accid Anal Prev* 92:219, 2016.

Heise RA. Alcohol and automobile accidents. *JAMA* 103:739, 1934.

Hels T, Lyckegaard A, Simonsen KW, Steentoft A, Bernhoft IM. Risk of severe driver injury by driving with psychoactive substances. *Accid Anal Prev* 59:346, 2013.

Hoiseth G, Austdal LE, Wiik E, Bogstrand ST, Mørland J. Prevalence and concentrations of drugs in older suspected drugged drivers. *Traffic Inj Prev* 18:231, 2017a.

Hoiseth G, Berg-Hansen GO, Oiestad AM, Bachs L, Mørland J. Impairment due to alcohol, tetrahydrocannabinol, and benzodiazepines in impaired drivers compared to experimental studies. *Traffic Inj Prev* 18:244, 2017b.

Hoiseth G, Middelkoop G, Mørland J, Gjerde H. Has previous abuse of flunitrazepam been replaced by clonazepam? *Eur Addict Res* 21:217, 2015.

Hoiseth G, Tuv SS, Karinen R. Blood concentrations of new designer benzodiazepines in forensic cases. *Forensic Sci Int* 268:35, 2016.

Holcomb RL. Alcohol in relation to traffic accidents. *JAMA* 111:1076, 1938.

Holmgren A, Holmgren P, Kugelberg FC, Jones AW, Ahlner J. Predominance of illicit drugs and poly-drug use among drug-impaired drivers in Sweden. *Traffic Inj Prev* 8:361, 2007.

Holmgren A, Holmgren P, Kugelberg FC, Jones AW, Ahlner J. High re-arrest rates among drug-impaired drivers despite zero-tolerance legislation. *Accid Anal Prev* 40:534, 2008.

Homel R. Random breath testing in Australia: Getting it to work according to specifications. *Addiction* 88 (Suppl):27S, 1993.

Houwing S, Hagenzieker M, Mathijssen R, Bernhoft IM, Hels T, Janstrup K, Van der Linden T, Legrand SA, Verstraete A. *Prevalence of Alcohol and Other Psychoactive Substance in Drivers in General Traffic, Part I: General Results* (DRUID Deliverable D 2.2.3. SWOV). Institute for Road Safety Research: Leidschendam, the Netherlands, 2011.

Hubicka B, Bergman H, Laurell H. Alcohol problems among Swedish drunk drivers: Differences related to mode of detection and geographical region. *Traffic Inj Prev* 8:224, 2007.

Hubicka B, Laurell H, Bergman H. Criminal and alcohol problems among Swedish drunk drivers—Predictors of DUI relapse. *Int J Law Psychiatry* 31:471, 2008.

Huestis MA, Barnes A, Smith ML. Estimating the time of last cannabis use from plasma Δ9-tetrahydrocannabinol and 11-nor-9-carboxy-Δ9-tetrahydrocannabinol concentrations. *Clin Chem* 51:2289, 2005.

Huestis MA, Verstraete A, Kwong TC, Mørland J, Vincent MJ, de la Torre R. Oral fluid testing: Promises and pitfalls. *Clin Chem* 57:805, 2011.

Impinen A, Rahkonen O, Karjalainen K, Lintonen T, Lillsunde P, Ostamo A. Substance use as a predictor of driving under the influence (DUI) rearrests: A 15-year retrospective study. *Traffic Inj Prev* 10:220, 2009.

Impinen A, Makela P, Karjalainen K, Haukka J, Lintonen T, Lillsunde P, Rahkonen O, Ostamo A. The association between social determinants and drunken driving: A 15-year register-based study of 81,125 suspects. *Alcohol Alcohol* 46:721, 2011.

Jantos R, Schuhmacher M, Veldstra JL, Bosker WM, Skopp G. Bestimmund der Blut/Serum Verhältnisse verschiedener forensisch relevanter Analyten in authentischen Proben. *Archiv Kriminolog* 227:188, 2011.

Jones AW. Top ten defence challenges among drinking drivers in Sweden. *Med Sci Law* 31:229, 1991.

Jones AW. Measuring alcohol in blood and breath for forensic purposes—A historical review. *Forensic Sci Rev* 8:13, 1996.

Jones AW. Medicolegal alcohol determination—Blood- or breath-alcohol concentration? *Forensic Sci Rev* 12:23, 2000.

Jones AW. Driving under the influence of drugs in Sweden with zero concentration limits in blood for controlled substances. *Traffic Inj Prev* 6:317, 2005.

Jones AW. Perspectives in drug discovery. 12. Cocaine. *TIAFT Bulletin* 43:7, 2013.

Jones AW, Neri A. Age-related differences in blood ethanol parameters and subjective feelings of intoxication in healthy men. *Alcohol Alcohol* 20:45, 1985.

Jones AW, Neri A. Age-related differences in the effects of ethanol on performance and behaviour in healthy men. *Alcohol Alcohol* 29:171, 1994.

Jones AW, Larsson H. Distribution of diazepam and nordiazepam between plasma and whole blood and the influence of hematocrit. *Ther Drug Monit* 26:380, 2004.

Jones AW, Holmgren A. What non-alcohol drugs are used by drinking drivers in Sweden? Toxicological results from ten years of forensic blood samples. *J Safety Res* 43:151, 2012.

Jones AW, Holmgren A. Amphetamine abuse in Sweden: Subject demographics, changes in blood concentrations over time, and the types of coingested substances. *J Clin Psychopharmacol* 33:248, 2013.

Jones AW, Holmgren A, Kugelberg FC. Concentrations of scheduled prescription drugs in blood of impaired drivers: Considerations for interpreting the results. *Ther Drug Monit* 29:248, 2007.

Jones AW, Holmgren A, Kugelberg FC. Driving under the influence of cannabis: A 10-year study of age and gender differences in the concentrations of tetrahydrocannabinol in blood. *Addiction* 103:452, 2008.

Jones AW, Kugelberg FC, Holmgren A, Ahlner J. Five-year update on the occurrence of alcohol and other drugs in blood samples from drivers killed in road-traffic crashes in Sweden. *Forensic Sci Int* 186:56, 2009.

Jones AW, Holmgren A, Ahlner J. High prevalence of previous arrests for illicit drug use and/or impaired driving among drivers killed in motor vehicle crashes in Sweden with amphetamine in blood at autopsy. *Int J Drug Policy* 26:790, 2015.

Jongen S, Vuurman EF, Ramaekers JG, Vermeeren A. The sensitivity of laboratory tests assessing driving related skills to dose-related impairment of alcohol: A literature review. *Accid Anal Prev* 89:31, 2016.

Jongen S, Vermeeren A, van der Sluiszen NN, Schumacher MB, Theunissen EL, Kuypers KP, Vuurman EF, Ramaekers JG. A pooled analysis of on-the-road highway driving studies in actual traffic measuring standard deviation of lateral position (i.e., "weaving") while driving at a blood alcohol concentration of 0.5 g/L. *Psychopharmacology* (Berl) 234:837, 2017.

Kalant H. Research on tolerance: What can we learn from history? *Alcohol Clin Exp Res* 22:67, 1998.

Kane G. The methodological quality of three foundational law enforcement drug influence evaluation validation studies. *J Negat Results Biomed* 12:16, 2013.

Karjalainen K, Lintonen T, Impinen A, Makela P, Rahkonen O, Lillsunde P, Ostamo A. Mortality and causes of death among drugged drivers. *J Epidemiol Community Health* 64:506, 2010.

Karjalainen K, Lintonen T, Impinen A, Lillsunde P, Makela P, Rahkonen O, Haukka J, Ostamo A. Socio-economic determinants of drugged driving—A register-based study. *Addiction* 106:1448, 2011.

Karjalainen K, Lintonen T, Joukamaa M, Lillsunde P. Mental disorders associated with driving under the influence of alcohol and/or drugs: A register-based study. *Eur Addict Res* 19:113, 2013.

Karjalainen K, Haukka J, Lillsunde P, Lintonen T, Makela P. The arrest of drivers under the influence as a predictor of subsequent social disadvantage and death. *Drug Alcohol Depend* 137:114, 2014.

Karjalainen K, Haukka J, Lintonen T, Joukamaa M, Lillsunde P. The use of psychoactive prescription drugs among DUI suspects. *Drug Alcohol Depend* 155:215, 2015.

Karinen R, Hoiseth G. A literature review of blood concentrations of new psychoactive substances classified as phenethylamines, aminoindanes, arylalkylamines, arylcyclohexylamines, and indolalkylamines. *Forensic Sci Int* 276:120, 2017.

Kataja M, Penttila A, Tenhu M. Combining the blood alcohol and clinical examination for estimating the influence of alcohol. *Blutalkohol* 12:109, 1975.

Kenntner-Mabiala R, Kaussner Y, Jagiellowicz-Kaufmann M, Hoffmann S, Kruger HP. Driving performance under alcohol in simulated representative driving tasks: An alcohol calibration study for impairments related to medicinal drugs. *J Clin Psychopharmacol* 35:134, 2015.

Kim JH, Mooney SJ. The epidemiologic principles underlying traffic safety study designs. *Int J Epidemiol* 45:1668, 2016.

Kouri T, Siloaho M, Pohjavaara S, Koskinen P, Malminiemi O, Pohja-Nylander P, Puukka R. Preanalytical factors and measurement uncertainty. *Scand J Clin Lab Invest* 65:463, 2005.

Kriikku P, Wilhelm L, Jenckel S, Rintatalo J, Hurme J, Kramer J, Jones AW, Ojanpera I. Comparison of breath-alcohol screening test results with venous blood alcohol concentration in suspected drunken drivers. *Forensic Sci Int* 239:57, 2014.

Kristoffersen L, Strand DH, Liane VH, Vindenes V, Tvete IF, Aldrin M. Determination of safety margins for whole blood concentrations of alcohol and nineteen drugs in driving under the influence cases. *Forensic Sci Int* 259:119, 2016.

Krotulski AJ, Mohr ALA, Friscia M, Logan BK. Field detection of drugs of abuse in oral fluid using the Alere™ DDS®2 mobile test system with confirmation by liquid chromatography tandem mass spectrometry (LC-MS/MS). *J Anal Toxicol* 42:170, 2018.

Kuypers KP, Legrand SA, Ramaekers JG, Verstraete AG. A case-control study estimating accident risk for alcohol, medicines and illegal drugs. *PLoS One* 7:e43496, 2012.

Lacey JH, Kelley-Baker T, Berning A, Romano E, Ramirez A, Yao J, Moore C, Brainard K, Carr K, Pell K, Compton R. *Drug and Alcohol Crash Risk—A Case Control Study* (DOT HS 812 117). US National Highway Traffic Safety Administration: Washington, DC, 2015.

Lacey JH, Kelley-Baker T, Berning A, Romano E, Ramirez A, Yao J, Compton R. *Drug and Alcohol Crash Risk: A Case-Control Study* (Report No. DOT HS 812 355). US National Highway Traffic Safety Administration: Washington, DC, 2016.

Lader M. History of benzodiazepine dependence. *J Subst Abuse Treat* 8:53, 1991.

Lader M. Benzodiazepines revisited—Will we ever learn? *Addiction* 106:2086. 2011.

Langel K, Gjerde H, Favretto D, Lillsunde P, Oiestad EL, Ferrara SD, Verstraete AG. Comparison of drug concentrations between whole blood and oral fluid. *Drug Test Anal* 6:461, 2014.

Launiainen T, Ojanpera I. Drug concentrations in post-mortem femoral blood compared with therapeutic concentrations in plasma. *Drug Test Anal* 6:308, 2014.

Laurell H. Effects of small doses of alcohol on driver performance in emergency traffic situations. *Accid Anal Prev* 9:191, 1977.

Legrand SA, Houwing S, Hagenzieker M, Verstraete AG. Prevalence of alcohol and other psychoactive substances in injured drivers: Comparison between Belgium and The Netherlands. *Forensic Sci Int* 220:224, 2012.

Legrand SA, Isalberti C, der Linden TV, Bernhoft IM, Hels T, Simonsen KW, Favretto D, Ferrara SD, Caplinskiene M, Minkuviene Z, et al. Alcohol and drugs in seriously injured drivers in six European countries. *Drug Test Anal* 5:156, 2013.

Legrand SA, Gjerde H, Isalberti C, Van der Linden T, Lillsunde P, Dias MJ, Gustafsson S, Ceder G, Verstraete AG. Prevalence of alcohol, illicit drugs and psychoactive medicines in killed drivers in four European countries. *Int J Inj Contr Saf Promot* 21:17, 2014.

Lerner BH. *One for the Road*. The Johns Hopkins University Press: Baltimore, MD, 2011.

Liljestrand G. Till frågan om läkarundersökning rörande alkoholpåverkan. *Tirfing* 34:97, 1940.

Lillsunde P, Gunnar T. Drugs and driving: The Finnish perspective. *Bull Narc* 57:213, 2005.

Liu RH. Important considerations in the interpretation of forensic urine drug test results. *Forensic Sci Rev* 4:51, 1992.

Lopez-Munoz F, Ucha-Udabe R, Alamo C. The history of barbiturates a century after their clinical introduction. *Neuropsychiatr Dis Treat* 1:329, 2005.

Macht DI. The history of opium and some of its preparations and alkaloids. *JAMA* 64:477, 1915.

Margot P. The role of the forensic scientist in an inquisitorial system of justice. *Sci Justice* 38:71, 1998.

Marillier M, Verstraete A. Driving under the influence of drugs. *WIREs Forensic Sci* e1326, https://doi.org/10.1002/wfs2.1326 (Accessed March 23, 2019).

Marques PR, Tippetts AS, Voas RB. Comparative and joint prediction of DUI recidivism from alcohol ignition interlock and driver records. *J Stud Alcohol* 64:83, 2003.

Martin TL, Solbeck PA, Mayers DJ, Langille RM, Buczek Y, Pelletier MR. A review of alcohol-impaired driving: The role of blood alcohol concentration and complexity of the driving task. *J Forensic Sci* 58:1238, 2013.

Maurer HH. Systematic toxicological analysis of drugs and their metabolites by gas chromatography-mass spectrometry. *J Chromatogr* 580:3, 1992.

Maurer HH. Systematic toxicological analysis procedures for acidic drugs and/or metabolites relevant to clinical and forensic toxicology and/or doping control. *J Chromatogr B Biomed Sci Appl* 733:3, 1999.

Maurer HH, Meyer MR. High-resolution mass spectrometry in toxicology: Current status and future perspectives. *Arch Toxicol* 90:2161, 2016.

Maurer HH. Mass spectrometry for research and application in therapeutic drug monitoring or clinical and forensic toxicology. *Ther Drug Monit* 40:389, 2018.

Mbughuni MM, Jannetto PJ, Langman LJ. Mass spectrometry applications for toxicology. *EJIFCC* 27:272, 2016.

McBay AJ. Barbiturate poisoning. *N Engl J Med* 273:38, 1965.

McKnight AJ, Langston EA, McKnight AS, Lange JE. Sobriety tests for low blood alcohol concentrations. *Accid Anal Prev* 34:305, 2002.

Mellanby E. Alcohol and alcoholic intoxication. *Brit J Inebriety* 17:157, 1920.

Meyer GM, Maurer HH, Meyer MR. Multiple stage MS in analysis of plasma, serum, urine and in vitro samples relevant to clinical and forensic toxicology. *Bioanalysis* 8:457, 2016.

Montgomery MR, Reasor MJ. Retrograde extrapolation of blood alcohol data: An applied approach. *J Toxicol Environ Health* 36:281, 1992.

Mørland J, Steentoft A, Simonsen KW, Ojanpera I, Vuori E, Magnusdottir K, Kristinsson J, Ceder G, Kronstrand R, Christophersen A. Drugs related to motor vehicle crashes in northern European countries: A study of fatally injured drivers. *Accid Anal Prev* 43:1920, 2011.

Moskowitz H, Burns M, Ferguson S. Police officers' detection of breath odors from alcohol ingestion. *Accid Anal Prev* 31:175, 1999.

Moskowitz M, Fiorentino D. *A Review of the Literature on the Effects of Low Doses of Alcohol on Driving-Related Skills* (DOT HS 809 028). US National Highway Traffic Safety Administration: Washington, DC, 2000.

Musto DF. Opium, cocaine and marijuana in American history. *Sci Am* 265:40, 1991.

Musto DF. Cocaine's history, especially the American experience. *Ciba Found Symp* 166:7, 1992.

National Safety Council. *A History of the Committee on Alcohol and Other Drugs*. https://www.nsc.org/Portals/0/Documents/NSCDocuments_Advocacy/NSChistoryofCAOD.pdf (Accessed March 23, 2019).

Nedahl M, Johansen SS, Linnet K. Postmortem brain-blood ratios of amphetamine, cocaine, ephedrine, MDMA and methylphenidate. *J Anal Toxicol*, 43:378–384, 2019.

Neutel CI. Risk of traffic accident injury after a prescription for a benzodiazepine. *Ann Epidemiol* 5:239, 1995.

O'Hanlon JF. Driving performance under the influence of drugs: Rationale for, and application of, a new test. *Br J Clin Pharmacol* 18 (Suppl 1):121S, 1984.

Orriols L, Delorme B, Gadegbeku B, Tricotel A, Contrand B, Laumon B, Salmi LR, Lagarde E. Prescription medicines and the risk of road traffic crashes: A French registry-based study. *PLoS Med* 7:e1000366, 2010.

Orriols L, Luxcey A, Contrand B, Gadegbeku B, Delorme B, Tricotel A, Moore N, Salmi LR, Lagarde E. Road traffic crash risk associated with benzodiazepine and z-hypnotic use after implementation of a colour-graded pictogram: A responsibility study. *Br J Clin Pharmacol* 82:1625, 2016.

Page TE. The drug recognition expert officer: Signs of drug impairment at roadside. In Mayhew DR, Dussault C (Eds): *Proceedings—16th International Conference on Alcohol, Drugs and Traffic Safety*. Montreal, Canada, p. 311, 2002.

Papoutsis I, Nikolaou P, Spiliopoulou C, Athanaselis S. Different aspects of driving under the influence of benzodiazepines. *Med Sci Law* 56:159, 2016.

Pehrsson A, Blencowe T, Vimpari K, Langel K, Engblom C, Lillsunde P. An evaluation of on-site oral fluid drug screening devices DrugWipe 5+ and Rapid STAT using oral fluid for confirmation analysis. *J Anal Toxicol* 35:211, 2011.

Penttila A, Tenhu M. Clinical examination as medicolegal proof of alcohol intoxication. *Med Sci Law* 16:95, 1976.

Petridou E, Moustaki M. Human factors in the causation of road traffic crashes. *Eur J Epidemiol* 16:819, 2000.

Poon R, Hodgson BT, Hindberg I, Rowatt C. Evaluation of three pocket-size breath alcohol analyzers. *Can Forensic Sci Soc J* 20:19, 1987.

Porath-Waller AJ, Beirness DJ. An examination of the validity of the standardized field sobriety test in detecting drug impairment using data from the drug evaluation and classification program. *Traffic Inj Prev* 15:125, 2014.

Ramaekers JG. Drugs and driving research in medicinal drug development. *Trends Pharmacol Sci* 38:319, 2017.

Ramaekers JG, Kauert G, van Ruitenbeek P, Theunissen EL, Schneider E, Moeller MR. High-potency marijuana impairs executive function and inhibitory motor control. *Neuropsychopharmacology* 31:2296, 2006a.

Ramaekers JG, Moeller MR, van Ruitenbeek P, Theunissen EL, Schneider E, Kauert G. Cognition and motor control as a function of Δ9-THC concentration in serum and oral fluid: Limits of impairment. *Drug Alcohol Depend* 85:114, 2006b.

Rasanen P, Hakko H, Jarvelin MR. Early-onset drunk driving, violent criminality, and mental disorders. *Lancet* 354:1788, 1999.

Rasmussen N. Making the first anti-depressant: Amphetamine in American medicine, 1929–1950. *J Hist Med Allied Sci* 61:288, 2006.

Robertson MD, Drummer OH. Responsibility analysis: A methodology to study the effects of drugs in driving. *Accid Anal Prev* 26:243, 1994.

Ross HL. Prevalence of alcohol-impaired driving: An international comparison. *Accid Anal Prev* 25:777, 1993.

Roth A. The uneasy case for marijuana as chemical impairment under a science-based jurisprudence of dangerousness. *Calif Law Rev* 103:841, 2015.

Rubenzer SJ. The standardized field sobriety tests: A review of scientific and legal issues. *Law Hum Behav* 32:293, 2008.

Rubenzer SJ. Judging intoxication. *Behav Sci Law* 29:116, 2011.

Schnabel E, Hargutt V, Krüger H-P. *Meta-Analysis of Empirical Studies Concerning the Effects of Alcohol on Safe Driving* (DRUID 6th Framework Programme). University of Wuerzburg: Wuerzburg, Germany, 2010.

Schulz M, Schmoldt A. Therapeutic and toxic blood concentrations of more than 800 drugs and other xenobiotics. *Pharmazie* 58:447, 2003.

Schulze H, Schumacher MB, Urmeew R, Auerbach K, Alvarez J, Bernhoft IM, De Gier H, Hagenzieker M, Houwing S, Knoche A, et al. *Driving Under the Influence of Drugs, Alcohol and Medicines in Europe—Findings from the DRUID Project.* Publications Office of the European Union: Luxembourg, 2012.

Schwope DM, Bosker WM, Ramaekers JG, Gorelick DA, Huestis MA. Psychomotor performance, subjective and physiological effects and whole blood delta(9)-tetrahydrocannabinol concentrations in heavy, chronic cannabis smokers following acute smoked cannabis. *J Anal Toxicol* 36:405, 2012.

Seferaj S, Ullah S, Tinglev A, Carlsson S, Winberg J, Stambeck P, Beck O. Evaluation of a new simple collection device for sampling of microparticles in exhaled breath. *J Breath Res* 12:036005, 2018.

Selesnick S. Alcoholic intoxication its diagnosis and medicolegal implications. *JAMA* 110:775, 1938.

Sharma S. Barbiturates and driving. *Accid Anal Prev* 8:27, 1976.

Sigel E, Steinmann ME. Structure, function, and modulation of GABA(A) receptors. *J Biol Chem* 287:40224, 2012.

Simonsen KW, Linnet K, Rasmussen BS. Driving under the influence of alcohol and drugs in the eastern part of Denmark in 2015 and 2016: Abuse patterns and trends. *Traffic Inj Prev* 19:468, 2018.

Skopp G, Potsch L. Cannabinoid concentrations in spot serum samples 24 to 48 hours after discontinuation of cannabis smoking. *J Anal Toxicol* 32:160, 2008.

Skopp G, Schmitt G, Potsch L. Plasma-to-blood ratios of congener analytes. *J Anal Toxicol* 29:145, 2005.

Skurtveit S, Christophersen AS, Mørland J. Female drivers suspected for drunken or drugged driving. *Forensic Sci Int* 75:139, 1995.

Smith JA, Hayes CE, Yolton RL, Rutledge DA, Citek K. Drug recognition expert evaluations made using limited data. *Forensic Sci Int* 130:167, 2002.

Sneader W. *Drug Discovery—A History.* Wiley: Chichester, UK, p. 468, 2005.

Snenghi R, Forza G, Favretto D, Sartore D, Rodinis S, Terranova C, Nalesso A, Montisci M, Ferrara SD. Underlying substance abuse problems in drunk drivers. *Traffic Inj Prev* 16:435, 2015.

Stanton MD. Drugs, Vietnam, and the Vietnam veteran: An overview. *Am J Drug Alcohol Abuse* 3:557, 1976.

Steentoft A, Simonsen KW, Linnet K. The frequency of drugs among Danish drivers before and after the introduction of fixed concentration limits. *Traffic Inj Prev* 11:329, 2010.

Strand MC, Gjerde H, Mørland J. Driving under the influence of non-alcohol drugs—An update. Part II: Experimental studies. *Forensic Sci Rev* 28:79, 2016.

Strand MC, Mørland J, Slordal L, Riedel B, Innerdal C, Aamo T, Mathisrud G, Vindenes V. Conversion factors for assessment of driving impairment after exposure to multiple benzodiazepines/z-hypnotics or opioids. *Forensic Sci Int* 281:29, 2017.

Strand MC, Vindenes V, Gjerde H, Mørland JG, Ramaekers JG. A clinical trial on the acute effects of methadone and buprenorphine on actual driving and cognitive function of healthy volunteers. *Br J Clin Pharmacol* 85:442, 2018.

Stuster J. Validation of the standardized field sobriety test battery at 0.08% blood alcohol concentration. *Hum Factors* 48:608, 2006.

Tan KR, Rudolph U, Luscher C. Hooked on benzodiazepines: $GABA_A$ receptor subtypes and addiction. *Trends Neurosci* 34:188, 2011.

Thomas RE. Benzodiazepine use and motor vehicle accidents. Systematic review of reported association. *Can Fam Physician* 44:799, 1998.

Thornton WW. While under the influence of intoxicating liquor. *Indiana Law J* 4:123, 1928.

Tiscione NB, Alford I, Yeatman DT, Shan X. Ethanol analysis by headspace gas chromatography with simultaneous flame-ionization and mass spectrometry detection. *J Anal Toxicol* 35:501, 2011.

Tjaderborn M, Jonsson AK, Sandstrom TZ, Ahlner J, Hagg S. Non-prescribed use of psychoactive prescription drugs among drug-impaired drivers in Sweden. *Drug Alcohol Depend* 161:77, 2016.

UK Government. *An Act for Regulation the Sale of Intoxicating Liquors.* 1872. http://www.legislation.gov.uk/ukpga/1872/94/pdfs/ukpga_18720094_en.pdf (Accessed March 23, 2019).

UK Government. *Misuse of Drugs Act 1971.* https://www.legislation.gov.uk/ukpga/1971/38/pdfs/ukpga_19710038_en.pdf (Accessed March 23, 2019).

UK Government. *Road Traffic Act, 1930.* http://www.legislation.gov.uk/ukpga/1930/43/pdfs/ukpga_19300043_en.pdf (Accessed March 23, 2019).

UK Government. *The Road Safety Act 1967 and Its Effect on Road Accidents in the United Kingdom rink,* 1967. https://www.icadtsinternational.com/files/documents/1969_055.pdf (Accessed May 27, 2019).

Ullah S, Sandqvist S, Beck O. A liquid chromatography and tandem mass spectrometry method to determine 28 non-volatile drugs of abuse in exhaled breath. *J Pharm Biomed Anal* 148:251, 2018.

US Drug Enforcement Administration (US Department of Justice). *Drug Scheduling.* https://www.dea.gov/drug-scheduling (Accessed March 23, 2019)

US National Highway Traffic Safety Administration (US Department of Transportation). *Impact of the Legalization and Decriminalization of Marijuana on the DWI System: Highlights from the Expert Panel Meeting* (Report No. DOT HS 812 430). US National Highway Traffic Safety Administration: Washington, DC, 2017.

Vainio A, Ollila J, Matikainen E, Rosenberg P, Kalso E. Driving ability in cancer patients receiving long-term morphine analgesia. *Lancet* 346:667, 1995.

Valen A, Bogstrand ST, Vindenes V, Gjerde H. Toxicological findings in suspected drug-impaired drivers in Norway —Trends during 1990–2015. *Forensic Sci Int* 280:15, 2017.

Verster JC, Roth T. Standard operation procedures for conducting the on-the-road driving test, and measurement of the standard deviation of lateral position (SDLP). *Int J Gen Med* 4:359, 2011.

Verstraete AG, Legrand S-A. *Drug Use, Impaired Driving and Traffic Accidents,* 2nd ed. Publications Office of the European Union: Luxembourg, 2014.

Vindenes V, Boix F, Koksaeter P, Strand MC, Bachs L, Mørland J, Gjerde H. Drugged driving arrests in Norway before and after the implementation of per se law. *Forensic Sci Int* 245:171, 2014.

Vindenes V, Jordbru D, Knapskog AB, Kvan E, Mathisrud G, Slordal L, Mørland J. Impairment based legislative limits for driving under the influence of non-alcohol drugs in Norway. *Forensic Sci Int* 219:1, 2012.

Voas RB, Fell JC. Strengthening impaired-driving enforcement in the United States. *Traffic Inj Prev* 14:661, 2013.

Voas RB, Tippetts AS, Fell JC. Assessing the effectiveness of minimum legal drinking age and zero tolerance laws in the United States. *Accid Anal Prev* 35:579, 2003.

Voas RB, Kelley-Baker T, Romano E, Vishnuvajjala R. Implied-consent laws: A review of the literature and examination of current problems and related statutes. *J Safety Res* 40:77, 2009.

Voas RB, Torres P, Romano E, Lacey JH. Alcohol-related risk of driver fatalities: An update using 2007 data. *J Stud Alcohol Drugs* 73:341, 2012.

Voas RB, DuPont RL, Shea CL, Talpins SK. Prescription drugs, drugged driving and per se laws. *Inj Prev* 19:218, 2013.

Voas RB, Tippetts AS, Bergen G, Grosz M, Marques P. Mandating treatment based on interlock performance: Evidence for effectiveness. *Alcohol Clin Exp Res* 40:1953, 2016.

Volkow N, Benveniste H, McLellan AT. Use and misuse of opioids in chronic pain. *Annu Rev Med* 69:451, 2018.

Walsh JM. *A State-by-State Analysis of Laws Dealing with Driving Under the Influence of Drugs* (DOT HS 811 236). US National Highway Traffic Safety Administration: Washington, DC, 2007.

Walsh JM, Verstraete AG, Huestis MA, Mørland J. Guidelines for research on drugged driving. *Addiction* 103:1258, 2008.

Widmark EMP. Eine Mikromethode zur Bestimmung von Äthylalkohol im Blut. *Biochem Z* 131:473, 1922.

Widmark EMP. *Principles and Applications of Medicolegal Alcohol Determinations*. Biomedical Publications: Davis, CA, p. 163, 1981.

Wigmore JG, Langille RM. Six generations of breath alcohol testing instruments: Changes in the detection of breath alcohol since 1930. An historical overview. *Can Soc Forensic Sci J* 42:276, 2009.

Wilhelmi BG, Cohen SP. A framework for "driving under the influence of drugs" policy for the opioid using driver. *Pain Physician* 15:ES215, 2012.

Williams PM. Current defence strategies in some contested drink-drive prosecutions: Is it now time for some additional statutory assumptions? *Forensic Sci Int* 293:e5, 2018.

Wolff K, Johnston A. Cannabis use: A perspective in relation to the proposed UK drug-driving legislation. *Drug Test Anal* 6:143, 2014.

Wolff K, Brimblecombe R, Forfar JC, Forrest AR, Gilvarry E, Johnston A, Morgan J, Osselton MD, Read L, Taylor D. *Driving Under the Influence of Drugs Report from the Expert Panal on Drug Driving*. Department of Transportation: London, UK, 2013.

World Health Organization. *Global Status Report on Road Safety 2018*. World Health Organization: Geneva, Switzerland, 2018.

Zuba D. Accuracy and reliability of breath alcohol testing by handheld electrochemical analysers. *Forensic Sci Int* 178:e29, 2008.

Zwicker TJ, Hedlund J, Northrup VS. *Breath Test Refusals in DWI Enforcement—An Interim Report* (DOT HS 809 876). US National Highway Traffic Safety Administration: Washington, DC, 2005.

Other Historical Events of Interest

II

Professor Robert F. Borkenstein

An Appreciation of His Life and Work*

2

DOUGLAS M. LUCAS

Contents

2.1 Introduction

In a 1985 paper, Professor Robert F. Borkenstein wrote about a former colleague:

> It is interesting just how much influence one person can have on a field. Just as Widmark was a 'one man army' in Sweden, a young American physician, Dr. Herman Heise, became a similar one man army in North America. (Borkenstein 1985)

No words could better have summarized Bob Borkenstein's influence on his chosen field of endeavor than his own words, as used to describe Dr. Heise.

* This chapter is an updated version of a review article previously published in *Forensic Science Review*: Lucas DM: Professor Robert F. Borkenstein—An appreciation of his life and work; *Forensic Sci Rev* 12(1/2):1; 2000.

In 1999, Dr. Herbert M. Simpson, former president and CEO of the Traffic Injury Research Foundation in Ottawa and a longtime colleague of Professor Borkenstein, described his friend thus (Simpson, Personal Communication, 1999):

> When most people in traffic safety hear the name Bob Borkenstein, they immediately think of the Breathalyzer. Some also recall his landmark study from Grand Rapids, Michigan in the 1960s, which provided real-world evidence of the risk of collision associated with different BACs (blood alcohol concentrations). This remarkably influential study continues to be widely cited today. A few others may think of Bob in the context of the International Council on Alcohol, Drugs and Traffic Safety, the organization he co-founded almost 70 years ago, which has fostered research cooperation and information sharing around the world. Those of us who know him personally think well beyond those impressive achievements. As someone who has known Bob for many years, I immediately think of two prominent attributes. The first of these is his genuine dedication and intellectual commitment to the field of alcohol, drugs and traffic safety. He has never been content to rest on his accomplishments, always looking for new issues and insights. The second attribute that impressed me is the scope of his thinking. He has never been content to think about the problem in traditional ways; he is always open to new perspectives.

"Genuine dedication," "intellectual commitment," and "innovative thinker" were perceptive summaries of Robert F. Borkenstein's professional persona, but there was much more to him than that. His friend and collaborator for over 50 years, the late Professor Kurt Dubowski, an international scientific celebrity in his own right, had this to say about his colleague:

> ... a superb career-long teacher and mentor to thousands of students at all levels, a talented and highly successful (rare!) inventor, an inveterate world traveller (to all five continents, I believe), a world class researcher (whose major opus, the Grand Rapids Study, is still being cited, debated, and repeated after more than 35 years), an innovator and a highly effective, devoted, and generous leader and official of many professional organizations (two of which he reorganized repeatedly—the Committee on Alcohol and Other Drugs of the National Safety Council, and the International Council on Alcohol, Drugs and Traffic Safety—very probably keeping them alive and productive through his stewardship and contributions). (Dubowski, Personal Communication, 1999)

These summaries by two such distinguished researchers form an appropriate preface to this appreciation of the life and work of another. While essential biographical details will be included below, most of this review will consist of an appreciation of the significant accomplishments of a remarkable individual who actually became a legend in his own time. If Bob Borkenstein was not truly a genius, he was certainly the closest to it that most of us will ever have the privilege to meet.

2.2 Biographical Information

Robert Borkenstein was a prime example of the sort of person who achieved greatness from relatively humble beginnings. Born in Fort Wayne, Indiana, on August 31, 1912, Bob's grandparents were German speaking and, although he spoke both German and English by the time he entered grade school in Fort Wayne, he was actually more comfortable in German. (Some of his papers in later life were published in German.) Bob finished high school just at the onset of the Great Depression and, as a result, was unable to go on to college.

He had, however, developed a great interest and considerable skill in the rapidly advancing field of photography and therefore, in the early 1930s, he worked as a photographic technician in Fort Wayne. This involved leaving home early in the morning, picking up film to be developed from a variety of locations and businesses, returning to the studio/laboratory to develop the photos and then delivering the finished product to the clients later that day. The resultant long days nourished the incredible work ethic which persisted throughout his career. The income from this work was essential to the family since, during the Depression, funds were scarce. Darlena Lindsay, who Bob hired in 1991 as his office manager and later became his course coordinator, remembered him describing how as a child he would go to buy coal by the wheelbarrow load to heat the home since that was all the family could afford at any one time (Lindsay, Personal Communication, 1999).

Borkenstein's father, although lacking in much formal education, had the same inventive mind that Bob demonstrated. He became a successful building contractor who built several well-known buildings in Fort Wayne and served on the City Council (Faville, Personal Communication, 1999). As Bob was growing up, he and his father worked together on many projects. During his high school days, Bob and some of his friends built a robot which, although crude by today's standards, was remarkable for its time—and actually worked (Lindsay, Personal Communication, 1999).

During his career as a photographic technician, Robert experimented with color film (before Kodak marketed it extensively) and developed considerable expertise that served him well in his later work (Dubowski, Personal Communication, 1999). Indeed, according to an article in the Indianapolis Star in 1940 (Anonymous 1940), in collaboration with a colleague, he "developed a simplified color printing process which eliminates the black printing plate, which has a tendency to dull color brilliance." This process eliminated several steps in the engraving of color printing plates resulting in quicker production and higher fidelity. During this time, Bob also built two color cameras using an optical system similar to the Technicolor camera, demonstrating the creative and technical skills that were to mark him as a special individual throughout his entire career.

From 1936 to 1958, he served the people of Indiana in the Indiana State Police (ISP) laboratory, about which more will be described below.

In 1942/1943, Bob also used his color photographic skills to develop the Rex Optical Comparator for the inspection of precision parts using color discrimination. This was produced for him by Rex Laboratories in Indianapolis, the same company that he later used to produce the early models of the Breathalyzer. In a 1997 letter to Lord Bramall at the American Air Museum in Britain (Havard, Personal Communication, 1999), Bob described a wartime application of this device (he had received an invitation from the Queen to attend a ceremony at the US Air Force Cemetery in Cambridge where she was unveiling a memorial):

> I was approached by a firm which was producing bomb latches intended to hold bombs in the bays until they were released when the aircraft had reached their targets. There were numerous failures because of the lack of the necessary precision. They were spot-inspecting the stampings for quality. This was slow and difficult because of the 50× magnification required

> and the effects of even the slightest vibration. I introduced color (both actual and afterimage) into a novel system that showed more at 10× magnification than the traditional comparator showed at 50×. Moreover, it was rapid enough that every piece could be inspected. So I feel I had a small role in the success of these missions. (Borkenstein 1997)

The comparator was patented in Bob's name and the patent "was donated to the cause" (Borkenstein 1997).

Although never hampered in his efforts by his lack of advanced academic qualifications, Bob's continuing thirst for knowledge drove him to gradually accumulate science and foreign language credits at the Indiana University Extension Center in Indianapolis. He finally received his AB degree in 1958, the year he retired from the ISP and joined the faculty at IU as chairman of the department of Police Administration. It is remarkable, and a tribute to his outstanding abilities and character, that Bob became chairman of a department in a large university while only recently having obtained a Bachelor's degree from that very university. Furthermore, he was a pioneering director of a major forensic science laboratory for 20 years and invented a very widely used breath testing instrument, without any formal academic background in science. These remarkable achievements were capped with the award of an Honorary Doctor of Science degree by Wittenberg University in 1963 and, the one of which he was most proud, an Honorary LL.D. from IU in 1987. The latter is something virtually unheard of for a member of the IU faculty itself (Dubowski, Personal Communication, 1999).

During his long career, Robert Borkenstein was an active contributor to many professional associations including: the Indiana University Society for Advanced Study, Indiana University Transportation Research Center, American Academy of Forensic Sciences, Harvard Associates in Police Science, International Association of Chiefs of Police, Academy of Criminal Justice Sciences, Alliance for Traffic Safety, American Public Health Association, National Safety Council, as well as the two in which his leadership was most pronounced, the International Council on Alcohol, Drugs and Traffic Safety and the Committee on Alcohol and Other Drugs of the National Safety Council which he joined in 1939.

Professor Borkenstein published approximately 50 papers, in both English and German, in various international journals. Most, but not all, dealt with some aspect of alcohol and traffic safety.

Shortly after moving from Fort Wayne to Indianapolis and the ISP laboratory in 1938, Bob married Marjorie, his best friend and strongest supporter for 60 years. In October 1997, Bob suffered a massive and debilitating stroke, which put an end to his brilliant active career. He never returned to his office and received home care for the rest of his life. Marjorie died in December 1998 followed by Bob at the age of 89 on August 10, 2002.

2.3 The Laboratory Director

Bob's photographic skills, combined with his fundamental analytical and creative ability, prompted some friends who were members of the ISP in 1935 to seek his advice and assistance with their investigations. He spent many evenings and weekends helping his friends in the investigation of traffic accidents and other incidents but, at that time, had no intention of entering police work on a full-time basis.

As a result of this experience, however, in 1936 when the ISP decided to establish the Indiana State Police criminological laboratory in the basement of the State Capitol building, Borkenstein was a natural to be looked to for advice during the developmental stages. This was one of the first forensic laboratories in the United States. Sharon Faville, who was Bob's lab and teaching assistant at IU for 16 years and lived with Bob and Marjorie for 8 of those years, recalled him saying that, after the laboratory was actually in operation in Indianapolis, he was literally drafted to become a member of the staff, initially as a civilian clerk because he did not meet the minimum height requirements for a trooper (Faville, Personal Communication, 1999). His importance to the ISP became such that eventually the height requirements were waived and he became successively a corporal, sergeant, lieutenant, and eventually captain (Conley, Personal Communication, 1999).

Bob did not have any intention of making law enforcement his career and planned to return to his first love, photography, as soon as the laboratory was running smoothly. As is so often the case with young people's ideas, the plan to move on to other endeavors never reached fruition. He quickly recognized the great potential of the forensic sciences which needed to be exploited, so he stayed on until retirement as captain in charge of Laboratory Services in 1958 (Kraemer 1996). During his career in the lab, in addition to his innovations in breath testing for alcohol (which will be described below), Bob was a leader in advancing the use of photography, particularly color photography, in law enforcement. He designed and built small labs for photo and fingerprint development in many of the ISP posts. More remarkably, he actually designed and had built 300 4 × 5 cameras (at a cost of $35.00 each) to equip these facilities (Borkenstein 1943). Bob Conley, a retired commander of the ISP Laboratory Division, described these as the "Rex 4 × 5s" (Conley, Personal Communication, 1999), a further indication of Bob's confidence in the Rex Company.

During his career in the ISP, he also worked with John Larson on the development of the polygraph and, in 1957, published a paper with Larson on "The Clinical Team Approach to Lie Detection" (Borkenstein and Larson 1957). Bob also made significant contributions to the evaluation and improvement of the first major electronic speed measurement device in traffic law enforcement (Anonymous 1983).

2.4 The Inventor

2.4.1 Early Work on Breath Tests for Alcohol

The observation that small amounts of alcohol are excreted in breath was reported by Anstie as early as 1874 (Anstie 1874). Cushny subsequently reported, based on his work with cats, that:

> The exhalation of volatile substances (including alcohol) from the lungs is exactly analogous to their evaporation from solutions in water, and the pulmonary cells seem to be purely passive in the process. (Cushny 1910)

His observation that these substances obeyed Henry's Law established that the concentration of alcohol in blood could be predicted from the concentration in the alveolar air. Another important milestone in the history of breath alcohol analysis appeared in a 1927 paper by Bogen. He collected expired breath in a football bladder and made an analysis for alcohol by passing two liters of this breath through a solution of potassium dichromate in sulfuric acid. Bogen reported that:

> ...as soon as the disturbing factor of alcoholic liquor still in the mouth is removed, which occurs usually within fifteen minutes after imbibition, in the absence of hiccupping or belching, the alcoholic content of 2 liters of expired air is a little greater than that of 1 cc. of urine." Further, "... the alcoholic content of these excretions (urine and breath) may also be determined for the purpose of evaluating the degree of alcoholic intoxication." (Bogen 1927)

Shortly thereafter followed the most substantive work of the early years of breath testing, a major publication by Liljestrand and Linde in 1930 (Liljestrand and Linde 1930) showing that the time courses in the body of breath alcohol concentration (BrAC) and blood alcohol concentration (BAC) were similar and that 1 cc of blood contained as much alcohol as is contained in 2 liters of air at 31°C. Over many years of research, a consensus was reached that, for law enforcement purposes, a blood/breath ratio of 2100/1 was gradually accepted to be most practical. For a detailed review of the history of the development of breath and blood testing for alcohol, the reader is referred to a publication by Wayne Jones (Jones 1996).

Although much of the basic research on alcohol and its measurement had occurred in Europe, little further happened there with respect to the development of breath testing after Liljestrand and Linde's work. The construction of compact and practical breath alcohol instruments suitable for use by the police was not considered feasible at that time, therefore it was left to researchers in the United States to pursue further developments. The idea of developing a practical instrument for breath alcohol analysis came in 1931 from Professor Rolla N. Harger at the Medical School in Indiana University. Research on chemical tests for intoxication had begun to gather momentum during the late 1930s as a result of the work of Heise and others that demonstrated that excessive drinking was a major cause of road-traffic accidents. The end of prohibition in the United States in 1933 had undoubtedly contributed to this (Borkenstein 1985). Breath alcohol testing became a major focus of interest, in part because of the practical problems associated with sampling blood for law enforcement purposes not the least of which was its inherent intrusive nature. Other problems included the difficulty in locating physicians or other medical personnel willing to draw the blood, often in the middle of the night; the need to transport the subject to that location; the requirements for the preservation of the sample and maintaining the chain of continuity until the analysis could be performed; the necessity of having a qualified laboratory perform the analysis and, of major importance, the delay in the results of the analysis being available to the investigator. A device that would permit a properly trained police officer to obtain reliable results using a sample of breath overcame many of these difficulties and thus was very attractive.

The first practical instrument intended for use by the police for breath alcohol analysis was the Drunkometer developed by Prof. Harger (Harger et al. 1938). It was quickly followed, in 1941, by the Intoximeter (Jetter et al. 1941) and the Alcometer (Greenberg and Keaton 1941).

The Drunkometer used a sample of mixed expired breath collected in a balloon. This breath was passed through a dilute solution of potassium permanganate in sulfuric acid until the color was removed, which required a fixed quantity of ethyl alcohol, 0.169 mg. The approximate volume of breath required to reach this end point was determined by direct water displacement which provided a preliminary rapid semi-quantitative screening test. For quantitative results, the volume of breath required to decolorize the permanganate was passed through a tube of Ascarite to remove the CO_2. This tube was then weighed in a laboratory and the amount of CO_2 determined. The weight of the alcohol accompanying 190 mg of CO_2 in the breath was considered to be "very nearly equal to the weight of the alcohol in 1 cc. of the subject's blood" (Harger et al. 1938).

In 1937, while searching for practical input into the development and application of his new invention, it was natural for Prof. Harger to request the assistance of the ISP lab to field-test his prototype Drunkometer. This was Bob Borkenstein's introduction to breath testing and the beginning of a long professional association of two great minds. Together, in 1937/1938, they established a 44-hour lecture and laboratory course for the training of Drunkometer operators. Because the operation of the Drunkometer was quite subjective, carelessness could not be tolerated so they also set up a statewide system of field supervision and retraining (Borkenstein 1976). While perhaps not directly related, it is also not surprising that the first law in the United States defining driving under the influence of alcohol in terms of blood alcohol concentration was passed in 1939 in Indiana (Borkenstein 1976).

2.4.2 Development of the Breathalyzer

As described above, the Drunkometer, while deserving of great credit as a "first," was somewhat complicated and, not surprisingly, the reliability of it and the other first generation breath test devices was frequently challenged. Borkenstein recognized the validity of some of these challenges and, based on this background, developed the Breathalyzer, the first of the "second generation" of breath testing instruments. This device represented a significant improvement over the earlier ones and incorporated several unique features. It was compact, robust, simple to operate and, of greatest importance, produced reliable results. It was destined to change the approach of law enforcement to drinking-and-driving problems nationwide. This technological innovation enabled traffic enforcement authorities to determine and quantify BACs with sufficient accuracy to meet the demands of courtroom evidence and with an immediacy that dramatically increased the ability of the police to respond quickly to potentially dangerous traffic situations.

In an interview with a writer for the IU Alumni magazine in 1988, Bob recalled that:

> The Breathalyzer came out of all this because I became so very discouraged with the whole problem. An invention is not just an idea; it's an idea to fill a need or an anticipated need. Here was a tool that was needed. It was my interest in photography that led to the Breathalyzer. In color photography work, I had developed a number of instruments for measuring light and had developed a densitometer to make the methods more exact. I drew on these same basic principles to create an instrument that would be extremely stable and objective in measuring body alcohol. The Breathalyzer is so amazingly simple—two photo cells, two filters, a device for collecting a breath sample, about six wires. That's about all that's in it. I left out every nut, bolt, screw and wire that was not important. The strength of the Breathalyzer is its innate stability. It requires less skill on the part of the operator, and its life expectancy is unlimited. There's nothing to wear out. The Breathalyzer is so simple and direct that it will be hard to kill. (Schuckel 1988)

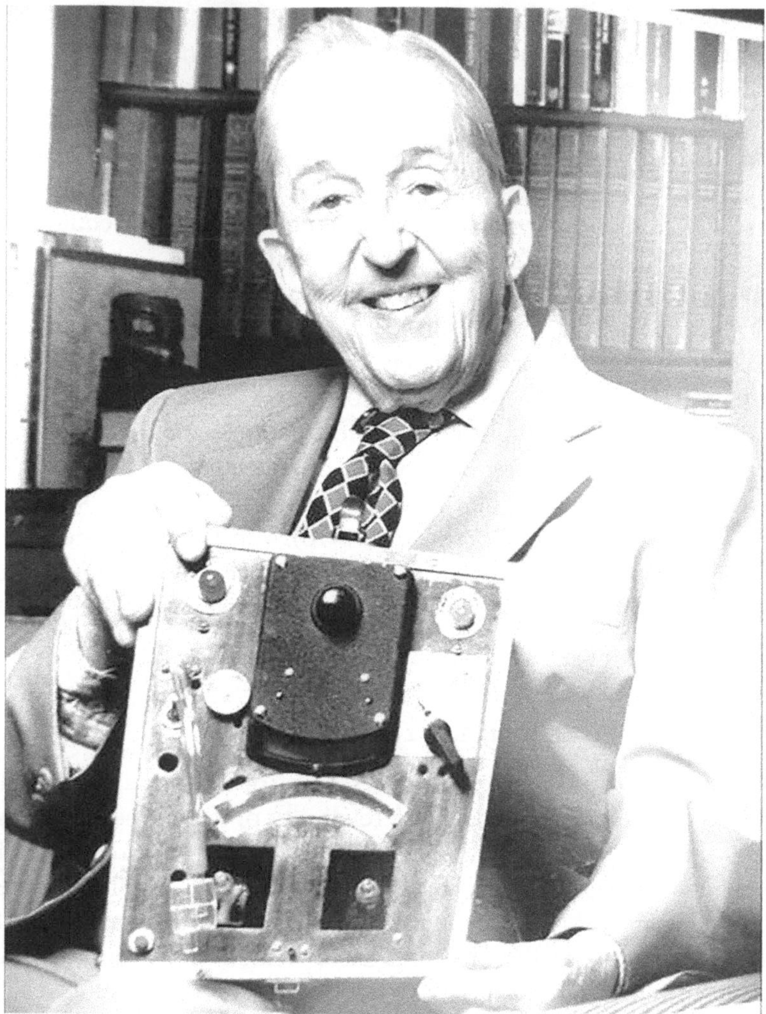

Figure 2.1 Professor Borkenstein holding the original prototype Breathalyzer instrument. (Photo taken in the early 1990s.)

Although it has long since been replaced by more modern instruments, the fact that the Breathalyzer was still in use in some jurisdictions 50 years or more after its invention confirmed Bob's prediction of its persistence (Figure 2.1).

Borkenstein had been thinking about the device for a long time, but it took only about two weeks, his annual ISP vacation in February 1954, to build a working model in the small, partial dirt-floor basement of 618 E. Third Street, his Indianapolis home. The "homemade" prototype Breathalyzer was contained in a wooden case with a sample chamber made from a 100-mL glass syringe with a cut-off portion of the plunger as the piston. Bob's longtime friend Bill Picton, formerly with the RCMP laboratory in Edmonton, Alberta, recalled visiting this "workshop" and being amazed at the almost primitive nature of the facility in which such an important invention had been conceived and developed:

> Bob Borkenstein showed that it was the forensic scientist and not the facilities that count. (Picton, Personal Communication, 1999)

The first public demonstration of the Breathalyzer was in October 1954 at the National Safety Congress in Chicago. This was described by George Larsen Jr. in *Traffic Digest and Review*:

> A new and significantly improved and simplified method of using breath to determine the degree of alcoholic influence was demonstrated last month before the Committee on Tests for Intoxication of the National Safety Council at the National Safety Congress in Chicago. Both the method and a lightweight compact device for using the method were developed by Lt. Robert F. Borkenstein, chief technician of the Indiana State Police and director of the ISP crime laboratory. Tests run by Lieutenant Borkenstein under varying conditions, many of which were observed by this writer, have given highly uniform results. In addition, other experts in the field such as Dr. R.N. Harger of the Indiana University School of Medicine and Dr. Ward Smith of the University of Toronto have run large numbers of tests with excellent results, according to reports they made to the Committee. (Larsen 1954)

Six prototype units were built based on the original model (a stainless steel cylinder with two holes at the appropriate level in the side replaced the glass syringe). These were field tested by various workers in the United States and Canada including Dr. Kurt Dubowski (at that time the first State Criminalist of the State of Iowa), Lloyd Shupe (of the Columbus, Ohio PD Laboratory), and Dr. Ward Smith (at the University of Toronto). After incorporating and testing their suggestions, 100 commercial instruments were built. These quickly found their way into practical police and courtroom use in many parts of the United States and Canada. The first commercially built instrument went to Grand Rapids, Michigan, and the second and third to the Province of Ontario (Borkenstein 1976).

2.4.3 The Design

Despite this considerable activity in the mid-1950s, a formal publication about the Breathalyzer did not appear in the peer-reviewed literature until 1961 (Borkenstein and Smith 1961). In addition to being so busy with this and other projects, one of the reasons for this delay was Borkenstein's hesitancy to publish since, as already described, he had minimal academic qualifications in science, particularly chemical analysis, and very limited experience in the preparation of a scientific paper. Bob finally was persuaded by his friends of the need to document his invention in the literature so he turned to Ward Smith to assist him with the preparation of the manuscript. By 1961, the Breathalyzer had been in use by the police in Ontario (under Smith's leadership) since 1956 so there was practical operational experience available to support the technical data in the paper.

The paper described the many unique and innovative features that were incorporated into Bob's design and which accounted for the Breathalyzer's wide acceptance, not only as a tool for law enforcement but also in scientific research.

2.4.3.1 The Sampling Device

Most of the "first generation" devices had relied on a sample of mixed expired air which required that an estimate be made of the proportion of alveolar air in the sample based on its CO_2 content. The sample in the Breathalyzer was collected using a modification of Haldane's method (Haldane and Priestley 1905). The breath was led into a stainless steel cylinder where it caused a piston to rise until it was above the level of two vent holes.

As long as the subject blew, the air was vented until, at the end of an expiration, the piston dropped to close the two vents thus capturing a fixed volume of the last portion of an expiration ("end-expiratory air").

The volume collected was equivalent to 52.5 mL at 34°C. (In their 1961 paper, Borkenstein and Smith used a temperature of 31°C as "the temperature at which the breath leaves the mouth." This was the temperature reported by Liljestrand and Linde in 1930 but later work by others confirmed 34°C as the more acceptable figure for this temperature.) This volume (52.5 mL) was 1/40th of 2100 mL and thus equivalent to 1/40th of one mL (25 µL) of blood. This was determined to be a sufficient volume to contain enough alcohol for an accurate determination and yet small enough to ensure uniform sampling of something approaching alveolar air.

In Borkenstein's original design, 100 mL had been collected using the glass syringe but he eventually became convinced that a smaller sample was practical and the final prototype had a vent slot cut in the syringe at the appropriate level. Because the 100 mL syringes broke quite regularly during this experimentation phase, their cost almost aborted the project prematurely (Dubowski, Personal Communication, 1999). That was not the only mishap during the development. Sharon Faville recalled almost burning down the home when "a hose slipped off the acetylene torch I was using to seal ampoules. Dr. B. rushed over to the tank and turned it off" (Faville, Personal Communication, 1999).

2.4.3.2 The Reagent

Using a very simple valve arrangement, the breath sample was passed through a glass ampoule containing acid dichromate, a common reagent for alcohol analysis. The ampoule served not only as a container for the reagent but also as the fixed length light path for the subsequent photometric measurement. One of the modifications made after the prototype was examined by Bob's colleagues was the composition of the reagent. The original dichromate concentration, which was based on Heise's and others' work with blood and urine samples, was too strong for the very small amounts of alcohol in a breath sample. (It must be remembered that Borkenstein's expertise was in photography, not chemistry. He was comfortable with color filters and photocells but not chemical stoichiometry.) Dubowski calculated a more appropriate concentration of 0.025% potassium dichromate in 50% sulfuric acid (Dubowski, Personal Communication, 1999).

In the early Breathalyzers, the reagent was heated to 50°C using an automobile cigarette lighter unit, but eventually a silver nitrate catalyst was added to the reagent and the heater was no longer required (Schuckel 1988). Under these conditions, the alcohol was quantitatively oxidized to acetic acid within 90 seconds. While many compounds may react with acid dichromate if introduced directly into the solution, when the sample was breath from a living person, considerable "biological specificity" was imparted to it. The analytical conditions (reagent concentration, temperature, and time) also provide some specificity for alcohol. Acetone, one of the chemicals that may be found on the breath of some living persons, does not react under these conditions. The reaction with ethyl alcohol remained virtually constant after 90 seconds. If methyl alcohol was present, a second reading after 10 minutes would have changed significantly from the first. In the early days, when many small hospitals in rural areas had minimal laboratory facilities, it was not unknown for them to request a Breathalyzer-equipped police officer to assist with the diagnosis of patients suffering from possible methyl alcohol-induced intoxication.

2.4.3.3 *The Photometer*

The truly unique and innovative design feature of the Breathalyzer was its photometric arrangement. This consisted of an incandescent visible light source (an automobile light bulb) on a moveable carriage between two similar ampoules (one "Test" and one "Reference"), two blue filters and two photocells wired in opposition through a simple galvanometer. The reaction between the acid dichromate and alcohol caused a quantitative decrease in the yellow color of the reagent and therefore, in accordance with the Beer-Lambert Law, a logarithmic increase in the blue light transmittance. If only one reagent ampoule, filter and photocell had been used (the conventional arrangement), the increments on the BAC scale would then have had to be logarithmic rather than linear.

Of greater importance, it would also have been necessary to use a potassium dichromate solution of exact, known strength. This would have presented a production quality control challenge because of the very weak solutions of potassium dichromate necessary to make the instrument sufficiently sensitive for the small amounts of alcohol actually being measured in a breath sample. With the photometric system in the Breathalyzer, the change in transmittance of the "Test" solution was measured by the distance through which the light source had to be moved to re-establish a null condition in the photoelectric circuit (the so-called "Bunsen Principle") (Dubowski, Personal Communication, 1999). This movement was automatically expressed in blood alcohol units (% w/v) on the instrument scale by a pointer driven across the scale by the movement of the lamp carriage. Because the galvanometer was always electrically and mechanically at "null" when readings were taken, indicating that the two photocells were receiving identical amounts of light through the ampoules and filters, the actual difference between the ampoules was determined by the position of the light required to attain this condition. Thus the intensity of the light source, its age, or changes in line voltage did not affect the results.

The photometric arrangement of the Breathalyzer also made the scale reading virtually independent of the concentration of dichromate. It thus allowed for a "Blank" test for possible contamination, a "Standard" test of the calibration and tests of two or more samples of breath from the subject, all with the same ampoule of reagent. Most users of the Breathalyzer incorporated these quality control checks into their operational protocols.

The linear BAC scale on the Breathalyzer was originally calibrated on a purely arithmetic basis. The factors in this calibration were the volume of the sample, the relationship between the concentrations of alcohol in breath and blood (1/2100), the quantitative relationship of the reaction between alcohol and acid dichromate, and the optical and spatial relationship between the movement of the light and the position of the pointer. These calculations were subsequently tested during practical evaluations and found to be valid.

2.4.4 Commercial Production

While it had never been Borkenstein's intention to patent his invention, he was persuaded by his friends and his attorney to do so. To pay the costs of this process he had to sell his dearly loved British sports car. The patent application was filed in 1954 and US, British, Canadian, Australian, Mexican, French, and German patents were eventually obtained. The royalties were assigned to the Indiana University Foundation (Kraemer 1996).

Commercial production was first arranged with Rex Metalcraft, a small company in Indianapolis. Bob was familiar with this company because it had produced his Optical Comparator and also the metal cases for Harger's Drunkometer (Dubowski, Personal

Communication, 1999). Being located in Indianapolis, Borkenstein was able to closely monitor the quality of the production. The actual manufacturing and distribution rights had been purchased by the Stephenson Corporation of Red Bank, New Jersey, a company which produced a variety of respiratory equipment and had also been the distributor of the Drunkometer. Although the early models of the Breathalyzer were manufactured by Rex, the Stephenson Corporation later turned to another company, Radio Frequency Laboratories in New Jersey, to redesign (with little or no input from Borkenstein) the electronic components of the Breathalyzer. The resultant RFL model was produced for only a few years and was quite unpopular with users because it was much more complicated to service than the original Rex model.

Stephenson reacted to the complaints about the RFL units and, with Borkenstein's substantial input, redesigned the Breathalyzer into the Model 800, which rapidly evolved into the Model 900. A 1969 replacement of the galvanometer in the Model 900 with an electronic unit converted the 900 into the Model 900A. This also was done without Borkenstein's advice and resulted in a brief furor in 1982 when an issue arose in the courts about the possibility of an effect on test results obtained with the 900A as a result of "radio frequency interference" (RFI). The amplification in the null meter of the 900A actually did result in fluctuations of the needle if a source of electromagnetic radiation (usually a police portable radio transmitter) was activated in very close proximity to a 900A. This effect was quite familiar to users of the instruments and was easily compensated for in their operations or with minor modifications to the electronics of the instrument. Nevertheless, it did, for a brief period, slightly tarnish the reputation of the Breathalyzer (Figure 2.2).

When the Stephenson Corporation was purchased by the Bangor Punta Corporation in the late 1960s, the Breathalyzer rights were assigned to one of that company's subsidiaries, Smith and Wesson (S & W). In addition to its engineering/manufacturing capability, S & W also had significant marketing contacts within the law enforcement community through their firearms and chemical crowd control agent sales. S & W designed (on their own) and briefly marketed the semi automated Model 1000 Breathalyzer. They also worked closely with Borkenstein on the development of the Model 2000, a microprocessor-controlled unit which used infrared (IR) absorption as the alcohol measurement technique. Bob had started thinking about an IR unit in the early 1970s and, although the Model 2000 was produced as a prototype in the early 1980s, it was never marketed. Despite this, his interest in IR devices for breath testing persisted and he assisted his friend Werner Adrian with the development of a prototype IR breath alcohol analyzer which became the progenitor of the BAC Verifier and eventually the BAC Datamaster (Dubowski, Personal Communication, 1999).

S & W continued to manufacture the Breathalyzer until 1984 when the rights for the Models 900 and 900A were sold to National Draeger Corporation (rights to the Model 2000 were not included in this transaction) (Blasi and Ryser, Personal Communication, 1999). Draeger also worked closely with Bob in the late 1980s/early 1990s to develop the Model 900B, a semi automated version of the 900A. It used the same sampling device, reagent and photometer arrangement as the Model 900A but incorporated a timer to turn on the light after 90 seconds, a microprocessor-controlled motor to drive the lamp carriage and an internal printer. It too was never marketed, primarily because the market had moved on to instruments that did not require the use of a chemical reagent.

Draeger continued to produce the Model 900A until late 1997. The final five instruments were sold in early 1999. In all, over 30,000 of the various models of the Breathalyzer

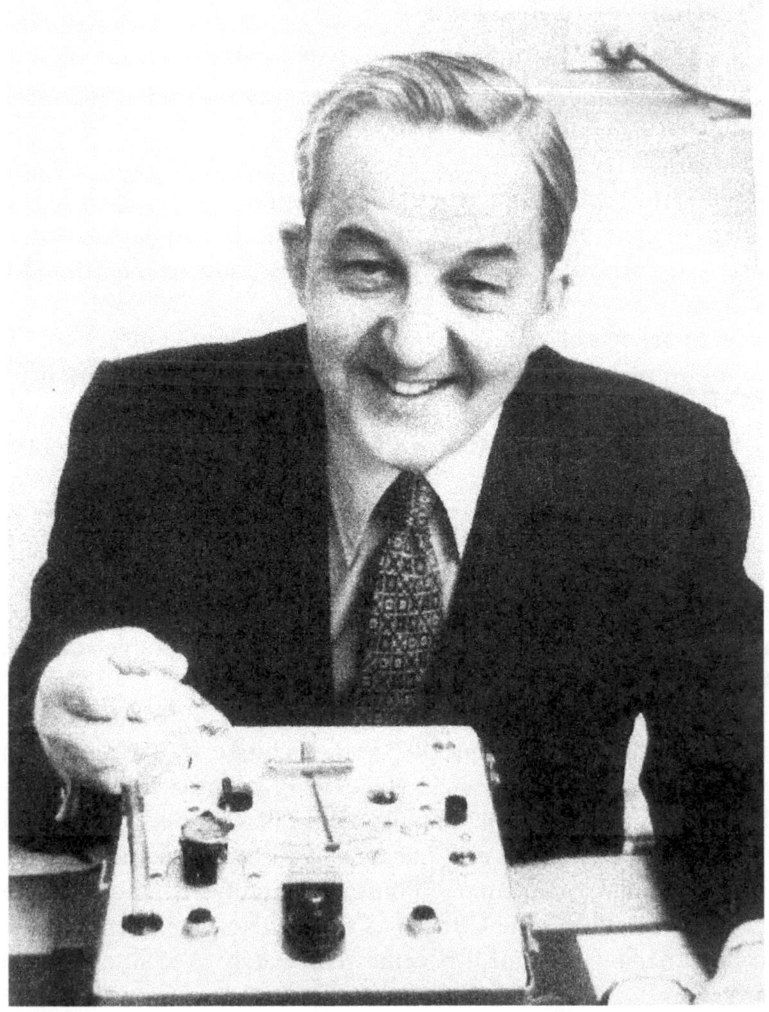

Figure 2.2 Professor Borkenstein checking one of the Series 900 Breathalyzer instruments.

were built and sold between 1955 and 1999, a remarkable record for any piece of equipment, particularly an analytical instrument. The Breathalyzer was, at one time, used in almost every state in the United States and Australia as well as every province in Canada (where it was often referred to as "the Borkenstein" in the courts to differentiate it from other devices; although the spelling "Breathaly**z**er" as opposed to "Breathaly**s**er" was a registered name, the name had become generic among the general public for any breath testing device with little attention paid to the specifics of the spelling).

Despite the introduction of third generation instruments in the 1970s and early 1980s, by 1985, 30 years after its introduction, the Breathalyzer was still being used in 24 states in the United States and in Canada. By 1999, 150 were still in use in New York, 950 in New Jersey, and about 1,500 in Canada (Blasi and Ryser 1999). It is difficult, if not impossible, to think of any item of scientific equipment, other than the microscope, that has had such a prolonged and important application in forensic science. The Breathalyzer can surely be considered to be to law enforcement what the Douglas DC-3 was to air transport.

2.4.5 The Breathalyzer in Research

The significant role of the Breathalyzer as a reliable tool for measurement of BAC was not restricted to law enforcement. It also found its way into scientific research into the effects of alcohol on behavior. Research in this area had slowed considerably during World War II but the explosion in motor vehicle registrations and use which followed in the late 1940s/early 1950s brought with it a dramatic increase in highway fatalities which rekindled interest in drinking/driving research and legislation (Borkenstein 1985). The fortuitous arrival on the scene of the Breathalyzer facilitated much of this research.

One of the early reports of such usage was a paper by Drew et al. (1959), "Effect of Small Doses of Alcohol on a Skill Resembling Driving." Although primarily dealing with the effects of alcohol on driving simulator tests, in this project Drew compared the results of the then existing breath testing methods with blood and urine tests and stated:

> The results from the Breathalyzer were good enough to warrant its consideration from a practical point of view.

This was a remarkable statement by investigators in a country that had theretofore viewed breath testing with skepticism, and it therefore attracted considerable attention in England and elsewhere.

The Breathalyzer was used in epidemiological studies by McCarrol and Haddon in New York City (McCarrol and Haddon 1962) and, of course, by Borkenstein himself in his massive Grand Rapids Study (Borkenstein et al. 1964). It was used in studies by the Royal Canadian Mounted Police of the effect of alcohol on driving ability as measured by road tests (Coldwell 1957) and by Smith and Lucas in 1966 in the classic Canadian Television Network (CTV) television documentary "Point Zero Eight." Although unpublished in the conventional sense, this 30-minute Christmas season television film had a major impact on legislation in Canada. Copies of it became very widely used internationally in driver education courses.

The Breathalyzer gave rise to a large body of literature concerned with its design, applications, limitations, and characteristics. Studies were performed in Switzerland, Germany, Australia, France, Italy, and Canada, particularly in the late 1950s and 1960s. Countless correlation studies between Breathalyzer results and blood tests were conducted. Some of these directly impacted on legislation in various countries. For example, in Australia, a study was done in the Australian Capital Territory in 1969, details of which were included in a "Report on Breath Analysing Equipment for Drivers of Motor Vehicles." This report stated:

> Having taken evidence from medical officers, scientists, police officers, and others experienced in the use of this equipment, the Committee is satisfied that the Breathalyzer is an accurate instrument providing a reliable method of measuring blood alcohol concentration in the human body.

This led to the adoption of the Breathalyzer as the only official instrument in the Australian Capitol Territory. Other Australian states followed this lead and the Breathalyzer became the standard instrument for law enforcement and court evidence in Australia for many years (Borkenstein 1976).

Similarly, in 1967/1968 Canada's Parliament gave careful consideration to the Breathalyzer as a device which would make it practical to enact enforceable legislation establishing a 0.08% "legal limit" based primarily on mandatory breath testing. In a letter to Prof. Borkenstein at that time, Mr. P. J. Farmer of the Canada Safety Council stated:

> The outcome of much soul-searching was that the Parliamentary Committee agreed that the provision of breath samples was neither an invasion of privacy nor self-incrimination. This and the fact that the Breathalyzer was considered reliable and the simplest way to measure blood alcohol content pretty much dictated that the .08 (%) legislation be tied to breath testing for legal determination of blood alcohol content. (Borkenstein 1976)

In fact, the Canadian legislation enacted in 1969 was widely referred to as "The Breathalyzer Law" and a large legal reference book is entitled *Breathalyzer Law in Canada* (McLeod et al. 1986).

A sidelight to the legislation in Canada was that it originally included a clause requiring the police to offer to collect a sample of breath for the use of the defendant before they could demand a breath test for evidential purposes. This clause was based on work that Borkenstein had done in the mid-1960s on a method for collecting the alcohol from a sample of breath for later analysis. He had been working with tubes packed with calcium chloride (later calcium sulfate) as an adsorbent and in fact, with Dubowski published a paper on this work in 1977 (Borkenstein and Dubowski 1977). Problems with production of tubes that would meet Bob's standards for quality persisted and the project never achieved commercial viability. The "sample for the accused" clause in the Canadian Criminal Code was therefore never proclaimed and was eventually removed from the Code.

Typical of similar activity in the various states in the United States, W. E. Smith in California published a paper in 1969, "Breathalyzer Experience under the Operational Conditions Recommended by the California Association of Criminalists" (Smith et al. 1969). In it he said:

> It is concluded that the Breathalyzer meets the standards of good law enforcement when operated in accordance with the operational disciplines recommended by the California Association of Criminalists.

The Breathalyzer became one of the first instruments to be placed on the 1974 Approved Products List issued by the National Highway Traffic Safety Administration of the Department of Transportation (Borkenstein 1976).

2.4.6 The Breathalyzer and the Law

There were hundreds of appellate court decisions bearing directly on the Breathalyzer, none of which were successful in attacking the scientific/analytical principles on which it was based. Reversals did, of course, occur but were based on improper use or on circumstances such as untrained operators, lack of evidence of the quality of the solution in the ampoules, lack of evidence of allowing sufficient time for mouth alcohol to disappear, civil liberties issues, and biological variables. Suffice it to say, the Breathalyzer weathered over half a century of scrutiny by law, medicine and science and survived, paving the way for later generations of instruments.

One of the major legal challenges, *State v. Downie*, occurred in New Jersey in 1989. This case concerned the reliability of the Breathalyzer and particularly its reliance on the 1/2100 breath/blood ratio to convert the BrAC to the BAC. Borkenstein marshaled an impressive array of expert witnesses (including this author), of whom he was the most persuasive, to present data in support of the Breathalyzer. The court ruled in favor of the use of the Breathalyzer in law enforcement and there were few significant challenges afterward. Boris Moczula, one of the prosecutors in the Downie case, described his first contact with Professor Borkenstein as follows (Moczula, Personal Communication, 1999):

> I had previously known him only by reputation. Influenced by his status as a giant in the forensic scientific community, I expected to greet a man of imposing physical size. How surprising to find such a diminutive individual, with the ever-present sparkle in his eye.

Prosecutor Moczula was also impressed (although it came as no surprise to Bob's friends) that the Professor insisted on receiving no compensation for his testimony in order that no one could suggest that his testimony was influenced by anything other than the science. He described an example of Bob's expertise as a witness:

> At a point in the litigation when defense attacks on the Breathalyzer's components were particularly intense, Doctor Borkenstein offered this simple analogy as explanation and encouragement: "If we focus upon the individual parts of a bumblebee, no one would expect such a cumbersome insect to be airborne. Yet the bumblebee flies." Several months later, when I first notified him of the court's favorable decision, I ended my correspondence with these same words: "The bumblebee flies." (Moczula, Personal Communication, 1999)

It has been said of Professor Borkenstein that, "He was not only one of the founding fathers of breath alcohol testing but also the attending pediatrician" (Jones, Personal Communication, 1999) and, perhaps even its geriatrician!

2.5 The Researcher

At a Symposium on Alcohol and Road Traffic conducted at Indiana University in 1958 chaired by Prof. Borkenstein, a panel of seven distinguished international experts approved the following statement:

> As a result of the material presented at this Symposium, it is the opinion of this Committee that a BAC of 0.05% will definitely impair the driving ability of some individuals and, as the BAC increases, a progressively higher proportion of such individuals are so affected, until at a BAC of 0.10%, all individuals are definitely impaired. (Borkenstein 1985)

This statement was soon endorsed by the National Safety Council, the American Medical Association, the International Association of Chiefs of Police and the Junior Bar Association, among others.

While immensely pleased with the fact that he was able to persuade such a panel of experts to agree on anything (including where to have lunch), the statement had required an all night session to draft (Shupe, Personal Communication, 1999), the discussions convinced Borkenstein of the need for a major research project to consolidate the bits and pieces of data on which the statement was based. The Grand Rapids Study, funded by the

US Public Health Service and the Licensed Beverage Industries of New York, was the result (Borkenstein et al. 1964). Without question, this research performed in 1962/1963 became the most influential epidemiological study of the role of alcohol in traffic accidents. On this topic, Dr. John Havard, longtime Secretary of the British and the Commonwealth Medical Associations and for over forty years one of Bob's closest friends, commented:

> What has always been so remarkable about Bob is the breadth of his knowledge of so many disciplines, particularly law and public health. He recognized the importance of the epidemiological approach to mortality and morbidity from road accidents, long before it had occurred to traditional epidemiologists, and it was his realization of the potential of the digital computer in advancing knowledge in this field that was such an influential factor in developing the Grand Rapids Study. This at a time when distinguished medically qualified epidemiologists were asking me what was meant by the epidemiology of road accidents. (Havard, Personal Communication, 1999)

The Grand Rapids Study was a large-scale roadside survey designed to assess the risk of a driver being involved in a crash as a function of the BAC. The concentration of alcohol in blood was estimated indirectly by taking samples of breath at the roadside in special plastic bags for later analysis with the Breathalyzer. The BAC of the drivers involved in accidents was compared with the BACs of a large control group of drivers passing the site of the accident on the same week day and the same time of day as the accident group. In this way, the risk of being involved in a crash was plotted as a function of BAC. As later described by Borkenstein himself:

> This study was designed to explode the monolith of the 'drunken driver' into as many components as practicable so that target groups could be identified. It was also designed to compare the alcohol factor to other factors involved in traffic accidents, or parametric to them. It was not originally designed to generate countermeasures or to estimate the relative risk of driving while intoxicated; however, the data by their nature suggest an exponentially increasing relative risk curve which was calculated from the data as an afterthought. This relative risk curve has been the basis of much controversy because of the under-representation of drinking drivers in accidents at 0.03% BAC. In spite of this, it has found its way into countless papers, books and educational material. (Borkenstein et al. 1974)

As principal investigator of the study, Bob demonstrated the wide scope of his detailed thought processes, his analytical mind and his innovative problem-solving ability. Not content to pick the most convenient site (Bloomington or perhaps Indianapolis), he researched and selected one that would meet his broad criteria and which would ensure the validity of the findings. Some of the factors involved in the selection of Grand Rapids were its size (large enough to have a sufficient sample of accidents for statistical validity), freedom from extreme seasonal population fluctuations, a good balance of heavy and light industry, commerce and educational institutions, a good accident records system, and a progressive police department. In addition, and not inconsequentially, the population demographics closely reflected those of the entire United States at that time.

Another matter which contributed to the significance of this research was the fact that it studied the role of alcohol not only in drivers who were involved in crashes, but also the involvement of drinking drivers at the same locations and in similar circumstances, who did not experience crashes. The one, by itself, was not significant without the other.

Borkenstein also recognized the importance to the study of obtaining the cooperation of the drivers being interviewed. There were a number of potentially sensitive matters in the questionnaire used for the interviews which required subjects to provide information of a personal nature. Bob identified another organization within his own University that had considerable experience with asking intimate questions of large numbers of people, the Kinsey Institute for Sex Research. Since, for some, "drunken" driving can have a stigma attached to it similar to that placed on socially unacceptable sexual practices, the Kinsey results suggested a risk that Borkenstein's investigation might find drinking and driving to be, for some, acceptable behavior unless it was discussed seriously by the interviewees. Staff members of the Institute for Sex Research were therefore asked to train the members of the research team who would conduct the interviews in Grand Rapids. This training proved to be of immense value to them and thus to the study (Borkenstein et al. 1974).

The BAC "legal limit" of 0.08%, which became so widely accepted internationally, was derived principally from the Grand Rapids Study and included other factors such as age, socioeconomic status, and education that interact with alcohol as accident causation factors at concentrations below 0.08%. The study concluded, however, that this competition diminishes and appears to disappear as BACs exceed 0.08% (Borkenstein 1985). The impact on public policy both in North America and in Europe was exemplified by events in England. In 1967, Barbara Castle, the Minister of Transport, while launching the Drink/Drive publicity campaign associated with the new Road Safety Act of 1967, stated:

> In recent years research has further increased our knowledge of the effects of alcohol on drivers. The most important contribution was Professor Borkenstein's study at Grand Rapids, Michigan, involving over 12,000 drivers. The results confirmed a good deal of earlier research, which by itself had remained inconclusive, and also gave more precise information than ever before about the increased accident risk at various blood-alcohol levels. Faced with the need to strengthen the law, and armed with this new scientific evidence, we decided that it would be right to lay down a blood-alcohol level above which it should be illegal to drive. The level has been set at 80 mg/100 ml (0.08% BAC) and to exceed it is to commit an offence. (Borkenstein 1985)

Also in 1967, at the seventeenth meeting of the Council of Ministers of the European Conference of Ministers of Transport, it was resolved that the member countries adopt a BAC not higher than 0.08% in legislation (Borkenstein 1985). Reference has been made above to Canada and Australia where legislation was very much influenced by the study. This policy also found its way into most states in the United States, which adopted a 0.08% BAC as the dividing point above which driving is prohibited by law.

The Grand Rapids Study became a cornerstone of traffic alcohol control legislation in the United States and abroad, and in the highway safety standards of the US Department of Transportation.

2.6 The Professor

Although the Breathalyzer and the Grand Rapids Study exemplify Bob's outstanding abilities as an inventor and as a researcher, some would say his most impressive achievements were associated with his career as a teacher. Sharon Faville, who worked closely with Bob for 16 years, described him thus:

> ... a compassionate, caring human being whose commitment to service assisted many young students and colleagues to develop their talents and careers. Teaching for Dr. B was both a passion and a mission. He challenged students to think independently and shared the analytical tools he used himself. He inspired creativity and critical thought. At a commencement address, he spoke to graduates about the 'indissoluble residue' they would take from their university experience: the process of learning to learn, of critical thought and investigation. (Faville, Personal Communication, 1999)

Robert Borkenstein's initial association with IU occurred when he joined the ISP Laboratory. The ISP Academy was located in Bloomington and became affiliated with the University in 1936/1937. It was the first police academy to be directly associated with a university, although the cadets were housed in tents during their stay. Lectures were held in the Chemistry Building auditorium. Because of his position in the Laboratory, Bob had a close association with the Police Academy as a lecturer and, through this, with members of the faculty of the Law School who also lectured at the Academy. In addition, the Laboratory occasionally required assistance from the IU Medical School in Indianapolis and so he developed associations with this faculty as well (Anonymous 1983).

Eventually, some of the Academy courses evolved into university credit courses and a Department of Police Administration was established in the Faculty of Arts and Sciences. Several attempts were made to recruit Bob into this department on a full-time basis but he resisted these efforts until 1958, when he retired from the ISP. The associate dean of Arts and Sciences was then finally able to persuade Bob to become an associate professor and chairman of the Department of Police Administration. At that time there were only two other similar programs in the United States, one at the University of California at Berkeley and the other at Michigan State University (Kraemer 1996).

As the new chairman of the Department, Professor Borkenstein's initial goals were to strengthen the faculty, to attract better students and, perhaps most challenging, to actually persuade some in the University that this department deserved to be based within the university. Eventually he succeeded but it took time. He distinguished his department's program from the Police Academy program by convincing the university senior faculty that, while the Academy effectively taught the "how", his department taught the "why." He insisted that the program become multidisciplinary, drawing on resources in psychology, political science, sociology, law, philosophy, and other disciplines. The curriculum was thus knit into the entire fabric of arts and sciences. In 1970, the department changed its name to Department of Forensic Studies and in 1985 it became the Department of Criminal Justice (Kraemer 1996).

Eventually Prof. Borkenstein was also able to develop a Master's and finally a Ph.D. program. The department had developed from one of only three in the United States, in a very humble and simple beginning without much acceptance in the academic environment, to one that contributed significantly to the university and the community it served.

Not content with having established a viable university department, Bob was very interested in ensuring that the resources of the department were made available to the community. He therefore formed the Center for Studies of Law in Action ("law" and "action" are words not often used in the same phrase) as a means of collecting relevant information from the field and disseminating it to practitioners. The philosophy of the center was to expose practitioners to academic developments while at the same time exposing faculty members to the real world from time to time to learn what problems they needed to work on. For example, in one of its most successful programs, the center brought qualified people from all over the country to Bloomington to learn the latest concepts in the supervision of programs for alcohol testing of drivers and the techniques that are used to carry out these tests. Resource people from around the world interacted with these practitioners to try to develop solutions to a major societal problem. This course, established in 1958 as Supervision of Chemical Tests for Alcohol with 11 students, is now known as the Robert F. Borkenstein Course on Alcohol and Highway Safety. It is offered twice a year and typically has 40 to 50 students. Boris Moczula, following his association with Prof. Borkenstein in the Downie case, became one of the instructors in the course. He said about it:

> I would marvel at how class members scurried for the opportunity to speak to him (Borkenstein) or be photographed with him. He greatly enjoyed the interaction and unpretentiously honored all requests. (Moczula, Personal Communication, 1999)

A second course, Effects of Drugs on Human Performance and Behavior, was established in 2002.

In summary, Prof. Borkenstein converted the Department of Police Administration from a traditional police training program to a multi-disciplinary teaching, research, and service center that rapidly achieved national prominence for its pioneering insistence on the integration of a liberal arts core into professional training in criminal justice. His vision established the department as one of the few in the field that is truly of university caliber, with emphasis on research and scholarship as well as teaching and service. Bob served as chairman until 1971 and continued as a professor in the department until his retirement from the university in March, 1987. He continued to hold the position of professor emeritus and director emeritus of the Center for Studies of Law in Action until his death in 2002.

2.7 The Laureate

For over 60 years, Robert F. Borkenstein was an international leader in the forensic sciences, criminal justice education, and traffic safety. His extensive research on highway safety established this field as an area for scientific research as well as social concern, and he served as a consultant in many countries around the world. He was most famous for his contributions to the understanding and control of alcohol impairment in traffic accidents, and his research and numerous publications on this subject are well known to the international forensic science and traffic law community. As might be expected, he was also the recipient of many awards and other honors. Among these were:

- The Liberty Bell Award from the Indiana Bar Association "for outstanding contribution to public understanding of the law," 1966;
- A Special Citation from the Ministry of the Interior of the Republic of China (Taiwan), 1970;
- The Distinguished Service to Traffic Safety Award of the National Safety Council, 1982;
- The Award of Merit of the Association for the Advancement of Automotive Medicine, 1982;
- A Distinguished Service Award in Recognition of Service to the State of Alaska, 1983;

- Induction into the Safety and Health Hall of Fame International, 1988;
- A Special Minister of Justice's Award, Government of Canada, 1992;
- The Gerin Medal of the International Association for Accident and Traffic Medicine, 1992;
- A Special Presidential Award of the International Council on Alcohol, Drugs and Traffic Safety, 1995; and
- The National Association of Governors' Highway Safety Representatives Award, 1996.

While each of these was special, Bob would probably have acknowledged two others as being particularly close to his heart. These were the prestigious Widmark Award of the International Committee (now Council) on Alcohol, Drugs, and Traffic Safety (ICADTS) awarded in Toronto in 1974, and the Robert F. Borkenstein Award established by the National Safety Council in recognition of his lifetime of work in the area of alcohol and drugs in relation to traffic and transportation.

The Widmark Award was established in honor of Professor Erik M. P. Widmark of the University of Lund, Sweden, whose comprehensive research during the first half of the twentieth century touched on all aspects of the pharmacology of alcohol and its quantitative estimation in body materials. He was the first person to apply the then contemporary knowledge to the problem of transportation safety. This award is the highest honor that the ICADTS can confer on individuals who have made outstanding contributions to the basic knowledge of alcohol and other mood-altering drugs and have applied to traffic safety problems. Each laureate must have contributed significantly and must have achieved international recognition over a sustained period of many years. These are demanding criteria. The first recipient was Bob's colleague, Prof. Rolla Harger, in 1965. This award was so special to Bob because he was a founding member of the ICADTS, serving as president from 1969 to 1986, and its driving force for over 40 years. He chaired the Widmark Awards Committee from 1986 to 1992. Of Bob's importance to ICADTS, Dr. John Havard wrote:

> He is one of the few people I know who has won international fame and yet has found time, as he so often has, to encourage and to help young workers in his many fields of interest. There are a number of well-known figures working in the field of alcohol and road accidents today who owe their success to his insistence, as a long serving member and as president of ICADTS, that priority should be given to helping young workers and, in particular, to making it possible for them to participate in its international conferences. (Havard, Personal Communication, 1999)

The Borkenstein award honors Bob's active participation in many of the activities of the National Safety Council for almost 60 years, including chairmanship of the Committee on Alcohol and Other Drugs. The first of these awards was presented to Professor Borkenstein himself on October 26, 1989. It was a source of great pride to him that his name was being used to honor the recipients, most of whom, until recent years, were close colleagues and good friends and all of whom still consider it to be one of their greatest honors because it is named after a person for whom they have enormous respect.

In addition to these formal awards, Bob was honored by invitations to present papers to national and international conferences on law enforcement, traffic safety and forensic sciences in Austria, Australia, Canada, the Republic of China (Taiwan), England, Finland, France, Germany, The Netherlands, Puerto Rico. Sweden, Switzerland, and New Zealand.

He served on the editorial boards of *Alcohol, Drugs and Traffic Safety*, *Forensic Science Review*, and *Journal of Traffic Medicine* as well as serving as a consulting editor for *Blutalkohol*.

2.8 The Person

All of the above describes many of the truly outstanding contributions that Robert F. Borkenstein has made to his chosen profession and particularly to traffic safety. What it does not adequately present, however, is the enormous impact of his persona on friends, students, colleagues and associates. His mind was always working; many of his colleagues described one of his outstanding characteristics as always working on a new project. His enthusiasm for these projects could be overwhelming. While discussing some of the activities of the Department of Criminal Justice in 1996, he enthused:

> I'm excited about it, I'm really excited about the years to come. (Kraemer 1996)

A journalist who interviewed Bob in 1988 described him thus:

> He is a reporter's dream. He automatically answers Who? What? When? Where? and How? It's as if he's methodically going through in his mind how the material should be presented and in what order—much like he must do when conducting an experiment or devising an invention. (Schuckel 1988)

Although deeply committed to his work, Bob was not a "one trick pony." He was equally at home in a snowball fight at his Divide, Colorado cabin as he was in the meeting rooms of international professional organizations. He and Marjorie were deeply caring, thoughtful, gracious and consummate hosts at magnificent dinner parties at 821 South High Street in Bloomington and at the Colorado cabin. These locations became the "crossroads of the world of alcohol and traffic safety and professional policing on a truly international scale" (Dubowski, Personal Communication, 1999). Lloyd Shupe described one of these occasions when:

> Bob asked a group of us to stop at his home for what he called a "Meeting of the Young Bucks with the Old Farts." The young bucks were Ward Smith, Kurt Dubowski, Jim Osterburg, and me. The old farts were Rolla Harger, Charlie Wilson, Clarence Muehlberger, and Raphael Ruenes (from Havana). (Shupe, Personal Communication, 1999)

Despite himself qualifying by 1999 as an "old fart," Bob's friends always looked upon him as a "young buck."

Bob was very much a hands-on host at these affairs. Kurt Dubowski remembered:

> He personally prepared his special punch in ample quantities and arranged the cheese platter just so, after hours of personally shopping for the right ingredients in Chicago, Indianapolis, or Bloomington. (Dubowski, Personal Communication, 1999)

The Professor also had a recreational as well as a professional interest in good wine. Bill Picton remembered a discussion about wine with Bob during which Bill mentioned that there was a winery in Edmonton, a city known more for its snow and cold winter weather (its football team is named "the Eskimos") rather than for its viniculture:

> Upon my departure, Bob presented me with a bunch of plastic grapes for use by the Edmonton winery. (Picton, Personal Communication, 1999)

Darlena Lindsay described how she and Bob had lunch together in Bob's office every day he was there. They took turns preparing it. The conversations, usually one-sided, covered an amazing range of topics with Bob's encyclopedic knowledge and range of interests never failing to amaze her. She recalled:

> If anything came up that he didn't know at that time, he would by the next day. He loved the theatre and dancing and, as an adult, took up fencing, the only sport he had any use for. (Lindsay, Personal Communication, 1999)

In these lunchtime conversations, Bob described his travels and the many wonderful places he had been, Vienna and Paris being his favorites.

His telephone bills must have been enormous; if he did not invent the term "networking," he certainly was one of its foremost practitioners. Many of his colleagues all over the world would describe his calls, arriving straight out of the blue, sometimes to discuss whatever was Bob's issue of the moment, or sometimes just to talk. This author's calls almost invariably arrived early (for him) on Saturday mornings, including one Saturday that happened to be Christmas day. John Havard described this characteristic:

> One of the most remarkable facts about Bob was the wide range of eminent people in different countries who count him among their friends. Around 1962, I was trying to interest a very large and important government department in Britain about a certain problem, and was having no luck whatsoever in getting anyone in authority to listen to me. I was astonished when the distinguished chief of the department (later ennobled as Lord ---) phoned me personally explaining that he had heard that Bob was visiting London and had given my number as a contact. He asked me to make it clear that he insisted that Bob stayed with him in London. (Havard, Personal Communication, 1999)

Marjorie was a highly talented artist who fostered Bob's interest in art. One of her pieces, of which he was particularly proud, was an interesting collage made from component parts of old Breathalyzers. It hung prominently on his office wall at IU. They had no children but shared a love for their beautiful cabin on the side of a mountain near Divide, Colorado, which they visited whenever possible until they found it necessary to give it up in 1996. Some of Bob's most creative thoughts were developed in the peace and solitude of the Rockies.

2.9 Conclusion

As a forensic scientist, one might assume that Bob Borkenstein would have considered that the solution to the problem of alcohol and traffic safety rested with technology and better ways of measuring BAC. As a police officer, he might have seen the answer in greater enforcement of stricter laws. As an educator, perhaps public information was the route to follow. While each of these has a role to play, such single solution approaches were not how he thought. A much broader approach is required. In a plea for more creative thinking, Bob proclaimed to an international audience in 1985:

> Perhaps we have been too optimistic in believing that the media, public information meetings, driver education schools and other means of disseminating information would solve the problem of understanding and would gain support of the public. This has been a dismal failure. I read over most of the papers I have written on this general subject during the past 30 years. In nearly every one of them I stated that the weakest link in attacking this problem has been public support. What we perceive as low-level action against the drunken driver is probably a direct result of lack of public support. We can inform and we can enforce and as a result change behavior through fear for a while. But when we fail to change attitudes, regression is bound to occur. (Borkenstein 1985)

In 1985, John Havard described one of Bob's legacies in the following way:

> If I was asked to identify the person who has made the biggest contribution toward the reduction of death and disability from motor accidents associated with alcohol, I would have no hesitation in identifying Bob. (Havard 1988)

The first words in this appreciation of Robert F. Borkenstein's life and work were those of Dr. Herb Simpson; it is therefore fitting that the final words also be his:

> His spirit, enthusiasm and dedication inspired me very early in my career and I think fondly of his influence, not only in the field of traffic safety, but on me personally. (Simpson, Personal Communication, 1999)

There are hundreds of others, including this author, who could only add "Amen."

Acknowledgments

The nature of this type of article is such that it depends on the willingness of many people to share their recollections and memories. The contributions of Robert Conley, Kurt Dubowski, Sharon Faville, John Havard, Wayne Jones, Boris Moczula, William Picton, Lloyd Shupe, and Herb Simpson are gratefully acknowledged. Much of the material for this article was derived through personal access to Prof. Borkenstein's papers in his office at Indiana University. The cooperation of Darlena Lindsay in guiding me through that material and her diligence in seeking out items that might answer my many questions could not have been more complete or more efficiently provided. Without all of these, this article would not have been possible. Dr. Ray Liu and *Forensic Science Review* made this trip to IU possible.

References

Anonymous. Borkenstein develops better color prints. *Indianapolis Star* July 18, 1940.
Anonymous. Robert F. Borkenstein receives doctor of laws degree. *Indiana's Finest*, 1983.
Anstie FE. Final experiments on the elimination of alcohol from the body. *Practitioner* 13:15, 1874.
Bogen E. Drunkenness: A quantitative study of acute alcoholic intoxication. *JAMA* 89:1508, 1927.

Borkenstein RF, Crowther RF, Shumate RP, Ziel WB, Zylman R. *The Role of the Drinking Driver in Traffic Accidents* (Research Report to the Injury Control Program, U.S. Public Health Service, Department of Health, Education and Welfare. Washington, DC), 1964.

Borkenstein RF, Crowther RF, Shumate RP, Ziel WB, Zylman R. The role of the drinking driver in traffic accidents (The Grand Rapids Study). *Blutalkohol* 11(Suppl) 1:9, 1974.

Borkenstein RF, Dubowski KM. A breath alcohol adsorption tube compatible with head space gas chromatography for blood alcohol analysis. *J Traf Med* 5:29, 1977.

Borkenstein RF, Larson JA. The clinical team approach to lie detection. In Leonard VA (Ed), *Academy Lectures on Lie Detection*. Charles C. Thomas: Pullman, WA, 1957.

Borkenstein RF, Smith HW. The Breathalyzer and its applications. *Med Sci Law* 2:13, 1961.

Borkenstein RF. A brief history of breath alcohol programs. Unpublished manuscript, 1976.

Borkenstein RF. *Address to Association for the Advancement of Automotive Medicine*. Seattle, WA, 1988.

Borkenstein RF. Historical perspective: North American traditional and experimental response. *J Stud Alcohol* (Suppl) 10:3, 1985.

Borkenstein RF. Letter to Field Marshal Lord Bramall. June 25, 1997.

Borkenstein RF. The Breathalyzer: A brief history. Unpublished manuscript.

Borkenstein RF. The camera as a witness. *International Photographer*, February 5, 1943.

Carson V. Professor combats drunken driving. *Indianapolis Star* March 2, 1983.

Coldwell BB. *Report on Impaired Driving Tests*. Crime Detection Laboratory, Royal Canadian Mounted Police: Ottawa, Canada, 1957.

Cushny AR. On the exhalation of drugs by the lungs. *J Physiol* 46:17, 1910.

Drew GC, Colquhoun WP, Long HA. *Effect of Small Doses of Alcohol on a Skill Resembling Driving*. Her Majesty's Stationery Office: London, UK, 1959.

Greenberg LA, Keator FW. Portable automatic apparatus for indirect determination of the concentration of alcohol in the blood. *J Stud Alcohol* 2:57, 1941.

Haldane JS, Priestley JG. The regulation of the lung ventilation. *J Physiol* 32:225, 1905.

Harger RN, Lamb E, Hulpieu HR. A rapid chemical test for intoxication employing breath. *JAMA* 110:779, 1938.

Havard JDJ. *Letter to Robert H. Cannon, National Science Foundation*. June 22, 1988.

Jetter WW, Moore M, Forrester GC. Studies in alcohol. IV. A new method for the determination of breath alcohol. *Am J Clin Path (Tech Suppl)* 5:75, 1941.

Jones AW. Measuring alcohol in blood and breath for forensic purposes: A historical review. *Forensic Sci Rev* 8:13, 1996.

Kraemer P. Interview of Prof. Robert Borkenstein. Indiana University Oral History Research Center: Bloomington, IN, May 22, 1996.

Larsen G. Institute report on new breath test method. *Traffic Dig Rev* 2:2, 1954.

Liljestrand G, Linde P. Über die ausscheidung des alkohols mit der exspirationsluft. *Scand Arch Physiol.* 60:273, 1930.

McCarrol RF, Haddon W Jr. A controlled study of fatal motor vehicle accidents in New York City. *J Chronic Dis* 15:811, 1962.

McLeod RM, Takach JD, Segal MD (eds.). *Breathalyzer Law in Canada*. Carswell: Toronto, Canada, 1986.

Schuckel K. Borkenstein's Breathalyzer. *Indiana Alumni* June 12, 1988.

Smith WE, Harding DM, Biassotti AA, Finkle BS, Bradford LW. Breathalyzer experiences under the operational conditions recommended by the California Association of Criminalists. *J Forens Sci Soc* 9:58, 1969.

Epidemiology of Alcohol-Related Accidents and the Grand Rapids Study*

3

PATRICIA F. WALLER (1932–2003)†

Contents

3.1 Introduction

The association between alcohol and injury was recorded in the writings of ancient Egypt (Waller 1985) and was referred to in the Proverbs of the Old Testament (Old Testament). The relationship of alcohol to difficulties in transportation has been noted by Borkenstein, Trubitt, and Lease (Borkenstein et al. 1963), who refer to the problems experienced by a drunken Noah in his ark during the Flood, as well as later accounts of drunken charioteers

* This chapter is an updated (format only) version of a review article previously published in *Forensic Science Review*: Waller PF: Epidemiology of alcohol-related accidents and the Grand Rapids Study; *Forensic Sci Rev* 12:107; 2000

† C. Rinehart and D. A. Sleet: A Tribute—Patricia Fossum Waller, PHD (1932–2003); *Inj Prev* 9:295; 2003.

in ancient Rome. They also note, however, that it was the advent of mechanical transportation that thrust the role of alcohol into the limelight. Rail transport preceded the automobile, and in 1899 the American Railway Association prohibited drinking while on duty.

With the appearance of the private motor vehicle, alcohol assumed an unprecedented importance in serious and fatal injury. Motor vehicles had not been on the roads long before it was recognized that alcohol was a factor in their crashes. In 1904 the *Quarterly Journal of Inebriety* included the following item:

> We have received a communication containing the history of twenty-five fatal accidents occurring to automobile wagons. Fifteen persons occupying these wagons were killed outright, five more died two days later, and three persons died later. Fourteen persons were injured, some seriously. A careful inquiry showed that in nineteen of these accidents the drivers had used spirits within an hour or more of the disaster. The other six drivers were all moderate drinkers, but it was not ascertained whether they had used spirits preceding the accident. The author of this communication shows very clearly that the management of automobile wagons is far more dangerous for men who drink than for driving of locomotive on steel rails. Inebriates and moderate drinkers are the most incapable of all persons to drive power motor wagons. The general palsy and diminished power of control of both reason and senses are certain to invite disaster in every attempt to guide such wagons. The precaution of railroad companies to have only abstainers guide their engines will soon extend to the owners and drivers of these new motor wagons. (US Department of Transportation 1968)

Although the relationship between alcohol and motor vehicle crashes was recognized, there was no objective scientific evidence of the magnitude or nature of the problem. In 1961 the Public Health Service sponsored a National Conference on Alcohol and Traffic Safety, based on five prior working conferences. Five major topics were covered, including Behavioral and Physiological Effects of Alcohol; Chemical Testing, Enforcement, and Legal Problems; Statistics and Experimental Design; Social Psychological Factors; and Motivational and Educational Aspects. A subsequent publication compiled the major papers and conclusions from this conference, and it is of interest to compare what was known at that time with what has occurred since. J. H. Fox, in a paper addressing drinking and driving as a public health concern (Fox 1963), posed four questions that needed to be answered in order to develop and implement a systematic prevention effort. These were

1. Is the ingestion of alcohol prior to driving a factor in traffic accidents? That is, can it be demonstrated that drinking prior to driving increases the likelihood of being involved in a traffic accident?
2. If so, how does the drug—alcohol—affect driving behavior so as to increase the chances of an accident occurring? That is, is there evidence to indicate that driving behavior deteriorates under the effect of the drug, and at what dosage?
3. What are the cultural patternings and social psychological factors which predispose toward drinking-driving? That is, are there social forces which channelize human behavior so as to create the situation in which drinking and driving occur in close temporal proximity?
4. If it is determined that the use of alcohol is a significant factor in traffic accidents, the question arises, what, if anything can be done about it? (pp. 249–250 in Ref. (Fox 1963)).

Although drinking and driving is a major health problem throughout the industrialized world, the primary focus of this presentation is on the United States, where systematic data, including alcohol data, have been compiled on all fatal traffic crashes for most of the past two decades. However, it is assumed that information on the relationship between alcohol use and probability of traffic crash would be relevant across international boundaries.

3.2 The Grand Rapids Study

Even at the time of Fox's writing, considerable information was available to answer the first two questions, and much more evidence has since accumulated. The first study that compared alcohol use in drivers in crashes with that of drivers using the same roads was reported in 1938 (Holcomb 1938). Comparison of the two driver groups showed that 25% percent of the crash-involved drivers had elevated BACs (0.10% or higher) compared to only 2% of those on the same roads but not in crashes, and 14% of crash-involved drivers had measured at or above 0.15% BAC, compared to only 0.15% of comparison drivers. This study clearly showed the elevated crash risk associated with alcohol use. However, the numbers of drivers involved were relatively small, 270 crash-involved drivers and 1,750 comparison subjects. Also, all the crash-involved drivers were injured to the extent that they required hospitalization. For the crash-involved drivers, alcohol involvement was measured using urine samples, but breath samples were used for the comparison drivers. The sample of crash-involved drivers was collected over a three-year period, while comparison drivers were obtained over a one-week period in the spring. Besides alcohol information, only information on age and sex was included. Nevertheless, this study was an important forerunner of later efforts to determine the role of alcohol in traffic crashes.

Although a number of subsequent studies strongly suggested that alcohol increases the likelihood of being in a crash, it was the landmark study conducted by Dr. Robert Borkenstein and his colleagues (1964), that clearly put to rest any doubts concerning the relationship between drinking and motor vehicle crashes. This study, known as the Grand Rapids Study, documented the relative risk of causing a crash as a function of objectively measured blood alcohol concentration (BAC). The full range of crashes was included rather than focusing solely on injured drivers. A total of 5,985 crash-involved drivers and 7,589 comparison drivers provided information. Unlike more limited previous studies, the Grand Rapids Study obtained, in addition to measures of alcohol, extensive background information on both crash-involved drivers and other drivers on the road at the same crash sites and at a time and day corresponding to those at which the crashes occurred. In addition to BAC, data collected included age, annual mileage, years of education, race, marital status, occupation, drinking frequency, and sex. Almost 96% of crash-involved drivers and almost 98% of comparison drivers cooperated with the study by providing the requested data.

Although the Grand Rapids Study was conducted in an urban area, a subsequent effort conducted in Vermont (Perrine et al. 1971) and covering the entire state found essentially the same relative risk of crash as a function of BAC. Today it is generally accepted by both the public and the authorities that higher BACs increase crash risk, but it took many years to achieve this widespread acknowledgment. When public perceptions were modified, however, the Grand Rapids Study was critical in bringing about the change.

The Grand Rapids Study made two critical contributions to the traffic safety field and to the literature on alcohol and driving. The first was an undisputed demonstration, based on a sizable data base, that elevated BACs are associated with elevated crash risk.

The second important contribution was the feasibility of a relatively inexpensive, objective, non-invasive measure of blood alcohol concentration, namely, the Breathalyzer, a measure that could be used by non-medical personnel.

3.2.1 Blood-Alcohol Concentration and Crash Risk

As in the case of Fox's first question, there was considerable information relevant to his second question, evidence that clearly showed the impairing effects of alcohol on psychological and physiological functioning. Numerous studies documented apparent effects of alcohol on reaction time, motor skills, nystagmus, sensory phenomena, and intellectual processes, but the studies were vulnerable to criticism on methodological grounds, and findings often appeared to be based more on belief than objective evidence (Carpenter 1963). Since 1963 a large literature has accumulated that shows that alcohol does indeed impair many behaviors essential to safe driving.

It is Fox's third question, concerning the social forces that affect the probability of drinking and driving, that has scarcely been investigated even yet. Reasons for this failure are many, but some will be discussed later in this paper.

Fox's final question, concerning what can be done to reduce drunken driving, has generated considerable effort and even some enlightenment, although much of the effort was characterized more by political considerations than by scientific rigor. Even so, considerable information has been accumulated that identifies measures that appear to be effective. These will be addressed in more detail elsewhere.

The Grand Rapids Study generated what may be the most often presented graph in the literature on alcohol and driving, the Grand Rapids graph illustrating the relative risk of causing a crash as a function of BAC (Figure 3.1). Careful inspection of this graph shows

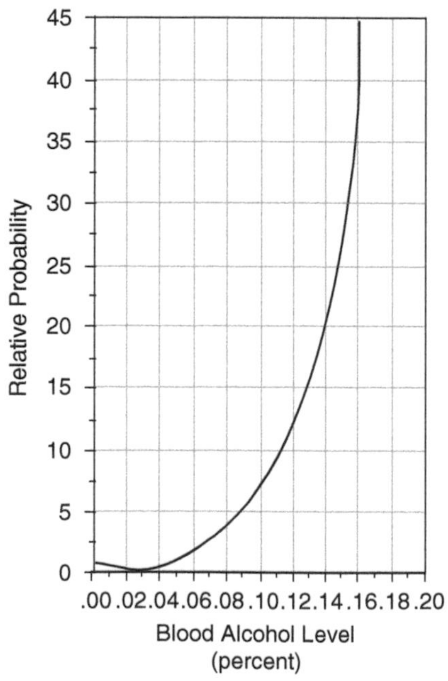

Figure 3.1 Relative probability of causing a crash as a function of BAC. (Reproduced from Borkenstein, R.F. et al., *Blutalkohol*, 11, 1974.)

that at about 0.02% BAC the relative probability of causing a crash is slightly lower than at zero BAC. This phenomenon became known as the "Grand Rapids Dip" and gave rise to speculation that a small amount of alcohol may actually improve performance. However, subsequent analyses by Hurst (1973) of the Grand Rapids data showed that the "dip" was an artifact created by the type of drinker likely to be detected in the comparison driving population. Hurst categorized drivers on the basis of reported frequency of drinking. When relative crash risk was examined within drinking-frequency group, he found that the risk of crash increased for *all* groups as BAC increased. However, those who were daily drinkers were more likely to be detected with low levels of alcohol and were more practiced drinkers and probably more practiced drivers. Hurst's initial analyses by drinking-frequency category did not extend beyond 0.09% BAC, but most drinking drivers who get into difficulty have much higher BACs.

Subsequently Hurst analyzed data from several studies, extending some of the relative risk curves to above 0.20% BAC (cited in Ref. (Hurst et al. 1994)). From these analyses he arrived at three conclusions. First, drivers who drink frequently are at lower risk of crash at a given BAC than are drivers who drink less frequently. Second, at any drinking frequency, crash risk increases with increasing BAC. Third, the findings greatly underestimate crash risk for drivers in general, in that they are based primarily on drivers who regularly drink and drive.

3.2.2 Chemistry-Based Enforcement

Borkenstein's development of the Breathalyzer enabled a relatively inexpensive objective means of measuring blood alcohol concentration (Voas and Lacey 1989). The use of the Breathalyzer eliminated the need for blood samples, thus greatly facilitating the task of determining blood alcohol level and greatly increasing the public acceptance of procuring the measure. Because of the evidence from the Grand Rapids Study that elevated BACs were associated with enormous increases in crash risk, it was possible to move from subjective judgments of impairment to an objective criterion. Just as speed limits do not take into consideration how proficient a driver may be at high speeds, it could be argued that it is irrelevant how skillful a driver may be at a BAC of 0.15%. The objective relative risk is unacceptably high. Once such evidence was made available, and objective, inexpensive, non-invasive measures of BAC could be obtained, the foundation was laid for legislation to implement uniform approaches to drunken driving.

Although legislation was slow to take advantage of the information provided in the Grand Rapids Study, nevertheless the study laid the groundwork for BAC-based legal limits for defining impairment and *per se* laws. The increasing ease of use and decreasing cost of pre-arrest breath tests enabled the implementation of sobriety checkpoints. These and other countermeasures were possible because of the early work of Borkenstein and his colleagues. It is difficult to overestimate the significance of Borkenstein's work when considering the history of drunken driving in the United States and elsewhere.

In light of the enormous progress that has been made since these early studies were conducted, it is difficult to realize how little solid evidence was available at the time to clearly establish the role of alcohol in traffic crashes and injuries. In general it was known that alcohol impairs judgment, as well as performance, and indeed this relationship had been observed since time immemorial. However, the extent to which alcohol actually made a difference in risk of crash and injury simply was not established.

3.3 Trends in Mileage and Drinking

3.3.1 Increasing Mileage

By the 1960s in the United States, and certainly in the two succeeding decades, both drinking and driving were increasing. In 1960 the annual vehicle miles driven was estimated to be 719 billion. This number had risen to 1,120 billion by 1970 and 1,521 billion by 1980. By 1990 it was up to 2,148 billion (National Safety Council 1998). These numbers are gross estimates at best, based on such information as gallons of fuel purchased. Nevertheless, the overall trends may be considered accurate.

3.3.2 Alcohol Consumption

Per capita consumption of alcohol in the United States is perhaps even more difficult to establish. Like vehicle mileage, it is based on sales data. Per capita consumption remained fairly steady in the decade preceding the 1960s, but began to rise in the early 1960s. It rose steadily, reaching a peak in 1980 and 1981, after which it began to decline (Williams et al. 1997). Thus, during the 1960s and 1970s, both alcohol consumption and mileage were increasing steadily. Although alcohol consumption began to decrease in the 1980s, per capita consumption was still 2.25 gallons of pure alcohol in 1993. This average per capita consumption occurs even though significant proportions of the population are abstainers, about 30% of men and 40% of women (US National Institute on Alcohol Abuse and Alcoholism 1997).

3.3.3 Alcohol Consumption and Drinking and Driving

Given these high rates of mileage driven and alcohol consumption, it should not be surprising that drinking and driving was not taken seriously by most of the population. It was considered more or less a "folk crime," something that happens and that should be taken in stride. Especially among young males, such behavior was considered more or less normal, part of the natural coming-of-age process in our society. Although strict penalties were enacted in some jurisdictions, they were seldom imposed.

In the late 1960s the author was present at a governor's luncheon focused on highway safety. The issue of drunk driving was especially highlighted, and the governor admonished the judges in the room for accepting plea bargains that reduced the driving under the influence charge to reckless driving. An elderly judge sitting at my table explained to me why judges were guilty of allowing the reduced charge. He said that whenever he convicted someone of drunk driving, almost invariably the person appealed for a jury trial. Because so many jurors at some point drove after drinking, their reaction was, "There, but for the grace of God, go I." And they failed to convict. With the conviction for reckless driving, at least the drunk driver was convicted of something, and the judicial system was not wasting its resources on a futile effort. In other words, judges could not "make the system work" in the absence of public support.

3.4 The Federal Program

The creation of a federal program in highway safety in 1966 gave rise to new efforts to reduce drunken driving. In the early 1970s the National Highway Traffic Safety Administration implemented Alcohol Safety Action Programs (ASAPs), community-based programs that incorporated enforcement, education, and treatment (see Ref. (Ross 1992) for a discussion). Unfortunately, the mixture of responsibility for program implementation as well as program evaluation, with strong pressures to show success, rendered objective evaluation of most of these programs virtually impossible. It was also extremely difficult to conduct these programs in ways that would allow reasonable interpretation of the findings. In any event, they had no appreciable impact on the overall magnitude of the problem.

Drunken driving remained a high priority of NHTSA, even when strong efforts to eliminate the agency resulted in drastic cutbacks of their programs. One of the most useful tools in defining the magnitude of the problem, as well as evaluating the impact of countermeasures, is the Fatality Analysis Reporting System (FARS, originally the Fatal Accident Reporting System). This reporting system compiles extensive data on every fatal traffic crash in the nation. Initiated in 1975, it took several years before the data were sufficiently reliable to conduct meaningful analyses. Furthermore, it took even longer for the alcohol data to become reliable (about 1982). The availability of this data file has been enormously useful in establishing what is happening in this field.

Because usable information on alcohol involvement was not available until 1982, it is not really feasible to use the data to track changes in alcohol-related fatal crashes prior to that time. However, the data on per capita consumption of pure alcohol (regardless of whether in the form of beer, wine, or hard liquor) indicate that in the US it peaked in 1981 and has steadily declined since then. There are no clear reasons for this decline, but it is relevant to note that the changes in per capita consumption varied across beverage type. The greatest decline occurred in consumption of spirits, that is, hard liquor. Consumption of wine actually continued to increase, peaking in 1986 and declining somewhat thereafter through 1993, when it was still as high as it had been in 1977. Figure 3.2 shows these changes (based on data reported in Ref. (Williams et al. 1997)).

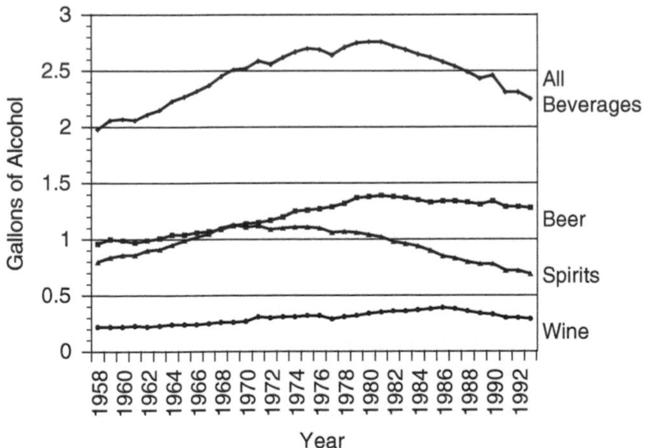

Figure 3.2 Per capita alcohol consumption (pure alcohol), age 15+, United States, 1958–1993. (Based on data reported in Williams, G.D. et al., *Apparent Per Capita Alcohol Consumption: National, State, and Regional Trends, 1977–1992,* Surveillance Report No. 35. National Institute on Alcohol Abuse and Alcoholism, Division of Biometry and Epidemiology, Rockville, MD, 1997.)

3.4.1 Beverage of Choice and Drunken Driving

Differential consumption of alcohol by beverage type is of importance in the consideration of drunken driving. In the very late 1960s, per capita consumption of spirits actually exceeded per capita consumption of beer, but for most years beer consumption has exceeded that of either spirits or wine. Furthermore, the Grand Rapids Study, as well as many studies since, reported that beer was overrepresented in crashes, as well as in drivers with high BACs. Beer remains the beverage of choice for drinking drivers. In contrast, wine does not appear to be a major factor in crashes. Whether this difference reflects differences in how the two beverages are used (e.g., with meals versus without meals) or those who choose one beverage over the other is not clear. The Grand Rapids Study reported an *under* representation in the crash population of drivers who reported spirits as their beverage of choice, compared to an overrepresentation of those who preferred wine or beer. However, beer was vastly overrepresented as the beverage of choice for those who were crash-involved.

While per capita consumption of each of the three beverage types has decreased in recent years, the slower decrease in beer consumption is of particular significance for drunken driving. Beer is the beverage that is most strongly promoted in conjunction with sports, including racing, where race cars prominently display major brands on their cars as they drive at high speeds. This clear distinction in how beer is promoted compared to distilled liquor may convey misconceptions on the part of the public in the relative risk associated with each.

Furthermore, the fact that alcohol in the form of beer has not shown the consumption decline seen for hard liquor suggests that any changes in drunken driving cannot be attributable simply to changes in overall alcohol consumption, since the beverage of choice for drinking drivers has not changed appreciably.

3.4.2 Changing BAC Rates in Fatal Crashes

Figure 3.3 is based on data from the FARS file for 1982 through 1997 (National Safety Council 1998), and shows changes in the proportion of drivers in fatal crashes with BACs of 0.10% or higher. It can be seen that all age groups have shown significant declines in their proportion of drivers with high BACs. Especially notable is the 16 to 20-year-old group, one that has been targeted by specific countermeasures such as the National Minimum Drinking Age (NMDA) and Zero Tolerance laws. (The NMDA established a nationwide minimum age of 21 for legal purchase and/or possession of alcohol, and the Zero Tolerance laws established severe penalties for drivers under age 21 who were found to have BACs above zero or 0.02%.) However, it can be seen that the two age groups that remain major problems are the 21 through 24 and 25 through 34. These drivers are of legal age for drinking and have proved remarkably resilient to countermeasures. They are not easily reached, since even those who continue their education beyond high school are not easily located. They continue to represent a major challenge to traffic safety.

Even so, drivers age 21 through 34 have shown marked decreases in alcohol positive drivers from 1982 to 1997. Indeed, it is the next oldest group, age 35 through 44, that has shown the smallest decreases of all. Although their rates are lower than those age 21 through 34, they have remained relatively unchanged over time.

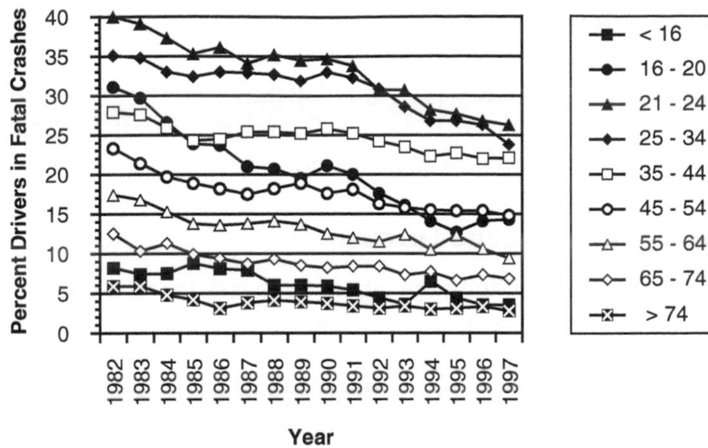

Figure 3.3 Proportion of drivers in fatal crashes with BAC of 0.10 percent or higher, United States, 1982–1997. (Based on data reported in US National Highway Traffic Safety Administration, *Traffic Safety Facts 1997*, US National Highway Traffic Safety Administration, Washington, DC, 1998.)

When patterns over time are examined by driver sex, it can be seen that there has been a decrease for both males and females in fatal crashes. Figure 3.4 shows these changes from 1982 to 1996 (National Safety Council 1997).

It can also be seen in Figure 3.4 that the vast majority of drivers testing positive for alcohol are at BACs of 0.10% or above, 76% for men and 72% for women in 1996. These percentages have decreased somewhat from 1982, when they were 78% and 74%, respectively. Nevertheless, it appears that for both men and women, most drinking drivers in fatal crashes are not moderate drinkers.

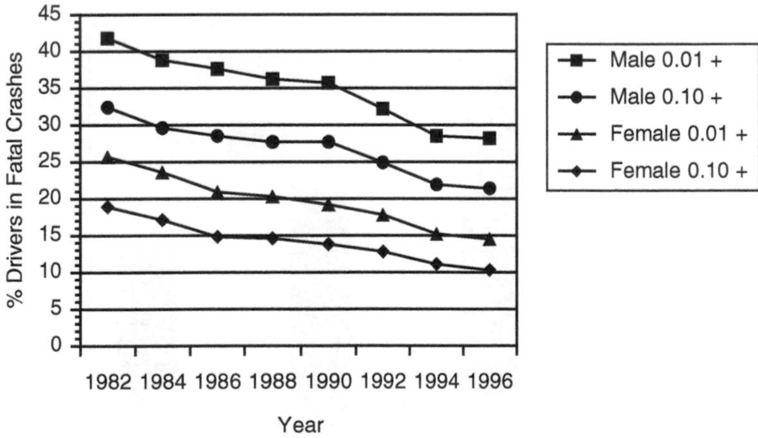

Figure 3.4 Percent of drivers in fatal crashes testing positive for alcohol, by sex, 1982–1996. (Based on data reported in US National Highway Traffic Safety Administration, *Traffic Safety Facts 1997*, US National Highway Traffic Safety Administration, Washington, DC, 1998.)

3.5 Potential Problem Populations

These data also mask certain potential problems that may materialize over time. These issues concern women drivers and older drivers. The Grand Rapids Study identified these two groups as being at higher crash risk at specified BACs.

3.5.1 Women and Drinking and Driving

At the time of the Grand Rapids Study, the higher crash risk for women was generally attributed to their relative inexperience in driving (and possibly in drinking, as well). However, that explanation is much less tenable today. Women still drive fewer miles than men, but they have significantly narrowed the gap. In 1990 women age 16–64 drove an average of over 10,000 miles annually, representing a 51.5% increase over their 1983 mileage of 6,722. By contrast, men increased their mileage only 14.5%, from 15,370 to 17,602 (Rosenbloom 1997).

Women have also changed their driving patterns. Indeed, the major changes in travel in the United States that occurred in the 1970s and 1980s was attributable primarily to changes in women's travel behavior (Pisarski 1992). Women are currently more likely to be driving at times and places where alcohol is involved, thus increasing their exposure to risk.

There is also some evidence that alcohol may differentially affect the driving performance of women. The higher crash risk reported in the Grand Rapids Study was confirmed in a study reported in 1972 (Carlson 1972) and more recently (Zador 1991). In the latter study, it was found that risk of being the driver in a nighttime single vehicle fatal crash at a BAC of 0.05 to 0.09%, compared to the risk at zero alcohol, was highest for young drivers (16–20), next for those age 21–24, and lowest for those age 25 and over, indicating that age and probably driving experience lowered crash risk at a given BAC. However, much more striking are the gender differences seen in all three age groups. For the youngest group, males showed an elevated risk of over 18-fold, but females showed a 54-fold increase. For drivers age 21 through 24, the corresponding figures were 11.8 for males and over 35 for females; and for ages 25 and older, the figures were 8.6 for males and 25.5 for females. Figure 3.5 illustrates these findings.

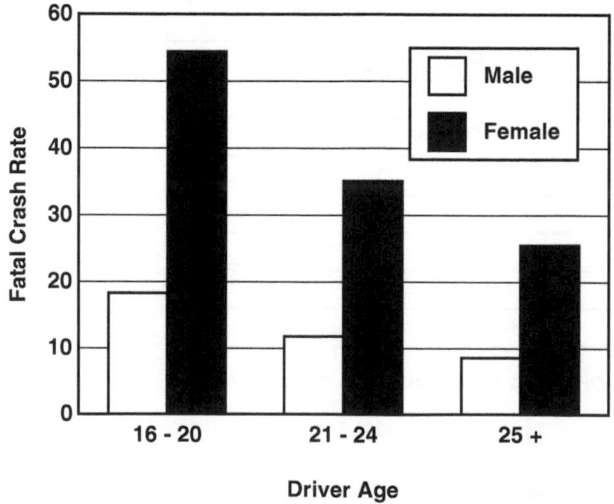

Figure 3.5 Relative risk of fatal single-vehicle crash at BAC 0.05–0.09 percent compared to zero alcohol. (Based on data reported in Zador, P.L., *J. Stud. Alcohol.*, 52, 302, 1991.)

At all ages, alcohol greatly increases the risk of being the driver in a single vehicle fatal crash. The overall relative risk declines with age, but the risk for females is about three times that for males in every age group.

These differences can no longer be attributable to relative driving inexperience on the part of women. Their annual mileage is sufficiently high that they should be proficient drivers, no longer in the learning stages where alcohol may be expected to be more impairing (Waller 1995, 1997). Avant has reported gender differences in the effect of alcohol on the ability to detect simulated traffic signs, with women more impaired than men (Avant 1990). It is true that women still consume much less alcohol than men, taking into consideration differences in weight and body composition. Whether these persistent differences in crash risk may be related to less experience in drinking remains to be determined.

Note should be taken of a marked concern worldwide about the increased presence of women in the drinking-driving population (Fell 1987; Popkin 1991; Valverius 1989). Women were becoming an increasing proportion of drinking drivers. In the U.S., in 1982 women represented 12.9% of all drivers in fatal crashes who tested positive for any alcohol, and 12.3% of such drivers with BACs of 0.10 or higher. By 1997, women were 16.6% of all drivers in fatal crashes who tested positive for any alcohol, and 15.6% of those with BACs of 0.10% or higher, indicating that women have, indeed, increased as a proportion of drinking drivers in fatal crashes.

However, closer analyses indicated that both men and women were decreasing their drunken driving, and that in the United States, based on drivers in fatal crashes, women were showing *greater* reductions than men in the proportion of those who were found to be legally intoxicated. If the proportion of crashes that are alcohol-related is considered, men have shown a decrease of 37% in their proportion of drivers in fatal crashes who have a BAC of 0.10% or higher, from 32.4% to 20.3%. During the same period, women have shown a decrease of 45.5%, from 18.9% to 10.3%.

Why, then, are women increasing as a proportion of all drinking drivers? The apparent discrepancy is attributable to the marked increase in both the amount of driving conducted by women and by their marked increase in fatal crashes. In 1982, 44,370 male drivers were in fatal crashes, compared to 10,675 women. In 1997 men had dropped to 40,658, but women had increased to 14,846. Thus, the proportion of drivers in fatal crashes who were male dropped from 80.6% to 73.3%, while women correspondingly raised their proportions from 19.4% to 26.7%. Consequently, even though women are a higher proportion of all drinking drivers in fatal crashes, they have actually decreased their proportion of drinking driving crashes at a higher rate than have men (based on data reported in Ref. (National Safety Council 1998)).

For drivers in fatal crashes both men and women, and drivers of all ages, have shown decreases in those who have been drinking. These decreases represent a decrease in absolute numbers as well as in proportions of all drivers in fatal crashes. Even though women have shown greater proportional decreases than men, their even greater increase in fatal crashes in general results in their increasing as a proportion of all drivers who test positive for alcohol.

3.5.2 Older Drivers and Drinking and Driving

A second population warranting attention is the older driver. The rapid expansion of this segment of the population has been recognized, and in the last decade there has been a burgeoning literature on the topic. However, very little has been ascertained concerning the effects of alcohol in relation to driving in this age group.

Older drivers are underrepresented in the drunken driving population. It has been reported fairly consistently that the major age group contributing to the problem is those age 21 through 24, 25 through 34, and 35 through 44. These age groups have both the largest absolute numbers of drivers in fatal crashes, and the highest proportions who test positive for alcohol. In 1997, almost half of drivers in this age group who were in fatal crashes tested positive for alcohol, compared to only 13.3% of those age 55 and higher. However, for both older and younger drivers, most of the alcohol-positive drivers are at BAC 0.10% or higher—82% to 86% for drivers age 21 through 44, and 72.8% for those age 55 and older. Older drivers are less likely to be alcohol involved, but those that do drink and drive are usually at an elevated BAC.

The concern about older drivers is based on three factors. First, there is evidence that alcohol may have greater impairing effects on the performance of older persons. Analyses of data from the Grand Rapids Study suggest that high BACs may be more detrimental to older drivers, but the numbers are sparse and not significant. However, other studies show that tasks requiring divided attention are increasingly difficult with increasing age and that alcohol has greater effects on more complex tasks. Thus, it may be anticipated that alcohol will have more detrimental effects on the performance of older drivers (Waller 1998).

Second, as discussed earlier, alcohol appears to increase crash risk more for women than for men. Women are increasing their proportion of the older driver population, through both increased licensure rates and increased mileage driven (Waller 1997). Between 1983 and 1990 women age 16 through 64 increased their mileage driven 51.5% compared to 14.5% for men in the same age group. Women age 65 and older showed almost identical increases—51.8%, compared to 30.8% for older men (Rosenbloom 1997). Interestingly, it is the older population that is showing the greatest increases in mileage driven. However, women live longer than men, and consequently they will account for a greater part of older driver mileage. To the extent that alcohol is more impairing for women, as well as more impairing for the elderly, this is an issue in need of monitoring.

Third, although drinking and driving is not a great problem among older drivers today, there may be cohort effects that would change this picture in the future. In the National Institute on Alcohol Abuse and Alcoholism's Eighth Special Report to Congress on Alcohol and Health (US National Institute on Alcohol Abuse and Alcoholism 1994) it is reported that

> … drinking patterns of middle age may be maintained into older age to a greater extent than previously appreciated and… some of the changes in drinking observed among the elderly may reflect those taking place in society as a whole rather than being an age-specific effect (p. 23).

If middle-age drinkers, and especially middle-age women who drink, persist in these patterns into old age, there may be a greater proportion of older drinking drivers in the future than is true today. Longitudinal studies indicate that drinking decreases with increasing age, but those who continue to drink often drive at high BACs. In 1997, for fatally injured drivers who were alcohol positive, of those age 55 through 64, 76.6% had BACs of 0.10% or higher. For those age 65 through 74 and those age 75 and higher, the proportions were 74.8% and 57.6%, respectively (National Safety Council 1998). At all ages, those drivers who are alcohol positive and fatally injured usually have BACs above the legal limits.

3.6 Alcohol and Pedestrian Casualties

Any discussion of alcohol and traffic safety should at least note the role of alcohol in pedestrian casualties. Pedestrians continue to represent a significant proportion of traffic fatalities—12.6% in 1998, although this proportion is decreasing. A small but carefully executed early study in Manhattan compared 50 consecutive cases of fatally injured adult pedestrians with 200 pedestrians comprising a comparison group systematically recruited at the same sites and at the same times of day and days of week. Of the fatally injured pedestrians, 74% had been drinking, compared with 33% of the comparison pedestrians. Furthermore, the fatally injured pedestrians were characterized by higher BACs than the comparison group (Haddon et al. 1961). Pedestrian fatalities generally fall into three categories—namely, the young (children), the elderly, and the intoxicated. The latter are usually neither young nor old. Fatally injured pedestrians have also shown a decrease in the proportion testing positive for alcohol. In 1982, 46.9% of fatally injured pedestrians age 14 and older had been drinking. By 1997 this proportion had dropped to 37.9%, a decrease of 19.2%. However, these proportions are still high, and considerably higher than those for drivers, indicating that simply addressing drunken driving is not an adequate approach to reducing alcohol-related traffic casualties.

3.7 Trends Over Time

3.7.1 Citizen Action Groups

Since the early 1980s, drinking driving has decreased markedly. In this author's opinion, the major catalyst for this change has been the citizen action groups. Remove Intoxicated Drivers (RID), begun in 1978, and Mothers Against Drunk Driving (MADD) begun in 1980, have served to mobilize the forces that were already working to combat the problem. As indicated earlier, the evidence was well established of the elevated risk of crash and serious or fatal injury associated with drinking and driving. What was lacking was widespread public awareness and motivation to change things. The citizen action groups filled that gap and provided the support and pressure to enact stricter laws and to see that they were enforced.

Although, from the outset, RID was taking a broader perspective, initially much of the focus was on penalties for the apprehended offender. Perhaps the broader approach was not feasible at the outset. RID's efforts were thwarted because their stand against blatant alcohol advertising to youth led to the media's refusal to publicize their efforts. In any event, MADD, as well as RID, spoke with a legitimacy that could not be denied by legislators and others. Mobilizing the victims and their families to carry the message and publicizing their efforts, these groups brought about changes that had been dismissed by many of the traffic safety professionals as impossible to achieve in the United States.

3.7.2 Declines in Drunken Driving

The FARS data are valid for alcohol only since 1982, but since that year there has been a steady decline for both men and women in the proportion of fatal crashes involving alcohol. Although total number of such crashes has not always declined, the proportion of fatal crashes involving alcohol has been markedly reduced. Declines in such crashes have been seen for every age group and for both sexes (Figures 3.3 and 3.4). Given the magnitude of the drinking driving problem and the extent to which it was ingrained in the society, these changes are nothing short of miraculous. They are a testimony to what can be accomplished when public interest is aligned with scientific evidence and sound evaluation to address a significant social problem. It should be added that national leadership was also a critical component of the degree of success.

3.7.3 Persistent Problem Populations

This is not to dismiss the magnitude of the task that remains. Drunken driving remains a major public health problem. Drivers age 21 through 34 remain a very significant problem. Furthermore, at all ages those who are drinking and driving tend to be at high BACs. Based on 1998 FARS data available on the Internet, over three-fourths of alcohol-positive drivers in fatal crashes for whom alcohol test results are available were at or above 0.10% BAC. And of those measuring that high, almost half are at 0.20% BAC or higher (49.3% males and 48.2% females in 1998 (US National Highway Traffic Safety Administration 1999). This persistence of high BACs among those who are in alcohol-related fatal crashes argues for a broad-based comprehensive approach to the problem of drunken driving.

3.8 Comprehensive Countermeasures

Traditionally the response to drunken driving has been to focus on the offender. Initially efforts were devoted primarily to enforcement, adjudication, and punishment. Ross has repeatedly stressed the need for swiftness and certainty of punishment, in addition to sufficient severity to have meaning (Ross 1982). These measures are essential for any effective program. However, they do not come into play until after a problem has developed. Preventive measures need to be based on the recognition that drinking and driving is a characteristic of the society and not simply of individuals. Consequently, effective countermeasures must address both individual perpetrators and the larger community. This approach goes beyond traditional traffic safety programs and includes pricing and availability, advertising and marketing, education, judicial and administrative proceedings, alternative transportation programs, and improved traffic records systems.

This approach is consistent with a model developed by Skinner (1990) describing the spectrum of drinkers, whereby a large proportion of the population drinks (but not heavily) and experiences no alcohol-related problems. (Since the majority of the adult population drives, it is assumed that most of those who drink also drive.) A somewhat smaller segment of the population drinks more and may experience mild to moderate alcohol-related problems. A still smaller segment drinks substantially and experiences more severe alcohol-related problems. However, the argument is made that modifying the early part of this continuum will have an impact on the size of the group that eventually experiences serious problems. Conversely, simply dealing with the most severe problems will not be very effective. While it is important to recognize and treat the smaller group of offenders, to change the ongoing magnitude of the problem requires broader measures applied earlier and to the larger population.

It appears that this is what is happening with drunken driving. As countermeasures were extended to address not just the severe offender but also the broader spectrum of drinkers, as well as potential drinkers, the entire population shifted. The Surgeon General's Workshop on Drunk Driving, conducted in 1988, took a broad-based approach to the problem, and, incidentally, was actually taken to court for going beyond the traditional programs in public education, enforcement, and punishment (US Department of Health and Human Services 1989). Nevertheless, the broader view of the problem has persisted, with changes occurring that are probably essential for reductions in drunken driving but which also reduce other alcohol-related social problems. Abstention rates have increased as per capita consumption of alcohol has decreased, with a corresponding decrease in the proportion of fatally injured drivers with any detectable alcohol, from 38.9% in 1982 to 23.7% in 1997. For males the decrease has been from 41.8% to 26.6%, and for females from 25.7% to 14.5%. At the same time, the proportion of alcohol-positive drivers who are at or above 0.10% BAC remains relatively unchanged, at around 75%.

3.9 Conclusion

While drunken driving remains a major societal problem, incredible progress has been made over the past 35 years, and particularly in the last two decades. The Grand Rapids Study was a critical factor in clearly defining the role of the drinking driver in traffic crashes and ensuing injury, as well as clearly demonstrating the feasibility of obtaining an objective chemistry-based measure of blood alcohol concentration. The citizen action groups provided a catalyst for unleashing the body of knowledge accumulated on this problem, but without the pivotal work of Robert Borkenstein and his colleagues, and the research that proceeded from it, it is doubtful that the subsequent advocacy efforts could have accomplished what they did. Innumerable studies have been conducted since 1964 to refine our understanding of the role of alcohol in crashes and injury, but the Grand Rapids Study remains the major foundation on which subsequent programs have been developed and implemented.

References

Avant LL. Alcohol impairs visual presence/absence detection more for females than for males. *Percept Psychophys* 48:285, 1990.

Borkenstein RF, Crowther RF, Shumate RP, Ziel WB, Zylman R. The role of the drinking driver in traffic accidents (The Grand Rapids Study). *Blutalkohol* 11 (Suppl 1): 1–131, 1974 (First published 1964).

Borkenstein RF, Trubitt JH, Lease RJ. Problems of enforcement prosecution. In Fox BH, Fox JH (Eds.): *Alcohol and Traffic Safety* (Public Health Service Publication No. 1043). US National Institutes of Health: Bethesda, MD, pp. 137–189, 1963.

Carlson WL. Alcohol usage of the nighttime driver. *J Safe Res* 4:12, 1972.

Carpenter JA. Effects of alcohol on psychological processes. In Fox BH, Fox JH (Eds.): *Alcohol and Traffic Safety* (Public Health Service Publication No. 1043). US National Institutes of Health: Bethesda, MD, pp. 45–90, 1963.

Fell JC. Alcohol involvement rates in fatal crashes: A focus on young drivers and female drivers. *Proceedings—31st Proceedings of the American Association for Automotive Medicine.* American Association for Automotive Medicine: Des Plaines, IL, pp. 1–30, 1987.

Fox JH. Drinking-driving—A public health concern. In Fox BH, Fox JH (Eds.): *Alcohol and Traffic Safety* (Public Health Service Publication No. 1043). US National Institutes of Health: Bethesda, MD, pp. 245–258, 1963.

Haddon W, Valien P, McCarroll JR, Umberger CJ. Controlled investigation of the characteristics of adult pedestrians fatally injured by motor vehicles in Manhattan. *J Chronic Dis* 14:655, 1961.

Holcomb RL. Alcohol in relation to traffic accidents. *JAMA* 111:1076, 1938.

Hurst PM, Harte D, Frith WJ. The Grand Rapids dip revisited. *Accid Anal Prev* 26:647, 1994.
Hurst PM. Epidemiological aspects of alcohol in driver crashes and citation. *J Safe Res* 5:130, 1973.
National Safety Council. *Accident Facts*™, ed.: National Safety Council: Itasca, IL, 1998.
Perrine MW, Waller JA, Harris LS. *Alcohol and Highway Safety: Behavioral and Medical Aspects.* US National Highway Traffic Safety Administration: Washington, DC, 1971.
Pisarski AE. *Travel Behavior Issues in the 90s.* Federal Highway Administration: Washington, DC, 1992.
Popkin CL. Drinking and driving by young females. *Accid Anal Prev* 12:37, 1991.
Old Testament. Proverbs 23:29–35.
Rosenbloom S. Trends in women's travel patterns, 1980/1983–1990. In Rosenbloom S (Ed.): *Women's Travel Issues.* US Federal Highway Administration: Washington, DC, pp. 7–26, 1997.
Ross HL. *Confronting Drunk Driving.* Yale University Press: New Haven, CT, 1992.
Ross HL. *Deterring the Drinking Driver: Legal Policy and Social Control.* Lexington Books: Lexington, MA, 1982.
Skinner HA. Executive summary: Spectrum of drinkers and intervention responses. Prepared for the IOM Committee for the Study of Treatment and Rehabilitation Services for Alcoholism and Alcohol Abuse, 1998. Cited in Institute of Medicine: *Broadening the Base of Treatment for Alcohol Problems.* National Academy Press: Washington, DC, p. 212, 1990.
US Department of Health and Human Services. *Surgeon General's Workshop on Drunk Driving* (Background Papers). US Department of Health and Human Services: Rockville, MD, 1989.
US Department of Health and Human Services. *Surgeon General's Workshop on Drunk Driving* (Proceedings). US Department of Health and Human Services: Rockville, MD, 1989.
US Department of Transportation. Alcohol and highway safety. Report to the U.S. Congress. US Government Printing Office: Washington, DC, Quoted in Jones RD, Joscelyn KD. *Alcohol and Highway Safety, 1978: Review of the State of Knowledge* (DOT HS 803-714). US National Highway Traffic Safety Administration: Washington, DC, pp. 1–2, 1968.
US National Highway Traffic Safety Administration. *Traffic Safety Facts 1997.* US National Highway Traffic Safety Administration: Washington, DC, 1998.
US National Highway Traffic Safety Administration. *Traffic Safety Facts 1998.* US National Highway Traffic Safety Administration: Washington, DC, 1999.
US National Institute on Alcohol Abuse and Alcoholism. Eighth special report to the U.S. Congress on alcohol and health (NIH Publication No. 94-3699). National Institutes of Health: Bethesda, MD, 1994.
US National Institute on Alcohol Abuse and Alcoholism. Ninth special report to the U.S. Congress on alcohol and health (NIH Publication No. 97-4017). National Institutes of Health: Bethesda, MD, 1997.
Valverius MR (Ed). Women, Alcohol, Drugs And Traffic, *Proceedings of the ICADTS International Workshop.* Almquist and Wiksell: Stockholm, Sweden, 1989.
Voas RB, Lacey JH. Issues in the enforcement of impaired driving laws in the United States. In U.S. Department of Health and Human Services: *Surgeon General's Workshop on Drunk Driving* (Working Papers). U.S. Department of Health and Human Services: Rockville, MD, pp. 136–156, 1989.
Waller JA. *Injury Control: A Guide to the Causes and Prevention of Trauma.* Lexington Books: Lexington, MA, p. 511, 1985.
Waller PF, Blow FC. Women, alcohol, and driving. In Galanter M (Ed.): *Recent Developments in Alcoholism*, Vol 12—*Women and Alcoholism.* Plenum Press: New York, pp. 103–123, 1995.
Waller PF. Alcohol, aging, and driving. In Gomberg ESL, Hegedus AM, Zucker RA (Eds.): *Alcohol Problems and Aging*, Research Monograph No. 33. National Institute on Alcohol Abuse and Alcoholism: Bethesda, MD, pp. 301–320, 1998.
Waller PF. Women, alcohol, and traffic safety. In Rosenbloom S (Ed.): *Women's Travel Issues*, FHWA-PL-97-024. US Department of Transportation: Washington, DC, pp. 479–499, 1997.

Williams GD, Stinson FS, Stewart SL, Dufour MC. *Apparent Per Capita Alcohol Consumption: National, State, and Regional Trends, 1977–1992*, Surveillance Report No. 35. National Institute on Alcohol Abuse and Alcoholism, Division of Biometry and Epidemiology: Rockville, MD. 1995. Quoted in Ninth Special Report to the US Congress on Alcohol and Health, p. 3, 1997.

Zador PL. Alcohol-related risk of fatal driver injuries in relation to driver age and sex. *J Stud Alcohol* 52:302, 1991.

The Analysis of Ethanol in Blood and Breath for Legal Purposes

4

A Historical Review*

A. WAYNE JONES

Contents

4.1 Introduction

4.1.1 Early Development

The first scientific investigations into the fate of alcohol in the human body can be traced back to the nineteenth century as reported in a substantive paper from 1874 (Anstie 1874). At that time the medical profession was divided on the question of what happened to alcohol in the body; was it a food, a drug, or a poison? An influential scientific paper from

* This chapter is an updated version of a review article previously published in *Forensic Science Review*: Jones AW: Methods for the analysis of ethanol in blood and breath for legal purposes—A historical review; *Forensic Sci Rev* 8:13; 1996.

France, which was cited and discussed in a book entitled, *Stimulants and Narcotics* (Anstie 1864), reached the following erroneous conclusion:

> The entire expulsion of all the alcohol taken into the body, in an unchanged form and within a short time, is certain, and that except indirectly (by modifying digestion) that substance has no alimentary properties.
> Alcohol is not, in any sense, a food and is neither transformed nor destroyed within the organism, but re-appears within a comparatively short time in the excretions being by them eliminated.

A British physician Dr. Francis Anstie (1833–1874) was one of the first to investigate what was happening to alcohol in the body, because he was concerned about the dangers of heavy drinking and drunkenness on public health during Victorian times (Baldwin 1977). Dr. Anstie used a chemical reagent consisting of 1 g $K_2Cr_2O_7$ and 300 mL of concentrated sulfuric acid—later known as Anstie's reagent—for the analysis of ethanol in body fluids. Although this analytical method was primitive by modern standards, it was sufficiently reliable to resolve the question of whether ethanol was metabolized in the body or excreted unchanged. Anstie found that the bulk of the dose of ethanol ingested was utilized in the body and "burnt-up" in the same way as ordinary foodstuffs and only a small fraction was excreted unchanged in breath, sweat, and urine (Anstie 1874). Ethanol is a source of energy for the body and during its metabolism 7.1 kcal per g are produced (Atwater and Benedict 1902).

Other early contributions to knowledge about alcohol and its actions in the organism came from France by Gréhant (1848–1910) and Nicloux (1873–1945) (Gréhant 1903; Nicloux 1896). Of special interest was a thesis from the University of Paris entitled *"Recherches expérimentales sur l'élimination de l'alcool dans l'organisme"* (Nicloux 1900). Professor Nicloux modified the Anstie method of alcohol analysis and went on to publish scores of articles about the distribution of ethanol in the body of living and deceased persons (Nicloux 1906).

Sir Edward Mellanby (1884–1955) a physician and pharmacologist from England investigated the disposition and fate of ethanol in human and animal experiments (Hawgood 2010). When ethanol was administration to dogs by stomach tube, ethanol was rapidly absorbed from the gut and peak blood-alcohol concentration (BAC) was reached between 10–60 minutes post-dosing. The results of Mellanby's research on alcohol were published in a monograph entitled, *Alcohol, Its Absorption into and Disappearance from the Blood under Different Conditions* (Mellanby 1919).

This monograph contained the first hint that ethanol was eliminated from the bloodstream at a constant rate independent of concentration in accordance with zero-order kinetics, which was confirmed in many later experimental studies (Wagner 1981). Mellanby also noticed that the impairment effects of ethanol were more pronounced on the rising limb of the BAC curve compared with the same BAC on the descending limb after absorption and distribution were completed (Mellanby 1920). This phenomenon was later referred to as the "Mellanby effect" and it reflected the development of acute tolerance to ethanol during a single exposure to the drug (Kalant 1998). The central nervous system seemingly adapts to the effects of ethanol and both behavioral and subjective feelings of intoxication disappear much faster than BAC decreases through metabolism and excretion (Holland and Ferner 2017).

The Mellanby effect, at least in part, was explained by the different concentrations of ethanol in the arterial (A) than venous (V) blood circulation. During the absorption phase A-BAC is higher than V-BAC by up to 0.03 g% after subjects drank a bolus dose. After equilibration in all body fluids is complete, which takes between 60 and 90 minutes after end of drinking the A-BAC and V-BAC are the same (Forney et al. 1964). In Mellanby's experiments ethanol was determined in venous blood samples, whereas ethanol is transported to the brain in arterial blood, which contains a higher concentration than the V-BAC measured.

A new study of A-V differences in ethanol concentrations with sampling times of blood extended for up to 6–7 hours post-dosing showed that A-BAC rose more rapidly and reached a higher concentration than V-BAC (Jones et al. 2004). A "crossover point" was reached by 60–90 minutes and thereafter A-BAC was always lower than V-BAC at all later times. These time-trends in A-V differences in BAC were confirmed when ethanol was taken orally or given by intravenous administration (Jones et al. 1997).

In the post-absorptive phase ethanol in the central blood compartment decreases through metabolism in the liver at a rate of ~0.015 g% per h and peripheral tissues compartments return ethanol with the venous blood. During the entire post-absorptive phase, provided no further drinking occurs, V-BAC is higher than A-BAC by about 0.005–0.008 g%.

Based on his experimental alcohol studies, Mellanby reached the following conclusion about the relationship between BAC and intoxication, which is highly relevant to consider because a person's BAC can be determined a lot more accurately than diminished performance.

> Now, although there is an unquestionable relationship between alcohol in the body and intoxication, it is not certain that the relation between the two is close enough to allow the latter to be strictly determined from the former. This fact would not be of much importance if there were as accurate a measure of intoxication as there is of alcohol in the blood, but this is not the case.

During the first half of the twentieth century, the undisputed leader in the field of forensic alcohol research was Erik Widmark (1889–1945), a professor of physiological chemistry at the University of Lund in Sweden; his research accomplishments spanned the first half of the twentieth century and his life and work have been reviewed elsewhere (Andreasson and Jones 1995; Jones 2017).

Already in 1914 Widmark suggested that the determination of ethanol in a person's urine would provide a useful clinical test to verify the signs and symptoms of drunkenness (Widmark 1914). In 1922 he presented a quantitative method for determination of ethanol in micro-volumes (~100 μL) of fingertip blood (Widmark 1922). This method of analysis was used to establish concentration-time profiles of ethanol in blood in men and women after they drank ethanol on an empty stomach or together with a meal (Widmark 1932). From this research the basic principles of ethanol pharmacokinetics were established including the Widmark parameters "β" (elimination rate from blood) and "rho" (volume of distribution), which are still widely used today in forensic casework (Jones 2017).

By the 1940s the state of knowledge about the actions of alcohol in the organism, including medicolegal aspects appeared in a book by Dr. Henry Newman (1907–1959), entitled *Acute Alcoholic Intoxication* (Newman 1941). Newman was professor of neurology at Stanford University, California and made many important contributions to research on alcohol before his untimely death at the age of 52 years. One chapter in Newman's book dealt with "the chemical diagnosis of drunkenness" and he gave a good account of the methods then available for quantitative analysis of ethanol in body fluids and how results should be interpreted. He also considered the development of tolerance to alcohol and underscored the difficulty in establishing a threshold BAC as a way to diagnose intoxication and as proof that a person was under the influence of alcohol from a legal point of view (Newman 1940).

Figure 4.1 shows twelve scientists who made important contributions to our knowledge about the analysis and interpretation of ethanol concentrations in blood and breath for clinical and forensic purposes; their year of birth and death and country of origin are included.

Francis E. Anstie
(1833-1874), UK
Arthur R. Cushny
(1866-1926), Scotland
Maurice Nicloux
(1873-1945), France
Edward Mellanby
(1884-1955), UK
Göran Liljestrand
(1886-1968), Sweden
Erik MP Widmark
(1889-1945), Sweden
Rolla N.Harger
(1890-1983), USA
Robert F.Borkenstein
(1912-2002),USA
Roger K. Bonnichsen
(1913-1986), Sweden
H. Ward Smith
(1914-1967), Canada
Kurt M. Dubowski
(1921-2017), USA
Gottfried Machata
(1925-2012), Austria

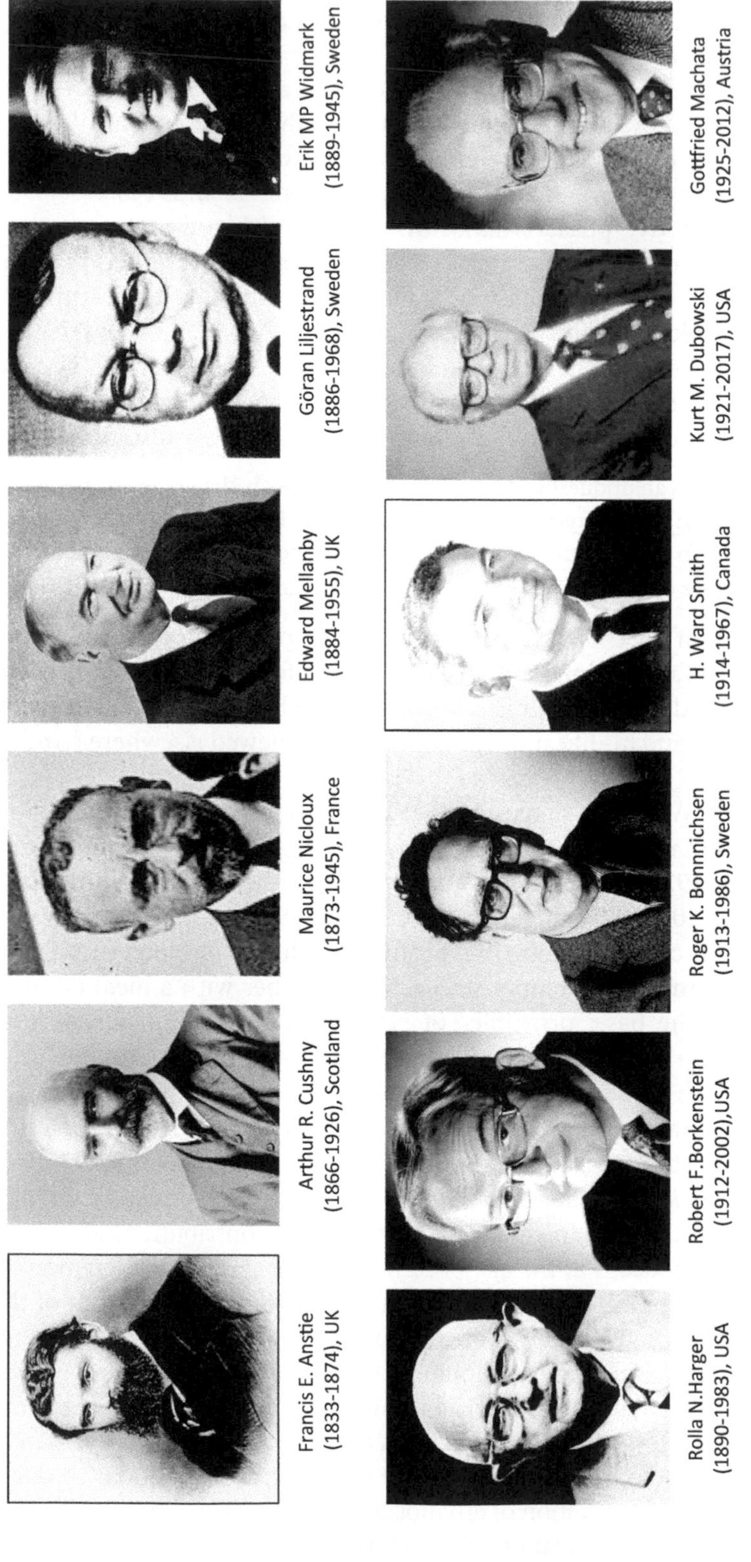

Figure 4.1 Twelve scientists who made significant contributions to the early development of analytical methods for determination of ethanol in blood and/or breath samples for legal purposes. Their year of birth and death are indicated along with the country where they worked.

4.1.2 Present Status

The analysis of alcohol in biological specimens, including breath, is one of the oldest and most well-established tests in forensic science and legal medicine (Wigmore and Langille 2009). Literally hundreds of publications describe a plethora of analytical approaches, techniques and procedures for quantitative analysis of ethanol in blood, breath and other biological specimens (Dubowski 1986; Friedemann and Dubowski 1959). Over the past 150 years, five basic analytical principles have been utilized for determination of ethanol; wet-chemistry oxidation, enzymatic oxidation, electrochemical oxidation, gas-liquid chromatography (GLC), and infrared (IR) spectrometry.

For the analysis of liquid samples, headspace (HS) GLC has become the gold standard procedure used in forensic laboratories worldwide for biological specimens from living and deceased persons (Machata 1975; O'Neal et al. 1996). Preparation of the specimen in readiness for analysis by headspace gas-liquid chromatography (HS-GLC) is simple and requires just three basic procedures:

1. Gently invert the evacuated tube containing the blood sample about 8–10 times to ensure that the red cells and plasma are mixed together.
2. Remove an aliquot (~100 µL) of blood specimen and dilute this with an aqueous solution of internal standard, such as *n*-propanol, in a fixed proportion, usually 1:10 to give an 11 times dilution. Eject the diluted blood into a small glass vial and make this airtight with a Teflon coated rubber stopper and crimped on aluminum cap.
3. Heat the glass vial with diluted blood to 50°C or 60°C until an equilibrium is reached before removing an aliquot of the vapor phase in equilibrium with the blood sample and injecting it into a gas chromatograph (GC) instrument fitted with flame ionization detector (FID). The sample of the air-phase can be removed with a gas-tight syringe or preferably by some automated GC sampling system, and several such instruments are available.

The HS-GLC method provides both a qualitative analysis based on retention times (RT), which is the time it takes for the volatile components to appear as a peak on the chromatogram. Quantitative analysis depends on intensity of the response (peak height or area) measured with a flame ionization detector (FID). The analytical results using HS-GLC are accurate and precise with a short analysis time, which permits ~100 blood specimens to be processed in a single analytical sequence (Dubowski 1977b).

The original packed GC columns used for separating volatile constituents in the blood are now replaced by capillary or wide-bore columns and these are produced commercially and made available by several manufactures, such as (www.restek.com), who offer columns dedicated to blood-alcohol analysis. Nevertheless, the traditional packed columns, such as polyethylene glycol on graphitized carbon black absorbent material denoted Carbopack B and C are still perfectly adequate for routine purposes and permit baseline separation of the ethanol peak from potential interfering substances.

Use of a mass spectrometric detector furnishes a higher analytical selectivity by identifying prominent mass fragments of ethanol in addition to RT of the components (Bonnichsen and Ryhage 1971). The electron impact mass spectrum of ethanol shows three prominent ions at m/z 31 (base peak), m/z 45 and m/s 46 (molecular ion). The continued use of HS-GLC with split sampling options and two different chromatographic systems is perfectly adequate for forensic purposes. Nevertheless, results of ethanol analysis by

HS-GLC are sometimes challenged when only RT is used to identify the substances emerging from the GC column. This has prompted some laboratories to introduce HS-GLC-MS methods for routine analysis of blood samples in drink-driving cases (Tiscione et al. 2011).

Methods based on enzymatic oxidation of ethanol with alcohol dehydrogenase (ADH) appeared in the 1950s and these were milder conditions were more selective for ethanol analysis than chemical oxidation procedures (Bonnichsen and Theorell 1951; Bücher and Redetzki 1951). Moreover, enzymatic methods could be automated, such as using a Technicon Auto-Analyzer, which was becoming increasingly necessary with the large increase in number people arrested for drunken driving during 1950s–1960s (Buijten 1975). Other enzymatic ADH procedures involved linking to secondary reactions of reduced co-enzyme nicotinamide adenine dinucleotide (NADH) producing a formazan dye, with an intense fluorescence and a highly sensitive analytical method (Caplan and Levine 1987; Cary et al. 1984).

The widely used enzyme multiplied immunoassay technique (EMIT) or fluorescence polarization immunoassay are easily adaptable to allow determination of ethanol in blood, urine, or plasma/serum specimens without any special pretreatment necessary (Kristoffersen and Smith-Kielland 2005). These robot-like batch analyzers are well proven in urine drug testing laboratories where a high throughput of samples takes place from drug-abuse treatment clinics or prison inmates, who are not permitted to drink alcohol or take psychoactive drugs.

The police authorities in most countries make use of roadside breath-testing with handheld electronic instruments as evidence of driver sobriety (Polissar et al. 2015). The large scale testing of motorists has been streamlined by use of so-called passive alcohol sensors (PAS) that don't require a disposable plastic mouthpiece and permit contact-free testing (Fell and Compton 2007). The device is held close to a person's mouth while they answer questions and a portion of the exhaled breath is aspirated into the instrument for analysis. A positive result is sufficient to give probable cause of alcohol influence and motivate further testing with more reliable methodology. The results from contact-free breath sampling are lower than the concentration in end-exhaled breath, but sufficient to evaluate driver sobriety in a non-invasive way (Foss et al. 1993).

Police in the state of Indiana were the first to use breath-alcohol instruments for evidential purposes in the form of the Drunkometer in 1938 (Harger et al. 1938). However, this instrument became more or less obsolete when the Breathalyzer was developed by Dr. Robert Borkenstein of Indiana University in 1954 (Borkenstein and Smith 1961). The Breathalyzer was easier to use by trained police officers and gave more reliable results and was approved throughout the United States, Australia, and Canada for legal purposes.

In the 1970s new and improved technology appeared for determination of ethanol in breath, as exemplified by infrared spectrometry (Harte 1971) and electrochemical oxidation (Jones et al. 1974). The research of Anstie (1867) and Bogen (1927) warned about conducting a breath-alcohol test within 15 minutes of the last drink, owing to risk for contamination from alcohol in the mucous surfaces of the oral cavity or regurgitation of stomach contents, which might cause false high readings (Gullberg 1992). Modern infrared breath-alcohol instruments are fitted with "slope detectors," which are intended to monitor the shape of the exhalation profile of ethanol (Lindberg et al. 2015). This allows detecting any unusual irregularity in the breath alcohol concentration (BrAC) during exhalation such as a waviness in the profile or a sudden change in slope might also indicate presence of alcohol in the mouth from recent drinking (Wigmore and Leslie 2001).

Prior to conducting an evidential breath-alcohol test a suspect should be observed for 15 minutes and not allowed to eat, drink or put anything in the mouth during this time.

The ability of slope detectors to identify presence of mouth alcohol is sometimes challenged, so a 15 min observation period also needs to be documented (Labianca 2018). In actual casework a much longer time than 15 min elapses from time of arrest, transport of the suspect to a police station, questioning and identification before an evidential breath test is administered. Yet another safeguard is to conduct two separate breath tests with every suspect 5–15 minutes apart and compare and contrast the two BrAC readings (Dubowski 1994).

Ethanol is the major organic constituent of exhaled breath after drinking alcoholic beverages, although it is sometimes alleged that other volatile substances were also present, such as acetone, which is produced naturally in the body. This has led to various ways of improving the analytical specificity in detecting ethanol, such as by use of two independent analytical principles or absorption of the IR radiation at multiple wavelengths (Caldwell and Kim 1997). Ethanol shows strong absorbance of IR radiation at wavelengths of 9.5 μM (C-O bond stretch) and 3.4 μM (C-H bond stretch) and inclusion of both enhances the confidence in detection of ethanol.

The Evidenzer, which is one of the latest generation of breath analyzers incorporates five IR filters at wavelengths in the range 3.3–3.5 μm and this instrument is currently used for legal purposes by police in Norway, Finland, Sweden and Ireland. After calibrating the instrument with ethanol vapors in the IR sampling chamber, all five filters are made to give the same response. Accordingly during testing of a suspect if one or more of the filters shows an aberrant IR absorption pattern this flags for the presence of an interfering substance. This might be attributed to acetone, isopropanol, diethyl ether, toluene, and/or butane according to tests done in apprehended drivers and verified by analysis of volatiles in blood (Jones and Andersson 2008).

Another way to enhance selectivity of breath-alcohol analysis is to use two independent analytical principles, such as IR absorption at 9.5 μM (C-O stretch) and electrochemical oxidation (Hartung et al. 2016). The first instrument to incorporate EC and IR methods was manufactured by Dräeger Inc., (Lübeck, Germany), christened Alcotest model 7110. This instrument was developed further resulting in models 7410 and the current version is Alcotest 9510.

In summary, after 1970 technological advances included analytical techniques such gas-liquid chromatography, IR spectrometry and electrochemical oxidation (Dubowski 1975). The instruments permitted automatic breath sampling, they could monitor the volume of breath exhaled, as well as the temperature at end exhalation. By monitoring the shape of the ethanol exhalation profile it was possible to detect if "mouth alcohol" was contaminating the breath specimen. Use of multiple IR wavelengths ensures high specificity of ethanol detection by flagging for presence of interfering substances (e.g., acetone). Quality assurance is enhanced if a calibration control check is done at the statutory BrAC limit (e.g., 0.08 g/210 L), and air from the room where the subject was tested is analyzed as a blank check along with a printed record of the test results for later use in court (Dubowski 1994).

4.2 Statutory Limits of Alcohol Concentration

4.2.1 Developments in Europe

Laws prohibiting the operation of a motor vehicle while under the influence of alcohol evolved fairly slowly compared with the expansion of motor transportation during the first decades of the twentieth century. As early as 1904 reports appeared showing that drivers of "motor wagons" were involved in fatal crashes after drinking spirits before driving (Crothers 1904). After prohibition was abolished in the United States, federal government became concerned about the threat to traffic safety owing to an increased prevalence of drunken driving. The authorities were anxious to develop better ways of testing for alcohol influence, such as by chemical analysis of ethanol in samples of blood, breath or urine (Borkenstein 1985).

In 1934 the Swedish government approved taking blood samples from suspects and BAC was introduced in evidence along with the results of a medical examination and clinical signs and symptoms of drunkenness. The BAC was considered more objective evidence of being under the influence of alcohol compared with subjective testimony from a police officer or a physician, which eventually culminated in a concentration *per se* law in 1941, set at a BAC of 0.08 g% (Andenaes 1988). Norway had already adopted a punishable BAC limit of 0.05 g% in 1936. The statutory alcohol limit for driving in Sweden was subsequently lowered to 0.05 g% in 1957 and then to 0.02 g% in 1990, where it stands today. There is also a more serious offence, referred to as aggravated drunken driver, if the BAC exceeds 0.10 g% with mandatory penalties including revocation of the driving permit for 24 months and short terms of imprisonment for up to 6 months.

Alcohol concentration *per se* laws simplified the evidence necessary to prosecute traffic offenders, because this legal framework meant it is not necessary to prove a driver was impaired by alcohol at the time of the offence. The lynchpin of the prosecution case was the accurate and precise determination of BAC or BrAC and whether this exceeds the statutory *per se* limits (Jones 1988).

It sometimes happened that the medical report about impairment of the suspect stood in conflict with the BAC, which caused problems for the courts and sometimes led to an acquittal. A government report in 1980 concluded that the determination of BAC was more objective evidence for over-consumption of alcohol and could also exonerate a suspect, who might be considered impaired for other reasons, such as a medical condition mimicking drunkenness. The compulsory examination of every suspect by a physician was therefore abandoned in 1981 and a registered nurse or phlebotomist was called to draw blood in drink-driving cases or an evidential breath-alcohol test was made.

After the Second World War motor transportation increased dramatically worldwide as did the prevalence of drunken driving and alcohol-related traffic crashes creating a major problem for public health and longevity (Hingson and Winter 2003). This prompted the British Medical Association (BMA) to appoint a committee of experts chaired by Sir Edward J. Wayne (1902–1990) to review the problem of drunken driving and to suggest ways to improve traffic safety by making prosecution more effective. The BMA committee produced several influential reports, such as "The Drinking Driver" (British Medical Association 1965) and another entitled "Relation of alcohol to road accidents" (British Medical Association 1960). The findings were important considerations when the British Road Traffic Act of 1967 was introduced, which represented a paradigm shift, by creating a statutory alcohol concentration *per se* limit of 80 mg% (0.08 g%) in blood. This made it a criminal offence to drive with a BAC of 0.08 g% or more regardless of whether the driver was impaired.

> To drive or attempt to drive a motor vehicle on a road or other public place having consumed alcohol in such a quantity that the proportion thereof in his blood or urine as ascertained from a laboratory test for which he subsequently provides a specimen exceeds the prescribed limit at the time he provides a specimen.

A prescribed alcohol limit was also set for urine samples at a concentration of 107 mg% (0.107 g%), which was an option for people who were not willing to provide blood for whatever reason, such as needle phobia (Rik 1996). Also in 1967, the UK police were allowed to test drivers at the roadside with a hand-held breath-alcohol screening device—Alcotest R80 tubes (Day et al. 1968).

Figure 4.2 shows a person blowing into an Alcotest tube and bag device and the chemical tubes after reaction with increasing amounts of alcohol in the breath. If the chemicals in the Alcotest tube changed color from yellow to green up to a graduation mark this indicated the driver's BAC was above the legal 0.08 g% limit. False positive and false negative rates were fairly high and the color change was difficult to observe in bad lighting conditions, but was an improvement over simply smelling alcohol on the driver's breath (Prouty and O'Neill 1971). Nevertheless, a positive roadside breath test was sufficient cause to arrest a driver for examination by a physician and sampling of blood or urine for laboratory analysis.

Prior to the 1967 Road-Traffic Act it was not mandatory for a driver to provide a sample of blood or urine for laboratory analysis. However, refusal to do so could be used in evidence when a driver was prosecuted for this traffic offence. The results of clinical tests of alcohol impairment constituted the main evidence put before the court in drink-driving cases in the UK at that time.

Setting the statutory BAC limit at 80 mg/100 mL (0.08 g%) was motivated by an epidemiological study of the risk of involvement in a crash in relation to the driver's BAC, which was done in Grand Rapids, Michigan 1963–1964 (Borkenstein et al. 1974). This was a case-controlled study comparing BAC of drivers involved in crashes with a matched control group of drivers on the same roads but not involved in crashes. Samples of breath were collected in self-sealing plastic bags and transported to a facility were a Breathalyzer 900 instruments was available. The test and control groups of drivers were matched for location and vicinity of the crash, age and gender, weekday, time of day and ethnicity. The results

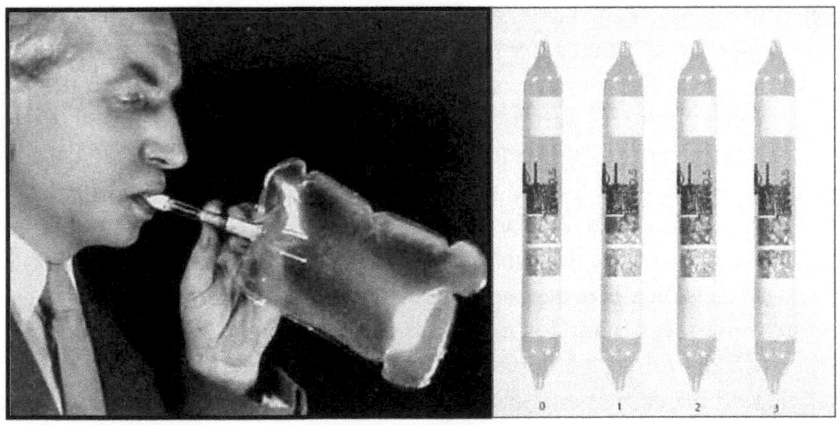

Figure 4.2 The chemical tube and bag device, developed in the mid-1950s in Germany was the first roadside breath-alcohol screening test. The left panel shows a breath sample being collected, and the right panel shows chemical tubes that contained potassium dichromate and sulfuric acid on silica gel. Shown to the right are detector tubes when no alcohol was detected in the breath and after reaction with increasing concentrations of ethanol. If the change in color from yellow to green extended up to a graduation mark in the middle of the tube this was a presumptive positive test.

were clearcut showing that as a driver's BAC increased above 0.04 g% the risk of involvement in a crash was definitely increased and the likelihood was appreciably higher as BACs passed 0.08 g%. Furthermore, drivers with BAC >0.08 g% were more likely to be involved in single-vehicle crashes and suffer more serious injuries.

When a driver opted to provide a urine sample instead of blood for analysis of alcohol, a necessary requirement was to collect two consecutive voids 30–60 minutes apart and the concentration in a second void was compared with the statutory UAC limit of 107 mg% (0.107 g%). Many studies verified a high correlation between UAC and BAC and the physiological principles of urine production were well established (Jones 2006). The setting of 80 mg% in blood and 107 mg% as being equivalent suggests that the urine/blood ratio of ethanol is 1.35:1 for a freshly voided specimen, although no attempt was made to calculate BAC from UAC was any individual case (Jones 2002). Sampling and analysis of urine in drink-driving cases is also an option in other countries including several US states. Indeed in some states the UAC was converted into the BAC for prosecution by assuming an average UAC/BAC ratio (Biasotti and Valentine 1985).

In the 1980s the instruments available for breath-alcohol analysis were much improved in terms of their analytical performance and ease of use by non-scientifically qualified personnel. The UK Home Office Forensic Science Service embarked on a rigorous laboratory testing of currently available breath-alcohol analyzers and determined accuracy and precision in relation to the coexisting BAC (Emerson et al. 1980). In 1983, the British government approved two evidential breath-alcohol analyzers, the Lion Intoximeter 3000 and Camic Breath Analyzer, which determined ethanol by IR absorptiometry. The Lion Intoximeter instrument was developed in the US (Intoximeters Inc.,) and was fitted with a single wavelength (3.4 μM) filter for absorption of IR radiation, which meant it was not completely specific for identification of ethanol in breath. The Lion Intoximeter was also fitted with a Taguchi semiconductor sensor, which was intended to indicate elevated concentrations of acetone in breath that might interfere with the ethanol reading.

The statutory BrAC limit for driving in UK was set at 35 μg/100 mL, which was derived from the existing 80 mg% BAC limit and dividing by a presumed mean blood/breath factor of 2300:1 (Emerson et al. 1980). Because of variations in blood/breath ratios of alcohol between subjects, a prosecution was not initiated until the BrAC was 40 μg/100 mL or more, which is 14% higher than the statutory BrAC limit of 35 μg/100 mL. Furthermore, each suspect provided two samples of breath and the lower of the two results was used for a prosecution, which gives additional benefit to the person being tested. Yet another safeguard was the option to give a sample of blood for analysis if BrAC was between 40 and 50 μg/100 mL. However, this particular option was abandoned in 2016, because it no longer served a useful purpose and was scientifically flawed because of the time it took before the blood sample was taken. No adjustment was made for metabolism of alcohol during this interval. A refusal to co-operate with providing a sample of blood, breath or urine represented a punishable offence that carried the same penalties as if the alcohol concentration had been above the legal limit for driving.

Shortly after evidential breath-alcohol testing was introduced for use by police authorities in UK (1983–1985) the results from the two approved instruments were challenged by defense lawyers and the news-media as being unreliable. In particular, the Lion Intoximeter 3000, which incorporated a single IR wavelength for determination of ethanol was considered suspect, owing to its lack of specificity. This particular instrument was also fitted with a semiconductor sensor (Taguchi or T-cell), which was intended to indicate if elevated concentrations of acetone were present in a person's breath. However, calibration of the T-cell was unstable and indicated elevated concentrations of acetone in breath far too often. This caused a lot of confusion, because the concentration of acetone in blood was insignificant and within normal limits (Jones et al. 1993).

The British government commissioned a survey of the performance of the two evidential breath-analyzers under the leadership of an independent expert Sir William Paton (1917–1993), a Fellow of the Royal Society and a distinguished pharmacologist from Oxford University (Cobb and Dabbs 1985). The conclusion from the Paton report was that results were acceptable and evidential breath testing was a reliable way to enforce drink-driving legislation. However, the T-cell (acetone detector) incorporated in the Lion Intoximeter 3000 instruments was faulty and disconnected.

The results from the Paton report established that the blood/breath ratio (BBR) of alcohol in apprehended drivers was between 2300:1 and 2400:1 and this supported adopting a 2300:1 ratio when the 35 µg/100 mL statutory BrAC limit for driving was introduced (Emerson et al. 1980). When the Paton report was published, one of the daily newspaper had a rubric "Own Goal for Drunk Drivers." Many other countries in Europe soon followed the lead set by the UK and evidential breath-alcohol testing was introduced in Austria and Holland in 1986, followed by Sweden in 1989.

4.2.2 Developments in North America

During the years of alcohol prohibition (1920–1933), the federal and state governments showed little interest in drunken driving and problems caused by alcohol-related crashes (Lerner 2011). Jurisprudence difficulties arose in defining "driving under the influence" in such a way that judges and jurors understood the seriousness of the problem. Traffic offenders were charged with drunken driving based on their own admissions of guilt, smell of alcohol on the breath and their general appearance and behavior, such as ability to walk a chalk line. Accordingly a successful prosecution was by no means certain and many offenders were acquitted if a case went to trial. An early definition of the phrase "under the influence of alcohol" in connection with driving came from the Supreme Court of Arizona in the case of Steffani v. State 42 Pac. (2nd) 615, which read as follows:

> The expression under the influence of intoxicating liquor covers not only all the well-known and easily recognized conditions, which is the result of indulging to any degree in intoxicating liquors, and which tends to deprive him of the clearness of intellect and control of himself which he would otherwise possess. If the ability of the driver of an automobile has been lessened in the slightest degree by the use of intoxicating liquors, then the driver is deemed to be under the influence of intoxicating liquor. The mere fact that the driver has taken a drink does not place him under the ban of the statute unless such drink has some influence upon him lessening in some degree his ability to handle said automobile.

An evaluation of the autopsy reports of drivers killed in motor-vehicle crashes showed a high prevalence of deceased with BAC >0.15 g% (Heise 1934). The first case-control study of BAC and crash risk was done in Evanston, Illinois and published in Journal of the American Medical Association in 1938 (Holcomb 1938). The BAC of drivers involved in crashes and in the non-crash control group was determined indirectly by analysis of breath with a Drunkometer instrument that had recently become available (Harger et al. 1938).

In the Evanston study, 47% of $n = 270$ drivers involved in crashes had consumed alcohol before driving and 14% of them had a BAC above 0.15 g%. Among 1750 control drivers, 12%

had consumed alcohol and 1.9% had a BAC above 0.15 g%. Up to a BAC of 0.05–0.06 g%, the risk of involvement in a crash was about the same as in non-drinking drivers. However, when BAC was above 0.1 g% the risk of involvement in a crash was increased 6 times, at 0.13 g% it was 10 times higher and at 0.15 g% 25 times greater risk compared with sober drivers.

Larger epidemiological surveys of the relationship between a driver's BAC and probability of involvement in a crash, such as the Grand Rapids Study, verified the higher crash risk (Borkenstein et al. 1974) as did a study from 2009 (Blomberg et al. 2009). The US states of Indiana and Maine were the first to stipulate a punishable BAC (0.15 g%) in 1939, although this was subsequently lowered to 0.10 g% and later to 0.08 g% in all 50 US states until Utah lowered its limit to 0.05 g% in December 2018.

One of the first researchers in the United States to draw attention to the problem of alcohol consumption and road-traffic safety was Dr. Herman Heise (1891–1984), who worked as a forensic pathologist (Heise 1934; Heise and Halporn 1932). During routine post-mortem examinations of victims of traffic crashes he noticed a much higher prevalence of alcohol in samples of the driver's blood and/or urine (Heise 1934). Dr. Heise was also an early spokesman for routine use of instruments for breath-alcohol testing to verify the signs and symptoms of drunkenness (Heise 1958). Along the lines already adopted in Sweden, the driver's BrAC or UAC was a more objective test of drunkenness and together with clinical signs and symptoms became the nucleus of a DUI prosecution in many US states (Heise 1969).

Abrogation of prohibition in 1933 prompted the US federal government to take a closer look at the question of drunken driving and the evidence necessary for a successful prosecution. In the intervening years the numbers of registered motor vehicle on the roads had increased astronomically. Taking samples of blood for forensic analysis of ethanol in drink-driving cases was hampered because of constitutional law and 4th Amendment rights of self-incrimination. Stopping a vehicle was considered a seizure and requesting samples of blood and urine for analysis was a search. It was voluntary to provide such specimens for analysis if there was probable cause to suspect a driver was impaired by alcohol and a refusal would be noted and used against the offender in trial, but no other penalty was imposed. Obtaining negative results from forensic analysis of blood or urine could help to exonerate a person suspected of drunken driving.

In 1953, New York became the first US state to adopt an implied consent law which meant that when a person is granted a driving permit, he or she indirectly also agrees to provide samples of blood, breath, urine, or saliva when asked to do so by a police officer if there is sufficient cause.

Much discussion and debate arose about what statutory BAC limit should be enforced. A special committee under the auspices of the American Medical Association addressed this question of medical and scientific evidence in the early 1940s. They formulated three demarcation zones depending on a driver's BAC as follows;

- Zone 1—BAC between 0.00% and 0.05% was considered as *prima facie* evidence that the person was not under the influence of alcohol.
- Zone 2—BAC between 0.05 and 0.15 g% was not *prima facie* evidence of under the influence but was admissible if physical signs and symptoms also indicated impairment.
- Zone 3—BAC above 0.15 g% was *prima facie* evidence of being under the influence of alcohol.

However, some prominent forensic scientists considered that a BAC of 0.15 g% was unacceptably high for most people who drink alcohol, and this led to a meeting of experts at Indiana University in Bloomington in 1958 to discuss the question of alcohol and road traffic safety. Delegates at the meeting arrived at the following statement, which was signed by seven scientists considered as leading authorities on the subject of alcohol and traffic safety:

> As a result of the material presented at this Symposium, it is the opinion of this Committee that a BAC of 0.05% will definitely impair the driving ability of some individuals, and as BAC increases, a progressively higher proportion of such individuals are so affected, until at a BAC of 0.10%, all individuals are definitely impaired.

The proceedings of the meeting was published in 1959 and ratified by other traffic safety organizations including the US National Safety Council Committee on Alcohol and other Drugs. The above statement prompted many US states to enact a statutory BAC limit for driving of 0.10 g%, which was later lowered to 0.08 g% where it remains today in 49 of 50 states.

Although breath-analysis was the primary means of testing driver sobriety, the results of the test were converted into the co-existing BAC, because DUI statutes referred to a punishable blood-alcohol concentration. Results from controlled drinking studies showed that BAC and BrAC were highly correlated and the average BBR was 2100:1 so BrAC × 2100 gave an estimate of the BAC. However, human alcohol dosing studies showed that the BBR was not a constant factor; it varied both between subjects and within the same subject over time and also depended on the particular breath-alcohol instrument used. This meant that prosecution evidence was often challenged because of alleged large variations in the BBR compared with the accepted 2100:1. The final result depended on the person's breathing pattern, body temperature, phase of ethanol metabolism and other physiological variables; in short the BBR was a moving target.

A more contemporary US scientist, who made a career-long contribution to research on blood- and breath-alcohol testing, was Professor Kurt M. Dubowski (1921–2017) from the University of Oklahoma (Jones 2018). The fruits of his research are contained in scores of published articles dealing with various aspects of human physiology, pharmacology and toxicology of ethanol and other drugs. The subject of Dr. Dubowski's PhD thesis (1949) form the Ohio State University was an evaluation of analytical methods for the determination of ethanol in biological specimens (Dubowski 1949).

In 1976 Dr. Dubowski and his colleague Dr. Morton Mason (1902–1985) published an important article on the subject of breath-alcohol analysis in Journal of Forensic Sciences (JFS), which dealt with the physiological principles and medicolegal applications of this technique (Mason and Dubowski 1976). They suggested that conversion of a measured BrAC into a presumed BAC for legal purposes should be abandoned and state legislators create two separate offences; namely a BAC limit of 0.08 g/100 mL (0.08 g%) or a BrAC limit of 0.08 g/210 L. The inclusion of 210 L of breath meant that 0.08 g ethanol in the numerator was the same regardless of the type of specimen (blood or breath) analyzed. Defense arguments, such as *"my client does not have a 2100 BBR"* became redundant because a limit of 0.08 g/210 L was written into the law.

The following quotation is taken from the JFS article cited above:

> We believe that the conversion of a breath quantity to a blood concentration of ethanol, for forensic purposes, should be abandoned and that the offense of driving while under the influence of alcohol should be statutorily defined in terms of the concentration of ethanol found in the breath in jurisdictions employing breath analysis. The breath sample should be obtained and analyzed only with instruments having capabilities which would require some extension of present federal standards for evidential breath-testing devices.

The results from controlled alcohol dosing studies showed that when a 2100:1 BBR was used to calibrate breath-alcohol instruments the venous BAC was underestimated by about

10% on average thus giving an advantage to the suspect (Harding and Field 1987; Harding et al. 1990). A more unbiased estimate of the BAC could be obtained if a BBR of 2300:1 had been used to calibrate the instrument or if BrAC was reported as g/230 L breath (Cowan et al. 2010).

In the 1980s when European nations began to consider using evidential breath-alcohol instruments for legal purposes, statutory BrAC limits were derived from existing BAC limits by dividing by a population average BBR of alcohol (Jones 2010). Unfortunately, there was no consensus reached as to the most appropriate BBR to use, which varied from 2000:1 to 2400:1.

In the UK a threshold BAC limit of 80 mg/100 mL was divided by a BBR of 2300:1 to give a statutory BrAC limit of 35 μg/100 mL. In other EU countries, the BAC of 0.05 g% was divided by a BBR of 2000 to give a statutory BrAC limit of 0.25 mg/L (Jones 2010). Furthermore, the concentration unit also differed between countries, such as μg/100 mL (UK and Ireland), mg/L (Sweden, Norway, and Finland), and μg/L (Belgium and Holland).

Table 4.1 compares the statutory BAC and BrAC limits adopted in various countries, the name of the evidential breath-alcohol instrument used and the assumed BBR when setting statutory BrAC limits for driving.

Table 4.1 Comparison of the Statutory Blood-Alcohol Concentration (BAC) and Breath-Alcohol Concentration (BrAC) Limits for Driving in Various Countries, the Evidential Breath-Analyzers Used for Legal Purposes and the Assumed Blood-Breath Ratio (BBR) of Alcohol

Country	BAC Limit[a]	BrAC Limit	Evidential Breath Analyzer	BBR of Ethanol
Sweden[b]	0.20 g/kg	0.10 mg/L	Evidenzer	2100
Finland[b]	0.50 g/kg	0.22 mg/L	Evidenzer	2400
Norway[b]	0.20 g/kg	0.10 mg/L	Evidenzer	2100
Switzerland[b]	0.50 g/kg	0.25 mg/L	Intoxilyzer 6000 Alcotest 9510	2100
Germany[b]	0.50 g/kg	0.25 mg/L	Alcotest 9510	2100
Ireland	50 mg%	22 μg%	Evidenzer	2300
UK[c]	80 mg%	35 μg%	Intoxilyzer 6000 Intox EC/IR BAC DataMaster	2300
Holland	0.50 mg/mL	220 μg/L	Alcotest 9510 Intox EC/IR BAC DataMaster	2300
Belgium	0.50 g/L	0.22 mg/L	Alcotest 9510	2300
Austria	0.50 g/L	0.25 mg/L	Alcotest 9510	2100
France	0.50 mg/mL	0.25 mg/L	Ethylométer	2000
US[d]	0.08 g% w/v	0.08 g/210 L	Intoxilyzer 8000 Intox EC/IR Alcotest 9510	2100
Canada	80 mg% w/v (0.08 g% w/v)	0.08 g/210 L	Intox EC/IR Alcotest 9510 Intoxilyzer 8000	2100

[a] Some countries enforce higher BAC and BrAC limits representing more serious traffic offences.

[b] Because BAC is in mass/mass units, a limit of 0.50 g/kg equals 0.53 g/L, so this influences the value of the BBR (density of blood is 1.055 g/mL on average).

[c] Scotland introduced a BAC limit of 50 mg% (BrAC limit = 0.22 μg% in 2015).

[d] The State of Utah lowered their statutory BAC limit from 0.08 g% to 0.05 g% in January 2019.

In actual DUI casework it is inevitably that some time elapses after an arrest before a suspect is tested for alcohol (Lewis 1987). The concentration of ethanol in blood is continuously changing and might have increased or decreased depending on time of the last drink in relation to the time of driving and sampling of blood or breath for analysis. If more than 60 minutes elapses after the last drink it is probably safe to assume the person was in the post-absorptive phase of the alcohol curve and that BAC was decreasing at a constant rate per hour of ~0.015 g% per h (Levine and Smialek 2000). In some US states the statutory BAC or BrAC limit refers to the time of an offence, which is usually taken to mean the time of driving or when an arrest was made. This necessitates making a back-calculation of the alcohol test result, which is sometimes a dubious practice because of the many assumptions that need to be made (Jones 2008). If the suspect's BAC or BrAC was below the statutory limit for driving at the time of sampling, the prosecution will often introduce expert testimony to calculate what the BAC or BrAC was at time of driving.

Because of the many variable factors involved a back-calculation should be done with caution taking the trouble to explain any necessary assumptions made. In some US states, to avoid having to back-calculate, if the blood or breath test is done within 2–3 hours of the time of driving the analytical result will be presumed to be not less than the value at the time of the offence. Samples taken longer than 2–3 hours after driving will need to be back extrapolated. Among the many factors to consider when such back-calculations are done are those listed below.

- Age, gender, and body weight of the suspect?
- Medical health, liver status and conditions related to rate of gastric emptying?
- Use of any medication at the time of drinking that might influence stomach emptying?
- Duration (start and end) of the drinking episode before driving?
- Beverage types and total quantity of alcohol consumed, pattern of drinking?
- Consumption of alcohol with or without food?
- Alcohol content of the last drink and time of completion of drinking before driving?
- Time between the last drink and time of the traffic stop?
- Time between traffic offence and time of blood draw or sampling breath?

Two other important things to consider are the elimination rate of ethanol from the body in that particular individual and the stage of alcohol absorption-distribution-elimination at the time of driving and sampling of body fluids for analysis. Biological variations in the elimination rate of ethanol can be overcome by assuming an adequately low value, such as 0.01 g% per h or by using a range of elimination rates, such as from 0.01 to 0.02 g% per h. The status of ethanol absorption, distribution, metabolism and excretion (ADME) in the body is more difficult to deal with and will depend on the pattern of drinking before driving, such as time of last drink, amount of ethanol contained in the drink, the fed-fasted state and time elapsed after end of drinking before a blood or breath sample was taken.

4.3 Blood-Alcohol Analysis in Europe

4.3.1 Wet-Chemistry Oxidation

The use of chemical analysis of alcohol in urine to support any clinical signs and symptoms of drunkenness has a long history, at least since 1914 (Widmark 1914). Sampling and analysis of urine was a lot more convenient than obtaining samples of venous blood with a syringe and needle, which was a much more invasive procedure. Analytical methods for determination of ethanol in body fluids had been introduced during the last decade of the nineteenth century by chemical oxidation with chromic acid (Nicloux 1900). The physiological principles of alcohol excretion was shown to occur by a passive diffusion process depending on the concentration in renal artery blood (Widmark 1918). Alcohol-induced or water-induced diuresis did not influence the urinary ethanol concentration (Widmark 1915). The experiments showed that the UAC reflected the BAC during the time that urine was formed in the kidney and collected in the bladder so the frequency of voiding and any urine retention were important considerations (Widmark 1930).

In 1922 Widmark developed a method for quantitative analysis of ethanol in small volumes (80–100 μL) of fingertip blood by a micro-diffusion method (Widmark 1922). The first page of the article, which appeared in a German language journal, is shown in Figure 4.3. The figure also shows a capillary tube before and after sampling blood, and the diffusion flask where the oxidation reaction occurs.

The blood sample (~100 μL) was obtained by pricking a fingertip or earlobe with a sterile lancet and capillary action draws blood into the S-shaped glass tubes, which are made airtight with small rubber stoppers. The inside glass surfaces of the capillaries were coated with a thin film of fluoride-oxalate mixture to prevent the blood from coagulating. The aliquot of blood analyzed was determined gravimetrically and ~100 mg

Biochemische Zeitschrift

Eine Mikromethode zur Bestimmung von Äthylalkohol im Blut.

Von

Erik M. P. Widmark.

(Medizinisch-chemisches Institut, Lund.)

(Eingegangen am 29. April 1922.)

Mit 3 Abbildungen im Text.

Eine Anzahl Probleme der Alkoholforschung stehen vor ihrer Lösung, sobald wir über eine hinreichend bequeme und genaue Methode zur Bestimmung der Alkoholkonzentration im Blute unter verschiedenen Versuchsbedingungen verfügen.

Die diesem Zwecke dienenden älteren Methoden, die allzu gut bekannt sind, um hier besprochen zu werden, haben alle den gemeinsamen Nachteil, daß sie zu große Blutmengen erfordern (mindestens 1—2 ccm), um beim Menschen oder kleineren Tieren in größerer Ausdehnung verwendet werden zu können.

Das Verfahren, durch Bestimmungen des Alkoholgehaltes im Urin indirekt die Veränderungen desselben im Blute zu ermitteln, hat sicherlich einen gewissen Vorteil[1]). Aber nicht unter allen Versuchsbedingungen tritt ein Diffusionsgleichgewicht zwischen Alkohol des Blutes und des Urins ein und besonders rasche Schwankungen der Blutalkoholkonzentration widerspiegeln sich nicht immer getreu in der des Urins.

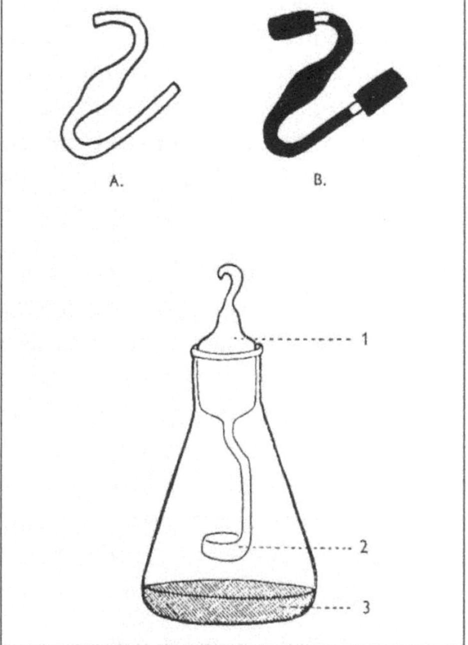

Figure 4.3 Title page of an article describing a micro-diffusion method for quantitative determination of ethanol in samples of fingertip blood (left panel). The right panel shows a capillary tube empty (A) and containing ~100 mg of blood (B) and below is shown a micro-diffusion flask with (1) ground glass stopper (2) cup to hold the weighed aliquot of blood, and (3) mixture of oxidizing agent (potassium dichromate and sulfuric acid) in excess.

was placed in the small cup connected to the ground glass stopper of the diffusion flask. The chromic acid was added to the flask, which was then kept in a water bath at 50°C for a few hours until the reaction was completed. Ethanol and other volatiles diffuse from the biological matrix and are oxidized by the chromic acid reagent. Ethanol gets oxidized via acetaldehyde to acetic acid and any remaining chromic acid reagent is determined by iodometric titration with standard sodium thiosulfate and starch indicator to detect an end-point.

The Widmark micro-diffusion method of blood-alcohol was approved and used for legal purposes in countries such as Germany, Denmark, Norway, and Sweden already in the 1940s–1950s. Because the required aliquot of blood was weighed on a torsion balance the concentration of ethanol was reported in units of mass/mass, mg/g or g/kg. This differs from the more common mass/volume units used today (g/L, g% or mg%) and values are not numerically the same, because the density of whole blood is 1.055 g/mL (Lentner 1981). This means that a statutory BAC limit of 0.08 g/100 mL existing in the United States is the same as 0.076 g/100 g blood and this has relevance when blood/breath ratios are calculated and compared between different countries (Table 4.1).

During the period 1900–1940 many investigators modified the basic chromic acid oxidation procedure, such as by varying the amount and/or concentration of the oxidizing agent, temperature of the reaction or alternative methods of volumetric analysis (Smith 1965). Some investigators preferred to extract ethanol by distillation, aeration, or protein precipitation rather than diffusion. Later on visible photometry was used to measure the reaction end-point and to calculate BAC by colorimetric procedures.

Some methods used acidified potassium permanganate as the oxidizing agent, which changed color from deep purple to colorless, although the reagent was unstable and had to be prepared fresh each time it was used. The plethora of wet-chemistry oxidation methods of alcohol analysis in blood and breath up until 1960 were the subject of a comprehensive review (Dubowski 1957; Friedemann and Dubowski 1959).

The main limitation of chemical oxidation was its lack of selectivity, because other volatile substances that might be present in blood, such as methanol, acetone, or diethyl ether were also oxidized giving false high ethanol concentrations. Additional tests were devised to check if blood or urine contained potential interfering substances, such as the Gerhardt's test for ketones. Accordingly, ferric chloride was added to a sample of urine and if there was a change to a wine-red color, this indicated that acetoacetate was present and presumably also acetone. In reality, the risk of chemical interference when the samples were taken from living subjects was much exaggerated in litigation when drunken drivers were prosecuted.

4.3.2 Enzymatic Oxidation

The next major advance in analytical methods for measuring alcohol in body fluids came in the early 1950s after the enzyme alcohol dehydrogenase (ADH) was prepared in a pure crystalline form (Bonnichsen and Wassen 1948). This enzyme soon became commercially available and was adopted as an in-vitro assay for determination of ethanol and results could then be compared with the older chemical oxidation methods (Bonnichsen and Theorell 1951). For example, elevated concentrations of acetone in blood did not interfere with the ADH method which was a problem when chromic acid oxidation methods were used for analysis.

The ADH-method of blood-alcohol analysis was developed by scientists in Sweden (Bonnichsen and Theorell 1951) and Germany in the early 1950s (Bücher and Redetzki 1951). Other aliphatic alcohols, such as methanol, *n*-propanol, and isopropanol, if these were present in blood did cross-react with the enzyme leading to false high ethanol concentrations. The ADH enzyme extracted from yeast was more specific than mammalian liver ADH (horse, pig and human), and was the preferred catalyst for forensic determinations of ethanol (Brink et al. 1954). The use of yeast ADH and optimization of the reaction conditions in terms of pH and incubation time meant that presence of methanol in the samples did not interfere with the assay of ethanol.

Scores of enzymatic oxidation methods have been described for analysis of serum, plasma, and urine without the need for any pretreatment apart from dilution (100–1,000 times) with buffer solution (pH 9.6) before starting the reaction. The co-enzyme nicotinamide adenine dinucleotide (NAD^+) is reduced to NADH in direct proportion to the concentration of substrate (ethanol) present. At room temperature completion of ethanol oxidation took about 60 min and the amount of NADH formed was measured by spectrophotometry at 340 nm.

Some of the early ADH methods required measuring the initial rate of the oxidation reaction which increases as a function of the amount of substrate present and therefore the concentration of alcohol. The more alcohol in the specimen analyzed the more NADH produced and the greater the absorption of UV light at 340 nm. A good early review of chemical and enzymatic methods applied to forensic alcohol analysis was published by Lundquist in 1959 (Lundquist 1959).

Increases in forensic laboratory workload made it obvious that some kind of automated analytical procedure was necessary and the ADH method was well-suited for this purpose, such as with Auto-Analyzer equipment and continuous flow procedures for monitoring the absorbance of NADH. The Auto-Analyzer was already used in clinical chemistry laboratories for determination of a wide range of biochemical constituents of the blood (Olsen 2012). In some forensic laboratories it was customary to use two independent methods, such as chromic acid oxidation and enzymatic oxidation and close agreement boosts confidence in the final result. High selectivity is especially important when dealing with postmortem specimens because other volatiles are produced after death that might interfere with non-specific chemical oxidation methods.

The isolation of ADH led to a deeper understanding of its biological function and stimulated a lot of research in factors influencing the metabolism of ethanol in humans (Jacobsen 1952). Among other things derivatives of pyrazole, such as 4-mthyl pyrazole were shown to act as enzyme inhibitors (Li and Theorell 1969).

4.3.3 Gas-Liquid Chromatography

In the late 1950s, the analytical technique of liquid-vapor chromatography was developed and this revolutionized the practice of analytical chemistry (James and Martin 1951). The early history of gas-liquid chromatography (GLC) and its applications was the subject of a review article (Bartle and Myers 2002). The first gas chromatograph was called a vapor fractometer, which refers to the separation of substances that can be vaporized and analyzed in the gas phase. These volatiles are mixed with a gas (the carrier gas) and transported through a long narrow column (made of glass, plastic or metal) containing the liquid stationary phase where the components were separated.

The mixture of volatile substances partition between the liquid stationary phase and an inert gas phase (nitrogen, helium or hydrogen). The liquid stationary phase is spread over an inert absorbent material creating a large surface area inside a coiled tube of about 2-m long and 3-mm inside diameter maintained at a constant temperature of 80°C–90°C. A complete or partial separation of the substances occur within the column and flow directly to a FID detector for quantitative analysis, which was highly sensitive for compounds containing carbon and hydrogen atoms in the molecule (Ettre 2002).

The introduction of GLC revolutionized the way that forensic science laboratories determined the concentrations of ethanol and other drugs in biological samples (Ettre 2003). The first publications describing application of GLC for a problem in forensic toxicology appeared in 1956 and concerned the separation and analysis of putrefaction products, mainly low-molecular weight aliphatic alcohols and aldehydes (Wolthers 1956). These substances were identified from their elution times by comparison with known authentic substances. Quantitative analysis after separation was done by enzymatic or chemical oxidation.

Scientists working in Europe were swift to take advantage of this new development and GLC methods were described for forensic blood-alcohol analysis by scientists in Austria (Machata 1962), Belgium (Heyndrickx et al. 1961), Czechoslovakia (Chundela and Janak 1960), and Sweden (Bonnichsen and Linturi 1962). Methods based on GLC were highly sensitive and specific and only a few microliters of the specimen were necessary for each determination. This new technology meant that ethanol was separated from the biological matrix, including water, in a single step prior to quantitative analysis by FID. Many papers were published between 1960 and 1980 describing new and improved materials for packing the GC columns or other ways of treating the blood specimens prior to injection onto the column for analysis. The GLC methods used in forensic science should be able to separate ethanol from closely related substances, e.g., methanol, acetaldehyde, acetone, and isopropanol within about 5 minutes. To protect the GC column from non-volatile constituents of the biological samples (e.g., fats, proteins etc.), ethanol was first separated by distillation or by precipitation of proteins with perchloric or trichloracetic acids before aliquots were injected onto the GC column for analysis.

Chundela and Janak (1960) suggested that the blood samples should be diluted 1:5 or 1:10 with an aqueous solution of an internal standard, such as another alcohol (*n*-propanol or *t*-butanol) to improve the analytical precision. Making a prior dilution of the blood with an internal standard (IS) meant that the exact volume of specimen injected into the GC instrument was not critical. For quantitative analysis the ratios of peak heights or peak areas (ethanol:IS) are plotted as a function of concentration of ethanol in known strength calibration standards. By measuring the ratios of ethanol to IS response compensates for any fluctuations in chromatographic operating conditions, e.g., gas flow rates, oven temperature, etc., during the time a long series of blood samples were being analyzed (Curry et al. 1966).

Inclusion of an internal standard increased reliability when manual injection of the specimen was done, because any between-injection variations in the exact volume of specimen was compensated by using the ratio of ethanol to *n*-propanol response for quantitative analysis (Jones 1977). According to several external proficiency trials done in the mid-1960s, some laboratories showed unacceptably large deviations from the all-laboratory mean value and the problem was traced to the technique used to inject samples into the GLC instrument and use of peak heights instead of peak areas for quantitative analysis. The results were much improved when blood samples were diluted with an internal standard and peak area ratios were measured with an electronic integrator (Emerson 2004).

A significant improvement in the methodology for GLC analysis of volatiles in blood came when the technique of headspace sampling was introduced (Machata 1964). Instead of injecting a small volume of liquid sample the vapor or air-phase in equilibrium with the liquid was analyzed. This meant that the column packing material (stationary phase) did not get contaminated with non-volatile substances in blood, such as fats and proteins (Hachenberg and Schmidt 1977). Moreover, headspace sampling methods could be automated and dedicated instruments became available from several manufactures that allowed up to 100 samples to be analyzed on each occasion (Machata 1975).

Table 4.2 contains brief methodological details summarizing the analytical methods used for determination of ethanol in blood and urine samples for forensic purposes; wet-chemical oxidation (1860–1950), enzymatic oxidation (1950–1960), GLC with liquid injection (1959–1970) and GLC by headspace sampling (1962–present).

4.4 Breath-Alcohol Analysis in Europe

4.4.1 Wet-Chemistry Oxidation

The research of Francis Edmund Anstie, already briefly mentioned, reported the first semi-quantitative analysis of ethanol in exhaled breath. During this work Anstie was astute enough to realize that the results were unreliable if done too soon after the end of drinking, owing to risk of contamination with high concentrations of alcohol in the oral mucosa (Anstie 1867). Accordingly, he gave the following warning about use of breath-alcohol analysis.

> It must not be tried during at least the first quarter of an hour after a dose had been taken for the mouth retains the characteristic smell even if the most moderate dose of any of the stronger smelling drinks for fully this time.

The Scottish pharmacologist Arthur Robertson Cushny (1866–1926) studied the exhalation of volatile substances through the lungs in a series of experiments with cats (Cushny 1910). He administered by intravenous infusion known amounts of acetone, chloroform, ether, ethyl acetate, methanol, and ethanol and the concentrations in expired air were measured and compared with the boiling point, volatility and solubility of the substances in water and reached the following conclusions;

> The exhalation of volatile substances from the lungs is exactly analogous to their evaporation from solutions in water, and the pulmonary cells seem to be purely passive in this process.
>
> The amount of any substance which is eliminated by exhalation is dependent not so much on its volatility as measured by the boiling point, but on its miscibility with water and its chemical affinity with water. The less the solubility and the more distant the affinity, the larger the amount exhaled.

This implies that the greater the solubility of the volatile substance in blood (which is 80–84% water) the less gets excreted with the breath and the lower is the air-blood partition coefficient. The solubility of the substances in the water fraction of blood is an important determinant of the amount exhaled (Jones 1983a).

Table 4.2 Chronological Development in the Analytical Methods Suitable for Blood-Alcohol Analysis

Time Period	Brief Details of the Analytical Method for Forensic Alcohol Determination
1860–1950	During ~100 years wet-chemistry methods of analysis dominated. Ethanol and other volatile substances in the blood were separated by diffusion, distillation, or aeration followed by oxidation with chromic acid (mixture of $K_2Cr_2O_7 + H_2SO_4$). The end-point of the reaction was determined either by volumetric analysis (titration) or in 1940s–1950s by photometric and colorimetry methods.
1950–1960	Enzymatic methods appeared in the early 1950s when liver alcohol dehydrogenase (ADH) was extracted and purified. The ADH enzyme derived from yeast proved to be more selective than mammalian ADH and yeast enzyme was widely used for this purpose. After precipitation of proteins in the blood or tissue by adding perchloric acid, the pH of the supernatant was adjusted to 9.6 with semicarbizide buffer, which contained NAD^+ coenzyme. The reaction was started by adding ADH and ethanol was oxidized to acetaldehyde with NAD^+ being simultaneously reduced to NADH. Quantitative analysis was done by monitoring the absorption of UV radiation by NADH at 340 nm.
1959–1970	Gas-liquid chromatography (GLC) and flame ionization detector (GLC-FID) was used for quantitative analysis of ethanol. An aliquot of blood or urine was diluted (1:5 or 1:10) with an aqueous solution of internal standard (*n*-propanol or *t*-butanol). Thereafter 1–5 μL of the diluted specimen was injected into the GLC instrument where it was vaporized and mixed with nitrogen as the carrier gas (mobile phase), before passage through a glass or stainless steel column containing a stationary liquid phase. The separation of volatile components occurred within the column and the effluent directed towards the FID detector for quantitation by measuring area under the peak response on a chromatogram. The time taken for a substance to elute through the column was known as its retention time (RT) and was used for qualitative analysis by comparison with RT of authentic substances.
1962–present	Instead of injecting a liquid sample, the GLC-FID method was adopted to work with the headspace (HS) vapor in equilibrium with the blood sample which was removed with gas tight syringe for analysis. An aliquot of the blood specimen (~100 μL) was first diluted (1:5 or 1:10) with internal standard (n-propanol) and the mixture then allowed to equilibrate at 50°C–60°C in an air-tight glass vial with rubber septum and crimped-on aluminum cap. After ~20–30 minutes, a portion of the headspace vapor above the blood was removed and injected into the GLC for analysis. Sensitivity of the analysis could be enhanced and matrix effects eliminated by saturating the diluted blood and ethanol standards with an inorganic salt, such as NaCl or K_2CO_3. HS-GLC evolved as the gold standard method and still today is used in most laboratories for the determination of ethanol and other volatiles in biological fluids.
	Some laboratories include headspace GLC analysis using both a FID and a mass spectrometric (MS) detector, which furnishes higher analytical selectivity. In addition to retention times, the electron impact mass fragments characteristic of ethanol are monitored, such as m/z 31 (base peak), m/z 45 and m/z 46 (molecular ion). With HS-GC-MS analysis deuterium labeled ethanol can be used as the internal standard.

The scientific basis of breath-alcohol analysis depends on Henry's law, which defines the relationship between concentration of a gas or volatile substance in the vapor phase in equilibrium with a liquid phase at a constant temperature (Henry 1803).

> At a constant temperature, the amount of gas that dissolves in a given type and volume of liquid is directly proportional to the partial pressure (concentration) of that gas in equilibrium with that liquid.

The high solubility of ethanol in water and blood means that only very small amounts of ethanol enter the alveolar air and are exhaled in the breath as it leaves the mouth.

Another early example of the analysis of volatile substances excreted in breath was acetone which was considered as a possible clinical test of the development of ketoacidosis in diabetic patients (Widmark 1917). This research on analysis of acetone in blood and breath was an important forerunner of the determination of ethanol as an indirect way to estimate the concentration in blood. The distribution ratio of acetone between blood and air in vitro was 300:1 at body temperature so 1 mL blood contained 300 times more acetone than the same volume of breath (Widmark 1920).

Research in pulmonary physiology and anesthesia helped to clarify many of the factors influencing gas exchange in the lungs, although ethanol is much more soluble in water than pulmonary gases (O_2, N_2, and CO_2) or the volatile inhalation anesthetics. During inhalation of ambient air and the subsequent exhalation ethanol equilibrates with the watery mucosa surfaces covering the upper respiratory tract (Hlastala 1998; Lindberg 2018). Accordingly, breathing pattern and the temperature and humidity of inhaled air will influence to some extent the concentration of ethanol in the expired breath (Jones 1982).

The physiological principles of ethanol excretion in breath and the relationship to BAC is well illustrated in a 1930 article published by two Swedish scientists shown in Figure 4.4 (Liljestrand and Linde 1930). Volunteer subjects were dosed with alcohol by mouth or per rectum and samples of venous blood and alveolar air were taken for analysis at various times after the end of drinking. The BrAC was BAC profiles followed a similar time course although the concentration in breath was about 2,000 times lower than the same volume of blood, which implies a 2000:1 blood/breath ratio.

The disposition and fate of ethanol in the body can be investigated by taking repetitive samples of blood or breath for analysis, although the two measurements agree more closely by plotting breath results as mg/2 L and blood results as mg/mL, hence a 2000:1

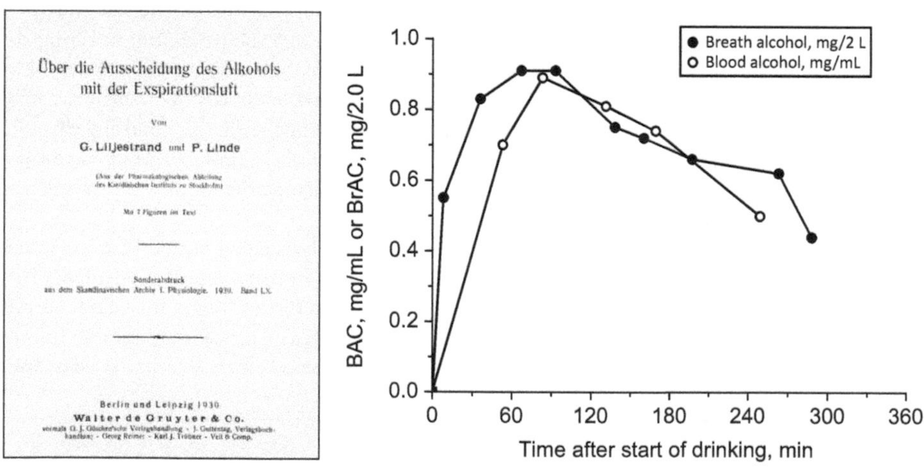

Über die Ausscheidung des Alkohols mit der Exspirationsluft

Von

G. Liljestrand und P. Linde

Sonderabdruck aus dem Skandinavischen Archiv f. Physiologie. 1930. Band LX.

Berlin und Leipzig 1930

Walter de Gruyter & Co.

vormals G. J. Göschen'sche Verlagshandlung - J. Guttentag, Verlagsbuchhandlung - Georg Reimer - Karl J. Trübner - Veit & Comp.

Figure 4.4 Title page from a seminal article by two Swedish scientists (Liljestrand and Linde) entitled "On the excretion of alcohol in the alveolar air" (left). They measured the blood/air partition ratio of ethanol in vitro and compared this with the blood/breath distribution ratio in vivo. The trace (right) shows concentration-time profiles of ethanol in venous blood and end-expired breath, with BrAC plotted as mg/2 L, thus assuming a 2000:1 blood/breath ratio (From Liljestrand, G. and Linde, P., *Skand. Arch. Physiol.*, 60, 273, 1930).

difference as shown in Figure 4.4. In the same article, the distribution ratio of ethanol in vitro between blood and air was close to 2000:1 when the equilibrium temperature was 31°C, which was considered to be the temperature of exhaled breath as it leaves the mouth (Liljestrand and Sahlstedt 1925).

A later study of the distribution of ethanol between water, blood and urine at various temperatures as a function of equilibrium temperature reported that the coefficient of ethanol solubility was ~6.5% per °C (Harger et al. 1950). Furthermore, the mean temperature of end-expired breath was found to be 34°C rather than 31°C when faster responding thermistors were used, which agrees well with more recent research reporting a breath temperature of 34.5°C (Cowan et al. 2010). The pattern of breathing (hypo- or hyperventilation) and fluctuations in the temperature and humidity of inhaled air also impact on the temperature of breath and therefore the exhaled ethanol concentration in addition to exchanges of ethanol between inhaled and exhaled air and the watery mucosa surfaces covering the upper airways (Hlastala 2010; Jones 1982).

Despite this early contribution to the physiology and practical application of breath-alcohol analysis, no further develops took place in Europe for many years. It seems that the Widmark micro-diffusion method of blood-alcohol analysis was fully accepted and had a proven reliability for forensic purposes. Moreover, obtaining the necessary blood samples for analysis was done by pricking a fingertip or earlobe puncture, which meant the required samples could be collected at police stations with little medical risk. The S-shaped capillary tubes used by Widmark that contained sodium fluoride as preservative and anticoagulant were easy to transport to a central laboratory for analysis.

In the early 1950s, research from Germany and Japan led to the development of methods for detecting various noxious gases and organic solvent vapors in the atmosphere. These were later adopted for analysis of certain gases in expired breath and a relatively simple device (Figure 4.2) for alcohol testing. The detector tube was packed with a mixture of potassium dichromate and sulfuric acid on crystals of silica gel, which changed in color from orange-yellow to green-blue if an oxidizing agent was present in the breath sample. Water vapor in the breath reacted with the sulfuric acid to generate heat to speed-up the chemical reaction.

The chemistry involved in this detector tube was obviously similar to the Widmark oxidation reaction already well established for the analysis of blood samples. In the early 1950s, a small tube-and-bag breath-analyzer called Alcotest was produced commercially in Germany. This simple device was highly practical as a means of screening drunk drivers at the roadside providing an immediate indication of the presence of alcohol. The Alcotest tube and bag device was approved for use in several European countries by the late-1950s as a more objective way to verify that a driver had consumed alcohol and was above the legal limit for driving.

A more sophisticated chemical tube and bag device for breath-alcohol analysis was developed in Japan in the mid-1950s and this system is still used to some extent for the testing of apprehended drivers (Kitagawa 1962). The person inflated a plastic bag with mixed-expired air and an exactly measured volume of breath was aspirated, using a hand held pump, through the detector tube to start a chemical reaction if there was alcohol in the breath. The tubes contained chromic acid crystals, which changed color from yellow to blue-green and the length of green stain in mm was used for quantitative analysis. After use, the detector tube could be preserved and if necessary presented as evidence in court when the person was prosecuted for a drunk driving offence.

In the early 1960s the Japanese inventor of the chemical detector tubes, Professor Tetsuzo Kitagawa (1907–1984) began collaboration with Dr. BM Wright, a biomedical engineer from England to develop a new more practical instrument for breath-alcohol analysis (Kitagawa and Wright 1962). Several prototype instruments were produced and although a reasonably good correlations was reported with BAC and the Breathalyzer instrument, the Kitagawa-Wright analyzer was never introduced into law enforcement practice (Begg et al. 1964).

4.4.2 Electrochemical Oxidation

In the early 1970s, the first hand-held breath-alcohol instrument that incorporated an electrochemical sensor for determination of ethanol appeared. This development work involved a collaboration between Lion Laboratories (Barry, Wales, UK), and scientists at the Department of Chemistry, University of Wales in Cardiff. Team leaders for this research included a chemist Dr. TP Jones (1935–2013) and a physiologist and bioengineer Dr. BM Wright (1912–2001) from the Medical Research Council in London. Figure 4.5 shows the first prototype instrument, which was christened "Alcolmeter" and this measured 11.5 × 6.0 × 2.5 cm and weighed only 180 g hence the designation "pocket model." The Alcolmeter aspirated a known volume (~1.5 mL) of breath as the test subject made a forced exhalation through a plastic mouthpiece tube fitted to the instrument (Jones et al. 1974).

The electrochemical oxidation of volatile alcohols had been described earlier as the detector for gas chromatographic analysis by scientists at the University of Innsbruck, Austria (Cremer et al. 1969). After drinking alcoholic beverages the only alcohol of interest in blood and breath is ethanol so the bulky GC equipment was unnecessary. The same electrochemical sensor was used as the detector for breath-alcohol analysis

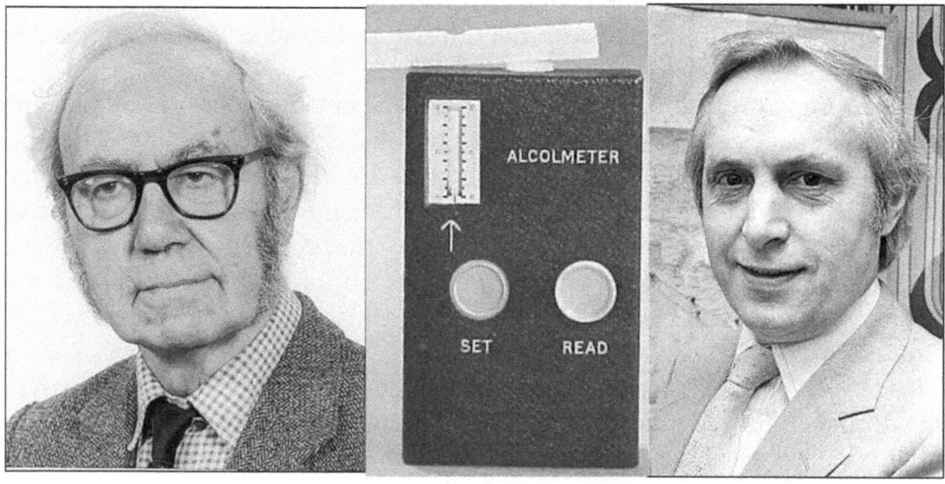

Figure 4.5 Two British scientists, Dr. TP Jones (chemist) and Dr. BM Wright (physiologist and bioengineer), led the development work on the first hand-held electronic breath analyzer incorporating an electrochemical detector (Alcolmeter Pocket Model) from 1972.

and the aspirating sampling system was highly reproducible and could also be adapted for determination of ethanol in blood and saliva by headspace sampling (Jones 1978b).

Since its inception in 1972, many different models of the Alcolmeter pocket model have appeared with different options for displaying results, such as analogue scale and pointer, color light diodes (green, amber and red), or pass, warn fail as well as digital display (Jones 1978e). One of the latest versions (Alcolmeter 400) automatically captures the required breath sample at the end of a prolonged exhalation and a printed record of the results is available for inclusion in the evidence package that goes to the crown prosecution service. Demographics of the person tested, the date, time and location of the test and the analytical result can be stored on-line and downloaded to a central computer for retrospective quality control if and when the results might be used for evidential purposes.

Many alternative hand-held instruments have since been developed that incorporate electrochemical oxidation for determination of ethanol in breath as shown in Figure 4.6.

Electrochemical detectors are reasonably specific for ethanol analysis, because neither acetone nor hydrocarbons (e.g., methane) if exhaled in human breath are oxidized at the electrode potential used (Kramer-Sarrett et al. 2017). However, other primary alcohols (methanol, *n*-propanol, isopropanol) undergo oxidation and might interfere with the ethanol response if these more toxic substances are ingested (Falkensson et al. 1989). Recent evaluations of handheld fuel-cell instruments show that they perform well for their intended purposes, which is primarily as a roadside screening test of driver sobriety (Zuba 2008).

Table 4.3 traces the chronological developments in instruments used as roadside breath-alcohol screening tests since the mid-1950s to the present time. The year is approximate and indicates when the various devices were advertised for sale or when they were mentioned or described in a scientific publication.

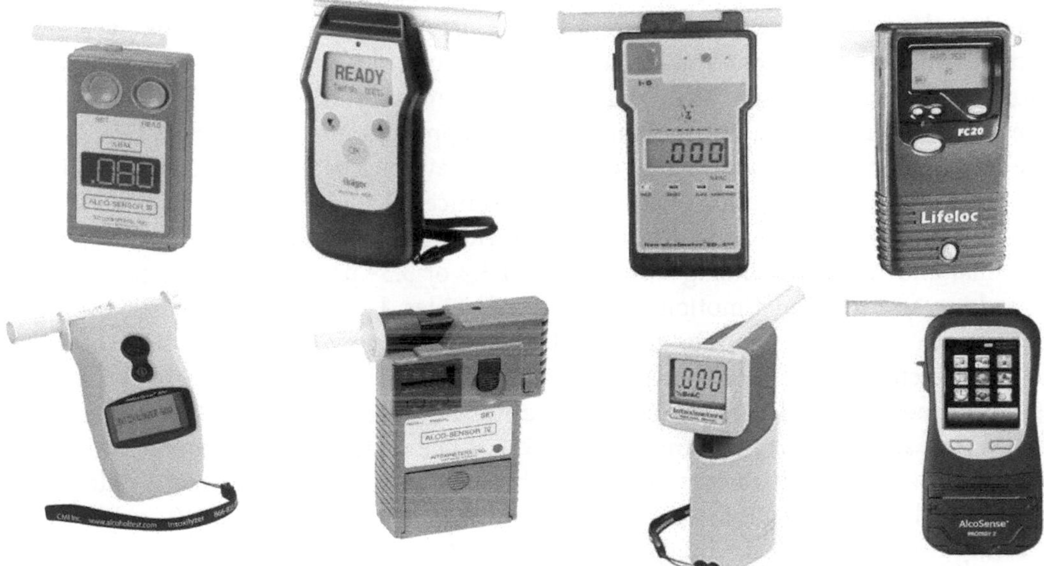

Figure 4.6 Examples of hand-held electronic instruments incorporating electrochemical sensors widely used in traffic-law enforcement as roadside screening tests for driver sobriety.

Table 4.3 Chronological Development of Hand-Held Instruments for Use as a Roadside Preliminary Breath-Alcohol Screening for Alcohol Influence

Year[a]	Preliminary Screening Test (country of origin)	Analytical Principle for the Determination of Ethanol
1953	Alcotest tube and bag (Germany)	Oxidation with $K_2Cr_2O_7 + H_2SO_4$ adsorbed on silica gel
1956	Kitagawa detector tube (Japan)	Oxidation with chromic acid on silica gel absorbent material
1969	Sober-meter (US)	Oxidation with $K_2Cr_2O_7 + H_2SO_4$ adsorbed on silica gel
1969	Alcolyser tubes (Wales, UK)	Oxidation with $K_2Cr_2O_7 + H_2SO_4$ adsorbed on silica gel
1972–74	Alcolmeter (Wales, UK)[b]	Electrochemical oxidation with a fuel-cell detector
1975	AlcoSensor (US)[b]	Electrochemical oxidation with a fuel cell detector
1978	ALERT J3A	N-type semiconductor (Taguchi cell)
1980	LifeLoc (US)	Electrochemical oxidation with a fuel-cell detector
1980–84	Alcotest (Germany)	Electrochemical oxidation with a fuel cell detector
1995[c]	Alcoodose 2 (France)	Infrared absorption at 9.4 μm

[a] The years are approximate and represent the first scientific report or when the device first became commercially available.

[b] The Alcolmeter device was re-designed and marketed in US as Alco-Sensor and gained wide acceptance and several different models soon became available.

[c] After 2000 a large number of hand-held instruments incorporating fuel-cell sensors and semi-conductors (Taguchi-cells) become available for purchase by the general public.

4.4.3 Infrared Spectrometry

Infrared (IR) spectrometry is a non-destructive analytical method first used for measuring alcohol and other volatiles in human breath in the mid-1960s (Stewart and Erley 1965). A practical instrument for breath-alcohol analysis based on infrared absorption at a single wavelength of 3.39 μM was described in 1971 (Harte 1971). Infrared technology is a well-established analytical technique because organic molecules absorb IR radiation in accordance with their molecular structure, functional groups and types of chemical bonding present. Quantitative analysis is accomplished by application of the Lambert-Beer law and the relationship between absorbance of certain IR wavelengths, the path length are directly proportional to concentration of absorbing substance.

The first two instruments to incorporate IR technology developed in Europe were Alcomat and Alcotest utilizing wavelengths of 3.4 or 3.39 μm, which correspond to C-H stretching and rotational motion of ethanol molecules. Later research focused on higher wavelength of 9.4 or 9.5 μm for greater selectivity corresponding to absorption of energy by the stretching of the C-O bonds in molecules of ethanol. The use of a higher wavelength (9.5 μm) meant that elevated breath acetone was no longer represented a problem as an interfering substance (Flores and Frank 1995). Some of the latest generation of evidential breath-alcohol instruments incorporate both IR and electrochemistry as detectors as exemplified by the Alcotest 7110, Mark III and later models such as 7310 and the more recently available Alcotest 9510 (Hartung et al. 2016).

The use of two independent analytical methods for analysis of ethanol is a desirable feature that gives more confidence in concluding that ethanol was indeed the volatile substance in the driver's breath (Hodgson and Taylor 2001). Yet another refinement in the breath-testing technology is ability to determine temperature of the end exhaled breath with thermistors located in the entrance of the breath-inlet tube. If a suspect happens to have a temperature on his or her breath above the assumed average value of 34°C, the instrument makes a correction to the alcohol content, by lowering the result by 6.5% per degree above 34°C (Schoknecht and Kophamel 1988).

The official method of blood-alcohol analysis used in Germany requires parallel determinations by two independent analytical methods, such as HS-GLC and ADH oxidation (Krause 2007). Many forensic experts were reluctant to accept the use of breath-alcohol analysis for legal purposes unless two independent analytical principles were incorporated into the instruments. The Dräger Company (Lübeck, Germany) took up this challenge and developed the Alcotest instrument, which uses both IR and EC detectors on the same sample of breath and results need to agree within certain pre-defined limits. A complicating factor is that ethanol determinations for legal purposes in Germany are done on serum and not on whole blood, although the statutory limits for driving are BAC. The serum ethanol concentration is converted to a BAC by dividing the mean of four separate determinations by a factor of 1.236 (Iffland et al. 1999). Using results of serum analysis to estimating BAC from BrAC. Both the serum/blood alcohol ratio and the blood/breath-alcohol varies between subjects although the latter is subject to more sources of physiological variation.

Extensive research began in Germany to establish a sound physiological basis for using breath-alcohol testing in law enforcement when drunken-drivers were prosecuted (Schoknecht et al. 1989; Zinka et al. 2009). The results verified previous work that showed that the BBR of alcohol had an inter-subject coefficient of variation of about 10%–12%, which is not excessive for a biological variable (Jachau et al. 2000; Jones 2016). The practical advantages of breath analysis compared with drawing blood for analysis were undeniable and Germany approved the use of this technology for prosecuting in minor road-traffic offences in 1998. However, if the evidential breath test showed a result above 0.55 mg/L (~1.1 g/kg in blood), which constitutes a more serious traffic offence, blood was taken and analyzed by two independent methods (ADH and HS-GLC) (Jachau and Musshoff 2009). The lower statutory alcohol limits for driving in Germany are 0.50 g/kg in blood or 0.25 mg/L in breath (Table 4.1), but to charge a person with a more serious offence (BAC > 1.1 g/kg) only blood-alcohol analysis is acceptable (Hartung et al. 2016).

4.5 Blood-Alcohol Analysis in North America

4.5.1 Wet-Chemistry Methods

The first analytical method for blood-ethanol in the United States was developed to assist with basic physiological research on alcohol and not medicolegal investigations and prosecution of drunken drivers (Benedict and Norris 1898). The first report that drinking before driving was dangerous and contributed to traffic fatalities appeared in 1904 (Crothers 1904). Proof that a driver was drunk at the time of the crash was more difficult to obtain. Urine became the first biological specimen used for analysis of alcohol, because it was available in large volumes and was easier to collect than removing blood from a vein. Taking a sample of the driver's blood was much more invasive and raised constitutional issues (4th Amendment rights) about unwarranted searches and seizures. By contrast, urine and breath were considered specimens that a person had voluntarily discarded and therefore more amenable for analysis of alcohol in criminal cases.

The first analytical methods were essentially minor modifications of the chromic acid oxidation procedures developed in Europe, such as Widmark's micro-diffusion method (Cavett 1938; Gettler and Freireich 1931; Harger 1935). The main problem with chemical oxidation methods is their limited specificity for identifying ethanol and various preliminary spot tests were necessary to exclude the presence of interfering substances, such as acetone, ether, acetaldehyde, paraldehyde, formaldehyde, acetone, methanol, and 2-propanol in the samples.

Volatile substances in urine or other biological specimen were extracted by steam distillation under acid conditions and at an alkaline pH, which removed any acids and bases present (Friedemann and Dubowski 1959). Some interfering substances, such as aldehydes and ketones, could be removed by placing a mercuric oxide scrubber between the blood sample and the condenser (Kozelka and Hine 1941). Such precautions were particularly important if ethanol was determined in autopsy blood specimens, because interfering volatiles might be produced in the body after death (Wolthers 1956). In the 1950s, the oxidation of ethanol with mixtures of dichromate-sulfuric acid continued to be used, but instead of volumetric analysis photometric methods were used instead (Smith 1965).

The large number of wet-chemistry oxidation methods of blood-alcohol analysis have been reviewed elsewhere (Friedemann and Dubowski 1959; Smith 1965). In the late 1940s, two scientists in North America devoted their PhD thesis to evaluate the methods suitable for blood alcohol analysis as tests for intoxication. One was Dr. H. Ward Smith (1914–1967) from Toronto, Canada, whose thesis was entitled *The Determination of Alcohol and Its Interpretation for Drivers* (Smith 1950). The other was Dr. Kurt M. Dubowski, whose 1949 PhD thesis from the Ohio State University was entitled *An Evaluation of Methods for Determination of Ethyl Alcohol in Biological Materials* (Dubowski 1949).

4.5.2 Gas Chromatographic Methods

The proceedings of a conference on analytical chemistry and applied spectroscopy was held in Pittsburg in 1958 and one of the presentations described a gas chromatograph fitted with a thermal conductivity detector for analysis of ethanol in blood after extraction with *n*-propyl acetate (Cadman and Johns 1958). Shortly afterwards the same investigators used a GLC method for analysis of other toxicological substances and the results were published in a peer-review journal (Cadman and Johns 1960). Another early GLC method separated ethanol from the biological matrix by distillation prior to the chromatography using a thermal conductivity detector (Fox 1958). The BAC was determined by comparison with a standard curve constructed from the analysis of known strength ethanol standards and peak height or peak areas for quantitative analysis.

The proceedings of a 1962 conference on the subject of alcohol and road traffic contained an article by David Lester (1916–1990) who described a GLC method for quantitative analysis of ethanol in biological samples by analyzing the vapor phase after equilibration at a controlled temperature (Lester 1962). This report appears to be the first application of headspace sampling applied to analysis of volatiles by GLC methods. The major advantage of headspace sampling was that the GC column does not become contaminated by non-volatiles substances in the blood, such as proteins, lipids and other endogenous compounds.

The development of HS-GLC was pioneered by the Perkin-Elmer instrument company and the first dedicated instrument Multifract F-40, dates from the early 1970s. This used a water bath to thermostat and equilibrate the samples, followed in 1984 model F-45, which made use of a heating block and 45 specimens could be analyzed in a single run. Other more recent versions have appeared including HS-100 and HS-110, which had positions for 110 specimens (Ettre 2001).

The sensitivity of HS-GLC method is increased by saturating the specimen with an inorganic salt, such as sodium chloride or sodium carbonate (Dubowski 1977b; Miller et al. 2004). The solubility of non-electrolytes in solution is lowered by adding substances that ionize and attract water molecules thus increasing the vapor pressure and concentration of ethanol in the headspace vapor (Watts and McDonald 1990). By saturating the biological specimen and the aqueous ethanol standards with an inorganic salt (NaCl or K_2CO_3), e.g., 0.5 mL blood or urine and 1 g salt, this permits measuring much lower concentrations and also any matrix effects and problems associated with varying amounts of water in the blood is eliminated. The GLC methods suitable for quantitative analysis of ethanol and other volatiles have been reviewed elsewhere (Cravey and Jain 1974; Jain 1971; Jain and Cravey 1972; Tagliaro et al. 1992).

4.6 Breath-Alcohol Analysis in North America

4.6.1 Wet-Chemistry Oxidation

An important historical article describing breath-alcohol analysis as a way to verify clinical signs and symptoms of intoxication was published in Journal of the American Medical Association (JAMA) in 1927 (Bogen 1927) The author was Dr. Emil Bogen (1896–1963) and he determined ethanol in breath and urine collected from patients admitted to a trauma unit for gross intoxication or enrolled in a clinic for detoxification. The patients were asked to inflate a football bladder with their breath and the alcohol content was determined by passage through a mixture of dichromate-sulfuric acid as an oxidizing agent. The change in color from yellow-orange Cr(VI) to various shades of green-blue Cr(III) was compared with a series of standard solutions of chromic acid after known amounts of ethanol had been added. These were kept in sealed glass tubes and used to make a visible comparison with the subject's breath sample thus providing a semi-quantitative method of ethanol determination.

The concentration of ethanol in breath of the detox patients was compared with results from the analysis of their urine and the degree of drunkenness. In this way Bogen established that the ethanol content in 2 L of breath was roughly equivalent to the amount in 1 mL of urine, which suggests a 2000:1 urine/breath ratio of ethanol. In conjunction with these early studies of breath-alcohol analysis the JAMA article contained the following warning about collecting the breath sample too soon after a recent drink or regurgitation of stomach contents;

> As soon as the disturbing factor of alcoholic liquor still in the mouth is removed, which occurs usually within fifteen minutes after imbibition, in the absence of hiccupping or belching, the alcoholic content of 2 L of expired air was a little greater than 1 cc urine.... The concentration of alcohol in the blood generally was about the same as that in the urine, but was sometimes a little lower.

In US states, taking blood samples from people suspected of impaired driving was considered a search and was not permissible unless this was done voluntarily. There were constitutional problems of self-incrimination and violation of 4th Amendment rights. This prompted efforts to develop methods for analysis of alcohol in breath, because people voluntarily discarded this type of biological specimen and could be used in evidence when a driver was charged with DUI. Professor Rolla N. Harger (1890–1983) at the department of pharmacology and toxicology at Indiana University began to develop such an instrument in 1931 and his paper was published in a scientific journal in 1938 (Harger et al. 1938).

An urgent need arose to gather objective and tangible evidence for criminal prosecution of traffic offenders, because drunken drivers were increasingly found culpable for road traffic crashes (Heise 1934; Heise and Halporn 1932). The use of breath analysis became a major focus avoiding practical and constitutional problems associated with obtaining blood samples, e.g., the long distances between towns where a doctor or trained phlebotomist might be available and willing to take the required samples. The law related to self-incrimination was also an obstacle and because breath was a non-invasive sampling procedure it was considered more acceptable than penetrating a vein with a needle.

Another major advantage of breath-testing over blood-testing was obtaining immediate information about the alcohol load in the body and whether a person was breaking the law by being above the legal limit. However, obtaining a proper sample of breath for analysis that reflected the concentration in end-expiratory air required considerable cooperation from the subject tested. Some instruments collected mixed-exhaled breath from the suspect and to estimate the proportion of alveolar air in the sample the CO_2 content was determined. This meant that the required breath sample could be obtained in a passive way and without violating a person's constitutional rights. Although the results obtained underestimated the actual concentrations of ethanol in alveolar air they gave evidence of gross intoxication.

The first generation of instruments for breath-alcohol analysis appeared in the late 1930s and early 1940s and were given names such as the Drunkometer (Harger et al. 1938), the Intoximeter (Jetter et al. 1941), and the Alcometer (Greenberg and Keator 1941). Each instrument was sufficiently portable and compact to be used at a police stations by trained officers. Both the Drunkometer and the Intoximeter contained an oxidizing agent made from a solution of potassium permanganate and sulfuric acid and this gave an immediate semi-quantitative indication of alcohol influence if the color changed from purple to colorless after reaction with ethanol in breath. For quantitative analysis a sample of the mixed expired air was trapped on magnesium perchlorate reagent for later analysis at a laboratory (Intoximeter). The amount of alveolar air in the breath sample analyzed was determined from the carbon dioxide content determined gravimetrically by weighing an Ascarite tube and assuming that alveolar air contained 5.5% v/v of this respiratory waste gas (CO_2).

Later version of the Drunkometer analyzed ethanol in rebreathed air, which meant that it was no longer necessary to measure CO_2 content. By rebreathing the initial exhalation about 5 times from a heated bag, the concentration of respiratory gases and other volatiles in breath approached the concentration in alveolar air and therefore the concentration in pulmonary blood entering the lungs (Jones 1983b).

The Alcometer device was designed to capture a sample of breath at the end of a prolonged exhalation (alveolar air) and the ethanol content was determined by oxidation with iodine pentoxide. This chemical reaction is not specific for ethanol and requires a high temperature to proceed in a short enough time. Furthermore, this reagent was unstable and problems were encountered when the instrument was shipped between different locations and its use in law enforcement was relatively short-lived.

The reliability of the first generation of breath-alcohol instruments devices was constantly being debated but the result was intended to support other evidence of driver impairment, such as clinical signs and symptoms. Much debate arose about the correct value of the BBR used to calculate BAC from BrAC and a re-evaluation was made of the three instruments available for breath-alcohol analysis. These tests were done under the auspices of the US National Safety Council, Committee on Alcohol and Other Drugs and the following conclusion was reached.

> The basic principle governing the operation of the three presently used breath alcohol methods (the Drunkometer, the Intoximeter, and the Alcometer) is the constant ratio existing between the concentration of alcohol in the alveolar air and the blood. Available information indicates that this alveolar air-blood ratio is approximately 1:2100. However, since each method involves different procedures, different empirical factors are involved in the calculation of concentrations of alcohol in the blood in each of the methods. It is the opinion of the subcommittee that the tests made on the Alcometer, the Intoximeter, and the Drunkometer, if conducted in the manner prescribed by the authors of the respective methods, will give comparable and reliable results for estimating the concentration of alcohol in the blood.

The next major advance in analytical technology for determination of alcohol in breath came with the invention of the Breathalyzer instrument, which was developed by Robert Borkenstein in 1954. This represented a significant improvement and was much easier to use by trained police officers and a single test only took about 5 minutes to complete including a control of the calibration. A scientific article dealing with the results of the Breathalyzer in relation to BAC was not published until 1961 (Borkenstein and Smith 1961).

The Breathalyzer captured a known volume of end-exhaled breath and ethanol was determined by oxidation with chromic acid contained in small glass ampoules. The reaction end-point and the concentration of ethanol was determined by photometry and balancing with an unopened ampoule containing the same strength chromic acid solution. An entire test sequence comprising the analysis of the subject's breath sample, an air-blank test, and control of the instrument calibration required 5 to 8 minutes to complete and nothing needed to be sent to a laboratory for analysis. The Breathalyzer instrument became widely used by police forces throughout the United States, Canada, and Australia when drunken drivers were tested. If the end-point of the chemical oxidation reaction was read on the photometer after exactly 90 seconds, other volatiles that might be present, such as methanol and acetone, did not cause an interference problem (Oliver and Garriott 1979).

The Breathalyzer instrument was evaluated and approved for use in Canada mainly thanks to the efforts of forensic scientist Dr. H. Ward Smith (1914–1967) from Toronto (Smith 1960, 1965). He developed a close collaboration with Professor Borkenstein and together they published the first scientific paper in 1961 describing the principles and operation of this Breathalyzer instrument (Borkenstein and Smith 1961). Others from Canada who contributed in various ways to acceptance of evidential breath-alcohol analysis were E.J. Fennell (British Columbia), W.R. Picton (Alberta), and D.M. Lucas (Ontario). Indeed, after Ward-Smith's untimely death aged 53 years from lung cancer he was succeeded by Lucas as chief forensic scientist in Toronto.

The Canadian Society of Forensic Sciences established an alcohol test committee to oversee the requirements necessary and develop performance standards for quality control of results of forensic blood- and breath-alcohol testing. Among other things, this committee drafted guidelines for evaluating new instruments and standards of performance in terms of their accuracy, precision and specificity when results were used to prosecute traffic offenders.

As early as 1956–1957 the Breathalyzer instrument was approved by the Royal Canadian Mounted Police in Toronto and later throughout the country (Coldwell and Grant 1963). Early research was initiated in Ottawa to compare ethanol concentrations in blood, breath, urine and saliva in drinking studies and to determine the relationship between BAC and impairment of body functions (Coldwell and Smith 1959; Coldwell and Grant 1963). The leader in this research effort was Dr. Blake B. Coldwell who wrote a comprehensive report of the results as a book (Coldwell 1957). The ethanol concentrations in biological fluids at various times post-drinking were compared with cognitive and psychomotor tests of impairment as well as on-the-road driving performance (Penner and Coldwell 1958).

4.6.2 Gas-Liquid Chromatography

The success afforded GC methods for blood-alcohol analysis led to this same analytical technique being applied to the analysis of breath samples. The first such instrument was reported at a conference on alcohol, drugs and driving held in Freiburg, Germany in 1969. This was the GC Intoximeter, which incorporated on-column gas sampling loop for capturing a breath aliquot (0.25 mL) kept warm in an oven and connected to the chromatographic column. The GC Intoximeter was fitted with a flame ionization detector (FID) for quantitative analysis of volatiles and the stationary phase was Porapak Q contained in a short (30 cm × 3 mm) stainless steel tube. Ethanol was separated on the column from other volatile substances, such as methanol, acetone, and isopropanol and the detector signals were plotted as a function of time on a strip-chart recorder.

Other breath volatiles could be identified on the chromatogram from their retention times in comparison with authentic standard substances. A pressurized gas cylinder contained a mixture of nitrogen and hydrogen served as fuel for the detector and carrier gas (mobile phase) with the required air for the FID being supplied by a small pump. A big advantage of the GC Intoximeter (GCI) was its FID detector, which was not sensitive to water vapor in the breath. A competing GC instrument known as Alco-Analyzer used a thermal conductivity detector, which gave a large response to water vapor and a longer time between repetitive tests. The GC Intoximeter won approval for forensic purposes in several US states and Canadian provinces. Its accuracy, precision and specificity were evaluated in detail under both in-vitro and in-vivo conditions (Jones 1978c, 1978d). Besides being able to sample and analyze breath directly, the GC Intoximeter could also capture breath in specially treated indium tubes. This provision for encapsulating and storing triplicate samples of breath for later confirmatory analysis was a novel feature of this instrument allowing the testing of drivers in remote locations. The indium tubes needed to be sent to a central laboratory for analysis of alcohol by the GC Intoximeter.

4.6.3 Infrared Spectrometry

In the late 1960s infrared (IR) spectrometry was used for monitoring respiratory and anesthetic gases, such as diethyl ether, in the expired air (Stewart and Erley 1963). Soon afterwards, this same methodology was applied to measure volatile substances in human breath, including ethanol (Guyton and Gravenstein 1990). By 1971, a new instrument for breath-alcohol analysis was described that incorporated an IR spectrometer suitable for use at police stations (Harte 1971). This new instrument was christened Intoxilyzer and within a short space of time was approved for law enforcement purposes in several US states.

Infrared spectrometry is currently the leading analytical technology incorporated into instruments for evidential breath-alcohol analysis for forensic purposes. The first IR instrument was Intoxilyzer 4011 although this had a large breath-sample chamber (600 mL) making it difficult to obtain end-exhaled breath from some individuals with low vital capacity (Harte 1971). Moreover, absorption of IR radiation was monitored at a single wavelength of 3.4 or 3.39 μm, which corresponds to the C-H bond stretching and rotational frequencies in ethanol molecules. Accordingly, other volatile substances in breath with C-H bonds, such as the methyl groups in acetone, which also absorb IR radiation and masquerade as ethanol, i.e., a non-specific response.

Measuring the absorption of IR radiation at a single wavelength is not considered sufficiently reliable for evidential purposes, because after prolonged periods of fasting, after eating low carbohydrate diets and in untreated diabetics breath-acetone concentrations are elevated (Dubowski and Essary 1984). The problem posed by acetone was solved by measuring the absorption of IR radiation at two different analytical wavelengths, e.g., 3.39 and 3.48 μm, and using a third reference wavelength (3.80 μm) where no absorption of IR energy by ethanol and acetone occurred (Dubowski and Essary 1983; Oliver and Garriott 1979).

For routine purposes IR absorptiometry proved a highly stable measuring system for analysis of ethanol and once the instrument was initially calibrated the response remained remarkably stable over time. However, a check of the instrument calibration was necessary in conjunction with every apprehended driver being tested. This was achieved by generating known strength air-alcohol vapors with the help of a wet-bath breath-simulator device. More recently pressurized tanks containing know-strength dry-gas alcohol standards have been used for the same purpose (Dubowski and Essary 1991, 1996). The analysis of a known strength ethanol standard either before, after and sometimes before and after a drunken driver is tested verifies the instrument was reporting accurate results.

The latest generations of infrared breath alcohol analyzers are highly selective for identification of ethanol molecules and if there are interfering substances these are either flagged or adjustments are made to the ethanol response (Jones and Andersson 2008). Acetone is an endogenous breath volatile and prolonged fasting, eating low carbohydrate diets or in poorly treated type I diabetes the concentrations increase in blood and exhaled breath (Krishan and Lui 2002). Infrared breath-alcohol analyzers with several wavelengths in the 3.3–3.4 μm range or at 9.5 μm can distinguish ethanol from acetone and either abort the test or make a correction to the result reported (Wallage and Bugyra 2017).

Several major developments in the technology of breath-alcohol analysis occurred in the 1970s when electrochemical oxidation, GLC, IR spectrometry, and metal-oxide semiconductors (Taguchi cell) were incorporated into various breath-alcohol analyzers for clinical, forensic and research purposes (Dubowski 1991; Wigmore and Langille 2009).

Table 4.4 classifies evidential breath-alcohol instruments into six different generations depending on when they were developed and used in traffic law enforcement.

Biological aspects of breath-alcohol testing was a hot research topic in the 1970s and raised concern about the need to monitor respiratory variables, such as breath temperature, exhaled volume and resistance to exhalation and the subject's breathing technique (Dubowski 1974). Although results of controlled drinking experiments found a high statistical correlation between BAC and BrAC, the BBR of alcohol varied widely both between subjects and also within subjects as a function of time after start of drinking (Alobaidi et al. 1976). These finding were considered problematic, because at the time breath-test results were always converted into BAC using a constant 2100:1 BBR.

Most studies showed that when BrAC was converted into BAC, the results were 10%–15% lower than the actual venous BAC if comparisons were made in the post-absorptive phase of the BAC curve (Jones and Andersson 1996, 2003). The mean BBR was closer to 2300:1 rather than 2100:1 in the post-absorptive phase and some nations adopted a higher BBR when their statutory BrAC limits were derived from existing BAC limits. Because a 2100:1 BBR gave a certain advantage to the person tested compared with measuring BAC, continued use of a 2100:1 ratio was deemed acceptable in criminal cases such as drunken driving (Mason and Dubowski 1976).

Physiological factors associated with sampling breath, such as variable exhaled breath volumes, interactions between water soluble ethanol and the mucous membranes of the upper airway is considered problematic when breath-alcohol testing is used for evidential purposes (Hlastala 2010; Hlastala and Anderson 2016). The pattern of breathing before providing a breath sample and the temperature and humidity of the ambient air breathed also impact on the BBR of alcohol (Jones 1982).

Table 4.4 Classification of Evidential Breath-Alcohol Instruments into Six Generations Depending on the Time Period When They Were Developed/Used for Legal Purposes—The Approximate Time Period (years), Name of the Instrument, and Brief Details of the Analytical Method for Analysis of Ethanol Are Shown

Generation (years[a])	Breath Analyzer	Scientific Principle for Analysis of Breath Ethanol
First (1938–1954)	Drunkometer[b] Intoximeter[b] Alcometer	• Oxidation with acidified potassium permanganate (Drunkometer and Alcometer) or iodine pentoxide (Alcometer)
Second (1953–1970)	Breathalyzer Photo-electric Intoximeter Ethanograph	• Oxidation with acidified potassium dichromate sulfuric acid mixture in glass ampoules, using photometry to detect an end-point
Third (1969–1974)	Intoxilyzer 4011 GC Intoximeter Alco-Analyzer	• IR absorptiometry at a single wavelength of 3.4 μm (Intoxilyzer) • GC separation on Porapak Q with FID detector for quantitation analysis (Intoximeter) • GC separation on Porapak Q and thermal conductivity detector for quantitation (Alco-Analyzer)
Fourth (1975–1980)	Intoximeter 3000 Intoxilyzer 5000 Alcomat BAC DataMaster Alcotest 7110	• Single wavelength IR (3.4 μm) and T-cell combined in same unit (Intoximeter) • Analysis by IR absorption at three wavelengths close to 3.4 μm (Intoxilyzer) • Analysis by infrared at 9.5 μm (Alcomat) • Dual wavelength IR analyzer at 3.39 μm and 3.48 μm (DataMaster) • Both IR analysis and electrochemical fuel cell detector (Alcotest)
Fifth (1980–2000)	Intoxilyzer 6000 Intox EC/IR Alcotest 7410 DataMaster DMT	• Multiple-wavelength IR analyzer around 3.4 μM (Intoxilyzer) • Electrochemical fuel cell detector for quantitative analysis and IR detector to monitor CO_2 and presence of mouth alcohol (Intoximeter) • Combined use of IR detector at 9.5 μM and electrochemical (fuel cell) detector (Alcotest)
Sixth (2000–2019)	Intoxilyzer 9000 Alcotest 9510 Evidenzer Intox DMT (dual sensor)	• Multiple IR wavelengths (Intoxilyzer) • Infrared detector (9.5 μm) and electrochemical detector (Alcotest) • Multiple five-filter IR wavelengths close to 3.3–3.5 μM (Evidenzer) • Infrared (9.5 μm and electrochemical detector [Intox DMT])

[a] Various prototype instruments might have appeared earlier than the dates shown.

[b] The Drunkometer and Intoximeter provided a qualitative result to ascertain if the BAC exceeded 0.15 g% by decolorization of acidified potassium permanganate. For quantitative analysis, the carbon dioxide content of the breath sample was analyzed to calculate the proportion of alveolar air in the sample collected assuming this was 5.5 vol%.

The Borkenstein Breathalyzer instrument analyzed ethanol in breath but reported the result as the person's BAC, which was considered suspect when new research showed appreciable inter- and intra-subject variations in the BBR of alcohol. A meeting of experts with international representation convened in Indianapolis (IN) in 1972 under the auspices of the US National Safety Council Committee on Alcohol and Other Drugs. On the agenda was a critical review of published research on the accuracy and precision of estimating BAC indirectly by analysis of breath and magnitude of biological variations in the BBR. After two days of discussion and deliberation the following statement was promulgated:

> The basic principle governing the design of breath alcohol instruments is that a physiological relationship exists between the concentration of alcohol in the expired alveolar air and in the blood. Available information indicates that 2.1 L of expired alveolar air contain approximately the same quantity of alcohol as 1 mL of blood. Continued use of this ratio in clinical and legal applications is warranted.

The expert statement was endorsed by US scientist (Borkenstein, Dubowski, Harger, and Forney) and with international support from Goldberg (Sweden) and Wright (UK). The continued use of the Breathalyzer instrument and the 2100:1 BBR was deemed acceptable because the results tended to underestimate the venous BAC, hence this gave a certain advantage to the person tested.

Beginning in the 1970s new technologies were applied to breath-alcohol analysis, including gas chromatography (Penton and Forrester 1970), infra-red spectrometry (Harte 1971) and electrochemical oxidation (Jones et al. 1974) and a new generation of instruments for roadside screening and evidential testing became available (Dubowski 1975).

One advantage of blood analysis over breath is that the specimen can be stored in a refrigerator and then re-analyzed if necessary if and when the result is challenged. Use of infrared analysis of ethanol is a non-destructive technique so the same specimen of breath could be captured and used for confirmatory analysis (Bergh 1985). Several US states required this option for storage of a breath specimen to allow a later confirmatory analysis at a forensic laboratory (Dubowski 1977). When the initial test was completed, the breath inside the infrared cell was pumped through a tube containing a chemical substance that absorbed the ethanol and other organic volatiles in the sample (Parker and Green 1990). The chemical tubes were filled with inert absorbent materials such as Tenax, calcium sulfate or silica gel, which could be shipped to a laboratory and analyzed by gas chromatography (Wilkinson et al. 1981). This re-analysis was practical but required knowledge of stability of ethanol during long-term storage. There were also administrative hurdles to mount, such as chain of custody etc. Since 2016 US states no longer require storage of breath samples for later analysis.

As more and more US states accepted concentration *per se* limits as evidence for prosecution less weight was given to results of clinical tests of impairment, although reliability of the chemical test evidence was continuously being challenged by defense attorney (Gullberg 2004; Jones 1991). With concentration *per se* statutes, the suspect's BAC or BrAC is the most important element in the prosecution case, but more difficult to challenge compared with oral testimony from the arresting police officer. This increasing importance of chemical analysis of ethanol as a test for intoxication led many defense attorney to undermine and criticise the analytical methods and the procedures used. Defense attorney became very knowledgeable about the science and law of blood- and breath-alcohol testing and adept at creating a reasonable doubt and winning an acquittal; see for example the website of the National College of DUI defense (https://ncdd.com/).

A large number of textbooks specializing in the defense and prosecution of impaired driving cases are available explaining the pros and cons of different types of evidence used under a concentration *per se* statute (Taylor and Oberman 2006). The aim seems to be to create a reasonable doubt in the minds of a judge and jury and hopefully win an acquittal for their client. Questions are raised about the qualifications and training of the person performing the breath- or blood-alcohol test, pre-analytical factors, such as observation/deprivation period of 15 minutes before conducting a breath-alcohol test, presence of interfering substances and much more (Bartell and McMurray 2017). Some law firms in UK and North America specialize in the this area of jurisprudence and are very knowledgeable about the disposition and fate of alcohol in the body and inherent problems when blood- or breath-alcohol concentrations are determined (Williams 2018). However, experience has shown that many defense arguments lack substance when subjected to experimental testing and independent scrutiny (Gullberg 2004; Jones 1991). The design of the Breathalyzer instrument required reading the result from an analogue scale calibrated to report the coexisting BAC, which assumed a population average 2100:1 BBR. The constancy of this calibration factor came under close scrutiny in the 1980s and culminated in litigation in the state of New Jersey in 1989 (State of NJ vs Andrew Downie et al.). Legal arguments were heard by a specially appointed judge and expert testimony was presented from scientists working in the United States, UK, Canada, and Sweden. The scientific literature dealing with blood and breath-alcohol testing was reviewed in depth and the magnitude of biological variations in the BBR were discussed and debated. The judge ruled in favor of the continued use of the Breathalyzer instrument in NJ and his opinion was later ratified in a judgment from the NJ Supreme Court.

The bulk of the expert testimony in the case indicated that use of the 2100:1 BBR gave a definite advantage to the suspect compared with measuring the co-existing venous BAC (Begg et al. 1964). It appeared that Breathalyzer® results underestimated venous BAC by about 10% on average unless testing was done during the absorption phase of the BAC curve (Jones 1978a). This follows because BrAC ran closer to the arterial BAC and not the venous BAC and significant arterio-venous differences in ethanol concentration existed during absorption (Lindberg et al. 2007). During the post-absorptive phase experimental evidence pointed towards a 2300:1 or 2400:1 BBR hence favoring the suspect compared with if venous blood was taken for laboratory analysis (Cobb and Dabbs 1985; Jones and Andersson 2003).

4.7 Concluding Remarks

This review has traced historical developments in the methods used for analysis of ethanol in blood and breath for legal purposes on two continents, North America and Europe. Historically, the determination of ethanol in blood and urine pre-dated the development of methods for breath-alcohol analysis. However, for legal purposes today use of evidential breath-alcohol analyzers are the primary means of generating evidence for prosecuting traffic offenders in most nations. With modern technology, the results of analysis of ethanol in breath are equally accurate, precise and selective for identification of ethanol as the use of HS-GLC-FID applied to blood analysis.

Table 4.5 lists some important milestones in development of methods for blood and breath-alcohol analysis and the scientists making these key contributions are also listed.

Table 4.5 Principal Development (1874–2000) in Methods Suitable for the Analysis of Ethanol in Blood and Breath for Clinical, Research and/or Forensic Purposes, the Scientists Involved with This Research and the Country Where They Worked

Year[a]	Scientists and Country Where the Development Work Was done	Brief Description of the Methodology Used to Determine Ethanol in Blood or Breath Samples
1874	Anstie (UK)	Used a mixture of $K_2Cr_2O_7 + H_2SO_4$ as oxidizing agent (chromic acid) for determination of ethanol by visual comparison of the color change with known ethanol standards.
1896	Nicloux (France)	Improved the potassium dichromate oxidation procedure for ethanol analysis making results more quantitative
1914	Widmark (Sweden)	Suggested the analysis of alcohol in urine would be a useful way to verify a clinical diagnosis of drunkenness.
1922	Widmark (Sweden)	Published a micro-diffusion method for quantitative analysis of alcohol in capillary blood samples (~100 µL) by oxidation with $K_2Cr_2O_7 + H_2SO_4$ in excess and determination of the end-point by iodometric titration.
1927	Bogen (US)	Analyzed breath samples by oxidation with a mixture of $K_2Cr_2O_7 + H_2SO_4$ and visible colorimetry for quantitation. He reported that the urine/breath ratio of alcohol was about 2000:1.
1930	Liljestrand/Linde (Sweden)	Determined the blood/air partition ratio of alcohol in-vitro and the blood/breath ratio of alcohol in-vivo. They found that the blood-breath ratio was ~2000:1 at 31°C (breath temperature).
1938	Harger (US)	Breath-alcohol was analyzed with the Drunkometer; ethanol in mixed expired air was oxidized with acidified potassium permanganate and a known volume also trapped on chemical absorbent material for later analysis of CO_2 content, which was used to determine proportion of alveolar air assuming this contained 5.5 vol%.
1941	Forrester Sr. (US)	Ethanol in breath was analyzed by oxidation with $KMnO_4$ to furnish an on-the-spot result and a portion of the sample was trapped on chemical absorbent (magnesium perchlorate) for later analysis at a laboratory.
1941	Greenberg/Keator (US)	Developed the Alcometer, which sampled breath at the end of a prolonged exhalation. The ethanol it contained was determined by oxidation with iodine pentoxide as oxidizing agent.
1951	Bonnichsen/Theorell (Sweden) Bücher/Redetzki (Germany)	The enzyme alcohol dehydrogenase (ADH) was extracted and purified from horse liver and used to determine blood-ethanol concentration in-vitro. Later methods used ADH from yeast, which proved more selective for the oxidation of ethanol.
1954	Borkenstein (US)	Developed the Breathalyzer device, which became widely used for law enforcement purposes in US, Canada and Australia; ethanol was oxidized with $K_2Cr_2O_7 + H_2SO_4$ and a photometric method for detection of the end-point.
1954	Grosskopf (Germany) Kitigawa (Japan)	Development a chemical detector tube containing $K_2Cr_2O_7 + H_2SO_4$ on silica gel for oxidation of ethanol, which was used as a roadside breath-alcohol screening test.
1956	Wolthers (Denmark)	First application of gas-phase chromatography for separation of volatile alcohols in post-mortem specimens.
1958	Cadman/Johns (US)	Described the use of gas chromatography for analysis of ethanol with thermal conductivity detector.

(*Continued*)

Table 4.5 (*Continued*) Principal Development (1874–2000) in Methods Suitable for the Analysis of Ethanol in Blood and Breath for Clinical, Research and/or Forensic Purposes, the Scientists Involved with This Research and the Country Where They Worked

Year[a]	Scientists and Country Where the Development Work Was done	Brief Description of the Methodology Used to Determine Ethanol in Blood or Breath Samples
1962	Lester (US) Machata (Austria)	Use of headspace sampling for analysis of blood by gas chromatography with flame ionization detector (FID).
1970	Penton/Forrester Jr (US)	Introduced a compact gas chromatograph with FID detector for breath-alcohol analysis and possibility of storage of breath samples in crimped indium tubing for later confirmatory analysis.
1971	Harte (US)	Described a compact single wavelength (3.39 μm) infrared breath-alcohol analyzer named Intoxilyzer, which was later further developed to become Intoxilyzer 5000 incorporating three different wavelengths for enhanced specificity.
1974	Jones/Jones/Williams/ Wright (UK)	Introduced the first hand-held electronic instrument for breath-alcohol analysis based on electrochemical oxidation of ethanol with a fuel cell detector (Alcolmeter pocket model).
2000	Andersson (Sweden)	In collaboration with Nanopuls AB, Andersson development a five-filter infrared analyzer (3.3–3.5 μm) for quantitative analysis of ethanol in expired breath (the Evidenzer), which is used for legal purposes in several countries.
2000	Olsson (Sweden)	A Swedish company (Servotek AB) developed an instrument for analysis of ethanol in breath that incorporated passive (contact free) sampling; a mouth piece was unnecessary. Infrared technology was used to measure ethanol, CO_2 and water vapor in a breath and ethanol content of the sample was adjusted to the concentration expected for saturation with water vapor at 37°C as present in alveolar breath.

[a] The year is approximate because the development, evaluation and publication of the research results is often spread over several years.

History has a clang of being old, but to understand any scientific discipline one needs to know its history and in this connection something about the various pioneers involved in this domain of forensic science. Early developments in the US mainly focused on methods of breath-analysis, such as the Breathalyzer® instrument developed by Robert Borkenstein in 1954 (Borkenstein 1985; Borkenstein et al. 1963). Fifty years of roadside breath-alcohol tests conducted by the police in UK was commemorated in 2017 to mark the 1967 road-traffic act when the 80 mg/100 mL (0.08 g%) concentration *per se* limit was introduced (Turnbridge 2017).

The technology available for breath-alcohol analysis has improved considerably since the days of the Breathalyzer instrument, mainly thanks to integrated circuits and the micro-processor chip, which revolutionized design and construction of electronic instruments (Dubowski 1991). The latest generation of evidential breath-alcohol analyzers are fitted with several quality control features including mouth alcohol detectors and ways to detect any interfering substances. After starting the instrument, the main task of the operator is to observe the suspect for at least 15 minutes and then encourage him or her to make a prolonged exhalation into the instrument through a mouth piece. The ethanol concentration is monitored during exhalation and samples captured for analysis after a minimum blow time, and flow rate is achieved to increase quality assurance of the results used for legal purposes (Dubowski 1991).

Since the early 1970s, the gold-standard method for forensic blood-alcohol analysis is HS-GLC-FID or HS-GLC-MS, both of which have excellent intra-laboratory and inter-laboratory precision with coefficients of variation of 2%–5% of the mean (Jones 2013).

When comparing contributions made by scientists in Europe and North America, one can see that US scientists were initially more interested in developing methods of breath-alcohol analysis, whereas in European countries blood or urine samples were specimens of choice for forensic analysis. The basic physiological principles of breath analysis as an indirect way to monitor BAC was first reported in a 1930 article written in German (Liljestrand and Linde 1930). However, at that time it was more practical to take samples of fingertip blood from arrested drivers rather than samples of their breath and shipping this type of specimen to a laboratory for analysis (Widmark 1922).

The UK was the first country in Europe to approve breath-alcohol analysis for evidential purposes in 1983 quickly followed by other EU nations, such as Holland in 1986 and Sweden in 1989. Statutory BrAC limits were introduced such as 35 µg/100 mL in UK equivalent to 80 mg% in blood assuming a BBR of 2300:1 (Cobb and Dabbs 1985). Other countries adopted different units of concentration for reporting statutory BAC and BrAC limits and BBRs ranging from 2000:1 to 2400:1 (see Table 4.1). However, blood-alcohol analysis will always be needed, because some suspects refuse to cooperate with the police in providing the required breath samples for analysis. Obtaining blood samples is a lot easier when people are injured in traffic crash and taken to hospital for emergency treatment. Many people of short stature, and/or respiratory dysfunction are unable to provide two consecutive end exhalations for the required duration of time, flow rate and pressure to satisfy requirements of the instrument (Honeybourne et al. 2000; Jones and Andersson 1996).

It remains an open question whether the enforcement of drunken driving statutes is more effective and economical when instruments for breath-alcohol analysis are used compared with taking blood samples for analysis at an accredited laboratory. However, a definite advantage of breath testing over blood sampling is that it gives immediate results so that decisions can be made to arrest a suspect, suspend the driving license and/or confiscate the vehicle or registration plates. However, if drivers are impaired by drugs other than alcohol, then blood samples are necessary for toxicological analysis.

References

Alobaidi TA, Hill DW, Payne JP. Significance of variations in blood: Breath partition coefficient of alcohol. *Br Med J* 2:1479, 1976.

Andenaes J. The Scandinavia experience. In Laurence MD, Snortum JR, Zimring FE (Eds.). *Social Control of the Drinking Driver.* The University of Chicago Press: Chicago, IL, 1988.

Andreasson R, Jones AW. Erik M.P. Widmark (1889–1945): Swedish pioneer in forensic alcohol toxicology. *Forensic Sci Int* 72:1, 1995.

Anstie FE. *Stimulants and Narcotics*. MacMillan: London, UK, 1864.

Anstie FE. Prognosis and treatment of certain diseases. *Lancet* 90:385, 1867.

Anstie FE. Final experiments on the elimination of alcohol from the body. *The Practitioner* 13:15, 1874.

Atwater WO, Benedict FG. An experimental inquiry regarding the nutritive value of alcohol. *Mem Natl Acad Sci* 8:235, 1902.

Baldwin AD. Anstie's alcohol limit, Francis Edmund Anstie 1833–1874. *Am J Public Health* 87:679, 1977.

Bartell DJ, McMurray MC. *Attacking and Defending Drunk Driving Tests.* James Publishing: Costa Mea, CA, 2017.

Bartle KD, Myers P. History of gas chromatography. *Trends Anal Chem* 21:547, 2002.

Begg TB, Hill ID, Nickolls LC. Breathalyzer and Kitagawa-Wright methods of measuring breath alcohol. *Br Med J* 1:9, 1964.

Benedict FC, Norris RS. The determination of small quantities of alcohol. *J Am Chem Soc* 20:293, 1898.

Bergh AK. Observations on ToxTrap silica gel breath capture tubes for alcohol analysis. *J Forensic Sci* 30:186, 1985.

Biasotti AA, Valentine TE. Blood alcohol concentration determined from urine samples as a practical equivalent or alternative to blood and breath alcohol tests. *J Forensic Sci* 30:194, 1985.

Blomberg RD, Peck RC, Moskowitz H, Burns M, Fiorentino D. The Long Beach/Fort Lauderdale relative risk study. *J Safety Res* 40:285, 2009.

Bogen E. Drunkenness: A quantitaive study of acute alcoholic intoxication. *J Am Med Assoc* 89:1508, 1927.

Bonnichsen RK, Wassen AM. Crystalline alcohol dehydrogenase from horse liver. *Arch Biochem* 18:361, 1948.

Bonnichsen RK, Theorell H. An enzymatic method for the microdetermination of ethanol. *Scand J Clin Lab Invest* 3:58, 1951.

Bonnichsen RK, Linturi M. Gas chromatographic determination of some volatile compounds in urine. *Acta Chem Scand* 16:1289, 1962.

Bonnichsen RK, Ryhage R. Determination of ethyl alcohol using gas chromatography mass spectrometry as a routine method. *Blutalkohol* 8:241, 1971.

Borkenstein RF. Historical perspective: North American traditional and experimental response. *J Stud Alcohol* 10:3–12, 1985.

Borkenstein RF, Smith HW. The Breathalyzer and its applications. *Med Sci Law* 2:13, 1961.

Borkenstein RF, Trubitt HJ, Lease RJ. Problems of enforcement and prosecution. In Fox BH, Fox JH (Eds.). *Alcohol and Traffic Safety* (Public Health Service Publication No 1043). US Department of Health, Education and Welfare: Washington, DC, 1963.

Borkenstein RF, Crowther RE, Shumate RP, Zeil WB, Zylman R. The role of the drinking driver in traffic accidents (the Grand Rapids Study). *Blutalkohol* 11(suppl 1):1–131, 1974.

Brink NC, Bonnichsen R, Theorell H. A modified method for the enzymatic microdetermination of ethanol. *Scand J Clin Lab Invest* 10:223, 1954.

British Medical Association. *Relation of Alcohol to Road Accidents.* British Medical Association: London, UK, 1960.

British Medical Association. *The Drinking Driver* (Report of a Special Committee). British Medical Association: London, UK, 1965.

Bücher T, Redetzki H. Eine spezifische photometrische Bestimmung von Äthylalkohol auf fermentivem. *Klin Wochenschr* 29:615, 1951.

Buijten JC. An automated ultramicro distillation technique for determination of ethanol in blood and urine. *Blutalkohol* 14:405, 1975.

Cadman WJ, Johns T. Gas chromatographic determination of ethanol and other volatiles from blood. *Pittsburgh Conference on Analytical Chemistry and Applied Spectroscopy*, Pittsburgh, 1958.

Cadman WJ, Johns T. Applications of the gas chromatograph in the laboratory of criminalistics. *J Forensic Sci* 5:369, 1960.

Caldwell JP, Kim ND. The response of the Intoxilyzer 5000 to five potential interfering substances. *J Forensic Sci* 42:1080, 1997.

Caplan YH, Levine B. Evaluation of the Abbott TDx-radiative energy attenuation (REA) ethanol assay in a study of 1105 forensic whole blood specimens. *J Forensic Sci* 32:55, 1987.

Cary PL, Whitter PD, Johnson CA. Abbott radiative energy attenuation method for quantifying ethanol evaluated and compared with gas-liquid chromatography and the Du Pont ACA. *Clin Chem* 30:1867, 1984.

Cavett JW. The determination of alcohol in blood and other body fluids. *J Lab Clin Med* 23:543, 1938.

Chundela B, Janak J. Quantitative determinations of ethanol besides other volatile substances in blood and other body liquids by gas chromatography. *J forensic Med* 7:153, 1960.

Cobb PGW, Dabbs MDG. *Report on the Performance of the Intoximeter 3000 and Camic Breath Evidential Instruments During the Period 16 April 1984 to 15 October 1984*. Her Majesty's Stationery Office: London, UK, 1985.

Coldwell BB (Ed.). *Report on the Impaired Driver*. Queen's Printer and Controller of Stationery. Ottawa, Canada, 1957.

Coldwell BB, Smith HW. Alcohol levels in body fluids after ingestion of distilled spirits. *Can J Biochem Physiol* 37:43, 1959.

Coldwell BB, Grant GL. A study of some factors affecting the accuracy of the breathalyzer. *J Forensic Sci* 8:149, 1963.

Cowan JM, Burris JM, Hughes JR, Cunningham MP. The relationship of normal body temperature, end-expired breath temperature, and BAC/BrAC ratio in 98 physically fit human test subjects. *J Anal Toxicol* 34:238, 2010.

Cravey RH, Jain NC. Current status of blood alcohol methods. *J Chromatogr Sci* 12:209, 1974.

Cremer E, Gruber HL, Huck H. Electro-chemical detector for the gas chromatographic determination of alcohols and aldehydes. *Chromatographia* 2:197, 1969.

Crothers TD. Editorial. *Q J Inebriety* XXV1:308, 1904.

Curry AS, Walker GW, Simpson GS. Determination of ethanol in blood by gas chromatography. *Analyst* 91:742, 1966.

Cushny AR. On the exhalation of drugs by the lungs. *J Physiol* 40:17, 1910.

Day M, Muir GG, Watling J. Evaluation of 'Alcotest R80' reagent tubes. *Nature* 219:1051, 1968.

Dubowski KM. *An Evaluation of Methods for the Determination of Ethyl Alcohol in Biological Materials* (PhD Thesis). The Ohio State University: Columbus, OH, 720 p, 1949.

Dubowski KM. Some major developments related to chemical tests for intoxication. *Police* 2:54, 1957.

Dubowski KM. Biological aspects of breath-alcohol analysis. *Clin Chem* 20:294, 1974.

Dubowski KM. Recent developments in breath alcohol analysis. In Israelstam S, Lambert S (Eds.), *Proceedings—6th International Conference on Alcohol, Drugs and Traffic Safety*, Addiction Research Foundation: Toronto, ON. 483 p, 1975.

Dubowski KM. Collection and later analysis of breath-alcohol after calcium sulfate sorption. *Clin Chem* 23:1371, 1977a.

Dubowski KM. *Manual for Analysis of Ethanol in Biological Liquids*. US National Highway Traffic Safety Administration: Washington, DC, 1977b.

Dubowski KM. Recent developments in alcohol analysis. *Alc Drugs Driving* 2:13, 1986.

Dubowski KM. *The Technology of Breath Alcohol Analysis*. US Department of Health and Human Services: Rockville, MD, 1991.

Dubowski KM. Quality assurance in breath-alcohol analysis. *J Anal Toxicol* 18:306, 1994.

Dubowski KM, Essary NA. Response of breath-alcohol analyzers to acetone. *J Anal Toxicol* 7:231, 1983.

Dubowski KM, Essary NA. Response of breath-alcohol analyzers to acetone: Further studies. *J Anal Toxicol* 8:205, 1984.

Dubowski KM, Essary NA. Evaluation of commercial breath-alcohol simulators: Further studies. *J Anal Toxicol* 15:272, 1991.

Dubowski KM, Essary NA. Vapor-alcohol control tests with compressed ethanol-gas mixtures: Scientific basis and actual performance. *J Anal Toxicol* 20:484, 1996.

Emerson VJ. *Alcohol Analysis*, 2nd ed. Royal Society of Chemistry: Cambridge, UK, 2004.

Emerson VJ, Holleyhead R, Isaacs MD, Fuller NA, Hunt DJ. The measurement of breath alcohol. The laboratory evaluation of substantive breath test equipment and the report of an operational police trial. *J Forensic Sci Soc* 20:3, 1980.

Ettre LS. Headspace-gas chromatography: An ideal technique for sampling volatiles present in non-volatile matrices. *Adv Exp Med Biol* 488:9, 2001.

Ettre LS. The invention, development and triumph of the flame ionization detector. *LC-GC Europe* 15:364, 2002.

Ettre LS. Comments on the early history of gas chromatographic methods for oil analysis. *J Chromatogr A* 993:217, 2003.

Falkensson M, Jones AW, Sorbo B. Bedside diagnosis of alcohol intoxication with a pocket-size breath-alcohol device: Sampling from unconscious subjects and specificity for ethanol. *Clin Chem* 35:918, 1989.

Fell JC, Compton C. Evaluation of the use and benefit of passive alcohol sensors during routine traffic stops. *Annu Proc Assoc Adv Automot Med* 51:437, 2007.

Flores AL, Frank JF. *The Likelihood of Acetone Interference in Breath Alcohol Measurement* (DOT HS 806 922). US National Highway Traffic Safety Administration: Washington, DC, 1995.

Forney RB, Hughes FW, Harger RN, Richards AB. Alcohol distribution in the vascular system: Concentration of orally administered alcohol in blood from various points in the vascular system, and in rebreathed air, during absorption. *Q J Stud Alcohol* 25:205, 1964.

Foss RD, Voas RB, Beirness DJ. Using a passive alcohol sensor to detect legally intoxicated drivers. *Am J Public Health* 83:556, 1993.

Fox JE. Gas chromatographic analysis of alcohol and certain other volatiles in biological material for forensic purposes. *Proc Soc Exp Biol Med* 97:236, 1958.

Friedemann TE, Dubowski KM. Chemical testing procedures for the determination of ethyl alcohol. *J Am Med Assoc* 170:47, 1959.

Gettler AO, Freireich AW. Determination of alcoholic intoxication during life by spinal fluid analysis. *J Biol Chem* 92:199, 1931.

Greenberg LA, Keator FW. Portable automatic apparatus for indirect determination of the concentration of alcohol in the blood. *Q J Stud Alcohol* 2:57, 1941.

Gréhant N. Nouvelles recherchres sur l'alcoolisme aigu. *Comp Rend Soc Biol* 52:894, 1903.

Gullberg RG. The elimination rate of mouth alcohol: Mathematical modeling and implications in breath alcohol analysis. *J Forensic Sci* 37:1363, 1992.

Gullberg RG. Common legal challenges and responses in forensic breath alcohol determination. *Forensic Sci Rev* 16:91, 2004.

Guyton DC, Gravenstein N. Infrared analysis of volatile anesthetics: Impact of monitor agent setting, volatile mixtures, and alcohol. *J Clin Monit* 6:203, 1990.

Hachenberg H, Schmidt AP. *Gas Chromatographic Headspace Analysis*. Heyden & Sons: London, UK, 1977.

Harding P, Field PH. Breathalyzer accuracy in actual law enforcement practice: A comparison of blood- and breath-alcohol results in Wisconsin drivers. *J Forensic Sci* 32:1235, 1987.

Harding PM, Laessig RH, Field PH. Field performance of the Intoxilyzer 5000: A comparison of blood- and breath-alcohol results in Wisconsin drivers. *J Forensic Sci* 35:1022, 1990.

Harger RN. A simple micromethod for the determination of alcohol in biological material. *J Lab Clin Med* 20:746, 1935.

Harger RN, Lamb EB, Hulpieu HR. A rapid chemical test for intoxication employing breath a new reagent for alcohol and a procedure for estimating the concentration of alcohol in the body from the ratio of alcohol to carbon dioxide in the breath. *J Am Med Assoc* 110:779, 1938.

Harger RN, Raney BB, Bridwell EG, Kitchel MF. The partition ratio of alcohol between air and water, urine and blood: Estimation and identification of alcohol in these liquids from analysis of air equilibrated with them. *J Biol Chem* 183:197, 1950.

Harte RA. An instrument for the determination of ethanol in breath in law-enforcement practice. *J Forensic Sci* 16:493, 1971.

Hartung B, Schwender H, Pawlik E, Ritz-Timme S, Mindiashvili N, Daldrup T. Comparison of venous blood alcohol concentrations and breath alcohol concentrations measured with Draeger Alcotest 9510 DE Evidential. *Forensic Sci Int* 258:64, 2016.

Hawgood BJ. Sir Edward Mellanby (1884–1955) GBE KCB FRCP FRS: Nutrition scientist and medical research mandarin. *J Med Biogr* 18:150, 2010.

Heise HA. Alcohol and automobile accidents. *J Am Med Assoc* 103:739, 1934.

Heise HA. Chemical tests for intoxication. *Rocky Mt Med J* 55:46, 1958.

Heise HA. Breath and urine alcohol. Practical considerations of simultaneous determinations. *Rocky Mt Med J* 66:37, 1969.

Heise RA, Halporn B. Medicolegal tests of drunkenness. *Penn Med J* 36:190, 1932.

Henry W. Experiments on the quantity of gases absorbed by water, at different temperatures, and under different pressures. *Philos Trans R Soc* 93:29, 1803.

Heyndrickx A, Vandenbussche E, Coulier V. Determination of ethyl- and methylalcohol in blood by gas chromatography: Distribution of ethyl alcohol in a human foetus. *J Pharm Belg* 16:334, 1961.

Hingson R, Winter M. Epidemiology and consequences of drinking and driving. *Alcohol Res Health* 27:63, 2003.

Hlastala MP. The alcohol breath test: A review. *J Appl Physiol* 84:401, 1998.

Hlastala MP. Paradigm shift for the alcohol breath test. *J Forensic Sci* 55:451, 2010.

Hlastala MP, Anderson JC. Alcohol breath test: Gas exchange issues. *J Appl Physiol (1985)* 121:367, 2016.

Hodgson BT, Taylor MD. Evaluation of the dräger alcotest 7110 MKIII dual C evidential breath alcohol analyzer. *Can Soc Forensic Sci J* 34:95, 2001.

Holcomb RL. Alcohol in relation to traffic accidents. *J Am Med Assoc* 111:1076, 1938.

Holland MG, Ferner RE. A systematic review of the evidence for acute tolerance to alcohol: The "Mellanby effect". *Clin Toxicol* (Phila) 55:545, 2017.

Honeybourne D, Moore AJ, Butterfield AK, Azzan L. A study to investigate the ability of subjects with chronic lung diseases to provide evidential breath samples using the Lion Intoxilyzer 6000 UK breath alcohol testing device. *Respir Med* 94:684, 2000.

Iffland R, West A, Bilzer N, Schuff A. Zur Zuverlässigkeit der Blutalkoholbestimmung: Das verkeilungsverhältnis des Wassers zwischen Serum und Vollblut. *Rechtsmedizin* 9:123, 1999.

Jachau K, Musshoff F. Beweissichere Atemalkoholanalytik in Deutschland. *Rechtsmedizin* 19:445, 2009.

Jachau K, Schmidt U, Wittig H, Römhild W, Krause D. Zur Frage der Transformation von Atem- in Blut-alkoholkinentrationen. *Rechtsmedizin* 10:96, 2000.

Jacobsen E. The metabolism of ethyl alcohol. *Pharmacol Rev* 4:107, 1952.

Jain NC. Direct blood-injection method for gas chromatographic determination of alcohols and other volatile compounds. *Clin Chem* 17:82, 1971.

Jain NC, Cravey RH. Analysis of alcohol. II. A review of gas chromatographic methods. *J Chromatogr Sci* 10:263, 1972.

James AT, Martin AJ. Liquid-gas partition chromatography. *Biochem J* 48:vii, 1951.

Jetter WW, Moore M, Forrester GC. Studies in alcohol. IV. A new method for the determination of breath alcohol: Description and examination of the perchlorate method for breath-alcohol determinations. *Am J Clin Pathol* 11:75, 1941.

Jones AW. Micro-technique of sample dilution for determination of alcohol in blood by gas chromatography. *Analyst* 102:307, 1977.

Jones AW. Variability of the blood:breath alcohol ratio in vivo. *J Stud Alcohol* 39.1931, 1978a.

Jones AW. A rapid method for blood alcohol determination by headspace analysis using an electrochemical detector. *J Forensic Sci* 23:283, 1978b.

Jones AW. The precision and accuracy of a gas chromatograph intoximeter breath alcohol device part I—*in-vitro* experiments. *J Forensic Sci Soc* 18:75, 1978c.

Jones AW. The precision and accuracy of a gas chromatograph intoximeter breath alcohol device part II—*in-vivo* experiments. *J Forensic Sci Soc* 18:81, 1978d.

Jones AW. Evaluation of breath alcohol instruments. II: *In vivo* experiments with alcolmeter pocket model. *Forensic Sci* 12:11, 1978e.

Jones AW. How breathing technique can influence the results of breath-alcohol analysis. *Med Sci Law* 22:275, 1982.

Jones AW. Determination of liquid/air partition coefficients for dilute solutions of ethanol in water, whole blood, and plasma. *J Anal Toxicol* 7:193, 1983a.

Jones AW. Role of rebreathing in determination of the blood-breath ratio of expired ethanol. *J Appl Physiol Respir Environ Exerc Physiol* 55:1237, 1983b.

Jones AW. Enforcement of drink-driving laws by use of "per se" legal alcohol limits: Blood and/or breath concentration as evidence of impairment. *Alc Drugs Driving* 4:99, 1988.

Jones AW. Top ten defence challenges among drinking drivers in Sweden. *Med Sci Law* 31:229, 1991.

Jones AW. Reference limits for urine/blood ratios of ethanol in two successive voids from drinking drivers. *J Anal Toxicol* 26:333, 2002.

Jones AW. Urine as a biological specimen for forensic analysis of alcohol and variability in the urine-to-blood relationship. *Toxicol Rev* 25:15, 2006.

Jones AW. Biochemical and physiological research on the disposition and fate of ethanol in the body. In Garriott JC (Ed.), *Medicolegal Aspects of Alcohol*, 4th ed. Lawyers & Judges Publishing: Tuscon, AZ, 2008.

Jones AW. The relationship between blood alcohol concentration (BAC) and breath alcohol concentration (BrAC) a review of the evidence (Road safety web publication no 15). Department of Transport: London, UK, 2010.

Jones AW. Blood alcohol analysis by gas chromatography—Fifty years of progress. In Verstraete A (Ed.), *TIAFT—Our First 50 Years*. Academia Press: Gent, Belgium, 2013.

Jones AW. Evidential breath alcohol analysis and the venous blood-to-breath ratio. *Forensic Sci Int* 37, 2016.

Jones AW. Profiles in forensic toxicology Professor Erik Widmark (1889–1945). *TIAFT Bull* 47:10, 2017.

Jones AW. Profiles in forensic toxicology: Professor Kurt M. Dubowski (1921–2017). *TIAFT Bull* 48:8, 2018.

Jones AW, Andersson L. Variability of the blood/breath alcohol ratio in drinking drivers. *J Forensic Sci* 41:916, 1996.

Jones AW, Andersson L. Comparison of ethanol concentrations in venous blood and end-expired breath during a controlled drinking study. *Forensic Sci Int* 132:18, 2003.

Jones AW, Andersson L. Determination of ethanol in breath for legal purposes using a five-filter infrared analyzer: Studies on response to volatile interfering substances. *J Breath Res* 2:026006, 2008.

Jones AW, Sagarduy A, Ericsson E, Arnqvist HJ. Concentrations of acetone in venous blood samples from drunk drivers, type-I diabetic outpatients, and healthy blood donors. *J Anal Toxicol* 17:182, 1993.

Jones AW, Norberg A, Hahn RG. Concentration-time profiles of ethanol in arterial and venous blood and end-expired breath during and after intravenous infusion. *J Forensic Sci* 42:1088, 1997.

Jones AW, Lindberg L, Olsson SG. Magnitude and time-course of arterio-venous differences in blood-alcohol concentration in healthy men. *Clin Pharmacokinet* 43:1157, 2004.

Jones TP, Jones AW, Williams PM. Some recent developments in breath alcohol analysis. *The Police Surgeon* 6:80, 1974.

Kalant H. Research on tolerance: What can we learn from history? *Alcohol Clin Exp Res* 22:67, 1998.

Kitagawa T. Detector tubes for analysis of alcohol in breath. In Havard JD (Ed.), *Alcohol and Traffic Safety*. British Medical Association: London, UK, 1962.

Kitagawa T, Wright BM. A quantitative detector-tube method for breath-alcohol estimation. *Br Med J* 2:652, 1962.

Kozelka FL, Hine CH. Method for determination of ethyl alcohol for medicolegal purposes. *Ind Eng Chem Anal Ed* 13:905, 1941.

Kramer-Sarrett M, Lin E, Chua KS, Picketshote N, Resaie A, Pimentel M. Examination of the effects of breath hydrogen and methane levels on the EC/IR II. *Can Soc Forensic Sci J* 50:125, 2017.

Krause D. Guidelines for determining the blood alcohol concentration (BAC) in blood for forensic purposes. *Blutalkohol* 44:273, 2007.

Krishan S, Lui SM. A study of acetone interference in Intoxilyzer® 5000C. *Can Soc Forensic Sci J* 35:159, 2002.

Kristoffersen L, Smith-Kielland A. An automated alcohol dehydrogenase method for ethanol quantification in urine and whole blood. *J Anal Toxicol* 29:387, 2005.

Labianca DA. Non-foolproof nature of slope detection technology in the Dräger Alcotest 9510. *Forensic Tox* 36:222, 2018.

Lentner C. *Geigy Scientific Tables—Units of Measurement. Body Fluids. Composition of the Body. Nutrition*. CIBA-GEIGY: Basel, Switzerland, 1981.

Lerner BH. *One for the Road*. The Johns Hopkins University Press: Baltimore, MD, 2011.

Lester D. The concentration of apparent endogenous ethanol. *Q J Stud Alcohol* 23:17, 1962.

Levine B, Smialek JE. Status of alcohol absorption in drinking drivers killed in traffic accidents. *J Forensic Sci* 45:3, 2000.

Lewis KO. Back calculation of blood alcohol concentration. *Br Med J* (Clin Res Ed) 295:800, 1987.

Li TK, Theorell H. Human liver alcohol dehydrogenase: Inhibition by pyrazole and pyrazole analogs. *Acta Chem Scand* 23:892, 1969.

Liljestrand G, Sahlstedt AV. Temperatur und Feuchtigkeit der ausgeatmeten Luft. *Skand Arch Physiol* 25:94, 1925.

Liljestrand G, Linde P. Über die Ausscheidung des Alkohols mit der Exspirationsluft. *Skand Arch Physiol* 60:273, 1930.

Lindberg L. A review of basic physical properties and physiological mechanisms involved in alcohol airway exchange processes and the alcohol breath test. *Blutalkohol* 55:395, 2018.

Lindberg L, Brauer S, Wollmer P, Goldberg L, Jones AW, Olsson SG. Breath alcohol concentration determined with a new analyzer using free exhalation predicts almost precisely the arterial blood alcohol concentration. *Forensic Sci Int* 168:200, 2007.

Lindberg L, Grubb D, Dencker D, Finnhult M, Olsson SG. Detection of mouth alcohol during breath alcohol analysis. *Forensic Sci Int* 249:66, 2015.

Lundquist F. The determination of ethyl alcohol in blood and tissues. In Glick D (Ed.), *Methods of Biochemical Analysis*. Interscience: New York, 1959.

Machata G. Routineuntersuchung der Blutalkoholkonzentration mit dem Gaschromatographen. *Mikrochim Acta* 50:691, 1962.

Machata G. Über die gaschromatographische Blutalkoholbestimmung, Analyse der Dampfphase. *Mikrochim Acta* 52:262, 1964.

Machata G. The advantages of automated blood alcohol determination by head space analysis. *Z Rechtsmed* 75:229, 1975.

Mason MF, Dubowski KM. Breath-alcohol analysis: Uses, methods, and some forensic problems—Review and opinion. *J Forensic Sci* 21:9, 1976.

Mellanby E. Alcohol: *Its Absorption into and Disappearance from the Blood Under Different Conditions*. Her Majestey's Stationary Office: London, UK, 1919.

Mellanby E. Alcohol and alcoholic intoxication. *Brit J Inebriety* 17:157, 1920.

Miller BA, Day SM, Vasquez TE, Evans FM. Absence of salting out effects in forensic blood alcohol determination at various concentrations of sodium fluoride using semi-automated headspace gas chromatography. *Sci Justice* 44:73, 2004.

Newman HW. Alcohol tolerance: Its importance in relation to chemical tests for drunkenness. *Cal West Med* 52:9, 1940.

Newman HW. *Acute Alcoholic Intoxication*. Stanford University Press: Palo Alto, CA, 1941.

Nicloux M. Dosage de l'alcool éthylique dans des solutions où cet alcool est dilué dans des proportions comprises entre 1/500 et 1/3000. *Comp Rend Soc Biol* 48:841, 1896.

Nicloux M. *Recherches Expérimentales Sur l'élimination de l'alcool dans l'organisme* (MD Thesis). University of Paris: Paris, France, 1900.

Nicloux M. Simplification de la méthode de dosage de l'alcool dans le sang et dans les tissus. *Comp Rend Soc Biol* 60:1034, 1906.

O'Neal CL, Wolf CE 2nd, Levine B, Kunsman G, Poklis A. Gas chromatographic procedures for determination of ethanol in postmortem blood using t-butanol and methyl ethyl ketone as internal standards. *Forensic Sci Int* 83:31, 1996.

Oliver RD, Garriott JC. The effects of acetone and toluene on Breathalyzer® results. *J Anal Toxicol* 3:99, 1979.

Olsen K. The first 110 years of laboratory automation: Technologies, applications, and the creative scientist. *J Lab Autom* 17:469, 2012.

Parker KM, Green JL. Delayed ethanol analysis of breath specimens: Long-term field experience with commercial silica gel tubes and breathalyzer collection. *J Forensic Sci* 35:1353, 1990.

Penner DW, Coldwell BB. Car driving and alcohol consumption: Medical observations on an experiment. *Can Med Assoc J* 79:793, 1958.

Penton JR, Forrester MR. A gas chromatographic breath analysis system with provisions for storage and delayed analysis of samples. *Proceedings—5th International Conference on Alcohol and Traffic Safety*. Schulz Förlag: Freiburg, Germany, 1970.

Polissar NL, Suwanvijit W, Gullberg RG. The accuracy of handheld pre-arrest breath test instruments as a predictor of the evidential breath alcohol test results. *J Forensic Sci* 60:482, 2015.

Prouty RW, O'Neill B. *An Evaluation of Some Qualitative Breath Screening Tests for Alcohol*. Insurance Institute for Highway Safety: Washington, DC, 1971.

Rik KJ. Blood or needle phobia as a defence under the Road Traffic Act 1988. *J Clin Forensic Med* 3:173, 1996.

Schoknecht G, Kophamel B. Das Temperaturproblem bei der Atemalkoholanalyse. *Blutalkohol* 25:345, 1988.

Schoknecht G, Fleck K, Kophamel B. Die Zuverlässigkeit von Atemalkoholmessgeräten. *Blutalkohol* 26:71, 1989.

Smith HW. *The Determination of Alcohol and Its Interpretation for Drivers* (PhD Thesis). University of Toronto: Toronto, ON, 150 p, 1950.

Smith HW. Drinking and driving. *Crim Law Q* 3:65, 1960.

Smith HW. Methods for determining alcohol. In Curry AS (Ed.), *Methods of Forensic Science*, Vol 4. Interscience: New York, 1965.

Stewart RD, Erley DS. Detection of toxic compounds in humans and animals by rapid infrared techniques. *J Forensic Sci* 8:31, 1963.

Stewart RD, Erley DS. Detection of volatile organic compounds and toxic gases in humans by rapid infrared techniques. In Stoleman A (Ed.), *Progress in Chemical Toxicology*, Vol 2. Academic Press: New York, , 1965.

Tagliaro F, Lubli G, Ghielmi S, Franchi D, Marigo M. Chromatographic methods for blood alcohol determination. *J Chromatogr* 580:161, 1992.

Taylor L, Oberman S. *Drunk Driving Defense*. Wolters Kluwer: Austin, TX, 2006.

Tiscione NB, Alford I, Yeatman DT, Shan X. Ethanol analysis by headspace gas chromatography with simultaneous flame-ionization and mass spectrometry detection. *J Anal Toxicol* 35:501, 2011.

Turnbridge R. *Fifty Years of the Breathalyser—Where Now for Drink Driving*? Parliamentary Advisory Council for Transport: London, UK, 2017.

Wagner JG. History of pharmacokinetics. *Pharmacol Ther* 12:537. 1981.

Wallage HR, Bugyra IM. Interferent detect on the Intoxilyzer® 8000C in an individual with an elevated blood acetone concentration due to ketoacidosis. *Can Soc Forensic Sci J* 50:157. 2017.

Watts MT, McDonald OL. The effect of sodium chloride concentration, water content, and protein on the gas chromatographic headspace analysis of ethanol in plasma. *Am J Clin Pathol* 93:357. 1990.

Widmark EMP. Om alkoholens öfvergång i urinen samt om en enkel, kliniskt användbar metod för diagnosticering af alkoholförekomst i kroppen. *Upsala Läkareförenings Förhandlingar N F* 19:241, 1914.

Widmark EMP. Über die Konzentration des genossenen Alkohols in Blut und Ham unter verschiedenen Ulmständen. *Scand Arch Physiol* 33:85, 1915.

Widmark EMP. Acetonkoncentrationen i blod, urin och alveolärluft (MD Thesis). University of Lund: Lund, Sweden. 1917.

Widmark EMP. Eine Modifikation der Niclouxschen Methode zur Bestimniung von Äthylalkohol. *Scand Arch Physiol* 35:125, 1918.

Widmark EMP. Studies in the acetone concentration in blood, urine, and alveolar Air. III: The elimination of acetone through the lungs. *Biochem J* 14:379, 1920.

Widmark EMP. Eine Mikromethode zur Bestimmung von Äthylalkohol im Blut. *Biochem Z* 131:473, 1922.

Widmark EMP. Zur Frage nach dem übergang des Alkohols in den Harn durch Diffusion. *Biochem Z* 218:445, 1930.

Widmark EMP. *Die theoretischen Grundlagen und die praktische Verwendbarkeit der gerichtlich-medizinischen Alkoholbestimmung.* Urban & Schwarzenberg Verlag: Berlin, Germany, 140 p, 1932.

Wigmore JG, Leslie GM. The effect of swallowing or rinsing alcohol solution on the mouth alcohol effect and slope detection of the intoxilyzer 5000. *J Anal Toxicol* 25:112, 2001.

Wigmore JG, Langille RM. Six generations of breath alcohol testing instruments: Changes in the detection of breath alcohol since 1930. An historical overview. *Can Soc Forensic Sci J* 42:276, 2009.

Wilkinson DR, Sockrider DW, Bartsch CL, Kataoka YG, Zettle JR. The trapping, storing, and subsequent analysis of ethanol in in-vitro samples previously analyzed by a nondestructive technique. *J Forensic Sci* 26:671, 1981.

Williams PM. Current defence strategies in some contested drink-drive prosecutions: Is it now time for some additional statutory assumptions? *Forensic Sci Int* 293:e5, 2018.

Wolthers H. Vapour fractometry (gas chromatography): separation of primary, aliphatic alcohols (C_1–C_5) in dilute, aqueous solutions: description of a simple experimental apparatus. *Acta Med Leg Soc* (Liege) 9:325, 1956.

Zinka B, Gilg T, Eisenmenger W. Münchener Fälle der Länderstudie 2006 zum Beweiswert der Atemalkoholanalys im strafrechtlich relevanten Konzentrationsbereich. *Blutalkohol* 46:1, 2009.

Zuba D. Accuracy and reliability of breath alcohol testing by handheld electrochemical analysers. *Forensic Sci Int* 178:e29, 2008.

Forensic Issues Involving Alcohol

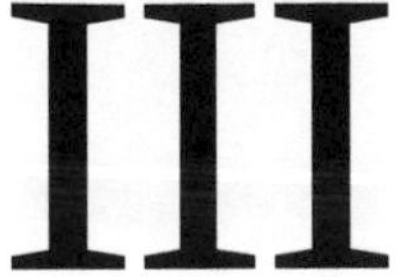

Use of Punishable Limits of Blood- and Breath-Alcohol Concentration in Traffic-Law Enforcement

5

Some Advantages and Limitations*

A. WAYNE JONES

Contents

* This chapter is an updated version of a review article previously published in *Forensic Science Review*: Jones AW: Medical alcohol determination—Breath- or blood-alcohol concentration; *Forensic Sci Rev* 12(1/2):23; 2000.

5.1 Introduction

Daily consumption of alcohol in moderation (1–2 units or 8–16 g ethanol) is not a danger to a person's health or well-being, because the blood-alcohol concentration (BAC) reached is fairly low <0.3 g/L (0.03 g%). By contrast, over-consumption of alcohol impairs body functioning and a person's ability to perform skilled tasks, such as driving deteriorates. Heavy drinking and drunkenness are responsible for considerable morbidity and mortality in society, including blunt or sharp force trauma, drownings, suicides, as well as accidents in the home, on the roads and in the workplace (Cherpitel 2007; Holmgren and Jones 2010; Pajunen et al. 2018).

Road-traffic fatalities represent the leading cause of death in people under the age of thirty (WHO 2018). Postmortem examination of drivers killed in traffic crashes found that between 20% and 50% had consumed alcohol before the crash and that their BAC at autopsy was above the statutory limits for driving (0.02–0.08 g%) in different countries (Jones et al. 2009). Impaired driving after use of psychoactive substances other than alcohol is also a growing problem for traffic safety as evidenced by roadside-surveys and crash statistics (Ahlner et al. 2014; Brady and Li 2014; Gjerde et al. 2011).

Alcohol acts as a depressant of the central nervous system (CNS), and the degree of impairment is tightly linked with the amount consumed (the dose), the speed of drinking, and the BAC reaching the brain (Evans et al. 1974; Weafer and Fillmore 2012). Among other things, a person's peripheral vision deteriorates, reaction times are slower, judgment is impaired and people are more likely to take risks as BAC approaches 0.05–0.08 g% (Ferrara et al. 1994; Moskowitz and Fiorentino 2000). Epidemiological surveys of road traffic crashes, such as the Grand Rapids Study, established a quantitative relationship between a driver's BAC and the probability of being involved in a crash (Blomberg et al. 2009; Borkenstein 1974). In 1967 the UK government introduced a statutory *per se* BAC limit for driving of 80 mg/100 mL (0.08 g%) based on the results of this important Grand Rapids Study (Jones 1988b). This represented a paradigm shift in the way that drunken drivers were prosecuted, because clinical signs and symptoms of impairment were no longer necessary (Penttila and Tenhu 1976; Voas and Fell 2013).

Measuring the concentration of ethanol in blood and other biological specimens requires relatively simple analytical procedures and the results are accurate, precise, and fit for forensic purposes (Seto 1994; Tagliaro et al. 1992). Alcohol tops the list of toxic substances identified in blood samples from apprehended drivers and victims of sudden, unnatural and suspicious deaths, according to forensic autopsies and toxicology reports (Jones and Holmgren 2009a). Accordingly, the determination of ethanol in blood and other biological specimens represents a large part of the workload at forensic science and toxicology laboratories worldwide (Jones 2016).

Forensic alcohol research is tightly linked with the determination of ethanol in biological specimens for legal purposes, and with studies on the disposition and fate of ethanol in the body and interpretation of BAC in relation to signs and symptoms of intoxication. This chapter updates an earlier review article dealing with the pros and cons of breath-alcohol versus blood-alcohol analysis in forensic science and legal medicine when drunken drivers are prosecuted (Jones 2000).

5.2 Historical Background

5.2.1 Alcohol and Traffic Accidents

The dangers of operating a motor vehicle (motor wagons) after consumption of alcohol were recognized early in the history of motorized transportation, as evidenced by an editorial appearing in *The Quarterly Journal of Inebriety* (Crothers 1904):

> We have received a communication containing the history of twenty-five fatal accidents occurring to automobile wagons. Fifteen persons occupying these wagons were killed outright, five more died two days later, and three died a few weeks after the accident, making twenty-three persons killed. Fourteen persons were injured, some seriously. A careful inquiry showed that in nineteen of these accidents the drivers had used spirits within an hour or more of the disaster. The other six drivers were all moderate drinkers, but it was not ascertained whether they had used spirits preceding the accident. The author of this communication shows very clearly that the management of automobile wagons is far more dangerous for men who drink than the driving of locomotives on steel rails. Inebriates and moderate drinkers are the most incapable of all persons to drive motor wagons. The general palsy and diminished power of control of both the reason and senses are certain to invite disaster in every attempt to guide such wagons. The precaution of railroad companies to have only total abstainers guide their engines will soon extend to the owners and drivers of these new motor wagons. The following incident illustrates this new danger: A recent race between the owners of large wagons, in which a number of gentleman took part, was suddenly terminated by one of the owners and drivers, who persisted in using spirits. His friends deserted him, and in returning to his home his wagon ran off a bridge and was wrecked. With the increased popularity of these wagons, accidents of this kind will rapidly multiply, and we invite our readers to make notes of disasters of this kind.

Despite these early warning signs of a pending danger of driving after consumption of spirits there was no effective legislation to deal with the drinking driver. The British Licensing Act (UK Government 1872) had made it an offense to be "*drunk while in charge on any highway or other public place of any carriage, horse, cattle, or steam engine,*" but it was not until 1925 that the statute was extended to apply to mechanically propelled vehicles.

The evidence necessary for a successful prosecution of drunken drivers rested on admissions of alcohol consumption by the driver, the smell of alcohol on the breath and eye-witness reports about the driving incident. The evidence available was improved when the suspect was examined by a physician or police surgeon to document various clinical signs and symptoms of drunkenness (British Medical Association 1927). The results of the medical examination also helped to distinguish alcohol intoxication from a medical condition that might have mimicked drunkenness, such as low-blood sugar, epilepsy, or other neurological or psychiatric disorder.

The examination of arrested drivers was improved when the various clinical tests administered became more standardized and classified as mild, moderate, or severe intoxication. The examining physician might also be called to testify in court as an expert witness and therefore subjected to cross examination. Experience showed that many suspects were acquitted because of the subjective nature of the medical evidence; the defense council often argued that a pathological state or illness had simulated the effects of alcohol intoxication, thus raising a reasonable doubt and an acquittal.

Table 5.1 Percentage of Individuals Judged Under the Influence of Alcohol Based on Clinical Signs and Symptoms When Examined by Seven Different Physicians in Relation to Blood-alcohol Concentration (BAC)

	Physician Number and the Percentage Considered Impaired Based on Clinical Tests[a]						
BAC g%	1	2	3	4	5	6	7
0.00–0.049	0% (0)	25% (4)	0% (1)	50% (2)	0% (2)	0% (1)	25% (4)
0.05–0.099	100% (4)	50% (4)	78% (9)	50% (2)	60% (5)	0% (0)	25% (4)
0.10–0.149	91% (21)	92% (12)	77% (22)	86% (14)	57% (14)	63% (16)	43% (21)
0.15–0.199	100% (32)	97% (34)	100% (34)	94% (34)	83% (35)	69% (39)	77% (38)
0.20–0.249	100% (30)	100% (30)	100% (27)	93% (30)	100% (31)	79% (29)	95% (22)
0.25–0.299	100% (10)	100% (13)	100% (8)	86% (14)	100% (10)	100% (7)	90% (10)
>0.30	100% (2)	100% (2)	100% (1)	100% (3)	100% (2)	100% (1)	100% (1)

[a] Seven different physicians each examined 100 apprehended drivers without knowledge of their BAC and recorded any signs and symptoms of alcohol influence using various clinical tests of drunkenness. The number of suspects at each BAC interval is shown in brackets.

Table 5.1 shows the outcome from a clinical examination of arrested drivers in Sweden (Liljestrand 1940). Seven physicians each examined 100 individuals suspected of drunken driving. The physicians conducted a clinical examination and administered a questionnaire before reaching a conclusion whether the person was impaired by alcohol or not. In general, the higher the BAC the greater percentage of suspects considered under the influence of alcohol. However, there was a lot of variation between different physicians in the intermediate BAC ranges. For example, between 0.10 and 0.15 g% one physician judged 91% of those examined as impaired by alcohol, whereas another considered only 43% of people impaired at this same BAC range.

5.2.2 Chemical Tests for Intoxication

The problem of alcohol intoxication and transportation started to attract attention from the US federal government after prohibition was abolished in 1933, because in the intervening years (1920–1932) ownership of private motor vehicles had increased astronomically (Blocker 2006; Borkenstein 1985). The US government was concerned about the dangers for traffic safety when alcohol became a legal recreational drug. Representatives of the US Department of Justice (Bureau of Prohibition) wrote to the Swedish expert on the subject of alcohol and traffic safety (Professor Erik MP Widmark) asking about the reliability of scientific tests of drunkenness (Andreasson and Jones 1996a). The letter from the US government read in part as follows:

> Such tests in our various states vary from smelling the offender's breath to making him walk a chalk line, but no scientific test apparently is applied.
> We are particularly anxious to know what the alcoholic content of the blood must be before a person can be described as being under the influence of alcohol. Some median line must have been established on one side of which an offender is not under the influence of liquor and on the other side of which he may be said to be intoxicated. Just what that line is we should like to know.

Early in the twentieth century, scientists in Europe focused attention on determination of ethanol in body fluids as an objective way to confirm that a person was drunk thus corroborating any clinical signs and symptoms of alcohol influence (Nicloux 1906; Widmark 1914). Finding a high concentration of ethanol in blood or urine would also help to distinguish alcohol intoxication from a medical condition mimicking drunkenness, such as head injuries, metabolic disorder, hypoglycemia, or a cerebral infarction (stroke) or mental confusion, amnesia, or a manic state (British Medical Association 1965).

A veritable pioneer in forensic medical alcohol research during the first half of the twentieth century was Professor Erik Widmark (1889–1945) who is shown in Figure 5.1.

Widmark investigated analytical and physiological aspects of alcohol in living and deceased persons and the fruits of this research were published in a 1932 monograph, written in German entitled *"Die theoretischen Grundlagen und die praktische Verwendbarkeit der gerichtlich-medizinischen Alkoholbestimmung"* (Widmark 1932). This book was translated into English 50 years later and re-published in 1981 and the title page is shown in Figure 5.1. The life and work of Widmark including his many contributions to alcohol research and traffic safety have been reviewed in depth elsewhere (Andreasson and Jones 1995, 1996b).

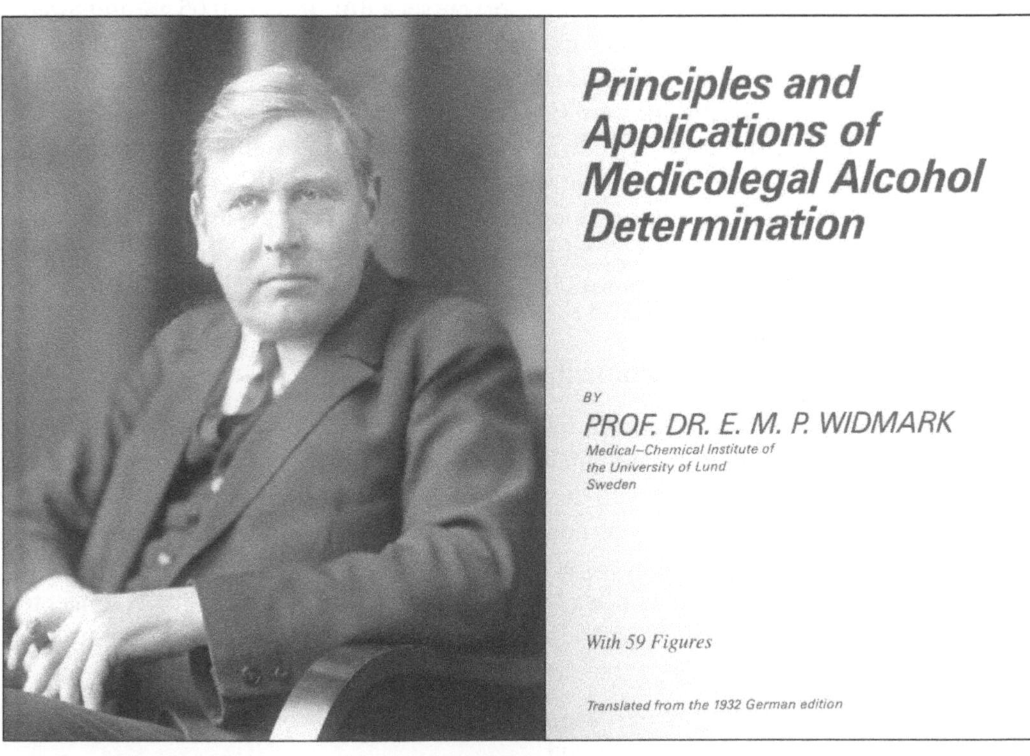

Principles and Applications of Medicolegal Alcohol Determination

BY

PROF. DR. E. M. P. WIDMARK

Medical–Chemical Institute of the University of Lund Sweden

With 59 Figures

Translated from the 1932 German edition

Figure 5.1 Photograph of Erik MP Widmark (1889–1945), who was appointed Professor of Medical and Physiological Chemistry at the University of Lund (Sweden) in 1920. The title page of the English translation (in 1981) of his famous German monograph, which was first published in 1932, is shown at the right.

In 1922 Widmark published a micro-diffusion method for quantitative analysis of ethanol in samples of fingertip blood (Widmark 1922). This analytical method became quickly accepted as a routine procedure for clinical, forensic and research purposes. Ethanol and other volatiles in blood were separated by diffusion in a closed glass flask heated to a temperature of 50°C containing a mixture of potassium dichromate and strong sulfuric acid in excess. After the oxidation of ethanol was complete, the amount of dichromate remaining was determined by iodometric titration and the BAC was calculated.

Blood samples from apprehended drivers were taken at a police station with the aid of specially constructed S-shaped glass capillaries by pricking a fingertip and drawing ~100 µL of blood into the tube. Six capillaries were filled with blood and four were analyzed and the other two kept in reserve. If the four results agreed within 0.025 g% this was deemed acceptable precision. The BAC used for prosecution was obtained by subtracting 0.014 g% from the mean of the four determinations, which is an allowance for analytical uncertainty. The prosecution BAC was stated as being not less than that value reported with a high degree of statistical certainty (99.9%).

The Widmark micro-diffusion method was highly reliable and ethanol concentrations as low as 0.005 g% could be determined with acceptable accuracy and precision. The results of an early inter-laboratory proficiency test of this method are shown in Table 5.2 based on analysis done at laboratories in Sweden, Norway, and Denmark. The good reliability of the Widmark method made it possible for countries like Norway (in 1936) and Sweden (in 1941) to introduce statutory BAC limits for driving. Norway set a BAC limit of 0.05 g% and Sweden 0.08 g%, which was later lowered to 0.05 g% (in 1956) and then to 0.02 g% (1990).

Although urine specimens were easier to collect than blood and also available in larger volumes the urine-alcohol concentration (UAC) is more difficult to relate to BAC and brain exposure to ethanol at the time of voiding (Widmark 1915). Ethanol concentrations in urine reflect the BAC during the time that specimen is formed in the kidneys and stored in the bladder until voided (Biasotti and Valentine 1985). In individual cases, a person might not have emptied the bladder for several hours and during this time the BAC decreases through metabolism in the liver, whereas the UAC was much higher (Jones 2002).

5.2.3 Clinical Tests for Alcohol Influence

Until 1980 every apprehended driver in Sweden was examined by a physician and results from a clinical examination were presented in evidence together with the measured BAC. Often there were discrepancies between the physician's report and the ethanol concentration in blood and this sometimes led to acquittals, despite a BAC *per se* statute. The appearance and demeanor of the suspect was noted along with measurements of pulse rate, pupil size and reaction to light, degree of ataxia when standing upright, slurred speech, finger-finger test, picking up small objects from the floor, and ability to walk straight (Penttila and Tenhu 1976).

Table 5.2 Results from an Early Inter-laboratory Proficiency Test of Blood Alcohol Analysis Using the Widmark Micro-diffusion Method

Blood Sample	Laboratory in Denmark, g%	Laboratory in Norway, g%	Laboratory in Sweden, g%
A	0.087	0.086	0.087
B	0.140	0.139	0.141
C	0.186	0.183	0.188

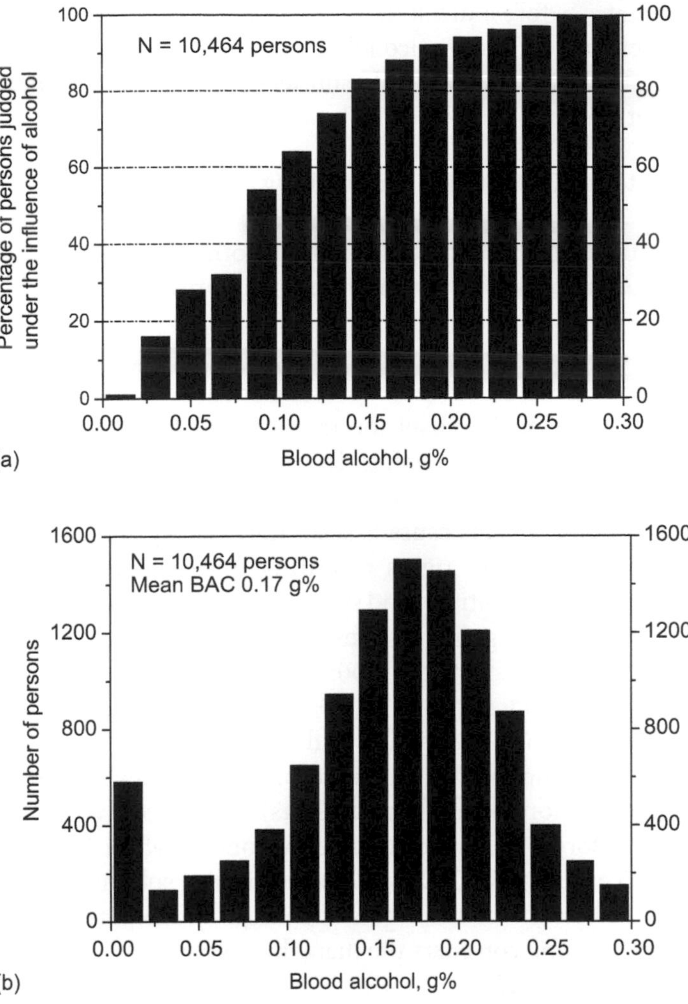

Figure 5.2 (a) Upper plot shows the relationship between percent of drivers judged impaired by alcohol in relation to their blood-alcohol concentration (BAC). After being arrested by the police, each person was examined by a physician, who performed clinical tests of drunkenness. (b) The lower plot shows a frequency distribution of BAC in this same population of apprehended drivers.

The suspects were questioned about recent use of alcohol or other drugs and then a conclusion was reached about the degree of impairment and whether this was slight, moderate or severe. At the end of the examination a blood sample was taken for toxicological analysis. Information from the clinical examinations showed only a weak correlation with the driver's BAC according to studies by several investigators (Widmark 1930; Wolff 1956).

Figure 5.2 (upper part) plots the percentage of individuals (apprehended drivers) deemed under the influence of alcohol in relation to their BAC, which ranged from below 0.05 to above 0.30 g%. About 15% of individuals were considered impaired at a mean BAC of 0.03 g%, 33% at 0.07 g%, 55% at 0.11 g%, and 94% at 0.21 g%. The lower plot in Figure 5.2 shows the distribution of BAC in apprehended drivers in Sweden with a mean of 1.6 g/kg (0.16 g%), and median 1.7 g/kg (0.17 g%). During a prosecution for drunken driving, the BAC was also converted into the amount of liquor (40 vol%) absorbed and distribution in all body fluids and tissues, because this information was easier to comprehend by lay people (Wolff 1956).

In the United States before a drink-driving suspect is arrested, the police require evidence that the person is impaired by alcohol. This requires doing certain behavioral tests, commonly referred to as standardized field sobriety tests (SFSTs), at the roadside in close proximity to time of driving (Burns 2003). These tests included:

- Walking heel-to-toe in a straight line, turning and walking back, while following directions;
- Standing on one-leg for 30 seconds holding the other leg outstretched; and
- Examination of the person's eyes and measuring presence of any horizontal gaze nystagmus.

The results of performing SFSTs and failures in one or more of the tests provide the necessary probable cause or reasonable suspicion that a suspect is impaired by alcohol before making an arrest and doing further testing. This might entail administering an evidential breath-alcohol test or sampling blood for toxicological analysis.

The need to establish probable cause is seemingly deeply rooted in US constitutional law and the Fourth Amendment rights regarding unreasonable searches and seizures (Stuster 2006). However, the sensitivity and specificity of field sobriety tests are limited and both false positive and false negative responses were common especially when BAC was close to the 0.08 g% limit (Hlastala et al. 2005). The reliability of SFSTs to detect impairment at a lower BAC threshold, such as 0.05 g% has not been established.

In many EU nations, and in Australia and New Zealand, the police authorities are allowed to stop drivers at random without any suspicion that they had been drinking (Peek-Asa 1999). The use of random breath testing (RBTs) is an effective way to detect impaired drivers when low statutory BAC or breath-alcohol concentration (BrAC) BrAC limits are enforced, such as 0.05 g% or 0.05 g/210 L. Asking a driver to submit to a RBT is not much of an infringement of the person's human rights and integrity compared with drawing a blood sample for analysis when one considers the many lives saved by removing drunken drivers from the roads (Ferris et al. 2013).

5.3 Statutory Limits of Alcohol in Blood and Breath

The first blood-alcohol concentration *per se* statutes were introduced in 1936 in Norway and 1941 in Sweden. This legal framework made it a crime to drive with a BAC above the prescribed limit regardless of whether the driver showed signs and symptoms of behavioral impairment (Jones 1988a). Most nations worldwide now enforce concentration *per se* limits, although these vary four-fold (0.02–0.08 g%) depending more on political forces, social and cultural norms regarding drinking and driving rather than results of traffic safety research (Fell and Voas 2006b).

A concentration *per se* law creates a razor-sharp difference in outcome in borderline cases and small differences in BAC, which lack any pharmacologic significance, could make the difference between punishment and/or acquittal. A person's BAC is continuously changing depending on the absorption, distribution and metabolism of ethanol, which shows considerable biological variation. This means that the timing of the blood draw or the breath-alcohol test in relation to time of driving is an important consideration for people near a prescribed alcohol limit (Jones 1988a). When evidential breath-alcohol

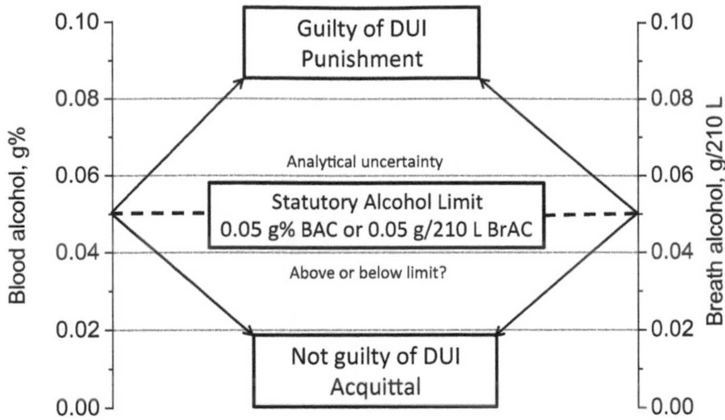

Figure 5.3 Schematic diagram illustrating the consequences of a blood- or breath-alcohol concentration *per se* law and the importance of uncertainty of analytical measurement for those close to a statutory limit.

analyzers are used to test offenders, the way the person exhales into the instrument, including duration of exhalation can alter the final ethanol concentration in the breath by 10-15% (Anderson and Hlastala 2019; Jones 1982).

Figure 5.3 shows the effect of analytical uncertainty in a graphical way and underscores the importance of making an allowance to the final result in borderline cases.

The statutory concentration limits of alcohol in blood and breath currently enforced in different countries are given in Table 5.3. In addition, many countries enforce higher BAC limits that represent a more serious offense with enhanced penalties for those convicted. In Sweden, for example, a BAC exceeding 1.0 mg/g (~0.10 g%) or a BrAC above 0.50 mg/L is referred to as aggravated drunken driving and a person's driving permit can be withdrawn for 24 months and even imprisonment is a possible sentence. However, these stiffer penalties have done little to deter the hard-core drinking driver; because recidivism rates are often as high as 30% within a few years of a first offense (Ahlner et al. 2016).

The threshold limits of BrAC have been derived from the pre-existing BAC limits by assuming a population average breath-to-blood conversion factor. However, no consensus was reached about the most appropriate blood/breath ratio (BBR) to use in the calculation and this varied between countries: 2300:1 (the UK and the Netherlands), 2100:1 (Sweden, Norway, and Finland), 2000:1 (France, Austria, and Poland), and 2100:1 in the US and Canada (Jones 2010a). Since the breath-alcohol limit and the blood/breath factor were fixed by statute, this avoids any legal discussion and debate in individual cases about biological variations in BBR (Jaffe et al. 2013). However, some European countries continue to convert BrAC into the presumed BAC for legal purposes (e.g., Poland, Spain, and Italy).

The statutory BAC and BrAC limits shown in Table 5.3 are arranged depending on whether the various countries use mass/mass or mass/volume concentration units for BAC. Because density of blood is 1.055 g/mL on average (Lentner 1981), a BAC of 0.50 g/kg is the same as 0.53 g/L or 0.053 g%. When BBRs are calculated, mass/volume units must be used for both BAC and BrAC. Accordingly in a country where the statutory BAC is 0.50 g/L and the statutory BrAC is 0.25 mg/L, the BBR is (0.50/0.25) × 1000 = 2000:1. However, if a country has a statutory BAC limit of 0.50 g/kg (0.53 g/L) and a BrAC limit of 0.25 mg/L, the corresponding BBR is (0.53/0.25) × 1000 or 2120:1. In countries where

Table 5.3 Statutory Concentration *per se* Limits of Alcohol in Blood and Breath in Various Countries Worldwide Depending on Whether Mass/mass (m/m) or Mass/volume (m/v) Units of Blood-Alcohol Concentration (BAC) Are Used

Country	Statutory Blood-Alcohol Limit[a]	Statutory Breath-Alcohol Limit[b]	Assumed Blood/Breath Ratio of Alcohol
European Nations Where Mass/mass Units Are Used for Statutory BAC[c]			
Denmark	0.50 g/kg	0.25 mg/L	2100
Norway	0.20 g/kg	0.10 mg/L	2100
Sweden	0.20 g/kg	0.10 mg/L	2100
Finland	0.50 g/kg	0.22 mg/L	2400
Germany	0.50 g/kg	0.25 mg/L	2100
Switzerland	0.50 g/kg	0.25 mg/L	2100
Other EU Nations Where Mass/volume Units for Statutory BAC Operate			
Poland	0.20 g/L	0.10 mg/L	2000
France	0.50 g/L	0.25 mg/L	2000
Belgium	0.50 g/L	0.22 mg/L	2300
The Netherlands	0.50 g/L	0.22 mg/L	2300
England & Wales	80 mg%	35 µg%	2300
Scotland	50 mg%	22 µg%	2300
Ireland	50 mg%	22 µg%	2300
Austria	0.50 g/L	0.25 mg/L	2000
Spain	0.50 g/L	0.25 mg/L	2000
Italy	0.50 g/L	0.25 mg/L	2000
Portugal	0.80 g/L	0.40 mg/L	2000
Other Countries Worldwide Where Mass/Volume Units for BAC Operate			
Australia[d]	0.05 g%	0.05 g/210 L	2100
Canada[d]	0.08 g%	0.08 g/210 L	2100
Japan	0.30 g/L	0.15 mg/L	2000
New Zealand	50 mg%	250 µg/L	2300
US (49 states)[d]	0.08 g%	0.08 g/210 L	2100
US (Utah)[d]	0.05 g%	0.05 g/210 L	2100

[a] In some countries, lower BAC limits might apply to young novice drivers (<21 y) or drivers of commercial vehicles.

[b] These BrAC limits were calculated from the pre-existing BAC limits assuming a population average BBR of alcohol, hence BrAC = BAC/BBR.

[c] Density of whole blood = 1.055 kg/L, hence 0.50 g/kg = 0.53 g/L.

[d] In these countries, the g/210 L breath assumes a BBR of 2100:1.

results of evidential breath-alcohol tests are reported as BAC the instrument is pre-calibrated with the accepted BBR of alcohol.

5.4 Alcohol in the Body

After drinking beer, wine, or spirits, the alcohol (ethanol) contained in these beverages is absorbed from the stomach and intestines (duodenum and jejunum) and enters the portal venous blood flowing through the liver (Kalant 1996a). Ethanol easily passes biological membranes and distributes into the total body water compartment. At equilibrium, the concentrations of ethanol in different body fluids and tissues are proportional to their water content, because ethanol does not bind to plasma proteins nor is it very soluble in lipids. Absorption of ethanol is a passive diffusion process along concentration gradients, so one would expect that ethanol in stronger drinks, such as liquor is absorbed faster than weaker beverages, such as wines and beer (Berggren and Goldberg 1940). This has been verified by experiments showing that C_{max} is higher and t_{max} shorter when subjects drank the same dose of ethanol as vodka (40 vol%) compared with table wine (12.5%) or beer (5%) (Mitchell et al. 2014). A slower absorption of ethanol from beer might be explained by its carbohydrate content, which is known to delay gastric emptying (Jones 1991b). Factors influencing gastric emptying are important determinants of ethanol absorption into the blood, because of a large surface area provided by the villi and microvilli (Cortot et al. 1986).

Eating a meal during or before drinking slows the absorption of alcohol because food in the stomach dilutes ethanol in the drink and also delays gastric emptying and under these conditions, the peak BAC is appreciably less compared with drinking the same quantity of ethanol on an empty stomach (Jones and Jönsson 1994; Kalant 2000; Watkins and Adler 1993). Hyperglycemia slows and hypoglycemia accelerates gastric emptying, which means that time of day when drinks are taken, and other factors influencing blood-glucose level e.g., carbohydrate-deficient diets, pregnancy, and diabetes, are important considerations (Schvarcz et al. 1995). Smoking cigarettes was reported to delay opening of the pyloric sphincter, thereby slowing the rate of absorption of ethanol into the portal blood (Johnson et al. 1991).

Many environmental, genetic and medical factors combine to influence the disposition and fate of ethanol in the body as reflected in the peak BAC reached and rate of clearance of ethanol from the bloodstream (Li et al. 2001). After absorption, alcohol is distributed throughout all body fluids and tissues in proportion to their water content (Endres and Gruner 1994). Drinking alcohol on an empty stomach is usually associated with rapid absorption and an early occurring peak BAC, because stomach emptying is faster and absorption is more effective from the duodenum and jejunum, owing to larger absorption surface area (Jones et al. 1991).

The BAC reached after drinking depends not only on the rate of absorption but also on the person's body weight, liver weight, and particularly the ratio of fatty tissue to lean tissue mass. A person with more fat per kg body weight will generate a higher BAC for a given dose of ethanol than a leaner person, because ethanol is less soluble in lipids compared with water. Because women generally have more fatty tissue per kg of body weight and therefore less body water there are gender differences to consider (Lucey et al. 1999). Accordingly, females are exposed to higher BAC than men for the same dose of alcohol per kg of body weight. This might be important for gender-related differences in organ and tissue damage resulting from heavy drinking (Milic et al. 2018).

After absorption from the gut, the concentration of ethanol in the portal circulation, liver, heart, and lungs are initially higher than in the peripheral venous blood returning to the heart, owing to extraction of some of the ethanol by the skeletal muscles and other peripheral tissues rich in water. The consequence of this is an arterial-venous difference in BAC, the magnitude of which decreases as absorption proceeds. In the post-absorptive phase when ethanol is fully equilibrated in all body fluids the venous BAC is slightly higher than the arterial BAC, by 0.001 to 0.005 g% and the A-V difference becomes negative

(Jones et al. 2004). As ethanol is progressively cleared from the central blood compartment it is replaced by ethanol from tissue-water entering the venous blood returning to the heart, which explains the slightly higher concentration compared with arterial blood. For the entire post-absorptive period, provided no further ethanol is consumed, the V-BAC remains higher than the A-BAC.

The elimination of alcohol from the body begins immediately after drinking and the principal alcohol-metabolizing enzyme is hepatic alcohol dehydrogenase (ADH), which converts ethanol into acetaldehyde, a highly toxic metabolite which is swiftly transformed into acetate by aldehyde dehydrogenase (ALDH) (Zakhari 2006). Most of the acetate produced during ethanol oxidation leaves the liver and becomes oxidized mainly in muscle tissue into carbon dioxide and water, the end products of ethanol catabolism. The alcohol-metabolizing enzymes (ADH and ALDH) display racial and genetic variations and a multitude of isoenzymes exist with characteristic substrate specificity, K_m and V_{max} values and different intrinsic activity (Agarwal and Goedde 1992).

Hormonal influences, such as testosterone concentrations in blood increase the activity of alcohol metabolizing enzymes (Erol et al. 2019). This suggests that women metabolize ethanol slightly faster than men, which would result in enhanced production of the toxic acetaldehyde metabolite (Quertemont et al. 2005). The pharmacokinetic profiles of ethanol were not much influenced by the female menstrual cycle (Mumenthaler et al. 1999); however, women reach a higher BAC than men for the same dose/kg of ethanol ingested, owing to less body water and a smaller distribution volume (Kalant 2000).

The higher sensitivity of Asian populations (Chinese, Japanese, Koreans) to alcohol is related to a genetic defect in the hepatic enzyme for metabolism of acetaldehyde, mitochondrial ALDH (Agarwal and Goedde 1992). In these individuals blood acetaldehyde concentrations are appreciably higher than in Caucasians with normal ALDH activity (Mizoi et al. 1987). The higher acetaldehyde content of blood during ethanol metabolism triggers a host of unpleasant effects including nausea, tachycardia, and breathing difficulties (Mizoi et al. 1989). These clinical manifestations are similar to those seen when people treated with the alcohol-sensitizing drug Antabuse (which inhibits ALDH) drink alcohol (Crabb et al. 1993; Peachey and Sellers 1981).

Another important alcohol-metabolizing enzyme (CYP2E1) is located in the microsomal fraction of the liver cell and becomes involved in the oxidation of ethanol when BAC is between 0.06-0.08 g% which is close to the K_m value of the enzyme (Lieber 1991). After a period of continuous heavy drinking, the CYP2E1 enzyme is inducible, which might explain why alcoholics can eliminate alcohol faster from the blood than moderate consumers (Jones and Sternebring 1992; Keiding et al. 1983). An enhanced activity of CYP2E1 after chronic drinking via enzyme induction has negative consequences leading to adverse drug-ethanol interactions, such as with acetaminophen, organic solvents, and environmental chemicals that produce toxic metabolites (Weathermon and Crabb 1999).

An important consideration when analytical methods of blood- and breath-alcohol concentration are compared and contrasted is whether the results can be used to study the disposition and fate of ethanol in the body regardless of the biological specimen analyzed (Dettling et al. 2006). The time-course of BAC and BrAC should agree well for a wide range of drinking conditions and pharmacokinetic parameters derived from them must be comparable regardless of whether blood or breath was analyzed (Pavlic et al. 2007).

5.5 Pharmacokinetics of Ethanol

The subject of pharmacokinetics is concerned with the absorption, distribution, metabolism, and excretion (ADME) processes and how these can be described in quantitative terms (Dettling et al. 2008). Ethanol is determined in specimens of whole blood or plasma taken at various times post-dosing and a concentration-time (C-T) curve is plotted for evaluation in a quantitative way (Holford 1987). C-T profiles can also be constructed after analysis of ethanol in other biological specimens, such as breath, saliva, and urine and a pharmacokinetic analysis done with these data (Rowland and Tozer 1995). A prerequisite for use of breath analysis is that the target drug is volatile, such as an anesthetic gas, or an organic solvent, such as acetone or ethanol. These substances pass from the pulmonary-capillary blood into the alveolar air and are exhaled from the lungs in breath (Beauchamp 2011).

Knowledge about the pharmacokinetics of ethanol pre-dates that of most other drugs, because analytical methods for BAC determinations were available in the 1920s (Widmark 1922). The C-T profiles were evaluated in mathematical terms by defining a set of parameters that represent ADME processes already in the 1930s (Widmark 1932). During and for some time after drinking the BAC rises until a peak maximum concentration in blood is reached (C_{max}), which usually takes between 10 and 60 minutes after the end of drinking (t_{max}). In the post-peak phase of the C-T profile BAC decreases at a constant rate per unit time (β-slope) independent of the starting BAC according to a zero-order kinetic model and rate constant (k_0) (Jones 2011).

Later studies showed that the linear elimination phase lasted until the BAC had decreased to between 0.01–0.02 g% and thereafter became curvilinear. As more sensitive analytical methods became available in the 1950s, such as enzymatic oxidation, the entire post-absorptive elimination phase looked more like a hockey stick rather than a straight line (Lundquist and Wolthers 1958). The enzyme mainly responsible for ethanol metabolism, hepatic ADH, has a Michaelis constant (K_m) between 0.005–0.01 g% BAC. Accordingly, at a BAC of twice this concentration the enzyme is saturated with substrate at BAC above 0.01–0.02 g%—hence zero-order kinetics. Later work verified these earlier findings when GLC methods were applied to ethanol analysis enabling the determination of endogenous concentrations in blood (Wilkinson et al. 1975).

The entire BAC profile in the post-absorptive phase looks more like a hockey stick rather than a straight line in accordance with Michaelis–Menten saturation kinetics (Wagner et al. 1989). The BAC time course is therefore best described by Michaelis–Menten kinetics rather than zero-order kinetics (Wagner 1973). However, because the BACs encountered in forensic toxicology are from 0.02 to 0.5 g% the Widmark zero-order model is appropriate for most of the questions arising in routine casework (Brick 2006).

Figure 5.4 shows a typical blood-alcohol profile obtained after a healthy male subject drank a moderate dose of ethanol (0.68 g/kg) on an empty stomach. The method used to calculate the volume of distribution of ethanol (r-factor) and the disappearance rate from blood (β-factor) are shown on the plot. This male subject had a V_d for ethanol of 0.64 L/kg and an elimination rate from blood (β-slope or k_0) of 0.015 g% per hour, both of which are important pharmacokinetic parameters for ethanol (Jones 2010b; Maskell et al. 2019). The maximum BAC reached (C_{max}) is probably the best indication of the initial impairment

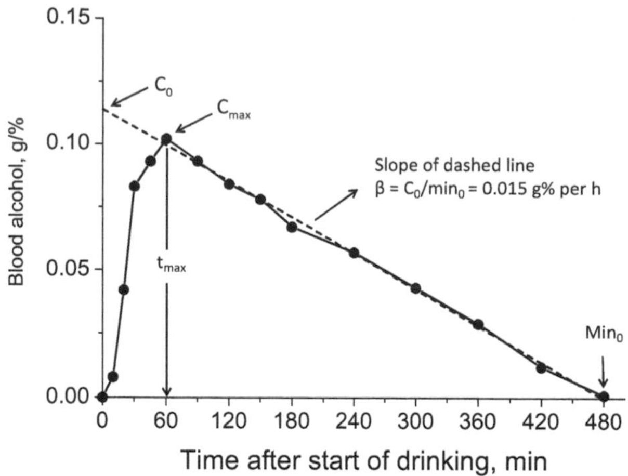

Figure 5.4 A typical blood-alcohol concentration-time profile in one male subject who drank 0.68 g ethanol per kg body weight as neat whisky on an empty stomach. The zero-order elimination rate of ethanol from blood was calculated as shown on the graph, being 0.015 g% per h.

effects on body functions and area under the concentration-time curve (AUC) reflects the duration of exposure of the body organs and tissue to ethanol.

Figure 5.5 shows examples of concentration-time profiles of ethanol in capillary blood and end-expired breath after three male subjects drank neat whisky on an empty stomach. The C-T profiles are clearly very similar when derived from analysis of blood or breath samples; BAC is g/100 mL and BrAC g/210 L to allow a direct comparison. The relatively slow rate of absorption (plot a) or rapid absorption (plots b and c) was well characterized regardless of whether blood or breath was analyzed. These curves are representative examples from a larger controlled drinking study involving 21 healthy men (Jones 1978c). The near simultaneous specimens of fingertip blood and end-expired breath were analyzed for up to seven hours post-dosing (Jones 1984). Ethanol was determined in breath by means of a GLC method (GC Intoximeter) and in capillary blood by an automated enzymatic oxidation method (Buijten 1975; Jones 1978c).

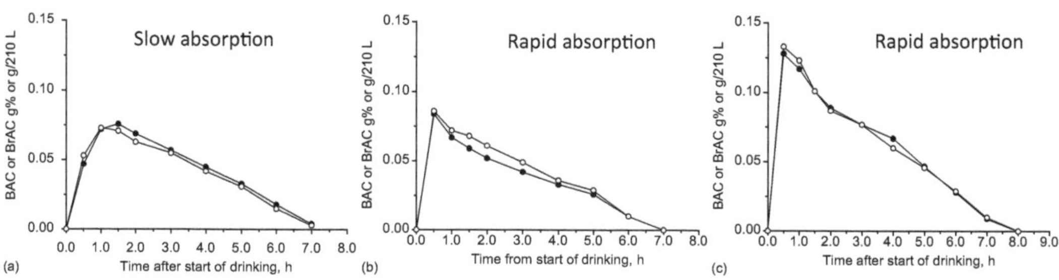

Figure 5.5 (a–c) Concentration-time profiles of ethanol in blood (•) and breath (○) after three subjects drank a moderate dose of ethanol as neat whisky on an empty stomach. The absorption, distribution, and elimination phases of the curves can be monitored equally well from repetitive analysis of ethanol in blood or breath samples.

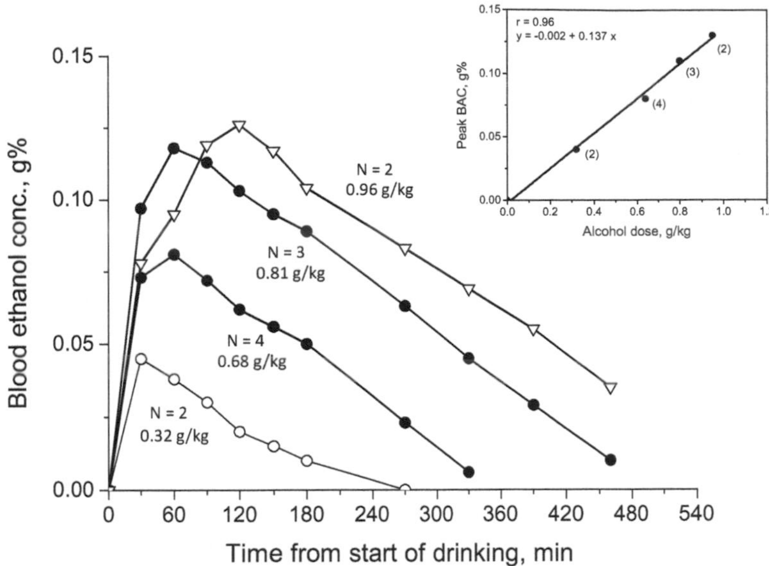

Figure 5.6 Mean blood-alcohol profiles obtained after healthy men consumed increasing doses of ethanol (0.32, 0.68, 0.81, or 0.96 g per kg body weight) as neat whisky on an empty stomach. After the highest dose of alcohol, one subject vomited at 60 minutes post-drinking. The insert graph shows a strong correlation (r = 0.96) between the dose of ethanol consumed and the peak concentration determined in blood.

The shapes of C-T profiles after increasing doses of ethanol consumed as neat whisky on an empty stomach are shown in Figure 5.6 (Gullberg and Jones 1994). The relationship between dose and peak BAC was highly correlated (r = 0.96) as shown by the small insert graph in Figure 5.6. Both the peak BAC and AUC increased with increasing dose of ethanol consumed and it took longer to eliminate all the ethanol from the body after higher doses. Regardless of the dose ingested, there was a linear declining phase (zero-order kinetics) running parallel indicating similar disappearance from blood over this range of ethanol doses.

Another alcohol dosing study was done (0.54, 0.68, and 0.85 g/kg) to compare C-T profiles of ethanol in capillary blood and breath as a function of time after drinking ended. The ethanol concentrations at 60 minutes post-dosing and areas under the C-T profiles were measured and compared for BAC and BrAC. Breath ethanol concentration was determined with an electrochemical analyzer Alcolmeter (Lion Laboratories PLC: Barry, Wales, UK) and BAC was determined by an enzymatic oxidation method (Jones 1985). Figure 5.7 shows close agreement between BAC and BrAC at 60 minutes from start of drinking (40 minutes after end of drinking) and the same was observed for AUC. The pharmacokinetic profiles for breath-alcohol ran on a slightly lower level than the concentrations in capillary blood as verified by smaller AUCs for each dose administered.

Taken together, the results from hundreds of controlled drinking studies involving oral ingestion of ethanol show that the pharmacokinetic profiles in blood and breath are very similar during ADME processes (Mumenthaler et al. 2000). However, making such

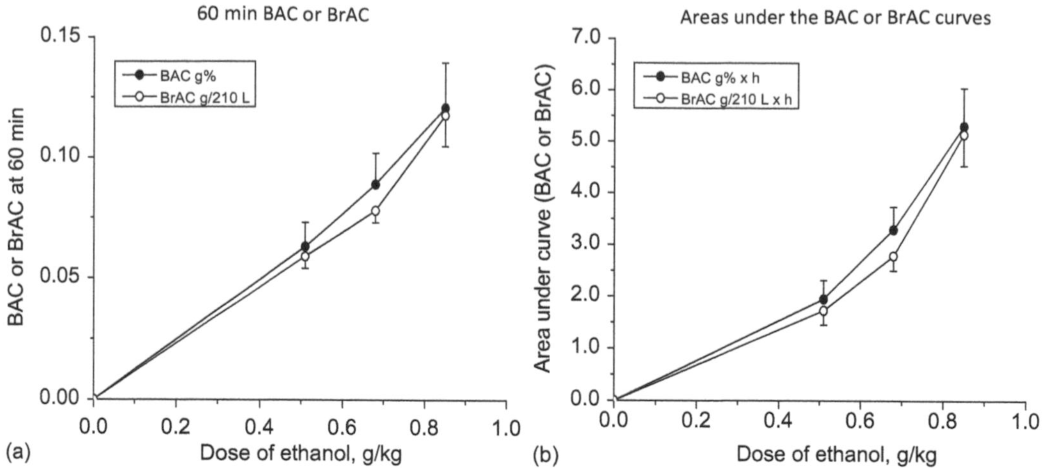

Figure 5.7 (a) Close agreement between blood- and breath-alcohol concentration at 60 min after the end of drinking (left frame) after three doses of ethanol (0.54, 0.68, or 0.81 g/kg) was ingested as neat whisky on an empty stomach. (b) The right frame shows a similar close agreement for area under the concentration-time curves of ethanol in blood and breath.

a comparison requires that BrAC is expressed in units of g/210 L instead of mg/L, owing to the roughly 2000 time lower concentration of ethanol in breath compared with blood (Jones 1978d).

5.5.1 Arterio-Venous Differences

Studies of arterial-venous differences in drug concentrations and pharmacokinetics in humans are scarce (Chiou 1989). For a drug like ethanol, one can expect to find arterio-venous (A-V) differences being more pronounced across organs and tissues with a low ratio of blood flow to tissue mass, such as skeletal muscles, which contain about half the total body water (Kalant 2000). During the time ethanol is being consumed and for some time afterwards the concentration in the arterial blood is higher than in venous blood, owing to uptake of ethanol by tissue water. The venous blood draining the tissue and returning to the heart has a lower concentration of ethanol than arterial blood (Payne et al. 1966). When the absorption of ethanol is complete and there is equilibration in all the body fluids and tissues, the arterial and venous blood concentrations should be the same for a brief instant. For those tissues with a rich blood supply, such as the brain, lungs, and kidney, the arterial-venous differences in ethanol concentration will be small or negligible.

After drinking alcoholic beverages, the concentration of ethanol is highest in the stomach and intestine and in the portal venous blood transporting ethanol to the liver. From the liver ethanol is taken via the hepatic vein to the heart, the lungs, back to the heart and throughout the entire systemic circulation. As drinking continues and more ethanol gets absorbed into the blood and distributed into body water, the A-V differences become progressively smaller. When ingestion ends and the rate of absorption gradually becomes slower that rate of distribution and metabolism, the BAC profile enters the post-peak declining phase (Kaltenbach et al. 1998).

A-V differences in ethanol concentration are shown in Figure 5.8 for one subject who drank 0.60 g ethanol per kg body weight as a bolus dose. Blood samples were taken from

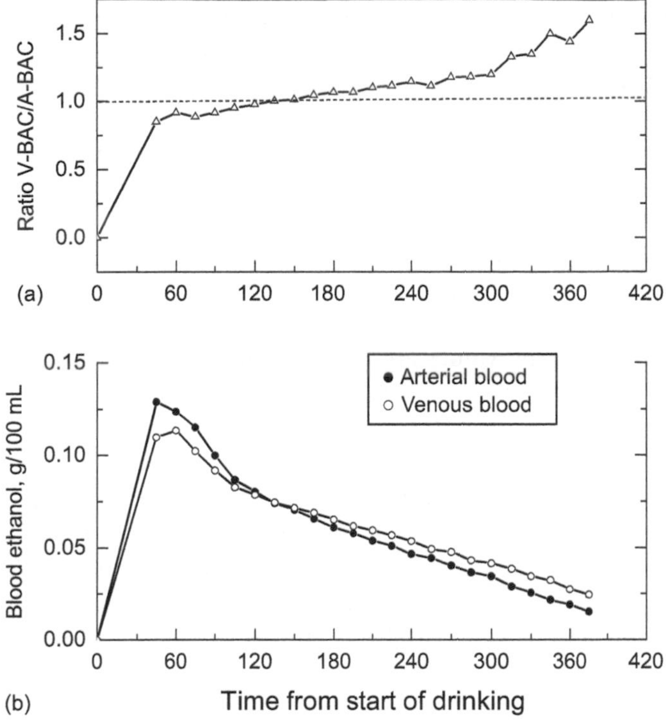

Figure 5.8 Relationship between the concentration of ethanol in blood samples taken from a radial artery (A-BAC) and a cubital vein (V-BAC) after a person drank 0.60 g ethanol/kg body weight. Blood was drawn from indwelling catheters located on the same arm. (a) The upper plot shows V-BAC/A-BAC ratios plotted as a function of sampling time after end drinking and (b) the lower plot shows the actual concentration-time profiles.

a radial artery and a cubital vein for up to seven hours post-dosing (Jones et al. 2004). Arterial BAC rose more rapidly and reached a higher concentration than venous BAC. After about 90–120 minutes a crossover point was reached and thereafter venous BAC was higher than the arterial BAC. As ethanol was gradually cleared from the central (arterial) compartment through metabolism in the liver, ethanol returns from tissue water to the venous blood, which now is slightly higher than arterial BAC. The upper part of Figure 5.8 shows that the A-V differences in ethanol concentration are continuously changing over time throughout the ADME of ethanol.

Ethanol enters the alveolar air sacs by passive diffusion from the pulmonary blood circulation and together with respiratory gases enters the breath. The alveolar BrAC should mirror the concentration of ethanol in arterial blood rather than the venous BAC returning to the heart from the tissues. The high solubility of ethanol in water and blood meant that its blood/air partition coefficient at 37°C is 1800:1, much higher than for other gases and volatile substances (Jones 1983). After passage through the lungs, the oxygenated blood returns to the heart before being pumped throughout the entire systemic circulation and brain to cause impairment of performance and behavior. As measures of diminished psychomotor performance after drinking alcohol, arterial BAC and BrAC are preferred to venous BAC, which has a lower concentration during the absorption phase. Arterial-venous differences are particularly marked after rapid drinking on an empty stomach, which favors rapid absorption into the blood. After ethanol is equilibrated in all body fluids and tissues the A-V differences are much less pronounced and venous BAC is now slightly higher than arterial BAC (Jones et al. 2004).

The commonly accepted blood/breath ratio of alcohol is 2100:1 and this was determined when subjects were tested during the post-peak phase of the BAC curve (Harger et al. 1950). Later studies showed that the BBR depended to some extent on the time after drinking when the samples were analyzed (Alobaidi et al. 1976). During the absorption phase, the BBR was less than 2100:1 and in the post-absorptive phase was 2300:1, which is mainly accounted for by differences between arterial and venous BAC. Accordingly, if a 2100:1 BBR is used to estimate venous BAC before ethanol is fully equilibrated in all body fluids and tissues the resulting values are too high, because BrAC is closer to arterial BAC rather than venous BAC (Martin et al. 1984).

In forensic practice, it is doubtful if many individuals are arrested by the police for drunken driving during the absorption phase of the BAC curve (Jones 1990b). Moreover, it might be argued that if a person consumes alcohol while driving, or if the BAC is still in the absorption phase then the impairment effects of alcohol on driving performance are more pronounced compared with tests made in the post-absorptive phase (Weafer and Fillmore 2012). Under these circumstances, the BrAC is probably a more reliable indicator of exposure of the brain to alcohol and deleterious effects of the drug (Holland and Ferner 2017).

5.6 Alcohol-Induced Impairment

Alcohol, like the general anesthetics, depresses the central nervous system (CNS), resulting in sedation and narcosis in a dose-dependent manner (Rubenzer 2011). After drinking moderate quantities of alcohol to reach a BAC of 0.03 g%, a person becomes more talkative, experiences feelings of mild euphoria, especially during the rising phase of the BAC profile. As more alcohol is consumed and the BAC increases, above 0.08 g% the impairment of body functions is more evident; reaction times are slower, divided attention tasks are more difficult, gait is unsteady and speech is slurred. At BACs of 0.15 g% many people have lost self-control and need help in standing and walking straight, some might exhibit aggressive behavior and are difficult to reason or rationalize with (Ziporyn 1985).

Unlike other CNS depressants such as barbiturates or benzodiazepines or even anesthetic gases, much larger quantities of ethanol must be consumed to cause narcosis and impairment of body functions. This follows from the high solubility of ethanol in water and the fact body water comprises 50%–60% of body weight, leading to massive dilution of the dose ingested. The impairment effects of drinking alcoholic beverages must have been recognized thousands of years ago and caused problems for public health then as it is today (Room et al. 2005). Over-consumption of alcohol is particularly dangerous when skilled tasks, such as driving are performed (Canfield et al. 2014).

The first suspicion that a motorist is under the influence of alcohol or drugs usually comes from observations about the manner of driving or involvement in a crash. After eye-to-eye contact with the driver and depending on his or her behavior, the answers to questions and any smell of alcohol on the breath, slurred speech, etc., raises a suspicion of impaired driving. The arresting police officer might then administer a battery of field-sobriety tests which normally includes: (a) walking and turning, (b) one-leg stand,

(c) finger-to-nose, and (d) horizontal gaze nystagmus (HGN) (Burns 2003). In some jurisdictions, the police are permitted to perform a roadside breath-alcohol test to confirm initial suspicions of drunken driving (Kriikku et al. 2014). Depending on the results, the suspect is cautioned, arrested and taken for more rigorous testing, which might entail an evidential breath-alcohol test or a blood sample for toxicological analysis. If the driver is suspected of being under the influence of drugs other than alcohol then a physician or police surgeon is instructed to make a clinical examination (Penttila and Tenhu 1976). In the United States and other nations police officers are specially trained in recognizing the signs and symptoms of impairment associated with certain psychoactive substances and these individuals are referred to as "drug recognition experts" and are expected to examine arrested drivers (Page 2002).

People behave differently after consumption of the same dose of ethanol, depending on many factors, such as their personality, pattern of drinking, type of alcoholic beverage, fed vs fasted state, mental health, age and gender, etc. The same amount of alcohol consumed by the same individual on different occasions can produce different signs and symptoms of alcoholic influence. A major stumbling block to using behavioral tests as evidence of impairment is different complexity of the tasks performed, the experience of the examining physician or police officer and the development of tolerance to ethanol and whether the BAC curve was in the rising phase or the declining at the time tests were made (Morris et al. 2017).

5.6.1 Development of Tolerance

Tolerance to the effects of alcohol has been recognized for centuries and anecdotes about people who "can hold their liquor" or "who never seem to get drunk" are illustrations of this phenomenon (Kalant 1998). Human beings show enormous variation in their response to ethanol and other drugs of abuse. Besides innate differences caused by genetic and hereditary factors, people develop tolerance to the pharmacological effects of ethanol and other drugs after repeated usage, so that the brain adapts to the untoward effects (Kalant 1996b). Alcohol intoxication is not always visible and people with high BAC, such as 0.3 g% might not exhibit overt signs and symptoms of impairment (Brick and Erickson 2009). Indeed, physicians have declared people sober despite high BAC, indicating the development of tolerance to alcohol (Olson et al. 2013).

Widmark recognized two kinds of alcohol tolerance: (a) consumption tolerance, and (b) concentration tolerance (Widmark 1981). Consumption tolerance means that after a given consumption of alcohol, widely different concentrations are reached in the blood owing to different patterns of absorption, distribution, and elimination as well as any gender, body weight, and body water differences. The inter-individual differences in organ and tissue damage caused by alcohol and susceptibility to alcohol dependence is probably more related to consumption tolerance. Concentration tolerance, on the other hand, is related to the first appearance of symptoms of alcohol influence at a particular threshold BAC. The intensity of these symptoms can differ widely among different people despite the same BAC being reached.

Another aspect of tolerance to alcohol is acute tolerance (Holland and Ferner 2017), which was already noted by Mellanby (1920), who found that the degree of impairment was greater at a given venous BAC on the rising portion of the blood alcohol curve than at the same concentration on the descending limb of the BAC curve. A higher arterial

Table 5.4 Percentages of Subjects Judged to Be Under the Influence of Alcohol According to the Time After End of Drinking When They Were Examined by Physicians Who Looked for Signs and Symptoms of Drunkenness

	Percentage of Subjects Judged to Be Under the Influence of Alcohol		
Blood Alcohol, g%[a]	BAC Still Rising	1.0–1.5 hours Post-Peak	2.0–2.5 hours Post-Peak
0.012–0.050	50% (40/80)	NA[b]	0% (0/4)
0.051–0.080	57% (47/83)	5% (1/18)	0% (0/28)
0.081–0.100	66% (33/49)	4% (1/23)	4% (1/24)
0.101–0.120	77% (40/52)	36% (8/22)	21% (4/19)
0.121–0.140	69% (29/42)	38% (8/21)	15% (3/20)
0.141–0.160	91% (30/33)	NA[b]	NA[b]

[a] Subjects drank 0.75, 1.0, or 1.25 g/kg body weight as a bolus dose on an empty stomach.
[b] NA = not applicable because there were no subjects with BACs at these specific times after drinking.

BAC during absorption might explain some of the acute tolerance development, but there is a generalconsensus among behavioral scientists that acute tolerance develops almost immediately after administration of alcohol and that this effect is independent of the dose (Forney et al. 1964). A faster rate of change in BAC on the ascending limb of the BAC curve is an important consideration for the degree of intoxication and the development of acute tolerance (Morris et al. 2017).

Table 5.4 makes a comparison of clinical signs and symptoms of alcohol impairment and BAC on the rising and declining limbs of the blood-alcohol curve. The volunteers drank a bolus dose of ethanol (0.75, 1.0, or 1.25 g/kg), and samples of venous blood were taken for analysis at various times post-dosing. Each subject was examined by a physician and a battery of behavioral tests was administered at or near to when blood was taken for determination of ethanol. The physicians were required to decide whether the subjects they had examined were "under the influence of alcohol" or not (Alha 1951).

The results in Table 5.4 make it clear that a larger proportion of subjects were judged as impaired during the rising phase of the BAC curve compared with tests done 1–1.5 and 2–2.5 hours after drinking ended. One can also see that the mean BAC when samples were taken on the post-peak phase of the BAC curve were higher than during the absorptive phase. By 1–2.5 hours post-dosing most subjects had entered the post-absorptive phase of the BAC curve and had adapted to the acute effects of alcohol on brain functioning (Alha 1951). This phenomenon is a good illustration of the development of acute tolerance to the effects of a drug during a single exposure (Martin and Moss 1993).

Alcohol influences sensory, motor, and cognitive functions in a dose-dependent manner as reflected in greater impairment after increasing doses and higher BAC (Goldberg 1943). The idea of using some computer-based performance testing of traffic offenders to determine degree of impairment is hard to defend, because baseline or pre-drinking results are unavailable for that person. The eye movements, such as gaze nystagmus, are sensitive to effects of alcohol and other drugs although measuring these in a reliable way require considerable training and co-operation from the subject tested. Many people arrested for drunken driving are obstreperous and not willing to cooperate with the police in conducting the necessary clinical tests of impairment. The quantitative analysis of ethanol in samples of blood or breath therefore represents the most reliable and objective way to prove over-consumption of alcohol and evidence for prosecution in impaired driving cases. The measured BAC or BrAC can also be used to calculate the amount of alcohol in the body and the total amount consumed if the time of starting to drink is known (Jones and Holmgren 2009b).

5.7 Methods of Analyzing Alcohol in Blood and Breath

Qualitative and quantitative determination of ethanol in body fluids represents the most frequently requested chemical analysis at forensic toxicology laboratories since the 1950s (Wigmore and Langille 2009). The analytical technology available for ethanol determination in blood and breath is accurate, precise, and specific for identifying ethanol. The chronological development of various methods of forensic blood-alcohol analysis are summarized in Table 5.5.

5.7.1 Blood-Alcohol Methods

The first methods of blood-alcohol analysis appeared more than 100 years ago and although by modern standards these procedures were rather primitive, they at least took the guesswork out of deciding whether a person had over-indulged in alcoholic beverages (Nicloux 1906). The first analytical procedures required that ethanol was first separated from the biological matrix either by diffusion, distillation, or aeration prior to its analysis by chemical oxidation with chromic acid. Otherwise, the proteins in the biological matrix could be precipitated by adding perchloric acid and determination of ethanol in the supernatant after centrifugation. The principal oxidizing agent used was a mixture of potassium dichromate and strong sulfuric acid in excess (Harger 1935). The amount of oxidizing agent remaining after reacting with ethanol was determined by volumetric analysis using sodium thiosulfate and iodometric titration (Widmark 1922). The main drawback of the wet-chemistry

Table 5.5 Chronological Development of the Analytical Methods Used for Determination of Ethanol in Blood for Legal Purposes

Time Period	Analytical Principles Used for the Determination of Ethanol in Blood
1900–1950	Chemical oxidation of alcohol with mixtures of potassium dichromate and sulfuric acid after separation of volatiles from the biological matrix by diffusion, distillation, or aeration.
1950–1960	Enzymatic oxidation of ethanol with alcohol dehydrogenase (ADH) extracted from yeast.[a] Separation of ethanol by diffusion or analysis of the supernatant after protein precipitation. The coenzyme nicotinamide adenine dinucleotide (NAD^+) becomes quantitatively reduced in the reaction to NADH which is monitored at a wavelength of 340 nm.
1960–1970	Gas chromatography (packed columns)[b] and flame ionization detector with direct injection of the blood sample after dilution (1:10) with an internal standard (*n*-propanol).
1972–2000	Headspace gas chromatography (packed columns)[b] with flame ionization detector by sampling the vapor phase in equilibrium with the blood sample after dilution (1:10) with an internal standard (*n*-propanol or *t*-butanol) and heating to 50°C or 60°C.
1985–2000	Headspace gas chromatography-mass spectrometry was used for identification of ethanol by its mass fragments *m/z* 31 (base peak), 46 (molecular ion), and 45 on electron impact.

[a] Various modifications of the ADH method are used to complement results from analysis by gas chromatography and thus two different analytical principles for ethanol determination. The ADH method for ethanol can be incorporated into immunoassay methods for the determination of drugs of abuse, e.g., enzyme multiplied immunoassay technique (EMIT).

[b] Capillary or wide bore columns are now more commonly used for blood-alcohol analysis by gas chromatography.

oxidation methods was their lack of specificity, because other organic volatiles, if present in the blood specimen (e.g., acetone, methanol, ether), were also oxidized, resulting in artificially high BAC results (Friedemann and Dubowski 1959).

In the 1950s, enzymatic oxidation, a much milder procedure, was introduced when the alcohol dehydrogenase (ADH) enzyme had been isolated and purified from horse liver and yeast (Bonnichsen and Wassen 1948). ADH methods were more selective for the identification of ethanol, because acetone in the blood or urine did not represent a problem because it was not a good substrates for oxidation by ADH. By optimizing the conditions of the enzymatic reaction in relation to pH, reaction time, temperature, and source of the enzyme, higher specificity was achieved because oxidation of methanol occurred very slowly under these conditions (Bonnichsen and Theorell 1951). Furthermore, learning the necessary analytical procedures was a lot easier for technicians with ADH methods compared with chemical oxidation and titrimetric analysis. Larger batches of specimens could be analyzed daily with the ADH method, and this was becoming increasingly necessary considering the higher prevalence of drunken driving arrests during the 1950s–1960s. The ADH method of blood-alcohol analysis lent itself to automation and various Auto-Analyzer systems from Technicon, which were already being used in clinical chemistry laboratories were adapted for ethanol determinations (Buijten 1975).

Since the early 1960s, gas chromatography (GC) has been the forensic method of choice for determination of ethanol and other volatiles in biological samples (Curry et al. 1966). GC methods furnish both a qualitative screening analysis and a quantitative determination in the same analytical run. Unknown substances are identified from their retention time RT (the time from injection to appearance of the peak) and comparison with the RT of authentic standard substance. Finding coincident retention times when the same sample is analyzed with two or more different chromatographic systems (i.e., different stationary phases in the column) furnishes very strong evidence for positive identification of the unknown volatile substance (qualitative analysis). Quantitative analysis requires measuring the area under the resulting peak on the chromatogram and comparing this with a calibration curve constructed from analysis of known strength ethanol standards under the same conditions.

Computer-aided analytical methods and dedicated chromatographic work-stations are now available in forensic laboratories for blood-alcohol analysis. These permit more rapid data handling including multiple point calibration curves, non-linear curve fitting, on-line statistical analysis and quality assurance of the results used for legal purposes along with control charts (Jones and Schuberth 1989).

GC methods with flame ionization detector (FID) are highly sensitive for determination of low-molecular-weight alcohols, and 1–2 μL of blood specimen is sufficient for a single determination. Problems caused by blood proteins clogging the micro-syringes or the inlet to the chromatographic column is avoided by dilution of the specimen 1 + 10 with an internal standard (*n*-propanol or *t*-butanol) before injection and use of a glass pre-column placed before the analytical column (Jones 1977). Otherwise, blood-proteins can be removed by precipitation with acids or organic solvents and the supernatant analyzed or ethanol can be removed from the blood by distillation prior to analysis. However, these approaches were rather time consuming and unnecessary and are unnecessary with modern methods used today.

The current analytical methods used in forensic laboratories involves GC analysis and a technique known as headspace (HS) sampling—hence the so-called HS-GC method, which is ideally suited for determination of volatile organic substances

(Anthony et al. 1980). In brief, an aliquot of whole blood (100 μL) is first diluted 1 + 10 with *n*-propanol as an internal standard and the mixture is allowed to equilibrate in an air-tight container kept at 50°C or 60°C (Watts and McDonald 1987). After reaching vapor-liquid equilibration, which normally requires 20–30 minutes of heating at constant temperature, an aliquot of the vapor phase is removed with a gas-tight syringe and injected into the gas chromatograph (Machata 1975).

Figure 5.9 is a schematic showing the setup for headspace sampling along with GC analysis of blood-ethanol using *n*-propanol as an internal standard. A portion of the equilibrated air-phase above the blood sample is removed with a gas-tight syringe and injected into the GC for analysis. When large numbers of samples have to be determined, some automated sampling system is desirable and such equipment is available from several manufacturers. Up to 110 samples can be determined by HS analysis in the same analytical run. The results of HS-GC analysis of blood-ethanol are highly accurate and precision as verified by inter-laboratory proficiency tests; the between laboratory coefficients of variation (CV) are about 2%–5% and within-run precision show CVs of 0.50%–1.0% (Jones 2013).

Pre-analytical factors are also important to consider in connection with blood sampling for forensic purposes including chain of custody consideration such as:

- Qualifications and experience of the person charged with drawing blood, whether physician, nurse, phlebotomist, laboratory technician, or police officer;
- Swabbing (disinfection) of the skin at the venipuncture site should not be done with ethanol or isopropanol even though risk of carry-over of alcohol to the blood is very unlikely (Lippi et al. 2017);

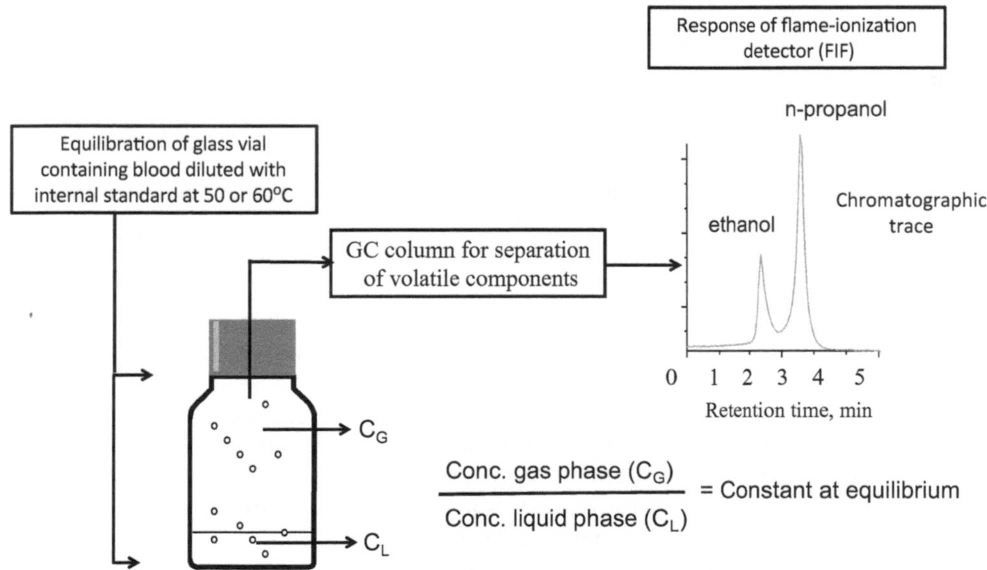

Figure 5.9 Schematic diagram showing analytical setup necessary for gas chromatographic headspace analysis of ethanol in blood after dilution with *n*-propanol as an internal standard. The headspace sampling vial is shown along with a chromatogram containing a peak for ethanol and another for *n*-propanol.

- Type of evacuated tubes; expiry date, nominal volume, color of stopper, glass or plastic, and amount of sodium fluoride preservative and anticoagulant present (Jones and Ericsson 2016);
- Number of inversion of the blood tubes after sampling to ensure adequate mixing and dissolution of the chemical preservatives to avoid formation of clots;
- Control proper labeling of the tubes with name of suspect, date and time, and mode of transport and/or shipment to the laboratory;
- Use of security tapes or other tamper proofing procedures to ensure specimen integrity?
- Where the packages refrigerated during transport and how much time elapsed from sampling to arrival and registration at the laboratory?
- Inspection of the tubes on arrival; volume of blood to air space in the tube (Jones and Fransson 2003); and
- Stability of ethanol in blood during storage at the laboratory (Shan et al. 2011).

5.7.2 Breath-Alcohol Methods

The methods available for measuring ethanol in breath have undergone enormous improvements over the past 75 years since the Breathalyzer was developed. These developments are summarized in Table 5.6 in roughly chronological order between the years 1938 and 2019.

Like methods of blood-alcohol analysis, the concentration of ethanol in breath was determined by chemical oxidation with potassium dichromate, potassium permanganate,

Table 5.6 Chronological Development in Analytical Methods for Determination of Alcohol in Breath for Legal Purposes

Time Period	Analytical Principles and Instruments Used for the Determination of Ethanol in Breath
1938–1950	Chemical oxidation with potassium permanganate (Drunkometer and Intoximeter) to give an immediate, but qualitative result followed by storage of a portion of mixed expired air for laboratory analysis and quantitation determination of ethanol after calculating the proportion of alveolar air from its CO_2 content (Drunkometer, Intoximeter). The Alcometer instrument captured a sample of end-exhaled breath and ethanol was determined by oxidation with iodine pentoxide.
1954	Chemical oxidation of ethanol with potassium dichromate + sulfuric acid and photometry for detecting the endpoint (Breathalyzer).
1969–1970	Gas chromatography with thermal conductivity detector (AlcoAnalyzer) or flame ionization detector (GC Intoximeter).
1971	Single wavelength infrared absorptiometry at 3.39 or 3.4 μM (Intoxilyzer 4011).
1972–1980	Hand-held electrochemical (fuel cell) analyzers such as Alcolmeter SD-2, or 400, AlcoSensor III and IV and the Alcotest 7110, 7410, or 9510.
1980	Infrared spectrometry at a single wavelength of 3.4 μM (Intoximeter 3000) or at three wavelengths 3.39–3.42 μM (C–H) bond stretching frequency (Intoxilyzer 5000 and DataMaster) or at 9.5 μM for (C–O) bond stretching (Alcotest 7110, 7410, 9510).
1990s	Dual sensor technology incorporating both electrochemical oxidation (fuel cell) and infrared absorption at 9.5 μM (Alcotest 7110, 7310, and 9510).
2000s	Small compact mass spectrometers, although developed and commercially available are rarely used for analysis of ethanol and forensic testing.
2010s	Contact-free quantitative analysis of ethanol in breath using water vapor as an internal standard enabling rapid analysis without the need for making a prolonged exhalation or attaching a mouth piece to the instrument (Grubb et al. 2012).

or iodide pentoxide as oxidizing agents. The first generation of instruments were the Drunkometer, the Alcometer, and the portable Intoximeter. These devices were operated by trained police officers and gave an indication of the driver's BAC, although by modern standards the results could only be considered semi-quantitative (Friedemann and Dubowski 1959).

A breakthrough came with development of the Breathalyzer instrument by Robert F. Borkenstein in 1954, which incorporated several novel features compared with its predecessors (Borkenstein and Smith 1961). It was more robust, simpler to use (making it easier to train police operators), and exhibited a remarkable long-term stability when used in the field under diverse conditions. The Breathalyzer instrument gave results within a couple of minutes of sampling breath, and by the 1960s was firmly established and used in law enforcement in US states, Canada, and Australia. When BAC was compared with BrAC determined with the Breathalyzer, the results were 10%–15% low—thus erring on the side of the person being tested (Begg et al. 1964). The Breathalyzer instrument was also used in epidemiological research to determine risk of a driver being involved in a crash, such as the Grand Rapids Study from 1965 (Borkenstein 1974).

In the early 1970s several new technologies were introduced for breath-alcohol analysis including gas chromatography (Penton and Forrester 1970), infrared (IR) spectrometry (Harte 1971), and electrochemical oxidation (Jones et al. 1974). The advent of microprocessors brought about a revolution in the size and construction of instruments for breath-alcohol analysis. Small hand-held breath-alcohol analyzers became widely used, primarily for roadside screening of motorists, such as the Alcolmeter pocket model (Lion Laboratories PLC, Barry, UK), the Intoxilyzer (CMI Inc., Owensbro, KY), the AlcoSensor (Intoximeter Inc., St. Louis, MI), and the Alcotest (Draeger Safety Inc., Breathalyzer Division, Durango, CO). These are hand-held devices and all of them incorporate electrochemical oxidation for determination of alcohol (fuel-cell) sensors (Zuba 2008). Different display options are available including pass-warn-fail format or green-amber-red colored light diodes and also a digital readout giving results to two or three decimal places (Poon et al. 1987).

For the purposes of quantitative evidential breath-alcohol analysis, infrared spectroscopy has emerged as the most reliable and stable technology (Martin 2011). The infrared absorption spectrum of ethanol shows distinct absorption bands close to 3.4 µM corresponding to C-H bond stretching and also at 9.5 µM corresponding to the C-O stretching frequencies. The original single-wavelength IR breath-alcohol instruments, e.g., Intoxilyzer 4011 (CMI Inc.) and Intoximeter 3000 (Intoximeter Inc.), are not considered sufficiently selective for identification of ethanol. The Intoxilyzer model EN (CMI Inc.), the DataMaster (National Patent Analytical Systems Inc., Mansfield, OH), and the Evidenzer (Nanopuls AB, Sweden) incorporate multiple wavelength IR filters (Jones and Andersson 2008; Martin 2011).

The number of infrared filters has increased from one to three and later from three to five, mainly to counteract defense challenges suggesting that various interfering substances might exist in human breath leading to false high ethanol readings (Jones and Andersson 2008). The endogenous volatile substance in breath that might be at an elevated concentration is acetone (Dubowski and Essary 1983; Jones 1988a) but this can be distinguished from ethanol with one extra IR filter (Krishan and Lui 2002). Under most circumstances, the concentrations of acetone in blood and breath are too low to be considered a serious problem when breath-analysis is used for forensic purposes (Jones et al. 1993; Wallage and Bugyra 2017). However, in untreated diabetics or after prolonged fasting or eating low carbohydrate foods, abnormally high concentrations of acetone circulate in the blood and concentrations in breath are also elevated.

Other potential interfering substances include various aliphatic alcohols, such as methanol and isopropanol, industrial chemicals and organic solvents subject to abuse, e.g., toluene, gasoline, glue, or butane gas. After sniffing or inhaling these substances, there is a definite risk of interference with IR analyzers if testing is done shortly after exposure ends (Chan 2018; Denney 1990). The longer the time elapsed after inhalation of the solvents, the lower the risk of interference, because of a rapid washout of these low-boiling volatiles from the lungs. The available evidence suggests that normal occupational exposure to organic solvent vapors does not constitute a problem jeopardizing reliability and continued use of evidential breath-alcohol analyzers based on infrared absorption.

One of the latest generation of breath instruments is the Alcotest 9510 (Draeger Safety Inc., Lübeck, Germany), which incorporates both IR absorptiometry at 9.5 μM and electrochemical (EC) oxidation for identification and quantitative analysis of ethanol (Hartung et al. 2016). Use of two independent methods of analysis furnishes higher selectivity for identification of ethanol in the breath. Another of the latest generation of breath-test instruments is the Intox EC/IR (Intoximeters Inc., St. Louis, MO). This device also incorporates dual technology although IR is used as a detector for end-exhaled air and presence of mouth alcohol, whereas EC is used for quantitative determination of ethanol. The IR detector monitors both ethanol and CO_2 during a prolonged exhalation, and calculating and comparing the two signals gives an indication that uncontaminated end-exhaled breath is entering the instrument. Mouth alcohol arises from breath testing is done too soon after the end of drinking or if the subject might have regurgitated stomach contents containing alcohol just before exhalation (Lindberg et al. 2015; Modell et al. 1993).

When the first generation of instruments for breath-alcohol analysis appeared, including the Breathalyzer, the statutory *per se* limits of BAC or BrAC did not exist in most US states. Moreover, if the person's BAC or BrAC was above a statutory limit for driving this was taken as a presumption of guilt and most weight of evidence was given to results of clinical and behavioral tests of impairment (Jones 1988a). The lowering of threshold alcohol limits for driving and the increasing enforcement of concentration *per se* statutes directed more attention on the reliability of the methods used to determine a driver's BAC or BrAC (Gullberg 2004; Taylor and Oberman 2006).

When using results of breath-alcohol analysis in a criminal prosecution, all aspects of the testing protocol including preparation of the subject and quality assurance of the analytical results must be well-documented (Dubowski 1994). The following are important considerations:

- At least 15 minutes should elapse after an arrest before starting the breath-alcohol test procedure.
- The suspect should be observed and not left alone during the 15 minutes before the test.
- Prior to the sampling of breath the subject should not have engaged in strenuous exercise for at least 5 minutes.
- There should be no hypo- or hyper-ventilation before making a prolonged exhalation into the breath-alcohol analyzer.
- The suspect's mouth should not have come into contact with alcohol from consumption, emesis, or regurgitation for at least 15 minutes before the tests.

- The suspect should not be allowed to eat any food, chew gum, or drink water or soft-drinks within 15 minutes of the breath-alcohol testing.
- At least two separate breath specimens should be collected and analyzed at an interval of between 5 and 15 minutes apart.
- At least one calibration control test done before, after, or between the two subject tests is necessary.

5.8 Comparing Blood- and Breath-Alcohol Concentration

The Breathalyzer was designed and intended as an indirect and non-invasive way to estimate the coexisting BAC (Borkenstein and Smith 1961). This required calibration of the instrument with an assumed average blood/breath ratio of alcohol of 2100:1. However, the BBR is not a constant factor and various both between and within subjects owing to analytical, biological, and instrumental factors (Alobaidi et al. 1976; Jones 1978b). Moreover, different breath-alcohol instruments, owing to inherent design features, such as the resistance to exhalation, the type of mouthpiece used, and the parameters set for accepting a breath sample, such as volume discarded before sampling, impacted on the value of the BBR (Mulder and Neuteboom 1987). Among the physiological factors were the stage of ethanol metabolism, the breathing pattern before exhalation, pulmonary diseases, body temperature, and the person's age, height, and vital capacity were all relevant (Jones 1990a).

The biological variability in the BBR of alcohol was not considered a serious problem when the results were used as supporting evidence of alcohol intoxication. During the early years of using chemical tests of intoxication the main evidence for prosecution was the testimony and observations made by the arresting police officer and the results of a medical examination of the suspect. However, with the advent of concentration *per se* laws much more weight is given to the accuracy, precision and reliability of the BAC or BrAC determinations.

As discussed above, the existence of A-V differences in ethanol concentration make the BBR a moving target varying from less than 2100:1 during absorption phase shortly after end of drinking towards 3000:1 or more late in the post-absorptive phase (Jones 2010). This BBR dilemma was solved by defining a statutory BrAC limit separate from the statutory BAC depending on whether the suspect submitted to a breath or blood test. Accordingly, in the United States the BAC limit of 0.08 g% was equivalent to 0.08 g/210 L in breath (Mason and Dubowski 1976). When evidential breath-alcohol instruments were adopted in EU nations, the preexisting statutory BAC limits were divided by an assumed BBR to arrive at a statutory BrAC.

The approval of new methods or instrument intended for evidential breath-alcohol analysis requires extensive validation under in-vitro and in-vivo conditions (Hodgson 2008; Martin 2011). The precision and accuracy of the results need to be documented before acceptance for legal purposes. Higher standards of performance are necessary for evidential instruments compared with hand-held devices intended for roadside screening (Zuba 2008).

Human alcohol dosing studies should include people of different age, gender, and lung capacities, both smokers and non-smokers. This permits evaluating easy of providing the required specimen of breath and prevalence of failing make a continuous exhalation for the required time (Hlastala and Anderson 2007). Duplicate analysis is essential and these should be taken 5–10 minutes apart and the signed differences between duplicate results used to calculate the analytical precision as a function of ethanol concentration in the breath (Gullberg 1987). From the results of near simultaneous sampling and determination of BAC and BrAC, a scatter plot is constructed with BAC on the x-axis and BrAC plotted on the y-axis. Although this type of data is commonly evaluated by linear regression analysis, there are other statistical methods available when two methods of measurement are compared as described below (Gullberg 1991).

5.8.1 Regression and Correlation Analysis

The traditional way to compare results of nearly simultaneous measurements of BAC and BrAC is to construct a scatter plot and use a linear regression analysis to evaluate the data (Twomey and Kroll 2008). Careful consideration should be given to the concentration units for reporting BAC and BrAC when such comparisons are made. In the United States BAC is reported as grams of alcohol per 100 mL blood and BrAC as grams of alcohol per 210 L breath, which implies that the BBR is 2100:1 (0.08 g/100 mL divided by 0.08 g/210 L = 2100:1).

Figure 5.10 gives an example of such a scatter plot obtained with Intoxilyzer 5000 a quantitative infrared analyzer approved for testing drivers apprehended in Sweden. After they had failed a roadside breath-alcohol screening test the suspects were expected to undergo an evidential breath-alcohol test (Jones and Andersson 1996). In this particular comparison, breath was tested first and venous blood taken between 15–120 minutes later and analyzed in triplicate by headspace gas chromatography. The BrAC is plotted as the dependent y-variate and is regressed against the BAC plotted as the independent x-variate, which seems justified because errors in BAC determination are usually less than BrAC measurements.

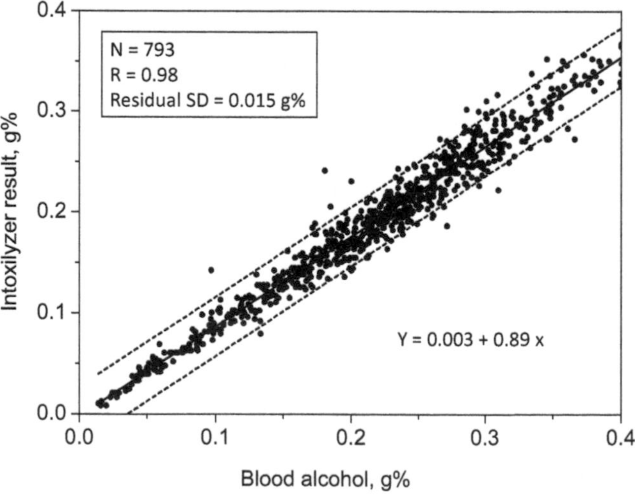

Figure 5.10 Scatter plot showing a high correlation (r = 0.98) between the concentration of ethanol in venous blood and end-exhaled breath samples in apprehended drivers. Ethanol in breath was determined with a quantitative infrared breath-analyzer (Intoxilyzer 5000) and blood-ethanol was determined by headspace gas chromatography. The analysis of breath samples was always done first and the blood samples were taken between 10 and 60 minutes later. The metabolism of ethanol between the times of sampling blood and breath was corrected for by assuming an average elimination rate from blood of 0.019 g% per h.

The blood- and breath-alcohol concentrations were highly correlated ($r = 0.98$) over a wide range of ethanol concentrations from 0.01 to 0.40 g% However, a high correlation does not necessarily mean a good agreement, because both constant and proportional biases arise that can distort the agreement (Ludbrook 2010b; Stockl et al. 1998). The existence of a constant bias, if present, is indicated by the value of the y-intercept which was −0.002 ± 0.0014 g/210 L (±SE) and this was not significantly different from zero ($t = 1.4$, $p > 0.05$). However, a proportional bias was established because the regression coefficient was 0.892 ± 0.0063 (±SE) and this differed from unity ($t = 17.1$, $p < 0.001$). This proportional bias in the breath-alcohol readings indicate that the instrument gives results about 11% less than venous BAC on average. The Intoxilyzer 5000S therefore tends to under-report BAC, erring on the side of the suspect. In absolute terms, the BAC-BrAC difference will be larger at higher blood-alcohol concentration, e.g., 0.011 g/210 L at 0.10 g% and 0.022 g/210 L at 0.20 g%.

The random variation in the breath-alcohol readings is represented by the residual standard deviation, which is a measure of the scatter of the data points around the linear regression line (Linnet 1999). Although a few outliers were present (points most distant from the regression line), the residual standard deviation (SD) was 0.015 g/210 L. This standard deviation applies at the mean BAC and BrAC of 0.202 g% and 0.187 g/210 L, respectively. One also notes that the magnitude of scatter around the regression line tends to increase as the concentration of ethanol in blood and breath increases. The random variations in the BrAC can be expressed as a coefficient of variation (residual SD/Mean BrAC) × 100 to give a CV% of 8.0% so 95% of the results agree within ±16% (1.96 × residual SD). However, the Intoxilyzer 5000S showed a proportional bias reading lower than the venous BAC by about 11% on average as indicated by a regression coefficient of 0.89 (Jones and Andersson 1996).

5.8.2 Method of Differences

A recommended statistical method to evaluate results of method comparison studies is referred to as a Bland–Altman plot, named after two British statisticians who described this approach in a paper published in the Lancet (Bland and Altman 1986). The individual differences between results for each comparison are calculated along with their mean and standard deviation. Whether the mean difference differs from zero can be evaluated by a Student t-test. A graph is then constructed with each difference in concentration (BrAC-BAC) plotted on the y-axis and the mean concentration by the two methods plotted on the *x*-axis. The 95% limits of agreement (±1.96 × SD) are calculated and plotted as dashed lines above and below the mean difference line (Ludbrook 2010a).

An example of a Bland and Altman plot utilizing results of blood and breath analysis is shown in Figure 5.11 with data obtained from a controlled drinking study; BAC was determined by HS-GC and BrAC was measured with a hand-held instrument with digital display, Alcolmeter S-D2 (Jones and Jönsson 1993). The mean bias between blood and breath test results was close to zero (0.0004 g%) and the variability (SD of differences) was 0.009 g%, which means that 95% of differences between Alcolmeter S-D2 and BAC are expected to range from −0.018 g% below to +0.018 g% above the mean bias of 0.0004 g%. Over the range of concentrations of alcohol encountered in this study from 0 to 0.10 g% there was no indication that the magnitude of the BAC and BrAC differences depended on the concentration.

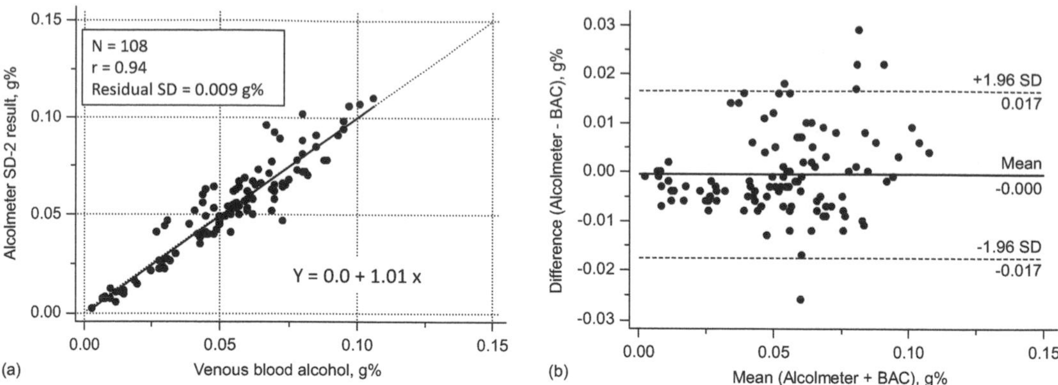

Figure 5.11 Correlation-regression analysis of blood- and breath-alcohol concentrations (a) compared with using a Bland and Altman plot (b). The mean difference between breath- and blood-alcohol is an indication of the bias between the two measurements, which happened to be zero in this study. The standard deviation (SD) of the differences can be used to calculate upper and lower limits of agreement, with 95% of all results falling within the limits ± 1.96 × SD (±0.017 g%).

Agreement between two methods of measuring the same quantity is sometimes done by calculating a Pearson's correlation coefficient, although finding a high correlations close to unity indicates strong association, but not necessarily a good agreement (Bland and Altman 1999).

5.8.3 Calculating Blood/Breath Ratios of Alcohol

Another approach to evaluate closeness of agreement between BAC and BrAC results is to calculate individual blood/breath ratios of alcohol along with their mean and standard deviation (Alobaidi et al. 1976; Jones 1978b). However, care is needed when ratios are calculated at low BAC (<0.02 g%), because the size of the ratios are exaggerated. A low absolute difference is associated with a high BBR when BAC is less than 0.02 g%. The variance of the measurements in absolute units (g% or g/210 L) tends to increase as the concentration of alcohol in the specimens increases. However, when expressed as coefficients of variation (CV%, (SD/Mean) × 100), the results are highest at low concentrations of ethanol. This relationship between CV% and concentration has ramifications when blood/breath ratios are calculated and compared. The approximate CV% of the BAC/BrAC ratio is calculated as $[(CV_{BAC})^2 + (CV_{BrAC})^2)^{1/2}$ which suggests large relative variation at low ethanol concentrations.

Figure 5.12 is a plot of BAC vs BrAC in two people who drank 0.80 g ethanol per kg body weight in 30 minutes. The concentration-time profiles show good agreement for absorption and post-absorption phases (Figure 5.12, lower plot). However, the blood/breath ratios of ethanol (upper plot) change continuously as a function of time after drinking. For the first 60 minutes after the end of drinking BBRs are mostly less than 2100:1 and then increase to exceed 2300:1 as the BAC curve enters the declining phase and by seven hours after drinking end they increase to 3400:1 as BAC deceases toward 0.01 g%.

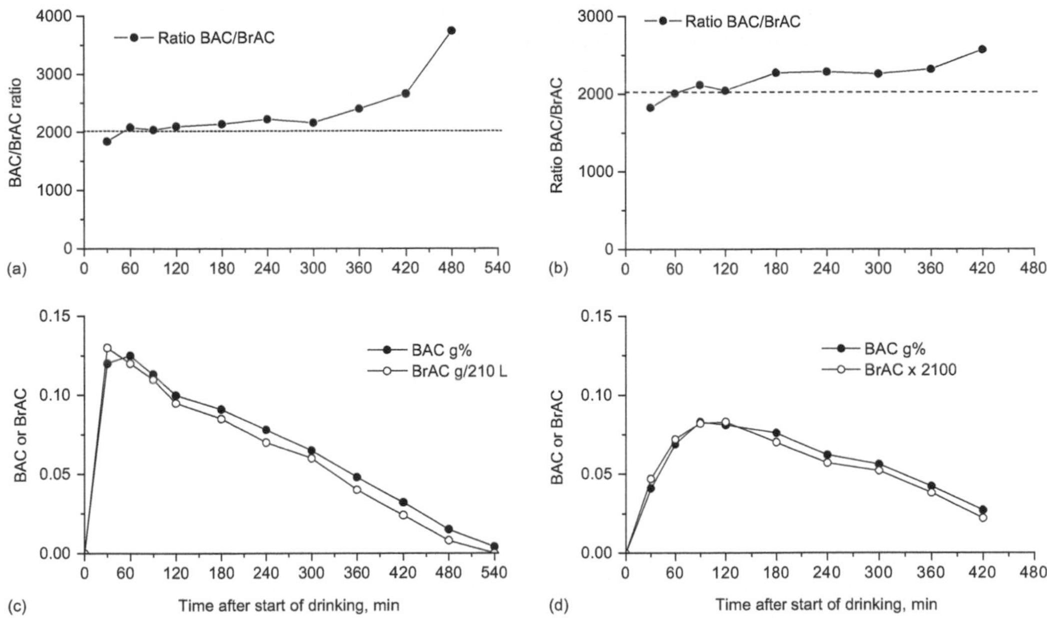

Figure 5.12 Concentration-time profiles of ethanol in venous blood and end-expired breath in two subjects after they drank 0.80 g alcohol per kg body weight diluted with orange juice. Blood ethanol was analyzed by an enzymatic oxidation method and breath-alcohol by a gas chromatograph (GC) Intoximeter Mk II instrument. The top frames (a and b) show how the blood/breath ratios of alcohol vary in relation to sampling time after end of drinking and the bottom frames (c and d) show concentration-time profiles.

The results of this experiment show that the blood/breath ratio of alcohol is a moving target and the main reason is that BrAC follows more closely the arterial BAC and not venous BAC as discussed elsewhere (Lindberg et al. 2007).

5.8.4 Blood- and Breath-Alcohol Parameters

The equivalence between BAC and BrAC for forensic purposes, such as in drink-driving cases can be further assessed by calculating pharmacokinetic parameters and comparing these statistically for any significant differences. This was done in drinking experiments with 21 men who consumed 0.68 g/kg ethanol as whisky on an empty stomach (Jones 1978a). Breath was analyzed using a GC Intoximeter both before and after fingertip blood was taken for determination of ethanol. The resulting mean BAC and BrAC were plotted and the resulting C-T profiles used to determine important pharmacokinetic parameters. Parameters such as maximum BAC and BrAC, time of reaching the peak, the area under the curves, time elapsed to reach zero concentrations and the elimination rates of ethanol from blood and breath were calculated (see Table 5.7).

The good agreement between pharmacokinetic parameters of ethanol shown in Table 5.7 supports the introduction of evidential breath-test instruments as a replacement for BAC measurements. Table 5.7 also shows good agreement between the main kinetic

Table 5.7 Comparison of the Pharmacokinetic Parameters Derived from Concentration-Time Profiles of Ethanol in Venous Blood and End-Expired Breath—Ethanol in Breath Was Determined with the MK II GC Intoximeter and in Capillary Blood by an Automated ADH Method

Alcohol Parameter[a]	Blood-Ethanol Profiles[b]	Breath-Ethanol Profiles[c]
Peak BAC or BrAC	0.091 ± 0.016 g%	0.097 ± 0.04 g/210 L
Concentrations at 40 min post-drinking	0.082 ± 0.014 g%	0.084 ± 0.015 g/210 L
Time to peak[d]	38 min (range 10–120)	36 min (range 10–100)
Time to zero alcohol (extrapolated)	494 ± 38 min	488 ± 38 min
Rate of elimination of alcohol from blood or breath	0.012 ± 0.0011 g% per h	0.012 ± 0.0012 g/210 L/h
Estimated (extrapolated) ethanol concentration at time of dosing	0.100 ± 0.006 g%	0.099 ± 0.007 g/210 L
Elimination rate of alcohol from the whole body	83 ± 6.4 mg/kg/h	84 ± 6.7 mg/kg/h
Area under concentration-time curves (0–420 min)	22.1 ± 2.4 g% × min	21.9 ± 2.4 g/210 L × min
Apparent volume of distribution	0.69 ± 0.04 L/kg	0.69 ± 0.05 L/kg[e]

[a] Values shown are Mean±SD for $n = 21$ male subjects who drank 0.68 g/kg ethanol as neat whisky on an empty stomach.
[b] Ethanol in blood was determined by an enzymatic method.
[c] Ethanol in breath was determined with an MK II gas chromatograph intoximeter.
[d] Timed from end of drinking, which lasted 20 minutes.
[e] Not strictly applicable owing to the kind of units used to report breath-alcohol concentration.

parameters of ethanol including peak concentrations reached, elimination rate, volume of distribution, and area under the curves.

5.9 Dealing with Uncertainty in Analytical Results

Quality assurance and certain scientific safeguards are necessary when results of forensic blood- and/or breath-alcohol analysis are used as the sole evidence for prosecution in a drink-driving case (Dubowski 1994). As mentioned before, an essential requirement with breath testing is to wait at least 15 minutes after the last drink before a person is tested. This alcohol deprivation and observation period is essential to avoid contamination of the breath sample with so-called mouth alcohol (Sterling 2012). This refers to residual alcohol in the oral cavity from the alcoholic drink, because the initial concentrations in the mucous surfaces are higher than expected until about 15 min after end of drinking (Modell et al. 1993). The time necessary for removal of this "mouth alcohol" has been well studied and shown to require up to 15 minutes after finishing a drink (Gullberg 1992). During an evidential breath-alcohol test, the subject should always be made to provide two separate exhalations about 5–10 minutes apart (Gullberg 1987). Close agreement between the two results supports the absence of a "mouth alcohol effect." Other quality assurance requirements include the analysis of ambient air in the room where the person was tested and also a calibration control check of the instrument, before or after or between the two subject tests (Dubowski 1994). A host of other quality assurance procedures and controls are sometimes required when breath-alcohol instruments are used for evidential purposes. Defense arguments directed against BrAC results increasingly focus on accuracy, precision and selectivity of the analytical method used. Other common targets for defense attack are physiological and/or environmental factors or alleged response to interfering substances (Gullberg 2004).

Methods used for determination of ethanol in blood are not subjected to the same vigorous attack and criticism as methods of breath-alcohol analysis (Jones 1991). This might be accounted for by the fact that blood samples are analyzed at a forensic laboratory by trained scientists whereas breath testing is done by a trained police officer. Furthermore, there is a biological component of variation inherent in sampling and analysis of breath, which makes a significant contribution to the overall variation (Gullberg and McElroy 1992).

Pre-analytical factors need consideration with all types of clinical and forensic laboratory methods and their contribution can be minimized by adopting a standardized sampling procedure (Lippi et al. 2013). On arrival at the laboratory, the tubes of blood should be carefully inspected, making a note of any unusual appearance, such as the presence of clots or any obvious dilution that might have occurred (e.g., when samples are taken from victims of traffic accidents receiving intravenous fluids to counteract shock) (Riley et al. 1996). Inspection of the blood specimen is an important first step in the analytical procedure. Prior to analysis the specimen tubes with blood should be inverted 8–10 times to ensure mixing of plasma and red cells. Alternatively, a batch of specimen tubes is mechanically rotated for a few minutes before aliquots of blood are removed and diluted with internal standard in preparation for quantitative analysis of ethanol.

All determinations of BAC for legal purposes should be done in duplicate or triplicate and ideally these assays undertaken by different technicians working independently with different sets of GC equipment (Jones and Schuberth 1989). Calibration of the GC requires use of known strength ethanol standards purchased from a traceable source and covering the range of BAC encountered in casework. During an analytical run other ethanol standards should be included every fifth or tenth blood sample for quality control purposes and derived from a different source than those used to calibrate the GC equipment.

The concentration of ethanol in the blood samples as received is assumed to be identical with that flowing through the vein of the suspect at the time of sampling. Despite these precautions, the analytical measurements have inherent uncertainty, owing to random and systematic variations or bias in the procedures. Regular participation in external proficiency trials has become an important part of laboratory accreditation. Although such procedures are well established for laboratory analysis of blood samples they are just beginning to be developed for breath-alcohol instruments.

In contrast to the measurement of BAC, the determination of alcohol in the exhaled breath is more prone to biological variations (Dubowski 1975). Two separate and consecutive breath samples and the differences between the duplicates gives a measure of the analytical precision. Two separate exhalations should be analyzed 5 and 10 minutes apart and not multiple measurements on the same exhalation profile. With modern breath-testing technology, the results are reported to three decimal places (Gullberg 2015). The mean of the duplicate or triplicate determination gives the best estimate of the person's BrAC at the time of testing.

The closeness of agreement between the results of duplicate measurements, which should not exceed a critical value, e.g., 0.02 g/210 L is important for acceptance as forensic evidence. Every breath-alcohol test should be preceded by a simulator control test with a known strength air-alcohol standard at 0.08 g/210 L if this is the statutory limit for driving. In some jurisdictions, a test of instrument accuracy is done once before and once after the subject is tested. The difference between the two simulator test results is another quality control window with a maximum permissible differences of ±10%, or from 0.072 to 0.088 g/210 L at a target value of 0.08 g/210 L.

The analysis of air-alcohol standards (from wet-bath simulator or pressurized tubes) should accompany every subject test and is proof that the instrument was correctly calibrated at the time (Dubowski 1994). The analysis of room-air as alcohol-blank is done between the subject and simulator tests and should meet pre-set requirements, e.g., 0.002 g/210 L maximum deviation. The development of an external proficiency program for use with evidential breath-alcohol instruments might entail periodically analyzing an alcohol solution in the simulator without disclosing the expected instrument result or analyzing an alcohol-air mixture from a dry-gas standard (Gullberg and Logan 2006).

In most jurisdictions when the police administer an evidential breath-alcohol test, the standard operating procedure (SOP) requires that duplicate determination are made and the lower of the two results is the value used for prosecution. Furthermore, the third decimal place is frequently truncated so that 0.109 g/210 L becomes 0.10 g/210 L. However, these allowances are not much benefit to a person when the duplicate test results agree to the third decimal, as they often do with current generation breath-alcohol instruments (Gullberg 2015). In other instances, a prosecution might not be made unless the actual BrAC was 0.01 or 0.02 g/210 L above the prescribed statutory limit for driving. Accordingly, if the statutory BrAC limit was 0.08 g/210 L, a prosecution is initiated if the result is above 0.10 g/210 L, the 0.02 g/210 L difference acting as a guard band decision rule. In the UK the statutory BrAC for driving is 35 μg/100 mL but a prosecution is not made unless the lower of two results is 40 μg/100 mL or more (14% higher).

Instead of these somewhat arbitrary approaches of giving "the benefit of the doubt" to a suspect, a more scientific way makes use of statistical methods and probability calculations. The amount deducted from the mean of duplicate test results is calculated in such a way that the final result for prosecution can be stated with a confidence of 99% or 99.9% as being not less than the true BrAC (Gullberg 2012). The principles of quality assurance and calculating an acceptable level of risk of making incorrect decisions with compliance at a threshold limit has been described for forensic blood-alcohol analysis and it should be perfectly feasible to implement the same system with evidential breath alcohol testing (Jones and Schuberth 1989).

Table 5.8 shows a print-out from an evidential breath-alcohol analyzer that includes a deduction for uncertainty in the measurements. With a 15% deduction from the mean of two consecutive measurements it can be stated that the suspect's true BrAC is not less than this result used for prosecution with 99.9% confidence. This leaves only a 1 in 1000 chance that the prosecution result is higher and this is only of interest around some threshold value, such as the statutory limit for driving. In civil litigation less stringent standards of legal proof are required, such as a preponderance of the evidence. In this type of case it might be appropriate to report a mean BrAC result.

Table 5.8 Example of a Print-out When an Evidential Breath-Alcohol Analyzer Was Used by the Police as Evidence for Prosecuting Alcohol Impaired Drivers

Sequence of Testing	Instrument Reading
Room air blank	0.000 g/210 L
Calibration control test[a]	0.078 g/210 L
Room air blank	0.000 g/210 L
First subject test[b]	0.105 g/210 L
Room air blank	0.000 g/210 L
Second subject test[b]	0.115 g/210 L
Room air blank	0.000 g/210 L
Calibration control test[a]	0.081 g/210 L
Mean breath alcohol	0.110 g/210 L
Allowance for uncertainty[c]	0.015 g/210 L
Prosecution value[d]	0.095 g/210 L

[a] Results from the calibration control test must be within the "target value" of the ethanol standard (0.080 g/210 L) to be deemed acceptable, such as within ± 0.005 to 0.008 g/210 L.

[b] The duplicate subject breath-test results must agree to within a certain pre-defined margin, such as 0.02 g/210 L to be accepted for legal purposes.

[c] The actual allowance made for uncertainty depends on the mean concentration of ethanol in the breath sample. This requires a prior knowledge of the relationship between standard deviation (SD) of ethanol analysis with that particular evidential breath instrument. The SD tends to increase with concentration of ethanol in breath so a larger deduction is necessary for suspects with high alcohol levels to achieve the same statistical confidence of 99.9% for all suspects.

[d] The concentration of alcohol in the suspect's breath at the time of testing was at not less than 0.095 g/210 L with a statistical certainty of 99.9%.

5.10 Conclusions

Legislators debate and decide on the statutory BAC or BrAC limits for driving, and hopefully their decisions reflect the best available scientific evidence about impairment of the driver and the risk of involvement in a traffic crash (Fell and Voas 2006a). However, the statutory BAC limits for driving differ four-fold between countries (0.02–0.08 g%) and so does the corresponding BrAC limits, because the latter were derived from the existing BAC limits by assuming a population average BBR of alcohol. However, there was no consensus when this important ratio was decided upon and values ranged from 2000 to 2400 in different countries. In Australia, Canada, and the United States, the assumed BBR was 2100:1 chosen in part on the understanding that it gave a certain advantage to the suspect compared with the analysis of ethanol in samples of venous blood (Jones 2010).

In tests with apprehended drivers a linear regression analysis showed that venous BAC was underestimated by about 10%–15% when a 2100:1 BBR was used to report BrAC results (Jones and Andersson 2003). In several controlled drinking studies when comparisons were made in the post-absorptive phase of the BAC curve a closer agreement between BAC and BrAC was achieved using a 2300:1 BBR (Emerson et al. 1980). Direct comparison of BAC and BrAC in apprehended drivers resulted in a mean BBR closer to 2400:1 (Cobb and Dabbs 1985; Jones and Andersson 1996). The higher BBR observed when apprehended drivers are tested probable stems, at last in part, from a failure to obtain an end exhaled breath sample for analysis. Sampling the breath before a person reaches a vital capacity exhalation means that BrAC is lower than expected and the resulting BBR is skewed toward high values. Some countries (e.g. France, Germany, Spain, and Portugal) opted to use a BBR of 2000:1, which would underestimate the venous BAC and give even more benefit to the person tested (Jones 2010).

The technology currently available for evidential breath-alcohol testing is probably as good as it can be for its intended purpose. Modern instruments incorporate microprocessors and allow continuous monitoring of the exhalation profile of ethanol, automated sampling on reaching an end-exhalation, control of the instrument's calibration as proof of accuracy etc. The accuracy and precision of ethanol determinations done with modern breath-alcohol analyzers matches that obtained with HS-GC methods applied to blood samples with coefficients of variation of 1%–2% at the threshold 0.08 g% limit in blood or 0.08 g/210 L in breath (Gullberg 2003).

One source of variation often neglected is the pre-analytical factors associated with obtaining the proper sample; the analytical result is only as good as the specimen received for analysis and this applies to both blood and breath samples (Zamengo et al. 2014). In a typical DUI prosecution, the results of breath-alcohol analysis are challenged by the defense more often than BAC results. There are probably several reasons for this, such as the fact a trained police officer is responsible for the evidential breath-alcohol test, whereas laboratory technicians or university-trained chemists perform the blood-alcohol analysis.

There is no doubt that results of breath-alcohol analysis are more prone to biological variations owing to different patterns of breathing into the instrument and breath-to-breath physiological variation, such as lung function, vital capacity and breath- and body- temperature (Jones 1982). Duplicate determinations of BAC are usually done on aliquots of blood removed from the same evacuated tube and the sampling variation is therefore minimal. The variation in analytical results would increase if blood from different sampling sites was analyzed, such as left and right arm cubital veins (Jones et al. 1989). Only with this type of experimental design can the magnitude of sampling variation between blood and breath be properly compared and contrasted.

Scores of studies verify a high correlation between BAC and BrAC over a wide range of ethanol concentrations from 0.01 to 0.50 g%. Indeed, the association between BAC and BrAC is much stronger than the correlation between BAC and various measures of cognitive or psychomotor impairment after drinking alcohol. Furthermore, a strong quantitative relationship exists between a driver's BrAC and the risk of involvement in a road traffic crash, whereas similar relationships have not been demonstrated for impairment of body functions (Blomberg et al. 2009). The non-invasive nature of sampling breath makes it more convenient than sticking a needle in a person's vein to draw a sample of venous blood for analysis.

Although the BrAC can be used to calculate the co-existing BAC, such a conversion requires that the BBR of alcohol is known. In forensic casework this is unnecessary, because most jurisdictions enforce statutory BrAC limits alongside their BAC limits. Discussions about variability in the BBR of alcohol are irrelevant, because the value was fixed by the legislator when the drink-driving statutes were written. Many studies showed that use of a 2100:1 BBR gave results about 10–15% less than the coexisting venous BAC (Cowan et al. 2010). If a person is tested when actively absorbing alcohol then the BrAC (g/210 L) is expected to be higher than the venous BAC (g%), owing to arterio-venous differences in ethanol pharmacokinetics (Jones et al. 2004). Because not many drivers are thought to be still absorbing alcohol when they are breath tested, this is not a major problem impinging on reliability of BrAC measurements (Levine and Smialek 2000).

The continued use of BAC or BrAC measurements as evidence for the prosecution of traffic offenders is strongly supported under a *per se* statute. The choice between the two specimens (blood v breath) has certain advantages and limitations as outlined in Table 5.9.

Table 5.9 Some Advantages and Limitations of the Use of Blood- and/or Breath-Alcohol Analysis in Law Enforcement as Evidence for the Prosecution of Traffic Offenders

Sampling and Analysis of Blood-Alcohol	Sampling and Analysis of Breath-Alcohol
Chain-of-custody, transport, and storage of the sample before arrival at the laboratory is important to document.	Chain-of-custody is not an issue with evidential breath alcohol analysis.
Blood specimens can be taken from living and deceased persons.	Sampling of breath is possible only from people who are prepared and capable of making a prolonged exhalation.
Blood samples can be taken regardless of state of health or consciousness of the drunk-driving suspect, such as hospitalized victims of traffic crashes.	Some individuals with respiratory dysfunction (asthma or chronic obstructive pulmonary disease) cannot meet the requirement of making a prolonged exhalation for at least 6 seconds.
Analysis of drugs other than alcohol is possible and often desirable because of drug-impaired driving legislation and concentration *per se* or zero tolerance laws.	Although non-alcohol drugs can be determined in breath, the results are difficult to interpret and don't correlate to concentrations determined in blood.
Confirmatory analysis of the result is easily done on stored blood samples although the ethanol concentrations decrease slightly over time.	Methods are available to store breath samples for later confirmatory analysis, but this procedure is more troublesome and no longer practiced.
Blood samples can be analyzed for various biomarkers that indicate a person is a heavy or problem drinker and in need of treatment.	Searching for biochemical markers of alcoholism is not possible with breath analysis, although "breath biopsy" is becoming much used in clinical medicine.
Results of blood alcohol analysis are usually obtained 3–7 days after the road-traffic offence.	On-the-spot results of alcohol concentration in breath is obtained, which allows making decisions about arrest and confiscating of the driving permit and differentiating ethanol intoxication form other conditions that mimic drunkenness.
Invasive sampling procedure, some people claim to suffer from needle phobia.	Non-invasive sampling procedure, but cooperation from the suspect is required.
Physician, nurse or phlebotomist is required to take blood sample.	Trained police officers operate the breath-alcohol instruments.
The blood specimen for analysis is normally taken from a driver 1–2 hour after the time of the traffic offense.	Breath samples for alcohol analysis can be obtained closer to the time of driving, even at the roadside.
The concentration of ethanol in blood is not influenced by the method of sampling or whether it had undergone hemolysis, although clotted samples present a problem.	The breath-alcohol concentration is influenced by the subject's breathing maneuver before exhalation, hypo-ventilation increases and hyper-ventilation decreases the ethanol content in breath.
Blood samples can be taken during or any time after drinking starts. Ethanol-based swabs should not be used to clean the needle puncture site.	Results of breath analysis are not valid if done within the first 15 min after the last drink, owing to presence of mouth alcohol leading to false high readings.
The concentration of alcohol in arterial blood is higher than venous blood during absorption phase and slightly lower in the post-absorptive period.	The arterial blood ethanol concentration and the breath ethanol concentration are in much closer agreement during the absorption and post-absorptive phases of the blood-ethanol curve.

The concentration-time course of BrAC follows more closely the arterial BAC rather than the venous BAC during ADME of ethanol in the body, especially during the absorption phase of the BAC curve (Lindberg et al. 2007). During the consumption of alcohol and for some time afterwards (absorptive phase) the arterial BAC rises rapidly and is distinctly higher than the venous BAC. After about 60–120 minutes a crossover point is reached when arterial and venous BAC are the same. Ethanol is cleared from the central blood compartment by metabolism in the liver and replaced by ethanol in venous blood draining the tissues, which has a slightly higher ethanol concentration during the post-absorptive phase (Jones et al. 2004).

Both BAC and BrAC results are equally valid as objective ways to prove whether a person is in breach of the drink-driving legislation and exceeds a statutory alcohol limit. Under a concentration *per se* statute some consideration should be given to possible analytical variations, because in borderline cases this could mean the difference between punishment and/or acquittal (see Figure 5.3). The uncertainty of the results could be illustrated by reporting a mean ethanol concentration along with a confidence interval that encompass 95%, 99%, or 99.9% of all possible concentrations, assuming a normal distribution (Gullberg 2012).

It would also be acceptable to make a deduction from the mean concentration of ethanol and report this lowered result as being not less than the true BAC or BrAC with a high degree of probability, such as 95%, 99%, or 99.9%, depending on the amount subtracted from the mean concentration. In practice, this might require subtracting between 6% and 15% from the mean BrAC depending on the accuracy and precision of the analytical method used. Making a percentage deductions seems more appropriate because the SD of analysis increases with the concentration of ethanol in the breath sample (Gullberg 2006).

Alternatively, a mean BAC or BrAC could be reported along with a range of values within which the true concentration is likely to exist with 95%, 99%, or 99.9% confidence limits depending on the standard of proof necessary; whether beyond a reasonable doubt or preponderance of the evidence. Reporting the analytical results along with their uncertainty would allow the trier of fact to judge the strength of the evidence and draw the appropriate conclusions in drink-driving cases.

References

Agarwal DP, Goedde HW: Pharmacogenetics of alcohol metabolism and alcoholism; *Pharmacogenetics* 2:48; 1992.

Ahlner J, Holmgren A, Jones AW: Prevalence of alcohol and other drugs and the concentrations in blood of drivers killed in road traffic crashes in Sweden; *Scand J Public Health* 42:177; 2014.

Ahlner J, Holmgren A, Jones AW: Demographics and post-mortem toxicology findings in deaths among people arrested multiple times for use of illicit drugs and/or impaired driving; *Forensic Sci Int* 265:138; 2016.

Alha AR: Blood alcohol and clinical inebriation in Finnish men: A medico-legal study; *Ann Acad Sci Fenn* 26:1; 1951.

Alobaidi TA, Hill DW, Payne JP: Significance of variations in blood: Breath partition coefficient of alcohol; *Br Med J* 2:1479; 1976.

Anderson JC, Hlastala MP: The alcohol breath test in practice: Effects of exhaled volume; *J Appl Physiol*; 126:1630; 2019.

Andreasson R, Jones AW: Erik M. P. Widmark (1889–1945): Swedish pioneer in forensic alcohol toxicology; *Forensic Sci Int* 72:1; 1995.

Andreasson R, Jones AW: Historical anecdote related to chemical tests for intoxication; *J Anal Toxicol* 20:207; 1996a.
Andreasson R, Jones AW: The life and work of Erik M. P. Widmark; *Am J Forensic Med Pathol* 17:177; 1996b.
Anthony RM, Sutheimer CA, Sunshine I: Acetaldehyde, methanol, and ethanol analysis by headspace gas chromatography; *J Anal Toxicol* 4:43; 1980.
Beauchamp J: Inhaled today, not gone tomorrow: Pharmacokinetics and environmental exposure of volatiles in exhaled breath; *J Breath Res* 5:037103; 2011.
Begg TB, Hill ID, Nickolls LC: Breathalyzer and Kitagawa-Wright methods of measuring breath alcohol; *Br Med J* 1:9; 1964.
Berggren SM, Goldberg L: The absorption of ethyl alcohol from the gastrointestinal tract as a diffusion process; *Acta Physiol Scand* 1:246; 1940.
Biasotti AA, Valentine TE: Blood alcohol concentration determined from urine samples as a practical equivalent or alternative to blood and breath alcohol tests; *J Forensic Sci* 30:194; 1985.
Bland JM, Altman DG: Statistical methods for assessing agreement between two methods of clinical measurement; *Lancet* 1:307; 1986.
Bland JM, Altman DG: Measuring agreement in method comparison studies; *Stat Methods Med Res* 8:135; 1999.
Blocker JS Jr: Did prohibition really work? Alcohol prohibition as a public health innovation; *Am J Public Health* 96:233; 2006.
Blomberg RD, Peck RC, Moskowitz H, Burns M, Fiorentino D: The Long Beach/Fort Lauderdale relative risk study; *J Safety Res* 40:285; 2009.
Bonnichsen RK, Wassen AM: Crystalline alcohol dehydrogenase from horse liver; *Arch Biochem* 18:361; 1948.
Bonnichsen RK, Theorell H: An enzymatic method for the microdetermination of ethanol; *Scand J Clin Lab Invest* 3:58; 1951.
Borkenstein RF: The role of the drinking driver in traffic accidents (the Grand Rapids Study); *Blutalkohol* 11:1; 1974.
Borkenstein RF: Historical perspective: North American traditional and experimental response; *J Stud Alcohol* Suppl 10:3; 1985.
Borkenstein RF, Smith HW: The Breathalyzer and its applications; *Med Sci Law* 2:13; 1961.
Brady JE, Li G: Trends in alcohol and other drugs detected in fatally injured drivers in the United States, 1999–2010; *Am J Epidemiol* 179:692; 2014.
Brick J: Standardization of alcohol calculations in research; *Alcohol Clin Exp Res* 30:1276; 2006.
Brick J, Erickson CK: Intoxication is not always visible: An unrecognized prevention challenge; *Alcohol Clin Exp Res* 33:1489; 2009.
British Medical Association: Test for drunkenness; *Br Med J* i:53; 1927.
British Medical Association: *The Drinking Driver—Report of a Special Committee*; British Medical Association: London, UK; 1965.
Buijten JC: An automated ultramicro distillation technique for determination of ethanol in blood and urine; *Blutalkohol* 14:405; 1975.
Burns M: An overview of field sobriety test research; *Percept Mot Skills* 97:1187; 2003.
Canfield DV, Dubowski KM, Cowan M, Harding PM: Alcohol limits and public safety; *Forensic Sci Rev* 26:9; 2014.
Chan K: The response of the Intox EC/IR II to isopropanol and isopropanol/ethanol mixtures; *Can Forensic Sci Soc J* 51:67; 2018.
Cherpitel CJ: Alcohol and injuries: A review of international emergency room studies since 1995; *Drug Alcohol Rev* 26:201; 2007.
Chiou WL: The phenomenon and rationale of marked dependence of drug concentration on blood sampling site: Implications in pharmacokinetics, pharmacodynamics, toxicology and therapeutics (Part I); *Clin Pharmacokinet* 17:175; 1989.

Cobb PGW, Dabbs MDG: *Report on the Performance of the Intoximeter 3000 and Camic Breath Evidential Instruments During the Period 16 April 1984 to 15 October 1984*; Her Majesty's Stationery Office: London, UK; 1985.

Cortot A, Jobin G, Ducrot F, Aymes C, Giraudeaux V, Modigliani R: Gastric emptying and gastrointestinal absorption of alcohol ingested with a meal; *Dig Dis Sci* 31:343; 1986.

Cowan JM, Burris JM, Hughes JR, Cunningham MP: The relationship of normal body temperature, end-expired breath temperature, and BAC/BrAC ratio in 98 physically fit human test subjects; *J Anal Toxicol* 34:238; 2010.

Crabb DW, Dipple KM, Thomasson HR: Alcohol sensitivity, alcohol metabolism, risk of alcoholism, and the role of alcohol and aldehyde dehydrogenase genotypes; *J Lab Clin Med* 122:234; 1993.

Crothers TD: Editorial; *Q J Inebriety* XXV1:308; 1904.

Curry AS, Walker GW, Simpson GS: Determination of ethanol in blood by gas chromatography; *Analyst* 91:742; 1966.

Denney RC: Solvent inhalation and "apparent" alcohol studies on the Lion Intoximeter 3000; *J Forensic Sci Soc* 30:357; 1990.

Dettling A, Fisher F, Böhler S, Ulrichs F, Schuff A, Skopp G, Von Meyer L, Graw M, Haffner HT: Grundlagen der Pharmakokinetik des Ethanols anhand von Atemalkoholkonzentrationen. Teil 1 Anflutung und Gipfelkonzentrationen; *Blutalkohol* 43:257; 2006.

Dettling A, Witte S, Skopp G, Graw M, Haffner HT: A regression model applied to gender-specific ethanol elimination rates from blood and breath measurements in non-alcoholics; *Int J Legal Med* 123:381; 2008.

Dubowski KM: Studies in breath-alcohol analysis: Biological factors; *Z Rechtsmed* 76:93; 1975.

Dubowski KM, Essary NA: Response of breath-alcohol analyzers to acetone; *J Anal Toxicol* 7:231; 1983.

Dubowski KM: Quality assurance in breath-alcohol analysis; *J Anal Toxicol* 18:306; 1994.

Emerson VJ, Holleyhead R, Isaacs MD, Fuller NA, Hunt DJ: The measurement of breath alcohol: The laboratory evaluation of substantive breath test equipment and the report of an operational police trial; *J Forensic Sci Soc* 20:3; 1980.

Endres HG, Gruner O: Comparison of D_2O and ethanol dilutions in total body water measurements in humans; *Clin Investig* 72:830; 1994.

Erol A, Ho AM, Winham SJ, Karpyak VM: Sex hormones in alcohol consumption: A systematic review of evidence; *Addict Biol* 24:157; 2019.

Evans MA, Martz R, Rodda BE, Kiplinger GF, Forney RB: Quantitative relationship between blood alcohol concentration and psychomotor performance; *Clin Pharmacol Ther* 15:253; 1974.

Fell JC, Voas RB: Mothers Against Drunk Driving (MADD): The first 25 years; *Traffic Inj Prev* 7:195; 2006a.

Fell JC, Voas RB: The effectiveness of reducing illegal blood alcohol concentration (BAC) limits for driving: Evidence for lowering the limit to.05 BAC; *J Safety Res* 37:233; 2006b.

Ferrara SD, Zancaner S, Giorgetti R: Low blood alcohol concentrations and driving impairment. A review of experimental studies and international legislation; *Int J Legal Med* 106:169; 1994.

Ferris J, Mazerolle L, King M, Bates L, Bennett S, Devaney M: Random breath testing in Queensland and Western Australia: Examination of how the random breath testing rate influences alcohol related traffic crash rates; *Accid Anal Prev* 60:181; 2013.

Forney RB, Hughes FW, Harger RN, Richards AB: Alcohol distribution in the vascular system. Concentration of orally administered alcohol in blood from various points in the vascular system, and in rebreathed air, during absorption; *Q J Stud Alcohol* 25:205; 1964.

Friedemann TE, Dubowski KM: Chemical testing procedures for the determination of ethyl alcohol; *J Am Med Assoc* 170:47; 1959.

Gjerde H, Christophersen AS, Normann PT, Mørland J: Toxicological investigations of drivers killed in road traffic accidents in Norway during 2006–2008; *Forensic Sci Int* 212:102; 2011.

Goldberg L: Quantitative studies on alcohol tolerance in man; *Acta Physiol Scand* 5(Supp 16):1; 1943.

Grubb D, Rasmussen B, Linnet K, Olsson SG, Lindberg L: Breath alcohol analysis incorporating standardization to water vapour is as precise as blood alcohol analysis; *Forensic Sci Int* 216:88; 2012.
Gullberg RG: Duplicate breath testing: Statistical vs forensic significance of differences; *J Forensic Sci Soc* 27:315; 1987.
Gullberg RG: Duplicate breath alcohol analysis: Some further parameters for evaluation; *Med Sci Law* 31:239; 1991.
Gullberg RG: The elimination rate of mouth alcohol: Mathematical modeling and implications in breath alcohol analysis; *J Forensic Sci* 37:1363; 1992.
Gullberg RG: Breath alcohol measurement variability associated with different instrumentation and protocols; *Forensic Sci Int* 131:30; 2003.
Gullberg RG: Common legal challenges and responses in forensic breath alcohol determination; *Forensic Sci Rev* 16:91; 2004.
Gullberg RG: Estimating the measurement uncertainty in forensic breath-alcohol analysis; *Accred Qual Assur* 11:562; 2006.
Gullberg RG: Estimating the measurement uncertainty in forensic blood alcohol analysis; *J Anal Toxicol* 36:153; 2012.
Gullberg RG: How many digits should be reported in forensic breath alcohol measurements? *J Anal Toxicol* 39:411; 2015.
Gullberg RG, McElroy AJ: Identifying components of variability in breath alcohol analysis; *J Anal Toxicol* 16:208; 1992.
Gullberg RG, Jones AW: Guidelines for estimating the amount of alcohol consumed from a single measurement of blood alcohol concentration: Re-evaluation of Widmark's equation; *Forensic Sci Int* 69:119; 1994.
Gullberg RG, Logan BK: Results of a proposed breath alcohol proficiency test program; *J Forensic Sci* 51:168; 2006.
Harger RN: A simple micromethod for the determination of alcohol in biologic material; *J Lab Clin Med* 20:746; 1935.
Harger RN, Forney RB, Barnes HB: Estimation of the level of blood alcohol from analysis of breath; *J Lab Clin Med* 36:306; 1950.
Harte RA: An instrument for the determination of ethanol in breath in law-enforcement practice; *J Forensic Sci* 16:493; 1971.
Hartung B, Schwender H, Pawlik E, Ritz-Timme S, Mindiashvili N, Daldrup T: Comparison of venous blood alcohol concentrations and breath alcohol concentrations measured with Draeger Alcotest 9510 DE Evidential; *Forensic Sci Int* 258:64; 2016.
Hlastala MP, Polissar NL, Oberman S: Statistical evaluation of standardized field sobriety tests; *J Forensic Sci* 50:662; 2005.
Hlastala MP, Anderson JC: The impact of breathing pattern and lung size on the alcohol breath test; *Ann Biomed Eng* 35:264; 2007.
Hodgson BT: The validity of evidential breath alcohol testing; *Can Soc Forensic Sci J* 41:83; 2008.
Holford NH: Clinical pharmacokinetics of ethanol; *Clin Pharmacokinet* 13:273; 1987.
Holland MG, Ferner RE: A systematic review of the evidence for acute tolerance to alcohol—the "Mellanby effect"; *Clin Toxicol (Phila)* 55:545; 2017.
Holmgren A, Jones AW: Demographics of suicide victims in Sweden in relation to their blood-alcohol concentration and the circumstances and manner of death; *Forensic Sci Int* 198:17; 2010.
Jaffe DH, Siman-Tov M, Gopher A, Peleg K: Variability in the blood/breath alcohol ratio and implications for evidentiary purposes; *J Forensic Sci* 58:1233; 2013.
Johnson RD, Horowitz M, Maddox AF, Wishart JM, Shearman DJ: Cigarette smoking and rate of gastric emptying: Effect on alcohol absorption; *Br Med J* 302:20; 1991.
Jones AW: Micro-technique of sample dilution for determination of alcohol in blood by gas chromatography; *Analyst* 102:307; 1977.

Jones AW: The precision and accuracy of a gas chromatograph intoximeter breath alcohol device part II—in-vivo experiments; *J Forensic Sci Soc* 18:81; 1978a.

Jones AW: Variability of the blood: Breath alcohol ratio *in vivo*; *J Stud Alcohol* 39:1931; 1978b.

Jones AW: Evaluation of breath alcohol instruments. II: In vivo experiments with alcolmeter pocket model; *Forensic Sci* 12:11; 1978c.

Jones AW: How breathing technique can influence the results of breath-alcohol analysis; *Med Sci Law* 22:275; 1982.

Jones AW: Determination of liquid/air partition coefficients for dilute solutions of ethanol in water, whole blood, and plasma; *J Anal Toxicol* 7:193; 1983.

Jones AW: Interindividual variations in the disposition and metabolism of ethanol in healthy men; *Alcohol* 1:385; 1984.

Jones AW: Electrochemical measurement of breath-alcohol concentration: Precision and accuracy in relation to blood levels; *Clin Chim Acta* 146:175; 1985.

Jones AW: Breath acetone concentrations in fasting male volunteers: Further studies and effect of alcohol administration; *J Anal Toxicol* 12:75; 1988a.

Jones AW: Enforcement of drink-driving laws by use of "per se" legal alcohol limits: Blood and/or breath concentration as evidence of impairment; *Alc Drugs Driving* 4:99; 1988b.

Jones AW: Physiological aspects of breath-alcohol measurement; *Alc Drugs Driving* 6:1; 1990a.

Jones AW: Status of alcohol absorption among drinking drivers; *J Anal Toxicol* 14:198; 1990b.

Jones AW: Concentration-time profiles of ethanol in capillary blood after ingestion of beer; *J Forensic Sci Soc* 31:429; 1991a.

Jones AW: Top ten defence challenges among drinking drivers in Sweden; *Med Sci Law* 31:229; 1991b.

Jones AW: Medicolegal alcohol determination—Blood- or breath-alcohol concentration? *Forensic Sci Rev* 12:23; 2000.

Jones AW: Reference limits for urine/blood ratios of ethanol in two successive voids from drinking drivers; *J Anal Toxicol* 26:333; 2002.

Jones AW: Evidence-based survey of the elimination rates of ethanol from blood with applications in forensic casework; *Forensic Sci Int* 200:1; 2010a.

Jones AW: *The Relationship Between Blood Alcohol Concentration (BAC) and Breath Alcohol Concentration (BrAC)—A Review of the Evidence* (Road Safety Web Publication no 15); Department of Transport: London, UK; 43 p; 2010b.

Jones AW: Pharmacokinetics of ethanol—Issues of forensic importance; *Forensic Sci Rev* 23:91; 2011.

Jones AW: Blood alcohol analysis by gas chromatography—Fifty years of progress; In Verstraete A (Ed.): *TIAFT—Our First 50 Years*; Academia Press: Gent, Belgium; 2013.

Jones AW: Alcohol: Breath analysis; In Payne-James J, Byard RW (Eds.): *Encyclopedia of Forensic and Legal Medicine*, 2nd ed; Elsevier: Oxford, UK; 2016.

Jones AW, Schuberth J: Computer-aided headspace gas chromatography applied to blood-alcohol analysis: Importance of online process control; *J Forensic Sci* 34:1116; 1989.

Jones AW, Sternebring B: Kinetics of ethanol and methanol in alcoholics during detoxification; *Alcohol Alcohol* 27:641; 1992.

Jones AW, Jönsson KÅ: Determination of ethanol in breath and estimation of the blood alcohol concentration with Alcolmeter S-D2; In Utzelmann G, Berghaus G, Kroj G (Eds.): *Proceedings —12th International Conference on Alcohol, Drugs and Traffic Safety*; Verlag TUV: Köln, Germany; 1993.

Jones AW, Jönsson KÅ: Food-induced lowering of blood-ethanol profiles and increased rate of elimination immediately after a meal; *J Forensic Sci* 39:1084; 1994.

Jones AW, Andersson L: Variability of the blood/breath alcohol ratio in drinking drivers; *J Forensic Sci* 41:916; 1996.

Jones AW, Andersson L: Comparison of ethanol concentrations in venous blood and end-expired breath during a controlled drinking study; *Forensic Sci Int* 132:18; 2003.

Jones AW, Fransson M: Blood analysis by headspace gas chromatography: Does a deficient sample volume distort ethanol concentration? *Med Sci Law* 43:241; 2003.

Jones AW, Andersson L: Determination of ethanol in breath for legal purposes using a five-filter infrared analyzer: Studies on response to volatile interfering substances; *J Breath Res* 2:026006; 2008.

Jones AW, Holmgren A: Age and gender differences in blood-alcohol concentration in apprehended drivers in relation to the amounts of alcohol consumed; *Forensic Sci Int* 188:40; 2009a.

Jones AW, Holmgren A: Concentration distributions of the drugs most frequently identified in post-mortem femoral blood representing all causes of death; *Med Sci Law* 49:257; 2009b.

Jones AW, Ericsson E: Decreases in blood ethanol concentration during storage at 4°C for 12 months were the same for specimens kept in glass and plastic tubes; *Pract Lab Med* 4:76; 2016.

Jones AW, Jönsson KÅ, Jorfeldt L: Differences between capillary and venous blood-alcohol concentrations as a function of time after drinking, with emphasis on sampling variations in left vs right arm; *Clin Chem* 35:400; 1989.

Jones AW, Jönsson KÅ, Neri A: Peak blood-ethanol concentration and the time of its occurrence after rapid drinking on an empty stomach; *J Forensic Sci* 36:376; 1991.

Jones AW, Sagarduy A, Ericsson E, Arnqvist HJ: Concentrations of acetone in venous blood samples from drunk drivers, type-I diabetic outpatients, and healthy blood donors; *J Anal Toxicol* 17:182; 1993.

Jones AW, Lindberg L, Olsson SG: Magnitude and time-course of arterio-venous differences in blood-alcohol concentration in healthy men; *Clin Pharmacokinet* 43:1157; 2004.

Jones AW, Kugelberg FC, Holmgren A, Ahlner J: Five-year update on the occurrence of alcohol and other drugs in blood samples from drivers killed in road-traffic crashes in Sweden; *Forensic Sci Int* 186:56; 2009.

Jones TP, Jones AW, Williams PM: Some recent developments in breath alcohol analysis; *The Police Surgeon* 6:80; 1974.

Kalant H: Current state of knowledge about the mechanisms of alcohol tolerance; *Addict Biol* 1:133; 1996b.

Kalant H: Pharmacokientics of ethanol: Absorption, distribution, and elimination; In Beglieter H, Kissin B (Eds.): *The Pharmacology of Alcohol and Alcohol Dependence*; Oxford University Press: New York; 1996a.

Kalant H: Research on tolerance: What can we learn from history? *Alcohol Clin Exp Res* 22:67; 1998.

Kalant H: Effects of food and body composition on blood alcohol curves; *Alcohol Clin Exp Res* 24:413; 2000.

Kaltenbach ML, Vistelle R, Hoizey G, Lamiable D, Zbierski L: Arterio-venous ethanol levels in blood and plasma after intravenous injection in rabbits; *Alcohol* 15:319; 1998.

Keiding S, Christensen NJ, Damgaard SE, Dejgard A, Iversen HL, Jacobsen A, Johansen S, Lundquist F, Rubinstein E, Winkler K: Ethanol metabolism in heavy drinkers after massive and moderate alcohol intake; *Biochem Pharmacol* 32:3097; 1983.

Kriikku P, Wilhelm L, Jenckel S, Rintatalo J, Hurme J, Kramer J, Jones AW, Ojanpera I: Comparison of breath-alcohol screening test results with venous blood alcohol concentration in suspected drunken drivers; *Forensic Sci Int* 239:57; 2014.

Krishan S, Lui SM: A study of acetone interference in Intoxilyzer® 5000C; *Can Soc Forensic Sci J* 35:159; 2002.

Lentner C: *Geigy Scientific Tables—Units of Measurement: Body Fluids: Composition of the Body. Nutrition*; CIBA-GEIGY: Basel, Switzerland; 1981.

Levine B, Smialek JE: Status of alcohol absorption in drinking drivers killed in traffic accidents; *J Forensic Sci* 45:3; 2000.

Li TK, Yin SJ, Crabb DW, O'Connor S, Ramchandani VA: Genetic and environmental influences on alcohol metabolism in humans; *Alcohol Clin Exp Res* 25:136; 2001.

Lieber CS: Hepatic, metabolic and toxic effects of ethanol: 1991 update; *Alcohol Clin Exp Res* 15:573; 1991.

Liljestrand G: Till frågan om läkareundersökning rörande alkoholpåverkan; *Tirfing* 34:97; 1940.

Lindberg L, Brauer S, Wollmer P, Goldberg L, Jones AW, Olsson SG: Breath alcohol concentration determined with a new analyzer using free exhalation predicts almost precisely the arterial blood alcohol concentration; *Forensic Sci Int* 168:200; 2007.

Lindberg L, Grubb D, Dencker D, Finnhult M, Olsson SG: Detection of mouth alcohol during breath alcohol analysis; *Forensic Sci Int* 249:66; 2015.

Linnet K: Necessary sample size for method comparison studies based on regression analysis; *Clin Chem* 45:882; 1999.

Lippi G, Becan-McBride K, Behulova D, Bowen RA, Church S, Delanghe J, Grankvist K, Kitchen S, Nybo M, Nauck M, et al.: Preanalytical quality improvement: In quality we trust; *Clin Chem Lab Med* 51:229; 2013.

Lippi G, Simundic AM, Musile G, Danese E, Salvagno G, Tagliaro F: The alcohol used for cleansing the venipuncture site does not jeopardize blood and plasma alcohol measurement with head-space gas chromatography and an enzymatic assay; *Biochem Med* (Zagreb) 27:398; 2017.

Lucey MR, Hill EM, Young JP, Demo-Dananberg L, Beresford TP: The influences of age and gender on blood ethanol concentrations in healthy humans; *J Stud Alcohol* 60:103; 1999.

Ludbrook J: Confidence in Altman-Bland plots: A critical review of the method of differences; *Clin Exp Pharmacol Physiol* 37:143; 2010a.

Ludbrook J: Linear regression analysis for comparing two measurers or methods of measurement: But which regression? *Clin Exp Pharmacol Physiol* 37:692; 2010b.

Lundquist F, Wolthers H: The kinetics of alcohol elimination in man; *Acta Pharmacol Toxicol* (Copenh) 14:265; 1958.

Machata G: The advantages of automated blood alcohol determination by head space analysis; *Z Rechtsmed* 75:229; 1975.

Martin CS, Moss HB: Measurement of acute tolerance to alcohol in human subjects; *Alcohol Clin Exp Res* 17:211; 1993.

Martin E, Moll W, Schmid P, Dettli L: The pharmacokinetics of alcohol in human breath, venous and arterial blood after oral ingestion; *Eur J Clin Pharmacol* 26:619; 1984.

Martin TL: An evaluation of the Intoxilyzer® 8000C evidential breath alcohol analyzer; *Can Soc Forensic Sci J* 44:22; 2011.

Maskell PD, Jones AW, Savage A, Scott-Ham M: Evidence based survey of the distribution volume of ethanol: Comparison of empirically determined values with anthropometric measures; *Forensic Sci Int* 294:124; 2019.

Mason MF, Dubowski KM: Breath-alcohol analysis: uses, methods, and some forensic problems—Review and opinion; *J Forensic Sci* 21:9; 1976.

Mellanby E: Alcohol and alcoholic intoxication; *Brit J Inebriety* 17:157; 1920.

Milic J, Glisic M, Voortman T, Borba LP, Asllanaj E, Rojas LZ, Troup J, Kiefte-de Jong JC, van Beeck E, Muka T et al.: Menopause, ageing, and alcohol use disorders in women; *Maturitas* 111:100; 2018.

Mitchell MC Jr, Teigen EL, Ramchandani VA: Absorption and peak blood alcohol concentration after drinking beer, wine, or spirits; *Alcohol Clin Exp Res* 38:1200; 2014.

Mizoi Y, Adachi J, Fukunaga T, Kogame M, Ueno Y, Nojo Y, Fujiwara S: Individual and ethnic differences in ethanol elimination; *Alcohol Alcohol* 1:389; 1987.

Mizoi Y, Fukunaga T, Ueno Y, Adachi J, Fujiwara S, Nishimura A: The flushing syndrome after ethanol intake caused by aldehyde dehydrogenase deficiency in Orientals; *Acta Med Leg Soc* (Liege) 39:481; 1989.

Modell JG, Taylor JP, Lee JY: Breath alcohol values following mouthwash use; *J Am Med Assoc* 270:2955; 1993.

Morris DH, Amlung MT, Tsai CL, McCarthy DM: Association between overall rate of change in rising breath alcohol concentration and the magnitude of acute tolerance of subjective intoxication via the Mellanby method; *Hum Psychopharmacol* 32; 2017.

Moskowitz M, Fiorentino D: A review of the literature on the effects of low doses of alcohol on driving-related skills (DOT HS 809 028); US National Highway Traffic Safety Administration: Springfield, VA, 2000.

Mulder JA, Neuteboom W: The effects of hypo- and hyperventilation on breath alcohol measurements; *Blutalkohol* 24:341; 1987.

Mumenthaler MS, Taylor JL, O'Hara R, Fisch HU, Yesavage JA: Effects of menstrual cycle and female sex steroids on ethanol pharmacokinetics; *Alcohol Clin Exp Res* 23:250; 1999.

Mumenthaler MS, Taylor JL, Yesavage JA: Ethanol pharmacokinetics in white women: Nonlinear model fitting versus zero-order elimination analyses; *Alcohol Clin Exp Res* 24:1353; 2000.

Nicloux M: Simplification de la méthode de dosage de l'alcool dans le sang et dans les tissus; *Comp Rend Soc Biol* 60:1034; 1906.

Olson KN, Smith SW, Kloss JS, Ho JD, Apple FS: Relationship between blood alcohol concentration and observable symptoms of intoxication in patients presenting to an emergency department; *Alcohol Alcohol* 48:386; 2013.

Page TE: The drug recognition expert officer: Signs of drug impairment at roadside; In Mayhew DR, Dussault C (Eds.): *Proceedings—16th International Conference on Alcohol, Drugs and Traffic Safety*; Montreal, Canada; 2002.

Pajunen T, Vuori E, Lunetta P: Epidemiology of alcohol-related unintentional drowning: is postmortem ethanol production a real challenge? *Inj Epidemiol* 5:39; 2018.

Pavlic M, Grubwieser P, Libiseller K, Rabl W: Elimination rates of breath alcohol; *Forensic Sci Int* 171:16; 2007.

Payne JP, Hill DW, King NW: Observations on the distribution of alcohol in blood, breath, and urine; *Br Med J* 1:196; 1966.

Peachey JE, Sellers EM: The disulfiram and calcium carbimide acetaldehyde-mediated ethanol reactions; *Pharmacol Ther* 15:89; 1981.

Peek-Asa C: The effect of random alcohol screening in reducing motor vehicle crash injuries; *Am J Prev Med* 16:57; 1999.

Penton JR, Forrester MR: A gas chromatographic breath analysis system with provisions for storage and delayed analysis of samples; *Proceedings—5th International Conference on Alcohol and Traffic Safety*; Schulz Förlag: Freiburg, Germany; 1970.

Penttila A, Tenhu M: Clinical examination as medicolegal proof of alcohol intoxication; *Med Sci Law* 16:95; 1976.

Poon R, Hodgson BT, Hindberg I, Rowatt C: Evaluation of three pocket-size breath alcohol analyzers; *Can Forensic Sci Soc J* 20:19; 1987.

Quertemont E, Eriksson CJ, Zimatkin SM, Pronko PS, Diana M, Pisano M, Rodd ZA, Bell RR, Ward RJ: Is ethanol a pro-drug? Acetaldehyde contribution to brain ethanol effects; *Alcohol Clin Exp Res* 29:1514; 2005.

Riley D, Wigmore JG, Yen B: Dilution of blood collected for medicolegal alcohol analysis by intravenous fluids; *J Anal Toxicol* 20:330; 1996.

Room R, Babor T, Rehm J: Alcohol and public health; *Lancet* 365:519; 2005.

Rowland M, Tozer TN: *Clinical Pharmacokinetics—Concepts and Applications*, 3rd ed; Williams & Wilkins: Baltimore, MD; 1995.

Rubenzer S: Judging intoxication; *Behav Sci Law* 29:116; 2011.

Schvarcz E, Palmer M, Aman J, Berne C: Hypoglycemia increases the gastric emptying rate in healthy subjects; *Diabetes Care* 18:674; 1995.

Seto Y: Determination of volatile substances in biological samples by headspace gas chromatography; *J Chromatog A* 674:25; 1994.

Shan X, Tiscione NB, Alford I, Yeatman DT: A study of blood alcohol stability in forensic antemortem blood samples; *Forensic Sci Int* 211:47; 2011.

Sterling K: The rate of dissipation of mouth alcohol in alcohol positive subjects; *J Forensic Sci* 57:802; 2012.

Stockl D, Dewitte K, Thienpont LM: Validity of linear regression in method comparison studies: Is it limited by the statistical model or the quality of the analytical input data? *Clin Chem* 44:2340; 1998.

Stuster J: Validation of the standardized field sobriety test battery at 0.08% blood alcohol concentration; *Hum Factors* 48:608; 2006.

Tagliaro F, Lubli G, Ghielmi S, Franchi D, Marigo M: Chromatographic methods for blood alcohol determination; *J Chromatogr* 580:161; 1992.

Taylor L, Oberman S: *Drunk Driving Defense*; Wolters Kluwer: Austin, TX; 2006.

Twomey PJ, Kroll MH: How to use linear regression and correlation in quantitative method comparison studies; *Int J Clin Pract* 62:529; 2008.

UK Government: *Licensing Act. Intoxicating Liquor*; 1872; http://wwwlegislationgovuk/ukpga/1872/94/pdfs/ukpga_18720094_enpdf (Accessed July 27, 2019).

Voas RB, Fell JC: Strengthening impaired-driving enforcement in the United States; *Traffic Inj Prev* 14:661; 2013.

Wagner JG: Properties of the Michaelis-Menten equation and its integrated form which are useful in pharmacokinetics; *J Pharmacokinet Biopharm* 1:103; 1973.

Wagner JG, Wilkinson PK, Ganes DA: Parameters Vm' and Km for elimination of alcohol in young male subjects following low doses of alcohol; *Alcohol Alcohol* 24:555; 1989.

Wallage HR, Bugyra IM: Interferent detect on the Intoxilyzer® 8000C in an individual with an elevated blood acetone concentration due to ketoacidosis; *Can Soc Forensic Sci J* 50:157; 2017.

Watkins RL, Adler EV: The effect of food on alcohol absorption and elimination patterns; *J Forensic Sci* 38:285; 1993.

Watts MT, McDonald OL: The effect of biologic specimen type on the gas chromatographic headspace analysis of ethanol and other volatile compounds; *Am J Clin Pathol* 87:79; 1987.

Weafer J, Fillmore MT: Acute tolerance to alcohol impairment of behavioral and cognitive mechanisms related to driving: Drinking and driving on the descending limb; *Psychopharmacology* (Berl) 220:697; 2012.

Weathermon R, Crabb DW: Alcohol and medication interactions; *Alcohol Res Health* 23:40; 1999.

Widmark EMP: Om alkoholens öfvergång i urinen samt om en enkel, kliniskt användbar metod för diagnosticering af alkoholförekomst i kroppen; *Upsala Läkareförenings förhandlingar N F* 19:241; 1914.

Widmark EMP: Über die Konzentration des genossenen Alkohols in Blut und Ham unter verschiedenen Ulmständen; *Scand Arch Physiol* 33:85; 1915.

Widmark EMP: Eine Mikromethode zur Bestimmung von Äthylalkohol im Blut; *Biochem Z* 131:473; 1922.

Widmark EMP: Blodalkoholbestämning vid diagnosen av alkoholpåverkan; *Sv Läkartidningen* 27:690; 1930.

Widmark EMP: *Die theoretischen Grundlagen und die praktische Verwendbarkeit der gerichtlich-medizinischen Alkoholbestimmung*; Urban & Schwarzenberg Verlag: Berlin, Germany; 1932.

Widmark EMP: *Principles and Applications of Medicolegal Alcohol Determinations*; Biomedical Publications: Davis, CA; 163 p; 1981.

Wigmore JG, Langille RM: Six generations of breath alcohol testing instruments: Changes in the detection of breath alcohol since 1930. A historical overview; *Can Soc Forensic Sci J* 42:276; 2009.

Wilkinson PK, Wagner JG, Sedman AJ: Sensitive head-space gas chromatographic method for the determination of ethanol utilizing capillary blood samples; *Anal Chem* 47:1506; 1975.

Wolff E: The blood alcoohl test in motorists in the Scandinavian countries; *Acta Med Leg Soc* 11:11; 1956.

World Health Organisation: *Road Traffic Injuries*; World Health Organisation: Geneva, Switzerland; 2018.

Zakhari S: Overview: How is alcohol metabolized by the body? *Alc Res Health* 29:245; 2006.

Zamengo L, Frison G, Tedeschi G, Frasson S, Zancanaro F, Sciarrone R: Variability of blood alcohol content (BAC) determinations: The role of measurement uncertainty, significant figures, and decision rules for compliance assessment in the frame of a multiple BAC threshold law; *Drug Test Anal* 6:1028; 2014.

Ziporyn T: Definition of impairment essential for prosecuting drunken drivers; *J Am Med Assoc* 253:3509; 1985.

Zuba D: Accuracy and reliability of breath alcohol testing by handheld electrochemical analysers; *Forensic Sci Int* 178:e29; 2008.

Common Legal Challenges, Responses, and Court Decisions in Forensic Breath- and Blood-Alcohol Analysis*

ROD G. GULLBERG

Contents

* This chapter is an updated version of a review article previously published in *Forensic Science Review*: Gullberg RG: Examples of legal challenges and court decisions related to forensic breath-alcohol analysis; *Forensic Sci Rev* 16:91; 2004.

6.1 Introduction

During 2017, over 990,000 arrests occurred for driving while under the influence of alcohol (DUI) in the United States. This exceeded the number of arrests for other individual felonies including murder, rape, robbery, aggravated assault and burglary (US Federal Bureau of Investigation 2017). No other crime or civil proceeding impacts such a broad spectrum of society as does DUI. Although DUI may be a criminal offense or an infraction, depending on the jurisdiction, the focus here will be on the criminal context, where more significant defense challenges commonly occur. In response to increasing epidemiological evidence as well as political pressure, most jurisdictions continue to increase the penalties for a DUI conviction in an effort to address this significant public safety problem. In addition, many jurisdictions have revised their criminal and administrative statutes regarding DUI, which has added complexity to the issues. Revisions to "implied consent" statutes along with defining the offense as having a "*per se* breath or blood alcohol concentration" have resulted in prosecutions relying principally on breath or blood alcohol evidence in many jurisdictions. Since an individual's property and often livelihood are impacted by a DUI conviction, people are willing to incur significant expense for their defense. No other single offense brings the forensic science profession into contact with the legal system more than DUI.

The criminal defense community, therefore, has responded with a variety of challenges to this increasingly complex and specialized area of litigation. DUI defense is a highly specialized law practice today with an ever increasing focus on scientific and technical issues. These challenges have been directed primarily toward forensic breath alcohol analysis because over 90% of DUI cases involve breath alcohol evidence. As breath-test programs have advanced with regard to technology, protocols, biological and epidemiological research, data analysis, etc., the defense issues have expanded, becoming more sophisticated and focused. In view of *per se* legislation, breath and blood alcohol evidence is persuasive and compelling. Juries want to hear evidence of the alcohol concentration. It makes the decision easier when it can be based on an objective analytical result. Therefore, the defense is often focused on pretrial suppression hearings in an effort to preclude the "trier of the facts" (e.g., judge, jury, hearing officer, etc.) from hearing the objective analytical results. Many legal firms specializing in DUI defense have learned well the technology and mounted a host of technical and creative challenges (e.g., circuitry voltage values, causes of error records, susceptibility to radio frequencies, clock accuracy, error record percentages, software technical details, etc.). Forensic personnel in Washington State, for example, where over 20,000 persons were arrested for DUI and administered breath alcohol tests during 2017, encounter many of these challenges. Moreover, the defense community in Washington State has become technically well educated and networked in their efforts to scrutinize all program details including:

- Administrative rules
- Program policy/protocol manuals
- Maintenance records
- Technical instrument features
- Training outlines and records
- Phone call and e-mail records

- Prior court testimony
- Instrument software validation and approval
- The syntax of Implied Consent Rights (the missing semicolon defense), etc.

The purpose here is to present several of the most common defense challenges encountered with the presentation of forensic breath and blood alcohol evidence in DUI cases. We present only a small number of defense challenges due to space limitations. Many more examples exist that are often unique to different jurisdictions, owing to their unique legal and political contexts. Forensic personnel need to be alert to these challenges and carefully consider their relevance to the improvement of their programs. Indeed, program improvement can result from creative defense challenges. Although all of these challenges have been experienced in the State of Washington, most have also been encountered in other jurisdictions. Given the efficient network within the defense community, all of these issues along with many others are expected to eventually appear in all jurisdictions. Knowledge of these issues should assist other jurisdictions in program development, rule adoption, training, and case preparation. Since jurisdictions differ with regard to legislation, case law, instrumentation, protocols, administrative rules, resources, program policies, etc., several of the defense challenges experienced in one area may have little impact elsewhere. However, knowledge of challenges in one jurisdiction may assist in preparation elsewhere in an effort to minimize the impact. Finally, our overall objective should be to develop a forensic measurement program that provides analytical evidence that has the highest reliability and integrity possible. This often results from encountering and considering challenges to our program policy and procedures. It is recommended that a list of challenges faced by a jurisdiction be developed along with effective responses. Such a list would be very helpful to new personnel in their training. In addition to defense challenges, we must consider the challenges raised in the National Academy of Science report of 2009 (US National Research Council 2009). The report emphasized the importance of accreditation, proficiency testing, quality control, best practices, code of ethics, further research, etc. "An accredited laboratory has in place a management system that defines the various processes by which it operates on a daily basis, monitors that activity, and responds to deviations from the acceptable practices using a routine and thoughtful method." Such daily consideration would greatly improve our programs.

6.2 The Adversarial Legal Context

Responding to legal and procedural challenges is clearly a significant responsibility for forensic toxicologists. This responsibility must be faced with the highest level of transparency and integrity. A significant proportion of their time may be spent on legal matters including:

- Pretrial discussion with prosecutors or defense attorneys
- Providing pretrial discovery material
- Case preparation
- Testimony in hearings and in trials

For example, the forensic toxicologists in the Washington State Toxicology Laboratory, who prepare alcohol-water simulator solutions, spend approximately 80% of their court preparation time in regard to breath test cases and only 20% regarding blood or drug cases.

Forensic toxicology is among the "mandated sciences" where science finds itself applied in response to public policy and directives. Our scientific knowledge, however, is incomplete, our technology is limited, and our evidence is often subjective and open to interpretation. Breath alcohol measurement along with its legal support is an effort to provide more objective and reliable analytical evidence. Challenge, therefore, is to be expected (Pollack 1973). Indeed, our constitutional framework outlines an adversarial legal system, a crucible of challenge and controversy from which, ideally, truth emerges. Unlike that of the forensic scientist, the role of the defense is not to be objective or to advance scientific understanding, but to be an advocate. Moreover, this is often how we are made aware of weaknesses within our programs. We must never forget that every forensically sound program can be improved, which is often facilitated by legal challenge. Our objective should be to present the most reliable and informative analytical results possible and in a manner that promotes justice. We must also keep in mind that our results are intended for consideration by lay juries who need our clarity, integrity, and full-disclosure. Part of the objectivity and professionalism of science is to consider and weigh the criticisms raised by persons holding different views. Indeed, part of our professional responsibility is to ensure and demonstrate that the evidence we present is fit-for-purpose (e.g., suitable and relevant for its intended application).

6.3 Common Defense Challenges to Breath Alcohol Analysis

6.3.1 Uncertainty in Measurement Results

Per se legislation, prohibiting the operation of a motor vehicle by a person having a specified breath alcohol concentration (e.g., 0.08 g/210 L or more), has prompted defense attention on the measurement process, the analytical results and their uncertainty. Part of the defense strategy is to assert that breath alcohol results just above the prohibited limit could likely have been obtained from a subject, who in reality, had a true breath alcohol concentration below the limit. The argument is that excessive random or systematic error resulted in an aberrantly high result (a false-positive). Moreover, this argument will apply to all prohibited concentrations (e.g., 0.02 g/210 L for minors, 0.04 g/210 L for commercial motor vehicle operators, and 0.15 g/210 L for enhanced penalties).

Measurement uncertainty near the critical limits is a fair and relevant argument and should be raised by a responsible defense attorney. Breath alcohol analysis, like all measurements, possesses uncertainty. Forensic scientists must be prepared to acknowledge this and compute appropriate estimates. Figure 6.1 illustrates this issue by showing different hypothetical uncertainty intervals (A and B) that can arise in different measurement contexts for the same sample mean (0.088 g/210 L). This could be applied to any critical concentration. The question is, which uncertainty interval is correct for a particular case? Clearly, this would be relevant for the court to know. The defense would like to argue that B is correct while the prosecution would prefer to argue for A. It is not for the forensic witness to assert which interval should apply. We are simply to perform the computation. The jury weighs the evidence and makes the inference. The forensic scientist must

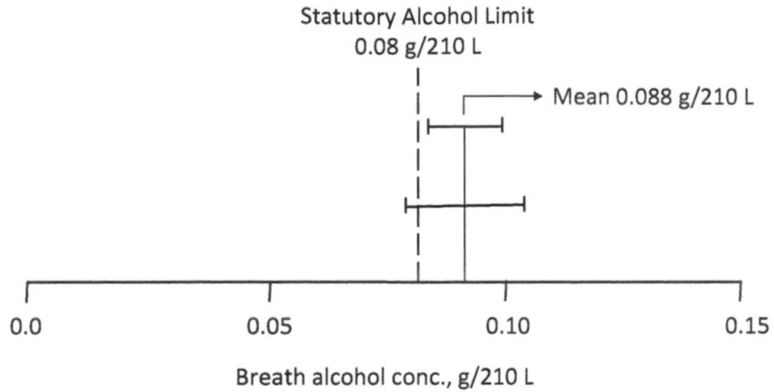

Figure 6.1 Illustration of 95% confidence intervals for measurement uncertainty of two systems having the same mean result of 0.088 g/210 L.

simply be prepared to compute and explain these intervals (e.g., a 95% confidence interval quantifying the uncertainty) based on estimates appropriate for their instrumentation and protocols. Duplicate breath analyses along with control measurements from a carefully managed and maintained program will provide reliable data for these calculations. Clearly, at some mean BrAC value, the lower 95%, 99%, or other selected confidence interval limit will fall below the critical limit. This reality of measurement must be acknowledged. However, it only impacts those results near the *per se* levels. Most concentrations, and confidence intervals, will be significantly greater than this. The approach taken by some European jurisdictions is to perform this calculation and then offer the evidence in the prosecution only if the lower 99% confidence interval limit exceeds the statutory limit. Finally, program accreditation will also require that measurement uncertainty be determined. Accreditation should be pursued by breath test programs in order to add integrity and informative value to their results. Accreditation, along with proficiency testing, should help address many common defense challenges by demonstrating compliance with important elements of quality control.

Preparation prior to trial is very important for this issue. The forensic scientist must have the relevant information and perform the computations before trial. The mathematical details should also be presented in court for the jury to see by the use of an easel along with clear explanation. The jury can then take the document for deliberation. These must also be disclosed to attorneys for both sides prior to trial so that all are aware of the computations along with their assumptions and limitations. Often, these results become the basis for a plea bargain or other agreed arrangement prior to trial. An additional consideration is the fact that modern computerized breath test instruments have the capacity to printout the measurement uncertainty on the document received at the completion of the test procedure. This capability should be requested by customers and pursued by manufacturers.

All of these details regarding measurement uncertainty must also be recorded in the program's SOP manual. In this way all forensic scientists will be consistent in their computational results. Moreover, the SOP manual must be completely available to the defense upon a discovery request. The manual should also be available on the program web site.

A court case from Idaho is unique regarding this issue of measurement uncertainty (*State v. Jones* 2016). While this case involved a blood sample, it is still relevant to breath alcohol analysis. The Supreme Court of Idaho denied the defendants request to introduce evidence of measurement uncertainty. The defendant's blood alcohol result was 0.207 g/100 mL. Idaho has a statute applying enhanced penalties for results over 0.20. The high court held "…the testing machine's margin of error was irrelevant." The offense is committed based on the instrument result and not what the blood, breath or urine concentrations were at the time of driving. There is no need to extrapolate or to show that the result reflects some reality in the human body.

In a case involving driver's license suspension, the Supreme Court of Idaho also ruled that measurement uncertainty was irrelevant (*Elias-Cruz v. Idaho Department of Transportation* 2012). Elias-Cruz was a minor arrested for DUI having a breath alcohol result of 0.021 and 0.020 g/210 L. Elias-Cruz desired to enter evidence that, considering the uncertainty of measurement, would put her breath alcohol results below 0.02. The high court ruled that "…a violation can be shown simply by the results of a test for alcohol concentration that complies with the statutory requirements… the margin of error in the testing equipment is irrelevant."

We come back to this issue of measurement uncertainty again in the later section on blood alcohol defense challenges. There we illustrate the calculations for determining uncertainty in both blood and breath alcohol measurements.

As we have shown above, the sampling of breath and the resulting difference in duplicate results contribute significantly to measurement uncertainty. For this reason, jurisdictions performing duplicate tests have criteria requiring specific agreement. In Wisconsin, the administrative rules require "…results in a test sequence within 0.02 g of alcohol per 210 L of breath shall be deemed to be an acceptable agreement." Gregory A. Mickelson (the defendant) was arrested for OWI (operating while intoxicated) and administered a breath alcohol test of two samples resulting in 0.176 and 0.156 g/210 L. The defendant argued that the difference of exactly 0.020 g/210 L did not comply with the administrative rules since the difference was not less than 0.02. Mickelson argued that the exact difference of 0.020 was not "within 0.02." He argued that "within" should require the two results to differ by less than 0.02. The Court of Appeals in Wisconsin reject the defendant's motion to suppress (*State v Mickelson* 2004).

6.3.2 Biased Results due to the Presence of an Interfering Substance

As early as 1927, Bogen recognized that acetone and other volatile organic compounds (VOC) were potential interfering substances in the potassium dichromate oxidation of breath alcohol (Bogen 1927). Except for the application of multiple filters, modern infrared instruments suffer from the same lack of specificity for ethanol. Not only is the endogenous production of acetone from diabetes or extreme fasting a potential concern, but the widespread potential for occupational exposure to VOCs in industry has also resulted in defense challenges. Moreover, the arguments have extended to gasoline exposure (Cooper 1981), fuel additives (Buckley et al. 2001), aerosol inhalers (Gomm et al. 1990), and even the over 100 VOC present in normal human breath (Krotoszkynski et al. 1977). Even though highly improbable for biasing a breath alcohol measurement, the implication that subjects may have some other VOCs in their breath presents a defense challenge requiring an effective response. Mostly, due to statutory construction and case law, this issue generally goes to the weight rather than admissibility.

Depending on the specific facts of the case, there are several approaches that the prosecution can take in response to this challenge. If the subject claims to be diabetic or fasting, then some evidence of medical diagnosis should be solicited. In these cases the prosecution may be able, through the forensic witness, to introduce some of the voluminous literature showing the extremely small probability that endogenous acetone will bias a breath alcohol measurement (Dubowski and Essary 1984; Flores and Frank 1985; Jones 1987; Jones et al. 1996). If the subject experienced occupational exposure, then the critical information to obtain includes:

- Duration of exposure
- Environment of exposure
- Use of respiratory protective equipment
- Materials exposed to
- Time between last exposure and breath alcohol test
- Observations of the arresting officer
- Possibility of chemicals on clothing
- Instrument features designed to detect interfering substances

The forensic witness should also be able to introduce some of the literature relating to occupational exposure (Gill et al. 1991a, 1991b, 1991c). In addition, some of the literature relates to specific breath test instruments (Caldwell and Kim 1997; Cowan et al. 1990; Logan et al. 1994). The observations of the arresting officer are also very important in this regard. They may reveal that the individual had organic material on their clothing, contributing to the VOC being inhaled just prior to breath sampling. An important question for the operator to routinely ask is whether the subject was exposed to any VOC in the last 24 hours. Depending on statutory construction, the subject may be deemed incapable of providing a breath sample and allow for the request of a blood sample under implied consent. Moreover, many VOCs do not yield normal breath alcohol exhalation curves as expected by the instrument during sample acquisition for alcohol. In addition to several other defense arguments, the response to this issue can be enhanced through implementing a sound breath test protocol including:

- 15-minute minimum pre-exhalation observation time
- Using only approved instruments employing specific features (i.e., dual technology, multiple filters)
- Trained operators
- External wet-bath simulator or dry gas controls
- Duplicate breath samples with acceptable agreement (Dubowski 1994).

One final possibility, depending on the facts of the case and agreement of all parties, is for the subject to be offered a reduced charge in exchange for the provision of breath samples following normal occupational exposure to the VOC. Such an experiment can be arranged for more than one occasion and has the potential to greatly advance our forensic understanding of potential interferences in measuring breath alcohol.

Several analytical approaches to this issue have also been advanced. Most infrared instruments employ multiple filters to improve the selectivity for ethanol. One instrument, the Alcotest 9510 (Drager, Inc.: Irvine, TX), employs dual technology (infrared and electrochemical), which also improves selectivity for ethanol since electrochemical technology is less susceptible to VOC. If the subject was administered a roadside pre-arrest breath test (PBT) using an electrochemical (fuel cell) device, the results can be compared to the subsequent evidential device and supplemented with appropriate expert testimony. Such admissibility of the PBT result may require a pre-trial evidentiary hearing (a Frye or Daubert hearing) (*Frye v United States* 1923; *Daubert v Merrell Dow Pharmaceuticals* 1993; Funk 2018). Those states, however, that require submission to a roadside PBT test may want to reconsider this in view of a 2010 Georgia case (*Olevik v. State* 2017). The Supreme Court of Georgia ruled that a driver was not required to submit to a roadside PBT test since it would be an act of compelled incrimination. Over 30 states appear to adhere to rules of evidence defined by Daubert while the rest follow Frye or some other legal case. The Frye court ruled basically that scientific evidence must be generally accepted in the relevant scientific community in order to be admissible. New or experimental methods considered to be marginal would not be admissible. This became known as the "general acceptance test." Daubert, on the other hand, was a more flexible standard allowing the judge to be the "gatekeeper" of scientific testimony by considering several criteria for scientific reliability. One required consideration is "the known or potential error rate of the method." In most US states, evidence for the reliability of the PBT or a new evidentiary breath test instrument will have to be presented in order to meet one of these court decisions (Funk 2018). Finally, the forensic scientist can determine the amount of vapor acetone necessary to produce a 0.01 g/210 L ethanol equivalent on the particular instrument and compare this to the biomedical literature on expected levels resulting from specific medical conditions.

6.3.3 Storage of Alcohol Simulator Solutions in Plastic Containers

Simulator solutions in Washington State, like most jurisdictions, are stored in both 500-mL and 1-gal polyethylene (plastic) bottles. The solutions are labeled with a batch number, reference value, date of preparation, expiration data and sealed with evidence tape. By administrative rules, they are not used beyond one year thereafter. Through the testimony of an expert witness, the defense may argue that volatile materials such as ethanol must be stored only in glass containers at 4°C. It would be helpful for a jurisdiction to experimentally test the shelf life of the solutions over a one-year period.

An effective response to this issue begins with a clearly written program policy regarding the preparation, storage, distribution, and use of simulator solutions. The policy should include:

- Preparation protocol;
- Testing protocol by an independent method and reporting its uncertainty (e.g., gas chromatography);
- Record documentation;
- Sealing (tamper proof), storage, labeling and shelf life;
- Installation protocol;
- Qualified personnel;
- Expiration date; and
- Homogeneity test, etc.

When these predefined and approved procedures are complied with, the admissibility of the evidence should follow with various arguments going to the weight of the evidence.

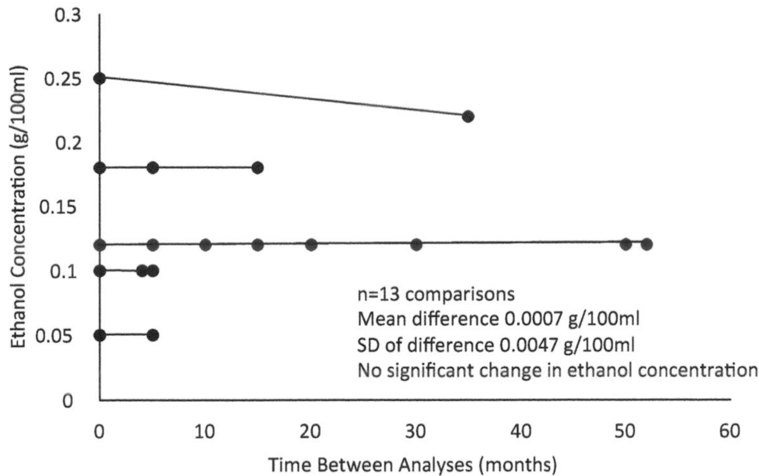

Figure 6.2 Change in ethanol concentration over time when stored in plastic bottles as determined by gas chromatography.

Evidence regarding the storage stability in plastic containers can be obtained where solutions stored in plastic bottles for varying periods of time are reanalyzed and compared to the original results. Figure 6.2 illustrates such results where the change between the first and subsequent analysis by gas chromatography is shown as a function of time. Figure 6.2 represents solutions stored both in 500-mL and 1-gal plastic containers. For solutions stored over time periods ranging from 4 to 53 months, the mean decrease was 0.0007 g/100 mL with a 95% confidence interval including zero. In addition, sequential plots of simulator results on specific breath test instruments using solutions stored over several months can also reveal analytical stability. This evidence should demonstrate that for alcohol simulator solutions, the loss occurring through polyethylene is immeasurable over reasonable time periods. In addition, the suitability of storing simulator solutions in polyethylene containers was recently verified in a study evaluating the change occurring over a one-year period (Dubowski et al. 2002). Moreover, an extreme example of testing alcohol solution stability in polyethylene bottles stored at room temperature for 26 years has been reported (Chow and Wigmore 2005). For bottled solutions at 0.04, 0.24 and 0.30 g/100 mL the percent changes ranged from –15.6 to +8.3. For a solution at 0.36 g/100 mL the maximum percent change was +39.1. While these extreme changes would not be forensically acceptable, the study demonstrates remarkable stability under extreme duration. The requirement to store volatiles in glass, therefore, may be appropriate for trace analysis, but is unnecessary for alcohol simulator solutions. Moreover, program personnel should be prepared to provide solution samples to the defense team for their independent analysis. In addition to advancing our forensic knowledge, objective measurement data are often the best way to evaluate the substance of some of these challenges.

One additional analysis that should be undertaken is a homogeneity test. Assume that 100 plastic bottles of solution are prepared and bottled. Select the first bottle prepared and sealed, then select the 25th percentile bottle, then the 50th percentile, and 75th percentile and finally the last bottle. Then perform n = 10 measurements on each bottle by gas chromatography. Then do a one-way ANOVA with the five sets of data. Acceptance of the null hypothesis that all five mean results are equal would provide strong evidence for the homogeneity of the 100 bottles prepared. Finally, it can be argued that storage of simulator solutions in polyethylene plastic is "customary to the discipline," of which the court should also be made aware.

6.3.4 Simulator Thermometer Accuracy and Traceability

The temperature of simulator solutions is critical to ensure the appropriate application of Henry's Law. Where the administrative rules require specific temperatures (i.e., 34°C ± 0.3°C), the uncertainty in temperature measurements becomes a basis for legal challenge. As with all analytical instruments, thermometer measurements have uncertainty. Moreover, their uncertainty does not necessarily directly affect a breath alcohol result. It would only influence the measurement of the simulator control standard. Use of the simulator to calibrate the instrument, however, would influence the accuracy of the breath test instrument on subsequent breath test results. This issue regards technical compliance with a foundational evidential requirement in the statue or administrative rules. In addition, there are several spin-off issues including:

- Position of immersion lines relative to the solution on partial-immersion mercury thermometers;
- Operator ability to read the thermometer accurately without parallax consideration;
- Acceptable protocols to establish traceability to NIST (NIST 2019);
- Admissibility of certification records from out-of-state labs that are not "regular business record exceptions to the hearsay rule," etc.

Challenges can also arise where the forensic protocols for establishing traceability do not conform to those recommended by NIST (Taylor and Kuyatt 1994).

Again, responding to this issue begins with a sound protocol for the periodic testing and documentation of simulator thermometers using a reference thermometer traceable to NIST. Moreover, these protocols should be part of the program SOP manuals and not within the administrative rules that govern evidence admissibility. SOP manuals are easier to revise when necessary compared to statute or administrative rules. The policy should include:

- A clear definition of traceability to be applied within the program
- Thermometer testing protocol
- Testing interval
- Accuracy required
- Documentation (to appear on the program web site)
- Testing/calibration required for the reference thermometer and its documentation, etc.

Documentation must be retained and provided to the defense regarding the traceability of simulator thermometer measurements up through the reference thermometer and ultimately to NIST. In addition, measurements at all levels should be done in replicate to allow for uncertainty estimates, as recommended by NIST.

Administrative rules requiring a specific solution temperature must be carefully written to minimize legal challenge. They should be written so the requirement is that the measurement result from a certified thermometer is within the expected value (e.g., 34°C ± 0.3°C), not that the solution itself must exist at a specified temperature. Like so many areas, carefully written administrative rules coupled with sound protocols should minimize the success of these challenges. The required simulator temperature is best retained in policy manuals while the required simulator measurement result remains in the administrative rules. Again, these issues should go to the weight and not admissibility of the evidence. Often, however, it will require the creation of a thorough legal record and appeal to an appellate court level for resolution of these highly technical matters (*City of Seattle v. Fawn Allison* 2002).

The State of New Jersey has recently faced significant challenges regarding simulator thermometers. The manufacturer of their Alcotest 9510 instruments (Drager Safety Diagnostics, Inc., Irvine, TX) has recommended that simulators use thermometers that are traceable to NIST when calibrating the Alcotest 9510 instrument. A Special Master was assigned to conduct a hearing and develop a record regarding the reliability/applicability of simulator thermometers. Following a lengthy hearing the Special Master concluded that "…failure to test the simulator solutions with the NIST traceable digital thermometer before calibrating an Alcotest machine [would] undermine or call into question the scientific reliability of breath tests subsequently performed on the Alcotest machine" (*State v. Cassidy* 2018). The Special Master further stated that "… the State failed to carry its burden of proving by clear and convincing evidence that the Alcotest was scientifically reliable without a NIST traceable temperature check. The court further held, "The party proffering the evidence need not show infallibility of the technique nor unanimity of its acceptance in the scientific community." This was an important and reasonable point to remember. The Special Master also found it compelling that the simulator thermometer was the only component independent of the 9510 instrument and not calibrated by Drager. On appeal, the State Supreme Court wrote a lengthy opinion (over 240 pages) holding in favor of the lower court and asserting that "Breath test results produced by Alcotest machines not calibrated using a NIST traceable thermometer are inadmissible."

6.3.5 Error/Repair Record History on a Particular Instrument

One of the advantages of computerized instruments and advanced technology is the ability to collect records of all tests. Many jurisdictions collect these data within their breath test programs (Carpenter and Turner 2003). Along with all other documentation maintained within the program, however, such data are subject to legal/public disclosure. Indeed, an adequate and responsible defense will require the review of these data along with all other relevant records maintained by the program regarding the instrument used in testing their client. Often the defense strategy is to laboriously introduce each document through the prosecution witness in an effort to portray the instrument as having a long history of maintenance problems. The database may also contain error records (e.g., simulator out of range, calibration error, system won't zero, radio frequency interference, etc.), which the defense will also want introduced in court. Finally, phone call complaint records received from instrument operators and maintained by communication facilities will also be requested and introduced if available.

Managing all of these data and records can be an overwhelming but very important responsibility. All of these records must be efficiently maintained and fully disclosed to the defense when requested. There can also be significant costs associated with providing this information including:

- Paper
- Computer media
- Personnel time
- Postage, etc.

In some cases, these costs, or a portion thereof, can be recovered from the requesting party. Moreover, some programs have experienced significant legal challenge with unfortunate consequences by either not fully disclosing all documents or giving the appearance of hiding or destroying information. Other than proprietary information owned by a manufacturer or the redaction of arrested subject identification, there should be no reason for failing to disclose all documents in the possession of breath test program personnel. Where jurisdictions lack resources to efficiently provide the requested information, arrangements might be made with libraries for their availability. The issue of discoverable records is best handled by developing a web site for the program. All records can be placed there, providing transparency and full disclosure. This can only benefit the program's integrity from the perspective of attorneys and courts alike.

The prosecution can respond in several ways to this challenge. When appropriate, it should be emphasized that all of the requested material was promptly provided or made available to the defense through the web site because there was nothing to hide. Having all material available on a web site should address the issue of timely response. The purpose of retaining this information from the program's perspective should also be explained, such as:

- Carefully document the performance of all instruments
- Document all calibration and certification records
- Document all repairs for program cost and maintenance history
- Provide summary statistics of DUI enforcement efforts
- Evaluate trends in DUI demographic data
- Project future program and public safety needs
- Provide data for research or legislative purposes

The court and jury will appreciate the need for data retention in our present "information age." Through the forensic witness, the prosecutor should also emphasize the independence of each subject test. For each subject, the instrument must fully complete all test criteria from beginning to end. If the system fails at any point, the test is aborted. Therefore, each completed test is independent of all others before or after in several respects. The forensic witness should be able to fully explain all steps of the test protocol and why there can be confidence in particular results. A carefully designed and easily interpretable breath test document is also important to illustrate the full compliance with the preapproved test procedure. Visual aids are also helpful for explaining technical details to the court. It will also be important for the forensic witness and prosecutor to review all records prior to trial so their explanation and impact are well understood. Here again, carefully worded administrative rules that clearly define a complete and valid breath test document as the sole required basis for evidence admissibility will mitigate much of the defense challenge.

Finally, when addressing the challenge of error records in the database, the prosecution can argue that not all subjects offered a breath test will produce a fully valid result. Indeed, there should be some small percentage (i.e., 5%) of tests that are not valid and admissible in court. If all tests appeared to be fully valid, one might question the forensic sufficiency of the program standards. The important instrumental feature in this regard is its design to abort or identify any test not fully compliant with predetermined quality-control parameters.

6.3.6 Computation of Widmark Estimates

The equation developed by E.M.P. Widmark has long been used by forensic toxicologists to provide an estimate of either the number of drinks necessary to yield a particular blood alcohol concentration (BAC) or the BAC resulting from consuming a specified number of drinks (Widmark 1981). Indeed, this is the most widely performed computation in forensic toxicology. Widmark's basic equation is:

$$N = \frac{Wr\left[BAC_t + \beta t\right]}{0.82\left[fl.oz.alcohol/drink\right]} \tag{6.1}$$

where N = number of drinks; W = body weight in ounces; r = volume of distribution in L/Kg; BAC_t = the BAC at time t in Kg/L; β = the linear elimination rate in Kg/L/hr; t = time since first drink in hr; and 0.82 = the density of ethanol in ounce/fluid ounce and fl.oz. alcohol is the fluid ounces of alcohol per drink.

A large body of research has evaluated all aspects of this equation and its forensic relevance (Friel et al. 1995a, 1995b; Reed and Kalant 1977; Thieden and Hunding 1991; Watson et al. 1981). Frequently, the defense approach is to have the forensic witness compute the BAC based on the subject's statement that he/she had only "two drinks." In this case the prosecution should have the witness now compute the number of drinks based on the breath alcohol result. It is important that the jury hear both computations. The defense emphasis is now on discrediting the measurement result due to the seemingly enormous amount of alcohol necessary to achieve the specific alcohol test level.

The approximation nature of the equation must be emphasized. The equation is a function of several random and uncertain (either measured or arbitrarily estimated) variables. This is why an uncertainty estimate (e.g., ±25%) should always accompany the result. Even Widmark provided an equation for an uncertainty estimate (Widmark 1981). If the defense introduces only the estimated BAC based on the subject's statement regarding what he/she had to drink, the prosecution should have the witness compute the number of drinks based on the actual breath alcohol results. Having done this, the question can be posed to the court regarding which computation is more realistic:

- The one based on information provided by an intoxicated subject when arrested; or
- The one relying on forensically acceptable analytical results.

Moreover, the prosecution should note that using BrAC in place of BAC in the equation would yield reduced estimates for the actual number of drinks since BrAC predominantly underestimates BAC (Harding et al. 1990). Ideally, the forensic witness should be prepared to perform all computations in front of the court for subsequent review and consideration. When the witness is aware that Widmark calculations will be an issue, they can come prepared with notes and computations. These notes, however, may end up being admitted into the record. Finally, when addressing the apparently large amount of alcohol necessary to achieve specific breath alcohol concentrations, it might be useful to introduce the fact that the average BrAC for those arrested for DUI is near 0.15 g/210 L and breath alcohol concentrations in arrested drivers range from zero to above 0.40 g/210 L (Gullberg et al. 1997). If the witness cannot address this in his/her testimony, the prosecutor might include it in closing argument. Clearly, people consume large amounts of alcohol to achieve these forensically relevant alcohol concentrations.

6.3.7 The Software within the Instrument

Modern breath alcohol instruments are computerized with microprocessor control and associated software or firmware. The software is often encoded within some form of EPROM (erasable programmable read-only memory) device. A lower-level language format, such as Assembly, is generally employed. The software may require approximately 24 kilobytes of memory and comprise over 150 pages of printed material. Since the software contains the instruction set necessary for controlling all instrument operations, including computation of the breath alcohol result, it is of significant interest to the defense and their experts. The defense will typically request the software to be provided in electronic and hard-copy format for review by its experts. Pretrial hearings will likely follow in which the defense experts highlight alleged weaknesses in the code. These alleged deficiencies are then introduced before the jury in subsequent trials in order to minimize the weight of the evidence. Such effort by the defense can be quite expensive.

An example of significant defense challenge to the instrument software is found in the New Jersey supreme court case of *State v Chun* et al. (2008). The record in this case was developed over four months of testimony before an appointed Special Master. The challenge was to the breath test results from the Alcotest 7110 MKIII-C (Drager Safety Diagnostics, Inc., Irvine, TX). Most of the defense challenge involved the software in the instrument with the major issues including in part:

- Software availability to the defense experts
- The relevance of using the blood-to-breath conversion factor of 2100 to 1
- The need to monitor and record the breath temperature
- The required breath volume was too much for the elderly
- Duplicate test agreement requirements
- The fuel cell drift algorithm
- Only the manufacture can make changes to the software
- A "buffer overflow error" influencing a third test where the first two did not agree
- The overall design of the software

While there were a few revisions required of the manufacturer, the Special Master judge hearing the case ruled in the state's favor on most of these and other issues. This case probably represents the most complete and exhaustive record challenging the admissibility of breath alcohol test results in drunk driving cases. There were over 8,300 pages of transcribed testimony, 13 witnesses, over 400 exhibits, and 41 days of testimony. There seemed to be "no stone unturned." The State Supreme Court of New Jersey agreed for the most part with the

Special Master's opinion and denied most of the defense challenges. Jurisdictions preparing for pre-trial evidentiary hearings would do well to review this case from New Jersey. In addition, breath test programs (along with manufacturers) need to be prepared to turn over the instrument software for defense expert review in the likely event that it is ordered by the court. A protective order can accompany the disclosure of the software code.

The software, along with certain other components, is a critical element within the total measurement system. The proper function of the software is best evaluated as part of the total system operation. Using known controls, duplicate samples, pre-exhalation observation time, trained operators, duplicate test agreement, sequential monitoring of critical analytical functions and validated instruments will evaluate the total measurement system and demonstrate the fitness-for-purpose of all integrated components, including the software. The prosecution should argue that a complete and successful breath test, with the accompanying document, ensures that all components of the measurement system were operating properly during that particular test run. Knowledge and review of the software should not be necessary to interpret the validity and integrity of a specific breath alcohol test result.

Manufacturers of breath test instruments are concerned that their software and its proprietary features might be disclosed to competitors. This is understandable in view of the developmental costs involved. Manufacturers should be made aware that the defense will likely subpoena the software as part of their defense. Protective orders can be obtained to provide some protection for the manufacturers. Moreover, some manufacturers also refuse to sell an instrument to anyone other than forensic or law enforcement personnel. Such practice seems to foster the impression that there is something to hide. It seems that such a policy by the manufacturer should be reconsidered.

Software versions can be formally approved and included within the administrative rules, following a thorough total system evaluation while operating within the instrument. The printout document for an individual should then reveal the software version employed for easy verification of its approval. This should help to ensure legal admissibility.

Prior to purchasing new instruments, jurisdictions should request that the manufacturer obtain independent testing and evaluation of the software. This will document that a reasonable effort was made to independently ensure its integrity. Breath test device manufacturers must also be made aware that their software, often proprietary, may be requested by the defense under discovery or court order. Protective orders can be employed to protect the manufacture's legitimate interests.

Defense experts may come from other specialized fields of computer and software application. Rarely is there a direct correspondence between the fitness-for-purpose in these other fields (e.g., Department of Defense, Federal Aviation Administration, etc.) and the needs of forensic breath alcohol measurement. Fitness-for-purpose is always determined within the context of the measurement's intended application (Magnusson and Örnemark 2014). Alleged errors in the code, however, should be carefully considered since software quality is an elusive concept, determined largely within the context of its intended application (Kitchenham and Pfleeger 1996).

The instrument software (among other related issues) was also a major defense challenge in a Massachusetts case (Commonwealth v. Ananias 2017). While this was a lower court opinion, there was an extensive record created along with a thoroughly detailed opinion of the judge hearing the case. As part of the defense challenge and request, the court ordered that the state provide two AlcoTest 9510 (Drager Safety Diagnostics, Inc., Irvine, TX) instruments to the defense for their evaluation. While this is a novel and unusual request, it may become more widespread. Moreover, there is probably no harm in allowing such a request and furthers the state's position of transparency and full disclosure. This case probably created the most extensive record regarding software issues. These issues included in part: coding style, error records, configuration files, bits, coding "best practices," initialized variables, rounding of results, general reliability, etc. The court seemed to comprehend the technical issues quite well and recognized the stylistic and elusive nature of writing code. Two different authors might write different code where both accomplish the same purpose. Another issue was the difference between the IR and EC results. The dual technology is designed to detect interfering substances. Drager allows a difference of up to 0.008 g/210 L. Several breath tests reported results where differences exceeded this value. The court also heard testimony regarding the potential for interfering substances to be measurable in human breath and the validity of the 2100:1 ratio. On these issues the court found the instrument to provide reliable and accurate breath alcohol results. The lack of providing complete discovery to the defense was also an issue. This is best addressed with the development of a program web site. In summary, the court found that the software, while not perfect, is adequate and reliable for its intended purpose. The defense also challenged several elements of the state laboratory's practices. Specifically, they challenged the issues of accreditation, measurement uncertainty, measurement traceability and the documentation of program protocols. The court denied the defense motion to suppress based on the first three issues here but not the fourth. The court found it necessary that the program become accredited. The court also found that the lab did not have adequate and approved protocols and records for their analytical practices. It was also required that protocols and records be stored and available on a web site. The court recognized that the lab was a "program in progress." Finally, evidence obtained after June 2011 (when the AlcoTest 9510 was introduced) would not be admissible. The court required that the State program comply with seven requirements before using breath test results in court. As a result of this "lack of protocols issue" most courts in Massachusetts are not admitting the breath test results to this day. This continues as a major legal dispute in the state. Despite this not being an appellate court decision, there was a large number of creative defense challenges from which to learn and consider.

It is also worth noting that the National Safety Council's Committee on Alcohol and Other Drugs has a position statement on instrument software: "It is the position of the National Safety Council Committee on Alcohol and Other Drugs that access to the Source Code of the software of an evidential breath alcohol analyzer is not pertinent, required, or useful for examination or evaluation of the analyzer's accuracy, scientific reliability, forensic validity, or other relevant characteristics, or of the trustworthiness and reliability of analysis results produced by the analyzer. These matters can be and have been fully assessed and examined by multiple other well established and recognized methods and procedures in common use worldwide; and many other adequate and appropriate means exist to challenge evidential breath alcohol analysis results." (US Department of Transportation National Highway Traffic Safety Administration 2013.)

6.3.8 Records Generated by Other Program Personnel

Records generated by program personnel are often critical to establishing the foundation for admissibility of breath test evidence. Such records might include:

- Instrument certification forms
- Simulator or dry gas control replacement records

- Thermometer certification records
- Repair or maintenance records, etc.
    - Training records
    - Personnel job descriptions
    - Experimental records
    - Instrument validation records

Where several individuals have similar responsibilities for a specific task, there will be occasions when the one performing the work is not able to testify during the trial. Often, the defense argues that the form is not admissible except through the individual who actually performed the specific work described on the document.

Admissibility of records generated by someone other than the one testifying is an issue addressed in the Sixth Amendment to the United States Constitution. The Sixth Amendment requires the right to be confronted by one's accusers. This is known as the "confrontational clause" of the Sixth Amendment. While several state courts in addition to the US Supreme Court have heard arguments and ruled on various aspects of this issue, it still remains controversial and unclear. Some US Supreme Court cases relevant here are:

- *Crawford v. Washington*; 3 t 541 U.S. 36 (2004)
- *Melendez-Diaz v. Massachusetts*; 557 U.S. 305, 309 (2009)
- *Bullcoming v New Mexico*; 564 U.S., 131 S. Ct. 2705 (2011)

It is important that the prosecutor make a good faith effort to obtain the in-court testimony of the author of the documents (i.e., breath test instrument certification or repair records). Where the author or originating technician is unavailable the prosecutor must show this and the reasons. This is an issue because even documents and records are considered "testimonial" and fall under the confrontational clause. The court ruled in favor of the defense in both the *Melendez-Diaz* and *Bullcoming* cases because live testimony from the analyst performing the analysis was not given in court. Even live testimony from the supervisor did not meet the confrontational requirement. The forensic scientists and the prosecutor need to study this issue carefully prior to trial in the event that the principle technician is not available. Laboratory practices may have to change to ensure more than one technician is involved in the testing processes.

Program documents should generally be admissible through qualified personnel as a "regular business record exception" to the hearsay rule. In order to meet one of the issues in *Melendez-Diaz* and *Bullcoming*, it should be emphasized that these regular program records are not kept with the specific purpose of prosecution in mind. Language to this effect might also be appropriately included in the program SOP. These qualified personnel should have "custodian of the records" as part of their responsibilities so they have access to the records and are able to describe the work reported on the forms as part of their normal duties. Personnel may need to submit copies to others so that all are able to handle the admissibility testimony in the event of someone's unavailability. Their job descriptions should also list "records custodian" as part of their responsibilities. Records not routinely generated within the program may not be admissible, except, perhaps, in pretrial admissibility hearings where evidentiary rules are often relaxed. However, even records generated by other agencies may be admissible as a component part along with documents that would be defined as a "regular business record exception."

6.3.9 Compliance with Pre-exhalation Observation Time

Virtually all jurisdictions performing evidential breath alcohol testing require that the subject be observed for a minimal time period (e.g., 15 or 20 minutes) prior to breath sample collection to ensure they place no foreign material in their mouth and allow the dissipation of "mouth alcohol," if any. The administrative rules generally contain the specific requirements and may vary among jurisdictions. Depending on the specific requirements, the defense may argue that the required observation was not complied with for a number of reasons including:

- The officer turned his/her back for a moment
- The officer was completing paperwork during the period
- The officer was preparing the instrument during the period
- The subject's mouth was not adequately checked at the beginning of the period
- The subject produced an undetected belch
- The subject regurgitated during the period
- The time period was not documented properly
- An exact 15-minute observation time may not be the case when considering the seconds digit, etc.

Similar to many others, this issue is best addressed with careful wording of the administrative rules and thorough training of operators. The rules must not be worded in such a way that strict compliance is impossible. Operators should be trained and prepared to testify that they used only one clock for the time determination—preferably the clock on the instrument, which will also correspond to the times printed on the document. Operators must be prepared to carefully document the time that observation began and avoid the appearance of "digit preference" (e.g., recording more 0s or 5s for the minute digit). Printout documents should show both the beginning of observation and the time of breath sampling. Instruments can also be programmed to require a minimum time period before sample provision and between samples. The operator/forensic scientist can also be prepared to discuss the exponential nature of the elimination rate of "mouth alcohol" and how the potential for bias decreases as a function of time and increasing end-expiratory BrAC (Gullberg 1992). Belching, detected or not, will not bias a test result because that portion of the exhaled breath, typically an earlier fraction of the exhaled stream, passes through the sample chamber and is replaced by the last portion of breath exiting the lungs.

6.3.10 Inconsistency between Reported Observations and BrAC

The DUI arrest case report will generally include a summary of the officer's observations regarding the driving, field sobriety tests, odor of alcohol and statements made by the subject. Often, the defense will suggest that the high BrAC (e.g., >0.15 g/210 L) is inconsistent with the uneventful description of the field sobriety test performance. Particularly when Widmark's estimation reveals a large number of drinks necessary, the defense will argue that the apparent inconsistency must be due to an inaccurate breath alcohol result.

Responding to this issue must begin with the arresting officer writing a very detailed and thorough report. Standard and computerized report formats can be helpful in this regard. All observations, beginning with the driving and including all aspects of the field sobriety tests, must be recorded in great detail. Moreover, reports must be factually unique to each subject while avoiding vague and generalized statements. On occasion, the defense may request several DUI case reports from the officer to use for comparison and suggest that the same information is recorded for all subjects. The forensic expert can respond with testimony regarding the tolerance developed with alcohol and how alcoholics are able to conceal many of the overt signs of impairment. The correlation between signs and symptoms of impairment and BrAC is ambiguous in some respects. Usually this issue goes to the weight of the evidence rather than the admissibility.

6.3.11 The "Rising BrAC" Defense

The measurement of alcohol in the human body is a dynamic process—it is constantly changing. During consumption the pharmacokinetic curve rises, reaches a peak after the end of consumption, followed by a linear decline. The general appearance of this pharmacokinetic curve is seen in Figure 6.3. Given this knowledge, the defense will often argue that while the subject was driving the alcohol concentration was prior to the peak and below the *per se* level. Later, at the time of the breath test the alcohol concentration was higher, near the peak. This basically argues that the subject was on the "rising" portion of the BrAC curve while driving. Many jurisdictions define the offense

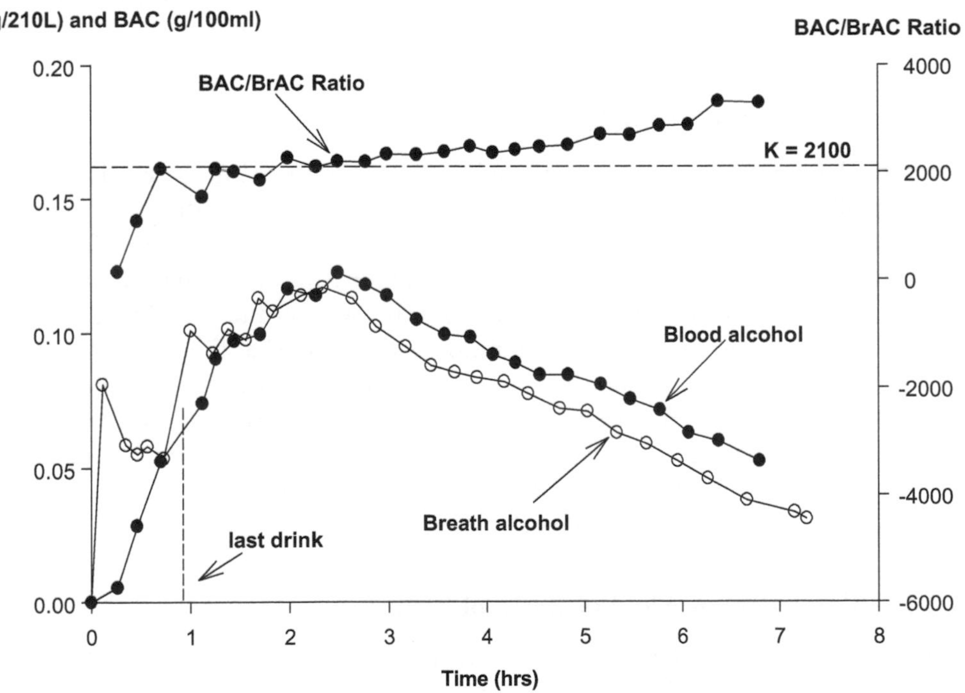

Figure 6.3 The pharmacokinetic curves of both blood and breath alcohol in one individual showing their relationship along with the blood/breath ratio.

of drunk driving as "driving while having a breath or blood alcohol concentration of 0.08 or more." Such language strictly requires that the concentration be determined at the time of driving. This never occurs. The breath test is usually administered at least one hour after driving.

Some research has attempted to address this issue by testing the breath at the roadside with a PBT device and then again, perhaps two hours later, at the time of the evidential test (Gullberg and McElroy 1992). While these results showed the unlikely case where the subsequent test was significantly higher than the roadside test, there still needs to be more research of this nature. The manner in which most jurisdictions have addressed this issue is by enacting what are referred to as "two-hour laws." Here the drunk driving offense is defined as having a 0.08 g/210 L or more within two hours of driving. Some jurisdictions have defined the offense to be within three hours. This legislative approach seems to be the most effective.

A case in the state of Idaho involved the "rising BrAC" defense (*State of Idaho v. Justin Keith Austin* 2018). Austin was arrested for DUI and claimed that he had consumed three drinks a short time before the stop. He then submitted to a breath alcohol test 30 minutes later with results of 0.085 and 0.086 g/210 L. His defense expert witness claimed that at the time of driving Austin's breath alcohol should have been 0.06 to 0.065 g/210 L. The Supreme Court of Idaho held that "…the alcohol concentration in a defendant's blood, breath, or urine at the time he or she was driving is irrelevant." Further, "…the statute does not require a defendant to have a blood alcohol level of 0.08 while driving." It is the result at the time of the test that defines the offense. There is no need to extrapolate to determine the alcohol concentration at the time of driving. This decision of the high court would apply equally to blood, breath or urine. Legislation such as Idaho's would easily handle the issues related to uncertainty, rising BAC and retrograde extrapolation.

6.3.12 Retrograde Extrapolation

Another challenging issue, closely related to the "rising BrAC defense" also considers the pharmacokinetics of alcohol in the body and is that known as "retrograde extrapolation." Where the test is administered one or more hours after driving, the state often wants to try and show that the breath alcohol concentration at the time of driving was over 0.08. This is of particular interest where the evidential test is below 0.08 and the "retrograde extrapolation" is an attempt to show the concentration was over 0.08 at the earlier time of driving. This practice is fraught with significant uncertainty. Where this computation is attempted it should be accompanied with its many assumptions. In response to this challenge, like the "rising BrAC defense," many jurisdictions have enacted "two-hour" laws. Again, these define the offense as having a 0.08 more within two hours of driving. This should preclude the need to perform any retrograde calculations.

6.3.13 Blood/Breath Alcohol Ratio of 2100:1

A very old defense challenge to breath alcohol analysis is the use of a blood-to-breath conversion factor of 2100:1. When breath alcohol instruments were first developed, the objective was to measure breath alcohol and convert it mathematically to a blood alcohol concentration. A great deal of experimental work was done to try and establish this conversion factor. It was determined that when the blood alcohol concentration

(BAC) was the same as (or nearly so) the breath alcohol concentration (BrAC) then the conversion factor from breath to blood was 2100. This is shown in the following equation:

$$K_{BAC/BrAC} = \frac{BAC\frac{g}{100\,mL}}{BrAC\frac{g}{210\,L}} = \frac{BAC}{BrAC} \bullet 2100 \tag{6.2}$$

Therefore, knowing that K = 2100, when BAC = BrAC we simply multiply a BrAC result by 2100 in order to obtain the corresponding BAC estimate. If BrAC = 0.10, for example:

$$2100 = \frac{BAC\frac{g}{100\,mL}}{0.10\frac{g}{210\,L}} \Rightarrow \frac{2100(0.10\,g)}{210000\,mL} = \frac{0.10\,g}{100\,mL} = BAC \tag{6.3}$$

We must remember that this relationship represents a ratio of measured blood alcohol and breath alcohol. This is not the blood/air partition coefficient determined from Henry's Law at the blood/air interface in the alveoli of the lungs (Jones 1983). Most of the historical data consisting of simultaneous paired blood and breath measurements were nearly equal when the blood was venous and measured as g/100 mL and the breath was end-expiratory and measured with g/210 L. In recent years and with better breath test instruments the blood-to-breath ratio is determined to be closer to 2300:1 (Jones and Andersson 1996). The water/air partition coefficient, however, is important to consider when calibrating breath test instruments with simulator devices. Where simulator solutions are prepared and measured to be considered standard reference materials, the ethanol concentration in solution (g/100 mL) should be divided by 1.23 to yield the vapor ethanol concentration in g/210 L. This is the value that should be used as the reference value when calibrating a breath test instrument (Gullberg 2005). This will yield a calibrated value that is biased slightly low by approximately 2.5%.

The value of this blood/breath conversion factor (2100) has been a widely employed defense argument for the last 80 years. However, it is only an issue where the DUI statutory language defines the offense as having a "blood alcohol concentration" of 0.08 or more. Such language requires the jury to interpret the breath alcohol result as a blood alcohol equivalent. This is where the conversion factor of 2100, and its associated uncertainty, becomes an issue. Such testimony before the jury can become quite complex and confusing. To avoid this problem, most jurisdictions have revised their statutory language to state that the offense occurs when the defendant has "either a breath alcohol of 0.08 g/210 L, or a blood alcohol of 0.08 g/100 mL." In this way there are two ways to commit the offense of drunk driving. The law expresses the offense clearly in terms of the specimen measured (breath or blood). The 2100:1 conversion factor should not be considered. The breath test instrument makes no assumptions about the conversion factor. It has been calibrated to simply compute the concentration in terms of g/210 L. The key here is to have statutory language that defines the offense in terms of the specimen measured.

This assumption of 2100:1 for the blood/breath ratio was the principle focus of the defense challenge before the Supreme Court of New Jersey in the case of *State v. Downie* et al. (1990). New Jersey had a *per se* DUI statute at the time defining the offense as having a "... blood alcohol concentration of 0.10% or more by weight of alcohol in the defendant's blood...." The instrument employed in New Jersey at the time was the Breathalyzer 900 series. Having to prove that the defendant has a specific alcohol concentration in their blood while having only a breath alcohol measurement, naturally resulted in a challenge focused on the use of 2100 for converting breath alcohol to blood alcohol. A lengthy pretrial hearing was held in which ten expert witnesses testified regarding the reliability of the 2100:1 ratio. The court noted at length in its opinion the fact that using the 2100:1 ratio actually resulted in a reduced estimate of the corresponding blood alcohol level. Figure 6.3 illustrates the pharmacokinetic relationship between blood and breath alcohol over time. We see how blood alcohol exceeds breath alcohol in the post-absorptive state. This evidence was compelling to the court in *State v. Downie*. In addition, the fact that two samples are obtained and the lower of the two are used for prosecution with the result truncated to two digits, also impressed the court. The court, in its opinion, seemed also to have a good comprehension of the physiology of alcohol pharmacokinetics and analysis. As a result the court ruled that the "...breathalyzer is a reliable and indispensable tool for law-enforcement purposes." Indeed, the court seemed to understand very well the voluminous technical testimony regarding the blood/breath relationship by concluding, "...we find unpersuasive the argument that blood should be the sure and ultimate measure of inebriation."

6.3.14 Mouth Alcohol Effect

Early in the development of breath alcohol instrumentation and analysis it was realized that a recent drink of an alcoholic beverage would yield a biased high result when sampling the breath shortly after consuming the drink. Over the years a number of studies have investigated this issue in order to determine how long the time should be to allow for the dissipation of alcohol from the oral cavity to avoid the bias (Fessler et al. 2008; Dubowski 1975; Sterling 2012; Lindberg et al. 2015; Caddy et al. 1978). It has been well established that a 15-minute observation time is more than enough to allow for the elimination of "mouth alcohol" and avoid a biased breath sample. Moreover, when there is already consumed alcohol in the subject's system, the time needed to allow for dissipation declines inversely as a function of the true end-expiratory breath alcohol (Gullberg 1992). If, for example, the individual has a true end-expiratory BrAC of 0.10 g/210 L due to the consumed alcohol, any mouth alcohol must decline only to the 0.10 g/210 L level to avoid a biased result. Fifteen minutes is more than enough time for subjects arrested for drunk driving since they have been consuming alcohol. This results from the fact that "mouth alcohol" is eliminated in an exponential manner and approaches asymptotically the value that is coming from the deep lungs due to consumption. This is also an issue when the subject might rinse the mouth with an alcohol containing mouth wash (Foglio-Bonda et al. 2015; Modell et al. 1993). This defense may be argued even where the subject was exposed to and inhaling air containing alcohol or other volatile organic compounds in a work environment (Campbell and Wilson 1986). Following occupational exposure, the volatile compounds are eliminated in an exponential manner. It would be important to ask the subject when their exposure ended since the time between exposure and sampling would be important. It is also important for the operator to note whether the subject had the odor of volatile organic compounds coming from their clothing. Inhaling this just prior to sample collection could be an issue. The best way to address this issue is to have the operator/police officer verify the subject's mouth is empty of any foreign material and then employ an observation period of at least 15 minutes before providing the first sample. The subject should not be allowed to introduce anything (even water) into the mouth during this observation period. This should be emphasized in training as part of the breath test protocol. The observation and sampling times should also be recorded by the operator. It is also important that the subject be kept under constant observation during this period so the operator can be sure that nothing was placed in the subject's mouth and no regurgitation of stomach contents occurs. A belch during this time should not be a problem because the gas brought from the stomach will be replaced by the end-expiratory sample coming from the lungs. The next best way to address this issue is to obtain two breath samples approximately two to three minutes apart. Their acceptable pre-determined agreement is evidence that there is no "mouth alcohol" bias.

Another issue related to "mouth alcohol" bias is the gastroesophageal reflux disease (GERD) defense. Here the defense argues that the individual experienced a GERD event and brought up raw alcohol from the stomach into the throat or oral cavity, resulting in a biased result. This seems to be anatomically disallowed because the final sample to reside in the instrument would be the last portion coming from the deep lungs, not the stomach. The other protection against this occurring is the "mouth alcohol detection" system of the instrument. Software in the instrument requires a normal breath exhalation profile which is uniquely different from a "mouth alcohol" profile. When this occurs, the test is aborted. Finally, the GERD defense fails when duplicate breath samples agree within the pre-determined value.

6.4 Additional Challenges

To be sure, many other legal challenges to breath alcohol analysis exist. We are constrained by time and space to cover them all. Many of these are unique to a particular jurisdiction because of their statutes, administrative rules, case law, instrumentation, etc. Several of these additional challenges include:

- The presence of tongue jewelry biased the result
- Error records or aborted tests require full recertification of the instrument
- Implied consent rights were inadequate (i.e., a missing semicolon defense)
- The discovery material provided was incomplete
- The instrument warranty provided by the manufacturer is inadequate
- The risk of bias due to other interfering sources such as radio frequency interference, endogenously produced alcohol, consuming bread products, the multitude of volatile organic compounds found in normal human breath, etc.
- Simulator devices have a vapor matrix more similar to human breath than dry gas standards
- Test bias due to gastroesophageal reflux disease (GERD)
- The threshold set for interference detection requires that this amount be subtracted from every subject's test result
- Drinking after the accident (hip-flask defense)

- Variation in sequential simulator control test results
- Variation observed between the subject's duplicate breath test results
- All possible analytical error percentages must be summed and then subtracted from the subject's results
- Failing to use a new mouthpiece for each separate exhalation
- Photographing the internal components of the instrument
- A request to borrow an instrument for evaluation
- Preservation of the breath sample for re-analysis

In addition, defense attorneys may request to photograph an instrument's location in an effort to compare with the officer's statements regarding compliance with pre-exhalation observation time. Again, these reflect only some of the multitude of challenges raised in DUI litigation. Moreover, many current challenges are only slight revisions of ones that have been in dispute for many years and often previously discredited. We must remember, however, that a particular set of jurors has likely not heard these issues before and the defense objective is to craft a specific issue that is compelling. The state forensic witness must be as prepared as possible to address these issues with a thorough knowledge of the literature and with integrity, always ready to answer "I do not know," and yet ready to learn for the next time that question is posed.

Most of these additional challenges, like the others, are best managed with carefully crafted administrative rules coupled with a forensically sound measurement protocol. The administrative rules must be drafted so that only the minimum requirements are specified. Extra detail should be left to policy manuals. A measurement protocol following sound forensic practice that is fit-for-purpose (Dubowski 1994) will surmount most of these additional defense challenges. In particular, duplicate breath samples will mitigate many of these challenges. Moreover, data collection systems can be used to generate plots that show evidence of statistical control for the instrument over time. Novel approaches to addressing the "hip-flask defense" through congener analysis, for example, have also been reported (Iffland and Jones 2002, 2003). Finally, much can be learned from networking with other jurisdictions experiencing similar challenges and considering their responses.

One additional feature that can significantly help address many of the defense challenges is the development of a breath test program web site. All of the program records, forms, SOP manual, training outlines, CVs of personnel, etc., can be placed there for the defense to freely obtain at any time. This would greatly demonstrate the program's transparency and integrity. Challenges regarding lack of disclosure should be eliminated. Moreover, there should be no appearance of withholding information helpful to the defense. Developing and maintaining such a site can be very laborious. It will likely require one individual fulltime to properly maintain such a system.

The prosecutor's approach to the case will clearly depend on whether the issue is a pretrial admissibility hearing or whether the issue will go to the weight in front of the jury. In either case, a close working relationship must be established between the forensic scientist and the prosecutor so that all technical aspects of the breath-testing program are understood and a complete record is established. A networking of prosecutors within or between jurisdictions, like that offered by the National District Attorneys Association (National District Attorneys Association 2019), is also helpful to address challenges.

Internet sites can also be developed where relevant court decisions and case briefs can be posted for other prosecutors to obtain. Sharing relevant information between jurisdictions can be very useful and facilitated in this way.

Prosecutors in the UK also face a number of defense challenges, many of which are similar to those outlined above (Williams 2018). Their drunk driving offense is defined by *per se* limits for three possible biological specimens: breath: 35 μg/100 mL breath, blood: 80 mg/100 mL blood and urine: 107 mg/100 mL urine. Prosecutors will hear the defense argument that the alcohol level was "rising" but below the *per se* limit at the time of driving. This has been addressed with a Statutory Assumption that the alcohol level in any of the biological specimens at the time of driving was the same as at the time of analysis. This has the same effect as a "two-hour law" in the United States. The defense in the UK also commonly challenges the apparent discrepancy between what the defendant says they had to drink and the estimated amount determined by Widmark's Equation 6.1. The defense also subpoenas a host of documents in an effort to find some potential error in the breath test instrument. Again, the development of a forensic program web site where all program records and documents would be available at any time to the defense would relieve the burden of providing the records by the prosecution. Finally, there is a proposal in the UK that statutory language should include a statutory assumption regarding the reliability of type-approved breath alcohol test instruments, similar to that provided for blood and urine analysis.

6.5 Common Defense Challenges to Blood Alcohol Analysis

Compared to forensic breath alcohol analysis, the analysis of blood alcohol is probably the next most common forensic measurement performed. In Washington State, approximately 90% of forensic measurement for alcohol is breath and 10% is blood. Many of the defense challenges to breath testing discussed earlier also apply to blood alcohol testing. Moreover, the suggested responses would be the same. Some of the similar challenges include: measurement uncertainty, interfering substances, use of certified reference materials, traceability, Widmark calculations, sixth amendment confrontation clause, program records, training of program personnel, "Rising BAC" defense, retrograde extrapolation, etc. Some of these corresponding issues are more easily addressed with blood alcohol. For example, interfering substances are addressed in the instrument technology. Gas chromatography (GC), generally considered to be the "gold standard" for ethanol quantitation in biological specimens, is more selective for ethanol than infrared. On the other hand, head space GC has a number of elements that can be challenged. These include in part: equilibration of samples by time and temperature, using materials such as sodium fluoride that can "salt out" the ethanol, dilution factors, internal standards, chain of custody issues, refrigeration, coelution problems, purging between samples to avoid carryover, matrix differences between blood samples and calibration solutions, GC columns and temperatures, quantifying the peak areas, etc. (Watts and McDonald 1987). Finally, one of the significant advantages of blood alcohol analysis over breath is the fact that a sample is retained and can be measured again at a later date by either the State expert or the defense expert. Our objective here is to comment on some of the most common defense challenges to blood alcohol measurement and suggest some responses.

6.5.1 Measurement Uncertainty

The need to determine and report measurement uncertainty is just as important for blood alcohol analysis as for breath alcohol (Barone and Vosk 2015). The same approach as discussed above for breath alcohol will apply for blood analysis. There are, however, several ways, including technical details, in which measurement uncertainty can be computed. There is no single best approach. As a result many analytical scientists find it difficult to determine and perform the correct computations (Kristiansen 2001). Several authors have discussed the importance of and different methods for computing measurement uncertainty in blood alcohol analysis (Sklerov and Couper 2011; Gullberg 2012; Wallace 2010; Kristiansen and Petersen 2004; Jones 1989). Moreover, this concept of measurement uncertainty is quite basic and should be straightforward for judges to comprehend and exercise their "gate keeping" responsibility under Daubert.

There are also case law regarding measurement uncertainty in blood alcohol analysis upon which we commented earlier under breath uncertainty. The Idaho State Supreme Court ruled in 2016 on such a case. (*State v. Jones* 2016). Jones (the defendant) was arrested for DUI and provided a blood sample which had an ethanol concentration of 0.207 g/100 mL with an uncertainty calculation of ±0.0103 g/100 mL. It was not clear how this uncertainty estimate was determined or by whom. Idaho has an enhanced penalty statute for results over 0.20 g/100 mL. Jones tried to introduce evidence of measurement uncertainty, arguing that the blood alcohol results could be below the 0.20 limit. The Supreme Court denied Jones motion and held that it was not error to exclude the measurement uncertainty. The high court held "… the testing machine's margin of error was irrelevant because the standard is no longer the concentration of alcohol in the driver's blood." The court further held "The equipment need not precisely measure the alcohol concentration in the person's blood (*Elias-Cruz v. Idaho Department of Transportation* 2012). The test need only be based upon the correct formula, and the equipment must be properly approved and certified." Moreover, while the Elias-Cruz case in the Idaho Supreme Court involved breath alcohol, the decision would apply equally to blood alcohol analysis.

We next present a common approach to computing measurement uncertainty found in the GUM document and illustrate its application for breath alcohol:

$$u_c = \bar{Y}\sqrt{\left[\frac{\frac{u_{Sampling}}{\sqrt{n_{Breath}}}}{\bar{Y}}\right]^2 + \left[\frac{\frac{u_{Analytical}}{\sqrt{n_{Analytical}}}}{\bar{X}}\right]^2 + \left[\frac{\frac{u_{Ref}}{\sqrt{n_{Ref}}}}{\overline{Ref}}\right]^2 + \left[\frac{\frac{Bias}{\sqrt{3}}}{\overline{Ref}}\right]^2} \quad (6.4)$$

where u_c = the combined uncertainty; $\bar{Y}$ = the mean breath alcohol result; $u_{Sampling}$ = the uncertainty due to the breath sampling component; n_{Breath} = the number of breath samples obtained (n = 2); $\bar{X}$ = the mean of the duplicate blood alcohol results; $u_{Analytical}$ = the analytical component of uncertainty; $n_{Analytical}$ = the number of measurements performed on the certified reference material (CRM); u_{Ref} = the uncertainty for the CRM found on the certificate of analysis; n_{Ref} = the number of measurements performed by the manufacturer of the CRM; $\overline{Ref}$ = the mean of the assigned reference value; Bias = the maximum observed bias when measuring the CRM.

Next, we employ the same general approach for computing the uncertainty in blood alcohol analysis as follows:

$$u_c = \overline{Y}\sqrt{\left[\frac{\frac{u_{Analytical}}{\sqrt{n_{Analytical}}}}{\overline{X}}\right]^2 + \left[\frac{\frac{u_{Ref}}{\sqrt{n_{Ref}}}}{\overline{Ref}}\right]^2 + \left[\frac{\frac{Bias}{\sqrt{3}}}{\overline{Ref}}\right]^2} \tag{6.5}$$

where $\overline{Y}$ = the mean blood alcohol result; $u_{Analytical}$ = the analytical component of uncertainty; $n_{Analytical}$ = measurements performed on the certified reference material (CRM); $\overline{X}$ = the mean of the replicate control standard results; u_{Ref} = the uncertainty for the CRM found on the certificate of analysis; n_{Ref} = the number of measurements performed by the manufacturer of the CRM; $\overline{Ref}$ = the mean of the assigned reference value; Bias = the maximum observed bias when measuring the CRM.

Employing Equation 6.5 we have made the following assumptions:

- All measurement results are random and normally distributed
- All measurement results are independent
- The computed confidence intervals will bracket the true population parameter (i.e., mean or difference) with 95% probability
- The measurement function is multiplicative

From Equation 6.5 we notice that there is no sampling component like there is for breath alcohol in Equation 6.4. Instead, we employ the duplicate results to compute the analytical component (the standard deviation) according to the following equation:

$$SD = \sqrt{\frac{\sum_{i=1}^{k} d_i^2}{2k}} \tag{6.6}$$

where d = the duplicate test difference; k = the number of individual duplicate results within the concentration interval.

Equation 6.5 does not include a sampling component because only one blood sample was obtained by the phlebotomist. The analytical component of the standard deviation in Equation 6.5 is due only to the measurement variation in the analyst's procedure and the gas chromatograph. The first term in Equation 6.5 comes from the uncertainty function developed for the duplicate blood alcohol results observed in Figure 6.4, which shows the uncertainty functions developed from Equation 6.6 for both breath and blood alcohol analyses. While assuming that the duplicate blood alcohol analyses includes all sources of variation in both the analytical and procedural components, it is important that each of the duplicate measurements fully involve all procedures independently. From Figure 6.4 we see that the breath alcohol uncertainty is significantly larger than that for blood. This results from the

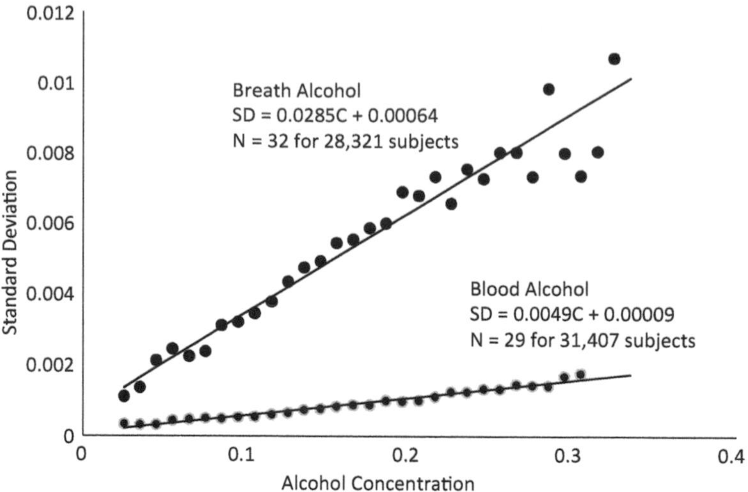

Figure 6.4 Uncertainty functions for both breath and blood alcohol analysis.

large variation in breath sampling due to the efforts of an intoxicated subject. The individual cannot influence the variation in the sampling of blood like they can for breath. The result will be that breath will have a larger confidence interval for its uncertainty estimate.

The equations observed in Figure 6.4 are least-squares linear fits to the data. Each point for both plots are standard deviation estimates for duplicate test means occurring within 0.01 bins. The standard deviations are determined from the differences between the duplicate results within each bin according to Equation 6.6.

We now illustrate the computation of the combined uncertainty for both breath and blood alcohol using the models in Figure 6.4 and Equations 6.4 and 6.5. The calculation first employs the equation for the uncertainty function for breath observed in Figure 6.4. From this equation we determine the standard deviation to be 0.00292 g/210 L for the sampling component.

$$u_{\text{Sampling}} = 0.0285(0.080) + 0.00064 = 0.00292 \text{ g/210 L} \tag{6.7}$$

We now incorporate the uncertainty estimates for the remaining three terms into Equation 6.4 and obtain Equation 6.8. We have included reasonable estimates for the three remaining terms simply to illustrate the calculations involved. Moreover, we assume our mean BrAC results are 0.080 g/210 L.

$$u_c = 0.080\sqrt{\left[\frac{\frac{0.00292}{\sqrt{2}}}{0.080}\right]^2 + \left[\frac{\frac{0.0008}{\sqrt{10}}}{0.080}\right]^2 + \left[\frac{\frac{0.0006}{\sqrt{2}}}{0.080}\right]^2 + \left[\frac{\frac{0.004}{\sqrt{3}}}{0.080}\right]^2} = 0.00314 \text{ g/210 L} \tag{6.8}$$

$$95\% \text{ Confidence Interval: } 0.080 \pm 1.96\,(0.00314) \Rightarrow 0.074 \text{ to } 0.086 \text{ g/210 L}$$

Equation 6.8 is simply combining the components of variation by the method of root sum of squares (RSS). These are actually coefficients of variation that are being summed. Next we employ Equation 6.5 along with the model in Figure 6.4 to compute the estimate of combined uncertainty for blood alcohol:

$$u_c = 0.080\sqrt{\left[\frac{\frac{0.00048}{\sqrt{2}}}{0.080}\right]^2 + \left[\frac{\frac{0.0006}{\sqrt{2}}}{0.080}\right]^2 + \left[\frac{\frac{0.004}{\sqrt{3}}}{0.080}\right]^2} = 0.00239 \text{ g/100 mL} \quad (6.9)$$

$$95\% \text{ Confidence Interval: } 0.080 \pm 1.96\,(0.00239) \Rightarrow 0.075 \text{ to } 0.085 \text{ g/100 mL}$$

The expanded uncertainty for these calculations is 0.00468 g/100 mL or 5.9%. This is similar to the expanded uncertainty of 4.8% found by other researchers (Hwang et al. 2017). Another study using an enzymatic method of analysis observed an expanded uncertainty of 19.74% (Ustundag and Huysal 2017). This large expanded uncertainty was probably due in part to using inter-laboratory (proficiency) test data for precision estimates and a bias estimate of 8.16%. From the computations above we see that the combined uncertainty (estimated by a 95% confidence interval) for both breath and blood alcohol results at a value of 0.08 are very similar. The blood alcohol confidence interval is only slightly less than for breath alcohol. Having the first term in both equations is very important since this is derived from the duplicate measurements. The variation associated with the duplicate measurements, for both breath and blood, will include many sources of variation. These sources will include procedural as well as analytical. The importance of performing duplicate analyses cannot be overemphasized and should be a requirement for program accreditation. The nature in which the duplicates are performed is also important. In most forensic cases, the duplicates will be performed by different analysts on different sets of instrumentation (Jones 1989). Forensic toxicologists performing blood alcohol analyses should be prepared to show the computations for Equation 6.9 in court whenever called to testify. Indeed, such computations determining measurement uncertainty will be a requirement for accreditation. In addition, the computation of Equation 6.9 should be part of the written report of blood alcohol results sent to the enforcement agency, prosecution, and defense. The computations of uncertainty illustrated here (or those selected by program administrators) should also be outlined in the program SOP and provided on the program web site. Moreover, not only is the uncertainty of blood alcohol analysis of importance but also the uncertainty associated with Certified Reference Materials used in calibration and accuracy checks (Gates et al. 2009). All personnel should be thoroughly trained in these computations so there is consistency in testimony. Personnel should also be provided the relevant literature on measurement uncertainty so they can document and justify the methods they employ.

Another method for computing measurement uncertainty is referred to as the "guard band" approach. This method can also be applied to either breath or blood alcohol analysis. Figure 6.5 illustrates the calculation. The upper limit for a 95% (or 99%) confidence interval is determined which is illustrated as the upper limit of the band. For the value of $K_{0.95} = 1.645$, if the mean of duplicate results exceeds this upper limit for

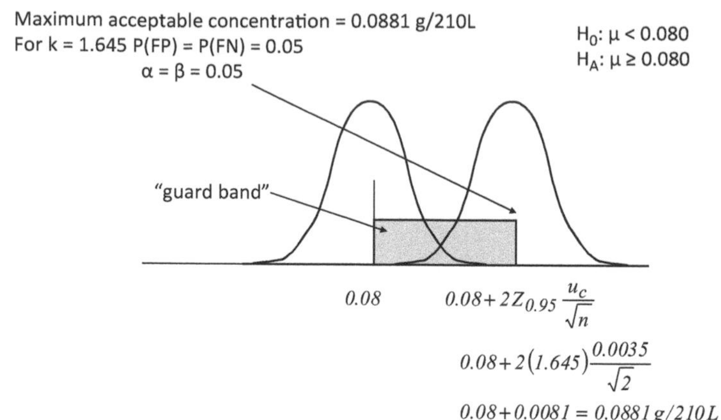

Figure 6.5 Measurement uncertainty determined by the method of using a "guard band."

the band then we can conclude that the true population mean is at least equal to 0.08 or more with 95% confidence. If $K_{0.995} = 2.575$ then we have 99.5% confidence. Figure 6.5 shows the standard deviation of 0.0035 g/210 L which, for illustration, is the estimated standard deviation for a single measurement of breath alcohol. For a blood alcohol measurement this standard deviation would be smaller and determined from the combined uncertainty for blood alcohol analysis. The false-positive and false-negative error probabilities are both 0.05. With this analysis we are testing the null hypothesis that the true mean breath alcohol is less than 0.08 g/210 L. The value of 2 in the equation of Figure 6.5 includes both false-positive and false-negative error probabilities. If our measurement exceeds the upper guard band limit we reject the null hypothesis and $p < 0.05$. Figure 6.5 shows that given the illustrated information we would not prosecute under a *per se* 0.08 law until we had a mean result of 0.089 g/210 L or larger. This guard band method is very similar to that employed in Sweden where the upper guard band limit corresponds to the 99.9% confidence interval limit for the mean of the duplicate results (Jones and Schuberth 1989). Their *per se* limit, however, is approximately 0.02 g/100 mL. A similar approach is applied in the UK where 6 mg/dL is subtracted from the mean of duplicate blood alcohol results if the mean is below 100 mg/dL and 6% is subtracted from the mean of results over 100 mg/dL (Walls and Brownlie 1985). This subtraction assumes a standard deviation of 2 mg/dL. Another study from the UK shows the technical detail of such calculations (Searle 2015). The UK also has case law supporting such a practice (Walker v Hodgins 1983). Denmark has a similar practice where 0.1 g/Kg is subtracted from blood alcohol results to account for their assumed combined uncertainty (Kristiansen and Petersen 2004).

Another case from the State of Idaho related to measurement uncertainty involved a urine sample collected from Van Camp (the defendant) containing two prescription drugs of cyclobenzaprine and Seroquel (*Idaho Transportation Department v. Johnathan P. Van Camp* 2012). A breath test showed no alcohol. The defendant's driver's license was suspended. On appeal the defendant argued that it was not shown that the two drugs were "intoxicating." The Supreme Court of Idaho ruled that under Idaho Code 18-8002A(7), "...the hearing officer shall not vacate the suspension unless one of the five listed grounds has been proven by a preponderance of the evidence." The only subsection of the statute that might have supported the defendant's argument was subsection (c) stating, "...the test results did not show ... the presence of drugs...." Since the test results did clearly show the presence of drugs the high court upheld the driver's license suspension.

Finally, a case from Michigan in 2011 was quite informative (People v. Jeffrey J. Jabrocki 2011). A blood sample from the defendant resulted in 0.303 and 0.298 g/100 mL. According to laboratory practice, the third digit is truncated and the results were reported as 0.29. While this was a case at only the district court level, the opinion was lengthy and very insightful. The court expressed concern that only the one result (0.29) was reported. In the end, the court denied the admissibility of the blood alcohol results. Measurement uncertainty is not new and accreditation organizations are requiring it for blood alcohol analysis. The opinion of this case is worth reading to better understand some of the defense arguments.

6.5.2 Blood Sampling: Alcohol Free Swab and Clotting

Providing our customers with the most reliable and valid blood alcohol results requires pre-analytical, analytical, and post-analytical considerations. A critical pre-analytical component is the sampling conducted by the phlebotomist. One important issue related to blood sampling is the use of an alcohol-free swab. Prior to venipuncture of the antecubital vein the skin is commonly cleansed with a swab containing isopropanol or isopropanol mixed with providone-iodine. A number of studies have measured blood samples obtained following the use of various antiseptic swabs and found no significant contamination effect (Kiyoyama et al. 2009; Shahar et al. 1990; Miller et al. 2007; McIvor and Cosbey 1990; Goldfinger and Schaber 1982). Even using an alcohol swab containing ethanol showed no significant measured results (Lippi et al. 2017). Another study tested blood from both arms, one treated with an alcohol swab and the other with alcohol free swab and found no significant effect (Tucker and Trethewy 2010). This two-arm study would be a more powerful study from a statistical design perspective. From a forensic program perspective, it would be important to specify in the SOP what type of swab is allowed. Then police officers would have to be trained on the swabbing material allowed. The prosecutor and forensic scientists will be held strictly to the details specified in the SOP or administrative rules. In a related study, the use of alcohol-containing hand sanitizers showed no measurable effect on measured blood or breath alcohol concentration (Wigmore 2009).

When police officers have authority to request a blood sample at the hospital, they generally provide the phlebotomist with a collection kit that contains two 10 mL gray-top vials, the needles, and equipment for venipuncture and paperwork to be completed. The gray-top vials are designed for forensic blood alcohol determination. They will contain an anticoagulant (20 mg of potassium oxalate) and an antibacterial (100 mg of sodium fluoride). Without an anticoagulant the blood will begin to clot in less than a minute. The tubes may be glass or plastic. Two types of needles may be used—a 25-gauge butterfly needle or a straight 21-gauge needle. The tubes contain a vacuum which will draw the blood once the needle is located within the vein. A date will be printed on the tubes which specifies the date the vacuum will be guaranteed effective for. Following sample collection it is recommended that the phlebotomist invert the tubes 8–10 times for thorough mixing with the materials. Following the blood collection in the two tubes, the police officer must ensure the forms are completed correctly and thoroughly. The information should include name of phlebotomist, location, date and time of collection, name of defendant, name of officer and any other information requested on the form. The sample kit should then be transported to the forensic toxicology lab as soon as possible. The chain of custody of the samples are very important. The names, date, times and location of all personnel handling the samples must be recorded.

The blood collection technique was an issue in a Florida case in 2018 (*John Goodman v. Florida Department of Law Enforcement* 2018). The blood collection kit contains a straight 21-gauge needle while the phlebotomist collecting Goodman's blood used a 25-gauge butterfly needle. The straight 21-gauge needle evacuates the blood directly into the vacutainer tube. The butterfly needle has an extra length of tubing connecting it to the vacutainer tube. The Florida Administrative Code Rules do not specify which type of needle can be used. They do specify, however, that an alcohol-free antiseptic must be used on the skin. Goodman argued further that the wrong needle type was used for him since the kit contained the other type.

Goodman further argued that clots formed and would as a result increase the blood alcohol concentration. This could occur with a butterfly type needle because of the extra time before the blood reaches the anticoagulant. The defendant also argues that the forensic toxicologists performing the blood alcohol analysis may not have correctly observed the existence of blood clotting. The Supreme Court of Florida denied all of the defendant's motions and upheld his conviction. Moreover, a study published in 1990 found that there was no significant difference between clotted blood and normal blood collected from the same subject and analyzed by gas chromatography (Senkowski and Thompson 1990). The program SOP, however, should specify the steps to be followed when encountering samples that display various degrees of clotting.

An issue related to needle size and clotting is hemolysis, which is the breakdown of red blood cells in the blood. This is thought to possibly occur by using too small of a needle (>21 gauge) or resulting from in vivo causes. One study showed that the commonly used needle size of >21 gauge was not a cause and the fact that head space gas chromatography uses headspace ethanol would not be affected by hemolysis (Tiscione 2015).

Another case from Wisconsin (*Wisconsin v. Patrick K. Kozel* 2017) involved the issue of phlebotomist authority. The statute stated in part that the individual drawing the blood sample must be a "…person acting under the direction of a physician." The training, qualifications and credentials of the phlebotomist were all entered into evidence. The Supreme Court of Wisconsin denied the defense motions and ruled that the phlebotomist was acting in compliance with the statute.

The use of hand sanitizer materials have also been evaluated (Brown et al. 2007). In this study volunteers rubbed their hands with either ethanol or isopropanol containing hand sanitizers 30 times in one hour. Within minutes of the last exposure they provided breath samples and blood samples. Ethanol was measured in the breath of some volunteers at 1 to 2 minutes post-exposure and 5 to 7 minutes in serum. The results were in the third digit and below levels of detection. No measurable isopropanol was observed. The transdermal passage of hand sanitizers do not appear to be a concern.

Forensic scientists are strongly urged to meet with local hospital personnel to discuss common issues and legal challenges. Such meetings should include the local prosecutors as well. Forensic program policies (SOP) should be shared with the hospital personnel so they are aware of policies that relate to blood sampling, storage, chain of custody and analytical methods. Likewise, the hospital policies should be shared with the forensic personnel. Policies, procedures, and legal challenges should be discussed and fully understood by all parties. There may also be hospital policies and records that could be placed on the program web site to improve the provision of discovery requests. These simple steps should significantly improve program performance and help ensure the provision of accurate and reliable blood alcohol results.

6.5.3 Measurement Units

The statutory language defining the offense of DUI in Illinois in 1996 was "...alcohol concentration means grams of alcohol per 100 mL of blood." Kevin Kotecki (defendant) was involved in an accident and transported to the hospital where a blood sample was obtained (*People v. Kotecki* 1996). The results of the alcohol analysis recorded on the hospital form was "153" This was apparently a sample analyzed in the hospital clinical lab and not obtained from a forensic analysis. The court took judicial notice that the recorded value of "153" was equivalent to 0.153. Additional notation on the hospital form stated under "UNITS MG/DL." The result was properly recorded as 153 mg/dL which corresponds to 0.153 g/100 mL. On appeal the Court of Appeals reject the defendant's motion and upheld the conviction of the trial court. This case illustrates the importance of attention to detail. Record all numerical results with the full information so there is no doubt. It is also a bit unusual that the prosecutor in this case relied only on the hospital (presumably a serum alcohol result) measured result. The forensic route of analysis would have been more complete and straightforward.

6.5.4 Blood Sample Stability Over Time

The time between blood collection and time of trial can be lengthy—often six months or more. Prior to trial, a common defense request is for a sample of the blood for their own arranged analysis. Or, the defense may request that the government lab perform the analysis again. In either case, it would be important to know how long the stored and refrigerated blood samples are stable and provide the same (or nearly so) blood alcohol concentration. Several studies have evaluated the stability of alcohol in whole blood stored over long periods of time (Shan et al. 2011; Jones 2007; Booker et al. 2009; Vance et al. 2015; Laurens et al. 2018). The decline in alcohol concentration seemed to be a function of headspace volume and temperature during storage. Another source of decrease in ethanol concentration over time is the chemical oxidation of ethanol to formaldehyde (Kristoffersen et al. 2006).

Ethanol can also be lost during storage due to microbial contamination and degradation (Dick and Stone 1987). Such can occur if the concentration of sodium fluoride is too low—there should be 100 mg. This issue can be addressed with a few basic procedures: Post-mortem blood sample should be analyzed separate from normal samples, samples should be stored at temperatures below 4°C, the concentration of sodium fluoride should be at least 2% w/v (100 mg) and use careful laboratory practice that avoids contamination of the samples. These steps should be clearly outlined in the program SOP. Moreover, ethanol can be lost from the sample simply during storage without preservatives for up to 180 days. In one study blood samples containing no preservatives but stored at −18°C showed significant decline in ethanol concentration over the 180 days (Stojiljkovic et al. 2016). In another study, blood vials filled at least half way and stored in unopened vials at room temperature for 5–10 years showed significant decreases of 0.01–0.05 g/dL (Tiscione et al. 2015). Refrigeration at 4°C or less along with minimal opening and near full vials appear to be basic steps to minimize alcohol loss.

Post-mortem blood samples have their own additional issues and challenges. The blood can arrive at the lab in various states of decomposition and clotting. Homogenization is often necessary. The time between death and sampling can also greatly influence the sample quality. In addition, temperature, cause of death and sample site can also greatly influence the condition and analytical results. The commonly used internal standard of n-Propanol may not be the best choice for post-mortem samples (Countryman et al. 2010). Unstoppered, leaking septum or frequent opening of gray-top tubes can also lead to a significant loss of alcohol, even within 30 minutes of exposure (Saracevic et al. 2014). These issues can result in a number of challenges from the defense. Forensic toxicologists need to be prepared for a variety of challenges. Several authors have addressed the issues associated with post-mortem samples.

6.5.5 "Salting Out Effect" due to Low Blood Volume

When blood is collected into the vacutainer tube it is mixed immediately with the antibacterial sodium fluoride. The salt sodium fluoride has the effect of increasing the volume of blood while decreasing the liquid portion of the blood sample. This forces more of the volatile ethanol into the headspace above the blood sample—the "salting out effect." Since the vapor headspace sample is measured for ethanol concentration in a headspace gas chromatograph, the increased concentration of ethanol in the headspace due to the presence of excess sodium fluoride relative to the blood volume may yield a biased result. The likelihood of this occurring may be increased by a low volume of blood (i.e., <2.5 mL in the 10 mL tube) compared to the 100 mg of sodium fluoride in the tube. This issue has been studied (Jones 1994) and found to result in no significant bias. In fact, the addition of more sodium fluoride resulted in decreased measured ethanol concentrations (Miller et al. 2004). The potential for an increase in headspace concentration is obviated by a dilution of 10 times with n-propanol (the common internal standard) and also by allowing sufficient time for equilibration to occur. This dilution reduces the sodium fluoride concentration in the sample and thus minimizes the difference in matrix effect comparing blood to calibrant aqueous solutions. It is important that the calibrant matrix be as similar to the blood sample matrix as possible. The concentration of ethanol in the diluted blood sample can now be accurately determined by comparing the headspace concentration to a calibration curve developed from the known ratio of solution to headspace ethanol concentrations. The diluted blood sample is now similar to the aqueous ethanol solutions used to develop the calibration curve. Moreover, even with a low blood volume in the tube the partitioning of ethanol between air and solution tends toward to the solution. Not much partitions into the headspace. Finally, in his study, Jones found that low blood volumes actually resulted in lower blood alcohol concentration by 2%–3%.

One court decision is relevant to this issue of blood volume. A superior court in the State of Delaware heard testimony regarding the volume of blood collected by the phlebotomist (*State of Delaware v. Lamontra R. Fountain* 2016). The rules for collection of blood samples stated "Using normal procedures, withdraw blood from subject (allow tube to fill to maximum volume)." While the gray-top tubes will hold a maximum volume of approximately 10.5 mL, the phlebotomist testified that she collected about 6 mL. While this was a very adequate volume for alcohol analysis by head space GC, the legal issue was with regard to the requirement in the rules. This is a clear example of how written rules and procedures will be applied very literally by the defense in order to show some shortcoming by the state. Your program will be held to every word and detail in the program SOP and any additional recording of rules and procedures. This is reflective of an issue in Washington State several years ago where a missing semicolon in the Implied Consent Rights resulted in several breath test results being suppressed. In the Delaware case state witnesses testified that 0.5 mL would be sufficient to obtain a valid blood alcohol result. The court seemed to comprehend the technical testimony and seemed inclined to rule in the state's favor until it heard testimony that the phlebotomist may have not followed some important steps. The phlebotomist testified that the needle was placed into the vacutainer tube prior to inserting into the vein. It was argued that this could lead to a loss of the vacuum as well as allow for contamination. Based on this the superior court in Delaware suppressed the blood alcohol results.

6.5.6 Expired Date on Gray-Top Tubes

There will be a date noted on the label on the gray top vacutainer tubes. This date refers to the vacuum seal. There is a guarantee by the manufacturer that the vacuum will remain until that date so that blood can be collected. The date does not refer to any chemical composition or other analytical features. To avoid this argument, police officers should ensure that the vial is not used after the noted date. Even though there is no analytical influence, it is a simple step to just avoid the issue entirely by ensuring the noted date is not past.

6.6 Additional Challenges

The issues presented above include a reasonable and objective response. There is not time or space to discuss all the possible defense challenges that could arise. Defense attorneys are very clever and creative. They work hard, as appropriate, for their clients, always seeking to develop some new and unique challenge that will persuade the jury with some reasonable doubt. Below we present, without response, several other possible challenges that have been heard by forensic scientists. The reader is encouraged to evaluate these issues and develop appropriate responses:

- The request of blood from a defendant requires a search warrant
- Defense request for a blood sample to be analyzed by their selected laboratory
- The State must show that the chemical in the tubes are correct
- Serum has a higher concentration than whole blood
- Interfering substances in the gas chromatograph analysis
- Foreign substances (i.e., tongue jewelry) in the mouth during exhalation
- Failure to use a new mouthpiece for the second breath sample
- Incorrect clock time on the instrument may bias the test result
- No control measurements performed at 0.02 g/210 L for the testing of minors

- Instrument software version used with the defendant was not the same as that used by the operator in training
- Download data containing the defendant's results were lost
- Use of unheated breath tube
- Officer at a "refusal hearing" was shown to have a large percentage of refusal occurrences
- Officer did not wait an additional 15 minutes where test showed the presence of "mouth alcohol"
- Uncertainty in Widmark calculations
- Airbag particulate matter may bias breath test result
- Printout document showing all required steps is lost before trial
- Operator complaint phone calls—discoverable record and contents
- Uncertainty in simulator thermometers
- Fittings and tubing attached to simulator now no longer approved by NHTSA
- Breath sampling requirements result in smaller individuals providing a deeper lung biased sample
- Breath instrument has higher number of failed tests compared to other instruments
- Repair forms with check boxes that are pre-checked
- Must redact the higher result and the third digit of the lower result for court
- Inadequate manufacturer warranty on the instrument
- Is 0.078 and 0.085 for either breath or blood in excess of the *per se* 0.080 statute?
- Defense may want to bring the instrument into the court room
- How does the manufacturer's calibration recommendations compare to that used by the state?
- Control standard depletion rate is unusual
- Infusion of fluids during surgery and before blood sampling for ethanol
- Industrial inhalation of ethanol and other volatile organic compounds

These and other issues along with their responses can be found elsewhere (US Department of Transportation 2013).

6.7 Conclusion

There exist several other potential defense challenges to both breath and blood alcohol analysis (Jones 1991; US National Highway Traffic Safety Administration 2013). Many factors contribute to the vigorous challenge of forensic alcohol evidence in the prosecution of drinking-and-driving cases. Owing to the significant penalties associated with a DUI conviction we should not be surprised by the vigilant defense effort. Forensic toxicologists should not be surprised, but rather expect and prepare for such challenge. After all, defendants are expecting the most knowledgeable and aggressive challenges possible on their behalf. Knowledge of the more common challenges, such as those discussed here, can help the toxicologist and program personnel prepare for such issues. For many of the issues, the prosecution response will be fairly uniform across jurisdictions. For others, the response will depend on local statutes, administrative rules, case law, policies, instrumentation, and procedures. In view of the multitude of possible legal challenges, the forensic scientist must remain professional, truthful, non-adversarial, transparent and as objective as possible. They should always be alert and carefully consider the challenges with the view of improving their programs and analytical procedures. Some challenges, clearly, are forensically meaningless. Others, however, may indeed be forensically relevant and reflect areas of our program that need revision. We must listen to, evaluate and accept criticism from colleagues and customers alike with a continual view toward improving our program confidence and integrity. Often a small change in policy, procedure or documentation will address and eliminate the challenge. The point is, we must be alert to these situations and prepare to change as part of our continual effort to improve the forensic quality, credibility and integrity of our numerical evidence.

References

Barone PT, Vosk, T: Breath and blood tests in intoxicated driving cases: Why they currently fail to meet basic scientific and legal safeguards for admissibility; *Mich Bar J* 94(7):30; 2015.

Bogen E: Drunkeness: Quantitative study of acute alcoholic intoxication; *J Am Med Assoc* 89:1508; 1927.

Booker R, Lehmann GP, Mitchell JD: Blood alcohol concentration in expired and non-expired approved containers stored at room temperature and under refrigeration for 21 days; *Can Soc Forensic Sci J* 42:260; 2009.

Brown TL, Gamon S, Tester P, Martin R, Hosking K, Bowkett GC, Gerostamoulos D, Grayson ML: Can alcohol-based hand-rub solutions cause you to lose your drivers license? Comparative cutaneous absorption of various alcohols; *Antimicrob Agents Chemother* 51:1107; 2007.

Buckley TJ, Pleil JD, Bowyer JR, Davis JM: Evaluation of methyl t-butyl ether (MTBE) as an interference on commercial breath-alcohol analyzers; *Forensic Sci Int* 123:111; 2001.

Caddy GR, Sobell MB, Sobell LC: Alcohol breath tests—Criteria times for avoiding contamination by mouth alcohol; *Behav Res Methods Inst* 10:814; 1978.

Caldwell JP, Kim ND: The response of the Intoxilyzer 5000 to five potential interfering substances; *J Forensic Sci* 42:1080; 1997.

Campbell L, Wilson HK: Blood alcohol concentrations following the inhalation of ethanol vapour under controlled conditions; *J Forensic Sci Soc* 26:129; 1986.

Carpenter DA, Turner GL: Recent advances in software data collection and evaluation; *Sixteenth Annual Conference of the International Association for Chemical Testing*; Cocoa Beach, FL; April 2003.

Chow BLC, Wigmore JG: Technical note: The stability of aqueous alcohol standard used in breath alcohol testing after twenty-six years storage; *Can Soc Forensic Sci J* 38:21; 2005.

City of Seattle v. Fawn Allison; 148 Wn.2d 75 (2002).

Commonwealth v. Ananias et al.; 1248CR001075, 32 (2017).

Cooper S: Infrared breath alcohol analysis following inhalation of gasoline fumes; *J Anal Toxicol* 5:198; 1981.

Countryman S, Kelly K, Fernandez C: Critical factors in selecting an internal standard for accurate determination of blood alcohols in post mortem samples, *Phenomenex Applications* (TN-2041); 2010; https://phenomenex.blob.core.windows.net/documents/2fc9aab0-d265–49f8-a7aa-e794a97a8a11.pdf (Accessed April 22, 2019).

Cowan JM, McCutcheon JR, Weathermon A: The response of the Intoxilyzer 4011AS-A to a number of possible interfering substances; *J Forensic Sci* 35:797; 1990.

Daubert v. Merrell Dow Pharmaceuticals; 509 U.S. 579 (1993).

Dick GL, Stone HM: Alcohol loss arising from microbial contamination of driver's blood specimen, *Forensic Sci Int* 34:17; 1987.

Dubowski KM, Essary NA: Response of breath-alcohol analyzers to acetone: Further studies; *J Anal Toxicol* 8:205; 1984.

Dubowski KM, Goodson EE, Sample M: Storage stability of simulator ethanol solutions for vapor-alcohol control tests in breath-alcohol analysis; *J Anal Toxicol* 26:406; 2002.

Dubowski KM: Quality assurance in breath-alcohol analysis; *J Anal Toxicol* 18:306; 1994.

Dubowski KM: Studies in breath-alcohol analysis: Biological factors; *Z Rechtsmed* 76:93; 1975.

Elias-Cruz v. Idaho Department of Transportation; 153 Idaho 200, 280 P.3d 703 (2012).

Fessler CC, Tulleners FA, Howitt DG, Richards JR: Determination of mouth alcohol using the Drager evidential portable alcohol system; *Sci Justice* 48:16; 2008.

Flores AL, Frank JF: *The Likelihood of Acetone Interference in Breath Alcohol Measurement* (US DOT NHTSA Technical Report: DOT HS 806 922); Washington, DC, September 1985.

Foglio-Bonda PL, Poggia F, Foglio-Bonda A, Mantovani C, Pattarino F, Giglietta A: Determination of breath alcohol value after using mouthwashes containing ethanol in healthy young adults; *Eur Rev Med Pharmacol* 19:2562; 2015.

Friel PN, Baer JS, Logan BK: Variability of ethanol absorption and breath concentrations during a large-scale alcohol administration study; *Alcohol Clin Exp Res* 19:1055; 1995a.

Friel PN, Logan BK, Baer J: An evaluation of the reliability of Widmark calculations based on breath alcohol measurements; *J Forensic Sci* 40:91; 1995b.

Frye v. United States; 293 F. 1013 D.C. Cir. (1923).

Funk C: *Daubert Versus Frye: A National Look at Expert Evidentiary Standards*; The Expert Institute: New York; 2018; https://www.theexpertinstitute.com/daubert-versus-frye-a-national-look-at-expert-evidentiary-standards/ (Accessed April 22, 2019).

Gates K, Chang N, Dilek I, Jian H, Pogue S, Sreenivasan U: The uncertainty of reference standards—A guide to understanding factors impacting uncertainty, uncertainty calculations, and vendor certifications; *J Anal Toxicol* 33:532; 2009.

Gill R, Hatchett SE, Broster CG, Osselton MD, Ramsey JD, Wilson HK, Wilcox AH: The response of evidential breath alcohol testing instruments with subjects exposed to organic solvents and gases: I. Toluene, 1.1.1-trichloroethane and butane; *Med Sci Law* 31:187; 1991a.

Gill R, Osselton MD, Broad JE, Ramsey JD: The response of evidential breath alcohol testing instruments with subjects exposed to organic solvents and gases: III. White spirit exposure during domestic painting; *Med Sci Law* 31:214; 1991b.

Gill R, Warner HE, Broster CG, Osselton MD, Ramsey JD, Wilson HK, Wilcox AH: The response of evidential breath alcohol testing instruments with subjects exposed to organic solvents and gases: II. White spirit and nonane; *Med Sci Law* 31:201; 1991c.

Goldfinger TM, Schaber D: A comparison of blood alcohol concentration using non-alcohol and alcohol-containing skin antiseptics; *Ann Emerg Med* 11:665; 1982.

Gomm PJ, Weston SI, Osselton MD: The effect of respiratory aerosol inhalers and nasal sprays on breath alcohol testing devices used in Great Britain; *Med Sci Law* 30:203; 1990.

Goodman v. Florida Department of Law Enforcement; 229 So. 3d 366 (2018).

Gullberg RG, Andersson L, Jones AW: Comparison of evidential breath alcohol testing and drinking driving demographics in Sweden and the State of Washington; *J Traffic Med* 25:77; 1997.

Gullberg RG, McElroy AJ: Comparing roadside with subsequent breath alcohol analyses and their relevance to the issue of retrograde extrapolation; *Forensic Sci Int* 57:193; 1992.

Gullberg RG: Determining the air/water partition coefficient to employ when calibrating forensic breath alcohol test instruments; *Can Soc Forensic Sci J* 38:205; 2005.

Gullberg RG: Estimating the measurement uncertainty in forensic blood alcohol analysis; *J Anal Toxicol* 36:153; 2012.

Gullberg RG: The elimination rate of mouth alcohol: Mathematical modeling and implications in breath alcohol analysis; *J Forensic Sci* 37:1363; 1992.

Harding PM, Laessig RH, Field PH: Field performance of the Intoxilyzer 5000: A comparison of blood- and breath-alcohol results in Wisconsin drivers; *J Forensic Sci* 35:1022; 1990.

Hwang R, Beltran J, Rogers C, Barlow J, Razatos G: Measurement of uncertainty for blood alcohol concentration by headspace gas chromatography; *Can Soc Forensic Sci J* 50:114; 2017.

Idaho Transportation Department v. Johnathan Paul Van Camp; https://law.justia.com/cases/idaho/supreme-court-civil/2012/38958.html (Accessed April 22, 2019).

Iffland R, Jones AW: Evaluating alleged drinking after driving—The hip-flask defense. Part 1. Double blood samples and urine-to-blood alcohol relationship; *Med Sci Law* 42:207; 2002.

Iffland R, Jones AW: Evaluating alleged drinking after driving—The hip-flask defense. Part 2. Congener analysis; *Med Sci Law* 43:39; 2003.

Jones AW, Andersson L, Berglund K: Interfering substances identified in the breath of drinking drivers with Intoxilyzer 5000S; *J Anal Toxicol* 20:522; 1996a.

Jones AW, Andersson L: Variability of the blood/breath alcohol ratio in drinking drivers; *J Forensic Sci* 41:916; 1996b.

Jones AW, Schuberth J: Computer-aided headspace gas chromatography applied to blood-alcohol analysis: Importance of online process control; *J Forensic Sci* 34:1116; 1989.

Jones AW: Are changes in blood-ethanol concentration during storage analytically significant? Importance of method imprecision; *Clin Chem Lab Med* 45:1299; 2007.

Jones AW: Breath-acetone concentrations in fasting healthy men: Response of infrared breath-alcohol analyzers; *J Anal Toxicol* 11:67; 1987.

Jones AW: Determination of liquid/air partition coefficients for dilute solutions of ethanol in water, whole blood, and plasma; *J Anal Toxicol* 7:193; 1983.

Jones AW: Differences between capillary and venous blood alcohol concentrations as a function of time after drinking, with emphasis on sampling variations in left vs right arm; *Clin Chem* 35:400; 1989.

Jones AW: Salting-Out effect of sodium fluoride and its influence on the analysis of ethanol by headspace gas chromatography; *J Anal Toxicol* 18:292; 1994.

Jones AW: Top ten defence challenges among drinking drivers in Sweden; *Med Sci Law* 31:229; 1991.

Kitchenham B, Pfleeger SL: Software quality: The elusive target; *IEEE Software*; pp 12–21; January 1996.

Kiyoyama T, Tokuda Y, Shiiki S, Hachiman T, Shimasaki T, Endo K: Isopropyl alcohol compared with isopropyl alcohol plus providone-iodine as skin preparation for prevention of blood culture contamination; *J Clin Microbiol* 47:54; 2009.

Kristiansen J, Petersen HW: An uncertainty budget for the measurement of ethanol in blood by headspace gas chromatography; *J Anal Toxicol* 28:456; 2004.

Kristiansen J: Description of a generally applicable model for the evaluation of uncertainty of measurement in clinical chemistry; *Clin Chem Lab Med* 39:920; 2001.

Kristoffersen L, Stomyhr LE, Smith-Kielland A: Headspace gas chromatographic determination of ethanol: The use of factorial design to study effects of blood storage and headspace conditions on ethanol stability and acetaldehyde formation in whole blood and plasma; *Forensic Sci Int* 161:151; 2006.

Krotoszkynski B, Gabriel G, O'Neill H: Characterization of human expired air: A promising investigative and diagnostic technique; *J Chromatogr Sci* 15:239; 1977.

Laurens JB, Sewell FJJ, Kock MM: Pre-analytical factors related to the stability of ethanol concentration during storage of ante-mortem blood alcohol specimens; *J Forensic Leg Med* 58:155; 2018.

Lindberg L, Grubb D, Dencker D, Finnhult M, Olsson SG: *Forensic Sci Int* 249: 66;2015.

Lippi G, Simundic A-M, Musile G, Danese E, Salvagno G, Tagliano F: The alcohol used for cleansing the venipuncture site does not jeopardize blood and plasma alcohol measurement with head-space gas chromatography and an enzymatic assay; *Biochemia Medica* 27:398; 2017.

Logan BK, Gullberg RG, Elenbaas JK: Isopropanol interference with breath alcohol analysis: A case report; *J Forensic Sci* 39:1107; 1994.

Magnusson B, Örnemark U (Eds): *Eurachem Guide: The Fitness for Purpose of Analytical Methods—A Laboratory Guide to Method Validation and Related Topics*, 2nd ed; 2014; https://www.eurachem.org/images/stories/Guides/pdf/MV_guide_2nd_ed_EN.pdf (Accessed April 22, 2019).

McIvor RA, Cosbey SH: Effect of using alcoholic and non-alcoholic skin cleansing swabs when sampling blood for alcohol estimation using gas chromatography; *Br J Clin Pract* 44:235; 1990.

Miller BA, Day SM, Vasquez TE, Evans FM: Absence of salting out effects in forensic blood alcohol determination at various concentrations of sodium fluoride using semi-automated headspace gas chromatography *Sci Justice* 44:73; 2004.

Miller MA, Rosin A, Levsky ME, Gregory TJ, Crystal CS: Isopropyl alcohol pad use for blood ethanol sampling does not cause false-positive results; *J Emerg Med* 33:9; 2007.

Modell JG, Taylor JP, Lee JY: Breath alcohol values following mouthwash use; *JAMA* 270:2955; 1993.

National District Attorneys Association: Alexandria, VA; http://www.ndaa.org/ (Accessed April 22, 2019).

NIST Policy on Metrological Traceability; https://www.nist.gov/traceability/nist-policy-metrological-traceability (Accessed April 22, 2019).

Olevik v. State; 806 SE 2d 505 (2017).

People v Jabrocki; Unpublished opinion of the 79th District Court, County of Mason, State of Michigan, decided September 30, 2011 (No. 08–5461-FD).

People v. Kotecki; 279 Ill. App. 3d 1006 (1996).

Pollack S: Observations on the adversary system and the role of the forensic scientist: "Scientific truth" v. "legal truth"; *J Forensic Sci* 18:173; 1973.

Reed TE, Kalant H: Bias in calculated rate of alcohol metabolism due to variation in relative amounts of adipose tissue; *J Stud Alcohol* 38:1773; 1977.

Saracevic A, Simundic AM, Dukic L: The stability of ethanol in unstoppered tubes; *Clin Biochem* 47:92; 2014.

Searle J: Alcohol calculations and their uncertainty; *Med Sci Law* 55:58; 2015.

Senkowski CM, Thompson KA: The accuracy of blood alcohol analysis using headspace gas chromatography when performed on clotted samples; *J Forensic Sci* 35:176; 1990.

Shahar E, Wohl-Gottesman BS, Shenkman L: Contamination of blood cultures during venipuncture: Fact or myth? *Postgrad Med J* 66:1053; 1990.

Shan X, Tiscione NB, Alford I, Yeatman DT: A study of blood alcohol stability in forensic antemortem blood samples; *Forensic Sci Int* 211:47; 2011.

Sklerov JH, Couper FJ: Calculation and verification of blood ethanol measurement uncertainty for headspace gas chromatography; *J Anal Toxicol* 35:402; 2011.

State of Delaware v. Lamontra R. Fountain; Superior Court (2016); https://law.justia.com/cases/delaware/superior-court/2016/1411013133.html (Accessed April 22, 2019).

State of Idaho v. Justin K Austin: 163 Idaho 378, 413 P.3d 778 (2017).

State v. Cassidy: 230 N.J. 232 (2018).

State v. Chun et al.: 194 NJ 54 Supreme Court (2008).

State v. Downie: 117 N.J. 450, 569 A.2d 242 (1990).

State v. Jones: 375 Pacific Reporter 3d 279 (Id. 2016).

State v. Mickelson: 680 N.W. 2d 832 (2004).

Sterling K: The rate of dissipation of mouth alcohol in alcohol positive subjects; *J Forensic Sci* 57:802; 2012.

Stojiljkovic G, Maletin M, Stojic D, Brkic S, Abenavoli L: Ethanol concentration changes in blood samples during medium-term refrigerated storage; *Eur Rev Med Pharmacol Sci* 20:4831; 2016.

Taylor BN, Kuyatt CE: *Guidelines for Evaluating and Expressing the Uncertainty of NIST Measurement Results* (NIST Technical Note 1297); 1994; http://physics.nist.gov/TN1297 (Accessed May 12; 2019).

Thieden HID, Hunding A: A new approach to the determination of ethanol elimination rate in vivo: An extension of Widmark's equation; *Pharmacol Toxicol* 68:51; 1991.

Tiscione N: The impact of hemolysis on the accuracy of ethanol determinations; *J Anal Toxicol* 39:672; 2015.

Tiscione NB, Vacha RE, Alford I, Yeatman DT, Shan X: Long-term blood alcohol stability in forensic ante-mortem whole blood samples; *J Anal Toxicol* 39:419; 2015.

Tucker A, Trethewy C: Lack of effect on blood alcohol level of swabbing venipuncture sites with 70% isopropyl alcohol; *Emerg Med Australas* 22:9; 2010.

US Department of Transportation National Highway Traffic Safety Administration: *Challenges and Defenses II: Claims and Responses to Common Challenges and Defenses in Driving While Impaired Cases* (DOT HS 811 707); 2013; https://ndaa.org/wp-content/uploads/Chalenges-and-Defenses-II.pdf (Accessed April 22, 2019).

US Federal Bureau of Investigation (US Department of Justice): *Crime in the United States*; 2017; https://ucr.fbi.gov/crime-in-the-u.s/2017/crime-in-the-u.s.-2017/tables/table-29 (Accessed April 22, 2019).

US National Research Council: *Strengthening Forensic Science in the United States: A Path Forward*; The National Academies Press Washington, DC; 2009.

Ustundag Y, Huysal K: Measurement uncertainty of blood ethanol concentration in drink-driving cases in an emergency laboratory; *Biochem Med* (Zagreb) 27(3):030708; 2017.

Vance CS, Carter CR, Carter RJ, Del Valle MM, Peña JR: Comparison of immediate and delayed blood alcohol concentration testing; *J Anal Toxicol* 39:538; 2015.

Walker v Hodgins; RTR 34, Crim LR 555 (1983).

Wallace J: Proficiency testing as a basis for estimating uncertainty of measurement: Applications to forensic alcohol and toxicology quantitations; *J Forensic Sci* 55:767; 2010.

Walls H, Bownlie A: *Drink, Drugs and Driving*, 2nd ed; Sweet and Maxwell Limited: London, UK; 1985.

Watson PE, Watson ID, Batt RD: Prediction of blood alcohol concentrations in human subjects; *J Stud Alcohol* 42:547; 1981.

Watts MT, McDonald OL: The effect of biologic specimen type on the gas chromatograph head-space analysis of ethanol and other volatile compounds; *Am J Clin Pathol* 87:79; 1987.

Widmark EMP: Principles and Applications of Medicolegal Alcohol Determination; *Biomedical Publications*: Davis, CA; 1981.

Wigmore JG: The Purell defence: Can the use of alcohol-containing hand sanitizers cause an elevated breath or blood alcohol concentration? *Can Soc Forensic Sci J* 42:147; 2009.

Williams PM: Current defense strategies in some contested drink-drive prosecutions: Is it now time for some additional statutory assumptions? *Forensic Sci Int* 293:e5; 2018.

Wisconsin v. Kozel; WI3, Wis.2d, N.W. 2d (2017).

7 Quality Assurance in Forensic Breath-Alcohol Analysis*

ROD G. GULLBERG

Contents

7.1 Introduction

Forensic breath alcohol analysis is employed primarily in the prosecution of drunk driving laws throughout the western world. Breath alcohol analysis is also employed in emergency medicine, largely overdose cases, where the physician needs an estimation of the state of intoxication before treatment. The medical application is generally characterized as giving less consideration to quality control compared to the forensic application. Compared to forensic personnel, health care professionals rarely go to court to be challenged regarding their measurement results. Moreover, within the forensic context, breath alcohol is determined far more often than blood alcohol. Breath alcohol is probably obtained in over 90%

* This chapter is an updated version of a review article previously published in *Forensic Science Review*: Gullberg RG: Methodology and quality assurance in forensic breath alcohol analysis; *Forensic Sci Rev* 12:49; 2000.

of the drunk driving cases, due largely to its less invasive nature and immediate results. Our focus in this chapter is on the level of quality control that should be employed in the forensic breath testing context.

Drunk driving is a serious criminal offense in most all jurisdictions. Conviction results in significant penalties affecting the retention of a driving license, financial loss, property loss as well as impacting one's career. In most jurisdictions, the statutory language defines the offense as having a specified breath alcohol concentration of 0.080 g/210 L or a blood alcohol concentration of 0.080 g/100 mL. This evidence generally possesses the most weight for the judge or jury to consider in determining guilt or innocence. While it is common for numerical information to be very persuasive to a lay jury and judge, it can also be very confusing when embellished with complex statistical detail. For this reason it is very important to simplify and clarify numerical testimony. When the statutory language specifies the offense in terms of a numerical result which in turn corresponds to the value presented in court, judges and juries are strongly inclined to convict. For this reason, defense attorneys often focus on pre-trial evidential hearings in an attempt to have the results suppressed from being introduced into evidence at trial. Moreover, forensic toxicology has not been one of the disciplines vigorously criticized in the *NRC* report and elsewhere (US National Research Council 2009; Mnookin 2018). This is partly due to the cautious position in forensic toxicology stating, "… an individual should be presumed to be devoid of drugs unless there is over-whelming scientific evidence to the contrary" (Wu et al. 1999). In addition, forensic toxicology has a much stronger research foundation and culture than many of the other disciplines generating pattern identification evidence. Therefore, attention to quality control is absolutely necessary to maintain and enhance this foundation of confidence in forensic toxicology.

Given this background, it is clearly imperative that the numerical results, the product we produce, possess the highest possible integrity and confidence (Wu et al. 1999). Quality control includes those practices and procedures that must ensure the highest possible reliability in the results presented to the court. This chapter will focus on the quality control necessary in the forensic application of breath alcohol analysis.

Quality control in forensic breath alcohol analysis consists of many elements that work in combination to ensure integrity of the final numerical results. Quality is largely determined in the process, not in the product (Deming 1986). Our purpose here is to identify these elements, explain them, and illustrate their contribution to the final analytical results presented in court. Moreover, our data should be analyzed in the context of its intended use. This helps to ensure fitness-for-purpose rather than just an abstract summarizing of the data. These elements of quality control that at a minimum are necessary to ensure fitness-for-purpose and highest analytical confidence include:

- Trained personnel
- Duplicate analyses where the full analytical method is repeated in its entirety
- Three digit analytical results
- SOP manuals outlining all aspects of the program for full disclosure and complete transparency
- The measurement of traceable reference control standards as part of the run for alcohol analysis
- Analytical calibration with traceable Certified Reference Materials
- Validated and approved instrumentation

- Documented chain of custody
- Program accreditation
- Proficiency test participation
- Reporting of measurement uncertainty (Huang 2014)
- Printout and electronic storage of all measurement results

It must be remembered that every program can be improved upon. Quality control is part of a daily attitude and practice that recognizes the forensic purpose and responsibility and continually seeks total program credibility and improvement. Our objective here is to draw attention to and promote the importance of rigorous quality control in the discipline of forensic breath alcohol analysis. The intended result is to present our analytical results with the highest level of confidence to the end users so they can make a fully informed decision.

7.1.1 Who Employs Our Measurement Results?

Before any relevant quality control program can be developed, we must know who we perform the measurements for. Who will be using our results to make important informed decisions and what is their expected level of analytical confidence. For the most part, the forensic toxicologist does not perform analytical measurements for their own interest and use. So who are the end-users of our measurement results? Identifying these individuals along with their specific needs will largely define the QC program we eventually develop. Once their needs are identified, these should be transformed into performance requirements. Measurement results are the product of our labor and the end-users may find multiple applications. Some of these end-user applications include: development of probable cause by law enforcement to arrest, prosecution of drunk driving cases, development of traffic safety programs, public safety research, legislative policy development, court decisions and case law, legal defense community, training of personnel, etc. Each of these customers has unique needs that our quality control programs must consider. The numerical information we provide must be of a high quality that fosters confidence for these end-users and their applied interests. For some customers the QC elements are minimal while for others the expected QC integrity is considerable. The program must produce information that is fit-for-purpose, a concept that answers the question: "Do the results meet the needs of the customer?" Our programs must foster, in the words of W. Edwards Deming, "… a long term relationship of loyalty and trust" (Deming 1986).

For the most part, our end users are non-scientists and do not appreciate the details of metrology and the need for quality control and technical detail. Surveys have shown that a significant proportion (23%) of the American public lacks basic quantitative literacy (they would be considered innumerate) (Reyna et al. 2009). An important part of quality control is educating these individuals who will ultimately use our analytical results to make important and informed decisions. They will be relying on forensic personnel to provide them the most reliable measurements possible. For this reason, it is very important that the forensic personnel meet with, discuss and educate these professional colleagues. These individuals include, in part: law enforcement, prosecutors, defense attorneys, judges, policy makers, etc. Discussing and explaining with all of these professionals should include full disclosure and transparency. Mutual support and the sharing of information is imperative between the forensic scientist and the broader community of professionals who apply the results we supply to them. Finally, regular surveys sent to these colleagues asking for input and clarification would be very useful for improving services and enhancing program integrity.

7.1.2 The Legal Context

Before implementing a quality control program we must thoroughly understand the legal context within which we operate. The analytical measurement of an individual's breath alcohol concentration is part of a multifactor legal context. There are legislated laws, administrative rules and case law relating to and defining all aspects of our programs. Legislative elements require legislative action and are not easily revised. Administrative rules are more easily revised. Finally, there are case law which will significantly influence and regulate a breath alcohol test program. Forensic personnel developing a quality control program must consider each of these legal elements along with discussion from legal experts.

One of the most important legislative elements is the definition of the drunk driving offense as driving a motor vehicle while having 0.08 g/210 L or more. This *per se* language clearly defines the offense while imposing strong legislative weight on the numerical results. Moreover, most jurisdictions have additional *per se* limits established in law such as 0.02 g/210 L for minors, 0.04 g/210 L for commercial drivers, and 0.15 g/210 L for enhanced penalties. Whether it can be shown that the individual exceeds each of these unique limits will largely depend on the quality control built into the analytical program. More specifically, the uncertainty surrounding each of these *per se* limits will be critical for the jury and/or judge to consider. Moreover, the law, administrative rules, or local case law will further define: the units of measurement, the number of digits reported, the approved analytical equipment, the performance of control standards and their acceptable results, the performance of duplicate testing along with required agreement, the training and qualification of personnel, legal admissibility of analytical results, the requirement to be in compliance with program policy (SOP), etc. Finally, a strong quality control program must be in full compliance with and in support of the legal context of the relevant jurisdiction.

7.2 Essential Components for Program Operation

7.2.1 Program Accreditation

A quality characteristic that is given significant weight by customers is program accreditation. This affiliation sets a program on a somewhat elite level in the mind of those using and interpreting our measurement results. While most end-users of our results are not aware of what is involved in accreditation, the accomplishment seems generally quite impressive. Accreditation granted by a reputable organization is basically the assurance that a program (and/or individual) has demonstrated a basic level of quality assurance in providing an analytical product that is fit-for-purpose and meets the needs of customers.

Most forensic breath test programs will seek accreditation through ASCLD Lab-International, which has adopted ISO/IEC 17025 (ISO 2005). A supplemental document published in 2007 is specific to breath alcohol test programs (ASCLD 2007, 2013). It is important that the requirements of ISO/IEC 17025 be initially complied with and then followed by the ASCLD/LAB 2007 document considered supplementary. Both documents must be used in association. The general requirements for such accreditation include in part: (a) record keeping, (b) program audits, (c) management reviews, (d) competency tests for personnel, (e) measurement traceability, (f) measurement uncertainty, and (g) reporting of results. Professional accreditation is such an important feature of a quality breath test program and should be pursued with diligence as a major objective.

In addition to program accreditation, there exist organizations that will certify or credential individual personnel. Such recognition will imply a high level of professionalism and expertise. These organizations may or may not be forensically oriented. A list of organizations and credentials offered to laboratory scientists and supervisors can be found on the web (Dilulio 2006). Forensic scientists and supervisors should pursue the credentialing of program personal. This can be added to their CVs and also presented in court to enhance their expertise. Personnel graduating from college in the laboratory sciences should pursue credentialing as part of their degree programs.

7.2.2 Measurement Uncertainty

One of the most important elements in developing a program's quality control is the determination and reporting of measurement uncertainty. "A measurement result is complete only when accompanied by a quantitative statement of its uncertainty. The uncertainty is required in order to decide if the result is adequate for its intended purpose and to ascertain if it is consistent with other similar results" (Taylor and Kuyatt 1994). Forensic measurements are used for making critical decisions in a legal context. Measurement uncertainty helps to evaluate the risk of making an incorrect decision. Measurement results accompanied by their uncertainty allow a jury to weigh the evidence presented as an analytical result. Measurement uncertainty largely determines the weight given to measurement results.

All measurements possess uncertainty regardless of their context (Horwitz 2003). The reality of uncertainty derives from limitations in our technology as well as our imperfect procedures. Quantitative measurement uncertainty is defined as: an interval symmetric about a measurement result which includes the true measurement objective (the measurand) with a high level of probability. Figure 7.1 illustrates this concept of quantitative measurement uncertainty expressed as a confidence interval.

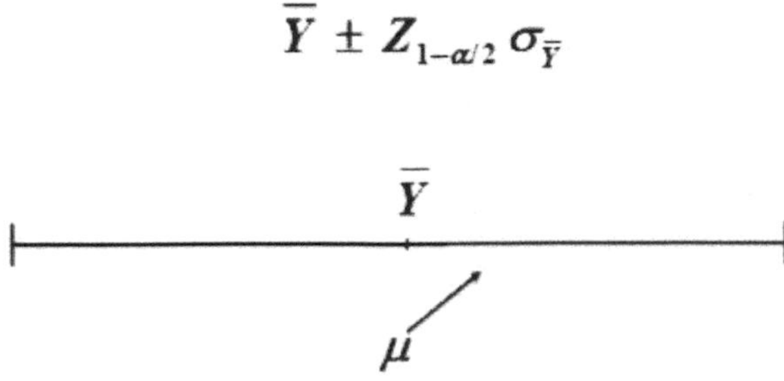

Figure 7.1 A confidence interval that is symmetric about a measurement result and within which the true measurement property (μ or population mean) will exist with a high level of probability.

The value of $\bar{Y}$ in Figure 7.1 represents the single or mean of replicate measurement results. The value of Z represents a coverage factor determined from a table of the Standard Normal Distribution. A value of $Z = 1.96$ will provide a 95% confidence interval while $Z = 2.57$ will provide a 99% confidence interval. The value of $\sigma_{\bar{Y}}$ represents the standard deviation of the $\bar{Y}$ value. Finally, μ represents the measurand, the true population mean.

Three principle elements have recently focused our attention on the issue of measurement uncertainty in forensic toxicology. These include:

- The National Research Council report of 2009 *Strengthening Forensic Science in the United States: A Path Forward* (US National Research Council 2009). The report stated: "All results for every forensic science method should indicate the uncertainty in the measurements that are made...."
- The US Supreme Court decision *Daubert vs Merrill Dow Pharmaceuticals* (Daubert 1993) which stated that one of its criteria for admissibility of scientific evidence was "...the technique's known or potential rate of error...."
- requirement for Accreditation under *ASCLD/LAB International* (ASCLD 2007): "...estimating uncertainty of measurement for all reported 'measurements that matter.'"

Measurement uncertainty is synonymous with measurement variation. The larger the variation the larger the uncertainty. The standard deviation quantifies variation and uncertainty. A large standard deviation means large variation. The more desirable small standard deviation means a smaller uncertainty. While there are several approaches to the estimation of measurement uncertainty (Kacker et al. 2007), we intend to focus on the commonly employed method of the root sum of squares (RSS). This determines the coefficient of variation for each included term, squares them and adds them for a combined estimate. This method will make the assumptions that the measurement function is multiplicative and all elements are independent. Our computation of measurement uncertainty will follow that outlined in the international metrology document: *Guide to the Expression of Uncertainty in Measurement (GUM)* (Bureau International des Poids et Mesures 2008). While there are several approaches to estimating measurement uncertainty, the *GUM* document, referred to as "the bottom-up approach," is widely recognized and endorsed by international metrology organizations. The basic procedure is to identify all components that contribute to uncertainty and combine them mathematically (RSS), yielding a combined uncertainty (i.e., standard deviation). The resulting combined uncertainty is a quantitative measure of variation and is represented by the $\sigma_{\bar{Y}}$ observed in Figure 7.1. Equation 7.1 shows the four principle components that influence uncertainty in breath alcohol analysis:

$$u_c = \bar{Y}\sqrt{\left[\frac{\frac{u_{Sampling}}{\sqrt{n_{Breath}}}}{\bar{Y}}\right]^2 + \left[\frac{\frac{u_{Analytical}}{\sqrt{n_{Analytical}}}}{\bar{X}}\right]^2 + \left[\frac{\frac{u_{Ref}}{\sqrt{n_{Ref}}}}{\overline{Ref}}\right]^2 + \left[\frac{\frac{Bias}{\sqrt{3}}}{\overline{Ref}}\right]^2} \tag{7.1}$$

where u_c (i.e., $\sigma_{\bar{Y}}$) is the combined uncertainty; $\bar{Y}$ is the mean breath alcohol result; $u_{Sampling}$ is the uncertainty due to the breath sampling component; n_{Breath} is the number of breath samples obtained (n = 2); $\overline{X}$ is the mean of the replicate control standard results; $u_{Analytical}$ is the analytical component of uncertainty; $n_{Analytical}$ is the number of measurements performed on the certified reference material (CRM); u_{Ref} is the uncertainty for the CRM found on the certificate of analysis; $\overline{Ref}$ is the mean of the assigned reference value; n_{Ref} is the number of measurements performed by the manufacturer of the CRM; Bias is the maximum observed bias when measuring the CRM.

Equation 7.1 is simply summing the components of variation by what is called the root sum of squares (RSS). Employing Equation 7.1 we have made the following assumptions:

- All measurement results are random and normally distributed
- All measurement results are independent
- The computed confidence intervals will bracket the true population parameter (i.e., mean or difference) with 95% probability
- The measurement function is multiplicative

If the measurement function were additive we would have added the variances of each term in a RSS calculation. If the measurement function were a mixture of multiplicative and additive terms then we would need to employ the method of error propagation derived from the Taylor series (Ku 1966). We estimate the uncertainty by first identifying the four terms in Equation 7.1. The first term (the sampling component) represents the variation contributed by the repeated measurement of the breath alcohol concentration (BrAC). The individual provides two independent breath samples approximately three minutes apart. This variation is determined from the development of an "uncertainty function" observed in Figure 7.2 (Thompson and Wood 2006). The uncertainty function in Figure 7.2 was determined from a set of duplicate data obtained from the Washington State Patrol breath alcohol test program.

The uncertainty function in Figure 7.2 is developed from n = 28,321 duplicate breath test results in Washington State during 2013. The equation observed in Figure 7.2 is a least-squares linear equation fit to the data. The data used for this analysis includes

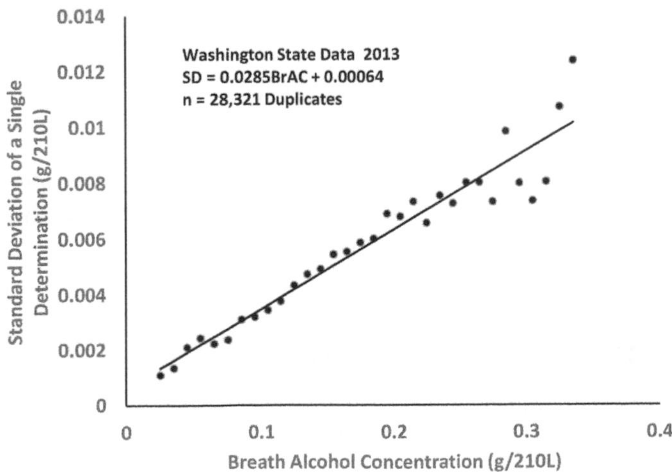

Figure 7.2 The uncertainty function for duplicate breath alcohol data obtained from the State of Washington during 2013.

even those duplicates which did not comply with the agreement standard in Washington State. The required agreement for admissible test results is that both measurements must be within ±10% of their mean. The data used to generate the uncertainty function in Figure 7.2 included some duplicates that did not comply with this required agreement. This was done in order to obtain an upper limit for the estimated variation. The equation of Figure 7.2 now provides a model with which to compute the first term ($u_{Sampling}$) in Equation 7.1. The points represent the variation (standard deviations) determined from the duplicate BrAC results. Each point is the standard deviation determined from all duplicate results having a mean result within a 0.010 g/210 L interval. The standard deviation is computed from:

$$SD = \sqrt{\frac{\sum_{i=1}^{k} d_i^2}{2k}} \tag{7.2}$$

where d is the duplicate test difference; k is the number of individual duplicate results within the concentration interval.

The uncertainty function in Figure 7.2 represents the variation associated with several components including: pre-analytical breathing pattern of the individual, exhalation pattern including flow rate and volume, analytical variation in the breath test instrument, over 28,000 individuals, 200 instruments statewide in different locations, over 3,000 police officer operators and approximately one year of time. All of these components ensure a large and conservative estimate of the uncertainty associated with the forensic analysis of breath alcohol concentration. From Figure 7.2 we clearly see that the variation is a linear function of concentration.

We now compute the combined uncertainty estimate for the four sources observed in Equation 7.1. We further assume the individual has provided a mean (n = 2) breath alcohol result of 0.080 g/210 L. The calculation first employs the equation for the uncertainty function of Equation 7.3 and observed in Figure 7.2. From Equation 7.3 we determine the standard deviation to be 0.00292 g/210 L for the sampling component.

$$u_{Sampling} = 0.0285(0.080) + 0.00064 = 0.00292\,g/210L \tag{7.3}$$

We now incorporate the uncertainty estimates for the remaining three terms in Equation 7.1 and obtain Equation 7.4. We have included reasonable estimates for the three remaining terms simply to illustrate the calculations involved.

$$u_c = 0.080\sqrt{\left[\frac{\frac{0.00292}{\sqrt{2}}}{0.080}\right]^2 + \left[\frac{\frac{0.0008}{\sqrt{10}}}{0.080}\right]^2 + \left[\frac{\frac{0.0006}{\sqrt{2}}}{0.080}\right]^2 + \left[\frac{\frac{0.004}{\sqrt{3}}}{0.080}\right]^2} = 0.00314\text{ g/210 L} \tag{7.4}$$

$$95\%\text{ Confidence Interval}: 0.080 \pm 1.96\,(0.00314) \Rightarrow 0.074\text{ to }0.086\text{ g/210 L}$$

The sample size of n = 10 for the second term in Equation 7.4 is simply illustrative of the number of measurements performed on the control standard in the field. There will be one or two control standard measurements performed with each individual administered the complete breath alcohol test. For the third term in Equation 7.4 we use the sample size of n = 2. Since we do not know exactly how many measurements were performed by the manufacturer of the reference control material, using n = 2 is the most conservative. For the fourth term in Equation 7.4 we assume the maximum observed bias when measuring the reference control material is 0.004 g/210 L. Although in our example of Equation 7.4 we have not corrected for the bias, this is possible to do if desired and is also a recommendation of the GUM document (Bureau International des Poids et Mesures 2008). Since we have not corrected for bias we include the uncertainty component observed as the fourth term in Equation 7.4. We further assume that all measurements were made at or near 0.080 g/210 L. Moreover, we are allowing some "double counting" of the uncertainty by including the second term in Equation 7.4. The second term is the analytical component which is already included in the first term—the sampling component. The duplicate measurements of breath include the analytical as well as all of the other components of variation noted above. Finally, we observe our 95% confidence interval to be 0.074 to 0.086 g/210 L. We conclude that we have bracketed the true population mean BrAC (μ) with 95% probability. This 95% confidence interval should now be reported along with the individual's duplicate BrAC results, each reported to three digits. Moreover, the modern computerized breath alcohol test instruments would be capable of printing this confidence interval on their printout documents. Vendors should be pressed to provide this feature. The software could be updated annually when new uncertainty functions are generated. This would avoid the need to perform these computations external to the instrument. The measurement results along with their confidence interval should also be accompanied by a textual statement regarding the explanation and interpretation of the results. Such an example is as follows:

> The mean measurement result was 0.0800 g/210 L (n = 2) with an expanded combined uncertainty of 0.00615 g/210 L assuming k = 1.96 and a normal distribution. An approximate 95% confidence interval for the true mean breath alcohol result is 0.0739 to 0.0862 g/210 L.

This could also be printed on the document at the time of the test.

As noted earlier, there are several ways to determine measurement uncertainty found in the metrology and analytical literature (Kacker et al. 2007). We have illustrated only one of those many possibilities. Program administrators need to determine the best approach for their unique programs while including input from colleagues and share holders. The approach selected must then be thoroughly outlined in their program SOP to allow for transparency and full disclosure. In addition, it is very important for the forensic toxicologist to acknowledge and testify to the reality and computation of measurement uncertainty. Being transparent regarding measurement uncertainty will only serve to enhance the integrity of the program.

As noted earlier, the model developed in Figure 7.2 shows a strong linear relation between variation and concentration. Higher breath alcohol concentrations tend to have larger differences between the duplicates. As a result, the duplicate test agreement criteria should account for this. Many jurisdictions require the agreement to be <0.02 g/210 L.

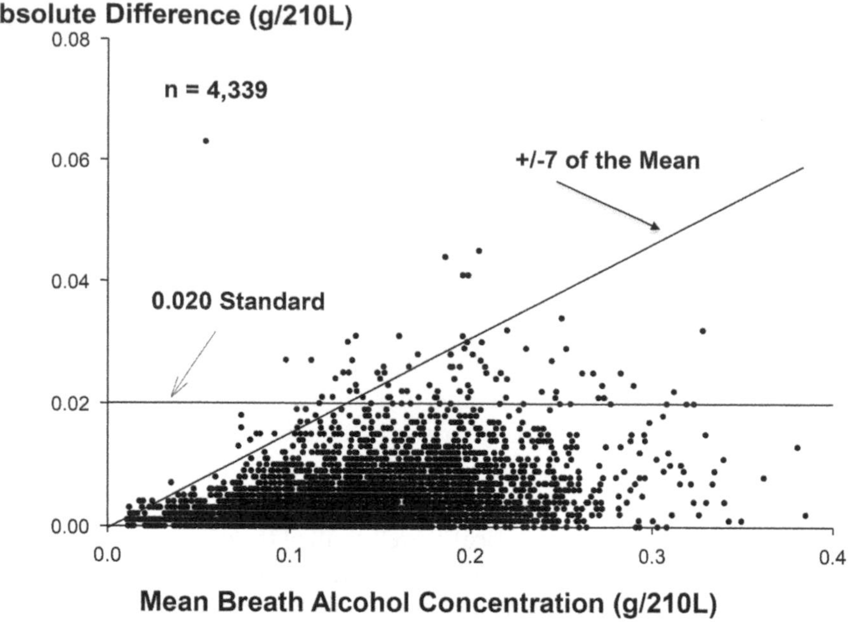

Figure 7.3 Plot of the absolute difference of duplicate tests against their mean. The increasing variation with concentration is clearly evident.

Having a constant like this would allow for many duplicate test results at higher concentration to be rejected. A better agreement criteria would be one that requires the two results to be within a specific proportion. This would allow a larger absolute difference as a function of concentration. For example, the two results could be required to agree within ±7% of their mean. Figure 7.3 shows the plot of absolute differences against their mean. This also reveals the increasing variation with concentration. We also see that the 0.020 criteria rejects many tests at higher concentrations. The ±7% criteria account for the increasing variation with concentration. A standard based on proportions seems to treat the data more objectively, allows for the reality of biological/sampling variation and provides better confidence. Moreover, there must be continual monitoring of all critical analytical systems within the instrument. When a critical tolerance or value setting is not correct (i.e., voltage settings, breath sample acceptance parameters, pre-sampling observation time, software check sum integrity, etc.), the test should be aborted and a record of the event preserved in memory. The operator would now be required to reinitiate the entire test protocol. Such error detection systems would be necessary to ensure analytical quality control.

An useful result of uncertainty estimation is the development of an uncertainty budget (Kristiansen and Petersen 2004). This identifies the percent of total uncertainty contributed by each component. In Table 7.1 we identify the proportion of total uncertainty contributed by each of the four components observed in Equation 7.4.

From Table 7.1 we see that the bias term contributes the most to total uncertainty. Part of this is due to how we selected the calculation of the bias contribution. As noted earlier there are several ways to deal with bias in measurement uncertainty. We chose a very conservative approach which assumes a rectangular distribution for the bias value.

Table 7.1 Proportion of Total Uncertainty Contributed by Four Components Observed in Equation 7.4

Component	Percent (%)
Breath sampling	38
Analytical	1
Reference standard	2
Bias	59
Total	100

Other methods of accounting for bias could have yielded a smaller proportion. Moreover, international metrological authorities have stated that those components that contribute less than one-third of the largest contributor may be eliminated (Ellison and Williams 2012). This would support our eliminating of the analytical and reference standard components in Table 7.1 from the total calculation. Given the forensic context of these results, we may be better served by continuing to include all of the terms. We have discussed here only a few examples for computing measurement uncertainty. Many other methods exist (Wallace 2010). These should be considered by program personnel in selecting the methods best suited to their individual program.

7.2.3 Proficiency Testing

Regular participation in a proficiency test program is one of the most important elements of quality control for a breath test program. Proficiency test participation is a way to ensure the analytical characteristics (i.e., accuracy and precision) of the program are of high quality and fit-for-purpose. Ideally, the analysis of breath samples should yield the same results across all methods, instruments, and program. This is the concept of comparability expressed as "Tested once, accepted everywhere" (Ellison et al. 2003). Participating in a proficiency test program allows for comparison among programs and the quantifying of measurement variation while enhancing confidence and quality control.

Proficiency testing, or inter-laboratory testing, has a long history in the analytical sciences (Sunderman 1992). The main objective is to allow for comparison between programs and also to study the variation across different methods all measuring the same material. Instrumentation, protocols and statistical methods have all advanced over the years and have added significant value to measurement results. There is a wide range of computational detail to which proficiency test results can be subjected. Some protocols and analysis are very basic while others compute a large number of performance criteria. The following is a suggested protocol and example set of analyses that would be very informative when evaluating program quality:

- Select the programs that will participate. Each should be an accredited forensic program.
- The coordinating program or source of the homogeneous reference material should prepare at least two reference materials (either gas standards or simulator

solutions) of different concentrations. The reference value of each material should be determined by some authoritative method such as headspace gas chromatography. Record the number of measurements, the mean, the standard deviation, and the uncertainty of the reference value.

- Dispense the reference material into containers marked with a coded value.
- Distribute the reference material containers to the participating programs in such a manner that the mode of transportation/delivery does not compromise the reference concentration value. In addition, deliver the materials along with a detailed protocol to be followed and data to be recorded by the participating program. Employ a standard data entry form for all participants.
- Each participating program should perform the same number of measurements (i.e., n = 10). The participants should note how the samples are introduced into the instrument (i.e., through the breath tube or through some other port). The participating program should record each of the replicate measurements to three decimal places along with the mean and standard deviation on a data entry form provided.
- Establish a date by which the results are to be returned to the coordinating program.
- The coordinating program should compute and plot the Q-Scores by two methods:

$$Q = \left[\frac{\overline{X}_i - R}{R}\right] \qquad Q = \left[\frac{\overline{X}_i - \overline{\overline{X}}_{Cons}}{\overline{\overline{X}}_{Cons}}\right] \tag{7.5}$$

where $\overline{X}_i$ is the mean result for the ith program; R is the reference value determined by the coordinating program; $\overline{\overline{X}}_{Cons}$ is the consensus mean value.

The results from Equation 7.5 are bias estimates. They could be multiplied by 100 to yield percent bias estimates. The consensus mean value is simply the mean of all the mean results from all participating labs. It should be an unbiased estimate of the reference value (R).

- Compute and plot Z scores:

$$Z = \left[\frac{\overline{X}_i - R}{\sigma}\right] \tag{7.6}$$

where σ is the fit-for-purpose or expected standard deviation that each program should obtain.

- Look for outliers (these need to be acknowledged in summary reports) and assess for normality employing, for example, QQ Plots (available in Microsoft Excel).
- The participating programs should not correct for bias in order to allow the coordinating program to determine between-program variability.

Incorporating these and other elements would result in a much more robust proficiency test program (Gullberg and Logan 2006).

Table 7.2 Hypothetical Results of Ten Participating Breath Test Programs

Program	Mean	SD[a]	n	Z Score
1	0.0782	0.0012	10	−1.8
2	0.0815	0.0014	10	1.5
3	0.0834	0.0008	10	3.4
4	0.0812	0.0008	10	1.2
5	0.0789	0.0009	10	−1.1
6	0.0780	0.0016	10	−2.0
7	0.0819	0.0014	10	1.9
8	0.0820	0.0008	10	2.0
9	0.0811	0.0014	10	1.1
10	0.0787	0.0007	10	−1.3

[a] Standard deviation.

The following is an illustration of a very basic analysis of results from a proficiency test. Table 7.2 shows the hypothetical results for ten participating breath test programs. Note that our mean is reported to four decimal places. This is one more than the three digit data values. The mean is more confident than the individual measurements. Each program was sent a 500 mL aliquot of the same simulator solution having a traceable reference value of 0.080 g/210 L. They were instructed to perform n = 10 measurements using one of their field evidential breath test instruments. Equation 7.6 was used to compute the Z score where the fit-for-purpose standard deviation (σ) is set to be 0.0010 g/210 L. One of the limitations of proficiency testing in forensic programs is that the measurements are not conducted "blind." It is hard to avoid knowing that the measurements are on standards known to have been received by a proficiency test organizer.

Figure 7.4 plots the Z score results where we see that all but program 3 had acceptable results within ±2 Z scores. Two Z scores are generally accepted in proficiency test programs. Programs with results between 2 and 3 Z scores should give attention to their analytical results. Z scores greater than 3 are considered unacceptable. Z score results can also be plotted in the format of Figure 7.5.

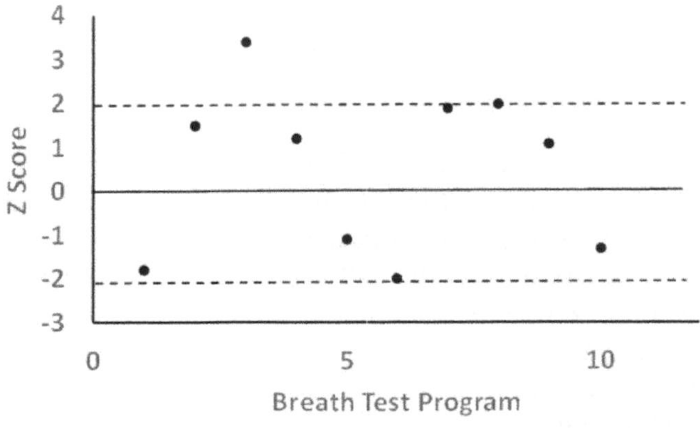

Figure 7.4 Plot of Z scores for the ten hypothetical breath test programs.

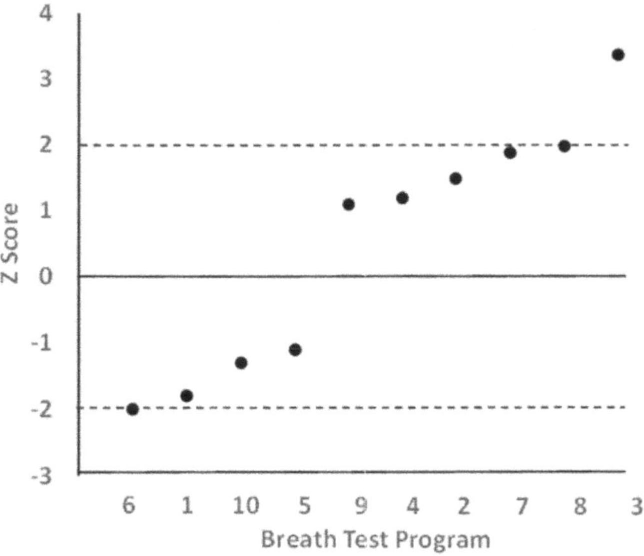

Figure 7.5 Sequential Plot of Z scores from smallest to largest for the hypothetical breath test program.

Ideally, the organizing program of the proficiency tests will have a traceable reference value (R in Equation 7.6) (Heydorn 2006; Kuselman 2006). If this is not available, then a consensus mean ($\overline{X}_{cons}$ in Equation 7.5) can be used which would be the mean of all program mean results and its uncertainty would be $\frac{\hat{\sigma}}{\sqrt{n}}$. Repeatability and reproducibility estimates can also be made with the results in Table 7.2. The bias determined from a consensus value would have greater uncertainty than a traceable reference value. The repeatability is the within program variation and is determined from the pooled variance of each program's standard deviation estimate. This is shown in Equation 7.7:

$$\hat{\sigma}_{repeatability} = \sqrt{\frac{\sum_{i=1}^{10}(n_i - 1)\sigma_i^2}{\sum_{i=1}^{10}(n_i - 1)}} = 0.00115\,g/210L \tag{7.7}$$

Equation 7.7 is simply a weighted estimate of the sample variance. Reproducibility is the between program variation and is estimated simply by finding the standard deviation of the n = 10 mean program results. This results in $\hat{\sigma}_{reproducibility} = 0.00188\,g/210L$. As expected the between-program variation (reproducibility) is larger than the within-program variation (repeatability). These Z score results should be made available to each programs set of customers (including accreditation bodies) so some evaluation of program fitness-for-purpose and analytical quality control can be evaluated.

We have focused on the Z score as a proficiency index. Another index suggested by some (Castelazo and Mitani 2012) is the Mean Squared Error (MSE) determined from:

$$MSE_{PT} = \overline{bias}^2 + \hat{\sigma}_{lab}^2 \tag{7.8}$$

where $\overline{bias}$ is the mean of all bias estimates; $\hat{\sigma}_{lab}^2$ is the between lab variance estimate.

From the MSE we now find the proficiency index R according to:

$$R = \frac{\sqrt{\overline{bias}^2 + \hat{\sigma}_{lab}^2}}{\sigma} \tag{7.9}$$

where σ is the fit-for-purpose or expected standard deviation as in the Z score.

Small values of R indicate better performance. The advantage of R over the Z score is that both bias and measurement variation are included in a single parameter. Another proficiency test index that incorporates the uncertainty is:

$$E_n = \frac{X_{lab} - X_{Reference}}{\sqrt{u_{lab}^2 + u_{Reference}^2}} \tag{7.10}$$

where X_{lab} and $X_{Reference}$ are the mean results for an individual lab and the Reference value; u_{lab}^2 and $u_{Reference}^2$ are the uncertainty (standard deviation) estimates for the individual lab and Reference value, respectively.

E_n values less than one are considered acceptable.

Participation in a proficiency test program is recommended at least annually and should be so stated in the program's SOP manual. Individual laboratories can coordinate the program by providing the samples and doing the data analysis to be reported back to the participants. On the other hand, organizations such as Collaborative Testing Services, Inc. (Collaborative Testing Services) and the College of American Pathologists are set up to be the coordinating agency and will provide their services and test materials. Their data is also available on the CTS web site for their materials which is convenient for further analysis. Moreover, they have correctly reported their Grand Mean and Standard Deviation estimates to four decimal places. In summary, participation in proficiency test programs is very important and adds significant value to a breath test program desiring to present measurement results of high quality and integrity. Further detail on developing a proficiency test program can be found elsewhere (ASTM guide 1973; Thompson and Wood 1993; ISO/IEC Guide 43-1 1997). Finally, a program could develop internal proficiency or audit testing for their personnel by providing control standards with unknown concentrations and having personnel perform calibration/quality assurance procedures.

7.2.4 The Breath Alcohol Test Protocol

The protocol employed in measuring an individual's breath alcohol is probably the most obvious and familiar to the customers of a breath test program. The program integrity and confidence is strongly dependent upon the breath test protocol and its associated printout document. This piece of evidence is highly probative and should be developed with careful thought and discussion. Moreover, it is important to keep in mind that this is a "forensic breath alcohol measurement," which sets it significantly apart from a routine clinical measurement.

Modern computerized breath test instruments will all produce a printout of the test results. Included in this printout are all of the critical steps that the instrument and operator accomplish. The order and clarity of this information and its relationship to the legal requirements is very important. The printout and the protocol it represents are critical to the legal admissibility of the test results along with a reflection of the program's overall quality control. For many program customers (juries, attorneys, judges, hearing officers, etc.) the printout document is the only piece of evidence observed from the program. Careful attention needs to be given to its contents and organization. Program customers should be thoughtfully involved in the development of this document. The advantage of a computer-controlled instrument is the ability to control this information regarding its order and detail. Moreover, a computer controlled instrument ensures a pre-designed protocol is followed, greatly reducing the operator involvement and risk of error.

A designed protocol for breath alcohol measurement should be given considerable attention and thought. Program customers should be involved as well for their input. Protocol development needs to consider the statutes and administrative rules governing the program, relevant case law, capabilities of the instrument, training level of personnel, and additional quality control objectives of the program. The following is a protocol proposal for the forensic measurement of breath alcohol:

- **At least a 15-minute pre-test observation period**: This ensures that any residual alcohol within the mouth will be eliminated and avoid biasing the result. A single key on the instrument should be pressed when the mouth check has occurred which in turn records the time and saves it to memory. This will subsequently appear on the test document. This avoids the issue of "terminal digit preference" which occurs when operators record the time themselves.
- **Data entry**: There should be pre-designed questions requiring the operator to respond in a determined format. Sufficient time should be allowed for data entry. Considerable thought should be given to the data entry questions and allowed responses. This is also where research interests of the program or customer personnel can be considered.
- **Blank test**: Here the instrument can purge its sample chamber, obtain a zero output signal and prepare for the next test. If the instrument is unable to perform this step an error message should appear and the test should be automatically aborted.
- **Internal Standard Check**: An electronic or physical internal standard (i.e., a quartz plate) can be tested with a required signal response.
- **Blank test**: Another blank test can be performed to ensure the output signal is zero in preparation for the next test. All of the blank tests ensure there is no carryover effect.
- **First Breath Sample Provision**: The individual is allowed to provide a breath sample at this time and there should be sufficient time to allow for this. The instrument should employ sampling criteria such as: minimum volume of 1.5 L, a minimum flow rate of, for example, 4 L/minute and a maximum allowed plateau for the breath alcohol exhalation curve. The sampling criteria may also be a form of "intelligent measurement." In other words, the sampling criteria could be programmed to depend on the subject's age, gender, weight, height, health, etc. For infrared instruments, the exhalation curve is a continuous signal output from the detector. Some fuel cell instruments have an infrared detector as

well, designed to monitor the exhalation curve and determine sampling criteria. When the sampling parameters are met the instrument analyzes the alcohol in the sample chamber and records the results. No result should be displayed, to avoid influencing the individual's further cooperation. During breath sampling the operator should continue to coach the individual by giving clear instructions, encouraging the individual to provide a full end-expiratory sample. This will also help ensure good agreement between the duplicate results. The full analytical procedure for the analysis of one individual is considered a "run" in breath alcohol analysis.

- **Blank test:** The sample chamber is purged and the output signal is zero.
- **External Control Standard:** An external control standard consisting of a simulator solution or gas standard is automatically sampled and analyzed by the instrument. This result must meet the predesigned requirements such as from 0.072 to 0.088 g/210 L for a 0.080 g/210 L standard. Or, the control limits could be determined from subsample means developed for X-bar control charts. If the result is not correct the test is aborted. These control standards can be regulated in a number of ways: only a specific number of tests allowed, only a set time period allowed, a concentration defined requirement to change standards, etc. If the standard measurement is not correct then no further tests should be allowed until the technician responds and evaluates the instruments proper working order. This avoids the bad practice of continual testing until the result is correct. Moreover, it would be useful to have different control standard concentrations over time. This would allow for evaluating bias at different concentrations. The required result could be programmed as a function of concentration (i.e., ±8%).
- **Blank test:** The sample chamber is purged and the output signal is zero.
- **Second Breath Sample Provision:** Apply the same criteria here as for the First Breath Sample above. When the sampling criteria are met, the instrument should automatically determine the agreement with the first sample. The required agreement between the two results must be pre-determined and encoded within the software. One suggestion for an acceptable agreement is that the two results both lie within ±7% of the mean of the two results. This would allow for a larger absolute difference at higher concentrations which occurs in breath alcohol analysis. Figure 7.3 shows a plot of absolute duplicate test differences against their mean along with approximate lines for a relative difference of ±7% and an absolute difference of 0.020 g/210 L. Such analysis and documentation should be part of program development to justify the selection of a specific test agreement value. If the two results do not agree, then the test should be aborted and a message indicating this to the operator. If the results are in agreement, then the result should again not be displayed.
- **Blank test:** The sample chamber is purged and the output signal is zero.
- **External Control Standard:** A second control standard measurement is performed with the same acceptance criteria as noted above. This control material may even be at a different concentration than the first control standard. One may be at a lower concentration (i.e., 0.080 g/210 L) while the second could be at a higher concentration (i.e., 0.200 g/210 L). This would provide increased confidence of accuracy at both relevant concentrations. Having duplicate breath alcohol results and duplicate external standard results also allows for the estimation of components of variance, comparing the breath to analytical sampling.

- **Blank test:** The sample chamber is purged and the output signal is zero. This is the final purge and blank test.
- **Printout Document:** The printout document should also contain the date, the individual's name and date of birth, the serial number of the instrument and the operator's signature and agency. Each of these identified steps will have criteria that must be met in order to conclude a fully valid and reliable test result has been produced. The breath test results are only shown on the printout document. Indeed, it is not assumed that every subject tested on the instrument will yield a fully valid test result. If every subject tested has a fully valid test, there would be some skepticism about the system's reliability. There should be some small percentage (i.e., 5%) of test results that do not meet all of the designed requirements. In these cases no printout should be produced and a record of test failure should be preserved for transfer to a host computer. The fact that some percentage of tests do not meet all of the required criteria yields confidence regarding system integrity and control. If all pre-determined analytical criteria have been met then the printout document can be generated. There should be enough copies for the individual, the operator and the prosecutor. All steps of the full test procedure should be retained in the memory of the instrument and downloaded to the host computer on a regular schedule. All analytical results on the document and in memory should include three digit results. If the agency so desires, the lowest of the two results could be truncated to two decimal places and indicated on the printout that this is the level for prosecution. Retaining the three digits on the document and in memory allows for a more thorough statistical analysis and full disclosure of the measurement results. The instrument could also have the capability of generating the measurement uncertainty and printing the 95% confidence interval on the document. If this is done, there should be some text that explains clearly the interpretation and meaning of measurement uncertainty. This explanation on the printout document might include, for example:

  The mean breath alcohol result was 0.0802 g/210 L (n = 2) with an expanded combined uncertainty of 0.0048 g/210 L assuming k = 2 and a normal distribution. An approximate 95% confidence interval for the true mean breath alcohol result is 0.0754 to 0.0850 g/210 L

This would in turn provide full disclosure and allow the prosecutor to determine more quickly if prosecution should be pursued. In addition, there should be the capability within the instrument or in the host computer to generate an additional printout document, should the original copies be lost. This feature should be provided for at any subsequent time. All of the features discussed here and others, regarding the breath test procedure, should be designed to achieve maximum quality control and confidence in the measurement results (Dubowski, 1960, 1994).

Any aborted test should provide a clear notification to the operator and require the entire test procedure to be accomplished again.

7.2.5 Program Personnel and Their Training

Critical to a robust breath alcohol test program and its integrity is the quality and expertise of its personnel. These individuals continually reflect the program to its customers, conveying its quality and integrity. These program personnel must be professionals, committed to the highest work ethic and integrity, always learning, and pursuing program improvement. Having such a reputation will greatly enhance the program's credibility and trust. Customer trust and loyalty will be the result of a program designed around transparency, integrity and professionalism. No case or measurement result is worth losing such valuable quality characteristics and reputation.

Every forensic breath test program will be designed differently. Each jurisdiction has its unique laws, administrative rules, case law, legal structure, facility and geographical limitations, agency design, political differences, etc. All of these must be considered in designing the responsibilities of program and personnel. Program personnel and their responsibilities might include, for example:

- **Instrument operators:** These may include police officers or individuals trained specifically for the purpose of operating the instruments and measuring the breath alcohol concentration.
- **Instrument technicians:** These individuals should first be trained as instrument operators and then also as instrument technicians. Their responsibility could include the annual calibration/certification of the instruments. They would also be responsible for repair of the instruments. In addition, they could be responsible for installing control standards (simulators or gas standards) on the field instruments at periodic times.
- **Instructors:** These individuals should first be instrument operators. They may or may not also be instrument technicians.
- **Supervisors:** These individuals should ideally be trained as operators, instructors and technicians. Such knowledge and background will allow them to supervise more directly and efficiently.
- **Administrators:** These are program directors who have authority to develop policy and write administrative rules. Ideally they would be trained at all levels of the program personnel.

Some programs may also choose to include laboratory scientists (i.e., toxicologists) who would be responsible for the preparation and testing of simulator solutions. The qualifications, training, responsibilities, and job description of each of the personnel listed above should be clearly and thoroughly documented in the program's SOP manual. Outlines and handouts for the training of these individuals should also be available on the program web site. Training needs to be directed toward the specific responsibilities of each individual. Exams and other performance measuring procedures should be retained by each individual's supervisor in a documentation book. Permits and certificates should be presented at the completion of the pre-designed training program which should then be made available on the web site to document the training program and qualifications. In addition, each member of the program should prepare and maintain a curricula vitae, which should also be on the program web site. Research and publication should be encouraged among all program personnel with the results being added to the CV. Personnel should also be encouraged to join and attend meetings of professional organizations. Finally, program administrators and supervisors should have full-time responsibilities and assignment within the breath test program.

7.3 Additional Components Helpful to Program Operation

7.3.1 Developing a Program Web Site

We live and work in a society with almost an unlimited amount of information. The challenge is to be able to obtain and use the relevant and reliable information and discard the unnecessary. Part of the challenge is the speed with which information (reliable or not) can be transferred from one individual to another. The internet has become the most widely used medium for this transfer and storage of information. Our forensic programs should take advantage of this important tool in order to better inform our customers with reliable information. At the heart of developing an useful web site is choosing what records to retain. Careful consideration needs to be applied here so that program records are relevant, useful and transparent to both customers and program personnel.

Forensic personnel understand very clearly the demands that defense counsel can make in preparation for trial or civil hearings. A long list of discovery requests are very common as defense attorneys prepare their case for court. Moreover, much of the requested material has already been provided to the same attorneys in previous cases. Complying with these requests can occupy the full-time effort of a secretarial staff. In addition to defense attorneys, there are many others who request and use material that we alone possess in our forensic breath test programs. We now want to discuss the elements that should be included in a web based breath alcohol test program. The information on the web site should be freely available to the entire public.

The following items are examples of material that should be incorporated and made available in a web-based program:

- **Contact information:** Phone numbers, email, address, hours, and names should all be easily accessed for the entire public to obtain.
- **Program personnel:** The names, titles, email, and hours of availability should be included for all program personnel. The CVs for all personnel should also be available. The CV should contain education, experience, publications, responsibilities, professional associations, credentials, etc.
- **Certificates of analysis (COA):** The COA should be available for all traceable control reference materials that are used in the program. This may include analytical records for the gas chromatograph (GC) where simulator solutions are prepared in house and traceability is developed through the GC.
- **Certification records:** Certificates should be available that indicate regular evaluation/calibration of equipment used in the program. This might include volt meters, traceable standardized thermometers, barometric pressure instruments, etc.
- **Records of calibration/certification:** Records of calibration and regular quality assurance regarding the breath test instruments must be available. These will show all measurement results at all concentrations along with information identifying the control materials used and their traceability. These records must also include the names of technicians performing the work along with dates and instrument serial numbers.
- **Repair and maintenance records:** Standardized forms must be prepared for all testing and maintenance procedures performed. Repair records must describe

the problems encountered, the diagnosis and repairs performed, dates, and time. Some of these may require re-calibration and quality assurance procedures before placing the instrument back in the field.

- **Breath test database:** For those programs that centrally collect data from the instruments, the data should be made readily available on the web site. Data should be easily available by typing in serial number and date frames. This data should not include names of subjects. While the rest seems readily discoverable, program managers may want to discuss inclusion and exclusion criteria with their legal counsel familiar with local case law and issues. The data should also be easily accessible for immediate transfer into software programs such as Microsoft Excel or other database management programs. Most will find this of great benefit when intending to do statistical analyses.
- **Program SOP manual:** All program policies and procedures should be incorporated into the SOP manual and made available on the web site. Dates that document revision and approval of policies must be clear. The SOP manual should contain all required policies, procedures and forms. The organizational chart should be included along with the classification of personnel and their job descriptions and regular assessment. Signatures of approval from program authorities must also be provided. The method for computing and reporting measurement uncertainty must also be included. Those programs obtaining or seeking accreditation should consult the accrediting agency regarding records and other information to be retained.
- **Training records:** Records of required training for personnel must be available. This should also include facsimiles of training certificates and/or permit cards for all program personnel. Training outlines and manuals that are approved by program authorities must also be available. This should not include, however, exams or scores obtained by program personnel. Training and classifications of personnel should also be defined in the program administrative rules and should be consulted when developing the web site.
- **Law and administrative rules:** The jurisdiction will likely have laws and administrative rules that legally define the program and its responsibilities. Copies of these should be made available or links could be provided to the jurisdiction's legal material that is typically available on the internet.
- **Published material/reports:** Where reports have been developed based on important experimental work, it would be useful to provided copies on the web site. This is particularly important where program personnel will frequently be testifying to this work. Selected peer reviewed publications could also be made available where it is particularly relevant to the program.
- **Tables of data and/or computations:** Any tables of data and/or computations that are used by the program personnel should be available. This might include temperature conversions, critical voltage calculations, water/air partition coefficients, statistical tables, measurement uncertainty calculations, Widmark calculations, etc.
- **Additional records to develop and preserve, including:** minutes of regular personnel meetings, program audit reports, test equipment calibration, instrument installation records, published research relevant to the program, corrections made to equipment and/or personnel along with corrective actions, record retention schedules etc.

Each breath test program is unique and defined locally by law, administrative rules, case law, equipment and program authorities. The items listed above are only examples to be considered by each program in view of their local considerations. Some programs may include several other items on their web site. Some items listed above may be unnecessary for some programs. Developing an useful web site will take a great deal of thought and discussion with key individuals. Moreover, when the web site is developed it will very likely require the management by a full-time individual. That individual will need to be responsible for polling the data from field instruments on a regular basis, adding/removing material from the web site, keeping it up to date and training people on how to use it properly. There will also be questions from the public that the web manager will need to address.

Developing a thorough and convenient web site will be well worth the effort. Besides saving a great deal of secretarial photocopying effort, program personnel and personnel from other jurisdictions will find it very helpful. Moreover, the web site makes the program more transparent. The integrity and quality control of the program will be enhanced through this effort in full disclosure.

7.3.2 Court Testimony

A breath test program's quality control and integrity is probably nowhere more evident than in the court testimony provided by its personnel. The admissibility of the breath test results in court is the final outcome of a long chain of pre-analytical, analytical, and post-analytical effort designed to produce high-quality, reliable, and probative measurement results. This is where the program customers are able to see and rely upon the best possible product we are able to produce. The clarity and integrity of the testimony of program personnel is critical to allow the judge or jury arrive at a complete and informed decision. Moreover, we are not saying that every test result will or should necessarily be admissible at trial. If there are issues that compromise the integrity of the results, then these results should not be admissible in a legal proceeding. A record of these failed tests should also be retained and available in view of providing full disclosure. There will indeed be some small proportion (i.e., 5%) of test results that are not acceptable and do not meet all of the criteria designed into the program. If every subject tested yielded results that met all acceptable criteria, there would, indeed should, be some question about the control limits of the program.

7.3.3 Program Research

Following the NAS report of 2009 (US National Research Council 2009) regarding deficiencies of the forensic sciences, there has been a flurry of critical publications. Most of these criticisms have been directed toward the pattern identification disciplines. Notably, these criticisms have not been directed toward forensic toxicology. This is largely due to the sound scientific foundation and research culture underlying forensic toxicology. This effort must continue with renewed effort and diligence.

Scientific research based on sound experimental design is the foundation on which our discipline can advance and acquire new knowledge. Some general elements that are foundational to good experimental design include:

- **Clear statement of the research question:** This is most commonly in the published introduction.
- **Informed/written consent:** This is absolutely necessary in human research studies.
- **Sample size:** Computing the appropriate sample size is necessary to avoid too few individuals and low power as well as too many individuals leading to a waste of resources. The appropriate size determined from published equations will be the most ethical.
- **Pre-determined statistical analysis:** This analysis must be appropriate to the study objectives. The response and predictor variables must be clearly defined. Analysis should include statistical hypothesis tests, effect size (Maher et al. 2013), and confidence intervals.
- **Identify the treatment and response variables:** Choose variables that are measurable and relevant to the research question. There may be primary and secondary end-points that must be identified in the design. Keep in mind that multivariate models are probably more representative of the real world than univariate models.
- **Identify the experimental units:** These are the units to which the treatments are applied.
- If the study is a randomized controlled trial (RCT) then explain how randomization was accomplished.
- Explain if double blinding was involved.
- Explain inclusion and exclusion criteria.
- Explain if study is a randomized controlled trial or an observational study. RCT allow for a causal inference while observational studies allow for association only. Some studies (i.e., the influence of alcohol on the risk of accident) would be unethical to perform as an RCT and can only be investigated through observational studies.

Finally, prior to publication authors must consult the journal's section on "Instruction for Authors" to be sure the format details are acceptable. This will help to obtain a positive review.

Experimentation can entail a number of different and unique characteristics. We have identified here only a few of the considerations necessary in designing an effective and meaningful study. Many excellent text books are available to help guide one through the process of skillful and relevant experimental design (Berger and Maurer 2002; Hicks 1973; Hulley and Cummings 1988; Box et al. 1978; Montgomery 1976). Studies should be designed with publication in view. For this reason, the journal's "Instructions for Authors" must be consulted and complied with. Publication provides the knowledge for the entire discipline and adds to everyone's enlightenment.

7.3.4 Analytical Evaluation

In addition to what we have discussed in some detail above, there are several tools available to evaluate other quality control aspects of a breath test program. For quality control to be effective, it must be measurable. All of these program features are designed and employed to avoid measurement error, either random of systematic, and thereby provide measurable quality. There will always be some non-zero probability of error—fallible humans and technology are involved at all levels. In view of this, our efforts must be directed to ensure our measurements are fit-for-purpose. Some additional considerations are shown below.

7.3.4.1 Method Validation

The purchase and employment of new instrumentation is part of all breath test programs. Before installing new instruments it is important to develop a plan for method validation. An important part of validation includes method comparison. A program probably has a history of analytical methods that are routinely accepted into court as evidence. It would be important to compare the new equipment to the old, approved equipment. One form of comparison could be done in the field by offering the defendant a voluntary test on the new instrument following the approved evidential instrument. This would provide data for comparison and also feedback from the operators on use of the new proposed instrument. The data would have to be provided in a discovery request. Several statistical techniques are available for this form of validation. Some include linear regression analysis, paired t-tests, Bland-Altman plots (Bland and Altman 1986), comparing blood to breath alcohol for the new instrument, compute measurement uncertainty, etc. It would also be useful to obtain duplicate breath alcohol data from a jurisdiction that has been using the new technology and generate an uncertainty function. Plotting the standard deviation against the mean through a large range using simulators or gas standards would also be informative. The validation plan and results should be maintained as part of the program SOP and also made available on the web site. Finally, one component of method validation should be participation in a proficiency test program prior to new instrument installation and field use.

7.3.4.2 Employ Control Charts for Existing Instruments

Control charts are visual tools that ensure the process is operating in statistical control with acceptable random variation. The chart also has the advantage of quickly identifying when the system is out of control. This occurs when warning or control limits are exceeded. Control charts are designed to monitor for "assignable causes" when an assignable error has occurred and for "random causes" when the variation is random and not due to some assignable source of error. Control charts are a very useful tool for quality control and can add confidence to the measurement process. The two most common types of control charts are the X-bar chart which monitors for shifts in the mean and R-bar control charts that monitor for variation. Figure 7.6 illustrates an X-bar control chart plotting means of four subsamples along with upper and lower control limits. This plot can be used to monitor accuracy due to shifts in the means. The control limits are determined from the mean of 25 subsample means. In Figure 7.6 we see a trend down which is characteristic of using simulator (alcohol in water) control standards. The last two results have exceeded the control limits and the system should be shut down, possibly in need of installing a new simulator solution. This example illustrates an instrument that is out-of-control and should automatically shut down, putting itself out of service until a technician can evaluate and correct the problem.

Warning limits for X-bar charts are generally determined from $\overline{X} \pm 2\sigma$ and the action (out-of-control) limits are found from $\overline{X} \pm 3\sigma$.

Figure 7.7 illustrates a range control chart which monitors variation. The lower control limit here is zero. Again, the last measurement exceeds the action limits indicating the need for intervention. Manufacturers of computerized breath test instruments should be

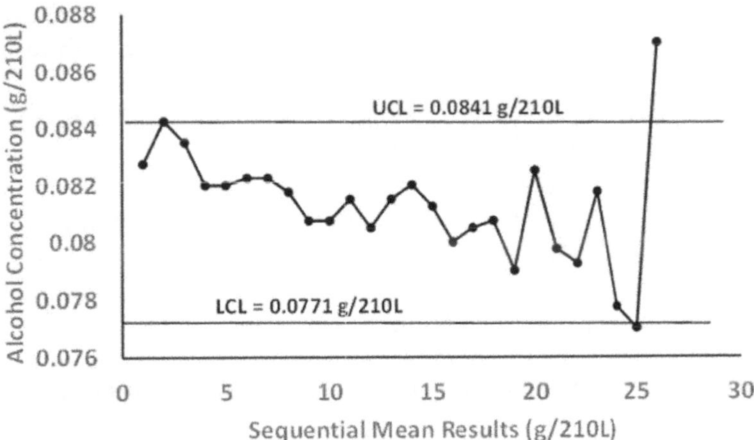

Figure 7.6 An X-bar control chart plotting sequential mean simulator results, each determined from a subsample size of four.

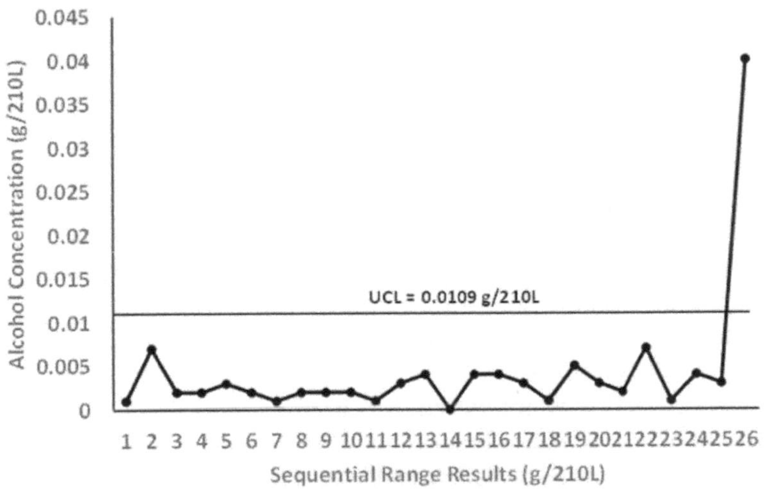

Figure 7.7 A range control chart plotting the range of sequential simulator results, each determined from a subsample size of four.

encouraged to write code that will automatically generate X-bar and range control chart data along with printout capability. This would be very informative for program personnel and end-users alike by alerting them to the need for intervention and by shutting down the system when necessary. While there are many types of control charts available, we have commented on only two very common ones. A classic text on control charts is available (Grant and Leavenworth 1988).

7.3.4.3 Preparation and Use of Control Standards

There are a number of control materials available with different levels of accuracy and integrity. Standard Reference Materials (SRM) of ethanol in water can be purchased directly from NIST or control materials can be prepared within the breath test program. Whatever level of quality chosen by the program, the SOP should define exactly what is used, their preparation and their reference values along with their uncertainty. Where a program develops its own internal quality control standards (i.e., simulator solutions) a test for homogeneity among the individual bottles should be done with results placed on the web site.

7.3.4.4 Pre-breath Test (PBT) Measurement

PBT measurement results are typically obtained at the roadside and provide an example of a screening test. We feel obliged to comment briefly on the use and interpretation of PBT results. PBT instruments can be very useful in assisting the arresting officer to obtain probable cause for the arrest. There should be a program of method validation in place before the use of PBT instruments also. This should be recorded in the SOP. As screening devices there is the potential for false-positive and false-negative results. A database of results from arrested drunk drivers should be obtained. A few well-trained officers could be assigned a few PBT instruments and then obtain roadside PBT results from arrested subjects voluntarily. These results could be compared to subsequent evidential instrument results. Several statistical analyses could be obtained. These results could be very helpful in a subsequent Frye hearing seeking admissibility of the PBT results. The PBT program should be developed and operated with as much quality control and integrity as possible.

7.3.4.5 Regular Instrument Calibration/Quality Assurance

There should be some regular time when each instrument is brought into the lab for an exhaustive evaluation. This should be a pre-determined protocol along with a regular schedule recorded in the program SOP. This may include, for example:

- Replicate tests (n = 10) at four different concentrations (i.e., 0.04, 0.08, 0.20, 0.30 g/210 L) using traceable control standards
- A maximum allowed bias of 5%
- A maximum allowed precision of 3% CV
- Capability of detecting an interferent (i.e., acetone)
- Capability of detecting Radio Frequency Interference
- Capability of completing correctly a full breath test analysis
- Capability of transferring data to the host computer
- Correct voltage settings on printed circuit boards, etc. Levels of Detection (LOD) and Levels of Quantitation (LOQ) could also be determined at this time from multiples of the standard deviation estimate at zero concentration. LOQ would be important to know in view of minor *per se* statutes of, for example, 0.02 g/210 L. These represent only a few of the possible features necessary to evaluate on perhaps an annual basis. Prepared forms noting all results should then be prepared and placed on the web site.

7.4 Conclusion

Many necessary and fit-for-purpose elements converge as part of a well-designed and pre-determined "quality control algorithm" to produce breath alcohol results capable of being presented with confidence and integrity in a forensic context. We have identified here only a few of the most important ones. Of the few we have discussed, program personnel certainly stands out as one of the most important. We cannot emphasize enough the importance of hiring quality personnel that have highest integrity along with a strong work ethic. Their willingness to state in court "I don't know," followed by their determination to find the answer, is so important. Moreover, these quality personnel must have a continual attitude of "learning to improve." Every good program can be improved upon. Acknowledging our weaknesses along with striving to improve provides the foundation for a program characterized by integrity and transparency.

Finally, we recommend the following elements in order for a program to meet the needs of their customers with quality, integrity, and fitness-for-purpose:

- Know the needs and purposes of your customers with a focus of providing them with the best possible service
- Know in detail the legal specifications and constraints of your program so your product is in full compliance
- Compliance with pre-determined criteria for analytical accuracy and precision
- Regular participation in proficiency testing
- Duplicate breath testing with preserved three-digit results
- Two control standards at different concentrations associated with each tested subject
- All program records and data preserved and available on a web site (see the Washington State Patrol web site at: http://www.wsp.wa.gov/breathtest/wdms_home.htm)
- Carefully selected and trained personnel with specified responsibilities and highest integrity
- Use of instruments that have been validated and determined to be in compliance with pre-determined analytical characteristics
- At least annual re-calibration and certification of breath test instruments
- Development of control charts for easy monitoring of statistical control

References

ASCLD/LAB-International: *ASCLD/LAB Policy on Measurement Uncertainty* (Document control number AL-PD-3060 Ver 1.1); 2013.

ASCLD/LAB International: Supplemental Requirements for the Accreditation of Breath Alcohol Calibration Laboratories; 2007; https://anab.qualtraxcloud.com/ShowDocument.aspx?ID=6862 (Accessed July 26, 2019).

ASTM International Committee e36 on Laboratory Accreditation: *Standard Guide for Proficiency Testing by Inter-Laboratory Comparisons*, Subcommittee E36-60 on Accreditation Systems; pp. 1–13; 1973.

Berger PD, Maurer RE: *Experimental Design*; Thomas Learning: Belmont, CA; 2002.

Bland JM, Altman DG: Statistical methods for assessing agreement between two methods of clinical measurement; *Lancet* 1:307; 1986.

Box GEP, Hunter WG, Hunter JS: *Statistics for Experimenters*; John Wiley & Sons: New York; 1978.

Bureau International des Poids et Mesures: *GUM: Guide to the Expression of Uncertainty in Measurement*; 2008; http://www.bipm.org/en/publications/guides/gum.html (Accessed July 26, 2019).

Castelazo I, Mitani Y: On the use of the mean squared error as a proficiency index; *Accred Qual Assur* 17:95; 2012.

Collaborative Testing Services, Inc.; https://cts-forensics.com/index-forensics-testing.php (Accessed July 26, 2019).

Daubert vs Merrill Dow Pharmaceuticals, Inc.; 509 U.S. 579 (1993).

Deming WE: *Out of the Crisis*; Massachusetts Institute of Technology: Cambridge, MA; p. 43; 1986.

Dilulio R: The science of credentialing scientists; 2006; http://www.clpmag.com/2006/07/the-science-of-credentialing-scientists/ (Accessed July 26, 2019).

Dubowski KM: Necessary scientific safeguards in breath alcohol analysis; *J Forensic Sci* 5:422; 1960.

Dubowski KM: Quality Assurance in Breath—Alcohol Analysis; *J Anal Toxicol* 18:306; 1994.

Ellison SLR, King B, Rösslein M, Salit M, Williams A (Eds): EURACHEM/CITAC Guide: Traceability in Chemical Measurements: A Guide to Achieving Comparable Results in Chemical Measurement; 2003; http://www.citac.cc/EC_Trace_2003.pdf (Accessed July 26, 2019).

Ellison SLR, Williams A (Eds): *EURACHEM/CITAC Guide: Quantifying Uncertainty in Analytical Measurement*, 3rd ed.; p. 16; 2012; https://www.eurachem.org/index.php/publications/guides/quam (Accessed July 26, 2019).

Grant EL, Leavenworth RS: *Statistical Quality Control*, McGraw-Hill: New York; 1988.

Gullberg RG, Logan BK: Results of a proposed breath alcohol proficiency test program; *J Forensic Sci* 51:168; 2006.

Heydorn K: The determination of an accepted reference value from proficiency data with stated uncertainties; *Accred Qual Assur* 10:479; 2006.

Hicks CR: *Fundamental Concepts in the Design of Experiments*, 2nd ed; Holt, Rinehart and Winston: New York; 1973.

Horwitz W: The certainty of uncertainty; *J AOAC Int* 86:109; 2003.

Huang H: Uncertainty-based measurement quality control; *Accred Qual Assur* 19:65; 2014.

Hulley SB, Cummings SR: *Designing Clinical Research*; Williams and Wilkins: Baltimore, MD; 1988.

International Organization for Standardization (ISO)/International Electrotechnical Commission (IEC): *ISO/IEC 17025 – General Requirements for the Competence of Testing and Calibration Laboratories*; 2005.

ISO/IEC Guide 43.1, *Proficiency Testing by Inter-Laboratory Comparisons*, 2nd ed; 1997.

Kacker R, Sommer K, Kessel R: Evolution of modern approaches to express uncertainty in measurement; *Metrologia* 44:513; 2007.

Kristiansen J, Petersen HW: An uncertainty budget for the measurement of ethanol in blood by headspace gas chromatography; *J Anal Toxicol* 28:456; 2004.

Ku HH: Notes on the use of propagation of error formulas; *J Res Natl Bur Stand Sec C* 70C:263; 1966.

Kuselman I: Comparability of analytical results obtained in proficiency testing based on a metrological approach; *Accred Qual Assur* 10:466; 2006.

Maher JM, Markey JC, Ebert-May E: The other half of the story: Effect size analysis in quantitative research; *CBE-Life Sci Educ* 12:345; 2013.

Montgomery DC: *Design and Analysis of Experiments*; John Wiley & Sons: New York, 1976.

Mnookin J: The uncertain future of forensic science; *Daedalus—The Journal of the American Academy of Arts and Sciences* 147:4; 2018.

Reyna VF, Nelson WL, Han PK, Dieckmann NF: How numeracy influences risk comprehension and medical decision making; *Psychol Bull* 135:943; 2009.

Sunderman FW: The history of proficiency testing/quality control; *Clin Chem* 36:1205; 1992.

Taylor BN, Kuyatt, CE: Guidelines for Evaluating and Expressing the Uncertainty (NIST Technical Note 1297); National Institute of Standards and Technology, Gaithersburg, MD; 1994; http://physics.nist.gov/Pubs/guidelines/TN1297/tn1297s.pdf (Accessed July 26, 2019).

Thompson M, Wood R: International harmonized protocol for proficiency testing of (chemical) analytical laboratories; *J AOAC Intl* 76:926; 1993.

Thompson M, Wood R: Using uncertainty functions to predict and specify the performance of analytical methods; *Accred Qual Assur* 10:471; 2006.

US National Research Council: *Strengthening Forensic Science in the United States: A Path Forward*; The National Academies Press: Washington, DC; 2009.

Wallace J: Ten methods for calculating the uncertainty of measurement; *Sci Justice* 50:182; 2010.

Wu AHB, Hill DW, Crouch D, Hodness CN, McCurdy HH: Minimal standards for the performance and interpretation of toxicology tests in legal proceedings; *J Forensic Sci* 44:516; 1999.

Pharmacokinetics of Ethanol

A Primer for Forensic Practitioners*

8

A. WAYNE JONES

Contents

* This chapter is an updated version of a review article previously published in *Forensic Science Review*: Jones AW: Pharmacokinetics of ethanol—Issues of forensic importance; *Forensic Sci Rev* 23:91; 2011.

8.1 Introduction

Biomedical research on alcohol (ethanol), including its disposition and fate in the human body, started in earnest in the 1920s when a reliable analytical method was developed to determine concentrations of the drug in blood and other biological specimens (Widmark 1922). Ethanol acts as a depressant of the central nervous system (CNS) and impairs cognitive and psychomotor functioning in a dose-dependent manner depending on the blood-alcohol concentration (BAC) reaching the brain. The ubiquitous use and abuse of alcoholic beverages in society makes ethanol the psychoactive substance most commonly encountered in forensic investigations of living and deceased persons (Jones and Holmgren 2009a).

Binge drinking and drunkenness are underlying factors in many types of criminal activity, including impaired driving, sexual assault, homicides, hooliganism, and domestic violence (Jones and Holmgren 2009b; Jones et al. 2008). In a recent survey of the relative dangerousness of recreational drugs on the individual and society, the legal drug ethanol topped the list ahead of heroin and crack cocaine (Nutt et al. 2010).

What happens to ethanol in the body after drinking alcoholic beverages belongs to the scientific discipline known as pharmacokinetics, which is a key sub-discipline of pharmacology and closely linked to pharmacodynamics, which deals with the action of drugs (Rowland and Tozer 1995). Reliable information about the factors influencing absorption, distribution, metabolism, and excretion (ADME) of ethanol is important in forensic science and legal medicine whenever alcohol-related crimes, such as drunken driving or drug-related sexual assault are investigated (Kerrigan 2010). An expert witness might be asked to estimate a person's BAC based on information provided about the number of drinks consumed or to perform a back-calculation of BAC to an early time point, such as the time of driving or when a road traffic crash occurred (Ferner and Norman 1996).

The relationship between a person's BAC and impairment of body functioning and ability to perform skilled tasks, such as driving, often need to be interpreted in a legal context when apprehended drivers are prosecuted (Kalant 1996a). Much depends on the dose of ethanol ingested and the factors influencing ADME processes as well as the development of tolerance to the impairing effects of ethanol consumption (Kalant et al. 1971). Forensic practitioners are often asked to calculate the amount of ethanol consumed from a measured BAC, which can be done with reasonable scientific certainty and knowledge of ethanol pharmacokinetics. More controversial is the question of back-calculating a person's BAC to an earlier point in time, such as the time of driving (Al-Lanqawi et al. 1992; Montgomery and Reasor 1992). When a back-calculation of BAC is done, this requires making certain assumptions about the ADME of ethanol and there is a lack of consensus on how this should be done in a criminal prosecution (Labay and Logan 2018; Lewis 1986).

This chapter reviews the disposition and fate of ethanol in the body from an historical perspective and gives an update of the many factors influencing ADME of ethanol in the human body. The pharmacokinetic parameters of ethanol were derived by the method described by Widmark including the apparent volume of distribution (V_d or rho factor) and the rate of elimination from the bloodstream (β or k_0) as well as from the whole body (B_{60}).

8.1.1 Historical Background

The word pharmacokinetics was obtained by combining two Greek words *"pharmakon"* meaning a drug or poison and *"kinesis"* which means movement (Wagner 1981). Pharmacokinetics is therefore concerned with the quantitative evaluation of concentration-time (C-T) profiles of drugs in blood, plasma, urine, or saliva after a specified route of administration (e.g., orally, intravenously, rectally, or subcutaneously).

The first appearance in print of the word pharmacokinetics was on page 244 in a book by Friedrich Dost (1910–1985), which was published in 1953 entitled *"Der Blutspiegel—Kinetik der Konzentrationsabläufe in der Kreislaufflüssigkeit"* (Dost 1953). An English translation of the book title is *"The Blood-profile—on the Kinetics of Concentration Changes in the Systemic Circulation."* In this book Dost derived mathematical formulas appropriate to describe the C-T profiles of endogenous and exogenous substances in blood or plasma after intra- and extra-vascular routes of administration (Dost 1968).

8.1.2 Erik MP Widmark

Knowledge about forensic pharmacokinetics of ethanol owes much to the pioneering research and publications of Erik MP Widmark (1889–1945), who was professor of physiological chemistry at the University of Lund in Southern Sweden (Jones 2009). Already in 1922 Widmark introduced a micro-diffusion method for the quantitative analysis of ethanol in blood, which made it possible to study the ADME of ethanol in the body (Widmark 1922). His dual qualifications in science and medicine and good grounding in mathematics put him in a strong position to make original contributions to knowledge about the pharmacokinetics of ethanol and other substances, such as acetone and methanol in body fluids.

The micro-diffusion method of blood-alcohol analysis was fully validated and subsequently used in several European countries as the official analytical method for legal purposes when drinking drivers were prosecuted (Andreasson and Jones 1996). Statutory blood-alcohol limits for driving were introduced in Sweden in 1941 (0.8 mg/g or ~0.08 g%) and in Norway in 1936 (0.5 mg/g or ~0.05 g%) (Jones 2000). However, it was not easy for a judge and jury to interpret the meaning of a person's BAC in relation to degree of impairment of skills necessary for safe driving and risk of a crash. It became a common practice to translate the BAC into number of centilitres of spirits (40% v/v) in the body at the time the blood sample was taken. With information about time of stating to drink it was also possible to calculate the total amount of ethanol a person had consumed. Various forensic calculations involving consumption of alcohol and the BAC reached were developed in the 1930s by Professor Erik Widmark (1889–1945) at the University of Lund (Sweden).

Table 8.1 gives a time-line of historical events leading to the development of pharmacokinetics with major focus on ethanol and the contributions by a selected number of pioneer workers in this field.

Widmark's seminal publication on the subject of ethanol pharmacokinetics appeared in a 1932 German monograph entitled *"Die theoretischen Grundlagen und die praktische Verwendbarkeit der gerichtlich-medizinischen Alkoholbestimmung"* (Widmark 1932). The importance of this work can be gleaned from that fact that it was translated into English in 1981 and entitled *"Principles and Applications of Medicolegal Alcohol Determination"* (Widmark 1981). The monograph contained 12 chapters dealing with the analysis ethanol, methanol and acetone in body fluids, the pharmacokinetic profiles of these substances,

Table 8.1 Principal Contributors to the Development of Knowledge About Pharmacokinetics (PK) with Special Reference to Ethanol PK and Forensic Applications

Year	Scientist	Brief Description of the Person's Contribution to Pharmacokinetics
1874	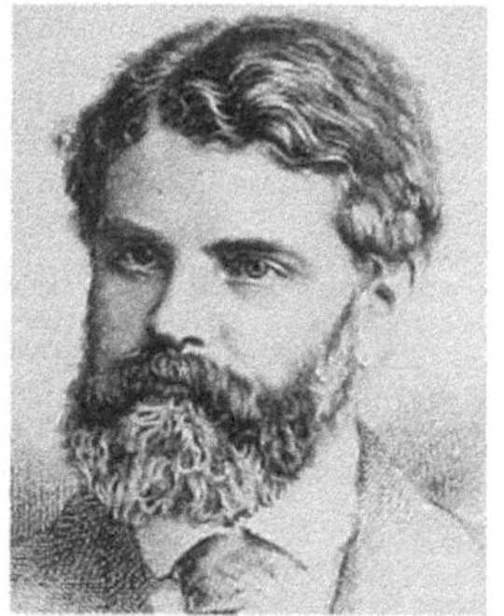 Francis Anstie (1833–1874)	British physician much concerned with public health in Victorian England and especially the problem caused by over-consumption of alcohol. He established a so-called "Anstie limit" which was the recommended daily dose of alcohol (1½ oz of 100% ethanol), corresponding to ~100 mL of 40 % v/v liquor (Baldwin 1977). He developed a method for quantitative analysis of ethanol in body fluids involving oxidation with a mixture of potassium dichromate and sulfuric acid. Using this method, Anstie showed that only a very small fraction of the alcohol a person consumed was eliminated from the body unchanged in breath and urine (Anstie 1874). Moreover, he wrote one of the first books on the subject of "Stimulants and Narcotics."
1919	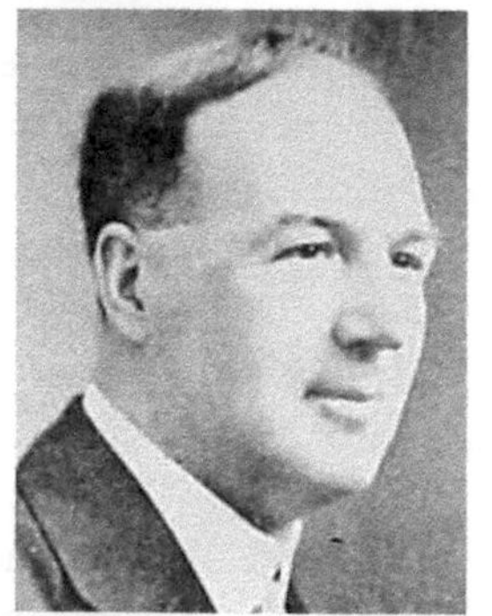 Edward Mellanby (1884–1955)	British physician and pharmacologist who studied the factors that influence blood-alcohol curves after drinking. Experimenting with humans and animals (dogs), Mellanby investigated the importance of dose administered and the type of beverage (beer and stout vs spirits) as well as the influence of food and milk in the stomach (Mellanby 1919). Mellanby was the first to suggest that alcohol was eliminated from blood by zero-order kinetics. He also studied impairment effects of ethanol in relation to BAC, reporting that this was more pronounced on the rising phase of the curve compared to the declining phase that develops later. This phenomenon reflects acute tolerance to ethanol during a single exposure to the drug and was referred to as the "Mellanby effect" (Mellanby 1920).
1932	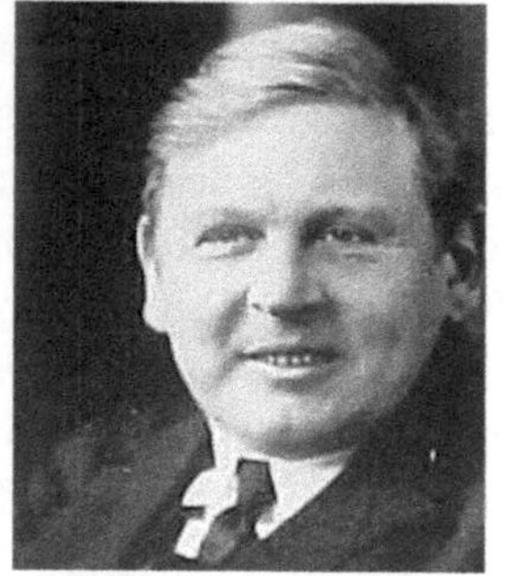 Eric MP Widmark (1889–1945)	Professor of Physiological Chemistry at the University of Lund in Sweden (Andreasson and Jones 1996), Widmark published seminal articles on the disposition and fate of acetone, ethanol and methanol in the body during the first half of the 20th century. His micro-diffusion method of blood-alcohol analysis was highly reliable and became used for legal purposes in some nations (Widmark 1922). The pharmacokinetics of ethanol was studied in men and women and the parameters β and rho were derived (Widmark 1932). Beta represented the rate of elimination of alcohol from the bloodstream and rho was the volume of distribution of ethanol. Widmark's German monograph from 1932 is considered a veritable classic for medicolegal studies on alcohol.

(Continued)

Table 8.1 (*Continued*) Principal Contributors to the Development of Knowledge About Pharmacokinetics (PK) with Special Reference to Ethanol PK and Forensic Applications

Year	Scientist	Brief Description of the Person's Contribution to Pharmacokinetics
1937	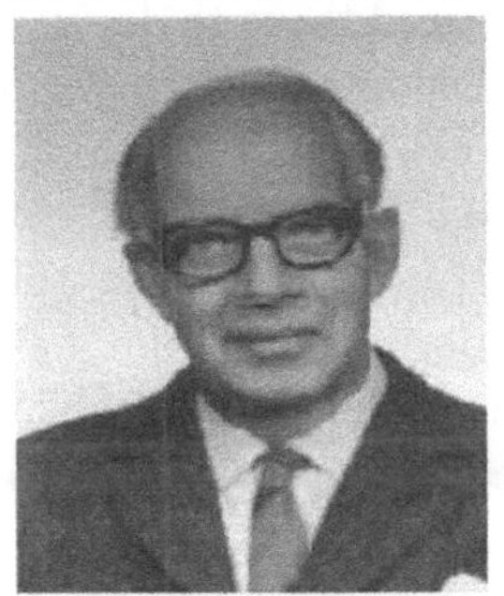 Torsten Teorell (1905–1992)	Professor of physiology and medical biophysics at the University of Uppsala in Sweden. He published two papers in 1937 that later became widely acclaimed as pioneer contributions to knowledge about compartment models and pharmacokinetics by intra and extra-vascular routes of administration (Teorell 1937a, 1937b). For this contribution Teorell is considered one of the founding fathers of pharmacokinetic theory, although he never concerned himself with what happened to alcohol in the body. The speed of distribution of drugs into the body fluids and tissues were discussed in relation to the route of administration and the new concept of compartment models.
1951	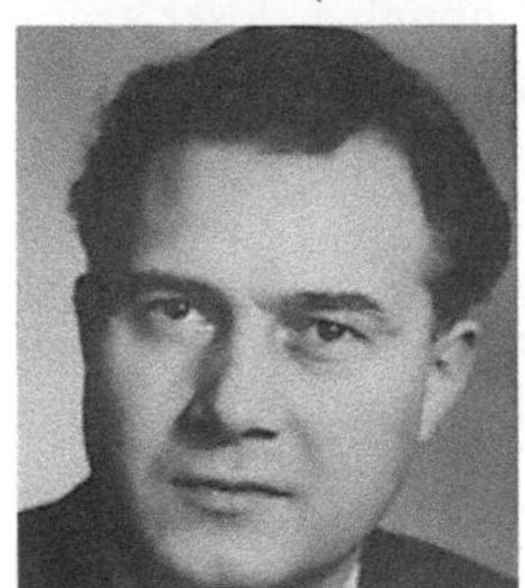 Antti Alha (1917–1989)	Antti Alha was a physician and forensic toxicologist from Helsinki, Finland who made extensive studies of human pharmacokinetics of ethanol in healthy men. He administered four different doses of ethanol (0.50–1.25 g/kg) and determined ethanol in blood by a chemical oxidation method. Pharmacokinetic parameters of ethanol were determined in relation to clinical signs and symptoms of drunkenness as a function of time after drinking (Alha 1951). The results of the drinking experiments appeared in a 92 page monograph, which unfortunately was not widely circulated, although it was an important contribution to knowledge about ethanol pharmacokinetics at the time.
1953	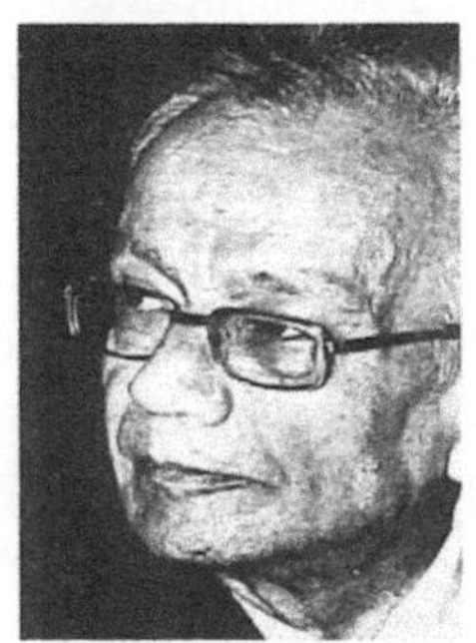 Friedrich H. Dost (1910–1985)	Professor Dost was a physician and pediatrician at the University of Giessen in Germany and is considered a pioneer in clinical pharmacokinetics of drugs. He is credited with coining the word pharmacokinetics, which first appeared in print in his famous book "Der Blutspiegel" in 1953 (Dost 1953). This reviewed all the available literature on the subject of clinical pharmacokinetics and the mathematical formula and equations necessary to describe the concentration-time profiles of endogenous and exogenous substances in blood and plasma using single and multiple compartment models.
1969	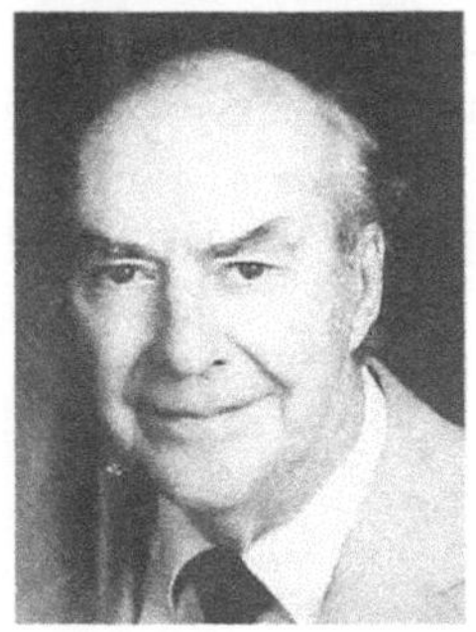 John G Wagner (1921–1998)	John Wagner was professor of pharmaceutics at the College of Pharmacy at the University of Michigan, USA. He wrote several books on the subject of biopharmacy and pharmacokinetics and was a strong proponent for use of the Michaelis–Menten equation or saturation kinetics to describe the C-T profiles of ethanol (Wagner 1973; Wagner et al. 1989). Wagner and his collaborators published many articles on the pharmacokinetics of ethanol including the effect of dose, eating solid food (Lin et al. 1976; Sedman et al. 1976), and oral vs intravenous administration in the fasting state (Wilkinson et al. 1976, 1977). Wagner verified that the area under the blood-alcohol curve increased more than proportionally with increasing dose, which is characteristic of non-linear kinetics.

the relationship between a person's BAC and the signs and symptoms of drunkenness, derivation of the parameters β and rho, and one chapter dealt with the synthesis of ethanol in the body after death (Widmark 1981).

In a series of human drinking experiments involving 20 men and 10 women Widmark plotted the pharmacokinetic profiles of ethanol in blood and used these to derive a set of kinetic parameters; β denoting the rate of elimination from the blood assuming zero-order kinetics, and the rho factor or distribution volume of ethanol. The latter parameter was found to be 0.55 (range 0.49–0.76) in women compared with a mean of 0.68 in 20 men (range 0.51–0.85). This gender difference was statistically highly significant ($p < 0.001$) and depends on the fact that the female body has less water per kg body weight than males, and thus a smaller volume (space) for dilution of the dose of ethanol ingested (Rosenfeld 1996).

The other important pharmacokinetic parameter is the rate of ethanol elimination from the blood in the post-absorptive phase, and this averaged 0.15 g/kg/h (SD 0.0336) for men and 0.156 g/kg/h (SD 0.0222) for women (Widmark 1981). This small gender difference was not considered statistically significant ($p > 0.05$), although a closer examination of the results, as well as many later studies, showed that the slope of the declining phase of the BAC curve was slightly steeper in women compared with men (Brick 2006; Dettling et al. 2007).

The early research done by Widmark was expanded to include experiments with another 20 women and 10 men (Osterlind et al. 1944). The Widmark rho factors (V_d) were updated to ~0.70 for men and ~0.60 for women, whereas the rate of elimination from blood of 0.15 g/kg/h was confirmed and considered to be independent of gender. Because the aliquots of blood analysed were weighed, the ethanol concentrations are in units of g/kg (same as mg/g), which meant that the rho factor, which is the ratio of ethanol dose (g/kg)/C_0 (mg/g) has no dimensions. This contrasts with the way BAC is reported in journal articles today, which is mostly in mass/volume units (g/L or g/100 mL) so a correction is necessary to the rho factors reported by Widmark. Taking the density of whole blood as 1.055 g/mL, a rho factor of 0.68 according to Widmark becomes 0.64 L/kg (see Table 8.3).

Some investigators failed to confirm the values of β and rho reported by Widmark, although this often depended on some departure from his stipulated experimental design, namely drinking a bolus dose of ethanol as neat spirits on an empty stomach. Others failed to appreciate that BAC was in mass/mass concentration units (mg/g or g/kg), which influences the values of β and rho by 5.5% (see later). Eating a meal before drinking, even a sandwich or snack, lowers the bioavailability of the dose of ethanol, which is important to consider when the rho factor is calculated as the ratio dose/C_0—values are abnormally high if part of the dose ingested undergoes first-pass metabolism and C_0 is lower than expected.

Ethanol pharmacokinetics and the various factors influencing ADME of this legal drug have been the subject of many previous review articles and some of these are worthy of note (Holford 1987; Holzbecher and Wells 1984; Kalant 1996b; Norberg et al. 2003; Wartburg Von 1989; Wilkinson 1980).

8.1.3 Properties of Ethanol

Ethanol is small polar molecule, which mixes with water in all proportions and distributes into the total body water space. Unlike many other drugs, there is no evidence that ethanol binds to plasma proteins and its solubility in lipids is insignificant compared with solubility in water. These special physico-chemical properties of ethanol require that

Table 8.2 Summary of the Major Physico-Chemical Properties of Ethanol

Property	Accepted Values
CAS-number[a]	64-17-5
Molecular weight	46.07 g/mol
Empirical formulae	C_2H_6O
Molecular formulae	CH_3CH_2OH (primary aliphatic alcohol)
Structural formulae	H_3C–CH_2–OH
Common name	Beverage or grain alcohol
Manufacture	Fermentation of starch, sugar or some other source of carbohydrate
Solubility in water	Mixes completely in all proportions
Boiling point	78.5°C at atmospheric pressure
Melting point	–114.1°C
Density	0.789 g/mL at 20°C
pK_a	15.9 at 25°C.
Dipole moment (polarity)	1.69 D
Dielectric constant (polarity)	24.3

[a] Chemical abstract service registry number.

large quantities must be consumed to raise the BAC to a level that elicits pharmacological impairment effects. Mild euphoria from ethanol is usually achieved after rapid drinking of about 20 g (20,000 mg) on an empty stomach. This compares with a standard dose of 10 mg morphine, 10 mg diazepam, 100 mg codeine or 1000 mg aspirin to obtain a desired therapeutic effect from these common medications. The main properties of ethanol are presented in Table 8.2.

8.1.4 Blood- and Breath-Alcohol Concentration Units

The standard operating procedure with the micro-diffusion method of blood-alcohol analysis required that the aliquots of whole blood (~100 mg) were weighed on a torsion balance, so the final analytical result was reported in units of mass/mass, actually mg/g or g/kg. With more modern analytical methods, such as gas chromatography, the aliquots of blood are measured by volume and the BAC is reported in units of mass/volume, such as g/100 mL (US), mg/100 mL (UK) or g/L and mg/mL (Europe). The connection between mass/mass and mass/volume is the density of whole blood, which on the average is 1.055 g/mL making a difference of 5.5% between mass/mass and mass/volume units (Lenter 1981). This should be considered when the pharmacokinetic parameters of ethanol (β and rho) are compared and contrasted with older studies, such as those published by Widmark. The values are slightly different and depend on whether the C-T profiles are constructed based on BAC in mass/mass or mass/volume units (see Table 8.3).

The statutory BAC limits for driving in the Nordic countries and in Germany are defined as per mille (parts per thousand) and this refers to mass/mass units, whereas most other nations report BAC as mass/volume (Andreasson and Jones 1996). Punishable limits of breath-alcohol concentration (BrAC) were introduced much later and expressed as mass/volume concentration units, so statutory BrAC limits were reported as mg/L, g/210 L or μg/L depending on the particular country (see Table 8.4).

Table 8.3 Widmark Factors, Rate of Elimination of Ethanol from Blood (β-slope) and Volume of Distribution (V_d) or Rho Factor for Male and Female Subjects When the Blood-Alcohol Concentration (BAC) Is Expressed in Mass/Mass (g/kg) or Mass/Volume (g/L) Units

	BAC (mass/mass)		BAC (mass/volume)[a]	
Pharmacokinetic Parameter	Men (n = 20)	Women (n = 10)	Men (n = 20)	Women (n = 10)
β-slope	0.150 ± 0.0336	0.156 ± 0.0222	0.158 ± 0.0354	0.164 ± 0.0234
Rho factor (V_d)	0.68 ± 0.085	0.55 ± 0.055	0.64 ± 0.081	0.52 ± 0.0521

[a] The density of whole blood is 1.055 g/mL on average so 1.0 g/L = 0.948 g/kg.

Table 8.4 Concentration Units Used in Various Countries for Reporting Blood-Alcohol Concentration (BAC) and Breath-Alcohol Concentration (BrAC) for Legal Purposes

Concentration Unit for Reporting BAC	Examples of Countries Where These Units Are Used	Concentration Unit for Reporting BrAC	Examples of Countries Where These Units Are Used
mg/g (g/kg)	Sweden, Denmark, Norway, Finland, Germany, Switzerland	mg/L	Austria, Sweden, Denmark, Norway, Finland, Germany, Spain and some other EU countries
mg/mL (g/L)	Austria, France, Holland, Spain, Belgium	µg/L	Holland, Belgium
mg/100 mL (mg%)	UK, Ireland, Canada, New Zealand	µg/100 mL	UK, Ireland
g/100 mL (g%)	US, Australia	g/210 L	USA, Australia

8.2 Alcohol in the Body

The disposition and fate of ethanol in the body is usually illustrated by plotting the concentrations determined in blood or plasma against the sampling times after start of drinking to give the concentration-time (C-T) profile. Hundreds of controlled drinking experiments with healthy men and women have been done over the years with consumption of ethanol in the form of beer, wine or spirits either on an empty stomach or after subjects had eaten a meal. The quantitative evaluation of BAC curves is done by defining a set of parameters, which underpins our current knowledge about human pharmacokinetics of ethanol.

Figure 8.1 shows a BAC profile for one healthy male subject who drank ethanol (0.68 g/kg) as neat whisky on an empty stomach (overnight fast). Also shown is the best-fitting straight line (dashed) drawn through selected data points on the post-absorptive declining phase of the BAC vs time curve. Extrapolating this straight line to intersect the y- and x-axes gives two important pharmacokinetic parameters, namely the y-intercept (C_0) and the x-intercept (min_0). These can be used to calculate the rate of elimination of ethanol from blood (k_0 or β-factor) and the distribution volume (V_d or rho factor), as shown within text boxes on the graph. Alternatively, the value of C_0 and β are the coefficients from a least-squares linear regression equation using selected C-T points on the post-absorptive declining phase.

Concentration-time curves of ethanol show several common features including a rising BAC immediately after drinking starts, which reflects the absorption of ethanol from the

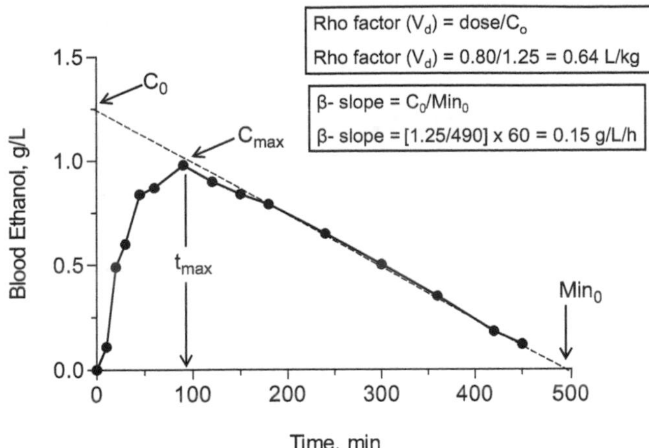

Figure 8.1 Typical blood-alcohol curve in one male subject after drinking 0.68 g ethanol per kg body weight as neat whisky on an empty stomach. Samples of capillary (fingertip) blood were taken for analysis of ethanol at repeated intervals and the pharmacokinetic parameters β-slope and rho factor were derived as shown in the text boxes.

stomach and intestine into the bloodstream. The ADME processes occur simultaneously but at different rates. As more time passes and the amount of ethanol remaining unabsorbed decreases, the rate of absorption becomes slower than the rate of clearance from the blood by metabolism and excretion. This marks the beginning of the post-absorptive phase and provided there is no further consumption of alcohol the BAC will continue to decrease at a more-or-less constant rate per unit time until reaching a BAC of 0.1–0.2 g/L.

The shapes of BAC curves show considerable inter-individual variations even under standardized drinking conditions, that is to say, when the same dose (gram per kilogram of body weight) is ingested as the same type of beverage in the same space of time. These variations are seen in Figure 8.2, which shows BAC curves for nine male subjects after they drank neat whisky on an empty stomach. Most of the inter-subject variation is seen during the first 120 minutes after start of drinking, which corresponds to the absorption phase.

The time-course of a drug in the body is usually discussed in terms of its rate of absorption, distribution, metabolism and excretion and one aim of pharmacokinetics is to describe these processes in quantitative terms. Table 8.5 illustrates ADME processes and the body organs involved in these processes.

8.2.1 Absorption

Absorption is the process by which a drug or poison passes from the site of administration into the bloodstream for distribution throughout all body fluids and tissues. Small amounts of ethanol can enter the blood by absorption through the mucous surfaces of the oral cavity, especially if a drink is held in the mouth for a sufficiently long time without swallowing. But for all practical purposes alcoholic drinks are swallowed and absorption from the gastro-intestinal canal occurs by a passive diffusion across the gut lumen, at rates that depend on the prevailing concentration gradient in accordance with Fick's law (Berggren and Goldberg 1940).

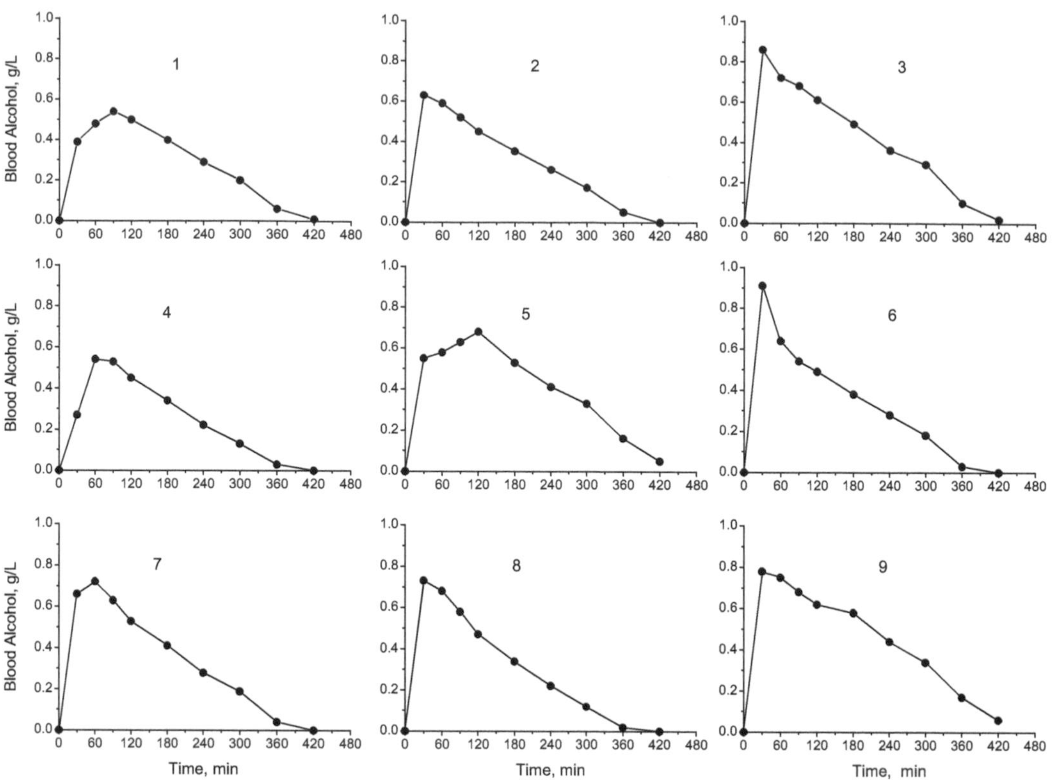

Figure 8.2 Examples of blood-alcohol profiles obtained in drinking experiments with nine healthy men who ingested the same dose of ethanol (0.68 g per kg body weight) as neat whisky on an empty stomach.

Table 8.5 Schematic Illustration of the Disposition and Fate of Ethanol in the Body Showing the Absorption, Distribution, Metabolism, and Excretion Processes and Organ Systems Involved

Stage	Organ System Involved	Comments About the Process
Absorption	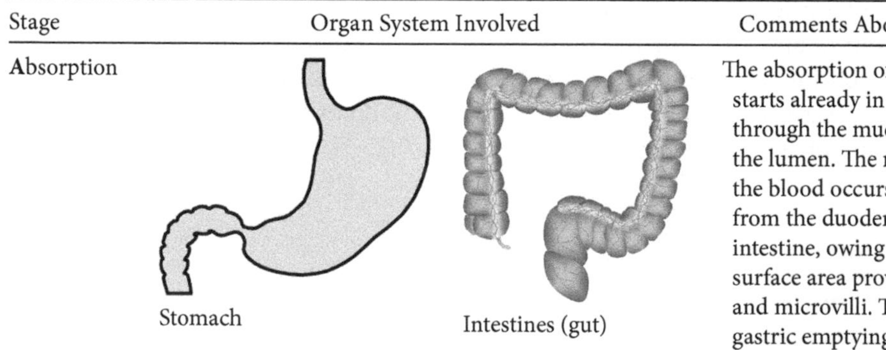	The absorption of ingested ethanol starts already in the stomach through the mucous surfaces of the lumen. The rate of uptake into the blood occurs much faster from the duodenum and small intestine, owing to the larger surface area provided by the villi and microvilli. The speed of gastric emptying is a major determinant of the rate of absorption of ethanol and hence C_{max} and t_{max} of the resulting blood-alcohol curve.

(Continued)

Table 8.5 (*Continued*) Schematic Illustration of the Disposition and Fate of Ethanol in the Body Showing the Absorption, Distribution, Metabolism, and Excretion Processes and Organ Systems Involved

Stage	Organ System Involved		Comments About the Process
Distribution	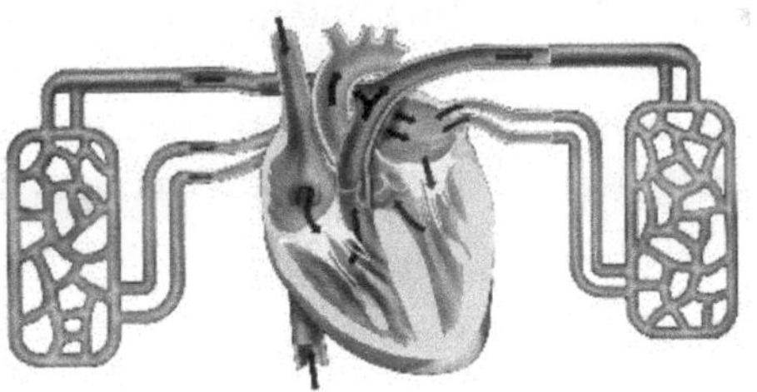 Arterial and venous blood circulation		After absorption from the gastro-intestinal tract, ethanol is transported throughout all body organs and tissues with the blood circulation. Ethanol passes freely across biological membranes and distributes into the total body water without binding to plasma proteins. However, a concentration gradient exists between the arterial (A) and venous (V) blood circulation with A > V during absorption and V > A during the post-absorptive period.
Metabolism	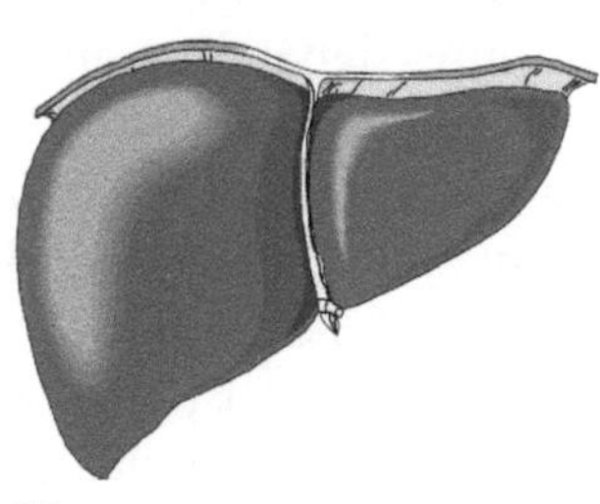 Liver		Ethanol enters the portal venous blood and is transported to the liver where oxidative enzymes e.g., alcohol dehydrogenase (ADH) starts to remove ethanol from the bloodstream. The ADH enzyme has a low k_m and is therefore saturated with substrate after the first couple of drinks (BAC > 0.20 g/L). For most forensic questions ethanol is eliminated from blood at a constant rate per unit time in accordance with zero-order kinetics.
Excretion	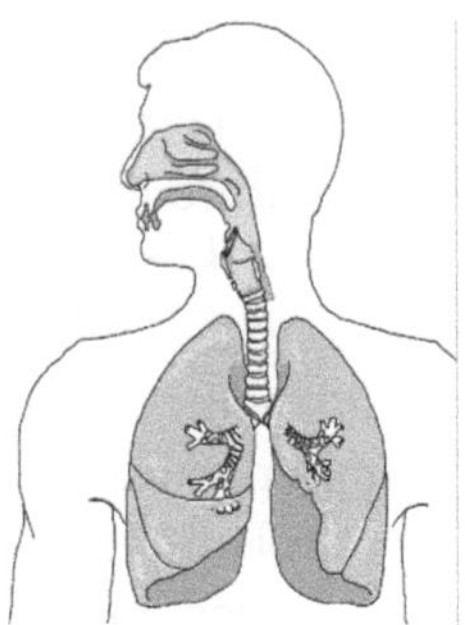 Lungs	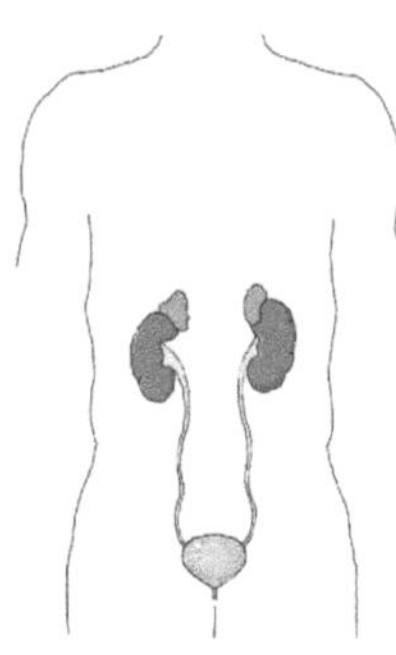 Kidneys	Only a small fraction (2%–10%) of the total dose of ethanol ingested is eliminated from the body unchanged via the lungs (breath) and kidneys (urine) and trace amounts in sweat. Excretion is a first-order process such that proportionally more of the ethanol gets eliminated unchanged after large doses are ingested to reach high BAC. Drinking massive amounts of water to cause diuresis or hyper-ventilation are not very effective ways of increasing the rate of ethanol clearance from the body.

Because ethanol is already in liquid form dissolution or solubilization is not necessary for absorption to occur, which means that the absorption time lag is negligible and ethanol is measurable in the blood immediately after drinking starts. The absorption of drugs taken in the form of tablets first require dissolution and the speed and extent of absorption depends on properties of the parent drug, such as its pKa and lipid solubility. This leads to a measurable lag-time before the active substance is detectable in the venous blood circulation. The absorption of ethanol is faster from the upper part of the intestines (proximal small bowel), owing to the larger absorption surface area provided by the villi and microvilli of the duodenum and jejunum.

8.2.1.1 Drinking Pattern and Dosage Form

The pattern of drinking (bolus or repetitive drinking), the concentration of ethanol in the drink and the presence of food in the stomach are major determinants of the speed of ethanol absorption into the blood. The time elapsed after the start of drinking before reaching C_{max} is denoted as t_{max} and the ratio of C_{max} to t_{max} gives a crude index of the rate of absorption of ethanol in g/L/h. Based on a large number of drinking studies, t_{max} usually occurs within 60 minutes after the end of drinking, although in any individual case this time might range from 5 minutes to 120 minutes depending on many variable factors.

An example of a BAC curve showing very rapid absorption of ethanol is shown in Figure 8.2 (subject 6), where an overshoot peak is evident and C_{max} is higher than expected for the dose of ethanol administered. The C_{max} is immediately followed by a diffusion plunge and during this time the excess ethanol in the blood re-equilibrates between the vascular system and the rest of the body water, a process that takes ~30–45 minutes. Another curve in Figure 8.2 (e.g., subject 5) shows an initial swift absorption with a marked rise in BAC, although this is followed by a much slower increase before reaching C_{max}. Under some circumstances the BAC profile shows no obvious C_{max} and instead a plateau develops, during which time the BAC remains more or less unchanged for 60–120 minutes before the rectilinear declining phase begins. Note that ethanol is still being metabolized even when the BAC remains unchanged for several hours.

The dosage form of ethanol corresponds to the nature of the drink consumed, whether whisky, gin, vodka, wine, beer, or even 95% v/v ethanol diluted with water (Gustafson and Kallmen 1988). In a German study BAC curves were not much different when 0.75 g/kg ethanol was consumed on an empty stomach as 4%, 8%, 20%, and 44% v/v dilutions with water (Springer 1972). This suggests that the volume of fluid in which ethanol is taken is less important for determining C_{max} and t_{max} provided the dose of ethanol remains the same. This seems to conflict with the notion of absorption being a passive diffusion process according to a concentration gradient, which emphasizes the role of other factors, such as efficacy of gastric emptying. Besides differences in ethanol content, alcoholic beverage differ in composition, such as the amount of carbohydrates and other constituents they contain, which also influences the rate of ethanol absorption into the blood by influencing gastric emptying (Wright and Cameron 1998).

8.2.1.2 Gastric Emptying

The single most important factor controlling the speed of absorption of ethanol into the bloodstream is the emptying rate of the stomach, which is controlled by the pyloric sphincter. The pylorus is normally almost totally closed, owing to tonic contraction of the pyloric muscle. Factors influencing stomach emptying and the pylorus valve are of paramount importance for how fast ethanol gets absorbed into the blood and the values of C_{max} and t_{max} on the resulting BAC curve.

8.2.1.3 Effects of Food

The presence of food in the stomach before drinking has a major influence on both rate and extent of absorption of ethanol as shown already by experiments done in the 1930s (Widmark 1941). The composition of the food in terms of macronutrients (carbohydrate, protein, or fat) seemed less important in delaying the rate of absorption of ethanol than the amount (bulk) of food eaten before drinking (Jones et al. 1997).

Figure 8.3 shows BAC profiles obtained in a cross-over study design experiment when four individuals drank the same dose of ethanol (0.80 g/kg) under fed or fasting conditions (Jones and Jonsson 1994b). Without exception, the curves in the fed state run on a lower level compared with the curves when alcohol was taken on an empty stomach. This give the impression that a smaller amount of alcohol had been administered after the meal, but this was not the case. The C_{max} was appreciably lower, the t_{max} occurred later and AUC was smaller when subjects had eaten a standardized breakfast before drinking. Moreover, in the fed state the BAC curves returned to zero about 1–2 hours earlier, which suggests an overall faster rate of ethanol metabolism. Because

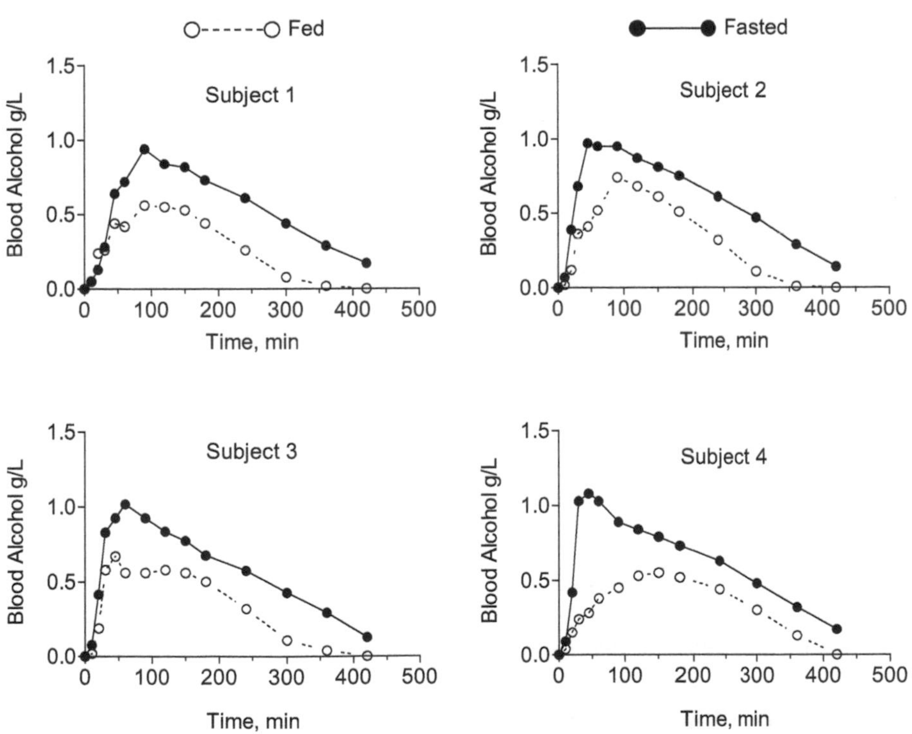

Figure 8.3 Cross-over experimental design (within-subjects) demonstrating the effect of drinking alcohol after eating a meal. The plots show food-induced lowering of blood-alcohol profiles in four healthy men after they drank ethanol (0.80 g/kg) as vodka diluted with orange juice either after an overnight fast or immediately after eating a standardized breakfast.

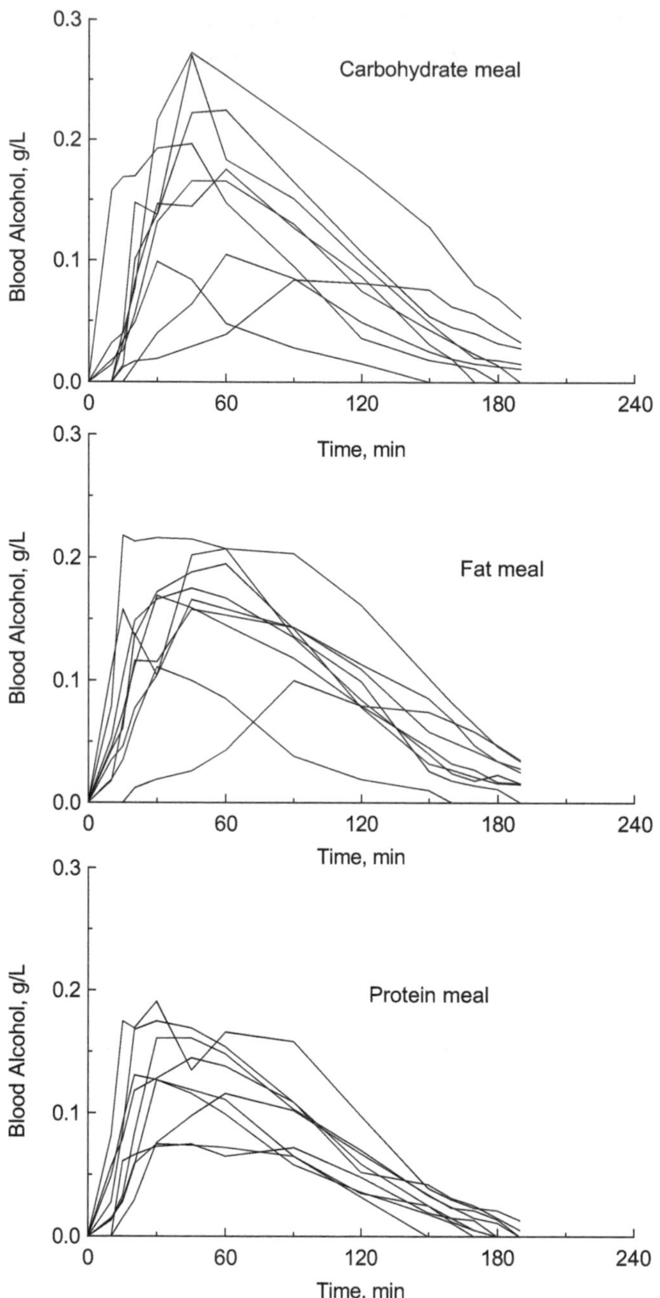

Figure 8.4 Highly variable shapes of blood-alcohol curves for nine subjects after they drank the same small dose of ethanol (0.30 g/kg) in 15 minutes after eating a standardized equicaloric fat-rich, carbohydrate-rich, or protein-rich meal.

the slopes of the rectilinear declining portions were not much different in the fed and fasting conditions, it seems that the accelerating effect of food on ethanol metabolism occurs during the absorption phase.

When small amounts of ethanol (e.g., 0.3 g/kg) were consumed after a meal the resulting BAC curves were highly variable as shown in Figure 8.4. Although C_{max}, t_{max} and

AUC can easily be calculated from the resulting BAC profiles it is not very practical to make a detailed pharmacokinetic evaluation and accomplish proper curve fitting to C-T data points on the post-absorptive phase. The examples of BAC curves shown in Figure 8.4 were obtained after ten healthy men drank a small dose of the ethanol (0.30 g/kg) diluted with orange juice in 15 minutes after they had eaten a standardized breakfast (Jones et al. 1997).

Other factors influencing gastric emptying include certain prescription drugs, anatomy of the gut, smoking cigarettes, surgical operations (gastric bypass), stress, and trauma as summarized in Table 8.6.

8.2.1.4 Rectal Administration

The speed and completeness of absorption of a drug depends on the route of administration, whether by mouth (orally), intravenously (parenterally) or by inhalation via the lungs, the skin (transdermal), or rectally. Alcohol is not absorbed through the intact skin to any measurable amount as demonstrated in two recent studies that confirmed the results from older work (Bowers et al. 1941; Hansen et al. 2010; Schrot et al. 2010). Ethanol can be given as an enema via the rectum as exemplified by the C-T profiles in Figure 8.5 depicting two

Table 8.6 Examples of the Most Important Factors Influencing the Rate of Absorption of Ethanol by Influencing Gastric Emptying

Slow Rate of Ethanol Absorption		Fast Rate of Ethanol Absorption	
Factor	References	Factor	References
Eating a meal before drinking alcohol	Sadler and Fox (2011), Sedman et al. (1976), Watkins and Adler (1993)	Drinking rapidly on an empty stomach, except when the subject suffers a pyloric spasm	Jones (1984)
Smoking cigarettes	Johnson et al. (1991)	Rapid ingestion of neat spirits as opposed to sherry, table wines, or various beers	Mitchell et al. (2014)
Taking medication that delays gastric emptying e.g., anticholinergic agents, antacids, aspirin; antispasmodic medicines, e.g., propantheline	Edelbroek et al. (1993)	Highly carbonated (CO_2) drinks and alcohol mixed with various sweeteners	Marczinski and Stamates (2013); Roberts and Robinson (2007); Wu et al. (2006)
Drinking beer with a high carbohydrate content compared with alcohol in form of neat spirits	Holford (1997)	Taking drugs that accelerate gastric emptying, such as cisapride, metoclopramide, erythromycin	Kechagias et al. (1999); Nimmo (1976); Oneta et al. (1998)
Trauma, shock, and massive blood loss and resuscitation fluids	Jones (2016)	Low blood sugar, type I diabetes (hypoglycemia)	Marathe et al. (2013); Russo et al. (2005)
Pyloric spasm if gastric mucosa is irritated by drinking neat spirits on empty stomach	Jones (1984)	Surgery to the gut, gastric bypass or gastrectomy	Klockhoff et al. (2002); Woodard et al. (2011)

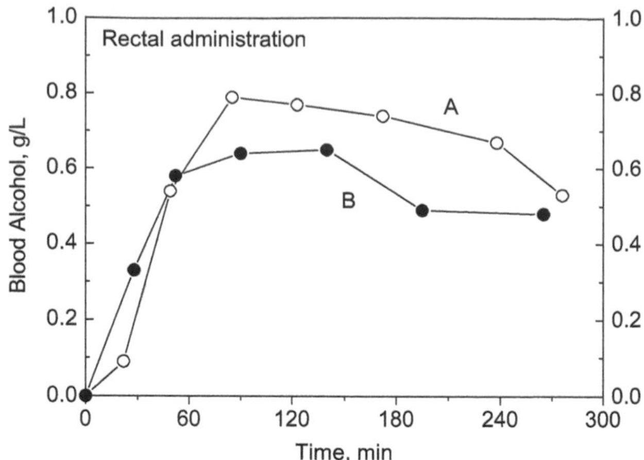

Figure 8.5 Blood-alcohol curves in two subjects (A and B) when the dose of ethanol was administered rectally over a time of 60 minutes. (From Liljestrand, G. and Linde, P., *Skand. Arch. Physiol.*, 60, 273, 1930.)

individuals denoted A and B (Liljestrand and Linde 1930). These curves were obtained after 45 g of ethanol was diluted to 300 mL with water and administered *per rectum* in the course of 35–40 minutes.

8.2.1.5 Pulmonary Inhalation

Absorption of alcohol into the bloodstream by inhalation via the lungs is not an effective way to raise the BAC for several good reasons. First, the ethanol contained in the inhaled air gets dissolved in the mucous surfaces covering the upper airway and leaves the lungs again with the next exhalation (Campbell and Wilson 1986; Kruhoffer 1983; Mason and Blackmore 1972). Second, very high concentrations of ethanol in the ambient air breathed are necessary, which are difficult to tolerate by humans (Lester and Greenberg 1951). Third, the amount of ethanol absorbed into the bloodstream via the lungs must exceed the hourly rate of ethanol metabolism, which is about 7–8 g/h. This makes it practically impossible for BAC (>0.1 g/L) to increase by breathing ethanol contained in the ambient air. The subject of alcohol inhalation and its impact on BAC was recently reviewed (MacLean et al. 2017).

If a person has an elevated BAC before entering a closed room or chamber containing ethanol in the atmosphere under these conditions, especially with high respiratory minute volumes e.g., after strenuous exercise, the ethanol absorbed by inhalation might balance the amounts lost by metabolism. If the blood-alcohol curve is in the post-absorptive declining phase when subjects inhale ethanol vapors, the slope of the declining phase will be less than expected (Kruhoffer 1983).

8.2.1.6 Absorption Kinetics

The absorption of ethanol into the blood is highly variable even when drinking occurs on an empty stomach. The peak BAC might occur 5–10 minutes after the end of drinking (Figure 8.2 curves 3, 6, 8, and 9) or as late as 120 minutes (curve 5) and such slow absorption, despite drinking neat spirits on an empty stomach, is probably explained by an ethanol-induced pyloric spasm.

The absorption of ethanol into the blood after oral ingestion is often considered to be a first-order process, but this is an over-simplification because of the variable and unpredictable nature of gastric emptying. The speed of absorption as reflected in the rate constant (min^{-1} or h^{-1}) is slower from the stomach (longer half-life) compared with the small intestine (shorter half-life), which makes it difficult to fit a pharmacokinetic model to the entire absorption process. In forensic science situations great care is needed when a statement is made about the absorption rate constant for ethanol for any given drinking scenario.

The BAC curve shown in Figure 8.6 was obtained in a 23 year-old male subject who drank 0.68 g/kg ethanol as neat whisky on an empty stomach resulting in a C_{max} at 100 minutes after the end of drinking. The C-T data points on the rising phase of the curve (Table 8.7) can be used to determine the absorption rate constant assuming first order kinetics by the graphic method of residuals.

The residuals method requires subtracting the BACs determined during the absorption phase from BACs at the same time points read from the dashed line extrapolated back to intersect the y-axis corresponding to the time of starting to drink (C_0). This gives a series of residual BACs, which on transformation to natural logarithms and plotted against sampling time (see insert graph in Figure 8.6) results in a straight line and least squares linear regression analysis of Ln residual BAC (y) and time (x) gave the equation ln y = 4.5 – 0.016x (r = 0.98). The regression coefficient is the first-order absorption rate constant ($k_{abs} = -0.016\ min^{-1}$), which corresponds to an absorption half-life of 43.3 minutes ($t_{½} = 0.693/k_{abs}$), indicating a slow rate of ethanol absorption for this individual, probably caused by a pyloric spasm after drinking neat whisky.

Experience from evaluating hundreds of BAC curves verifies the difficulty in determining a first-order absorption rate constant, especially when neat spirits are consumed on an empty stomach. Under these conditions the peak BAC might occur 10 minutes after end of drinking and the residual method is not applicable because of a lack of data points (Jones 1984). Instead, a more pragmatic approach is to divide C_{max} with t_{max} to give a rate

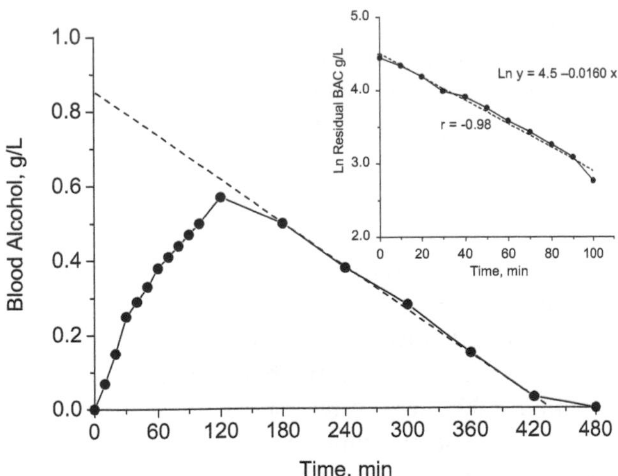

Figure 8.6 Blood-alcohol curve in a subject with slow rate of ethanol absorption as evidenced by a late occurring t_{max} (120 minutes post-dosing) showing how to derive a first-order absorption rate constant by the method of residuals (insert graph).

Table 8.7 Method of Determining First-Order Absorption Rate Constant of Ethanol Based on Actual Blood-Alcohol Concentrations (BAC) on the Absorption Phase of the Curve and Calculating Residuals (See Inset Graph in Figure 8.6)

	Blood-Alcohol Concentration[a]			
Time (min)	Actual	Extrapolated	Residual	Ln Residual
0	0	86	86	4.45
10	7	84	77	4.34
20	15	81	66	4.19
30	25	79	54	3.99
40	28	78	50	3.91
50	33	76	43	3.76
60	38	74	36	3.58
70	41	72	31	3.43
80	44	70	26	3.26
90	46	68	22	3.09
100	50	66	16	2.77

[a] BAC reported here in units of mg/100 mL to avoid negative logarithms.

of absorption as g/L/h. Moreover, in the real world people drink alcohol intermittently, sometimes over several hours as different types of drinks with or without food and the BAC successively increases for each additional drink taken. With this pattern of drinking, much of the total dose of alcohol is already absorbed into the blood during the drinking period and the peak BAC is reached shortly after finishing the last drink.

8.2.2 Distribution

After absorption from the stomach and intestines ethanol enters the portal venous blood and gets transported first to the liver, then to the right side of the heart and via the lungs, back to the heart and throughout the entire systemic circulation. The rate of equilibration of ethanol between the water fraction of the blood and the extra-cellular fluids and tissue depends on the cross-sectional area of the local capillary bed and blood flow per gram of tissue. Organs with a rich blood supply, such as the brain and kidney, equilibrate rapidly with ethanol in the blood, whereas bulky skeletal muscle with a lower ratio of blood flow to tissue mass equilibrates more slowly.

Total Body Water: Ethanol distributes into total body water and the concentration at equilibrium in the various body fluids and tissues depend primarily on their relative water contents. This means that sweat, saliva, cerebrospinal fluid (CSF), and urine, which are almost 100% water, have a higher concentration of ethanol than the blood, which is 80% w/w water (Buono 1999; Jones 1979, 1990; Mehrtens and Newman 1933). Likewise, the concentrations of ethanol in plasma and serum, which contain ~92% w/w water, are higher than an equal volume of whole blood. The plasma/blood distribution ratio averages about 1.15 with a 95% range from 1.10 to 1.20 (Charlebois et al. 1996; Winek and Carfagna 1987).

Gender Differences: Between 50% and 60% of a person's body weight is water, which on the average is higher in men than in women, because of gender differences in lipid (fat) content per kg body weight (Edelman et al. 1952; Goist and Sutker 1985; Jones and Neri 1985). The volume of blood is about 70–80 mL per kg body weight independent of gender, which corresponds to 4.9–5.6 L in a person weighing 70 kg. For a water soluble drug like ethanol the volume of distribution corresponds very closely with the total body water (TBW) as verified by isotope dilution experiments using ^2H_2O, ^3H_2O or H_2O^{18} as tracers (Endres and Gruner 1994; Norberg et al. 2001).

The larger the individual in terms of height and body weight the more body water space available for dilution of the ingested alcohol. For this reason in experimental alcohol research the dose of ethanol is almost always administered per kg body weight or per kg body water, which permits direct comparisons between different individuals with varying body weights.

Gender difference in TBW is the main reason that women reach a higher BAC than men for the same dose of ethanol administered per kg body weight. Differences in TBW are reflected in gender-related differences in volume of distribution, which averages 0.6 L/kg for women and 0.7 L/kg for men (Kwo et al. 1998; Marshall et al. 1983; Mumenthaler et al. 2000). The V_d for ethanol depends on the percentage of water in the whole body (usually 50%–60% of body weight) and the water content of the blood sample (usually 78%–82% w/w) needs to be considered when ethanol-dilution experiments are used to determine TBW (Loeppky et al. 1977; Watson 1989). If plasma or serum was used for analysis of ethanol and used to derive pharmacokinetic parameters the β-factor and rho factor would not be the same as those derived from analysis of whole blood. This follows because plasma or serum contains ~10%–20% (mean 15%) more water than whole blood and therefore concentrations of ethanol are higher (Jones et al. 1992). The y-intercept (C_0) of the plasma/serum C-T plot is ~15% higher so V_d calculated as dose/C_0 is correspondingly lower and the β-slope of the elimination phase is also steeper.

Several studies have looked specifically at blood-alcohol pharmacokinetics in women in relation to their age and body composition to complement the results from early studies by Widmark and others with male drinkers (Davies and Bowen 2000; Mumenthaler et al. 2000).

Body-Mass Index and Obesity: Body mass index (BMI) is the ratio of a person's weight in kg to the square of height in meters and has become widely used as a simple clinical index of obesity (Flegal et al. 2002; Seidell and Flegal 1997). The distribution volume of ethanol is expected to be lower in people with obesity compared with lean individuals, because ethanol is virtually insoluble in lipids and completely miscible in water. Table 8.8 attempts to relate a person's degree of obesity as reflected in BMI with the expected distribution volume (V_d) of ethanol for that individual. However, few if any drinking studies in obese individuals have been done so the values of V_d in Table 8.8 are intuitive, although not verified by experiment (Jones 2007). With the worldwide epidemic of obesity, the pharmacokinetics of drugs in obese individuals, including ethanol, deserves careful attention and more investigations (Cheymol 2000). Controlled drinking experiments in both obese and emaciated individuals are needed to determine the impact of extremes of body composition on the pharmacokinetic parameters β and rho.

Table 8.8 The Expected Distribution Volume of Ethanol (Widmark's Rho Factor) in Relation to a Person's Obesity as Reflected in a Body Mass Index (BMI)

Classification of Degree of Obesity	BMI, kg/m^2	Expected Distribution Volume of Ethanol (L/kg)
Underweight	<18.5	0.80–0.85
Normal weight	18.5–24.9	0.60–0.70
Pre-obese	25.0–29.9	0.50–0.60
Obese class I	30.0–34.9	0.40–0.50
Obese class II	35.0–39.9	0.30–0.40
Obese class III	>40	0.30–0.40

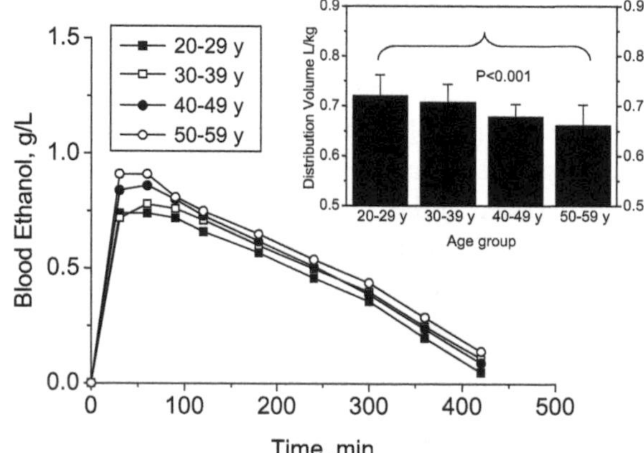

Figure 8.7 Mean blood-alcohol curves for four age groups of healthy men (20–59 years) after they drank a bolus dose of ethanol (0.68 g/kg) as neat whisky on an empty stomach. The insert graph shows that apparent distribution volume of ethanol V_d (mean ± SD) decreases with advancing age.

Age and Volume of Distribution: The influence of a person's age (20–60 years) on the distribution volume of ethanol is illustrated in Figure 8.7, which shows mean BAC curves for n = 48 healthy men (Jones and Neri 1985). The oldest age group (50–60 y) were on a higher level compared to younger subjects, giving higher value of C_0 and therefore lower V_d in the elderly (dose/C_0). The insert graph shows a statistically significant decrease in V_d as men age from 20 to 60 years as was verified by analysis of variance ($p < 0.001$). The mean ± SD value of V_d for the 48 healthy men was 0.69 ± 0.043 L/kg and the 95% range was from 0.604 to 0.776 L/kg. This range would probably be wider if subjects had been obese or emaciated (Table 8.9). In this same drinking study, the elimination rate of ethanol from blood (β-factor) was notcorrelated to a man's age between 20 and 60 years old ($p > 0.05$).

In summary, during the process of aging in men the proportion of water per kg body weight decreases, which results in a smaller body water space to dilute water-soluble drugs, such as ethanol (Chumlea et al. 2001). Since blood-water content remains more or less unchanged during ageing (80% w/w) this leads to a smaller volume of distribution in the elderly owing to a higher concentration of ethanol in blood for the same dose administered (Jones and Neri 1994; Lenter 1981).

Table 8.9 Influence of a Person's Age on the Volume of Distribution of Ethanol and the Rate of Elimination from Blood in Four Groups of Healthy Men after They Drank Neat Whisky (0.68 g/kg Ethanol) after an Overnight Fast

Age Group	n[a]	Volume of Distribution, L/kg (Widmark's rho factor)[b]	Rate of Ethanol Elimination From Blood, g/L/h (Widmark's β-factor)[c]
20–29 y	12	0.720 ± 0.042	0.126 ± 0.008
30–39 y	12	0.707 ± 0.036	0.122 ± 0.009
40–39 y	12	0.678 ± 0.026	0.130 ± 0.015
50–59 y	12	0.690 ± 0.043	0.126 ± 0.014

Source: Jones, A.W. and Neri, A., *Alcohol Alcohol*, 20, 45, 1985.
Note: Values shown are mean ± SD.
[a] Number of drinking subjects in each age group.
[b] Volume of distribution of ethanol decreases with age ($p < 0.001$).
[c] No significant change in rate of elimination from blood with increasing age ($p > 0.05$).

8.2.3 Metabolism

Most of the ingested ethanol (90%–98%) is removed from the body by oxidative metabolism, primarily in the liver and a very small fraction (<1%) is conjugated via the –OH group to produce the non-oxidative metabolites ethyl glucuronide and ethyl sulphate (Jones 2008b). The remainder of the dose administered (2%–8%) is eliminated unchanged by filtration in the kidney and excretion in the urine (Jones 2006). Small amounts (1%–2%) of ingested ethanol also undergo pulmonary excretion via the lungs and through the skin in the perspiration (Buono 1999).

8.2.3.1 Hepatic Enzymes ADH and ALDH

The two main enzymes involved in the metabolism of ethanol are Class I alcohol dehydrogenase (ADH), located in the cytosol fraction and Class II aldehyde dehydrogenase (ALDH) within the mitochondria (Crabb 1995; Edenberg 2007). A microsomal enzyme denoted CYP2E1 found within the smooth endoplasmic reticulum is also involved in oxidative metabolism of ethanol (Lieber 1997). Both ADH and CYP2E1 convert ethanol to acetaldehyde and this toxic metabolite is quickly oxidized to acetic acid by the action of low k_m ALDH (Agarwal and Goedde 1992; Morimoto and Takeshita 1996). The acetate produced during the catabolism of ethanol is transported away from the liver and is converted into the end products CO_2 and H_2O in the Krebs cycle (Mascord et al. 1992; Suokas et al. 1984). The complete breakdown of ethanol liberates energy, actually 7.1 kcal per gram (29.7 kJ) more than that obtained from ingestion of the same weight of protein and carbohydrate (Lieber 1994).

Figure 8.8 summarizes salient features of human metabolism of ethanol, including the oxidative and non-oxidative pathways and also the relative amounts excreted unchanged.

The hepatic metabolism of ethanol to acetaldehyde as well as subsequent conversion of the latter to acetic acid requires participation of the coenzyme nicotinamide adenine dinucleotide (NAD^+) (Zakhari 2006). During the oxidation of ethanol there is a shift in the redox state of the liver as NAD^+ is reduced to NADH, which has negative consequences for other NAD-dependent biochemical reactions. Among other things this accounts for ethanol-induced hypoglycemia, hyperlactacidemia and accumulation of fat in the liver of heavy drinkers and alcoholics (Lieber 1998).

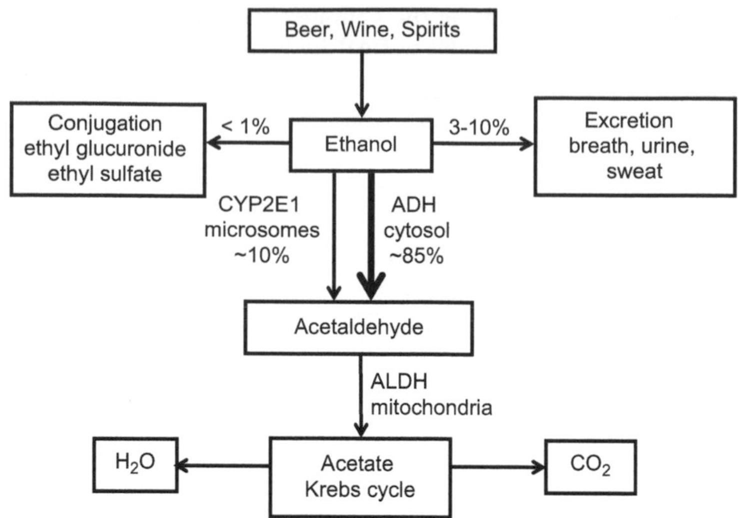

Figure 8.8 Schematic illustration of the disposition and fate of ethanol in the body showing both oxidative and non-oxidative metabolic pathways and the amounts of ethanol excreted unchanged.

8.2.3.2 Polymorphism of ADH and ALDH

Both ADH and ALDH are polymorphic enzymes that exist in multiple molecular forms and the various isozymes differ in catalytic activity and specificity for substrates (Edenberg 2007). One of the most widely studied polymorphisms occurs with ALDH, which exhibits marked racial and ethnic difference in catalytic activity. In 40%–50% of Asian populations the ALDH2 isoform has low or no enzymatic activity and this genetic trait makes those inheriting the ALDH2*2 allele are highly sensitive to drinking ethanol. These individuals flush in the face and neck, their blood pressure is lowered, there is an increase in heart rate caused by an accumulation in the blood of acetaldehyde produced during oxidation of ethanol. However, this genetic polymorphism of ALDH2 does not influence the BAC reached after drinking or the rate of elimination of ethanol from the blood stream (Wall et al. 1997). After moderate drinking the alcohol parameters β and rho in Asians were not much different from values observed in Caucasians and African Americans (Adachi et al. 1989; Tam et al. 2005; Thomasson et al. 1995). This means that the usual range of alcohol elimination rates (0.10–0.25 g/L/h) used for forensic purposes in Caucasians also applies to other racial groups.

8.2.3.3 Gastric ADH

The hepatic class I ADH has a low k_m (0.05–0.1 g/L) for ethanol as the substrate, which means that the enzyme is saturated after the first couple of drinks and ethanol is metabolized at a maximum velocity (Jornvall and Hoog 1995; Jornvall et al. 2000). Another variant of the ADH enzyme (class IV) having a much higher k_m is located in the gastric mucosa. Some investigators consider that gastric-ADH plays a prominent role in pre-systemic or first-pass metabolism of ethanol (Baraona et al. 1994a; Lieber et al. 1994). The finding of a lower activity of gastric ADH in women and alcoholics was said to make these individuals more vulnerable to the negative effects of drinking alcohol (Dohmen et al. 1996; Frezza et al. 1990). Opinions differ about the quantitative significance of gastric ADH in first-pass metabolism of ethanol and is difficult to distinguish from hepatic first-pass metabolism (Levitt 1993, 1994). Much seems to depend on the experimental conditions, particularly the dose of ethanol, the fed-fasting state of the subjects, and use of certain prescription drugs, such as histamine H_2-antagonists or aspirin (Furne and Levitt 1999; Levitt 1993; Toon et al. 1994). Very important in this connection is the speed of gastric emptying and a slower absorption increases the potential for first-pass metabolism to occur in the stomach and liver (Levitt and Levitt 1994; Oneta et al. 1998). From a large body of evidence the present consensus is that if pre-systemic first-pass metabolism of ethanol occurs at all then this is predominantly in the liver and not the gastric mucosa (Ammon et al. 1996; Caballeria et al. 1989).

8.2.3.4 *Microsomal Enzymes*

The CYP2E1 enzyme mentioned above has a higher k_m for ethanol as substrate (0.6–0.8 g/L) and becomes more important in clearance of ethanol from the blood after moderate to heavy drinking (Lieber 1997, 1999; Tanaka et al. 2000). Moreover, the CYP2E1 enzyme is inducible after periods of heavy drinking over weeks or months owing to a proliferation of the enzyme protein making this pathway more effective in the oxidation of ethanol and other drugs (Roberts et al. 1995; Takahashi et al. 1993). This explains the faster rates of ethanol metabolism observed in habituated individuals (alcoholics) during detoxification (Haffner et al. 1991; Keiding et al. 1983; Panes et al. 1993). However, the daily consumption necessary to induce the CYP2E1 enzyme leading to a faster rate of metabolism has not been established in humans (Oneta et al. 2002). In alcoholics during detoxification the average rate of elimination of ethanol from blood was 0.21 g/L/h although in some individuals the rate was no different from moderate drinkers (Brennan et al. 1995; Jones and Sternebring 1992).

The involvement of CYP2E1 in the metabolism of alcohol also accounts for a number of undesirable drug-alcohol interactions (Lieber 1997; Tanaka et al. 2000). For example, the widely used over-the-counter analgesic and antipyretic drug acetaminophen (paracetamol) is converted into a potentially toxic metabolite by CYP2E1 (Klotz and Ammon 1998; Lee et al. 1996). Accordingly, alcoholics with induced CYP2E1 activity should refrain from taking this medication because of the potential for hepatoxicity (Prescott 2000). The equation for CYP2E1 catalyzed oxidation of ethanol is shown below:

$$CH_3CH_2OH + NADPH + H^+ + O_2 \rightarrow CH_3CHO + NADP^+ + 2H_2O$$

An enzyme located in the peroxisomes (catalase) can, in theory, accomplish the oxidation of ethanol, at least under in-vitro conditions, whereas its role in-vivo is questionable (Crabb 1993; Zakhari 2006). The oxidative reaction requires the presence of hydrogen peroxide and not enough of this substance is available in-vivo. Therefore, for all practical purposes Class I ADH, Class II ALDH and CYP2E1 are the enzyme systems mainly responsible for in-vivo oxidative metabolism of ethanol in humans (Crabb et al. 1993, 2004; Li et al. 2001).

8.2.4 Excretion

A small fraction (2%–10%) of the amount of ethanol absorbed into the blood is excreted unchanged with the breath, the sweat, and the urine (Jones 2006; Pawan and Grice 1968).

Excretion is a first-order process so proportionally more of the drug is eliminated when larger doses or higher concentrations are reached in the blood (Kalant 1996b).

Urinary Excretion: The amounts of ethanol excreted in urine was studied after volunteers drank three doses of ethanol (0.51, 0.68, and 0.85 g/kg) on an empty stomach (Jones 1990). The volumes of urine voided at 60 minutes intervals were measured and from the concentration of ethanol the amount of drug excreted by the kidney was calculated. The results are shown in Table 8.10 and verify that only a small fraction of the dose of ethanol is cleared by glomerular filtration. For the highest dose of 0.85 g/kg the urinary excretion of ethanol represented only 2% of the total amount ingested.

Pulmonary Excretion: The amount of ethanol excreted via the breath depends on lung ventilation rate and the underlying blood-ethanol concentration as shown by the following theoretical calculation. If a person's BAC is 1.0 g/L and the blood/air ratio of ethanol at 37°C taken as 1800:1, then the alveolar air contains a concentration of 0.55 mg/L. In healthy individuals the respiratory minute volume at rest is about 6 L per minute for a tidal volume of 500 mL and 12 breaths per minute. Because ~30% of this breath is dead-space air and does not participate in gas exchange, the effective minute volume is 4.2 L per minute or 252 L per hour. Accordingly, at a BAC of 1.0 g/L (alveolar BrAC is ~0.55 mg/L) so about 139 mg (0.5 mg/L × 252 L) of ethanol is lost from the body per hour by exhalation. For a man with a body weight of 60–80 kg, this person eliminates about 6–8 g of 100% ethanol per hour from the entire body. So 139 mg of ethanol lost in the breath represents only 1.7%–2.3% of the total amount eliminated.

Sweat and Perspiration: A number of studies verify that trace amounts of ethanol are emitted from the body via the skin in perspiration, although the total quantity is trivial compared with the amount metabolized and excreted in urine and breath (Brown 1985; Buono 1999). However, the analysis of ethanol in sweat has found practical applications as a way to monitor abstinence in patients who must refrain from drinking as part of a rehabilitation program or as a condition of their employment (Marques and McKnight 2009; Swift 2000). Subjects are fitted with a tamper-proof skin-patch, which collects perspiration emitted over various periods of time before the patch is removed and any alcohol it collects is used to monitor abstinence from drinking (Phillips 1984).

Table 8.10 The Amounts of Ethanol Excreted in Urine after Three Increasing Doses of Ethanol Were Consumed as Neat Whisky on an Empty Stomach with (n = 16) Male Subjects at Each Dose

Ethanol Dose g/kg	Ethanol Dose in mL Whisky/kg[a]	Ethanol Excreted in Urine (mean ± SD)		Peak Diuresis (mL/min) Mean ± SD
		Grams of Ethanol	Percent of Dose	
0.51	1.5	0.29 ± 0.119	0.70 ± 0.290	2.56 ± 1.45
0.68	2.0	0.44 ± 0.246	0.80 ± 0.399	3.41 ± 2.26
0.85	2.5	1.00 ± 0.427	1.55 ± 0.501	6.12 ± 2.08

Source: Jones, A.W. *Forensic Sci Int*, 45, 217, 1990.

[a] Whisky 40% v/v ethanol.

8.3 Blood-Alcohol Profiles

Blood-alcohol curves in different individuals share certain common features (see Figure 8.2). The BAC increases immediately after the start of drinking until a peak or maximum concentration is reached, usually within 60 minutes of finishing the last drink. After the highest point on the BAC curve (C_{max}) a rectilinear declining phase starts, during which time the BAC decreases at a more or less constant rate until alcohol is no longer measurable in blood. The elevation and slope of the declining phase of the BAC depends on the relative rates of absorption, distribution and metabolism and examples of inter-subject variations are illustrated in Figure 8.2. The peak BAC occurs earlier if the gastric emptying is rapid often within 10–15 minutes after the end of drinking, although with a slow absorption the C_{max} might occur 120 minutes post-drinking.

8.3.1 Inter-individual Variations

Blood-alcohol curves show large inter-individual variations in C_{max} and t_{max} because these parameters are strongly dependent on the speed of gastric emptying, which differs widely between individuals depending on many factors. The magnitude of inter-individual variation in shapes of BAC profiles from two experimental protocols with different doses of ethanol is illustrated in Figure 8.9. In these two experiments the dose was administered according to the individual's body weight 0.68 g/kg in 48 subjects (upper plot) or 0.40 g/kg in 22 subjects (lower plot).

Curve A on the upper plot shows an unusually rapid absorption of ethanol from the gut with a clear-cut overshoot peak resembling BAC curves obtained when ethanol is given by intravenous infusion (see later) (Jones 1984). The C_{max} of the curve is higher than expected for the dose of ethanol administered and body weight of the individual. Such curves are not unusual when neat spirits are consumed on an empty stomach (overnight fast) as the pyloric sphincter opens to release ethanol into the duodenum and jejunum. The speed of absorption also determines the intensity of effects on the brain, as reflected in subjective and objective signs and symptoms of intoxication (Jones and Neri 1994; Martin and Moss 1993; Mitchell 1985).

Although drinking on an empty stomach curve B in Figure 8.9 exhibits a much slower absorption phase with a lower C_{max} and t_{max} occurring 100 minutes after end of drinking. Presumably in this case drinking neat whisky irritated the gastric mucosa and triggered a pyloric spasm so that ethanol was absorbed into the bloodstream through the stomach wall and not the proximal gut, where the absorption surface area is larger. Long experience with evaluating hundreds of controlled drinking experiments speaks against making a definitive statement about the time to reach C_{max} in any individual case.

Figure 8.9 (lower part) illustrates the large inter-individual variation in BAC profiles in experiments with 10 men and 12 women who drank a smaller dose of ethanol (0.4 g/kg) 2 hours after their last meal. Curve A and curve B on this plot also illustrates the large inter-subject differences in C_{max} and t_{max} reflecting highly variable rates of absorption despite the use of standardized drinking conditions.

Blood-alcohol curves also show intra-individual variations from drinking occasion to drinking occasion (Fraser et al. 1995; Passananti et al. 1990; Yelland et al. 2008). In a four-part cross-over study the rate of elimination of ethanol from blood varied as much between as within individuals as shown by analysis of variance (Jones and Jonsson 1994a).

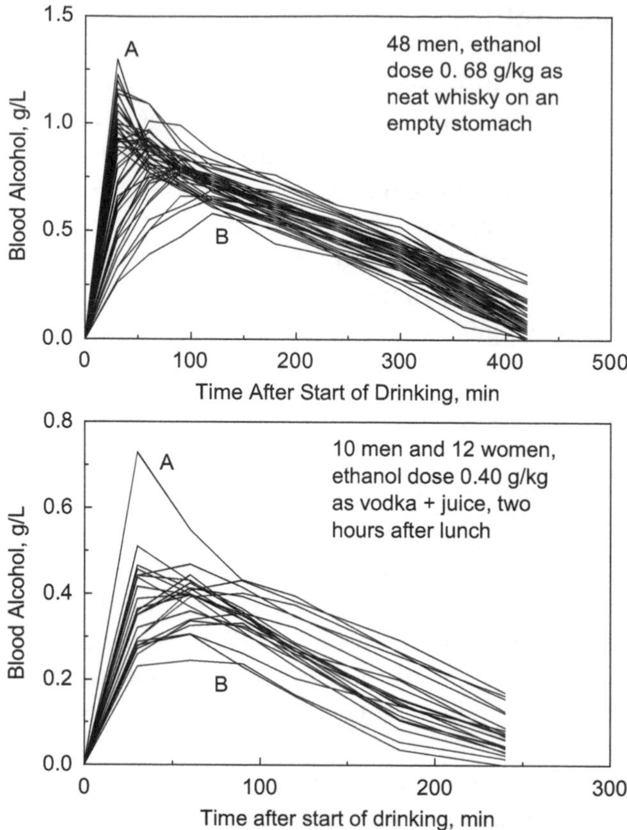

Figure 8.9 Inter-subject variation in blood-ethanol profiles for two drinking scenarios. The upper plot represents BAC curves in healthy men after they drank neat whisky on an empty stomach (n = 48 subjects). The lower plot shows BAC curves after a dose of 0.4 g/kg was ingested as pure ethanol (95% v/v) diluted with orange juice to ~20% v/v ~2 hours after eating lunch (n = 22 subjects, 10 men and 12 women).

This confirmed the results from an older drinking experiment when three volunteers drank the same dose of ethanol (0.50 g/kg) on ten occasions (Schonheyder et al. 1942). These observations speak against conducting drinking experiments in an attempt to reproduce blood-alcohol curves that might have existed in a drunken driver after the event. It is more prudent to work with a population average value of 0.15 g/L/h and a range from 0.10 g/L/h to 0.25 g/L/h, which should be appropriate for most individuals (Jones 2010).

8.3.2 Dose–Response Relationships

The relationship between dose of a drug and the pharmacokinetic or pharmacodynamic response is a cornerstone of pharmacology and therapeutics. In practice such studies are restricted in terms of the quantities (doses) that can safely and ethically be administered to human volunteers. Accordingly, in the many controlled drinking experiments the peak BAC is appreciably lower than the BAC observed in cases of acute alcohol poisonings and alcohol impaired drivers (Jones and Holmgren 2009b).

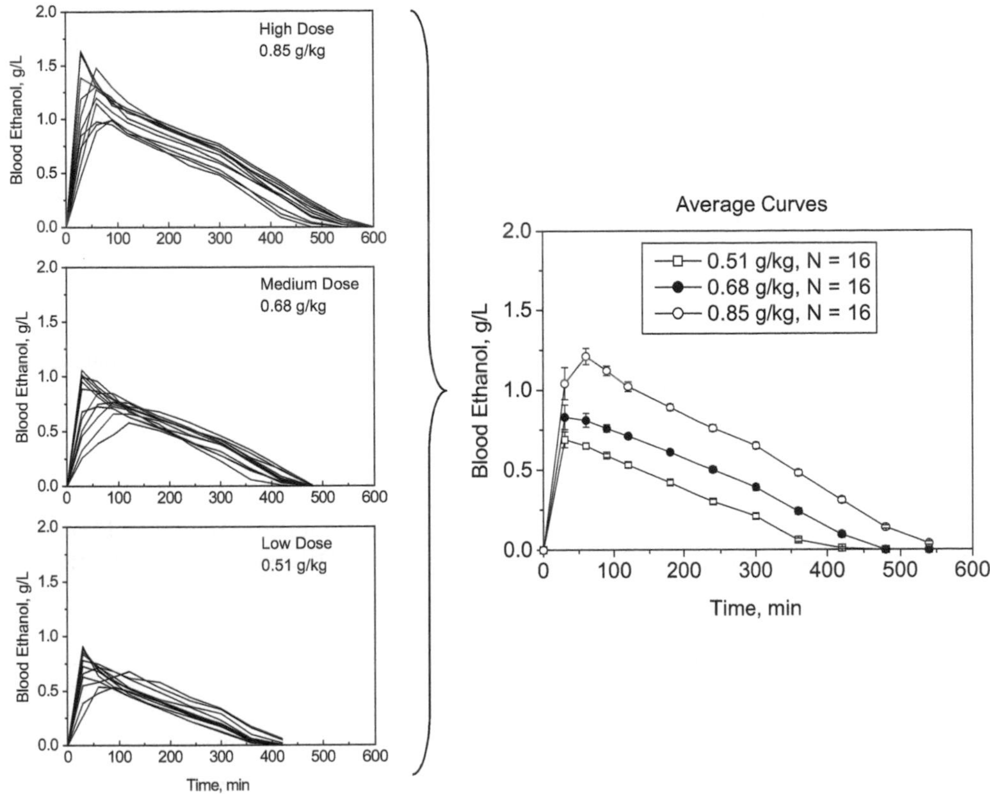

Figure 8.10 Inter-individual variations in blood-alcohol curves in 16 healthy men after they drank neat whisky on an empty stomach as three doses of ethanol (0.51, 0.68 or 0.85 g/kg). Also shown are the average BAC curves (± SD) for these same drinking conditions.

Figure 8.10 shows BAC curves in 16 male subjects who drank 0.51 g/kg, 0.68 g/kg or 0.85 g/kg ethanol as neat whisky at 9.00 am after an overnight fast. The inter-subject variations in BAC profiles are seen at each of the ethanol doses in the left part of the graph. An obvious increase in C_{max}, C_0, and AUC occurs with increasing ethanol dose as shown by the mean BAC curves (right part). When higher doses of ethanol were consumed (1.05 g/kg) as neat spirits in a drinking time of 30 minutes, some subjects experienced nausea and vomited and the experiment was stopped.

The pharmacokinetic parameters of ethanol from dose–response studies are presented in Tables 8.11 and 8.12. Both mean C_{max} and C_0 increased almost linearly with increasing dose of ethanol as might be expected (Table 8.11). However, the rate of elimination of ethanol from blood (β-slope) increased only slightly from 0.11 to 0.15 g/L/h with increasing ethanol dose, although a considerable overlap was found within each dosage interval. The distribution volume of ethanol (V_d or rho factor), depends primarily on a person's gender and body composition (fat:lean tissue) and was not influenced by the dose of ethanol administered.

Figure 8.11 shows the variation in C_{max} after subjects ingested four doses of ethanol as neat whisky on an empty stomach. Although the mean value of C_{max} increased with an increasing dose of ethanol ingested, there was a considerable overlap between the four doses.

Table 8.11 Dose–Response Study of Pharmacokinetic Parameters of Ethanol in Healthy Men after They Drank Neat Whisky on an Empty Stomach (10 h fast) in 15–25 minutes

Ethanol Dose, g/kg	n[a]	C_{max} g/L	t_{max} min[b] Mean (range)	β-slope g/L/h	C_0 g/L	V_d or Rho L/kg
0.51	16	0.75 ± 0.12	26 (10–100)	0.11 ± 0.01	0.75 ± 0.08	0.68 ± 0.06
0.68	16	0.91 ± 0.20	34 (10–100)	0.13 ± 0.02	0.98 ± 0.08	0.69 ± 0.05
0.85	16	1.31 ± 0.24[c]	31 (5–65)	0.15 ± 0.01[c]	1.34 ± 0.12[c]	0.64 ± 0.06[d]

Source: Jones, unpublished.

[a] n = number of drinking subjects per dose of ethanol.

[b] Timed from end of drinking.

[c] Statistically significant differences in C_{max}, β-slope and C_0 in relation to dose by analysis of variance.

[d] No statistically significant differences in V_d in relation to dose.

Table 8.12 Dose–Response Study of Pharmacokinetic Parameters of Ethanol in Healthy Men after They Drank Increasing Doses of Ethanol (94 vol%) Diluted to 30 % w/v with Water on an Empty Stomach (12 h fast) in ~5 min

Ethanol Dose, g/kg	n[a]	C_{max} g/L[b] (range)	t_{max} min[c] Mean (range)	β-slope g/L/h (range)	C_0 g/L (range)	V_d or Rho in L/kg (range)
0.25	12	0.54–0.89	48 (30–90)	0.095–0.148	0.57–0.86	0.58–0.75
0.75	31	0.68–1.28	53 (30–120)	0.084–0.222	0.96–1.51	0.49–0.78
1.0	33	1.00–2.02	76 (15–180)	0.105–0.243	1.18–1.93	0.52–0.84
1.25	33	1.30–2.30	84 (15–180)	0.074–0.190	1.59–2.28	0.55–0.79

Source: Alha, A., *Ann Acad Sci Fenn* A 26, 1, 1951.

[a] n = number of drinking subjects per dose of ethanol.

[b] Blood alcohol concentration was reported as g/kg (mass/mass) in the original article but converted to g/L in the table assuming density of whole blood was 1.055 g/mL, hence 1.0 g/kg = 0.948 g/L.

[c] Timed from end of drinking.

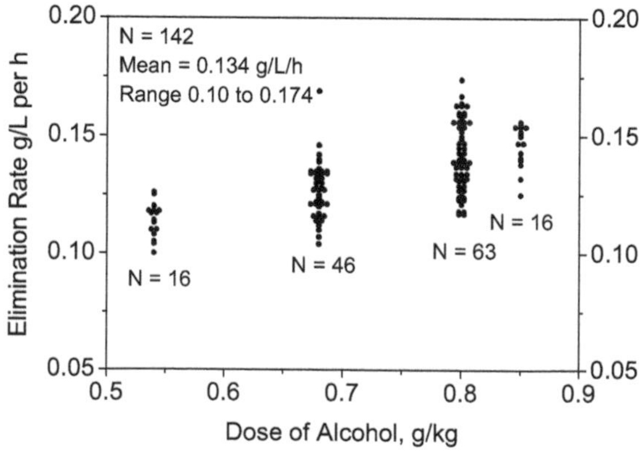

Figure 8.11 Scatter plots showing inter-individual variations in ethanol elimination rates from blood (β-slopes) after healthy men drank increasing doses of ethanol on an empty stomach.

The results of another dose–response study of ethanol pharmacokinetics involving 0.50 g/kg, 0.75 g/kg, 1.0 g/kg and 1.25 g/kg ethanol ingested as a 30% w/v solution in water within a drinking time of 5 minutes on an empty stomach (12-hour fast) are shown in Table 8.12. The pharmacokinetic parameters are shown as the range of values for each dose of ethanol consumed and there is clearly a considerable overlap for each dose ingested. The BACs in the original study were reported in mass/mass units, but converted in Table 8.12 to mass/volume units taking the density of blood as 1.055 g/mL (Alha 1951; Lenter 1981).

8.3.3 Intravenous Administration

In forensic science and toxicology alcoholic beverages are taken by mouth (oral ingestion) and ethanol contained in the drinks reach the systemic circulation after absorption from the gut. However, in some situations ethanol (8%–10% v/v) might be administered by intravenous infusion, such as in emergency medicine when patients are treated with ethanol as an antidote against methanol or ethylene glycol poisoning (Brent 2009). After the intravenous route of administration the bioavailability of ethanol is 100% because any first-pass metabolism that might occur in the liver or the gastric mucosa is avoided (Ammon et al. 1996; Cobaugh et al. 1999; Lisander et al. 2006; Shoaf 2000). The ratios of AUC for C-T profiles of drugs after oral and intravenous routes of administration provides basic information about the bioavailability of ethanol and other drugs.

Figure 8.12 depicts a blood-alcohol curve in one subject after a small dose of ethanol (0.4 g/kg) was given by constant rate intravenous infusion over 30 minutes. C_{max} occurred at the time the infusion pump was stopped and immediately after there was an abrupt decline in BAC, corresponding to a diffusion plunge as ethanol re-distributes between

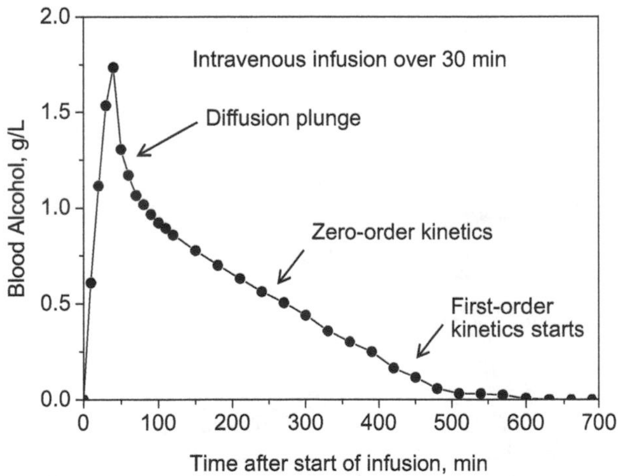

Figure 8.12 Example of a blood-alcohol curve when ethanol (0.6 g/kg) was administered by constant rate intravenous infusion over 30 minutes. Ethanol was given as a 10% v/v solution in isotonic saline and samples of venous blood were taken via an indwelling catheter at 5–10 minutes intervals during and after starting the infusion pump. The BAC curve shows an overshoot peak representing C_{max} followed by a diffusion plunge and then a rectilinear elimination phase (zero-order kinetics) until reaching a BAC of 0.1–0.2 g/L which marked the transition from zero-order to first-order kinetics.

the bloodstream and other body tissues and fluids. This re-distribution requires about 60 minutes after the infusion ended, because the half-life of the diffusion plunge after a rapid intravenous infusion was 10 minutes (Hahn et al. 1995).

Marked on the graph in Figure 8.12 is the transition point when the zero-order kinetics changes to first-order kinetics. The BAC curve in the entire elimination phase looks more like a hockey-stick rather than a straight line. This change over occurs as BAC drops below about 0.15–0.20 g/L when the ADH enzymes are no longer saturated with substrate. Below this concentration, the C-T profile is curvilinear and ethanol is elimination by first-order kinetics (see later). The intravenous route of administration avoids problems caused by variable gastric emptying, and any first-pass metabolism.

Figure 8.13 shows BAC curves after eight subjects received 0.3 g/kg ethanol by constant rate intravenous (i.v.) infusion over 30 minutes. The BAC curves showed inter-subject variations even when the ethanol was administered by i.v. infusion, which is probably related to different body composition, such as fat to lean tissue variations, because the dose of ethanol was administered per kg of body weight and not per kg of body water or lean body mass. After stopping the infusion pump the BAC curves decreased rapidly (diffusion plunge) and they might be influenced by muscular activity of the subjects or variations in blood flow to tissues or individual differences in hepatic enzyme activity.

8.3.4 Arterio-Venous Differences

Blood-ethanol concentration depends to some extent on where in the vascular system the sample is taken from, whether an artery, a capillary or a vein (Sedman et al. 1976). Studies have shown that arterial blood concentrations (A-BAC) are higher during the absorption phase of the BAC curve and the venous blood concentrations (V-BAC) are higher in the post-absorptive period (Martin et al. 1984; Wilkinson and Rheingold 1981). Some of the ingested ethanol gets taken up by tissue water, during each circulation of the blood, and

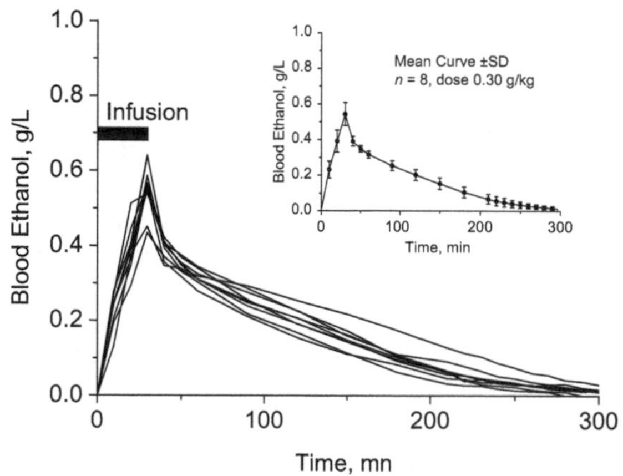

Figure 8.13 Inter-individual variations in concentration-time (C-T) profiles of ethanol after a dose of 0.30 g/kg was given by constant rate intravenous infusion. Intravenous administration removes any uncertainty about rate of gastric emptying, but C-T profiles still exhibit variations. The insert graph plots the changes in mean BAC (± SD) in relation to time after administration of ethanol.

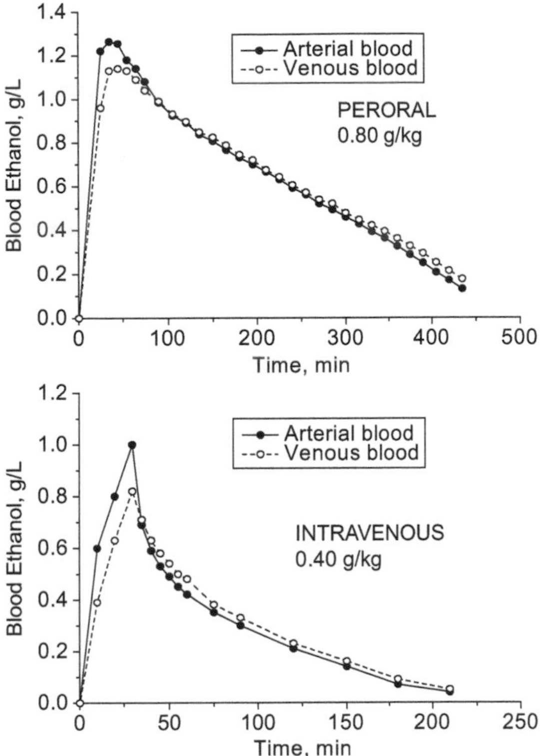

Figure 8.14 Concentration-time curves of alcohol in arterial (radial artery) and venous (cubital vein) blood after one male volunteer drank 0.8 g/kg ethanol (upper plot) or when a smaller dose (0.4 g/kg, 10% v/v) was given by intravenous infusion (lower plot) over 30 minutes.

initially muscle tissue is alcohol-free but holds a lot of water (Levitt 2004; Mather 2001). Accordingly, C-T profiles and some pharmacokinetic parameters will depend on whether arterial or venous blood was used to plot C-T profiles for pharmacokinetic analysis.

Figure 8.14 compares BAC profiles in blood from a radial artery and a cubital vein in two subjects after oral ingestion of alcohol (0.80 g/kg) and intravenous infusion (0.40 g/kg) of a smaller dose (Jones et al. 1997, 2004). The time allowed for drinking and infusion was 30 minutes. The BAC profiles are obviously different depending on the sampling site in the vascular system. During absorption from the gut or during infusion the A-BAC > V-BAC, whereas V-BAC > A-BAC during the post-absorptive period.

After oral ingestion A-V differences in concentration were maximum at the time the first blood sample was taken just 5 minutes post-dosing (Jones et al. 2004). Thereafter A-V difference decreased gradually as the time after drinking increased so by about 90 minutes post-dosing the A-V difference was zero. This marks the start of the post-absorptive phase of ethanol kinetics and at all later times the concentration of ethanol in venous blood was higher than in the arterial blood, owing to blood returning from peripheral tissues and metabolism occurring in the central liver compartment.

The temporal variations in A-V difference are illustrated in Figure 8.15 plotting A-V differences against time after the start of ethanol administration.

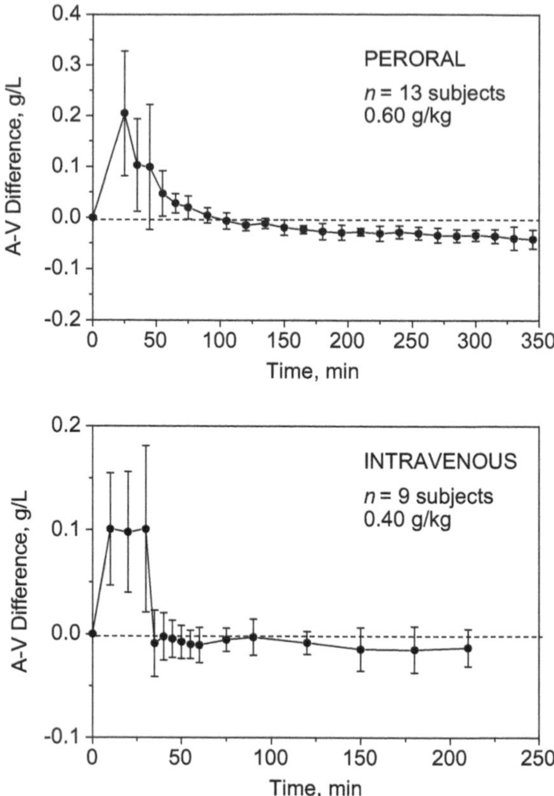

Figure 8.15 Temporal variations in arterial-venous differences in concentration of ethanol (mean ± SD) after subjects drank 0.6 g/kg ethanol (upper part) or when a smaller dose (0.4 g/kg) was given by intravenous infusion over 30 minutes (lower plot).

When ethanol was given as a constant rate intravenous infusion instead of by mouth an A-V difference was established almost immediately and remained constant (~0.1 g/L) during the infusion period (Jones and Andersson 2003). Within 5 minutes of stopping the infusion pump the A-V difference was abolished and at all later sampling times the concentration in venous blood exceed that in the arterial blood (negative A-V difference). The pharmacokinetic parameters of ethanol C_{max}, t_{max} and β-slope were slightly different when derived from analysis of venous or arterial blood as shown in Table 8.13.

Table 8.13 Comparison of Pharmacokinetic Parameters of Ethanol Derived from Arterial and Venous Blood-alcohol Curves after Healthy Men (n = 9) Drank 0.6 g Ethanol per kg Body Weight in 15 min

Blood Source	C_{max} g/L	t_{max} min Mean (median)	β-slope g/L/h	C_0 g/L	Rho Factor, V_d L/kg
Radial artery	0.98 ± 0.21	38 (35)	0.12 ± 0.017	0.75 ± 0.007	0.80 ± 0.084
Cubital vein	0.84 ± 0.18[a]	42 (35)	0.11 ± 0.019	0.75 ± 0.008	0.81 ± 0.099

Source: Jones, A.W. et al., *Clin Pharmacokinet* 43, 1157, 2004.

[a] Difference in mean arterial and venous blood alcohol concentration was statistically significant.

The existence of an A-V difference deserves consideration when results of breath-alcohol analysis are compared with venous BAC (Lindberg et al. 2007; Martin et al. 1984). The BrAC time course follows more closely the time course of arterial BAC rather than venous BAC, which means that temporal variations in A-V differences makes venous BAC/BrAC ratios about 1800:1 at 30 minutes after end of drinking increasing to 2100:1 by 60 minutes and being closer to 2300:1 or 2400:1 in the post-absorptive phase. When very low BACs are reached (<0.2 g/L) the venous BAC/BrAC ratio might exceed 3000:1, because arterial BAC reaches zero before venous BAC. In a controlled study of repetitive analysis of ethanol in breath, arterial and venous blood for up to 8 hours post-dosing, the arterial BAC/BrAC ratio was more or less constant during the absorption, distribution and elimination phases of ethanol kinetics (Lindberg et al. 2007).

8.3.5 Real-World Drinking Conditions

Most studies of the ADME of ethanol have involved the administration of moderate amounts of the drug as a bolus dose on an empty stomach, which is far removed from the real world, when people drink repetitively over several hours. In social situations people consume alcohol as beer, wine or spirits often together with food or snacks during social intercourse in pleasant surroundings. Limited information exists in the literature about shapes of BAC curves and the pharmacokinetics of ethanol under realistic social drinking conditions.

One notable exception was a drinking experiment done in Germany (Zink and Reinhardt 1984) in which the volunteers were allowed to drink massive amounts of alcohol more or less continuously for up to 10 hours. The BAC profiles were established unequivocally by frequent sampling and analysis of venous blood taken from an indwelling catheter at 15-minute intervals during and after drinking ended. The raw C-T data were available and used to re-evaluate the BAC curves and perform another pharmacokinetic evaluation (Jones et al. 2006). The BAC plots for four of the volunteers are shown in Figure 8.16.

Healthy male volunteers accustomed to heavy drinking were given alcoholic beverage of their choice, in the company of a girlfriend or spouse, and engaged in continuous drinking lasting 5–10 hours. The BAC curves rose continuously during the drinking to reach very high peak values, similar to those observed in forensic casework. In some of the subjects the peak BAC occurred even before the last drink was finished. It seems likely that so much alcohol was already absorbed and distributed in body fluids and tissues, that the amount contained in the last drink was not sufficient to increase the BAC any further.

Large discrepancies were found between the observed peak BAC and the expected BAC based on the Widmark equation and the total amount of ethanol consumed, the drinker's body weight and volume of distribution. The actual BAC was appreciably less than expected after assuming complete absorption and distribution of the entire dose. It is an open question what actually happened to the "missing alcohol" but most likely there was an appreciable first-pass metabolism or a more rapid metabolism taking place during the drinking period.

The rate of elimination from blood when derived from C-T points on the post-peak parts of the curves was in the range expected for moderate drinking, namely from 0.15 to 0.25 g/L/h (see Figure 8.16). The study by Zink and Reinhardt is unique to the forensic blood-alcohol literature and will probably never be duplicated considering the massive quantities of alcohol consumed by the volunteers.

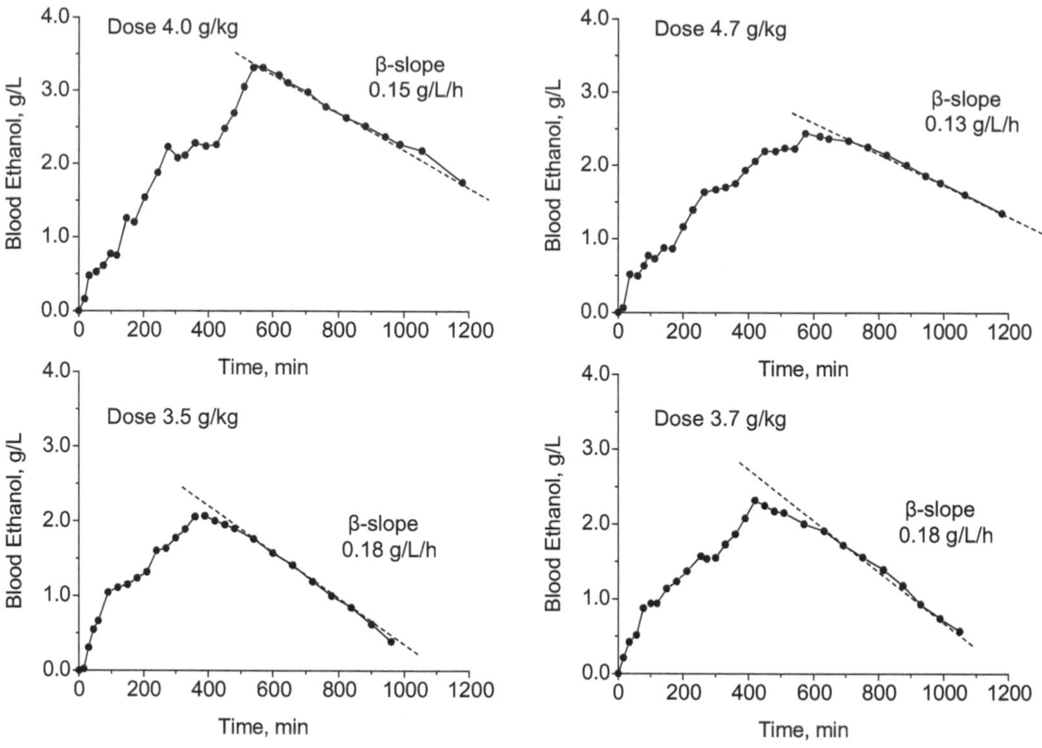

Figure 8.16 Blood-alcohol curves in four subjects after they drank massive amounts of ethanol under real-world conditions (Zink and Reinhardt 1984). The BAC rises steadily during the 8–12 hour drinking session before reaching a peak concentration (C_{max}) and then entering a post-absorptive elimination phase showing β-slopes calculated in the usual way.

8.3.6 Alcohol Clamp Experiments

Another approach to investigate ethanol pharmacokinetic involves use of a so-called alcohol clamp experiment (Ramchandani and O'Connor 2006; Ramchandani et al. 2006). This entails administrating a priming dose of ethanol by intravenous infusion to reach a pre-determined concentration in blood and then maintaining this concentration over several hours by infusion of ethanol in amounts that balance the losses through metabolism in the liver. In this type of experiment, the steady state concentration in blood is monitored by repetitive analysis of ethanol content in the exhaled air (Zoethout et al. 2008).

An example of the BAC profile obtained using the alcohol-clamp technique is depicted in Figure 8.17.

A good rule of thumb for the rate of infusion of ethanol to maintain a steady-state concentration in blood for a moderate drinker is 0.1 g/kg/h or 7 g per hour for a person with a body weight of 70 kg. Quantitative breath-alcohol instruments are ideal for use in alcohol-clamp experiments because they are non-invasive and give immediate feed-back about the arterial BAC allowing adjustments to the infusion. Using the alcohol-clamp method, various factors that influence metabolism of ethanol, such as eating a meal, can be investigated without the confounding influence of unpredictable rates of absorption from the gut and first-pass metabolism in the gastric mucosa or the liver (Ramchandani et al. 2001).

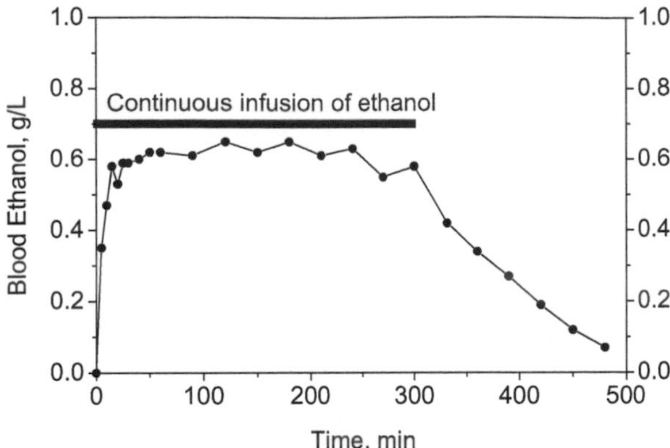

Figure 8.17 Example of the shape of a blood-alcohol curve during an alcohol-clamp experiment involving a priming dose of ethanol followed by constant rate infusion (~0.1 g/kg/h) to balance the ethanol cleared from the bloodstream through metabolism and excretion. (This trace was re-drawn from Zoethout, R.W. et al., *Br. J. Clin. Pharmacol.*, 66, 674, 2008.)

An alcohol-clamp experiment was used to study the effect of nutrients on the rate of ethanol metabolism. After reaching a steady-state concentration in breath the subjects ate a meal of known composition with differing proportions of fats, proteins or carbohydrates (Rogers et al. 1987). During and after eating the meal, the infusion rate of ethanol needed to be increased to maintain the same steady-state BAC, which suggests a food-induced acceleration in metabolism of ethanol. On stopping the infusion pump the rate of elimination of ethanol from blood can be determined in the usual way from C-T data points and linear regression analysis.

8.4 The Widmark Equation and Its Applications

When various blood-alcohol calculations are required in forensic science and legal medicine casework the traditional and the most well-proven approach is to make use of the Widmark equation or some minor modification thereof. This assumes a one-compartment pharmacokinetic model with zero-order elimination rate from blood provided BAC exceeds 0.20 g/L. Below this BAC the metabolizing enzymes are no longer fully saturated with substrate, which marks a transition over to first-order kinetics.

8.4.1 Basic Principles

From knowledge of chemical kinetics and reaction order, the rate equation for a zero-order process is given by the following differential equation:

$$-dC / dT = kC^0$$

This simplifies to $-dC/dT = k$, because $C^0 = 1$.

Integration of the above between the limits of C_0 and C_t and rearranging gives:

$$C_t = C_0 - \beta t$$

The coefficient β in this equation is the zero-order elimination rate constant that defines the linear decrease in concentration of ethanol in blood per unit time, such as g/L/h or g% per h depending on units used to report BAC. With drugs eliminated by zero-order kinetics the concept of elimination half-life ($t_{½}$) is not a very useful parameter, because it changes with the starting concentration. Replacing C_t in the above equation with $C_0/2$ and rearranging gives $t_{½} = C_0/2\beta$, which shows that $t_{½}$ is inversely proportional to the zero-order slope and directly proportional to the starting BAC or C_0.

For drugs metabolized by first-order kinetics $t_{½}$ is independent of dose and represents the time necessary for the concentration in blood or plasma, as well as the amount of drug in the body, to decrease by one half or 50%. In practice ~97% of a drug is eliminated from the body during a time corresponding to five half-lives.

The C_0 parameter in Figure 8.1 (y-intercept) represents the BAC reached if the entire dose of ethanol had been absorbed and distributed instantaneously into all body fluids and tissues without any metabolism or excretion occurring. Accordingly, the value of C_0 is higher than the value obtained by dividing the amount ingested (A) by the person's body weight in kilograms (A/kg). Ethanol distributes into all body fluids and tissues according to their relative water contents and blood-water is 78%–82% w/w, whereas total body water corresponds to 50%–60% of body weight.

The amount of alcohol absorbed and distributed in the body is easy to calculate from the concentration determined in blood using the Widmark equation and the important parameter referred to as the rho factor. This factor is multiplied by the person's body weight (kg) to give the reduced body mass (*die reduzierte Körpermasse*) as defined by Widmark, which represents the fraction of the body in which the drug is dissolved to give the same concentration as in the blood.

$$\text{BAC}\left(C_0\right) = \text{A}/\left(\text{kg} \times \text{rho}\right)$$

$$\text{A} = C_0 \times \text{kg} \times \text{rho}$$

Because ethanol mixes with total body water without binding to plasma protein the rho factor is related to the distribution of water between the blood and the rest of the body water.

$$\text{Rho factor} = \left(\text{alcohol in body}\right)/\left(\text{alcohol in blood}\right)$$

$$\text{Rho factor} = \left(\text{water in body}\right)/\left(\text{water in blood}\right).$$

The elimination rate of alcohol from the entire body, sometimes denoted B_{60}, is obtained by dividing the dose (g/kg) by the extrapolated time to reach zero BAC (min_0) as shown in Figure 8.1. The resulting value is usually reported as g/h or g/kg/h and agrees with the result obtained as the product of $\beta \times \text{rho} \times \text{body weight}$.

The main sources of uncertainty in the Widmark equation are the values of β and rho factors for the individual compared with reference values, usually taken as rho = 0.7 for non-obese men and 0.6 for women. Moreover, spurious results of such calculations are obtained if blood sampling is done before absorption and distribution of ethanol in all body fluids is complete. Any alcohol remaining unabsorbed in the stomach is not contributing to the BAC so the Widmark equation tends to overestimate the actual BAC. Moreover, if some of the ingested ethanol happens to undergo first-pass metabolism in the gastric mucosa or the liver this lower bioavailability skews the calculation of the rho factor as dose (g/kg)/C_0. Ideally, the dose of ethanol should be administered by intravenous infusion (100% bioavailability) when the rho factor or distribution volume is calculated.

8.4.2 Forensic Alcohol Calculations

The Widmark formula has four principal applications in forensic science and legal medicine:

- To estimate the amount of alcohol absorbed and distributed in all body fluids and tissues from the concentration determined in a sample of blood.
- To make a back extrapolation of a person's blood alcohol concentration from time of sampling blood to some earlier time, such as the time of driving.
- To estimate the total amount of alcohol a person has consumed after starting to drink until the time a blood sample was taken for analysis.
- To estimate the blood-alcohol concentration expected after drinking known quantities of ethanol, thus making a forward prediction of the BAC based on a given drinking scenario.

8.4.3 Amount of Alcohol in the Body

The Widmark equation is widely used to calculate the amount of alcohol absorbed and distributed in all body fluids and tissues from the concentration determined in a sample of blood as follows:

$$A = C_t \times \text{weight}\,(\text{kg}) \times \text{rho}$$

where A is the amount of ethanol in grams absorbed and distributed in the blood and all body fluids, C_t is the concentration of ethanol determined in a blood sample (mg/g or g/kg), weight is the body weight in kg and rho is the distribution factor for ethanol between the entire body and the blood. As discussed earlier, the value of the rho factor depends on age, gender and the individual's body composition especially degree of fat to lean body mass.

If there is any alcohol remaining unabsorbed in the stomach when the blood sample was taken it does not contribute to the BAC. For best results, this calculation should not be made until at least 90 minutes have elapsed after the last drink. Neither does the Widmark equation consider any pre-systemic metabolism that might occur in the stomach or the liver or both organs.

8.4.4 Amount of Alcohol Consumed

The Widmark equation ($C_t = C_0 - \beta t$) represents the elimination of alcohol from blood during the post-absorptive phase and is usually combined with the formula for the amount of alcohol in the body ($A = C_0 \times \text{kg} \times \text{rho}$) by eliminating C_0. This gives a useful formula that allows the total amount of alcohol consumed (A) to be calculated since starting to drink until the time of sampling blood.

$$A = kg \times rho \times (C_t + \beta t)$$

The above equation gives reliable estimates provided that the ethanol is ingested as a bolus dose on an empty stomach and blood samples are taken later than 90 minutes after end of drinking, so that alcohol is fully absorbed in all body fluids and tissues (Gullberg and Jones 1994; Wagner et al. 1990).

Similarly, an equation can be derived to allow calculating the BAC (C_t) expected after drinking a known quantity of alcohol (A):

$$C_t = A/(kg \times rho) - (\beta t)$$

The major source of uncertainty in both these equations derives from the parameters β and rho in relation to the values for a specific individual, which in practice is not known. A total uncertainty budget for use of the Widmark equation was published by Gullberg and was from 25% to 42% (2 × CV) depending on the question posed, whether the aim was to calculate the number of drinks consumed or the amount of alcohol in the body (Gullberg 2007).

The elimination rate of alcohol from the entire body averages about 0.1 g/kg body weight per hour corresponding to 7 g per hour for a person weighing 70 kg. This B_{60} parameter was found to be independent of gender because a lower rho factor in women is compensated by the slightly faster rate of elimination from blood (β) in females, so turnover rate or the product of β and rho is about the same for both sexes.

The total amount of alcohol consumed is easily derived from the BAC by first calculating the amount of ethanol in the body at the time of sampling blood ($A = C_t \times kg \times rho$) and then adding on the amount eliminated since the time of starting to drink (0.1 g/kg/h). This gives the grams of 100% ethanol, which if required can be converted into the number of drinks consumed, whether beer, wine or spirits depending on their alcohol content. Note that concentrations of alcohol in alcoholic beverages are expressed as % v/v, which needs to be converted to % w/v by multiplying by the density of ethanol 0.79 g/mL. Accordingly whisky, 40% (v/v); wine, 12% (v/v); and beer, 5% (v/v) correspond to 31.6% (w/v), 9.5% (w/v), and 4.0% (w/v), respectively.

8.4.5 Updating the Widmark Equation

The rho factor depends on a person's age, gender and body composition and was first determined in the 1930s in health volunteers, aged 19–40 years old, as the drinking subjects (20 men and 10 women). Body composition has changed over the years and in today's society there is a higher prevalence of obesity. This warrants re-consideration of the most appropriate rho factor to use when blood-alcohol calculations are requested for forensic purposes.

The question of altered body composition prompted Watson, Watson, and Batt (Watson et al. 1981) to update the Widmark equation. They did this by establishing a multiple regression equation with TBW as outcome variable and a person's age, height and weight as predictor variables. TBW was determined by isotope dilution and regressed on anthropometric measurements (age, height and weight) for a large population of healthy subjects (458 men and 265 women). These equations and the associated residual standard deviations for men and women and are given below:

$$\text{For man: TBW}\left(\text{L}\right) = 2.447 - 0.09516\ \text{age}\left(\text{y}\right) + 0.1074\ \text{height}\left(\text{cm}\right) + 0.3362\ \text{weight}\left(\text{kg}\right)$$

Residual standard deviation 3.78 L

$$\text{For woman: TBW}\left(\text{L}\right) = -2.097 + 0.1069\ \text{height}\left(\text{cm}\right) + 0.2466\ \text{weight}\left(\text{kg}\right)$$

Residual standard deviation 3.60 L

The TBW in liters derived from these equations is converted to percent of the person's body weight and then divided by the percent water in whole blood to give a subject-specific rho factor. The percentage water in blood varies little between individuals, although average values are slightly higher in women than in men because of gender differences in hematocrit value, being lower in women on average. Use of the above TBW equations to determine the rho factor gave results in good agreement with the values determined in controlled drinking experiments (Maskell et al. 2019).

Seidel et al. (2000) determined water content of blood in 256 women and 273 men by heating a portion to dryness and found mean ± SD (range) of 79.5% ± 0.97% (77%–82.8%) for women and 78.0% ± 1.14% (73.3%–87.7%) for men. These percentages are in % w/w and should be multiplied by the density of blood (1.055 g/mL) to give the water content in units of mass/volume; 83.9% (w/v) for women and 82.3% (w/v) for men on average.

$$V_d = \left(\%\ \text{water in body}\right) / \left(\%\ \text{water in blood}\right)$$

$$V_d = \left(\text{TBW/kg}\right) / 0.839\ \text{for women}$$

$$V_d = \left(\text{TBW/kg}\right) / 0.823\ \text{for men}$$

If an estimate of uncertainty in the calculation of TBW by the Watson, Watson, and Batt method is needed, this is given by ± (2 × SD), which represents a 95% range of values.

8.4.6 Other Updates

A vast body of literature on forensic aspects of alcohol is published in German language journals, such as *Blutalkohol* and *Zeitskrift für Rechtsmedizin*, which unfortunately is not widely appreciated or cited (Jones et al. 2006). A study by Seidel et al. (2000) was an attempt to update the Widmark equation and TBW was determined by a non-invasive bioelectrical impedance method in 273 men and 256 women. Accordingly, values of the rho factor (V_d) could be tailored to the height and weight of that specific individual; values for men (r_m) and women (r_w) are given by the equations below:

$$\text{Rho factor } r_m = 0.31608 - 0.004821 \text{ weight (kg)} + 0.004632 \text{ height (cm)}$$

$$\text{Rho factor } r_w = 0.31223 - 0.006446 \text{ weight (kg)} + 0.004466 \text{ height (cm)}$$

Drinking experiments were then performed in 30 women and 39 men to test the validity of the above equations showing a better agreement compared with average values derived by Widmark in the 1930s; rho = 0.68 for males and 0.55 for females.

Another useful update of the Widmark rho involved a consideration of the person's BMI (kg/m^2) and percent fat content of the body. Information is usually available to calculate a person's BMI and percentage of body weight composed of fat-free mass and fat as a percentage of body weight from tables of body composition and various nomograms. This information can be used to calculate a subject-specific rho factor for use in blood-alcohol calculations (Barbour 2001; Forrest 1986). In a controlled drinking experiment with male and female subjects of widely different BMI (16.0–35.9 kg/m^2), there was a strong negative correlation ($r = 0.78$ for females and $r = 0.66$ for males) between rho-factors from drinking experiments and the person's BMI (Maudens et al. 2014). The following equations were proposed as a way to estimate the rho factor from knowledge of the person's age, weight and BMI;

$$\text{Males (L/kg) rho factor } (V_d) = 0.8202 - 0.0090 \text{ BMI}$$

$$\text{Females (L/kg) rho factor } (V_d) = 0.7772 - 0.0099 \text{ BMI}$$

8.4.7 Retrograde Extrapolation

In some jurisdictions the prosecution of traffic offenders requires knowledge of the BAC existing at the time of driving, whereas blood (or breath) samples for alcohol analysis are usually obtained 1–2 hours later. This raises the tricky question of making a back-calculation of the person's BAC from the time of sampling blood to the time of driving, a process known as retrograde extrapolation or back calculation or simply back-tracking (Lewis 1986, 1987; Montgomery and Reasor 1992).

Other jurisdictions enforce a so-called 2- or 3-hour rule, which means that the measured BAC or BrAC is accepted as being not less than the measured values provided the samples were taken within 2 or 3 hours of the time of driving. If the blood sample, for some reason, was obtained outside this window, then the result would need to be calculated back to the recorded time of driving or traffic violation. Several important questions arise when back extrapolations are performed in criminal cases.

1. First, was any alcohol consumed after driving and before the blood or breath sample was taken, which if so must be considered and allowed for before a back calculation was done.
2. Second, the starting BAC should be the value after a deduction made for uncertainty in the analytical method used (random and systematic errors).
3. Third, a range of elimination rates of ethanol from blood should be used in the back calculation, such as a mean of 0.15 g/L/h and a range from 0.10 to 0.25 g/L/h. In apprehended drivers the mean elimination rate of alcohol was 0.19 g/L/h although in criminal cases to give a suspect the benefit it is common to work with a low elimination rate, such as 0.1 g/L/h.
4. Fourth, the BAC curve should be in the post-absorptive phase of the alcohol curve at the time of driving and at the time blood or breath were sampled. This assumption requires a careful consideration about the pattern of drinking including time of last drink and amount of ethanol it contained. Depending on available information some type of allowance might be necessary to adjust for contribution of ethanol in the last drink or existence of a BAC plateau if ethanol was consumed with food.

The rate of absorption of alcohol from the gut is highly variable making it uncertain whether a driver was in the post-peak phase of the BAC curve at the time of driving and at the time of blood sampling (Jackson et al. 1991). Experience has shown that the vast majority of people reach their peak BAC within 60 minutes after end of drinking a bolus dose. This time might be considerably shorter under real-world conditions with repetitive intake and when the last drink contained 12–14 g ethanol (Dufour 1999).

Assuming the person's BAC was in the post-peak phase at the time of driving and at the time of sampling blood then a backward extrapolation is a simple mathematical exercise as shown below:

$$C_1 = C_0 - (\beta \times t_1)$$

$$C_2 = C_0 - (\beta \times t_2)$$

In these equations, C_1 and C_2 are concentrations of alcohol in blood at sampling times of t_1 and t_2 on the declining phase of the BAC curve. Subtracting the two equations gives a general equation useful for retrograde extrapolation of BAC:

$$C_1 - C_2 = \beta \times (t_2 - t_1)$$

This equation simplifies to: $C_1 = C_2 + (\beta \times t_d)$ where C_1 is the BAC at the time of an offence, C_2 is BAC at time of sampling blood and td is the time difference in hours and β is the rate of elimination of alcohol from blood in g/L/h.

If time of driving was 90 minutes or more after the end of drinking it is safe to assume that a post-peak elimination phase had been reached. Under these circumstances making a back extrapolation is a simple matter as shown by the following example.

A road traffic crash (RTC) occurred at 2.00 am. The driver of the car was injured and a passenger was killed. A blood sample for ethanol analysis was obtained from the driver at 5.00 am, which showed an ethanol concentration of 0.30 g/L after making a deduction for analytical error (uncertainty). The police wanted to know whether the driver was above the statutory limit for driving (0.50 g/L) at the time of the crash, which was three hours before taking the blood sample. Investigations made by the police and statements from witnesses revealed that the driver had been drinking alcohol between 10.00 and 12:30 am. The last drink was finished at 12.30 am before driving home at 1.00 am.

Social drinking over a time of 2½ h (10–12.30) makes it reasonable to assume that ingested alcohol was absorbed and distributed in all body fluids and tissues by the time of the crash, which was 90 min after end of drinking. This supports the assumption of a post-absorptive BAC at time of the RTC (2.00 am) as well as at the time of sampling blood (5.00 am). Back calculation for three hours, assuming a low elimination rate of 0.1 g/L/h, shows that the driver's BAC at the time of the crash was at least 0.60 g/L (0.30 g/L + 0.10 g/L/h × 3), thus over the statutory limit for driving.

The highest court in Germany ratified back-calculations of BAC in drunk-driving cases to within 2 hours after the end of drinking if no information was available about the pattern of drinking and the amounts of alcohol consumed in the last drink. Accordingly, if a blood sample was taken 4 hours after the last drink the measured BAC could be back extrapolated for 2 hours, which would increase the actual BAC by at least 0.2 g/L (assumed elimination rate 0.1 g/L/h). If there was evidence indicating a normal social drinking pattern and conventional alcoholic beverages the back-calculation in German courts is done up to 1 hour after the end of drinking.

Drinking experiments to test the merits of back calculation by taking blood samples at 1.0 hour and 3.5 hours after the last drink have been published (Stowell and Stowell 1998). The BAC at 3.5 hours was then used to estimate the BAC at 1 hour assuming various rates of alcohol elimination from blood, such as 0.1 or 0.2 g/L/h. The BACs estimated 1 hour post-drinking agreed well with measured values when an average elimination rate of 0.15 g/L/h was used and in no case was the BAC over-estimated when a rate of 0.1 g/L/h was used.

The extent of the error in making a back estimation of BAC was investigated in another study of 24 subjects, who had consumed 0.71 g/kg ethanol as a bolus dose in 5 minutes (Al-Lanqawi et al. 1992). The mean C_{max} for these drinking conditions was 1.16 g/L (SD = 0.18 g/L) and the mean elimination rate of ethanol from *plasma* was 0.186 ± 0.026 g/L/h (± SD). This suggests a 95% range of elimination rates from plasma of 0.134 to 0.238 g/L/h (mean ± 2 × SD). Note that these values should be lowered by about 15% to correspond to the elimination rates of ethanol from whole blood (Jones 1993a).

The actual plasma-alcohol concentration at 4 hours and 6 hours post-dosing were used to estimate values at 1 hour post-dosing. Calculations used the average plasma elimination rate of 0.186 g/L/h (experimental mean), and the values of 0.15 g/L/h and 0.238 g/L/h. As expected the most unbiased estimates were obtained using the average rate (0.186 g/L/h) and the upper bound (0.238 g/L/h) gave the largest overestimate. The authors warn about assuming a single rate of elimination of alcohol from blood when back calculations are done for legal purposes.

In a study designed to mimic a typical Swedish dinner party, the volunteers drank ethanol (1.43 g/kg) over 90 minutes at the same time they were served food and under these conditions BAC reached plateau and remained unchanged for 1–2 hours. An important finding from this study was that 15 minutes after the end of drinking, despite eating a meal, the measured BAC was 80% of the final peak BAC (Jones and Neri 1991). This verifies that alcohol is absorbed from the stomach even under conditions when drinking occurs along with a substantial meal.

The various problems overshadowing a back extrapolation of BAC has prompted some jurisdiction to define the statutory BAC or BrAC as that existing at the time of the test. What constitutes a reasonable time after driving is a matter for the courts. After involvement in a traffic crash, a driver might leave the crash scene or is transported to hospital for emergency treatment. Under these circumstances a blood sample might not be obtained for several hours after the crash and at that time the BAC decreases below the statutory limit. Obviously the police authorities want to know whether the person was over the statutory limit for driving at the time of the crash (Jones 2011). Back extrapolation is often considered a dubious practice, because it requires so many assumptions about the ADME of alcohol and these need to be carefully explained to the court in each case.

8.4.8 Prospective Estimation

Forensic scientists are sometimes asked to calculate a persons' BAC based on information provided about the number of drinks consumed and the age, gender, and body weight of the individual. The Widmark equation is commonly used for these calculations but adjustments might be necessary to allow for less than 100% bioavailability of the dose of ethanol ingested.

Experiments have shown (see Figure 8.3) that when alcohol is ingested together with or after a meal the BAC curves run on a lower level and the apparent distribution volume (rho factor) calculated as dose (g/kg)/C_0 is abnormally high. If an expected BAC is calculated by use of the Widmark equation by plugging in a rho factor for the fasting state (0.68), the resulting BAC will be artificially too high.

Blood-alcohol parameters derived from BAC curves in the same individuals (cross-over design) after they drank ethanol (0.8 g/kg) in 30 minutes either on an empty stomach or after eating a standardized breakfast are shown in Table 8.14.

Table 8.14 Mean Blood-Alcohol Parameters (See Text for Details) Derived from a Drinking Experiment with 12 Healthy Men (Cross-Over Design) after They Consumed 0.80 g/kg Ethanol on an Empty Stomach (Overnight Fast) or Immediately after Eating a Standardized Breakfast

Drinking Condition	C_{max} g/L	t_{max} min[a]	C_0 g/L	V_d or Rho Factor L/kg	Min_0 min	β-slope g/L/h	B_{60} g/kg/h
Fed	0.62	120	0.97	0.82	393	0.15	0.123
Fasting	0.96[b]	45[b]	1.16[a]	0.69[b]	495[b]	0.14	0.097[b]

[a] Timed from end of drinking.

[b] Statistically significant difference between fed and fasting states.

The food-induced lowering of C_{max} and C_0 and a later occurring t_{max} and the abnormally high rho factor (dose/C_0) were statistically significant ($p < 0.001$). The rho factor (V_d) for ethanol depends primarily on an individual's age, gender and body composition, such as degree of adiposity. Accordingly, the rho factor can only take certain values and should not be the same when drinking occurs with or after a meal or on an empty stomach. In the fed state, some part of the dose of ethanol seemingly fails to reach the systemic circulation, probably because of an appreciable first-pass metabolism by enzymes located in the gastric mucosa or in the liver. The clearance rate of ethanol from blood in the fed state might be more than expected because of food-induced increase in liver blood flow (Hahn et al. 1994; Schmidt et al. 1992). Otherwise, some part of the dose of ethanol is bound to constituents of the food, such as the amino acids, and released over several hours at a slower rate than the actual elimination rate of ethanol from blood (0.15 g/L/h). Accordingly, the BAC curve exhibits a declining phase even when alcohol was still being absorbed from the stomach at a rate lower than 0.15 g/L/h.

If the rho factor for fasting conditions (e.g., 0.68 in men) is used to calculate C_t by means of the Widmark equation when alcohol was ingested with food the C_t is over-estimated.

$$A = C_t \times kg \times rho$$

$$C_t = A / (kg \times rho)$$

The above equation can be modified by lowering the dose of alcohol by 10%–20% to allow for pre-systemic metabolism if alcohol consumption had taken place together with or after a meal.

$$A \times f = C_t \times kg \times rho$$

$$C_t = (A \times f) / (kg \times rho) - (\beta \times t)$$

The factor "f" is less than unity (1.0) and compensates for the lower bioavailability of the ethanol dose in the fed state. Values of 0.9 or 0.8 might be appropriate depending on size of the meal and other considerations, as shown in the following example.

> Assume a young healthy male subject drank ethanol (0.80 g/kg) immediately after eating breakfast. What BAC would be expected at 90 min post-dosing? With a rho factor of 0.68 and an elimination rate of ethanol from blood of 0.15 g/L/h the estimated BAC (C_t) according to the Widmark equation is 0.95 g/L. Results from many drinking studies with food show a reduced bioavailability of the dose and requires some adjustment to the equation, such as, by use of the "f" factor assumed to be 0.80. The estimated BAC (C_t) at 90 post-dosing is now 0.72 g/L, which was in very good agreement with the value observed by experiment of 0.75 g/L.

The bioavailability of ethanol is 100% when the dose is given intravenously and close to 100% when neat spirits are consumed on an empty stomach (overnight 10 h fast). Both C_{max} and AUC are appreciably lower when ethanol is consumed together with or after a meal (see Figure 8.3 and Table 8.14). Furthermore, in forensic casework the reliability of blood-alcohol calculations is questionable when done using information provided by a person charged with a serious criminal offence, such as drunken driving. These individuals are rarely truthful about how much alcohol they had consumed and over what time period, although this is something for the courts to ponder over.

8.4.9 Hip Flask and Laced Drinks

The hip-flask drink also sometimes referred to as the glove-compartment drink implies the consumption of alcohol after driving or after involvement in a traffic crash. This defense argument has become increasingly common in some nations and has sometimes resulted in acquittals or a lesser charge being brought if graded penalties exist (Iffland and Jones 2003; Simic et al. 2004). In the UK the onus of proof in hip-flask cases rests on the suspect and his lawyers, who have to demonstrate to the court that it was the ethanol in the hip-flask drink that caused the person's BAC to be over the legal limit for driving.

In other nations the onus of proof in after-drink cases rests on the prosecution and unless the suspect is actually sitting behind the wheel of the vehicle there is a strong likelihood that he or she will claim consumption of alcohol after driving. Such claims tend to complicate the prosecution of traffic offenders and expert witnesses are required to evaluate the truthfulness of statements about drinking after driving and what it means for the BAC existing at the time of driving. The following example illustrates such an after-drink case.

After a minor road traffic crash, the driver of a motor vehicle claimed to have taken two gulps from a bottle of whisky, allegedly to calm the nerves. A roadside breath alcohol test on the driver was positive (statutory limit 0.50 g/L in blood) and a blood sample was taken 90 min later and was found to contain not less than 1.0 g/L ethanol after making a deduction for uncertainty. At trial the question about the after-drink arose and the court accepted that two swigs of whisky corresponded to 120 mL (40%, v/v; or 31.6%, w/v, which amounts to 38 g ethanol (100% v/v).

The man's body weight was 90 kg and because he was fairly obese (BMI = 30), instead of a distribution volume of 0.7 L/kg, the court accepted a V_d of 0.6 L/kg as being more appropriate in this case. The Widmark equation shows that the highest BAC from drinking 38 g ethanol after driving is 0.70 g/L [38/(90 × 0.6)]. Over the 1½ hour elapsed after the whisky was consumed some of the ethanol is metabolism in the liver. With a slow (0.10 g/L/h) or rapid (0.25 g/L/h) rate of metabolism the BAC could decrease by between 0.15 and 0.38 g/L over the 90 min between crash and time of blood sampling. The after-drink might therefore explain a BAC of 0.55 g/L (0.70–0.15) or 0.32 g/L (0.70–0.38), depending on slow or rapid rates of ethanol elimination from blood.

Before taking the two gulps of whisky after driving the BAC at the time of driving was either 0.45 g/L (1.0–0.55) or 0.68 g/L (1.0–0.32). If none of the alcohol contained in the after-drink was metabolized, which would benefit the suspect, the BAC at time of the crash would have been 0.30 g/L (1.0–0.70).

In this example complete absorption and distribution of the alcohol contained in the hip-flask drink is assumed, which is obviously to the suspect's advantage (Simic et al. 2004). If in reality some of the ethanol remained unabsorbed this has not contributed to the BAC. If there is an adjustment made to allow for the metabolism of some of the ethanol contained in the after drink then a low elimination rate is to the suspect's advantage (Iffland

and Jones 2002). The utility of double blood samples and urine/blood ratios of ethanol in evaluating the hip-flask drink was recently investigated in a controlled drinking experiment (Kronstrand et al. 2019).

A closely related argument in DUI litigation is the "laced drink" defense whereby the suspect alleges that his or her drink was spiked with vodka or some other strong alcoholic drink without altering the taste (Langford et al. 1999). And it was the extra alcohol from the vodka that caused the person's BAC to be above the legal BAC limit for driving. The BAC resulting from the amount of ethanol in the vodka added to the beer is easy to calculate by the Widmark equation and compared with the observed BAC. Also in the laced drink calculation some allowance is necessary for the metabolism of alcohol in the vodka, although this would not benefit the defendant in such cases.

8.5 Other Pharmacokinetic Models

Pharmacokinetics is the branch or sub-discipline of pharmacology that deals with absorption, distribution, metabolism and excretion of drugs and xenobiotics and how these processes can be described in quantitative terms. Compared with other psychoactive drugs massive quantities of ethanol are consumed (tens of grams) to cause impairment of body functions. Moreover, the hepatic enzyme systems that clear ethanol from the blood stream become saturated with substrate—hence zero-order kinetics for a large part of the BAC curve. At low BAC (<0.2 g/L) the enzymes are not fully saturated and the elimination kinetics changes to first-order.

8.5.1 First-order Kinetics

Most recreational drugs as well as prescription medication are eliminated from the body according to first-order kinetics (Rowland and Tozer 1995). This implies, among other things, that the rate of change in drug concentration in blood or plasma is directly proportional to the concentration existing at that time. The general rate equation for a first-order reaction is given below:

$$dC/dt = -kC$$

$$dC/C = -kdt$$

If this equation is integrated from $C = C_0$ at $t = 0$ and $C = C_t$ at a later time (t) one obtains the exponential function $C_t = C_0\ e^{-kt}$ corresponding to the C-T plot in Figure 8.18 (left part). Taking logarithms of this equation gives:

$$\text{Ln}\,C_t = \text{Ln}\,C_o - k_1 t$$

Plotting Ln C against time t gives a linear relationship as shown in Figure 8.18 (right part). In this equation the coefficients, k_1 is a first order rate constant and Ln C_0 is the y-intercept.

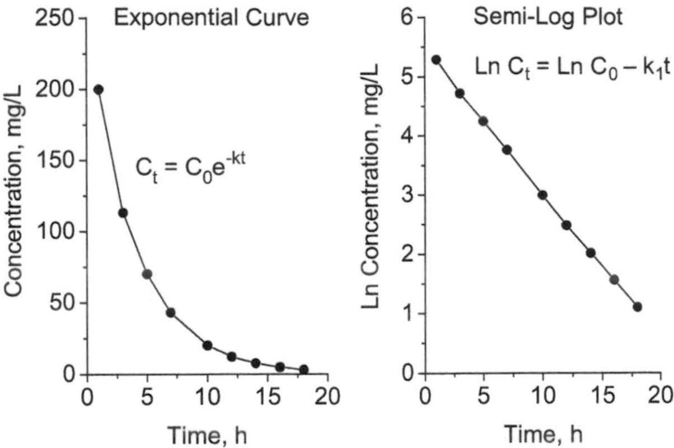

Figure 8.18 Concentration-time profiles for a drug eliminated according to first-order kinetics. The left trace shows an exponential decline after reaching C_{max} in blood and the right trace shows the effect of making a logarithmic transformation of drug concentrations, which is necessary to calculate the elimination rate constant (k_1) and half-life ($t_{½}$) of the drug.

The relationship between the half-life and the elimination rate constant for a first-order reaction is obtained by substituting $C_t = C_0/2$ into the above equation and re-arranging to give.

$$\mathrm{Ln}\,C_0/2 = \mathrm{Ln}\,C_0 - k_1t_{1/2}$$

$$k_1t_{1/2} = \mathrm{Ln}\,C_0 - \mathrm{Ln}\,C_0/2$$

$$k_1t_{1/2} = \mathrm{Ln}\,2$$

$$t_{1/2} = \mathrm{Ln}\,2/k_1 \text{ and because } \mathrm{Ln}\,2 = 0.693$$

$$t_{1/2} = 0.693/k_1$$

It has been suggested, although with very little scientific support, that at sub-lethal concentrations of ethanol in blood of 4–5 g/L (0.4–0.5 g/100 mL) the elimination kinetics might be first-order rather than zero-order (Hammond et al. 1973; Lindblad and Olsson 1976). This was first demonstrated in hospital emergency patients undergoing detoxification, but only a few blood samples were available for determination of ethanol making a proper kinetic analysis very difficult (Lamminpaa and Hoppu 2009). Moreover, at such very high BAC proportionally more ethanol is eliminated via the breath and urine because these are first-order kinetic processes.

8.5.2 Michaelis–Menten Kinetics

Evidence that the elimination kinetics of ethanol from blood might depend on the concentration in blood began to emerge in the early 1950s coinciding with the development of more sensitive enzymatic methods of analysis. With these so-called ADH-methods the concentrations in blood and the BAC curves could be followed to much lower levels. Other studies showed that the disappearance rate of ethanol from blood (β) was faster after subjects drank larger doses of ethanol and the zero-order slope tended to be steeper at higher starting BAC (Wilkinson 1980). These observation did not fit with the postulate of zero-order elimination kinetics of ethanol (Rangno et al. 1981). For drugs metabolized by saturation kinetics the area under the curve and the concentration of drug in blood changes more than proportionally with an increase in dose, which for some drugs has serious clinical implications (Ludden 1991; Wagner 1973, 1985).

Michaelis and Menten (M–M), a man and woman respectively, hypothesized the existence of an enzyme-substrate complex as a scientific basis to understand enzyme catalyzed biochemical reactions already in 1913 (Michaelis and Menton 1913). The M–M equation (see below) indicates that the velocity of the enzymatic reaction increases with substrate concentration but only up to a certain limiting value. This rate is denoted V_{max} and at higher concentration the enzyme is saturated with substrate and the reaction (oxidation) proceeds at maximum velocity. The substrate concentration at half maximum velocity ($V_{max}/2$) is denoted k_m and is a measure of the affinity of the enzyme for the substrate, being referred to as the Michaelis constant (Wagner et al. 1989).

$$-dC/dT = (V_{max} \times C)/(k_m + C)$$

For drugs eliminated by M–M kinetics the reaction rate (–dC/dT) is a function of both the substrate concentration (C) and the theoretical maximum reaction velocity V_{max}, and is inversely proportional to k_m the Michaelis constant for the particular enzyme involved. As substrate concentrations increase the binding sites on the enzyme become saturated and the enzymatic reaction occurs at maximum velocity (V_{max}). Table 8.15 illustrates the relationship between substrate concentration (BAC) and the rate of elimination from blood with different affinity of the enzyme for substrate as reflected by k_m values of 0.025, 0.05 or 0.10 g/L and a maximum reaction velocity of 0.22 g/L/h.

The application of the M–M equation to experimental C-T data for ethanol was first demonstrated by two Danish scientists in 1958 (Lundquist and Wolthers 1958). They obtained a good mathematical fit for ethanol concentrations-time profiles on the linear and the curvilinear portions of the curve. In their article the Michaelis constant for ethanol (k_m) was reported to be 2.03 mmol/L (0.09 g/L) and the maximum reaction velocity V_{max} was 0.22 g/L/h, the latter corresponds to the zero-order slope of the elimination phase (Lundquist and Wolthers 1958).

Table 8.15 Relationship between Concentration (BAC) and the Elimination Rate of Ethanol from Blood in a Capacity-Limited Enzymatic Reaction with V_{max} = 0.22 g/L/h and Assuming Three Different Michaelis Constants (k_m) of 0.025 g/L, 0.05 g/L and 0.10 g/L

	Elimination Rate g/L/h at k_m Values of		
Substrate Conc. (BAC) g/L	0.025 g/L	0.05 g/L	0.10 g/L
0.10	0.18	0.15	0.11
0.20	0.20	0.18	0.16
0.25	0.21	0.20	0.20
1.00	0.21	0.21	0.20
1.50	0.21	0.21	0.21
2.00	0.21	0.21	0.21

In the late 1970s, John G. Wagner (1921–1998) and his collaborators applied the M–M equation to blood-alcohol profiles and found convincing evidence of dose-dependent saturation kinetics (Wagner 1973; Wagner et al. 1989). The C-T plot looked more like a hockey stick rather than a straight line when plotted from high to very low BAC (<0.1 g/L). The relevance of considering such low BAC in routine forensic investigations of drunken drivers or alcohol-related trauma victims is questionable.

Figure 8.19 gives an example of a BAC curve when ethanol was given by intravenous administration and when blood samples were taken at short intervals of time down to very low BAC. The hockey stick shape of the C-T profile in the late post-absorptive phase of the curve is clearly evident.

Depending on the concentration of substrate (C), the M–M equation collapses into two limiting forms. When C is high compared with k_m the M–M equation becomes:

$$-dC / dt = V_{max}$$

When the substrate concentration (C) is low compared with k_m as the BAC drops below 0.1 g/L, the M–M equation becomes:

$$-dC / dt = (V_{max} \times C) / k_m = k_1 C$$

In the above equation $k_1 = V_{max}/k_m$ and this corresponds to the first-order elimination rate constant, which is directly proportional to the substrate concentration. The values of V_{max} and k_m can be determined graphically by use of the integrated form of the M–M equation as described in detail elsewhere (Wagner 1973; Wilkinson 1980). Strictly speaking the M–M equation applies when there is a single enzyme-substrate interaction although in practice various isoenzymes of ADH exist as well as the microsomal enzymes (CYP2E1). The latter have a higher k_m for ethanol as substrate of 0.6–0.8 g/L and its activity is boosted after periods of chronic daily drinking (Keiding et al. 1983).

Non-linear M–M kinetics can be considered as encompassing zero-order, which operates at moderate and high concentrations of substrate, and first-order kinetics that occur at low substrate concentrations. Although the M–M kinetic model provides a good fit to the entire post-absorptive elimination phase, spanning from high to very low BAC in forensic casework there is not much practical benefit compared the traditional use of a zero-order kinetic model. Figure 8.19 shows both the hockey stick shape of the BAC profile (left frame) and the result of a logarithmic transformation of BAC which makes it easier to observe the transition from zero-order to first-order, which occurs at a BAC of about 0.15–0.20 g/L

8.5.3 Pharmacokinetic Software

A number of different computer programs are available, which simplify making various pharmacokinetic calculations from concentration-time data collected from human and animal drug dosing studies. Some of these are fairly sophisticated e.g., WinNonLin, PharmaCalc and Boomer (Charles and Duffull 2001; Gabrielsson and Weiner 2000). Although this type of software is mainly intended for drug research and developments in the pharmaceutical industry they might also be used in academic and forensic research, including human pharmacokinetics of ethanol and other drugs (Norberg et al. 2003).

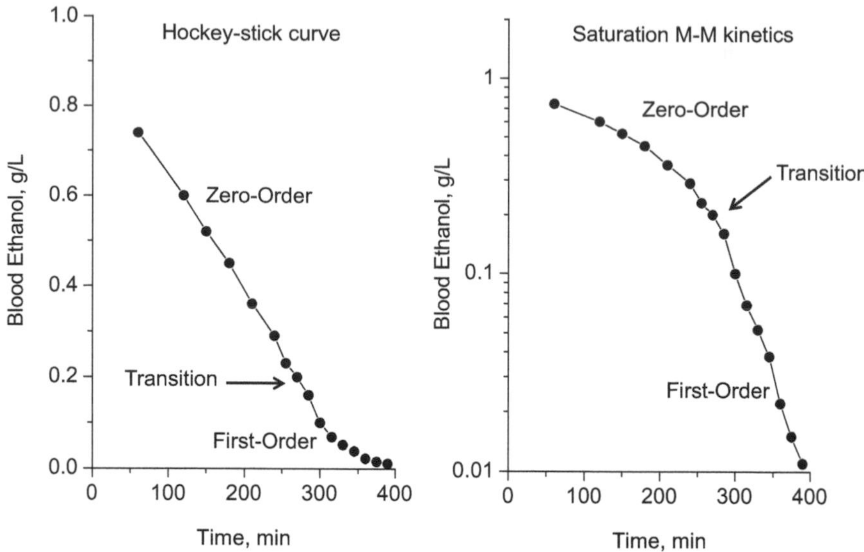

Figure 8.19 Post-absorptive phase of the concentration-time (C-T) profile of a drug eliminated by saturation kinetics. The left trace shows an exponential decline and a hockey-stick appearance of the C-T data points and transition from zero-order (high concentration) to zero-order kinetics at low concentrations. This pattern of elimination is characteristic of drugs that obey Michaelis–Menten (saturation) kinetics.

These software packages contain curve fitting algorithms and other procedures to evaluate concentration-time data for various input variables, such as dose, dosage interval, drug formulation and route of administration. The reliability of results generated by pharmacokinetic software and the uncertainty inherent in the parameter β and rho depends very much on the reliability of the C-T data gathered and used as the input values. Accurate and precise analytical methods and a careful consideration of pre-analytical factors are prerequisites to avoid the adage "junk in junk out."

The use of alcohol calculations in education and teaching of public health workers or for the training of police officers and forensic scientists is increasingly common (Davies and Bowen 2000). For this purpose nomograms and "know your limit" tables exist whereby users obtain an estimate of BAC from information about body weight, gender and number of drinks consumed. Caution is necessary when results from these alcohol nomograms are used to decide whether a person is "safe to drive" or is below a statutory alcohol limit and a confidence limits approach is recommended (Arstein-Kerslake 1986).

More sophisticated software packages have become available and are intended for making blood-alcohol calculations based on a person's age, body weight and gender, the pattern and duration of drinking, the type of drinks consumed and whether taken with or without food. Options exist for plotting the "expected" BAC curve based on certain assumptions about beta and rho. Examples of such programs include Easy-Alc, AlcoTrace, and AlcoGraph, although the validity and usefulness of this type of computer software using results with actual drinking experiments is hard to find in the literature (Posey and Mozayani 2007; Rockerbie and Rockerbie 1995).

A number of BAC calculators are available gratis over the Internet and operate together with spreadsheet programs, such as EXCEL (Zhang et al. 2017). The advantage and limitations of this software compared with a pen and paper and a hand-held calculator needs to be demonstrated (Hustad and Carey 2005). In most forensic situations, only a single measurement of the person's BAC or BrAC is available, which precludes the use of curve-fitting algorithms to derive pharmacokinetic parameters. Furthermore, information provided by a DUI suspect in a criminal prosecution regarding the number of drinks consumed is not sufficiently reliable to motivate making more detailed blood-alcohol calculations.

A computer program (PKQuest) was found useful in pharmacokinetic modeling and was applied to intestinal absorption of ethanol and first-pass metabolism (Levitt 2002, 2004). The same program was also used to compare the clinical pharmacokinetics of ethanol in venous and arterial blood based on actual experimental data and results seemed to be very satisfactory (Levitt 2004).

8.5.4 Pharmacokinetics in Alternative Specimens

In the field of clinical pharmacology and TDM, drugs are mostly determined in samples of plasma or serum, whereas in forensic science and toxicology whole blood is taken and used for toxicological analysis. Chemicals and other substances don't necessarily distribute evenly between the plasma and the erythrocyte fractions of whole blood, owing to varying degree of protein binding and the relative solubility in lipids compared to blood water (Jones and Larsson 2004; Jones et al. 1990).

Studies have shown that plasma and serum contain ~92% w/w water compared with whole blood, which is 80% w/w water, which suggests a plasma/blood distribution ratio of water and ethanol of 1.15 to 1 (92/80 = 1.15), which agreed well with values determined empirically in over 800 subjects (Iffland et al. 1999). The plasma/blood distribution ratio of ethanol varies between and within individuals depending on factors that influence the water content of specimens, such as the degree of hydration, hematocrit value, lipid content of serum, such as hyperlipidemia and disease states, such as anemia (Artiss and Zak 1987; Sharma et al. 1987).

The different amounts of water in different bio-fluids impacts on the slope of the C-T profiles depending on whether these were constructed from results of ethanol analysis in plasma/serum or whole blood (Jones et al. 1992). As mentioned earlier, the declining phase of the BAC curve is slightly steeper for plasma/serum resulting in a higher C_0 and lower calculated V_d (dose/C_0). Unfortunately, some published studies don't make it perfectly clear whether ethanol was determined in blood or serum/plasma. Blood-alcohol concentrations are mentioned but on closer inspection it becomes obvious that the investigators determined ethanol in plasma or serum, which obviously impacts on the pharmacokinetic parameters (Lekskulchai and Rattanawibool 2007).

There is a lot of interest among forensic toxicologists in analyzing ethanol and other drugs in alternative biological specimens, such as saliva (Gallardo et al. 2009). Figure 8.20 compares the mean C-T profiles of ethanol in saliva, breath, urine, and whole blood after 21 men drank 0.68 g/kg ethanol as a bolus dose on an empty stomach (Jones 1993b, 2006). The pharmacokinetic parameters were derived from individual C-T profiles of ethanol in different specimens and the results are presented in Table 8.16.

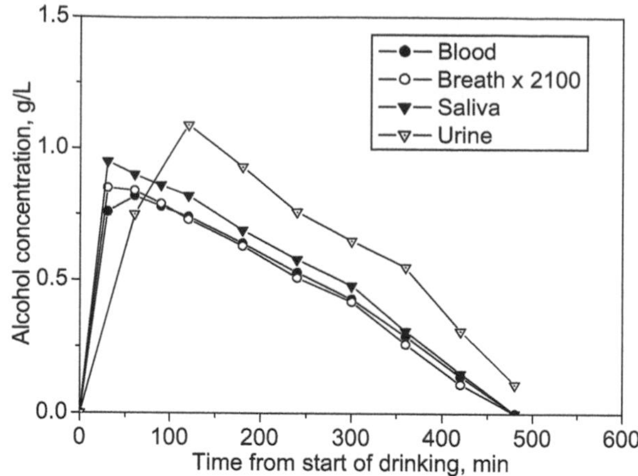

Figure 8.20 Mean concentration-time profiles of ethanol in blood, breath, urine, and saliva after 21 healthy men drank a moderate dose of ethanol (0.68 g/kg body weight) as neat whisky on an empty stomach. The ethanol concentrations in breath at each time point were multiplied by 2100 to allow making a direct comparison with the other biological specimens.

Table 8.16 Pharmacokinetic Parameters of Ethanol Derived from the Concentration-Time Profiles in Blood Compared with Plasma, Urine, and Saliva

	Ethanol Dose 0.60 g/kg[a]		Ethanol Dose 0.68 g/kg[b]		Ethanol Dose 0.68 g/kg[c]	
Parameter	Blood	Plasma	Blood	Urine	Blood	Saliva
C_{max} g/L	1.08 ± 0.17	1.20 ± 0.20	0.92 ± 0.16	1.08 ± 0.17	0.91 ± 0.16	1.09 ± 0.24
t_{max} min	60	60	54	129	38	44
β-slope or k_0 g/L/h	0.17 ± 0.04	0.19 ± 0.05	0.13 ± 0.06	0.16 ± 0.04	0.12 ± 0.01	0.13 ± 0.03
C_0 g/L	1.02 ± 0.09	1.12 ± 0.09	0.98 ± 0.06	1.40 ± 0.19	1.00 ± 0.06	1.10 ± 0.10
V_d or rho factor, L/kg	0.59 ± 0.05	0.54 ± 0.05	0.69 ± 0.05	0.48 ± 0.08	0.69 ± 0.04	0.66 ± 0.04

Sources: Jones, A.W., *Br. J. Clin. Pharmacol.*, 35, 669, 1993, Jones, A.W., *Clin. Chem.*, 39, 1837, 1993; Jones, A.W., *Toxicol. Rev.*, 25, 15, 2006; Jones, A.W. et al., *Eur. J. Clin. Pharmacol.*, 42, 445, 1992.

[a] Alcohol dose (0.60 g/kg, n = 15 subjects) given by a constant rate intravenous infusion over 60 min.

[b] Alcohol dose (0.68 g/kg, n = 30 subjects) after drinking neat whisky on an empty stomach in 20 min.

[c] Alcohol dose (0.68 g/kg, n = 21 subjects) after drinking neat whisky on empty stomach in 20 min.

The vast majority of pharmacokinetic studies of ethanol are based on sampling and analysis of blood, either capillary (fingertip), venous or arterial samples. By contrast, most forensic alcohol testing involves the use of evidential breath-alcohol instruments (Gullberg 2000). Translating the measured BrAC into the presumed BAC is not recommended because the BAC/BrAC ratio is not constant and varies depending on the stage of ethanol metabolism (Jones 1978). The concentration of alcohol in breath is more closely related to the arterial BAC rather than the venous BAC, as discussed earlier, even though statutory alcohol limits for driving are based on the analysis of venous blood (Lindberg et al. 2007).

The increasing use of breath-alcohol instruments for clinical and forensic purposes would gain a lot from more studies of pharmacokinetic parameters derived from repetitive breath-alcohol determinations (Fiorentino and Moskowitz 2013). The rate of ethanol elimination from breath should be used whenever a back calculation of the BrAC is done to time of driving and not making any conversion into BAC, owing to variability in the blood-breath alcohol relationship.

Table 8.17 shows a good overall agreement between mean and range of elimination rates of ethanol from breath (mg/L/h) in the four cited studies using two types of quantitative breath-alcohol instruments (Dettling et al. 2009; Jones and Andersson 2003; Pavlic et al. 2007). The slopes of the declining phase of the BrAC profiles were slightly steeper for females compared with males, in each study, which agrees with findings based on BAC curves (Dettling et al. 2007). The mean and range of elimination rates of ethanol from breath in Table 8.17 should be appropriate to use in a back-calculation (Haffner et al. 2003).

Most drunk-driving cases are prosecuted based on the concentration of ethanol in a suspect's breath and statutory BrAC limits are enforced in most countries, such as 0.08 g/210 L in USA or 35 μg/100 mL in UK (see Table 8.4). The increasing use of breath-alcohol testing for evidential purposes has prompted an investigation of inter- and intra-individual differences in C-T profiles of ethanol derived from analysis of exhaled air (Sadler and Fox 2011; Sadler and Lennox 2015). In this connection, the effect of eating a meal before drinking resulted in a lower C_{max} and C_0 as well as a smaller AUC for breath-alcohol curves compared with the fasting state, being in agreement with blood-alcohol curves (Kalant 2004).

Other body fluids used to construct C-T profiles of ethanol include lumbar cerebrospinal fluid and sweat, both of which show an appreciable time-lag compared with BAC profiles (Brown 1985; Buono 1999). The CSF and sweat curves had a higher C_{max} and later occurring t_{max} compared with BAC (Fleming and Stotz 1935; Mehrtens and Newman 1933). Distribution ratios of ethanol have also been investigated for tear fluid and blood and as expected the greater water content of tears (~100%) compared with blood (~80%) gave a mean tears-to-blood ratio of 1.25:1 (Buono 1999; Lund 1984).

Table 8.17 Elimination Rates of Ethanol from Breath Determined in Controlled Drinking Experiments in Healthy Male and Female Volunteers—Breath-Alcohol Concentrations Are in mg/L and Elimination Rates of Ethanol from Breath in mg/L/h

Investigators	Gender	n[a]	Mean Elimination Rate from Breath, mg/L/h	Lowest Value mg/L/h	Highest Value mg/L/h
Dettling et al. (2009)[b]	Male	96	0.080	0.049	0.112
	Female	81	0.092	0.065	0.124
Pavlic et al. (2007)[b]	Male	32	0.078	0.048	0.109
	Female	27	0.087	0.054	0.120
Jones and Andersson (2003)[c]	Male	9	0.075	0.068	0.083
	Female	9	0.087	0.070	0.103
Fiorentino and Moskowitz (2013)[c]	Male	84	0.071	0.030[d]	0.112[d]
	Female	84	0.086	0.039[d]	0.133[d]

[a] n = numbers of subjects.
[b] The evidential breath-alcohol analyzer used was Alcotest 7110 Mk III.
[c] The evidential breath-alcohol analyzer used was Intoxilyzer 5000S.
[d] Estimated from standard deviation (mean ± 3 × SD).

8.6 Concluding Remarks

Much is known about the pharmacokinetics of ethanol and the first systematic studies date back to the 1930s as exemplified by the work of Widmark in Sweden (Widmark 1932). Quantitative methods for the analysis of ethanol in blood and other body fluids were available long before other drugs and toxins could be determined reliably (Widmark 1922). After drinking alcoholic beverages, concentrations of ethanol in blood are 1,000–10,000 times greater than for other recreational drugs or prescription medication a person might ingest. The measured BAC is easy to convert into the amount of ethanol absorbed and distributed in all body fluids and tissues at the time of sampling. Because of the ubiquitous use and abuse of ethanol in society and the role of drunkenness in various types of crimes questions about the ADME of ethanol often arise when drunken drivers are prosecuted. Forensic investigators called to testify in court or to write expert opinions need to understand the basic principles of ethanol pharmacokinetics.

Ethanol is a legal drug, so drinking studies are easy to perform with health volunteers, although all experiments with human subjects need approval from an ethical review committee. The amounts of ethanol administered as a bolus dose are fairly low (0.3–1.0 g/kg) to avoid nausea and vomiting, which often occurs after larger amounts are consumed quickly on an empty stomach. In most controlled dosing studies, C_{max} of the BAC curve is between 0.8 and 1.2 g/L, which is considerable lower than the mean BAC in forensic casework, such as in apprehended drivers, being closer to a mean of 1.7 g/L (Jones and Holmgren 2009b).

The relevant scientific literature dealing with human pharmacokinetics of ethanol is spread throughout journals devoted to forensic science and legal medicine as well as clinical pharmacology and substance abuse research. This motivates preparation of comprehensive review articles to bring together this information making it more easily accessible to forensic practitioners as exemplified by a recent evidence-based survey of the elimination rates of ethanol from blood (Jones 2010).

Table 8.18 summarizes the results from many studies aimed at investigating factors that might influence ADME of ethanol. The results and conclusions from some of these could not be confirmed in later investigations, which means that more research is need to reach a definite conclusion. Much seems to depend on experimental design, dose of ethanol, the route and timing of administration and the number of subjects participating in the study. Pharmacokinetic parameters of ethanol should not be calculated when low doses (<0.3 g/kg) are administered, because the BAC reached barely saturates the hepatic metabolizing enzymes. A sufficient number of blood samples must also be taken on the post-absorptive phase to allow calculating the important C_0 parameter by back extrapolation.

Considerable research effort was devoted to study an alleged interaction between ethanol and drugs prescribed for hyper-acidity in the stomach, so-called histamine H_2-antagonists (e.g., cimetidine and ranitidine). This drug-alcohol interaction attracted a lot of attention when articles appeared in scientific journals suggesting that BAC was higher after drinking alcohol and taking this medication. The higher C_{max} was claimed to cause greater impairment of body functions and increased risk of being apprehended for impaired driving (Baraona et al. 1994b; DiPadova et al. 1992). The mechanism proposed to account for higher C_{max} was drug-induced inhibition of gastric alcohol dehydrogenase.

Table 8.18 Summary of Factors Influencing Absorption, Distribution, Metabolism, and Excretion (ADME) of Ethanol According to Human Dosing Studies Published in Peer-Reviewed Journals

Question Investigated	Brief Review of the Findings and Comments on the Relevance in Relation to Ethanol ADME	References
Phase of the menstrual cycle	Blood-alcohol parameters β and rho were not significantly different when drinking during the luteal and the follicular phases of the monthly menstrual cycle as verified by analysis of sex steroid hormones estradiol, progesterone, and testosterone in blood.	Correa and Oga (2004); Dettling et al. (2010); Lammers et al. (1995); Marshall et al. (1983) Mumenthaler et al. (1999)
Female gender	Less body water per kg body weight in women accounts for the lower V_d in the female gender. Activity of gastric ADH is also lower in women but the role of this enzyme in first-pass metabolism of ethanol is controversial. Nevertheless the rate of ethanol elimination from blood is slightly faster in women, which seems to be related to a larger liver mass per kg lean body weight.	Dettling et al. (2007); Kwo et al. (1998); Mishra et al. (1989); Mumenthaler et al. (2000); Thomasson (2000); Whitfield et al. (1990)
Sex steroid hormones	The concentrations of testosterone, estradiol and progesterone in serum from men and women influenced the elimination rate of ethanol from blood. Lower rates were seen in women with lower progesterone levels ($p < 0.05$). Other studies suggest low testosterone levels in men are associated with faster rates of ethanol elimination form blood.	Dettling et al. (2008); Hobbes et al. (1985); Mezey et al. (1988, 1989)
Age	During aging body water decreases, especially in men, which leads to a decrease in the volume of distribution of ethanol (lower rho factor). This leads to a higher BAC for a given dose/kg body weight. The rate of ethanol elimination form blood was the same for men aged between 20 and 60 years.	Bielefeld et al. (2015); Hein and Vock (1989); Jones and Neri (1985)
Sobering-up remedies (fructose and glucose)	Administration of carbohydrates, particularly fructose, is considered to accelerate the hepatic metabolism of ethanol. The experimental design, ethanol, dose and route and timing of administration in relation to intake of the sugars are important considerations. Ethanol mixed with sugars delays gastric emptying and lowers C_{max} and this has sometimes been confused with faster rates of ethanol metabolism.	Bode et al. (1979); Clark et al. (1973); Crow et al. (1981); Crownover et al. (1986); Mascord et al. (1988, 1991); Pavlic et al. (2007); Rogers et al. (1987); Soterakis and Iber (1975)

(Continued)

Table 8.18 (*Continued*) Summary of Factors Influencing Absorption, Distribution, Metabolism, and Excretion (ADME) of Ethanol According to Human Dosing Studies Published in Peer-Reviewed Journals

Question Investigated	Brief Review of the Findings and Comments on the Relevance in Relation to Ethanol ADME	References
Carbonated mixers	Variable effects observed on speed of absorption after drinking highly carbonated drinks, 14/21 subjects absorbed faster whereas 7/21 absorbed slower or showed no change. Much depends on gastric emptying.	Roberts and Robinson (2007); Wu et al. (2006)
Oxygenated drinks	No evidence exists that alcoholic drinks enriched with oxygen lead to a faster rate of elimination from blood. A recent study published this notion but was later criticized for several reasons. On closer examination there was confusion between use of zero-order and first-order kinetics when the BAC curves were evaluated.	Baek et al. (2010); Hyvarinen et al. (1978); Laakso et al. (1979); Lachenmeier and Rehm (2010); Rhee et al. (2013)
Kidney dysfunction	Blood-alcohol curves and the rate of elimination from blood were the same in patients undergoing hemodialysis compared with people having normal kidney functioning.	Jones and Hahn (1997)
Liver cirrhosis	Ethanol is metabolized primarily in the liver so damage to this organ (e.g., tissue necrosis) might be thought would slow the rate of elimination. However the abundance of hepatic ADH means that even in patients with cirrhosis sufficient enzyme is available for oxidative metabolism of ethanol.	Jones (2000); Lieber (1997); Winkler et al. (1969)
Gastric bypass surgery	Surgery to the gut (Roux-en-Y) for obesity leads to a higher C_{max} and earlier t_{max}, although the elimination rate from blood was not altered after surgery. By 30–40 min post-dosing the BAC was the same in operated and non-operated subjects serving as the control group. Nevertheless, operated patients should be warned about the risk of alcohol consumption and initial higher BAC.	Hagedorn et al. (2007); Klockhoff et al. (2002); Pepino et al. (2015); Steffen et al. (2013); Woodard et al. (2011)
Drugs used for treatment of gastric hyper-acidity (H_2 antagonists)	Cimetidine (Tagamet) and ranitidine (Zantac) were alleged to increases C_{max} after drinking ethanol by drug-induced inhibition of gastric ADH and the amelioration of gastric first-pass metabolism. This conclusion was later challenged by newer research, because much depends on the dose of ethanol administered and the fed-fasted state of the test subjects.	Brown and James (1998); Clemmesen et al. (1997); Fraser et al. (1991, 1992); Moody (2018)

This prevented the usual first-pass metabolism of ethanol in the gastric mucosa and led to an increased BAC and greater AUC after drinking (Caballeria et al. 1989; Lieber et al. 1994; Lim et al. 1993).

A critical review of these studies indicated that small numbers of subjects were involved (n = 6–8) and the doses of ethanol were very low (0.15–0.3 g/kg). Moreover this was consumed in the morning after the volunteers had eaten a fat-rich breakfast (DiPadova et al. 1992; Frezza et al. 1990). Experiments with more volunteers, higher doses of ethanol taken in the morning, at midday and/or in the evening failed to confirm the original reports (Toon et al. 1994). A review of the literature including meta-analysis failed to support the idea that Zantac or Tagamet impacted on the pharmacokinetics of ethanol (Fraser 1997; Fraser et al. 1991, 1993; Weinberg et al. 1998). Much seemed to depend on the dose of ethanol administered and whether this was consumed on an empty stomach or after a fat-rich meal. Eating a meal before drinking delays gastric emptying and leads to a highly variable absorption rate of ethanol into the blood and oxidation by hepatic metabolizing enzymes (Fraser et al. 1992; Levitt and Levitt 1994; Oneta et al. 1998; Wagner 1986).

The conventional way to determine bioavailability of a drug is by comparing AUC after oral and intravenous administration which is not appropriate for drugs metabolized by M–M kinetics, because the AUC does not increase in direct proportion to the dose and is strongly dependent on factors influencing liver blood flow (Dedrick and Forrester 1973; Wagner 1986). Moreover, after small doses of ethanol (e.g., 0.15–0.3 g/kg), especially in the non-fasted state, C_{max} is fairly low and highly variable. Finding small absolute differences between test and control treatments after small doses of ethanol and reaching a low BAC gives large percentage changes (Fraser et al. 1991; Julkunen et al. 1985; Lim et al. 1993). BAC curves are much more variable when subjects drink small doses of ethanol and C_{max} and AUC show appreciable variations (see Figure 8.4). In terms of experimental design many more drinking subjects would be necessary to achieve sufficient statistical power in order to detect the effect of a particular drug treatment (Wagner 1986).

The general consensus seems to be that cimetidine and ranitidine exert negligible influence on C_{max} reached after drinking compared with a placebo or no-drug control treatment (Fraser et al. 1993; Toon et al. 1994). The adverse interaction between drugs used to treat gastric hyperacidity is influenced by age, gender, and drinking habits of the individuals according to many articles published in high impact journals (DiPadova et al. 1992; Frezza et al. 1990). When larger doses of ethanol (0.6–0.8 g/kg) were ingested after one week of medication with H_2-antagonist drugs the effects on BAC profiles were small or negligible, which confirmed earlier findings (Fraser et al. 1992; Jonsson et al. 1992).

Drinking alcoholic beverages enriched with oxygen was reported to accelerate the rate of ethanol metabolism and relieve the hangover effects of an evening's heavy drinking (Baek et al. 2010). However, a closer examination of the article showed problems with interpreting BAC curves and a confusion between first-order and zero-order kinetics, so the conclusions must be considered suspect (Baek et al. 2010). This was commented upon in a letter to the editor, which pointed out a failure by other scientists to verify an accelerating effect of drinks enriched with oxygen on rate of ethanol metabolism (Laakso et al. 1979; Lachenmeier and Rehm 2010).

An important question that arises in forensic casework is the time required to reach the peak concentration in blood (C_{max}) after drinking and the rise in BAC after the last drink (Jones and Neri 1991; Jones et al. 1991). Much seems to depend on the pattern of drinking and the amount of ethanol contained in the last drink. In this connection, one needs to distinguish between rapid drinking on an empty stomach and social drinking spread over several hours. After a bolus dose the C_{max} usually occurs within 60 minutes (median) after the end of drinking, but in any individual case this might range from 5 to 120 minutes (Jones et al. 1991). Longer absorption times than 120 minutes are unlikely unless a pyloric spasm occurred and absorption occurred primarily through the gastric mucosa and not the upper small intestine (Jones et al. 1991). During real-world drinking with repeated intake over several hours, some individuals might have reached their peak BAC before finishing the last drink (Zink and Reinhardt 1984). Most of the ethanol gets absorbed into the blood stream during the drinking period and only the amount contained in the last drink might remain unabsorbed.

In Table 8.19 the rates of elimination of alcohol from blood are classified as slow, moderate, rapid, or ultra-rapid and the circumstances or conditions under which such rates might be observed is presented. Elimination rates from the blood (g/L/h) and the entire body (g/h) are shown. The latter is another important pharmacokinetic parameter, often denoted B_{60}, and assumes a man with body weight 70 kg and distribution volume of ethanol of 0.7 L/kg. The rates of ethanol elimination in Table 8.19 can be considered a physiological range based on cumulative knowledge from hundreds of controlled alcohol dosing studies and review of the scientific literature (Jones 2010). In any individual case,

Table 8.19 The Physiological Range of Elimination Rates of Ethanol from Blood and the Whole Body and Circumstances or Conditions under Which These Rates Might Be Observed in Practice

Elimination Rate of Ethanol	From Blood Stream g/L/h	From Whole Body g/h[a]	Circumstances or Conditions When Such Rates of Ethanol Elimination Might Be Observed
Slow	0.08 to 0.10	3.9 to 4.9	Malnourished individuals or people on low protein diets (Bode 1978) or suffering from advanced liver cirrhosis or portal hypertension. Administration of inhibitor of alcohol dehydrogenase 4-methyl pyrazole (fomepizole) (Brent et al. 2001).
Moderate	0.10 to 0.15	4.9 to 7.3	Healthy individuals after drinking moderate amounts of alcohol as a bolus dose on an empty stomach (10 h fast) to reach peak BACs of ~1.0 g/L (Jones 1984).
Rapid	0.15 to 0.25	7.3 to 12.3	Regular drinkers e.g., apprehended drivers and non-fasted individuals under social drinking conditions (Jones and Andersson 1996). Use of drugs or medication that boosts the activity of alcohol oxidative enzymes (e.g., CYP2E1). Intravenous administration of amino acids or carbohydrates, such as fructose (Lisander et al. 2006).
Ultra-rapid	0.25 to 0.35	12.3 to 17.1	Alcoholics during detoxification with high starting BAC > 2.0 g/L (Bogusz et al. 1977; Jones and Sternebring 1992). CYP2E1 enzyme activity is enhanced owing to binge drinking. People genetically predisposed to a more rapid metabolism of ethanol owing to hypermetabolic state, burn trauma or treatment with certain drugs, such as dinitrophenol (Jones et al. 1997).

[a] Rate of elimination from whole body was calculated for a healthy male subject (70 kg body weight) with a distribution volume of ethanol of 0.70 L/kg.

the rate of alcohol elimination from blood might range from a very low value of 0.10 g/L/h to a high of 0.35 g/L/h, which is a 3.5 fold range. However, the vast majority of people will show elimination rates from blood within the range 0.10–0.25 g/L/h (2.5 fold range) and a mean of 0.15 g/L/h is a good average rate for moderate drinkers and recommended for use in various BAC calculations.

The elimination rate of ethanol from blood has not been determined in drunken drivers in an unequivocal way i.e., by repetitive blood sampling and determining the slope of the post-absorptive elimination phase. However, useful, information can be gleaned by taking double or triple blood samples over a few hours and use these BACs for evaluation. With two consecutive blood samples 60 minutes apart the elimination rate is given by (BAC_1 – BAC_2) per hour. Validity of the resulting rate assumes that zero-order elimination kinetics operates and that the person was in the post-absorptive phase when the first blood sample was taken (Neuteboom and Jones 1990; Schweitzer 1968; Simic and Tasic 2007).

In a study of alcohol elimination rates in a population of 1,090 drinking drivers using double blood samples, a mean rate of 0.19 ± 0.05 g/L/h (± SD) was obtained with a 95% range from 0.09 to 0.29 g/L/h (Jones and Andersson 1996). In a sub-sample (n = 21) of traffic offenders with very high starting BAC (mean 4.05 g/L) the mean ethanol elimination rate from blood was 0.34 g/L/h (range 0.20–0.61 g/L/h) (Jones 2008a). The faster elimination rates in this population of drinkers probably stems from enzyme induction, because many traffic offenders are alcoholics with an enhanced capacity to dispose of ethanol, owing to induction of the microsomal CYP2EI enzyme (Keiding et al. 1983). The elimination rates of <0.1 g/L or >0.35 g/L are unrealistic and are probably bogus, owing to uncertainty about the position of the BAC curve when the first sample of blood was taken.

In most forensic cases blood or breath samples are available for analysis at only one time point, which means that nothing is known about the position of the blood-alcohol curve (absorptive, plateau, or post-absorptive) nor the pharmacokinetic parameters rho-factor and β-slope. During the prosecution of traffic offenders, the courts might require answers to questions such as:

- How much alcohol was ingested by the suspect to account for the prosecution BAC or BrAC result?
- Does the suspect's statement about his or her drinking agree with the result of the forensic blood or breath-alcohol analysis?
- What influence, if any, did drinking alcohol after driving have on the prosecution BAC or BrAC?
- The suspect claims his drink was spiked with vodka; what influence would this have had on the prosecution BAC or BrAC?

Questions such as these can be answered with a reasonable degree of scientific certainty because of the underlying knowledge base gleaned from hundreds of published and peer-reviewed alcohol dosing studies since the 1930s. Variations in BAC profiles and associated pharmacokinetic parameters of ethanol are much better characterized than for other psychoactive substances encountered in forensic casework.

Most human ethanol dosing studies have involved intake of a bolus dose ingested on an empty stomach and not repetitive drinking over several hours (Jones 1984). More studies would be welcomed to characterize BAC curves and derive pharmacokinetic parameters under real-world drinking conditions. The ideal experimental design should entail repeated intake of different types of alcoholic beverage (beer, wine, and/or spirits) with or without concomitant food intake. Values of C_{max} and t_{max} along with the increase in BAC before reaching C_{max} under social drinking conditions would provide useful information in forensic casework. One such study has already been mentioned, namely consumption of large amounts of alcohol for 6–12 hours and constucting blood-ethanol profiles from repetitive sampling at 15–30 minute intervals during and after drinking ended (Zink and Reinhardt 1984). Under these drinking conditions, the bioavailability of the dose of ethanol was decreased appreciably and the results from this unique study were the subject of a re-evaluation and further discussion in a peer-reviewed journal (Jones et al. 2006).

When blood-alcohol calculations are required in forensic casework, such as during the prosecution of traffic offenders, it is important to consider the magnitude of inter- and intra-individual variations in the pharmacokinetic parameters β and rho (Jones and Jonsson 1994a; Sadler and Lennox 2015). These factors vary between subjects and also within subjects on different drinking occasions, owing to variability in ADME processes (Norberg et al. 2003). The various assumptions made when BAC calculations are necessary for legal purposes should be carefully considered and explained when writing expert statements, or affidavits or testifying in court as an expert witness (Brick 2006; Gullberg 2007).

References

Adachi J, Mizoi Y, Fukunaga T, Ogawa Y, Imamichi H: Comparative study on ethanol elimination and blood acetaldehyde between alcoholics and control subjects; *Alcohol Clin Exp Res* 13:601; 1989.

Agarwal DP, Goedde HW: Pharmacogenetics of alcohol metabolism and alcoholism; *Pharmacogenetics* 2:48; 1992.

Alha A: Blood alcohol and clinical inebriation in Finnish men; *Ann Acad Sci Fenn* A 26:1; 1951.

Al-Lanqawi Y, Moreland TA, McEwen J, Halliday F, Durnin CJ, Stevenson IH: Ethanol kinetics: Extent of error in back extrapolation procedures; *Br J Clin Pharmacol* 34:316; 1992.

Ammon E, Schafer C, Hofmann U, Klotz U: Disposition and first-pass metabolism of ethanol in humans: Is it gastric or hepatic and does it depend on gender? *Clin Pharmacol Ther* 59:503; 1996.

Andreasson R, Jones AW: The life and work of Erik M. P. Widmark; *Am J Forensic Med Pathol* 17:177; 1996.

Anstie FE: Final experiments on the elimination of alcohol from the body; *The Practitioner* 13:15; 1874.

Arstein-Kerslake GW: A confidence interval approach to the development of blood-alcohol concentration charts; *J Safety Res* 17:129; 1986.

Artiss JD, Zak B: Problems with measurements caused by high concentrations of serum solids; *Crit Rev Clin Lab Sci* 25:19; 1987.

Baek IH, Lee BY, Kwon KI: Influence of dissolved oxygen concentration on the pharmacokinetics of alcohol in humans; *Alcohol Clin Exp Res* 34:834; 2010.

Baldwin AD: Anstie's alcohol limit, Francis Edmund Anstie 1833–1874; *Am J Public Health* 87:679; 1977.

Baraona E, Gentry RT, Lieber CS: Bioavailability of alcohol: Role of gastric metabolism and its interaction with other drugs; *Dig Dis* 12:351; 1994a.

Baraona E, Gentry RT, Lieber CS: Blood alcohol levels after prolonged use of histamine-2-receptor antagonists; *Ann Intern Med* 121:73; 1994b.

Barbour AD: Simplified estimation of Widmark "r" values by the method of Forrest; *Sci & Justice* 41:53; 2001.

Berggren SM, Goldberg L: The absorption of ethyl alcohol from the gastro-intestinal tract as a diffusion process; *Acta Physiol Scand* 1:245; 1940.

Bielefeld L, Auwarter V, Pollak S, Thierauf-Emberger A: Differences between the measured blood ethanol concentration and the estimated concentration by Widmark's equation in elderly persons; *Forensic Sci Int* 247:23; 2015.

Bode JC: The metabolism of alcohol: Physiological and pathophysiological aspects; *J R Coll Physicians Lond* 12:122; 1978.

Bode JC, Bode C, Thiele D: Alcohol metabolism in man: effect of intravenous fructose infusion on blood ethanol elimination rate following stimulation by phenobarbital treatment or chronic alcohol consumption; *Klin Wochenschr* 57:125; 1979.

Bogusz M, Pach J, Stasko W: Comparative studies on the rate of ethanol elimination in acute poisoning and in controlled conditions; *J Forensic Sci* 22:446; 1977.

Bowers RV, Burleson WD, Blades JF: Alcohol absorption from the skin in man; *Q J Studies Alc* 3:31; 1941.

Brennan DF, Betzelos S, Reed R, Falk JL: Ethanol elimination rates in an ED population; *Am J Emerg Med* 13:276; 1995.

Brent J: Fomepizole for ethylene glycol and methanol poisoning; *N Engl J Med* 360:2216; 2009.

Brick J: Standardization of alcohol calculations in research; *Alcohol Clin Exp Res* 30:1276; 2006.

Brown DJ: The pharmacokinetics of alcohol excretion in human perspiration; *Meth Find Exptl Clin Pharmacol* 7:539; 1985.

Brown AS, James OF: Omeprazole, ranitidine, and cimetidine have no effect on peak blood ethanol concentrations, first pass metabolism or area under the time-ethanol curve under 'real-life' drinking conditions; *Aliment Pharmacol Ther* 12:141; 1998.

Buono MJ: Sweat ethanol concentrations are highly correlated with co-existing blood values in humans; *Exp Physiol* 84:401; 1999.

Caballeria J, Frezza M, Hernandez-Munoz R, DiPadova C, Korsten MA, Baraona E, Lieber CS: Gastric origin of the first-pass metabolism of ethanol in humans: Effect of gastrectomy; *Gastroenterology* 97:1205; 1989.

Campbell L, Wilson HK: Blood alcohol concentrations following the inhalation of ethanol vapour under controlled conditions; *J Forensic Sci Soc* 26:129; 1986.

Charlebois RC, Corbett MR, Wigmore JG: Comparison of ethanol concentrations in blood, serum, and blood cells for forensic application; *J Anal Toxicol* 20:171; 1996.

Charles BG, Duffull SB: Pharmacokinetic software for the health sciences: Choosing the right package for teaching purposes; *Clin Pharmacokinet* 40:395; 2001.

Cheymol G: Effects of obesity on pharmacokinetics implications for drug therapy; *Clin Pharmacokinet* 39:215; 2000.

Chumlea WC, Guo SS, Zeller CM, Reo NV, Baumgartner RN, Garry PJ, Wang J, Pierson RN, Jr., Heymsfield SB, Siervogel RM: Total body water reference values and prediction equations for adults; *Kidney Int* 59:2250; 2001.

Clark ER, Hughes IE, Letley E: The effect of oral administration of various sugars on blood ethanol concentrations in man; *J Pharm Pharmacol* 25:319; 1973.

Clemmesen JO, Ott P, Sestoft L: The effect of cimetidine on ethanol concentrations in fasting women and men after two different doses of alcohol; *Scand J Gastroenterol* 32:217; 1997.

Cobaugh DJ, Gibbs M, Shapiro DE, Krenzelok EP, Schneidrer SM: A comparison of the bioavailability of oral and intravenous ethanol in healthy male volunteers; *Acad Emerg Med* 6:984; 1999.

Correa CL, Oga S: Effects of the menstrual cycle of white women on ethanol toxicokinetics; *J Stud Alcohol* 65:227; 2004.

Crabb DW: *Recent Developments in Alcoholism—The Liver.* Vol. 11. New York: Plenum Press; 1993:207.

Crabb DW: Ethanol oxidizing enzymes: Roles in alcohol metabolism and alcoholic liver disease; *Prog Liver Dis* 13:151; 1995.

Crabb DW, Dipple KM, Thomasson HR: Alcohol sensitivity, alcohol metabolism, risk of alcoholism, and the role of alcohol and aldehyde dehydrogenase genotypes; *J Lab Clin Med* 122:234; 1993.

Crabb DW, Matsumoto M, Chang D, You M: Overview of the role of alcohol dehydrogenase and aldehyde dehydrogenase and their variants in the genesis of alcohol-related pathology; *Proc Nutr Soc* 63:49; 2004.

Crow KE, Newland KM, Batt RD: The fructose effect; *N Z Med J* 93:232; 1981.

Crownover BP, La Dine J, Bradford B, Glassman E, Forman D, Schneider H, Thurman RG: Activation of ethanol metabolism in humans by fructose: importance of experimental design; *J Pharmacol Exp Ther* 236:574; 1986.

Davies BT, Bowen CK: Peak blood alcohol prediction: An empirical test of two computer models; *J Stud Alcohol* 61:187; 2000.

Dedrick RL, Forrester DD: Blood flow limitations in interpreting Michaelis constants for ethanol oxidation in vivo; *Biochem Pharmacol* 22:1133; 1973.

Dettling A, Fischer F, Bohler S, Ulrichs F, Skopp G, Graw M, Haffner HT: Ethanol elimination rates in men and women in consideration of the calculated liver weight; *Alcohol* 41:415; 2007.

Dettling A, Skopp G, Graw M, Haffner HT: The influence of sex hormones on the elimination kinetics of ethanol; *Forensic Sci Int* 177:85; 2008.

Dettling A, Witte S, Skopp G, Graw M, Haffner HT: A regression model applied to gender-specific ethanol elimination rates from blood and breath measurements in non-alcoholics; *Int J Legal Med* 123:381; 2009.

Dettling A, Preiss A, Skopp G, Haffner HT: The influence of the luteal and follicular phases on major pharmacokinetic parameters of blood and breath alcohol kinetics in women; *Alcohol* 44:315; 2010.

DiPadova C, Roine R, Frezza M, Gentry RT, Baraona E, Lieber CS: Effects of ranitidine on blood alcohol levels after ethanol ingestion. Comparison with other H2-receptor antagonists; *J Am Med Assoc* 267:83; 1992.

Dohmen K, Baraona E, Ishibashi H, Pozzato G, Moretti M, Matsunaga C, Fujimoto K, Lieber CS: Ethnic differences in gastric sigma-alcohol dehydrogenase activity and ethanol first-pass metabolism; *Alcohol Clin Exp Res* 20:1569; 1996.

Dost FH: *Der Blütspiegel-Kinetic der Konzentrationsablaüfe in der Krieslauffüssigkeit*. Leipzig: G. Thieme; 1953.

Dost FH: *Grundlagen den Pharmacokinetik*. Leipzig: G. Thieme; 1968.

Dufour MC: What is moderate drinking? Defining "drinks" and drinking levels; *Alcohol Res Health* 23:5; 1999.

Edelman IS, Haley HB, Schloerb PR, Sheldon DB, Friis-Hansen BJ, Stoll G, Moore FD: Further observations on total body water. I. Normal values throughout the life span; *Surg Gynecol Obstet* 95:1; 1952.

Edelbroek MA, Horowitz M, Wishart JM, Akkermans LM: Effects of erythromycin on gastric emptying, alcohol absorption and small intestinal transit in normal subjects; *J Nucl Med* 34:582; 1993.

Edenberg HJ: The genetics of alcohol metabolism: Role of alcohol dehydrogenase and aldehyde dehydrogenase variants; *Alcohol Res Health* 30:5; 2007.

Endres HG, Gruner O: Comparison of D2O and ethanol dilutions in total body water measurements in humans; *Clin Investig* 72:830; 1994.

Ferner RE, Norman E: *Forensic Pharmacology—Medicines, Mayhem and Malpractice*. Oxford: Oxford University Press; 1996.

Fiorentino DD, Moskowitz H: Breath alcohol elimination rate as a function of age, gender, and drinking practice; *Forensic Sci Int* 233:278; 2013.

Flegal KM, Carroll MD, Ogden CL, Johnson CL: Prevalence and trends in obesity among US adults, 1999–2000; *J Am Med Assoc* 288:1723; 2002.

Fleming R, Stotz E: Experimental studies in alcoholism 1. The alcohol content of the blood and cerebroispinal fluid following oral administration in chronic alcoholism and the psychoses; *Arch Neurol Psychiat* 33:492; 1935.

Forrest ARW: The estimation of Widmark's factor; *J Forensic Sci Soc* 26:249; 1986.

Fraser AG, Prewett EJ, Hudson M, Sawyerr AM, Rosalki SB, Pounder RE: The effect of ranitidine, cimetidine or famotidine on low-dose post-prandial alcohol absorption; *Aliment Pharmacol Ther* 5:263; 1991.

Fraser AG, Hudson M, Sawyerr AM, Smith M, Rosalki SB, Pounder RE: Ranitidine, cimetidine, famotidine have no effect on post-prandial absorption of ethanol 0.8 g/kg taken after an evening meal; *Aliment Pharmacol Ther* 6:693; 1992.

Fraser AG, Hudson M, Sawyerr AM, Smith MS, Sercombe J, Rosalki SB, Pounder RE: Ranitidine has no effect on postbreakfast ethanol absorption; *Am J Gastroenterol* 88:217; 1993.

Fraser AG, Rosalki SB, Gamble GD, Pounder RE: Inter-individual and intra-individual variability of ethanol concentration-time profiles: Comparison of ethanol ingestion before or after an evening meal; *Br J Clin Pharmacol* 40:387; 1995.

Fraser AG: Pharmacokinetic interactions between alcohol and other drugs; *Clin Pharmacokinet* 33:79; 1997.

Frezza M, di Padova C, Pozzato G, Terpin M, Baraona E, Lieber CS: High blood alcohol levels in women. The role of decreased gastric alcohol dehydrogenase activity and first-pass metabolism; *N Engl J Med* 322:95; 1990.

Furne J, Levitt MD: Speed of gastric emptying and metabolism of ethanol; *Gut* 45:916; 1999.

Gabrielsson J, Weiner D: *Pharmacokinetic and Pharmacodynamic Data Analysis: Concepts and Applications*. 3rd ed. Stockholm: Swedish Pharmaceutical Press; 2000.

Gallardo E, Barrosa M, Queiroz JA: Current technologies and considerations for drug bioanalysis in oral fluid; *Bioanalysis* 1:637; 2009.

Goist KC, Jr., Sutker PB: Acute alcohol intoxication and body composition in women and men; *Pharmacol Biochem Behav* 22:811; 1985.

Gullberg RG: Methodology and quality assurance in forensic breath alcohol analysis; *Forensic Sci Rev* 12:49; 2000.

Gullberg RG: Estimating the uncertainty associated with Widmark's equation as commonly applied in forensic toxicology; *Forensic Sci Int* 172:33; 2007.

Gullberg RG, Jones AW: Guidelines for estimating the amount of alcohol consumed from a single measurement of blood alcohol concentration: Re-evaluation of Widmark's equation; *Forensic Sci Int* 69:119; 1994.

Gustafson R, Kallmen H: The blood alcohol curve as a function of time and type of beverage: Methodological considerations; *Drug Alcohol Depend* 21:243; 1988.

Haffner HT, Besserer K, Stetter F, Mann K: Die Äthanol Eliminationsgeschwindigkeit bei Alkoholikern unter besonderer Berücksichtigung der Maximalwertvariante der forensischen BAK Rückrechung *Blutalkohol* 28:46; 1991.

Haffner HT, Graw M, Dettling A, Schmitt G, Schuff A: Concentration dependency of the BAC/BrAC (blood alcohol concentration/breath alcohol concentration) conversion factor during the linear elimination phase; *Int J Legal Med* 117:276; 2003.

Hagedorn JC, Encarnacion B, Brat GA, Morton JM: Does gastric bypass alter alcohol metabolism?; *Surg Obes Relat Dis* 3:543; 2007.

Hahn RG, Norberg A, Gabrielsson J, Danielsson A, Jones AW: Eating a meal increases the clearance of ethanol given by intravenous infusion; *Alcohol Alcohol* 29:673; 1994.

Hahn RG, Norberg A, Jones AW: Rate of distribution of ethanol into the total body water; *Am J Ther* 2:50; 1995.

Hammond KB, Rumack BH, Rodgerson DO: Blood ethanol. A report of unusually high levels in a living patient; *J Am Med Assoc* 226:63; 1973.

Hansen CS, Faerch LH, Kristensen PL: Testing the validity of the Danish urban myth that alcohol can be absorbed through feet: Open labelled self experimental study; *Br Med J* 341:c6812; 2010.

Hein PM, Vock R: Alkoholtrinkversuche mit über 60 Jahre alten männlichen Personen; *Blutalkohol* 26:98; 1989.

Hobbes J, Boutagy J, Shenfield GM: Interactions between ethanol and oral contraceptive steroids; *Clin Pharmacol Ther* 38:371; 1985.

Holford NH: Clinical pharmacokinetics of ethanol; *Clin Pharmacokinet* 13:273; 1987.

Holzbecher M, Wells A: Elimination of ethanol in humans; *Can Soc Forensic Sci J* 17:182; 1984.

Hustad JT, Carey KB: Using calculations to estimate blood alcohol concentrations for naturally occurring drinking episodes: A validity study; *J Stud Alcohol* 66:130; 2005.

Hyvarinen J, Laakso M, Sippel H, Roine R, Huopaniemi T, Leinonen L, Hytonen V: Alcohol detoxification accelerated by oxygenated drinking water; *Life Sci* 22:553; 1978.

Iffland R, Jones AW: Evaluating alleged drinking after driving—The hip-flask defence. Part 1. Double blood samples and urine-to-blood alcohol relationship; *Med Sci Law* 42:207; 2002.

Iffland R, Jones AW: Evaluating alleged drinking after driving—The hip-flask defence. Part 2. Congener analysis; *Med Sci Law* 43:39; 2003.

Iffland R, West A, Bilzer N, Schuff A: Zur Zuverlässigkeit der Blutalkoholbestimmung. Das verkeilungsverhältnis des Wassers zwischen Serum und Vollblut; *Rechtsmedizin* 9:123; 1999.

Jackson PR, Tucker GT, Woods HF: Backtracking booze with Bayes—The retrospective interpretation of blood alcohol data; *Br J Clin Pharmacol* 31:55; 1991.

Johnson RD, Horowitz M, Maddox AF, Wishart JM, Shearman DJ: Cigarette smoking and rate of gastric emptying: Effect on alcohol absorption; *Br Med J* 302:20; 1991.

Jones AW: Variability of the blood:breath alcohol ratio in vivo; *J Stud Alcohol* 39:1931; 1978.

Jones AW: Inter- and intra-individual variations in the saliva/blood alcohol ratio during ethanol metabolism in man; *Clin Chem* 25:1394; 1979.

Jones AW: Interindividual variations in the disposition and metabolism of ethanol in healthy men; *Alcohol* 1:385; 1984.

Jones AW: Excretion of alcohol in urine and diuresis in healthy men in relation to their age, the dose administered and the time after drinking; *Forensic Sci Int* 45:217; 1990.

Jones AW: Back-estimation of blood alcohol concentration; *Br J Clin Pharmacol* 35:669; 1993a.

Jones AW: Pharmacokinetics of ethanol in saliva: Comparison with blood and breath alcohol profiles, subjective feelings of intoxication, and diminished performance; *Clin Chem* 39:1837; 1993b.

Jones AW, Hahn RG: Pharmacokinetics of ethanol in patients with renal failure before and after hemodialysis; *Forensic Sci Int* 90:175; 1997.

Jones AW: Medicolegal alcohol determinations—Blood or breath alcohol concentration? *Forensic Sci Rev* 12:23; 2000.

Jones AW: Urine as a biological specimen for forensic analysis of alcohol and variability in the urine-to-blood relationship; *Toxicol Rev* 25:15; 2006.

Jones AW: Body mass index and blood-alcohol calculations; *J Anal Toxicol* 31:177; 2007.

Jones AW: Ultra-rapid rate of ethanol elimination from blood in drunken drivers with extremely high blood-alcohol concentrations; *Int J Legal Med* 122:129; 2008a.

Jones AW: Biomarkers of acute and chronic alcohol ingestion. In: Garriott JC, ed. *Medicolegal Aspects of Alcohol*, Vol. 4. Tuscon: Lawyers & Judges Publishing Company; 2008b.

Jones AW: Erik MP Widmark—Bridged the gap between forensic toxicology and alcohol and traffic safety research; *Blutalkohol* 46:15; 2009.

Jones AW: Evidence based survey of the elimination rates of ethanol from blood with applications in forensic casework; Forensic Sci Int 200:1; 2010.

Jones AW: Biomarkers of recent drinking, retrograde extrapolation of blood-alcohol concentration and plasma-to-blood distribution ratio of alcohol in a case of driving udner the influence of alcohol; *J Forensic Leg Med* 18:213; 2011.

Jones AW: Pharmacokinetic parameters of ethanol and subjective feelings of intoxication in healthy men after they drank 0.54 g/kg, 0.68 g/kg and 0.85 g ethanol per kg body weight as neat whisky on an empty stomach; (unpublished work) 2020.

Jones AW, Neri A: Age-related differences in blood ethanol parameters and subjective feelings of intoxication in healthy men; *Alcohol Alcohol* 20:45; 1985.

Jones AW, Neri A: Evaluation of blood-alcohol profiles after consumption of alcohol together with a large meal; *Can Soc Forensic Sci J* 24:165; 1991.

Jones AW, Sternebring B: Kinetics of ethanol and methanol in alcoholics during detoxification; *Alcohol Alcohol* 27:641; 1992.

Jones AW, Jonsson KA: Between-subject and within-subject variations in the pharmacokinetics of ethanol; *Br J Clin Pharmacol* 37:427; 1994a.

Jones AW, Jonsson KA: Food-induced lowering of blood-ethanol profiles and increased rate of elimination immediately after a meal; *J Forensic Sci* 39:1084; 1994b.

Jones AW, Neri A: Age-related differences in the effects of ethanol on performance and behaviour in healthy men; *Alcohol Alcohol* 29:171; 1994.

Jones AW, Andersson L: Influence of age, gender, and blood-alcohol concentration on the disappearance rate of alcohol from blood in drinking drivers; *J Forensic Sci* 41:922; 1996.

Jones AW, Andersson L: Comparison of ethanol concentrations in venous blood and end-expired breath during a controlled drinking study; *Forensic Sci Int* 132:18; 2003.

Jones AW, Larsson H: Distribution of diazepam and nordiazepam between plasma and whole blood and the influence of hematocrit; *Ther Drug Monit* 26:380; 2004.

Jones AW, Holmgren A: Concentration distributions of the drugs most frequently identified in post-mortem femoral blood representing all causes of death; *Med Sci Law* 49:257; 2009a.

Jones AW, Holmgren A: Age and gender differences in blood-alcohol concentration in apprehended drivers in relation to the amounts of alcohol consumed; *Forensic Sci Int* 188:40; 2009b.

Jones AW, Hahn RG, Stalberg HP: Distribution of ethanol and water between plasma and whole blood; inter- and intra-individual variations after administration of ethanol by intravenous infusion; *Scand J Clin Lab Invest* 50:775; 1990.

Jones AW, Jonsson KA, Neri A: Peak blood-ethanol concentration and the time of its occurrence after rapid drinking on an empty stomach; *J Forensic Sci* 36:376; 1991.

Jones AW, Hahn RG, Stalberg HP: Pharmacokinetics of ethanol in plasma and whole blood: Estimation of total body water by the dilution principle; *Eur J Clin Pharmacol* 42:445; 1992.

Jones AW, Jonsson KA, Kechagias S: Effect of high-fat, high-protein, and high-carbohydrate meals on the pharmacokinetics of a small dose of ethanol; *Br J Clin Pharmacol* 44:521; 1997.

Jones AW, Norberg A, Hahn RG: Concentration-time profiles of ethanol in arterial and venous blood and end-expired breath during and after intravenous infusion; *J Forensic Sci* 42:1088; 1997.

Jones AW, Lindberg L, Olsson SG: Magnitude and time-course of arterio-venous differences in blood-alcohol concentration in healthy men; *Clin Pharmacokinet* 43:1157; 2004.

Jones AW, Wigmore JG, House CJ: The course of the blood-alcohol curve after consumption of large amounts of alcohol under realistic conditions; *Can Soc Forensic Sci J* 39:125; 2006.

Jones AW, Kugelberg FC, Holmgren A, Ahlner J: Occurrence of ethanol and other drugs in blood and urine specimens from female victims of alleged sexual assault; *Forensic Sci Int* 187:40; 2008.

Jonsson KA, Jones AW, Bostrom H, Andersson T: Lack of effect of omeprazole, cimetidine, and ranitidine on the pharmacokinetics of ethanol in fasting male volunteers; *Eur J Clin Pharmacol* 42:209; 1992.

Jornvall H, Hoog JO: Nomenclature of alcohol dehydrogenases; *Alcohol Alcohol* 30:153; 1995.

Jornvall H, Hoog JO, Persson B, Pares X: Pharmacogenetics of the alcohol dehydrogenase system; *Pharmacology* 61:184; 2000.

Julkunen RJ, Di Padova C, Lieber CS: First pass metabolism of ethanol—A gastrointestinal barrier against the systemic toxicity of ethanol; *Life Sci* 37:567; 1985.

Kalant H: Intoxication automatism: Legal concept vs scientific evidence? *Contemp Drug Prob* 23:631; 1996a.

Kalant H: Pharmacokinetics of ethanol: Absorption, distribution, and elimination. In: Beglieter H, Kissin B, eds. *The Pharmacology of Alcohol and Alcohol Dependence.* New York: Oxford University Press; 1996b:15.

Kalant H: Effects of food and body composition on blood alcohol levels. In: Preedy V, Watson R, eds. *Comprehensive Handbook of Alcohol Related Pathology*, Vol. 1; 2004:87.

Kalant H, LeBlanc AE, Gibbins RJ: Tolerance to, and dependence on, some non-opiate psychotropic drugs; *Pharmacol Rev* 23:135; 1971.

Kechagias S, Jonsson KA, Jones AW: Impact of gastric emptying on the pharmacokinetics of ethanol as influenced by cisapride; *Br J Clin Pharmacol* 48:728; 1999.

Keiding S, Christensen NJ, Damgaard SE, Dejgard A, Iversen HL, Jacobsen A, Johansen S, Lundquist F, Rubinstein E, Winkler K: Ethanol metabolism in heavy drinkers after massive and moderate alcohol intake; *Biochem Pharmacol* 32:3097; 1983.

Kerrigan S: The use of alcohol to facilitate sexual assault; *Forensic Sci Rev* 22:15; 2010.

Klockhoff H, Naslund I, Jones AW: Faster absorption of ethanol and higher peak concentration in women after gastric bypass surgery; *Br J Clin Pharmacol* 54:587; 2002.

Klotz U, Ammon E: Clinical and toxicological consequences of the inductive potential of ethanol; *Eur J Clin Pharmacol* 54:7; 1998.

Kronstrand C, Nilsson G, Cherma MD, Ahlner J, Kugelberg FC, Kronstrand R: Evaluating the hip-flask defence in subjects with alcohol on board: An experimental study; *Forensic Sci Int* 294:189; 2019.

Kruhoffer PW: Handling of inspired vaporized ethanol in the airways and lungs (with comments on forensic aspects); *Forensic Sci Int* 21:1; 1983.

Kwo PY, Ramchandani VA, O'Connor S, Amann D, Carr LG, Sandrasegaran K, Kopecky KK, Li TK: Gender differences in alcohol metabolism: Relationship to liver volume and effect of adjusting for body mass; *Gastroenterology* 115:1552; 1998.

Laakso M, Huopaniemi T, Hyvarinen J, Lindros K, Roine R, Sippel H, Ylikahri R: Inefficacy of oxygenated drinking water in accelerating ethanol elimination in humans; *Life Sci* 25:1369; 1979.

Labay L, Logan BK: Call for a scientific consensus regarding the application of retrograde extrapolation to determine blood alcohol content in DUI cases; *J Forensic Sci* 63:1602; 2018.

Lachenmeier DW, Rehm J: Letter to the editor in regard to Baek, Lee, and Kwon (2010): Influence of dissolved oxygen concentration on the pharmacokinetics of alcohol in humans: Does oxygenated alcohol reduce hangover? *Alcohol Clin Exp Res* 34:1671; 2010.

Lammers SM, Mainzer DE, Breteler MH: Do alcohol pharmacokinetics in women vary due to the menstrual cycle? *Addiction* 90:23; 1995.

Lamminpaa A, Hoppu K: First-order alcohol elimination in severe alcohol intoxication in an adolescent: A case report; *Am J Emerg Med* 27:128 e5; 2009.

Langford NJ, Marshall T, Ferner RE: The lacing defence: Double blind study of thresholds for detecting addition of ethanol to drinks; *Br Med J* 319:1610; 1999.

Lee SS, Buters JT, Pineau T, Fernandez-Salguero P, Gonzalez FJ: Role of CYP2E1 in the hepatotoxicity of acetaminophen; *J Biol Chem* 271:12063; 1996.

Lekskulchai V, Rattanawibool S: Blood alcohol concentration after one standard drink in Thai healthy volunteers; *J Med Assoc Thai* 90:1137; 2007.

Lenter C, ed: *Geigy Scientific Tables.* Basel: Ciba-Geigy; 1981.

Lester D, Greenberg LA: The inhalation of ethyl alcohol by man. I. Industrial hygiene and medicolegal aspects. II. Individuals treated with tetraethylthiuram disulfide; *Q J Stud Alcohol* 12:168; 1951.

Levitt DG: PKQuest: Measurement of intestinal absorption and first pass metabolism—Application to human ethanol pharmacokinetics; *BMC Clin Pharmacol* 2:4; 2002.

Levitt DG: Physiologically based pharmacokinetic modeling of arterial—Antecubital vein concentration difference; *BMC Clin Pharmacol* 4:2; 2004.

Levitt MD: Review article: Lack of clinical significance of the interaction between H2-receptor antagonists and ethanol; *Aliment Pharmacol Ther* 7:131; 1993.

Levitt MD: Antagonist: The case against first-pass metabolism of ethanol in the stomach; *J Lab Clin Med* 123:28; 1994.

Levitt MD, Levitt DG: The critical role of the rate of ethanol absorption in the interpretation of studies purporting to demonstrate gastric metabolism of ethanol; *J Pharmacol Exp Ther* 269:297; 1994.

Lewis KO: Back calculation of blood alcohol concentration; *Br Med J (Clin Res Ed)* 295:800; 1987.

Lewis MJ: Blood alcohol: The concentration-time curve and retrospective estimation of level; *J Forensic Sci Soc* 26:95; 1986.

Li TK, Yin SJ, Crabb DW, O'Connor S, Ramchandani VA: Genetic and environmental influences on alcohol metabolism in humans; *Alcohol Clin Exp Res* 25:136; 2001.

Lieber CS: Alcohol and the liver: 1994 update; *Gastroenterology* 106:1085; 1994.

Lieber CS: Cytochrome P-4502E1: Its physiological and pathological role; *Physiol Rev* 77:517; 1997.

Lieber CS: Hepatic and other medical disorders of alcoholism: From pathogenesis to treatment; *J Stud Alcohol* 59:9; 1998.

Lieber CS: Microsomal ethanol-oxidizing system (MEOS): The first 30 years (1968–1998)—A review; *Alcohol Clin Exp Res* 23:991; 1999.

Lieber CS, Gentry RT, Baraona E: First pass metabolism of ethanol; *Alcohol Alcohol Suppl* 2:163; 1994.

Liljestrand G, Linde P: Über die Ausscheidung des Alkohols mit der Exspirationsluft; *Skand Arch Physiol* 60:273; 1930.

Lim RT, Jr., Gentry RT, Ito D, Yokoyama H, Baraona E, Lieber CS: First-pass metabolism of ethanol is predominantly gastric; *Alcohol Clin Exp Res* 17:1337; 1993.

Lin Y, Weidler DJ, Garg DC, Wagner JG: Effects of solid food on blood levels of alcohol in man; *Res Commun Chem Pathol Pharmacol* 13:713; 1976.

Lindberg L, Brauer S, Wollmer P, Goldberg L, Jones AW, Olsson SG: Breath alcohol concentration determined with a new analyzer using free exhalation predicts almost precisely the arterial blood alcohol concentration; *Forensic Sci Int* 168:200; 2007.

Lindblad B, Olsson R: Unusually high levels of blood alcohol? *J Am Med Assoc* 236:1600; 1976.

Lisander B, Lundvall O, Tomner J, Jones AW: Enhanced rate of ethanol elimination from blood after intravenous administration of amino acids compared with equicaloric glucose; *Alcohol Alcohol* 41:39; 2006.

Loeppky JA, Myhre LG, Venters MD, Luft UC: Total body water and lean body mass estimated by ethanol dilution; *J Appl Physiol* 42:803; 1977.

Ludden TM: Nonlinear pharmacokinetics: Clinical Implications; *Clin Pharmacokinet* 20:429; 1991.

Lund A: The secretion of alcohol in the tear fluid; *Blutalkohol* 21:51; 1984.

Lundquist F, Wolthers H: The kinetics of alcohol elimination in man; *Acta Pharmacol Toxicol (Copenh)* 14:265; 1958.

MacLean RR, Valentine GW, Jatlow PI, Sofuoglu M: Inhalation of alcohol vapor: Measurement and implications; *Alcohol Clin Exp Res* 41:238; 2017.

Marathe CS, Rayner CK, Jones KL, Horowitz M: Relationships between gastric emptying, postprandial glycemia, and incretin hormones; *Diabetes Care* 36:1396; 2013.

Marczinski CA, Stamates AL: Artificial sweeteners versus regular mixers increase breath alcohol concentrations in male and female social drinkers; *Alcohol Clin Exp Res* 37:696; 2013.

Marques PR, McKnight AS: Field and laboratory alcohol detection with 2 types of transdermal devices; *Alcohol Clin Exp Res* 33:703; 2009.

Marshall AW, Kingstone D, Boss M, Morgan MY: Ethanol elimination in males and females: Relationship to menstrual cycle and body composition; *Hepatology* 3:701; 1983.

Martin CS, Moss HB: Measurement of acute tolerance to alcohol in human subjects; *Alcohol Clin Exp Res* 17:211; 1993.

Martin E, Moll W, Schmid P, Dettli L: The pharmacokinetics of alcohol in human breath, venous and arterial blood after oral ingestion; *Eur J Clin Pharmacol* 26:619; 1984.

Mascord D, Smith J, Starmer GA, Whitfield JB: Effect of oral glucose on the rate of metabolism of ethanol in humans; *Alcohol Alcohol* 23:365; 1988.

Mascord D, Smith J, Starmer GA, Whitfield JB: The effect of fructose on alcohol metabolism and on the [lactate]/[pyruvate] ratio in man; *Alcohol Alcohol* 26:53; 1991.

Mascord D, Smith J, Starmer GA, Whitfield JB: Effects of increasing the rate of alcohol metabolism on plasma acetate concentration; *Alcohol Alcohol* 27:25; 1992.

Maskell PD, Jones AW, Savage A, Scott-Ham M: Evidence based survey of the distribution volume of ethanol: Comparison of empirically determined values with anthropometric measures; *Forensic Sci Int* 294:124; 2019.

Mason JK, Blackmore DJ: Experimental inhalation of ethanol vapour; *Med Sci Law* 12:205; 1972.

Mather LE: Anatomical-physiological approaches in pharmacokinetics and pharmacodynamics; *Clin Pharmacokinet* 40:707; 2001.

Maudens KE, Patteet L, van Nuijs AL, Van Broekhoven C, Covaci A, Neels H: The influence of the body mass index (BMI) on the volume of distribution of ethanol; *Forensic Sci Int* 243:74; 2014.

Mehrtens HG, Newman HW: Alcohol injected intravenously its penetration into the cerebrospinal fluid in man; *Arch Neurol Psychiat* 30:1092; 1933.

Mellanby E: Alcohol: Its absorption into and disappearance from the blood under different conditions; Medical Research Committee (Series nr 13, HMSO): London, UK; 1919.

Mellanby E: Alcohol and alcoholic intoxication; *Brit J Inebriety* 17:157; 1920.

Mezey E, Oesterling JE, Potter JJ: Influence of male hormones on rates of ethanol elimination in man; *Hepatology* 8:742; 1988.

Mezey E, Hamilton B, Potter JJ: Effect of testosterone administration on rates of ethanol elimination in hypogonadal patients; *Alcohol* 6:331; 1989.

Michaelis L, Menton ML: Die Kinetik der Invertinwirking; *Biochem Z* 49:333; 1913.

Mishra L, Sharma S, Potter JJ, Mezey E: More rapid elimination of alcohol in women as compared to their male siblings; *Alcohol Clin Exp Res* 13:752; 1989.

Mitchell MC: Alcohol-induced impairment of central nervous system function: Behavioral skills involved in driving; *J Stud Alcohol Suppl* 10:109; 1985.

Mitchell MC Jr, Teigen EL, Ramchandani VA: Absorption and peak blood alcohol concentration after drinking beer, wine, or spirits; *Alcohol Clin Exp Res* 38:1200; 2014.

Montgomery MR, Reasor MJ: Retrograde extrapolation of blood alcohol data: An applied approach; *J Toxicol Environ Health* 36:281; 1992.

Moody DE: The inhibition of first-pass metabolism of ethanol by H_2-receptor antagonists: a tabulated review; *Expert Opinion on Drug Safety* 17:917; 2018.

Morimoto K, Takeshita T: Low Km aldehyde dehydrogenase (ALDH2) polymorphism, alcohol-drinking behavior, and chromosome alterations in peripheral lymphocytes; *Environ Health Perspect* 104 Suppl 3:563; 1996.

Mumenthaler MS, Taylor JL, O'Hara R, Fisch HU, Yesavage JA: Effects of menstrual cycle and female sex steroids on ethanol pharmacokinetics; *Alcohol Clin Exp Res* 23:250; 1999.

Mumenthaler MS, Taylor JL, Yesavage JA: Ethanol pharmacokinetics in white women: Nonlinear model fitting versus zero-order elimination analyses; *Alcohol Clin Exp Res* 24:1353; 2000.

Neuteboom W, Jones AW: Disappearance rate of alcohol from the blood of drunk drivers calculated from two consecutive samples; what do the results really mean? *Forensic Sci Int* 45:107; 1990.

Nimmo WS: Drugs, diseases and altered gastric emptying; *Clin Pharmacokinet* 1:189; 1976.

Norberg A, Sandhagen B, Bratteby LE, Gabrielsson J, Jones AW, Fan H, Hahn RG: Do ethanol and deuterium oxide distribute into the same water space in healthy volunteers? *Alcohol Clin Exp Res* 25:1423; 2001.

Norberg A, Jones AW, Hahn RG, Gabrielsson JL: Role of variability in explaining ethanol pharmacokinetics: Research and forensic applications; *Clin Pharmacokinet* 42:1; 2003.

Nutt D, King LA, Phillips LD: Drug harms in the UK: A multicriteria decision analysis; *Lancet* 376:1558; 2010.

Oneta CM, Simanowski UA, Martinez M, Allali-Hassani A, Pares X, Homann N, Conradt C, Waldherr R, Fiehn W, Coutelle C, Seitz HK: First pass metabolism of ethanol is strikingly influenced by the speed of gastric emptying; *Gut* 43:612; 1998.

Oneta CM, Lieber CS, Li J, Ruttimann S, Schmid B, Lattmann J, Rosman AS, Seitz HK: Dynamics of cytochrome P4502E1 activity in man: Induction by ethanol and disappearance during withdrawal phase; *J Hepatol* 36:47; 2002.

Osterlind S, Ahlen M, Wolff E: Investigations concerning the constants "beta" and "rho" according to Widmark especially in women; *Acta Pathol Microbiol Scand* Supp 54:489; 1944.

Panes J, Caballeria J, Guitart R, Pares A, Soler X, Rodamilans M, Navasa M, Pares X, Bosch J, Rodes J: Determinants of ethanol and acetaldehyde metabolism in chronic alcoholics; *Alcohol Clin Exp Res* 17:48; 1993.

Passananti GT, Wolff CA, Vesell ES: Reproducibility of individual rates of ethanol metabolism in fasting subjects; *Clin Pharmacol Ther* 47:389; 1990.

Pavlic M, Grubwieser P, Libiseller K, Rabl W: Elimination rates of breath alcohol; *Forensic Sci Int* 171:16; 2007.

Pawan GL, Grice K: Distribution of alcohol in urine and sweat after drinking; *Lancet* 2:1016; 1968.

Pepino MY, Okunade AL, Eagon JC, Bartholow BD, Bucholz K, Klein S: Effect of Roux-en-Y gastric bypass surgery: Converting 2 alcoholic drinks to 4; *JAMA Surgery* 150:1096; 2015.

Phillips M: Sweat-patch testing detects inaccurate self-reports of alcohol consumption; *Alcohol Clin Exp Res* 8:51; 1984.

Posey D, Mozayani A: The estimation of blood alcohol concentration—Widmark revisited; *Forensic Sci Med Pathol* 3:33; 2007.

Prescott LF: Paracetamol, alcohol and the liver; *Br J Clin Pharmacol* 49:291; 2000.

Ramchandani VA, O'Connor S: Studying alcohol elimination using the alcohol clamp method; *Alcohol Res Health* 29:286; 2006.

Ramchandani VA, Kwo PY, Li TK: Effect of food and food composition on alcohol elimination rates in healthy men and women; *J Clin Pharmacol* 41:1345; 2001.

Ramchandani VA, O'Connor S, Neumark Y, Zimmermann US, Morzorati SL, de Wit H: The alcohol clamp: Applications, challenges, and new directions—An RSA 2004 symposium summary; *Alcohol Clin Exp Res* 30:155; 2006.

Rangno RE, Kreeft JH, Sitar DS: Ethanol "dose-dependent" elimination: Michaelis-Menten v classical kinetic analysis; *Br J Clin Pharmacol* 12:667; 1981.

Rhee SJ, Chae JW, Song BJ, Lee ES, Kwon KI: Effect of dissolved oxygen in alcoholic beverages and drinking water on alcohol elimination in humans; *Alcohol* 47:27; 2013.

Roberts BJ, Song BJ, Soh Y, Park SS, Shoaf SE: Ethanol induces CYP2E1 by protein stabilization. Role of ubiquitin conjugation in the rapid degradation of CYP2E1; *J Biol Chem* 270:29632; 1995.

Roberts C, Robinson SP: Alcohol concentration and carbonation of drinks: The effect on blood alcohol levels; *J Forensic Leg Med* 14:398; 2007.

Rockerbie DW, Rockerbie RA: Computer simulation analysis of blood alcohol; *J Clin Forensic Med* 2:137; 1995.

Rogers J, Smith J, Starmer GA, Whitfield JB: Differing effects of carbohydrate, fat and protein on the rate of ethanol metabolism; *Alcohol Alcohol* 22:345; 1987.

Rosenfeld LM: Physiology of water; *Clin Dermatol* 14:555; 1996.

Rowland M, Tozer TN: *Clinical Pharmacokinetics—Concepts and Applications*. 3rd ed. Baltimore: Williams & Wilkins; 1995.

Russo A, Stevens JE, Chen R, Gentilcore D, Burnet R, Horowitz M, Jones KL: Insulin-induced hypoglycemia accelerates gastric emptying of solids and liquids in long-standing type 1 diabetes; *J Clin Endocrinol Metab* 90:4489; 2005.

Sadler DW, Fox J: Intra-individual and inter-individual variation in breath alcohol pharmacokinetics: The effect of food on absorption; *Sci Justice* 51:3; 2011.

Sadler DW, Lennox S: Intra-individual and inter-individual variation in breath alcohol pharmacokinetics: Variation over three visits; *J Forensic Leg Med* 34:88; 2015.

Schmidt V, Oehmichen M, Pedal I: Beschleunigte Ethanolelimination nach Bariumbreischluck—Humanexperimentelle Studie mit parenteraler Alkoholzufuhr; *Blutalkohol* 29:119; 1992.

Schonheyder F, Strange-Petersen O, Terkildsen K, Posborg-Petersen V: On the variation of the alcoholemie curve; *Acta Med Scand* 109:460; 1942.

Schrot M, Puschel K, Edler C: Berauscht vom Champagnerbad—Fehlanzeige: Keine Alkoholresorption durch die intakte Haut; *Blutalkohol* 47:275; 2010.

Schweitzer H: Statistische Untersuchungen zur Alkoholelimination an 1512 Doppelentnahmen; *Blutalkohol* 5:73; 1968.

Sedman AJ, Wilkinson PK, Wagner JG: Concentrations of ethanol in two segments of the vascular system; *J Forensic Sci* 21:315; 1976.

Seidell JC, Flegal KM: Assessing obesity: Classification and epidemiology; *Br Med Bull* 53:238; 1997.

Seidl S, Jensen U, Alt A: The calculation of blood ethanol concentrations in males and females; *Int J Legal Med* 114:71; 2000.

Sharma A, Artiss JD, Zak B: Solids as a consideration in legal measurements: Blood ethanol concentrtaion as a model; *Microchem J* 36:28; 1987.

Shoaf SE: Pharmacokinetics of intravenous alcohol: Two compartment, dual Michaelis-Menten elimination; *Alcohol Clin Exp Res* 24:424; 2000.

Simic M, Tasic M: The relationship between alcohol elimination rate and increasing blood alcohol concentration—Calculated from two consecutive blood specimens; *Forensic Sci Int* 172:28; 2007.

Simic M, Tasic M, Stojiljkovic G, Budakov B, Vukovic R: "Cognac alibi" as a drunk-driving defense and medico-legal challenge; *Med Law* 23:367; 2004.

Springer E: Blutalkoholkurven nach Gabe von wässrigen Aethanollösungen verschiedener Konzentrationen; *Blutalkohol* 9:198; 1972.

Steffen KJ, Engel SG, Pollert GA, Li C, Mitchell JE: Blood alcohol concentrations rise rapidly and dramatically after Roux-en-Y gastric bypass; *Surg Obes Relat Dis* 9:470; 2013.

Stowell AR, Stowell LI: Estimation of blood alcohol concentrations after social drinking; *J Forensic Sci* 43:14; 1998.

Suokas A, Forsander O, Lindros K: Distribution and utilization of alcohol-derived acetate in the rat; *J Stud Alcohol* 45:381; 1984.

Swift R: Transdermal alcohol measurement for estimation of blood alcohol concentration; *Alcohol Clin Exp Res* 24:422; 2000.

Takahashi T, Lasker JM, Rosman AS, Lieber CS: Induction of cytochrome P-4502E1 in the human liver by ethanol is caused by a corresponding increase in encoding messenger RNA; *Hepatology* 17:236; 1993.

Tam TW, Yang CT, Fung WK, Mok VK: Widmark factors for local Chinese in Hong Kong. A statistical determination on the effects of various physiological factors; *Forensic Sci Int* 151:23; 2005.

Tanaka E, Terada M, Misawa S: Cytochrome P450 2E1: Its clinical and toxicological role; *J Clin Pharm Ther* 25:165; 2000.

Teorell T: Kinetics of distribution of substances administered to the body. I. The extravascular modesof administration; *Archs Int Pharmacodyn Ther* 57:205; 1937a.

Teorell T: Kinetics of distribution of substances administered to the body. II. The intravascular modes of administration; *Archs Int Pharmacodyn Ther* 57:226; 1937b.

Thomasson HR: Alcohol elimination: Faster in women? *Alcohol Clin Exp Res* 24:419; 2000.

Thomasson HR, Beard JD, Li TK: ADH2 gene polymorphisms are determinants of alcohol pharmacokinetics; *Alcohol Clin Exp Res* 19:1494; 1995.

Toon S, Khan AZ, Holt BI, Mullins FG, Langley SJ, Rowland MM: Absence of effect of ranitidine on blood alcohol concentrations when taken morning, midday, or evening with or without food; *Clin Pharmacol Ther* 55:385; 1994.

Wagner JG: Properties of the Michaelis-Menten equation and its integrated form which are useful in pharmacokinetics; *J Pharmacokinet Biopharm* 1:103; 1973.

Wagner JG: History of phartmacokientics; *Pharmac Ther* 12:537; 1981.

Wagner JG: New and simple method to predict dosage of drugs obeying simple Michaelis-Menten elimination kinetics and to distinguish such kinetics from simple first order and from parallel Michaelis-Menten and first order kinetics; *Ther Drug Monit* 7:377; 1985.

Wagner JG: Lack of first-pass metabolism of ethanol at blood concentrations in the social drinking range; *Life Sci* 39:407; 1986.

Wagner JG, Wilkinson PK, Ganes DA: Parameters Vm' and Km for elimination of alcohol in young male subjects following low doses of alcohol; *Alcohol Alcohol* 24:555; 1989.

Wagner JG, Wilkinson PK, Ganes DA: Estimation of the amount of alcohol ingested from a single blood alcohol concentration; *Alcohol Alcohol* 25:379; 1990.

Wall TL, Peterson CM, Peterson KP, Johnson ML, Thomasson HR, Cole M, Ehlers CL: Alcohol metabolism in Asian-American men with genetic polymorphisms of aldehyde dehydrogenase; *Ann Intern Med* 127:376; 1997.

Wartburg Von J: Pharmacokinetics of alcohol. In: Crow KE, Batt RD, eds. *Human Metabolism of Alcohol*. Vol. 1. Boca Raton: CRC Press; 1989:9.

Watkins RL, Adler EV: The effect of food on alcohol absorption and elimination patterns; *J Forensic Sci* 38:285; 1993.

Watson PE, Watson ID, Batt RD: Prediction of blood alcohol concentrations in human subjects. Updating the Widmark Equation; *J Stud Alcohol* 42:547; 1981.

Watson PE. Total body water and blood alcohol levels: Updating the fundamentals. In: Crow KE, Batt RD, eds. *Human Metabolism of Alcohol*. Vol. 1. Boca Raton: CRC Press; 1989.

Weinberg DS, Burnham D, Berlin JA: Effect of histamine-2 receptor antagonists on blood alcohol levels: A meta-analysis; *J Gen Intern Med* 13:594; 1998.

Whitfield JB, Starmer GA, Martin NG: Alcohol metabolism in men and women; *Alcohol Clin Exp Res* 14:785; 1990.

Widmark EMP: Eine Mikromethode zur Bestimmung von äthylalkohol im Blut; *Biochem Z* 131:473; 1922.

Widmark EMP. *Die theoretischen Grundlagen und die praktische Verwendbarkeit der gerichtlich-medizinischen Alkoholbestimmung*. Berlin: Urban & Schwarzenberg; 1932:140 p.

Widmark EMP: The influence of glycocoll on the absorption and metabolism of ethyl alcohol; *Kungl Physiol Sällsk Lund Förhand* 12:1; 1941.

Widmark EMP. *Principles and Applications of Medicolegal Alcohol Determinations*. Davis: Biomedical Publications; 1981:163 p.

Wilkinson PK: Pharmacokinetics of ethanol: A review; *Alcohol Clin Exp Res* 4:6; 1980.

Wilkinson PK, Rheingold JL: Arterial-venous blood alcohol concentration gradients; *J Pharmacokinet Biopharm* 9:279; 1981.

Winek CL, Carfagna M: Comparison of plasma, serum, and whole blood ethanol concentrations; *J Anal Toxicol* 11:267; 1987.

Winkler K, Lundquist F, Tygstrup N: The hepatic metabolism of ethanol in patients with cirrhosis of the liver; *Scand J Clin Lab Invest* 23:59; 1969.

Woodard GA, Downey J, Hernandez-Boussard T, Morton JM: Impaired alcohol metabolism after gastric bypass surgery: A case-crossover trial; *J Am Coll Surg* 212:209; 2011.

Wright NR, Cameron D: The influence of habitual alcohol intake on breath-alcohol concentrations following prolonged drinking; *Alcohol Alcohol* 33:495; 1998.

Wu KL, Chaikomin R, Doran S, Jones KL, Horowitz M, Rayner CK: Artificially sweetened versus regular mixers increase gastric emptying and alcohol absorption; *Am J Med* 119:802; 2006.

Yelland LN, Burns JP, Sims DN, Salter AB, White JM: Inter- and intra-subject variability in ethanol pharmacokinetic parameters: Effects of testing interval and dose; *Forensic Sci Int* 175:65; 2008.

Zakhari S: Overview: How is alcohol metabolized by the body? *Alcohol Res Health* 29:245; 2006.

Zhang Y, Wu C, Wan J: Development and validation of a model to predict blood alcohol concentrations: Updating the NHTSA equation; *Addict Behav* 71:46; 2017.

Zink P, Reinhardt G: Der Verlauf der Blutalkoholkurve bei großem Trinkmengen; *Blutalkohol* 21:422; 1984.

Zoethout RW, van Gerven JM, Dumont GJ, Paltansing S, van Burgel ND, van der Linden M, Dahan A, Cohen AF, Schoemaker RC: A comparative study of two methods for attaining constant alcohol levels; *Br J Clin Pharmacol* 66:674; 2008.

Biomarkers for the Identification of Alcohol Use/Misuse*

9

FEDERICA BORTOLOTTI AND
FRANCO TAGLIARO

Contents

9.1 Introduction

Unlike the diagnosis of acute alcohol "intoxication" (or simply "intake"), which is based on the direct identification and quantification of ethanol in blood and/or in breath, the diagnosis of chronic alcohol intake is by far more complex, requiring different and integrated methodologies, depending also on the context in which the diagnosis has to be performed (clinical, psychiatric, forensic, administrative, …).

Nowadays, for identifying a condition of chronic alcohol use/misuse, two different approaches can be adopted, independently or in an integrated mode. The former is based on the administration of questionnaires, such as CAGE, AUDIT (etc.), while the latter is based on the use of clinical, chemical, and biochemical markers. The use of questionnaires is mainly aimed to understand if "alcohol" is a problem for the patient. Thus, it is particularly helpful in a clinical/psychiatric setting. On the other hand, in a forensic-administrative context, it is necessary to ascertain if the "alcohol use/misuse" of a subject becomes a problem for the family of the patient and/or for the community. In this context, a diagnosis of alcohol abuse may have very negative consequences for the subject (e.g., rejection of child custody, confiscation of the driving license, loss of certification of "fitness to work," ...); therefore, the use of questionnaires looks to be clearly insufficient and, sometimes, dangerous. For these

* This chapter is an updated version of a review article previously published in *Forensic Science Review*: Bortolotti F, Tagliaro F: Biomarkers for the identification of alcohol use/abuse: Update and critical review; *Forensic Sci Rev* 23:55; 2011.

reasons, only chemical and biochemical markers (linked to accurate clinical data) may guarantee the required diagnostic sensitivity, accuracy, and objectivity.

In the last decades, many researchers spent efforts not only to find new markers of alcohol abuse, but also to verify in real conditions the specificity and sensitivity limits of the existing biomarkers and to optimize the analytical methodologies for their determination.

The great attention dedicated by clinical and forensic researchers is proved by the several hundreds of papers published on this subject, which can be retrieved in the main databases (e.g., PubMed, Scopus, and Web of Science) using the key words "alcohol abuse" and "biomarkers." In addition, many books and monographies on this subject have been published. Among the most recent books, one, i.e., *Garriott's Medicolegal Aspect of Alcohol*, is worth mentioning, with particular regard to the chapter entitled "Biomarkers of Acute and Chronic Alcohol Ingestion" (Bertholf and Bazydlo 2014).

A general classification of the markers of alcohol abuse includes two sub-groups: "*trait markers*" and "*state markers.*"

9.1.1 The Trait Markers

The *trait markers* refer to genetically transmitted characteristics, such as a specific biochemical profile or a modified activity of an enzyme or of a neurotransmitter system, which would give a "genetic predisposition" toward alcohol abuse and alcoholism. Typical examples of trait markers are the aldehyde dehydrogenase enzyme (ALDH2) involved in the alcohol metabolism (Crabb et al. 2004; Edenberg 2007) and the monoamine oxidase enzyme (MAO) involved in the catabolism of biogenic amines, such as dopamine, norepinephrine and serotonin (Duncan et al. 2012; Matthews et al. 2014; Nedic Erjavec et al. 2014; Cervera-Juanes et al. 2016). A role in the propensity for alcohol abuse has also been suggested for the altered inhibition of the NMDA glutamate receptor or for the altered potentiation of the GABAa inhibitory receptor (Edenberg and Foroud 2006; Wu et al. 2010). Very recently, an altered expression of the FK506-binding protein (FKBP5), a negative regulator of the glucocorticoid receptor, was reported to be associated to alcohol drinking in an animal model suggesting a role of this protein in the tendency to alcohol misuse (Nylander et al. 2017).

The validation in clinical practice of one or more reliable trait markers would allow to identify the persons at risk to develop alcohol related problems, opening the way to act promptly with educational programs and/or with a psychological support and then, hopefully, preventing the occurrence of these harmful conditions.

9.1.2 The State Markers

The *state markers* are used as indicators of a present condition of alcohol abuse and can be classified as chemical or biochemical.

The traditional chemical markers of alcohol abuse are represented by ethyl alcohol and its congeners present in the alcohol containing beverages, such as methanol and isopropanol. The biochemical markers, on the other hand, stem from the biochemical changes induced by chronic or repeated alcohol intake.

The most typical biomarkers for the diagnosis of alcohol abuse include gamma-glutamyltransferase (GGT), mean corpuscular volume (MCV), liver enzymes (aspartate-transaminase (AST) and alanine-transaminase (ALT), and carbohydrate-deficient transferrin (CDT). However, in the latest two decades, several other molecules have been studied and, in limited cases, applied to the diagnosis of alcohol abuse. Among these compounds, it is worth mentioning the minor products of the non-oxidative metabolism of ethanol (i.e. ethyl glucuronide, fatty acid ethyl esters, phosphatidylethanol) and a side-product of the serotonin metabolism (i.e. 5-hydroxytryptophol).

The currently available biomarkers classified according to the biochemical changes and the different detection windows are summarized in Table 9.1.

The large number of biomarkers, as well as the heterogeneity of the published studies, make it difficult to cover, with even accuracy, the whole subject in a single chapter. For this reason, the present work is focused on a critical review of the most used biomarkers and "*candidate biomarkers.*" Readers interested in specific aspects of this topic may refer to some recently published reviews (Cabarcos et al. 2015; Jastrzębska et al. 2016; Niemelä 2016; Andresen-Streichert et al. 2018; Bortolotti et al. 2018).

9.2 Aspartate Aminotransferase and Alanine Aminotransferase

Aspartate aminotransferase (AST) and alanine aminotransferase (ALT) are cellular enzymes involved in amino acid metabolism. They are found in various bodily tissues, including liver, heart, skeletal muscle, kidneys, brain, and red blood cells, and are commonly measured in the clinical setting as markers of liver health.

The serum concentration of AST and ALT are reported to be significantly higher in heavy drinkers than in moderate drinkers and abstainers (Rosman and Lieber 1994; Alatalo et al. 2009). On this basis, measuring the activity of these enzymes in serum has long been applied in connection with the clinical diagnosis of alcohol abuse. However, taking into consideration that hepatocytes contain high amounts of ALT and AST, their changes are directly related to liver damage, which can depend also on factors different from alcohol abuse. A ratio of AST to ALT exceeding 2.0 has been proposed to differentiate alcohol-related from non-alcohol-related liver damage (Musshoff and Daldrup 1998; Niemelä and Alatalo 2010; Topic and Djukic 2013; Goug et al. 2015).

On the other hand, AST activity increases also in the presence of muscle disease and myocardial infarction. Moreover, a fast-food–based hyperalimentation has been reported to induce profound ALT elevations in less than 4 weeks (Kechagias et al. 2008). For the above-mentioned reasons, the diagnostic specificity of ALT and AST is considered as insufficient for using them in a forensic context. However, the low cost and ease of the determination of these liver enzymes and their wide availability mean that they are still applied for the diagnosis of alcohol abuse in the clinical context, at least in a preliminary diagnostic phase.

9.3 Mean Corpuscular Volume

Mean corpuscular volume (MCV), which refers to the average size of erythrocytes, increases after a period of 4–8 weeks of continuous and sustained alcohol intake (Bertholf and Bazydlo 2014). This increase mainly depends on three factors: (1) the toxic action of alcohol on the membrane viscosity of erythrocytes; (2) the toxic action of acetaldehyde on the red cell precursors in bone marrow; (3) the interference of ethanol on the intestinal absorption and metabolism of folic acid and vitamin B12. After cessation of drinking, the MCV values return to the normal range in 2–4 months.

Table 9.1 Biomarkers Used or Proposed to Be Used for the Diagnosis of Recent and Chronic Use/Abuse of Alcohol

Biomarker Type	Biomarker Name	Biochemical Changes	Detection Window	Diagnostic Specificity	Diagnostic Sensitivity
Non-oxidative metabolites of ethanol	Ethyl glucuronide (EtG)	Conjugation of ethanol with glucuronic acid by UDP-glucuronyltransferase	In blood and urine: hours-days; In hair: months	High	High
	Ethyl sulfate (EtS)	Conjugation of ethanol with sulfate by sulfo-transferase	Hours-days	High	High
	Fatty acid ethyl esters	Esterification of free fatty acids with ethanol by FAEE esterases	In blood: hours-days; In hair: months	High	High
	Phosphatidylethanol (PEth)	Transphosphatidylation from phosphatidylcholine in presence of ethanol catalyzed by phospholipase D	2–3 weeks	High	High
	Cocaethylene	Liver transesterification of cocaine in case of co-administration of ethanol	In blood: hours-days; In hair: months	High	Low–moderate
Acetaldehyde products	Acetaldehyde protein adducts	Non-enzymatic reaction of acetaldehyde with serum proteins via Schiff's base formation	Depends on half-life of serum proteins	Low–moderate	Moderate–high
	Salsolinol	Condensation reaction of dopamine with acetaldehyde	Unknown	Unknown	Low–moderate
Biomarkers of alcohol-related metabolic changes	Carbohydrate-deficient transferrin	Collective name of two minor glycoforms of transferrin (asialo and disialo-Tf) whose serum concentration increases after repeated and sustained alcohol intake	2–3 weeks	High	Moderate–high
	5-Hydroxytryptophol (5-HTOL)	Minor metabolite of serotonin formed during oxidation of alcohol which increases in urine in comparison to oxidative metabolite 5-hydroxyindolacetic acid, 5-HIAA	Days	Low–moderate	Moderate–high
Biomarkers of alcohol-related organ damages	Aspartate aminotransferase (AST), alanine aminotransferase (ALT)	Liver enzymes whose serum concentration increase after liver damage	Weeks	Low–moderate	Low–moderate
	Gamma glutamyltransferase (GGT)	Liver enzyme whose serum concentration increases after liver damage	Weeks	Low–moderate	Moderate–high
	Mean corpuscular volume (MCV)	Average size of red blood cells (increases after heavy drinking)	Months	Low–moderate	Low–moderate

A dose–response correlation between alcohol consumption and MCV has been reported. Subjects with moderate alcohol consumption (<40 g/day) show an increase in MCV of 1–2 fL in comparison to abstainers (Koivisto et al. 2006). For this reason, the use of MCV has been suggested as a good way to monitor drinking by a subject over a longer period of time. However, MCV shows limited sensitivity (40%–60%) and low specificity, with possible false-positive results in the presence of non-alcohol-related diseases (such as B12 vitamin and folic acid deficiency, non-alcohol-dependent liver diseases, hematological disorders, hypothyroidism, tobacco addiction, etc.) (Musshoff and Daldrup 1998; Takahashi et al. 2016). The limited sensitivity of MCV has been recently demonstrated by a study aimed at investigating a plausible association between elevated MCV and crash accidents correlated with alcohol abuse (Porpiglia et al. 2019). In that study the authors demonstrated that MCV values were found elevated in drivers involved in accidents only if driving under severe alcohol intoxication, being not significantly increased in individuals who tended to drive in a condition of low-to-moderate alcohol intoxication. On this basis, MCV, as well as AST and ALT, cannot be used in a forensic context. However, these biomarkers are still included in the first panel of blood tests used by clinicians in the diagnosis of alcohol abuse.

9.4 Gamma-Glutamyl Transferase

Gamma-glutamyl transferase (GGT) is a serum enzyme with a glycoprotein structure mainly produced by the liver. It plays a key role in the gamma-glutamyl cycle, a pathway for the synthesis and degradation of glutathione and xenobiotic detoxification. In the latest decades, several studies have been published reporting a correlation between alcohol intake and GGT increases. On this basis GGT, alone or in combination with AST, ALT, and MCV, is the most commonly used first-level laboratory medicine test for the diagnosis of chronic alcohol abuse.

The increase of GGT concentration in serum occurs after long-term excessive and repeated alcohol consumption (>60 g/day for several weeks), which causes liver damage and then leakage of GGT from the hepatocytes and rise of the related enzyme activity in serum (Rosman and Lieber 1994). After cessation of drinking, the GGT serum levels return to normal limits after 20–25 days.

The diagnostic specificity of this marker is fairly low, taking into consideration that its increase can occur also for non-alcoholic liver diseases such as hepatitis C, cirrhosis, or carcinoma (Helander et al. 1998) and for other diseases (e.g., atherosclerotic cardiovascular disease, metabolic syndrome, diabetes, pancreatitis, kidney failure, obesity). For this reason, GGT has been proposed as a disease marker also in different medical fields (Paolicchi et al. 2006; Puukka et al. 2006; Iqbal et al. 2010; Niemela and Alatalo 2010; Bozbaş et al. 2011; Endre et al. 2011; Wiegand et al. 2011; Onat et al. 2012).

Moreover, the increase of GGT can be caused by the chronic use of some therapeutic drugs, such as barbiturates, antiepileptics, and anticoagulants (Bertholf and Bazydlo 2014). Notwithstanding these limitations, GGT is still widely used as a biomarker of alcohol abuse in both forensic and clinical contexts also because its determination is fairly inexpensive and is carried out in all clinical chemistry laboratories (Musshoff and Daldrup 1998; Anton et al. 2002; Bean et al. 2009; Bianchi et al. 2010; Topic and Djukic 2013). On the other hand, GGT, because of its wide detection window (several weeks), may be very helpful in monitoring the abstinence of recovering alcoholics.

9.5 Carbohydrate-Deficient Transferrin

The term carbohydrate-deficient transferrin (CDT) refers to a group of minor glycoforms of transferrin (Tf) in which serum concentration increases after chronic/sustained alcohol intake. Transferrin, a glycoprotein responsible for binding iron and transporting it via blood throughout the body, is characterized by the presence of branched oligosaccharide chains containing acetylglucosamine, galactose, mannose, and sialic acid. The sialic acid residues, in terminal position, are the only charged moiety of the chain, conferring an ionic charge to the molecule. According to the number of sialic residues present in the transferrin molecules, different glycoforms have been identified, which in the serum of a normal subject are present in the following percentages: tetrasialo-Tf 75%–80%; pentasialo-Tf 10%–15%; trisialo-Tf 5%–10%; disialo-Tf 1%–2%; hexasialo-Tf 1%–2%; a-, mono-, hepta-, octasialo-Tf <1% (Bergen et al. 2001; Flahaut et al. 2003; Helander and Jones 2007).

On the basis of a general consensus, CDT includes asialo- and disialo-Tf. In serum of non-alcohol abusers, asialo-Tf is not measurable, whereas disialo-Tf is present at a concentration below 2% of total transferrin. After the ingestion of 60–80 g of alcohol per day for at least 10–15 days, firstly increases disialo-Tf followed by asialo-Tf, which usually becomes measurable when disialo-Tf concentration is around 3% of total transferrin (Bortolotti et al. 2018; Paterlini et al. 2019). On that point, it is worth mentioning that very recently the group of Tagliaro reported the possibility of detecting asialo-Tf also when disialo-Tf value is below 3% by applying a particular sample pre-treatment based on the use of PEG (Porpiglia et al. 2018a) and by using an optimized capillary electrophoresis method (Porpiglia et al. 2018b).

After cessation of drinking, the CDT value returns within normal limits after 2 or 3 weeks of abstinence (Arndt 2001; Helander et al. 2016; Bortolotti et al. 2018). The biochemical mechanism of the alcohol-related CDT increase has not been fully clarified. Some authors have proposed the hypothesis of a reduction of the activity of sialyltransferase (ST), galactosyltransferase (GT), and *N*-acetylglucosamine transferase (*N*-AGT), which are glycosyltransferases involved in transferrin carbohydrate side chain synthesis, induced by alcohol or by its first metabolite, acetaldehyde (Stibler and Borg 1991; Xin et al. 1995). Alternatively, a combined multistep process involving both protein transport and change in enzymes activity has been suggested (Sillanaukee et al. 2001).

CDT concentration is expressed as the percentage ratio of the sum of disialo-and asialo-Tf (when detectable) on the total transferrin. Because the CDT-related glycoforms, in particular disialo-Tf, are present also in normal subjects, in order to support the diagnosis of alcohol abuse it is necessary to establish a "cut-off" percent concentration, above which CDT values are considered "positive," i.e., indicative of excessive alcohol use. However, this value may depend on what average alcohol intake is accepted as "*normal*" in the population as well as on the analytical methods used to determine CDT. Taking into considerations that variability, CDT cut-off usually ranges from 1.8% to 2.5% (Delanghe and De Buyzere 2009).

First reported in 1978 by Helena Stibler et al. (1978) CDT is presently one of the most widely adopted biochemical markers of chronic alcohol abuse in both clinical and forensic environments. One of the main reasons for the great success of this marker is its high diagnostic specificity (when CDT is determined with reliable methods), which is reported to be close to 100%. In the 1990s, several papers were published reporting increased CDT concentrations caused by pathological conditions different from alcohol abuse (e.g., liver diseases, diabetes, hemocromatosis, and high BMI) as well as non-pathological factors (tobacco smoking, use of drugs such as antiepileptics, antihypertensives, and contraceptives) (Bortolotti et al. 2018). However, it is now well demonstrated that the reported false-positive results were produced by nonspecific interferents on the immunometric methods utilized by the majority of the laboratories working on CDT. These methods, indeed, were based on the separation of CDT from the prevalent non-CDT glycoforms of Tf by using anion-exchange disposable microcartridges followed by an immunochemical detection by using antibodies against whole-transferrin. Therefore, the selectivity of the analytical procedure was dependent only on the selectivity of the solid-phase extraction, which was intrinsically poor (Arndt and Keller 2004; Fleming et al. 2004). The use of sophisticated molecular separation techniques, such as capillary electrophoresis and high-performance liquid chromatography (HPLC), for the determination of CDT, which started to spread only in the latest two decades, brought to a very significant reduction of the reports of false-positive results (Bergström and Helander 2008a, 2008b; Helander and Kenan Modèn 2013).

Sometimes the CDT measurement can be difficult in case of severe liver diseases, such as cirrhosis. Even if Fagan et al. showed that in patients with chronic liver disease the CDT levels were not affected by the stage or etiology of liver diseases (2013), the group of Stewart, which published on this topic two papers, in 2010 and 2017, respectively, showed the occurrence of a poor chromatographic resolution of disialotransferrin from trisialotransferrin (the so-called "di-tri bridging") in a significant percentage (30%) of cirrhotic patients and, even if in a much lower percentage (<4%), in patients with severe hepatitis (Stewart et al. 2010a, 2017). According to the authors, the possible presence of "di-tri bridging" in severe liver diseases diminishes the diagnostic utility of CDT as a marker in this specific category of patients, even if it did not cause false positive results, since the abnormal profile could be easily identified by separation methods. In agreement with the above-mentioned study by Stewart et al. (2017), in a very recent Letter to the Editor of *Alcohol and Alcoholism*, Verbeek et al. (2018a) reported a study where CDT was determined by capillary electrophoresis (Sebia®) in 117 cirrhotic patients, showing a di-tri bridging in 38% of them. On this basis, the authors pointed out the need for caution when CDT is used to evaluate alcohol use in cirrhotic patients.

A condition different from alcohol abuse that increases the level of CDT, and which could be a factor that impacts on specificity of the marker, is represented by pregnancy. Indeed, the data of the recent literature (Kenan et al. 2011; Bianchi et al. 2011; Bakhireva et al. 2012), consistently with that coming from the direct experience of the authors of the present chapter, show that during a physiological pregnancy, the disialo-Tf levels gradually increase up to reaching—before the delivery—values next to, and sometimes higher, than the cut-off usually applied to distinguish between normal subjects and alcohol abusers: 1.61% ± 0.23 (Kenan et al. 2011); 1.53% ± 0.22 (Bianchi et al. 2011); 1.67% ± 0.28 (Bakhireva et al. 2012); 1.57% ± 0.24 (personal data of the authors of the chapter). Within a month after the delivery, CDT values come back to the normal values. This phenomenon, clearly, does not affect the specificity of CDT as marker of alcohol abuse, since pregnancy is usually a patent or, at least, a known condition. However, it is important to be aware of this condition when alcohol abuse is investigated in pregnant women.

The most important limit of CDT is represented by its diagnostic sensitivity, which looks fairly moderate in comparison to its specificity. In fact, this marker fails to identify occasional abuses or binge drinking behaviors (Delanghe and De Buyzere 2009).

Concerning this crucial point, however, it is worth emphasizing that the evaluation of the diagnostic sensitivity of CDT is a complicated issue, since the individual alcohol consumption, a necessary prerequisite to calculate this parameter, is usually based on personal reports of the subjects or on different questionnaires (scarcely reliable outside the clinical field) with a possible bias in the estimation of the alcohol intake. In addition, the limit between "*normal*" and "*abnormal*" daily alcohol intake in different regions and cultures may vary dramatically. Furthermore, in some studies the diagnostic performances of CDT are evaluated toward "*heavy drinkers*," whereas in others on "*light*," "moderate," or "*hazardous drinkers*" (Bortolotti et al. 2018). This background led to a great variability of CDT diagnostic sensitivity values, reported in the different papers. According to some authors it is very low (<40%), according other authors very high (>90%) (Whitfield et al. 2008; Bertholet et al. 2014; Fagan et al. 2014; Pisa et al. 2015). An overall evaluation leads to identify a mean value ranging from 50% to 70%.

Traffic medicine represents one of the main application fields of CDT. In particular, this marker is widely used to assess the physical fitness of subjects applying to regain driver's licenses after their confiscation for drunk driving (Morgan and Major 1996; Bjerre et al. 2001; Bortolotti et al. 2002; Seidl 2004; Bean et al. 2009; Bianchi et al. 2010; Maenhout et al. 2012). In the same context, CDT has also been used to investigate the prevalence of chronic alcohol abusers among drunk drivers apprehended and submitted to blood alcohol analysis (BAC) (Gjerde and Mørland 1987; Iffland et al. 1994; Appenzeller et al. 2005a, 2005b; Bortolotti et al. 2007, 2015; Bianchi et al. 2010). All these studies, even if performed by different research groups in different countries, consistently showed a statistically significant high prevalence of chronic alcohol abusers among drunk drivers in comparison to drivers with BAC within legal limits. On the basis of these data, the authors concluded that increased CDT revealed not only a condition of chronic alcohol abuse, but also an increased risk to drive under alcohol influence. These conclusions were confirmed by a study of Marques et al. (2010) in which 534 drivers, who were convicted of driving under the influence of alcohol (DUI), agreed to install an ignition interlock device to verify the risk of recidivism after re-licensing. In that study, program entry and follow-up blood samples were used to measure PEth, CDT and GGT. Program entry urine was analyzed for ethyl ETG and ETS. Entry hair samples were tested for FAEE and ETG. Except for FAEE, all alcohol biomarkers were related significantly to the inter-lock BAC test profiles; higher marker levels predicted higher rates of interlock BAC test failures.

Effective policies to early assess excessive alcohol intake or abuse of alcoholic substances in workers are quite recent. This looks surprisingly since the policies to prevent drug use/abuse (e.g., workplace drug testing) date back to the 1980s. For many years, the investigation of alcohol misuse in workplace has been based only on the random determination of BAC in subjects suspected to be alcohol abusers. This approach showed important limits mainly in terms of diagnostic sensitivity. In the latest years, a slight change of the approach occurred, as witnessed by the publication of some studies investigating the diagnostic performances of the markers of alcohol abuse, including CDT, in the workplace (Coccini et al. 2008; Fustinoni et al. 2009; Hermansson et al. 2010; Marques 2012). The results of these studies, even if still preliminary, suggest that CDT is effective in identifying the workers with alcohol misuse problems.

In the clinical context, CDT in longitudinal studies proved suitable for the identification of relapses after a period of abstinence. On this basis, CDT has been proposed for monitoring abstinence during detoxification treatments (Walter et al. 2001; Baros et al. 2008; Chatzipanagiotou et al. 2010). In addition, Anton et al. reported that an increase or a reduction of CDT value of 30% indicates a significant change of alcohol use in recovering alcoholics (Anton et al. 2002). Furthermore, CDT has been proposed for monitoring compliance to requested alcohol abstinence of patients after heart transplantation, for identifying the alcoholic origin of acute pancreatitis, epilepsy, and spontaneous intracranial hemorrhage, and for evaluating the severity of nervous anorexia (Skipworth and Pereira 2008; Bortolotti et al. 2018). More recently, the usefulness of CDT to detect and to stratify alcohol problems among injured patients admitted to hospital emergency departments has been discussed (Neumann et al. 2009; Stewart et al. 2010b). Also, CDT has been used to identify at the Intensive Care Unit the alcoholic patients with highest risk to develop complications, such as tracheobronchitis, pneumonitis, sepsis, or cardiac failure (Spies et al. 1995). Indeed, increased values of CDT at admission in trauma patients have been shown to be associated with an increased duration of stay at Intensive Care Units and with overall hospitalization (Spies et al. 1998; Fleming et al. 2009; McKinzie et al. 2010; Matar et al. 2017).

An increasing number of researchers have proposed the use of CDT as a marker of pathological conditions not correlated to alcohol abuse. Among them, the most well-known is the carbohydrate-deficient glycoprotein syndrome (CDGS), which refers to a group of severe neurological disorders characterized by genetic defects in protein glycosylation (Biffi et al. 2007; Pérez-Cerdá et al. 2008; Parente et al. 2010; Bortolotti et al. 2018; Chang et al. 2018).

Presently, the determination of CDT can be performed by immunometric methods and by separation techniques, such as capillary electrophoresis (CE) and HPLC (Helander et al. 2003; Bortolotti et al. 2005). The only immunoassay currently available is based on the use of specific antibodies against CDT-related glycoforms (Delanghe et al. 2007; Marti et al. 2008; Whitfield et al. 2008; Nomura et al. 2018) and consequently looks to be far more specific and reliable that the older immunoassays (using antibodies specific for whole Tf), which were reported to produce up to 30% of false-positive results (Alden et al. 2005). However, it should be pointed out that also the separation methods, based on CE and HPLC, when used for high-productivity screening, suffer from low resolution power (Schellenberg et al. 2008; Kenan et al. 2010). On the other hand, high-resolution CE and HPLC methods were both reported as confirmatory techniques. Between the two, HPLC adopts a detection wavelength specific for the ferric iron bound to the transferrin molecule (460 nm), whereas CE uses wavelengths of 200–214 nm at which all the proteins absorb the UV light.

The International Federation of Clinical Chemistry—CDT-Working group (IFCC-CDT-WG), in the frame of a long-time work on the standardization of CDT determination (Helander et al. 2016), in 2007 proposed the HPLC based methods as candidate reference methods for CDT determination because of the higher selectivity guaranteed by the detection at 460 nm in comparison to the detection at 200 nm of CZE-based methods. Later, the same group identified a candidate reference measurement procedure (HPLC cRMP) for serum CDT (Helander et al. 2010a). According to the HPLC cRMP, the serum sample, after iron-saturation with ferric nitrilotriacetic acid (FeNTA) and precipitation of lipoproteins, should be analyzed by a HPLC-UV–visible method. The chromatographic separation of the transferrin glycoforms should be performed on an anion-exchange column using salt gradient elution. The quantification of individual glycoforms should be achieved by monitoring the specific absorbance of the transferrin–iron complex at 470 nm. The method uses baseline integration for all peaks from asialo-until hexasialo-transferrin, and the amount of disialotransferrin is calculated as the relative amount (%)

to total transferrin, based on peak areas, whereby total transferrin represents the sum of the peak areas for asialo-until hexasialotransferrin. After a validation through a network of CDT reference laboratories, the HPLC cRMP has recently been approved by IFCC-CDT-WG (Weykamp et al. 2013).

It is widely recognized, however, that between CE and HPLC exists an excellent statistical correlation (Bortolotti et al. 2005; Helander et al. 2005; Quintana et al. 2009). Very recently, a novel and effective analytical approach for CDT determination was reported (Sorio et al. 2017). The method is based on the formation of a transferrin-terbium fluorescent adduct (Tf-Fluo). After the addition of terbium, the serum sample is analyzed by anion exchange HPLC hyphenated with a fluorescence detector (λ exc 298 nm and λ em 550 nm). According to the authors, the procedure provides a clear separation and identification of Tf glycoform peaks without any interfering signals, allowing selective Tf sialoforms analysis in human serum and other body fluids (e.g., cadaveric blood, cerebrospinal fluid, and dried blood spots).

On the basis of the above-mentioned data and taking into consideration the possible relevant legal and administrative consequences of a CDT positive result, it is highly recommended to confirm the results obtained with the use of screening methods by more reliable confirmatory techniques (Arndt and Kropf 2002; Bortolotti et al. 2018).

Some authors suggested the combined use of GGT and CDT in order to increase the overall diagnostic reliability of these markers, although differences in the underlying physio-pathological mechanisms and in their "*detection windows*" would not seem to support this approach. Among the papers dedicated to the evaluation of the validity of this association, it is worth mentioning the study of Sillanaukee and Olsson, who reported a meta-analysis of six different clinical studies on alcohol abusers and social drinkers ($n = 1{,}412$) in which the diagnostic value of CDT, GGT, AST, ALT, and MCV was evaluated (Sillanaukee and Olsson 2001). The authors, on the basis of a predictive function $[0.8 \ln(GT) + 1.3 \ln(CDT)]$ derived from the study, concluded that for discriminating between alcohol abusers and social drinkers the combined use of CDT and GGT was better than any of the single markers. However, these conclusions are in part not confirmed by a recent study by Bianchi et al. in which the investigators demonstrated that, at least in traffic medicine, the diagnostic power of CDT is higher than that of the combination of GGT and CDT, ascribing the difference from the results previously published to the use of outdated technology (Bianchi et al. 2010).

9.6 Ethyl Glucuronide and Ethyl Sulfate

The main pathway of alcohol metabolism, as it is well known, is its oxidation to acetaldehyde catalyzed by alcohol dehydrogenase (ADH), followed by a second oxidation step to acetate catalyzed by aldehyde dehydrogenase (ALDH). However, ethanol is also transformed into ethyl glucuronide (EtG) and ethyl sulfate (EtS), which stem from a minor non-oxidative metabolic reaction, based on the conjugation with glucuronic acid or with sulfate by UDP-glucuronyl transferase and by sulfo-transferase, respectively. According to a consistent body of literature, less than 1% of the total amount of alcohol ingested is transformed through this secondary metabolic pathway (Kissack et al. 2008; Palmer 2009). EtG and EtS, being direct metabolites of ethanol, in principle look to be highly specific indicators of alcohol intake. These compounds are detectable in serum up to 6 hours after alcohol disappearance from blood and in urine, depending on dosage, from 6 to 100 hours after alcohol ingestion (Høiseth et al. 2007; Halter et al. 2008; Walsham and Sherwood 2014). On these grounds, these ethanol metabolites have been proposed as short-term biomarkers of alcohol abuse when determined in serum, and as short- to medium-term markers, when they are determined in urine, in the clinical, forensic and occupational setting (Skipper et al. 2004; Gjerde et al. 2010; Bertholf and Bazydlo 2014; Bogstrand et al. 2015; Høiseth et al. 2015; Kilo et al. 2016; Fucci et al. 2017).

On the basis of the difficulties in correlating quantitatively and accurately the ingested dose of alcohol with EtG/EtS concentrations in urine, a very reasonable suggestion is to use these markers just to monitor abstinence from alcohol. In this frame, the determination of ethyl glucuronide in urine has been proposed to monitor the abstinence of the patients before and after the surgical intervention of liver transplant (Erim et al. 2007). Moreover, both EtG/EtS have been reported to verify the abstinence of alcohol dependents and heavy drinkers during inpatient and outpatient detoxification treatments and at follow-ups (Høiseth et al. 2009; Junghanns et al. 2009; Dahl et al. 2011; Lande et al. 2011; Mutschler et al. 2010; Lowe et al. 2015; Barrio et al. 2017; Armer et al. 2017; Barrio et al. 2018).

Also, the determination of EtG in urine has been suggested as a way to prove retrospectively a recent driving-under-influence episode (Wurst et al. 2008a). Although a sound body of literature supports the use of urine EtG/EtS as markers of recent alcohol intake, particular attention has to be paid to the possibility of "*positive*" results not related to consumption of alcohol. Indeed, these compounds might be present in urine because of inadvertent exposure to ethanol-containing products such as mouthwash, hand sanitizers, medications, and food (Costantino et al. 2006; Arndt et al. 2009; Karch 2009; Thierauf et al. 2009; Høiseth et al. 2010a; Reisfield et al. 2011; Gessner et al. 2016). Moreover, drinking non-alcoholic beer and wine, which contain trace amounts of ethanol, may lead to false-positive results (Musshoff et al. 2010; Thierauf et al. 2010a). It is worth mentioning that a recent study by Müller and Iwersen-Bergmann demonstrated that EtG can be contained in wine (in milligram amounts in a bottle of wine) as natural compound, whereas it was not detected in any of the other tested alcoholic beverages, such as distilled spirits, liqueurs, and beer (Müller and Iwersen-Bergmann 2018).

For the above-mentioned reasons, the determination of EtG and EtS in urine to monitor alcohol abstinence has to be cautiously performed, after informing the patients to be aware about the possibility of sources of ethanol in foods, medications, or cosmetics/sanitizers (SAMHSA 2006; Jatlow and O'Malley 2010).

Finally, some authors have described a post-collection synthesis of EtG by *E. coli* in urine that also contained ethanol (Helander et al. 2007). Indeed, ethanol can be formed by the fermentation of glucose present in urine and then conjugated to EtG by the glucuronidase activity of bacteria (Musshoff et al. 2010; Thierauf et al. 2010b; Crews et al. 2011). In order to stabilize EtG in urine, the use of collection tubes containing sodium azide has been proposed (Luginbühl et al. 2017).

The development of high-sensitivity GC-MS and LC-MS analytical methods led to the possibility of determining EtG in hair (hEtG) where it is present at concentrations of picograms per milligram. This new toxicological use of hair analysis, which began just for research purposes (Skopp et al. 2000; Alt et al. 2000), has later expanded its application in both clinical and forensic contexts. In practice, the analysis of hair for EtG has been proposed for the objective diagnosis of chronic abuse of alcohol, similar to what is widely applied for demonstrating the chronic use of illicit drugs (Jurado et al. 2004; Morini et al. 2009a; Morini et al. 2009b; Kronstrand et al. 2012). As it is well known, xenobiotics and their metabolites present in the blood circulation enter hair roots and become embedded by the actively proliferating cells of the germination center, being then permanently fixed into the keratinized hair shaft. From a knowledge of the kinetics of hair growth, which in the scalp hair is about 1 cm per month, it is possible, on the basis of the length of the hair sample analyzed and on its distance from the root, to infer something about the duration and time period of the abuse of alcohol or drugs.

In the latest decade, many authors focused their attention on hEtG, mainly because of the wide detection window (month/years) shown by this biomarker. The different research groups investigated the possibility to use hEtG, alone or in association to other biomarkers (Boscolo-Berto et al. 2014; Biondi et al. 2019), in different contexts, including clinical medicine (Oppolzer et al. 2016; Beckmann et al. 2016; Verbeek et al. 2018b), in utero exposure to alcohol (Gutierrez et al. 2015; Joya et al. 2016; Bager et al. 2017; Gomez-Roig et al. 2018), alcohol detoxification programs (Cappelle et al. 2018), traffic medicine (Marques et al. 2014; Lendoiro et al. 2018), and occupational medicine (Salomone et al. 2018).

The above-cited papers show that hEtG is a reliable biomarker of alcohol abuse in different contexts. However, it is important to mention that the evidences coming from more than 30 years of experience on the use of hair and other keratinized tissues for the diagnosis of chronic consumption of or exposure to illicit drugs unraveled several crucial issues (e.g., external contamination, non-linear correlation between dose and concentration, effect of hair treatments, inside hair degradation, etc.) elucidating the advantages and the limits of hair testing for drugs. Unfortunately, the transfer of this experience to the diagnosis of alcohol abuse by using hEtG shows analytical and interpretative limitations, particularly relevant because alcohol use (unlike use of illicit drugs), in most parts of the world, is legal. Therefore, the demarcation line between "*normal*" and "*pathological*" is quantitative, and not merely qualitative, as for illicit drugs. Another weakness of hEtG analysis is represented by the irregular concentration distribution among the different areas of the scalp and of the body (scalp vs. pubic hair) (Kintz et al. 2008; Kerekes et al. 2009). Other warnings come from reports of the possibility of an "internal contamination" of hair by EtG present in sweat (Pragst et al. 2010; Biondi et al. 2019).

In addition, different hair treatments, including thermal hair straightening, hair bleaching and permanent coloring, as well as exposure to chlorinated swimming pool water were shown to significantly affect EtG concentration in hair (Ettlinger et al. 2014; Crunelle et al. 2015; Petzel-Witt et al. 2018; Luginbühl et al. 2018).

On this basis, it will not be so easy to use the presence of EtG in the hair to discriminate between "*acceptable use*" and abuse of alcohol. The Society of Hair Testing (SoHT) has published a "Consensus," concerning the use of hair testing for inferring chronic excessive consumption of alcohol. The document has been revised four times since it was firstly adopted on June 16, 2009 (Kintz 2010). The latest revision was adopted by the members of the Society during the business meeting in Brisbane on August 29, 2016. In this document two cut-off values for discrimination between teetotalers or occasional low amount consumption and moderate alcohol drinking (low cut-off), and between non-excessive (abstinence up to moderate alcohol intake) and chronic excessive drinking (high cut-off value) were defined (Society of Hair Testing 2016). The cut-off levels were fixed at 7 pg/mg and 30 pg/mg, respectively.

On the basis of the above-described limits and taking also into consideration the absence of large multicenter population studies, the use of hEtG in forensic science practice as a marker of chronic alcohol abuse should be adopted with caution, unless its application is limited to monitoring long-term conditions of abstinence from alcohol, as suggested by some authors (Alberman et al. 2010, 2011; Liniger et al. 2010).

Alternative matrices in which EtG has also been determined are oral fluid (Hegstad et al. 2009; Hoiseth et al. 2010b) and sweat (Schummer et al. 2008; Selvam et al. 2016). An interesting matrix in which EtG has been determined is meconium. This matrix was used in order to investigate the intrauterine exposure of newborns to alcohol (Morini et al. 2008; Bakdash et al. 2010; Morini et al. 2010; Tarcomnicu et al. 2010; Eichler et al. 2016; Lamy et al. 2017; Biondi et al. 2019).

Very recently, also fingernails have been proposed as matrix in which EtG can be determined, in association or alternatively to hair, to evaluate chronic or repeated alcohol abuse (Cappelle et al. 2017; May et al. 2018; Paul 2019).

Finally, the determination of EtG and/or EtS in post-mortem samples, including blood, urine, and vitreous humor, has been proposed to test whether ethanol consumption had occurred prior to death (Keten et al. 2009; Hoiseth et al. 2010c; Thierauf et al. 2011; Hegstad et al. 2017) and in order to exclude postmortem ethanol formation (Krabseth et al. 2014).

Concerning the analytical aspects, the determination of EtG and EtS in blood, urine, and hair is usually carried by highly sensitive methods mostly based on LC-MS-MS technology (Bicker et al. 2006; Morini et al. 2007; Lamoureux et al. 2009; Al-Asmari et al. 2010; Favretto et al. 2010; Helander et al. 2010b; Palumbo et al. 2018; Biondi et al. 2019), although GC-MS and capillary electrophoresis methods have also been developed (Nováková and Krivánková 2008; Jung et al. 2009; Agius et al. 2010; Shi et al. 2010; Vignali et al. 2018). On the other hand, the availability of immunoassay methods for the determination of EtG in urine and plasma has been reported, allowing for a wider use of this biomarker (Bottcher et al. 2008; Fucci et al. 2017).

9.7 Fatty Acid Ethyl Esters

Fatty acid ethyl esters (FAEE) stem from the esterification of free fatty acids produced during breakdown of triglycerides. The reaction is catalyzed by FAEE esterases (Laposata 1998; Laposata et al. 2002).

FAEE, among which ethyl stearate, ethyl palmitate, ethyl oleate, and ethyl arachidonate can be mentioned, are present in blood, hair, and in various organs prone to suffer from alcohol-related damages, such as liver, pancreas, heart, and brain. On this basis, some authors hypothesized a direct role of these molecules in the toxic action of alcohol on tissues and organs (Yamazaki et al. 1997; Beckemeier and Bora 1998; Laposata and Lange 1986; Laposata 1998; Werner et al. 2001; Vonlaufen et al. 2007).

The concentration-time profile of FAEE in blood follows closely that of ethanol, even if FAEE show a longer elimination phase. Indeed, these metabolites are reported to be detectable in blood up to 24 hours in the case of acute intoxication (Doyle et al. 1997). On this basis, these minor metabolites of ethanol, when determined in serum, have been proposed as biochemical markers of recent alcohol consumption (Bisaga et al. 2005). On the other hand, in chronic alcohol abusers FAEE are detectable in serum up to 100 hours after the last alcohol intake (Borucki et al. 2007) suggesting the possibility of using these molecules also as "*intermediate term*" markers of alcohol abuse (Kaphalia et al. 2004) and to differentiate chronic abusers from binge drinkers (Soderberg et al. 2003).

In the latest two decades, many papers have been published on the determination of FAEE in hair, often in association with EtG, in order to gather more information about the drinking behavior of the subjects over the last months before the sample was collected (Auwarter et al. 2001; Hartwig et al. 2003; Wurst et al. 2004; Yegles et al. 2004; De Giovanni et al. 2007; Wurst et al. 2008b; Pragst et al. 2010; Süsse et al. 2010; Bertol et al. 2014).

This diagnostic approach shows important limits closely related to those discussed above for hEtG. Moreover, particular attention should be given to interferences from hair care products containing alcohol (Hartwig et al. 2003; De Giovanni et al. 2008; Gareri et al. 2011). In the above-mentioned "Consensus" adopted by the SoHT in 2016, the authors state that ethyl palmitate (E16:0) can be used autonomously for interpretation instead of the concentration sum of the four esters, ethyl myristate, ethyl palmitate, ethyl oleate, and ethyl stearate (ΣFAEE), as previously applied. In the same "Consensus," after evaluation of the data from seven laboratories, the E16:0 cut-off for abstinence assessment was defined at 0.12 ng/mg for the 0–3 cm segment and at 0.15 ng/mg for the 0–6 cm segment. The cut-off for chronic excessive drinking was fixed at 0.35 ng/mg for the 0–3 cm segment and at 0.45 ng/mg for the 0–6 cm segment (Society of Hair Testing 2016).

As well as for EtG, some authors proposed the determination of FAEE in the hair of mothers and newborns to investigate the *in-utero* ethanol exposure (Pragst and Yegles 2008; Wurst et al. 2008c; Kulaga et al. 2009, 2010; Shor et al. 2010). With the same purpose, the determination of FAEE in meconium has also been reported (Chan et al. 2003; Moore et al. 2003; Chan et al. 2004; Garcia-Algar et al. 2008; Bakdash et al. 2010; Kwak et al. 2010; Cabarcos et al. 2014; Himes et al. 2014).

From an analytical point of view, the determination of FAEE, after a preliminary isolation of the molecules from the matrix by solid-phase extraction, is usually performed by the determination and quantitation by GC-MS (Pragst et al. 2001; De Giovanni et al. 2007; Zimmermann and Jackson 2010). However, analytical methods based on HPLC-DAD (Auwärter et al. 2004) and LC-MS (Kwak et al. 2010) have also been reported.

9.8 Phosphatidylethanol

Phosphatidylethanol (PEth) is an aberrant phospholipid formed by the enzyme phospholipase D when blood-ethanol is elevated in preference to reacting with choline (Aradóttir et al. 2004). PEth does not refer to a single adduct, but rather, is the name of a family of phospholipids that are defined as having a nonpolar phosphor-ethanol head with a pair of fatty acid chains attached to the sn-1 and 2 positions (Holbrook et al. 1992). These chains are between 16 and 20 carbons long and can exhibit some degree of saturation along the chain. There can be a wide range of fatty acid chain lengths and degrees of saturation, allowing for a variety of PEth homologues (Gnann et al. 2010). It is considered a biomarker of alcohol abuse, as it can only be formed when there is ethanol in the blood (Varga et al. 1998), even if other adducts can also be formed in the presence of other primary alcohols (Seidler et al. 1996). Over time, PEth begins to build up in cellular compartments of the blood, with the 16:0/18:1 and 16:0/18:2 homologues having the highest overall contribution when extracted from the cell membranes of red blood cells (Leidl et al. 2008).

The half-life of this biomarker in blood, after cessation of drinking, is about 4 days. For these reasons, PEth has been proposed as a biomarker of fairly recent ethanol intake (Isaksson et al. 2011; Bertholf and Bazydlo 2014). Although the earliest papers on the formation of PEth following alcohol consumption date back to the late 1980s (Mueller et al. 1988; Rakhimov et al. 1988), the first studies on its application to real cases appeared only at the end of the 1990s, showing an elevated diagnostic specificity (Hansson et al. 1997; Varga et al. 1998). The following studies confirmed the diagnostic power of this marker highlighting also its high diagnostic sensitivity (>90%) in comparison with other markers of chronic alcohol abuse, such as GGT, CDT, and MCV (Aradóttir et al. 2006; Hartmann et al. 2007). On this basis, PEth has been proposed as a reliable marker of chronic alcohol abuse in both forensic and clinical contexts (Varga et al. 2000; Kip et al. 2008; Wurst et al. 2010; Marques et al. 2011; Helander et al. 2019), including the investigation of prenatal exposure to alcohol (Stewart et al. 2010c; Lunginbühl et al. 2019; Maxwell et al. 2019).

The cut-off to distinguish alcohol use from alcohol abuse is reported to be 0.7 µm. The concentrations found in the studied populations range from 0.2 to 10 µm (Aradóttir et al. 2006). There has been some, but not much work done on investigating the influences that sample storage has on the production of PEth in the presence of ethanol (Varga and Alling 2002).

An interesting application of PEth is its determination in postmortem tissues and blood, which was proposed to investigate the antemortem alcohol intake (Bendroth et al. 2008; Hansson et al. 2001; Rainio et al. 2008). However, Aradottir et al. showed a possibility of pre-analytical formation of PEth in blood from the alcohol present in it, even if the autopsy samples were stored at –20°C. To overcome this artifact, the authors suggest to perform the PEth extraction within hours of autopsy (Aradóttir et al. 2004).

There has been a recent increase in the amount of studies focusing on the use of dried blood spots (DBS) as a means of sample storage for PEth samples. Different research groups have employed these DBS cards and have shown that they are useful for the storage of PEth positive blood samples (Beck et al. 2018; Luginbühl et al. 2019; Nguyen and Fitzpatrick 2019). The cards have been also used in the detection of PEth in blood samples taken from newborns who were exposed to ethanol while in the womb (Bracero et al. 2017). PEth was able to be detected from a set of dried blood spot cards up to 6 months after the initial collection (Kummer et al. 2016).

The currently available analytical methods are based on the use of HPLC coupled with evaporative light scattering detection (Aradóttir et al. 2005) or with mass spectrometry (Gnann et al. 2009, 2010). In addition, a method based on nonaqueous capillary electrophoresis (NACE) hyphenated with mass spectrometry was reported to be robust and reliable (Nalesso et al. 2010). An alternative indirect diagnostic approach reported by Nissinen et al. is based on the determination in plasma of antibodies against PEth by using a chemiluminescent immunoassay (2012).

A critical issue in PEth analysis is the extraction of this biomarker from whole blood, since it is usually complex and time-consuming. There are a wide array of techniques for the extraction of phospholipids from red blood cells. Typically, a simple extraction using an alcohol such as butanol or blend of methanol-chloroform can be employed. Most methods involve the extraction of PEth from collected blood use a single or multi-step organic extraction followed by a drying step. Recently, however, dispersive extractions have been used to increase the efficiency from two to five times (Wang et al. 2017). Furthermore, a simple method based on an automated filtration with Phree™ Phospholipid Removal Plates (Phenomenex, California, USA), after protein precipitation with acetonitrile, has been proposed (Casati et al. 2019).

9.9 Conclusions

The biomarkers can provide objective and relevant information for the clinical and/or forensic diagnosis of alcohol abuse. However, they should be used intelligently not only for the formation of the diagnostic verdict, but also to distinguish among acute intoxication, recent use/abuse, relapse to heavy drinking, chronic abuse, alcohol dependence, and dangerous drinking, as well as to identify alcohol-related organ damages.

Notwithstanding the efforts to identify the "*perfect*" biomarker of chronic alcohol abuse, none of the above-described indicators can be reported to fulfill the requirements of sensitivity, specificity, and reliability that would be expected from a diagnostic tool in such a controversial and delicate matter as alcohol misuse.

Actually, since the sensitivity, specificity, and detection window of each biomarker vary substantially, the choice of any indicator should depend on the aim and context for which the diagnosis of alcohol abuse is required (e.g., clinical, fitness to obtain a driver's license, fitness to work, child custody, etc.).

Concerning the analytical aspects, it is worth highlighting the need, especially if the diagnosis of alcohol abuse is required in a forensic context, for confirming the analytical results by at least a second method based on chemical–physical principles different from those of the methods used for the screening, according to widely accepted rules of forensic toxicology.

Moreover, it should be defined the "error rate" of each diagnostic tool as well as of the entire diagnostic process, to meet one of the well-known prongs of the Daubert standard (Keierleber and Bohan 2005).

Finally, it is worth emphasizing that the clinical and/or forensic diagnosis of alcohol abuse cannot be based only on the information provided by the biomarkers but it has to come from the integration of anamnestic, clinical, instrumental, and laboratory data.

References

Agius R, Nadulski T, Kahl HG, Schräder J, Dufaux B, Yegles M, Pragst F: Validation of a headspace solid-phase microextraction-GC-MS/MS for the determination of ethyl glucuronide in hair according to forensic guidelines, *Forensic Sci Int* 196:3, 2010.

Al-Asmari AI, Anderson RA, Appelblad P: Direct determination of ethyl glucuronide and ethyl sulfate in postmortem urine specimens using hydrophilic interaction liquid chromatography-electrospray ionization-tandem mass spectrometry, *J Anal Toxicol* 34:261, 2010.

Alatalo P, Koivisto H, Puukka K, Hietala J, Anttila P, Bloigu R, Niemelä O:Biomarkers of liver status in heavy drinkers, moderate drinkers and abstainers; *Alcohol Alcohol* 44:199; 2009.

Albermann ME, Musshoff F, Madea B: Comparison of ethyl glucuronide (EtG) and fatty acid ethyl esters (FAEEs) concentrations in hair for testing abstinence, *Anal Bioanal Chem* 400:175, 2011.

Albermann ME, Musshoff F, Madea B: A fully validated high-performance liquid chromatography-tandem mass spectrometry method for the determination of ethylglucuronide in hair for the proof of strict alcohol abstinence, *Anal Bioanal Chem* 396:2441, 2010.

Alden A, Ohlson S, Pahlsson P, Ryden I: HPLC analysis of carbohydrate deficient transferrin isoforms isolated by the Axis Shield %CDT method, *Clin Chim Acta* 356:143, 2005.

Alt A, Janda I, Seidl S, Wurst FM: Determination of ethyl glucuronide in hair samples, *Alcohol Alcohol* 35:313, 2000.

Andresen-Streichert H, Müller A, Glahn A, Skopp G, Sterneck M: Alcohol biomarkers in clinical and forensic contexts, *Dtsch Arztebl Int* 115:309, 2018.

Anton RF, Lieber C, Tabakoff B: CDTect Study Group. Carbohydrate-deficient transferrin and gamma-glutamyltransferase for the detection and monitoring of alcohol use: Results from a multisite study, *Alcohol Clin Exp Res* 26:1215, 2002.

Appenzeller BM, Schneider S, Maul A, Wennig R. Relationship between blood alcohol concentration and carbohydrate-deficient transferrin among drivers, *Drug Alcohol Depend* 79:261, 2005a.

Appenzeller BM, Schneider S, Yegles M, Maul A, Wennig R. Drugs chronic alcohol abuse in drivers, *Forensic Sci Int* 155:83, 2005b.

Aradóttir S, Asanovska G, Gjerss S, Hansson P, Alling C. PHosphatidylethanol (PEth) concentrations in blood are correlated to reported alcohol intake in alcohol-dependent patients, *Alcohol Alcohol* 41:431, 2006.

Aradóttir S, Olsson BL. Methodological modifications on quantification of phosphatidylethanol in blood from humans abusing alcohol, using high-performance liquid chromatography and evaporative light scattering detection, *BMC Biochem* 6:18, 2005.

Aradóttir S, Seidl S, Wurst FM, Jönsson BA, Alling C. Phosphatidylethanol in human organs and blood: A study on autopsy material and influences by storage conditions, *Alcohol Clin Exp Res* 28:1718, 2004.

Armer JM, Gunawardana L, Allcock RL. The performance of alcohol markers including ethyl glucuronide and ethyl sulphate to detect alcohol use in clients in a community alcohol treatment programme, *Alcohol Alcohol* 52:29, 2017.

Arndt T, Gierten B, Güssregen B, Werle A, Grüner J. False-positive ethyl glucuronide immunoassay screening associated with chloral hydrate medication as confirmed by LC-MS/MS and self-medication, *Forensic Sci Int* 184:e27, 2009.

Arndt T, Keller T. Forensic analysis of carbohydrate-deficient transferrin (CDT): Implementation of a screening and confirmatory analysis concept is hampered by the lack of CDT isoform standards, *Forensic Sci Int* 146:9, 2004.

Arndt T, Kropf J. Alcohol abuse and carbohydrate deficient transferrin analysis: Are screening and confirmatory analysis required? *Clin. Chem* 48:2072, 2002.

Arndt T. Carbohydrate-deficient transferrin as a marker of chronic alcohol abuse: A critical review of preanalysis, analysis, and interpretation, *Clin Chem* 47:13, 2001.

Auwärter V, Kiessling B, Pragst F. Squalene in hair—A natural reference substance for the improved interpretation of fatty acid ethyl ester concentrations with respect to alcohol misuse, *Forensic Sci Int* 145:149, 2004.

Auwärter V, Sporkert F, Hartwig S, Pragst F, Vater H, Diefenbacher A. Fatty acid ethyl esters in hair as markers of alcohol consumption. Segmental hair analysis of alcoholics, social drinkers, and teetotalers, *Clin Chem* 47:2114, 2001.

Bager H, Christensen LP, Husby S, Bjerregaard L. Biomarkers for the detection of prenatal alcohol exposure: A review, *Alcohol Clin Exp Res* 41:251, 2017.

Bakdash A, Burger P, Goecke TW, Fasching PA, Reulbach U, Bleich S, Hastedt M, Rothe M, Beckmann MW, Pragst F, et al. Quantification of fatty acid ethyl esters (FAEE) and ethyl glucuronide (EtG) in meconium from newborns for detection of alcohol abuse in a maternal health evaluation study, *Anal Bioanal Chem* 396:2469, 2010.

Bakhireva LN, Cano S, Rayburn WF, Savich RD, Leeman L, Anton RF, Savage DD. Advanced gestational age increases serum carbohydrate-deficient transferrin levels in abstinent pregnant women, *Alcohol Alcohol* 47:683, 2012.

Baros AM, Wright TM, Latham PK, Miller PM, Anton RF. Alcohol consumption, %CDT, GGT and blood pressure change during alcohol treatment, *Alcohol Alcohol* 43:192, 2008.

Barrio P, Mondon S, Teixidor L, Ortega L, Vieta E, Gual A. One year clinical correlates of EtG positive urine screening in Alcohol-Dependent Patients: A survival analysis, *Alcohol Alcohol* 52:460, 2017.

Barrio P, Teixidor L, Ortega L, Lligoña A, Rico N, Bedini JL, Vieta E, Gual A. Filling the gap between lab and clinical impact: An open randomized diagnostic trial comparing urinary ethylglucuronide and ethanol in alcohol dependent outpatients, *Drug Alcohol Depend* 183:225, 2018.

Bean P, Roska C, Harasymiw J, Pearson J, Kay B, Louks H. Alcohol biomarkers as tools to guide and support decisions about intoxicated driver risk, *Traffic Inj Prev* 10:519, 2009.

Beck O, Kenan Modén N, Seferaj S, Lenk G, Helander A. Study of measurement of the alcohol biomarker phosphatidylethanol (PEth) in dried blood spot (DBS) samples and application of a volumetric DBS device, *Clin Chim Acta* 479:38, 2018.

Beckemeier ME, Bora PS. Fatty acid ethyl esters: Potentially toxic products of myocardial ethanol metabolism, *J Mol Cell Cardiol.* 30:2487, 1998.

Beckmann M, Paslakis G, Böttcher M, Helander A, Erim Y. Integration of clinical examination, self-report, and hair ethyl glucuronide analysis for evaluation of patients with alcoholic liver disease prior to liver transplantation, *Prog Transplant* 26:40, 2016.

Bendroth P, Kronstrand R, Helander A, Greby J, Stephanson N, Krantz P. Comparison of ethyl glucuronide in hair with phosphatidylethanol in whole blood as post-mortem markers of alcohol abuse, *Forensic Sci Int* 176:76, 2008.

Bergen HR, Lacey JM, O'Brien J F, Naylor S. Online single step analysis of blood proteins: The transferrin story, *Anal Biochem* 296:122, 2001.

Bergström JP, Helander A. HPLC evaluation of clinical and pharmacological factors reported to cause false-positive carbohydrate-deficient transferrin (CDT) levels, *Clin Chim Acta* 389:164, 2008a.

Bergström JP, Helander A. Influence of alcohol use, ethnicity, age, gender, BMI and smoking on the serum transferrin glycoform pattern: implications for use of carbohydrate-deficient transferrin (CDT) as alcohol biomarker, *Clin Chim Acta* 388:59, 2008b.

Bertholet N, Winter MR, Cheng DM, Samet JH, Saitz R. How accurate are blood (or breath) tests for identifying self-reported heavy drinking among people with alcohol dependence, *Alcohol Alcohol* 49:423, 2014.

Bertholf R, Bazydlo L. Biomarkers of acute and chronic alcohol ingestion. In Caplan YH, Goldberger BA (Eds), *Garriott's Medicolegal Aspects of Alcohol*, 6th ed., Lawyers & Judges Publishing Company: Tucson, AZ. Chapter 4, 2014.

Bertol E, Del Bravo E, Vaiano F, Mari F, Favretto D. Fatty acid ethyl esters in hair: Correlation with self-reported ethanol intake in 160 subjects and influence of estroprogestin therapy, *Drug Test Anal* 6:930, 2014.

Bianchi V, Ivaldi A, Raspagni A, Arfini C, Vidali M. Pregnancy and variations of carbohydrate-deficient transferrin levels measured by the candidate reference HPLC method, *Alcohol Alcohol* 46:123, 2011.

Bianchi V, Ivaldi A, Raspagni A, Arfini C, Vidali M. Use of carbohydrate-deficient transferrin (CDT) and a combination of GGT and CDT (GGT-CDT) to assess heavy alcohol consumption in traffic medicine, *Alcohol Alcohol* 45:247, 2010.

Bicker W, Lämmerhofer M, Keller T, Schuhmacher R, Krska R, Lindner W. Validated method for the determination of the ethanol consumption markers ethylglicuronide, ethylphosphate and ethylsulfate in human urine by reversed phase/weak anion exchange liquid chromatography-mass spectrometry, *Anal Chem* 78:5884, 2006.

Biffi S, Tamaro G, Bortot B, Zamberlan S, Severini GM, Carrozzi M. Carbohydrate-deficient transferrin (CDT) as a biochemical tool for the screening of congenital disorders of glycosylation (CDGs), *Clin Biochem* 40:1431, 2007.

Biondi A, Freni F, Carelli C, Moretti M, Morini L. Ethyl glucuronide hair testing: A review, *Forensic Sci Int.* 300:106, 2019.

Bisaga A, Laposata M, Xie S, Evans SM. Comparison of serum fatty acid ethyl esters and urinary 5-hydroxytryptophol as biochemical markers of recent ethanol consumption, *Alcohol Alcohol* 40:214, 2005.

Bjerre B, Borg S, Helander A, Jeppsson JO, Johnson G, Karlsson G. CDT a valuable marker of overconsumption of alcohol. Guidelines for its use in connection with automobile driver examination, *Lakartidningen* 98:677, 2001.

Bogstrand ST, Høiseth G, Rossow I, Normann PT, Ekeberg O. Prevalence of ethyl glucuronide and ethyl sulphate among patients injured when driving or at work, *Alcohol Alcohol* 50:68, 2015.

Bortolotti F, De Paoli G, Pascali JP, Tagliaro F. Fully automated analysis of Carbohydrate-Deficient Transferrin (CDT) by using a multicapillary electrophoresis system, *Clin Chim Acta* 380:4, 2007.

Bortolotti F, De Paoli G, Pascali JP, Trevisan MT, Floreani M, Tagliaro F. Analysis of carbohydrate-deficient transferrin: Comparative evaluation of turbidimetric immunoassay, capillary zone electrophoresis, and HPLC, *Clin Chem* 51:2368, 2005.

Bortolotti F, Micciolo R, Canal L, Tagliaro F. First objective association between elevated carbohydrate-deficient transferrin concentrations and alcohol-related traffic accidents, *Alcohol Clin Exp Res* 39:2108, 2015.

Bortolotti F, Sorio D, Bertaso A, Tagliaro F. Analytical and diagnostic aspects of carbohydrate deficient transferrin (CDT): A critical review over years 2007–2017, *J Pharm Biomed Anal* 147:2, 2018.

Bortolotti F, Tagliaro F, Cittadini F, Gottardo R, Trettene M, Marigo M. Determination of CDT, a marker of chronic alcohol abuse, for driving license issuing: Immunoassay versus capillary electrophoresis, *Forensic Sci Int* 128:53, 2002.

Bortolotti F, Trettene M, Gottardo R, Bernini M, Ricossa MC, Tagliaro F. Carbohydrate-deficient transferrin (CDT): A reliable indicator of the risk of driving under the influence of alcohol when determined by capillary electrophoresis, *Forensic Sci Int* 170:175, 2007.

Borucki K, Dierkes J, Wartberg J, Westphal S, Genz A, Luley C. In heavy drinkers, fatty acid ethyl esters remain elevated for up to 99 hours, *Alcohol Clin Exp Res* 31:423, 2007.

Boscolo-Berto R, Favretto D, Cecchetto G, Vincenti M, Kronstrand R, Ferrara SD, Viel G. Sensitivity and specificity of EtG in hair as a marker of chronic excessive drinking: Pooled analysis of raw data and meta-analysis of diagnostic accuracy studies, *Ther Drug Monit* 36:560, 2014.

Bottcher M, Beck O, Helander A. Evaluation of a new immunoassay for urinary ethylglicuronide testing, *Alcohol Alcohol* 43:46, 2008.

Bozbaş H, Yıldırır A, Karaçağlar E, Demir O, Ulus T, Eroğlu S, Aydınalp A, Ozin B, Müderrisoğlu H. Increased serum gamma-glutamyltransferase activity in patients with metabolic syndrome, *Turk Kardiyol Dern Ars* 39:122, 2011.

Bracero LA, Maxwell S, Nyanin A, Seybold DJ, White A, Broce M. Improving screening for alcohol consumption during pregnancy with phosphatidylethanol, *Reprod Toxicol* 74:104, 2017.

Cabarcos P, Álvarez I, Tabernero MJ, Bermejo AM. Determination of direct alcohol markers: A review, *Anal Bioanal Chem* 407:4907, 2015.

Cabarcos P, Tabernero MJ, Otero JL, Míguez M, Bermejo AM, Martello S, De Giovanni N, Chiarotti M. Quantification of fatty acid ethyl esters (FAEE) and ethyl glucuronide (EtG) in meconium for detection of alcohol abuse during pregnancy: Correlation study between both biomarkers, *J Pharm Biomed Anal* 100:74, 2014.

Cappelle D, Lai FY, Covaci A, Vermassen A, Crunelle CL, Neels H, van Nuijs ALN. Assessment of ethyl sulphate in hair as a marker for alcohol consumption using liquid chromatography-tandem mass spectrometry, *Drug Test Anal* 10:1566, 2018.

Cappelle D, Neels H, De Keukeleire S, Fransen E, Dom G, Vermassen A, Covaci A, Crunelle CL, van Nuijs ALN. Ethyl glucuronide in keratinous matrices as biomarker of alcohol use: A correlation study between hair and nails, *Forensic Sci Int* 279:187, 2017.

Casati S, Ravelli A, Angeli I, Durello R, Minoli M, Orioli M. An automated sample preparation approach for routine liquid chromatography tandem-mass spectrometry measurement of the alcohol biomarkers phosphatidylethanol 16:0/18:1, 16:0/16:0 and 18:1/18:1, *J Chromatogr A* 1589:1, 2019.

Cervera-Juanes R, Wilhem LJ, Park B, Lee R, Locke J, Helms C, Gonzales S, Wand G, Jones SR, Grant KA, et al. MAOA expression predicts vulnerability for alcohol use, *Mol Psychiatry* 21:472, 2016.

Chan D, Bar-Oz B, Pellerin B, Paciorek C, Klein J, Kapur B, Farine D, Koren G. Population baseline of meconium fatty acid ethyl esters among infants of nondrinking women in Jerusalem and Toronto, *Ther Drug Monit* 25:271, 2003.

Chan D, Klein J, Karaskov T, Koren G. Fetal exposure to alcohol as evidenced by fatty acid ethyl esters in meconium in the absence of maternal drinking history in pregnancy, *Ther Drug Monit* 26:474, 2004.

Chang IJ, He M, Lam CT. Congenital disorders of glycosylation, *Ann Transl Med* 6:477, 2018.

Chatzipanagiotou S, Kalykaki M, Tzavellas E, Karaiskos D, Paparrigopoulos T, Liappas A, Nicolaou C, Michalopoulou M, Zoga M, Boufidou F, et al. Alteration of biological markers in alcohol-dependent individuals without liver disease during the detoxification therapy, *In Vivo* 24:325, 2010.

Coccini T, Crevani A, Acerbi D, Roda E, Castoldi AF, Crespi V, Manzo L. Comparative HPLC and ELISA studies for CDT isoform characterization in subjects with alcohol related problems. Prospective application in workplace risk-prevention policy, *G Ital Med Lav Ergon* 30:119, 2008.

Costantino A, Digregorio EJ, Korn W, Spayd S, Rieders F. The effect of the use of mouthwash on ethylglucuronide concentrations in urine, *J Anal Toxicol* 30:659, 2006.

Crabb DW, Matsumoto M, Chang D, You M. Overview of the role of alcohol dehydrogenase and aldehyde dehydrogenase and their variants in the genesis of alcohol-related pathology, *Proc Nutr Soc* 63:49, 2004.

Crews B, West R, Gutierrez R, Latyshev S, Mikel C, Almazan P, Pesce A, West C, Rosenthal M. An improved method of determining ethanol use in a chronic pain population, *J Opioid Manag* 7:27, 2011.

Crunelle CL, Yegles M, De Doncker M, Dom G, Cappelle D, Maudens KE, van Nuijs AL, Covaci A, Neels H. Influence of repeated permanent coloring and bleaching on ethyl glucuronide concentrations in hair from alcohol-dependent patients, *Forensic Sci Int* 247:18, 2015.

Dahl H, Voltaire Carlsson A, Hillgren K, Helander A. Urinary ethyl glucuronide and ethyl sulfate testing for detection of recent drinking in an outpatient treatment program for alcohol and drug dependence, *Alcohol Alcohol* 46:278, 2011.

De Giovanni N, Donadio G, Chiarotti M. Ethanol contamination leads to fatty acid ethyl esters in hair samples, *J Anal Toxicol* 32:156, 2008.

De Giovanni N, Donadio G, Chiarotti M. The reliability of fatty acid ethylesters (FAEE) as biological markers for the diagnosis of alcohol abuse, *J Anal Toxicol* 31:93, 2007.

Delanghe JR, De Buyzere ML. Carbohydrate deficient transferrin and forensic medicine, *Clin Chim Acta* 406:1, 2009.

Delanghe JR, Helander A, Wielders JP, Pekelharing JM, Roth HJ, Schellenberg F, Born C, Yagmur E, Gentzer W, Althaus H. Development and multicenter evaluation of the N latex CDT direct immunonephelometric assay for serum carbohydrate-deficient transferrin, *Clin Chem* 53:1115, 2007.

Doyle KM, Cluette-Brown JE, Dube DM, Bernhardt TG, Morse CR, Laposata M. Fatty acid ethyl esters in the blood as markers for ethanol intake, *JAMA* 227:792, 1997.

Duncan J, Johnson S, Ou XM. Monoamine oxidases in major depressive disorder and alcoholism, *Drug Discov Ther* 6:112, 2012.

Edenberg HJ, Foroud T. The genetics of alcoholism: Identifying specific genes through family studies, *Addict Biol* 11:386, 2006.

Edenberg HJ. The genetics of alcohol metabolism: Role of alcohol dehydrogenase and aldehyde dehydrogenase variants, *Alcohol Res Health* 30:5, 2007.

Eichler A, Grunitz J, Grimm J, Walz L, Raabe E, Goecke TW, Beckmann MW, Kratz O, Heinrich H, Moll GH, et al. Did you drink alcohol during pregnancy? Inaccuracy and discontinuity of women's self-reports: On the way to establish meconium ethyl glucuronide (EtG) as a biomarker for alcohol consumption during pregnancy, *Alcohol* 54:39, 2016.

Endre ZH, Pickering JW, Walker RJ, Devarajan P, Edelstein CL, Bonventre JV, Frampton CM, Bennett MR, Ma Q, Sabbisetti VS, et al. Improved performance of urinary biomarkers of acute kidney injury in the critically ill by stratification for injury duration and baseline renal function, *Kidney Int* 79:1119, 2011.

Erim Y, Böttcher M, Dahmen U, Beck O, Broelsch CE, Helander A. Urinary ethylglucuronide testing detects alcohol consumption in alcoholic liver disease patients awaiting liver transplantation, *Liver Transpl* 13:757, 2007.

Ettlinger J, Kirchen L, Yegles M. Influence of thermal hair straightening on ethyl glucuronide content in hair, *Drug Test Anal* 1:74, 2014.

Fagan KJ, Irvine KM, McWhinney BC, Fletcher LM, Horsfall LU, Johnson LA, Clouston AD, Jonsson JR, O'Rourke P, Martin J, et al. BMI but not stage or etiology of nonalcoholic liver disease affects the diagnostic utility of carbohydrate-deficient transferrin, *Alcohol Clin Exp Res* 37:1771, 2013.

Fagan KJ, Irvine KM, McWhinney BC, Fletcher LM, Horsfall LU, Johnson LA, O'Rourke P, Martin J, Scott I, Pretorius CJ, et al. Diagnostic sensitivity of carbohydrate deficient transferrin in heavy drinkers, *BMC Gastroenterol* 14:97, 2014.

Favretto D, Nalesso A, Frison G, Viel G, Traldi P, Ferrara SD. A novel and an effective analytical approach for the LC-MS determination of ethyl glucuronide and ethyl sulfate in urine, *Int J Legal Med* 124:161, 2010.

Flahaut C, Michalski JC, Danel T, Humbert MH, Klein A. The effects of ethanol on the glycosylation of human transferrin, *Glycobiology* 13:191, 2003.

Fleming M, Bhamb B, Schurr M, Mundt M, Williams A. Alcohol biomarkers in patients admitted for trauma, *Alcohol Clin Exp Res* 33:1777, 2009.

Fleming MF, Anton RF, Spies CD. A review of genetic, biological, pharmacological, and clinical factors that affect carbohydrate-deficient transferrin levels, *Alcohol Clin Exp Res* 28:1347, 2004.

Fucci N, Gili A, Aroni K, Bacci M, Carletti P, Pascali VL, Gambelunghe C. Monitoring people at risk of drinking by a rapid urinary ethyl glucuronide test, *Interdiscip Toxicol* 10:155, 2017.

Fustinoni S, De Vecchi M, Bordini L, Todaro A, Riboldi L, Bertazzi PA. Validity of carbohydrate-deficient transferrine (CDT) in assessing chronic abuse of ethyl alcohol in urban public transport workers, *Med Lav* 100:359, 2009.

Garcia-Algar O, Kulaga V, Gareri J, Koren G, Vall O, Zuccaro P, Pacifici R, Pichini S. Alarming prevalence of fetal alcohol exposure in a Mediterranean city, *Ther Drug Monit* 30:249, 2008.

Gareri J, Appenzeller B, Walasek P, Koren G. Impact of hair-care products on FAEE hair concentrations in substance abuse monitoring, *Anal Bioanal Chem* 400:183, 2011.

Gessner S, Below E, Diedrich S, Wegner C, Gessner W, Kohlmann T, Heidecke CD, Bockholdt B, Kramer A, Assadian O, et al. Ethanol and ethyl glucuronide urine concentrations after ethanol-based hand antisepsis with and without permitted alcohol consumption, *Am J Infect Control* 44:999, 2016.

Gjerde H, Christophersen AS, Moan IS, Yttredal B, Walsh JM, Normann PT, Mørland J. Use of alcohol and drugs by Norwegian employees: A pilot study using questionnaires and analysis of oral fluid, *J Occup Med Toxicol* 5:13, 2010.

Gjerde H, Mørland J. Concentrations of carbohydrate-deficient transferrin in dialysed plasma from drunken drivers, *Alcohol Alcohol* 22: 271, 1987.

Gnann H, Engelmann C, Skopp G, Winkler M, Auwärter V, Dresen S, Ferreirós N, Wurst FM, Weinmann W. Identification of 48 homologues of phosphatidylethanol in blood by LC-ESI-MS/MS, *Anal Bioanal Chem* 396:2415, 2010.

Gnann H, Weinmann W, Engelmann C, Wurst FM, Skopp G, Winkler M, Thierauf A, Auwärter V, Dresen S, Ferreirós Bouzas N. Selective detection of phosphatidylethanol homologues in blood as biomarkers for alcohol consumption by LC-ESI-MS/MS, *J Mass Spectrom* 44:1293, 2009.

Gomez-Roig MD, Marchei E, Sabra S, Busardò FP, Mastrobattista L, Pichini S, Gratacós E, Garcia-Algar O. Maternal hair testing to disclose self-misreporting in drinking and smoking behavior during pregnancy, *Alcohol* 67:1, 2018.

Gough G, Heathers L, Puckett D, Westerhold C, Ren X, Yu Z, Crabb DW, Liangpunsakul S. The utility of commonly used laboratory tests to screen for excessive alcohol use in clinical practice, *Alcohol Clin Exp Res* 39:1493, 2015.

Gutierrez HL, Hund L, Shrestha S, Rayburn WF, Leeman L, Savage DD, Bakhireva LN. Ethylglucuronide in maternal hair as a biomarker of prenatal alcohol exposure, *Alcohol* 49:617, 2015.

Halter CC, Dresen S, Auwaerter V, Wurst FM, Weinmann W. Kinetics in serum and urinary excretion of ethylsulfate and ethylglucuronide after medium dose ethanol intake, *Int J Legal Med* 122:123, 2008.

Hansson P, Caron M, Johnson G, Gustavsson L, Alling C. Blood phosphatidylethanol as a marker of alcohol abuse: levels in alcoholic males during withdrawal, *Alcohol Clin Exp Res* 21:108, 1997.

Hansson P, Varga A, Krantz P, Alling C. Phosphatidylethanol in post-mortem blood as a marker of previous heavy drinking, *Int J Legal Med* 115:158, 2001.

Hartmann S, Aradottir S, Graf M, Wiesbeck G, Lesch O, Ramskogler K, Wolfersdorf M, Alling C, Wurst FM. Phosphatidylethanol as a sensitive and specific biomarker: Comparison with gamma-glutamyl transpeptidase, mean corpuscular volume and carbohydrate-deficient transferrin, *Addict Biol* 12:81, 2007.

Hartwig S, Auwärter V, Pragst F. Effect of hair care and hair cosmetics on the concentrations of fatty acid ethyl esters in hair as markers of chronically elevated alcohol consumption, *Forensic Sci Int* 131:90, 2003.

Hartwig S, Auwärter V, Pragst F. Fatty Acid ethyl esters in scalp, pubic, axillary, beard and body hair as markers for alcohol misuse, *Alcohol Alcohol* 38:163, 2003.

Hegstad S, Johnsen L, Mørland J, Christophersen AS. Determination of ethylglucuronide in oral fluid by ultra-performance liquid chromatography-tandem mass spectrometry, *J Anal Toxicol* 33:204, 2009.

Hegstad S, Kristoffersen L, Liane VH, Spigset O. EtG and EtS in autopsy blood samples with and without putrefaction using UPLC-MS-MS, *J Anal Toxicol* 41:107, 2017.

Helander A, Böttcher M, Dahmen N, Beck O. Elimination characteristics of the alcohol biomarker phosphatidylethanol (PEth) in blood during alcohol detoxification, *Alcohol Alcohol* 54:251, 2019.

Helander A, Husa A, Jeppsson JO. Improved HPLC method for carbohydrate-deficient transferrin in serum, *Clin Chem* 49:1881, 2003.

Helander A, Jones AW. Recent advances in biochemical tests for acute and chronic alcohol consumption. In Karch SB (Ed), *Drug Abuse Handbook*, 2nd ed., CRC Press: Boca Raton, FL, pp. 401–427, 2007.

Helander A, Kenan Modén N. Effect of transferrin glycation on the use of carbohydrate-deficient transferrin as an alcohol biomarker, *Alcohol Alcohol* 48:478, 2013.

Helander A, Kenan N, Beck O. Comparison of analytical approaches for liquid chromatography/mass spectrometry determination of the alcohol biomarker ethylglucuronide in urine, *Rapid Commun Mass Spectrom* 24:1737, 2010b.

Helander A, Olsson I, Dahl H. Postcollection synthesis of ethyl glucuronide by bacteria in urine may cause false identification of alcohol consumption, *Clin Chem* 53:1855, 2007.

Helander A, Vabö E, Levin K, Borg S. Intra- and interindividual variability of carbohydrate-deficient transferrin, gamma-glutamyltransferase, and mean corpuscular volume in teetotalers, *Clin Chem* 44:2120, 1998.

Helander A, Wielders J, Anton R, Arndt T, Bianchi V, Deenmamode J, Jeppsson JO, Whitfield JB, Weykamp C, Schellenberg F, et al. Standardisation and use of the alcohol biomarker carbohydrate-deficient transferrin (CDT), *Clin Chim Acta* 459:19, 2016.

Helander A, Wielders J, Anton R, Arndt T, Bianchi V, Deenmamode J, Jeppsson JO, Whitfield JB, Weykamp C, Schellenberg F, International Federation of Clinical Chemistry and Laboratory Medicine Working Group on Standardisation of Carbohydrate-Deficient Transferrin. Standardisation and use of the alcohol biomarker carbohydrate-deficient transferrin (CDT), *Clin Chim Acta* 459:19, 2016.

Helander A, Wielders JP, Jeppsson JO, Weykamp C, Siebelder C, Anton RF, Schellenberg F, Whitfield JB, IFCC Working Group on Standardization of Carbohydrate-Deficient Transferrin (WG-CDT). Toward standardization of carbohydrate-deficient transferrin (CDT) measurements: II. Performance of a laboratory network running the HPLC candidate reference measurement procedure and evaluation of a candidate reference material, *Clin Chem Lab Med* 48:1585, 2010a.

Helander A, Wielders JP, Te Stroet R, Bergstrom JP. Comparison of HPLC and capillary electrophoresis for confirmatory testing of the alcohol misuse marker carbohydrate-deficient transferrin, *Clin Chem* 51:1528, 2005.

Hermansson U, Helander A, Brandt L, Huss A, Rönnberg S. Screening and brief intervention for risky alcohol consumption in the workplace: Results of a 1-year randomized controlled study, *Alcohol Alcohol* 45:252, 2010.

Himes SK, Concheiro M, Scheidweiler KB, Huestis MA. Validation of a novel method to identify in utero ethanol exposure: Simultaneous meconium extraction of fatty acid ethyl esters, ethyl glucuronide, and ethyl sulfate followed by LC-MS/MS quantification, *Anal Bioanal Chem* 406:1945, 2014.

Høiseth G, Bernard JP, Karinen R, Johnsen L, Helander A, Christophersen AS, Mørland J. A pharmaco-kinetic study of ethylglicuronide in blood and urine: Applications to forensic toxicology, *Forensic Sci Int* 172:119, 2007.

Høiseth G, Fosen JT, Liane V, Bogstrand ST, Mørland J. Alcohol hangover as a cause of impairment in apprehended drivers, *Traffic Inj Prev* 16:323, 2015.

Høiseth G, Karinen R, Christophersen A, Mørland J. Practical use of ethylglucuronide and ethyl sulfate in postmortem cases as markers of antemortem alcohol ingestion, *Int J Legal Med* 124:143, 2010c.

Høiseth G, Morini L, Polettini A, Christophersen A, Mørland J. Blood kinetics of ethyl glucuronide and ethyl sulphate in heavy drinkers during alcohol detoxification, *Forensic Sci Int* 188:52, 2009.

Høiseth G, Yttredal B, Karinen R, Gjerde H, Christophersen A. Levels of ethyl glucuronide and ethyl sulfate in oral fluid, blood, and urine after use of mouthwash and ingestion of nonalcoholic wine, *J Anal Toxicol* 34:84, 2010a.

Høiseth G, Yttredal B, Karinen R, Gjerde H, Mørland J, Christophersen A. Ethylglucuronide concentrations in oral fluid, blood, and urine after volunteers drank 0.5 and 1.0 g/kg doses of ethanol, *J Anal Toxicol* 34:319, 2010b.

Holbrook P, Pannell L, Murata Y, Daly J. Molecular species analysis of a product of phospholipase D activation: Phosphatidylethanol is formed from phosphatidylcholine in phorbol ester- and bradykinin-stimulated PC12 cells, *J Biol Chem* 267:16834, 1992.

Iffland R, Balling MP, Borsh G, Herold C, Kaschade W, Loffler T, Schmidtmann U, Stettner J. Evaluation of an increased blood level of GGT, CDT, methanol, acetone and isopropanol in alcohol intoxicated automobile drivers alcoholism indicators instead of medical-psychological examination, *Blutalkohol* 31:273, 1994.

Iqbal A, Iftikhar U, Ali FA, Memon S, Zuberi N. Comparison of gamma glutamyltransferase in normal and in type 2 diabetics, *J Pak Med Assoc* 60:945, 2010.

Isaksson A, Walther L, Hansson T, Andersson A, Alling C. Phosphatidylethanol in blood (B-PEth): A marker for alcohol use and abuse, *Drug Test Anal* 3:195, 2011.

Jastrzębska I, Zwolak A, Szczyrek M, Wawryniuk A, Skrzydło-Radomańska B, Daniluk J. Biomarkers of alcohol misuse: Recent advances and future prospects, *Prz Gastroenterol* 11:78, 2016.

Jatlow P, O'Malley SS. Clinical (nonforensic) application of ethyl glucuronide measurement: Are we ready? *Alcohol Clin Exp Res* 34:968, 2010.

Joya X, Mazarico E, Ramis J, Pacifici R, Salat-Batlle J, Mortali C, García-Algar O, Pichini S. Segmental hair analysis to assess effectiveness of single-session motivational intervention to stop ethanol use during pregnancy, *Drug Alcohol Depend* 158:45, 2016.

Jung B, Caslavska J, Thormann W. Determination of ethyl glucuronide in human serum by capillary zone electrophoresis and an immunoassay, *J Sep Sci* 32:3497, 2009.

Junghanns K, Graf I, Pflüger J, Wetterling G, Ziems C, Ehrenthal D, Zöllner M, Dibbelt L, Backhaus J, Weinmann W, et al. Urinary ethyl glucuronide (EtG) and ethyl sulphate (EtS) assessment: valuable tools to improve verification of abstention in alcohol-dependent patients during in-patient treatment and at follow-ups, *Addiction* 104:921, 2009.

Jurado C, Soriano T, Giménez MP, Menéndez M Diagnosis of chronic alcohol consumption. Hair analysis for ethyl-glucuronide, *Forensic Sci Int* 145:161, 2004.

Kaphalia BS, Cai P, Khan MF, Okorodudu AO, Ansari GA. Fatty acid ethyl esters: Markers of alcohol abuse and alcoholism, *Alcohol* 34:151, 2004.

Karch SB. Ethanol-based hand cleansers, *J Forensic Leg Med* 16:497, 2009.

Kechagias S, Ernersson A, Dahlqvist O, Lundberg P, Lindström T, Nystrom FH, Fast Food Study Group. Fast-food-based hyper-alimentation can induce rapid and profound elevation of serum alanine aminotransferase in healthy subjects, *Gut* 57:649, 2008.

Keierleber JA, Bohan TL. Ten years after Daubert: The status of the states, *J Forensic Sci* 50:1154, 2005.

Kenan N, Husand S, Helander A. Importance of HPLC confirmation of problematic carbohydrate-deficient transferrin (CDT) results from a multicapillary electrophoresis routine method, *Clin Chim Acta* 411:1945, 2010.

Kenan N, Larsson A, Axelsson O, Helander A. Changes in transferrin glycosylation during pregnancy may lead to false-positive carbohydrate-deficient transferrin (CDT) results in testing for riskful alcohol consumption, *Clin Chim Acta* 412:129, 2011.

Kerekes I, Yegles M, Grimm U, Wennig R. Ethyl glucuronide determination: Head hair versus non-head hair, *Alcohol Alcohol* 44:62, 2009.

Keten A, Tumer AR, Balseven-Odabasi A. Measurement of ethyl glucuronide in vitreous humor with liquid chromatography-mass spectrometry, *Forensic Sci Int* 193:101, 2009.

Kilo S, Hofmann B, Eckert E, Göen T, Drexler H. Evaluation of biomarkers assessing regular alcohol consumption in an occupational setting, *Int Arch Occup Environ Health*. 89:1193, 2016.

Kintz P, Villain M, Vallet E, Etter M, Salquebre G, Cirimele V. Ethyl glucuronide: Unusual distribution between head hair and pubic hair, *Forensic Sci Int* 176:87, 2008.

Kintz P. Consensus of the Society of Hair Testing on hair testing for chronic excessive alcohol consumption 2009, *Forensic Sci Int* 196:2, 2010.

Kip MJ, Spies CD, Neumann T, Nachbar Y, Alling C, Aradottir S, Weinmann W, Wurst FM. The usefulness of direct ethanol metabolites in assessing alcohol intake in nonintoxicated male patients in an emergency room setting, *Alcohol Clin Exp Res* 32:1284, 2008.

Kissack JC, Bishop J, Roper AL. Ethylglucuronide as a biomarker for ethanol detection, *Pharmacotherapy* 28:769, 2008.

Koivisto H, Hietala J, Anttila P, Parkkila S, Niemelä O. Long-term ethanol consumption and macrocytosis: Diagnostic and pathogenic implications, *J Lab Clin Med* 147:191, 2006.

Krabseth H, Mørland J, Høiseth G. Assistance of ethyl glucuronide and ethyl sulfate in the interpretation of postmortem ethanol findings, *Int J Legal Med* 128:765, 2014.

Kronstrand R, Brinkhagen L, Nyström FH. Ethyl glucuronide in human hair after daily consumption of 16 or 32 g of ethanol for 3 months, *Forensic Sci Int* 215:51, 2012.

Kulaga V, Pragst F, Fulga N, Koren G. Hair analysis of fatty acid ethyl esters in the detection of excessive drinking in the context of fetal alcohol spectrum disorders, *Ther Drug Monit* 31:261, 2009.

Kulaga V, Shor S, Koren G. Correlation between drugs of abuse and alcohol by hair analysis: Parents at risk for having children with fetal alcohol spectrum disorder, *Alcohol* 44:615, 2010.

Kummer N, Lambert WE, Samyn N, Stove CP. Alternative sampling strategies for the assessment of alcohol intake of living persons, *Clin Biochem* 49:1078, 2016.

Kwak HS, Kang YS, Han KO, Moon JT, Chung YC, Choi JS, Han JY, Kim MY, Velázquez-Armenta EY, Nava-Ocampo AA. Quantitation of fatty acid ethyl esters in human meconium by an improved liquid chromatography/tandem mass spectrometry, *J Chromatogr B* 878:1871, 2010.

Lamoureux F, Gaulier JM, Sauvage FL, Mercerolle M, Vallejo C, Lachâtre G. Determination of ethyl-glucuronide in hair for heavy drinking detection using liquid chromatography-tandem mass spectrometry following solid-phase extraction, *Anal Bioanal Chem* 394:1895, 2009.

Lamy S, Hennart B, Houivet E, Dulaurent S, Delavenne H, Benichou J, Allorge D, Marret S, Thibaut F. Perinatal network of Upper-Normandy. Assessment of tobacco, alcohol and cannabinoid metabolites in 645 meconium samples of newborns compared to maternal self-reports, *J Psychiatr Res* 90:86, 2017.

Lande RG, Marin B, Chang AS. Clinical application of ethyl glucuronide testing in the U.S. Army, *J Addict Dis* 30:39, 2011.

Laposata EA, Lange LG. Presence of nonoxidative ethanol metabolism in human organs commonly damaged by ethanol abuse, *Science* 31:497, 1986.

Laposata M, Hasaba A, Best CA, Yoerger DM, McQuillan BM, Salem RO, Refaai MA, Soderberg BL. Fatty acid ethyl esters: Recent observations, *Prostaglandins Leukot Essent Fatty Acids* 67:193, 2002.

Laposata M. Fatty acid ethyl esters: Ethanol metabolites which mediate ethanol-induced organ damage and serve as markers of ethanol intake, *Prog Lipid Res* 37:307, 1998.

Leidl K, Liebisch G, Richter D, Schmitz G. Mass spectrometric analysis of lipid species of human circulating blood cells, *Biochimica Biophysica Acta* 1781:655, 2008.

Lendoiro E, de Castro A, Jiménez-Morigosa C, Gomez-Fraguela XA, López-Rivadulla M, Cruz A. Usefulness of hair analysis and psychological tests for identification of alcohol and drugs of abuse consumption in driving license regranting, *Forensic Sci Int* 286:239, 2018.

Liniger B, Nguyen A, Friedrich-Koch A, Yegles M. Abstinence monitoring of suspected drinking drivers: Ethyl glucuronide in hair versus CDT, *Traffic Inj Prev* 11:123, 2010.

Lowe JM, McDonell MG, Leickly E, Angelo FA, Vilardaga R, McPherson S, Srebnik D, Roll J, Ries RK. Determining ethyl glucuronide cutoffs when detecting self-reported alcohol use in addiction treatment patients, *Alcohol Clin Exp Res* 39:905, 2015.

Luginbühl M, Nussbaumer S, Weinmann W. Decrease of ethyl glucuronide concentrations in hair after exposure to chlorinated swimming pool water, *Drug Test Anal* 10:689, 2018.

Luginbühl M, Weinmann W, Al-Ahmad A. Introduction of sample tubes with sodium azide as a preservative for ethyl glucuronide in urine, *Int J Legal Med* 131:1283, 2017.

Luginbühl M, Weinmann W, Butzke I, Pfeifer P. Monitoring of direct alcohol markers in alcohol use disorder patients during withdrawal treatment and successive rehabilitation, *Drug Test Anal* 11:859, 2019.

Maenhout M, Baten G, De Buyzere ML, Delanghe JR. Carbohydrate deficient transferrin in a driver's license regranting program, *Alcohol Alcohol* 47:253, 2012.

Marques P, Hansson T, Isaksson A, Walther L, Jones J, Lewis D, Jones M. Detection of phosphatidylethanol (PEth) in the blood of drivers in an Alcohol ignition interlock Program, *Traffic Inj Prev* 12:136, 2011.

Marques P, Tippetts S, Allen J, Javors M, Alling C, Yegles M, Pragst F, Wurst F. Estimating driver risk using alcohol biomarkers, interlock blood alcohol concentration tests and psychometric assessments: Initial descriptive, *Addiction* 105:226, 2010.

Marques PR, Tippetts AS, Yegles M. Ethylglucuronide in hair is a top predictor of impaired driving recidivism, alcohol dependence, and a key marker of the highest BAC interlock tests, *Traffic Inj Prev* 15:361, 2014.

Marques PR. Levels and types of alcohol biomarkers in DUI and clinic samples for estimating workplace alcohol problems, *Drug Test Anal* 4:76, 2012.

Marti U, Joneli J, Caslavska J, Thormann W. Determination of carbohydrate-deficient transferrin in human serum by two capillary zone electrophoresis methods and a direct immunoassay: Comparison of patient data, *J Sep Sci* 31:3079, 2008.

Matar MM, Jewett B, Fakhry SM, Wilson DA, Ferguson PL, Anton RF, Sakran JV. Identifying chronic heavy alcohol use in emergency general surgery patients: A pilot study, *Trauma Surg Acute Care Open* 29:1, 2017.

Matthews BA, Kish SJ, Xu X, Boileau I, Rusjan PM, Wilson AA, Di Giacomo D, Houle S, Meyer JH. Greater monoamine oxidase a binding in alcohol dependence, *Biol Psychiatry* 75:756, 2014.

Maxwell S, Thompson S, Zakko F, Bracero LA. Screening for prenatal alcohol exposure and corresponding short-term neonatal outcomes, *Reprod Toxicol* 85:6, 2019.

May PA, Hasken JM, De Vries MM, Marais AS, Stegall JM, Marsden D, Parry CDH, Seedat S, Tabachnick B. A utilitarian comparison of two alcohol use biomarkers with self-reported drinking history collected in antenatal clinics, *Reprod Toxicol* 77:25, 2018.

McKinzie BP, Worrall CL, Simpson KN, Couillard DJ, Leon SM. Impact of elevated per cent carbohydrate-deficient transferrin at hospital admission on outcomes in trauma patients, *Am Surg* 76:492, 2010.

Moore C, Jones J, Lewis D, Buchi K. Prevalence of fatty acid ethyl esters in meconium specimens, *Clin Chem* 49:133, 2003.

Morgan MY, Major MG. The use of serum carbohydrate-deficient transferrin in the assessment of "high risk offenders" in Great Britain, *Alcohol Alcohol* 31:625, 1996.

Morini L, Marchei E, F, Garcia Algar O, Groppi A, Mastrobattista L, Pichini S. Ethyl glucuronide and ethyl sulfate in meconium and hair-potential biomarkers of intrauterine exposure to ethanol, *Forensic Sci Int* 196:74, 2010.

Morini L, Marchei E, Pellegrini M, Groppi A, Stramesi C, Vagnarelli F, Garcia-Algar O, Pacifici R, Pichini S. Liquid chromatography with tandem mass spectrometric detection for the measurement of ethyl glucuronide and ethylsulfate in meconium: new biomarkers of gestational ethanol exposure? *Ther Drug Monit* 30:725, 2008.

Morini L, Politi L, Acito S, Groppi A, Polettini A. Comparison of ethyl glucuronide in hair with carbohydrate-deficient transferrin in serum as markers of chronic high levels of alcohol consumption, *Forensic Sci Int* 188:140, 2009b.

Morini L, Politi L, Polettini A. Ethyl glucuronide in hair. A sensitive and specific marker of chronic heavy drinking, *Addiction* 104:915, 2009a.

Morini L, Politi L, Zucchella A, Polettini A. Ethlyglicuronide and ethylsulphate determination in serum by liquid chromatography-electrospray tandem mass spectrometry, *Clin Chim Acta* 376:213, 2007.

Mueller GC, Fleming MF, LeMahieu MA, Lybrand GS, Barry KJ. Synthesis of phosphatidylethanol—A potential marker for adult males at risk for alcoholism, *Proc Natl Acad Sci U S A* 85:9778, 1988.

Müller A, Iwersen-Bergmann S. Ethyl glucuronide in alcoholic beverages, *Alcohol Alcohol* 53:532, 2018.

Musshoff F, Albermann E, Madea B. Ethyl glucuronide and ethyl sulfate in urine after consumption of various beverages and foods—Misleading results? *Int J Legal Med* 124:623, 2010.

Musshoff F, Daldrup T. Determination of biological markers for alcohol abuse, *J Chromatogr B* 713:245, 1998.

Mutschler J, Grosshans M, Koopmann A, Mann K, Kiefer F, Hermann D. Urinary ethyl-glucuronide assessment in patients treated with disulfiram: A tool to improve verification of abstention and safety, *Clin Neuropharmacol* 33:285, 2010.

Nalesso A, Viel G, Cecchetto G, Frison G, Ferrara SD. Analysis of the alcohol biomarker phosphatidylethanol by NACE with on-line ESI-MS, *Electrophoresis* 31:1227, 2010.

Nedic Erjavec G, Nenadic Sviglin K, Nikolac Perkovic M, Muck-Seler D, Jovanovic T, Pivac N. Association of gene polymorphisms encoding dopaminergic system components and platelet MAO-B activity with alcohol dependence and alcohol dependence-related phenotypes, *Prog Neuropsychopharmacol Biol Psychiatry* 54:321, 2014.

Neumann T, Gentilello LM, Neuner B, Weiss-Gerlach E, Schürmann H, Schröder T, Müller C, Haas NP, Spies CD. Screening trauma patients with the alcohol use disorders identification test and biomarkers of alcohol use, *Alcohol Clin Exp Res* 33:970, 2009.

Nguyen VL, Fitzpatrick M. Should phosphatidylethanol be currently analysed using whole blood, dried blood spots or both? *Clin Chem Lab Med*, 57:617, 2019.

Niemelä O, Alatalo P. Biomarkers of alcohol consumption and related liver disease, *Scand J Clin Lab Invest* 70:305, 2010.

Niemelä O. Biomarker-based approaches for assessing alcohol use disorders, *Int J Environ Res Public Health* 13:166, 2016.

Nissinen AE, Laitinen LM, Kakko S, Helander A, Savolainen MJ, Hörkkö S. Low plasma antibodies specific for phosphatidylethanol in alcohol abusers and patients with alcoholic pancreatitis, *Addict Biol* 17:1057, 2012.

Nomura F, Kanda T, Seimiya M, Satoh M, Kageyama Y, Yamashita T, Yokosuka O, Kato N, Maruyama K. Determination of serum carbohydrate-deficient transferrin by a nephelometric immunoassay for differential diagnosis of alcoholic and non-alcoholic liver diseases, *Clin Chim Acta* 485:181, 2018.

Nováková M, Křivánková L. Determination of ethyl glucuronide in human serum by hyphenation of capillary isotachophoresis and zone electrophoresis, *Electrophoresis* 29:1694, 2008.

Nylander I, Todkar A, Granholm L, Vrettou M, Bendre M, Boon W, Andershed H, Tuvblad C, Nilsson KW, Comasco E. Evidence for a link between Fkbp5/FKBP5, early life social relations and alcohol drinking in young adult rats and humans, *Mol Neurobiol* 54:6225, 2017.

Onat A, Can G, Örnek E, Çiçek G, Ayhan E, Doğan Y. Serum γ-glutamyltransferase: Independent predictor of risk of diabetes, hypertension, metabolic syndrome, and coronary disease, *Obesity* (Silver Spring) 20:842, 2012.

Oppolzer D, Barroso M, Gallardo E. Determination of ethyl glucuronide in hair to assess excessive alcohol consumption in a student population, *Anal Bioanal Chem* 408:2027, 2016.

Palmer RB. A review of the use of ethyl glucuronide as a marker for ethanol consumption in forensic and clinical medicine, *Semin Diagn Pathol* 26:18, 2009.

Palumbo D, Fais P, Calì A, Lusardi M, Bertol E, Pascali JP. Novel zwitterionic HILIC stationary phase for the determination of ethyl glucuronide in human hair by LC-MS/MS, *J Chromatogr B* 1100:33, 2018.

Paolicchi A, Emdin M, Passino C, Lorenzini E, Titta F, Marchi S, Malvaldi G, Pompella A. B-Lipoprotein and LDL associated serum glutamyltransferase in patients with coronary atherosclerosis, *Atherosclerosis* 186:80, 2006.

Parente F, Ah Mew N, Jaeken J, Gilfix BM. A new capillary zone electrophoresis method for the screening of congenital disorders of glycosylation (CDG), *Clin Chim Acta* 411:64, 2010.

Paterlini V, Porpiglia NM, De Palo EF, Tagliaro F. Asialo-transferrin: Biochemical aspects and association with alcohol abuse investigation, *Alcohol* 78:43, 2019.

Paul R. Alcohol markers in hair: an issue of interpretation, *Forensic Sci Med Pathol*, 15:281, 2019.

Pérez-Cerdá C, Quelhas D, Vega AI, Ecay J, Vilarinho L, Ugarte M. Screening using serum percentage of carbohydrate-deficient transferrin for congenital disorders of glycosylation in children with suspected metabolic disease, *Clin Chem* 54:93, 2008.

Petzel-Witt S, Pogoda W, Wunder C, Paulke A, Schubert-Zsilavecz M, Toennes SW. Influence of bleaching and coloring on ethyl glucuronide content in human hair, *Drug Test Anal* 10:177, 2018.

Pisa PT, Vorster HH, Kruger A, Margetts B, du Loots T. Association of alcohol consumption with specific biomarkers: A cross-sectional study in South Africa, *J Health Popul Nutr*, 33:146, 2015.

Porpiglia NM, Bortolotti F, Dorizzi RM, Micciolo R, Tagliaro F. Critical evaluation of the association between elevated mean corpuscular volume and alcohol-related traffic accidents: A retrospective study on 6244 car crash cases, *Alcohol Clin Exp Res* 43:1528, 2019.

Porpiglia NM, De Palo EF, Savchuk SA, Appolonova SA, Bortolotti F, Tagliaro F. A new sample treatment for asialo-Tf determination with capillary electrophoresis: An added value to the analysis of CDT, *Clin Chim Acta* 483:256, 2018a.

Porpiglia NM, Savchuk SA, Appolonova SA, Bortolotti F, Tagliaro F. Capillary Electrophoresis (CE) vs. HPLC in the determination of asialo-Tf, a crucial marker for the reliable interpretation of questioned CDT increases, *Clin Chim Acta* 486:49, 2018b.

Pragst F, Auwaerter V, Sporkert F, Spiegel K. Analysis of fatty acid ethylesters in hair as possible markers of chronically elevated alcohol consumption by headspace solid-phase microextraction (HS-SPME) and gas chromatography-mass spectrometry (GC-MS), *Forensic Sci Int* 121:76, 2001.

Pragst F, Rothe M, Moench B, Hastedt M, Herre S, Simmert D. Combined use of fatty acid ethyl esters and ethyl glucuronide in hair for diagnosis of alcohol abuse: Interpretation and advantages, *Forensic Sci Int* 196:101, 2010.

Pragst F, Yegles M. Determination of fatty acid ethyl esters (FAEE) and ethyl glucuronide (EtG) in hair: A promising way for retrospective detection of alcohol abuse during pregnancy? *Ther Drug Monit* 30:255, 2008.

Puukka K, Hietala J, Koivisto H, Anttila P, Bloigu R, Niemelä O. Additive effects of moderate drinking and obesity on serum gamma-glutamyl transferase activity, *Am J Clin Nutr* 83:1351, 2006.

Quintana E, Montero R, Casado M, Navarro-Sastre A, Vilaseca MA, Briones P, Artuch R. Comparison between high performance liquid chromatography and capillary zone electrophoresis for the diagnosis of congenital disorders of glycosylation, *J Chromatogr B* 877:2513, 2009.

Rainio J, De Giorgio F, Bortolotti F, Tagliaro F. Objective post-mortem diagnosis of chronic alcohol abuse—A review of studies on new markers, *Leg Med* (Tokyo) 10:229, 2008.

Rakhimov MM, Almatov KT, Mirtalipov DT, Kasimova GM, Khodzhaeva NI. Formation of phosphatidylethanol in alcoholic intoxication, *Vopr Med Khim* 34:101, 1988.

Reisfield GM, Goldberger BA, Crews BO, Pesce AJ, Wilson GR, Teitelbaum SA, Bertholf RL. Ethyl glucuronide, ethyl sulfate, and ethanol in urine after sustained exposure to an ethanol-based hand sanitizer, *J Anal Toxicol* 35:85, 2011.

Rosman AS, Lieber CS. Diagnostic utility of laboratory tests in alcoholic liver disease, *Clin Chem* 40:1641, 1994.

Salomone A, Bozzo A, Di Corcia D, Gerace E, Vincenti M. Occupational exposure to alcohol-based hand sanitizers: The diagnostic role of alcohol biomarkers in hair, *J Anal Toxicol* 42:157, 2018.

SAMHSA (Center for Substance Abuse Treatment). The role of biomarkers in the treatment of alcohol use disorders, *Substance Abuse Treatment Advisory* 5:1, 2006.

Schellenberg F, Mennetrey L, Girre C, Nalpas B, Pagès JC. Automated measurement of carbohydrate-deficient transferrin using the Bio-Rad %CDT by the HPLC test on a Variant HPLC system: Evaluation and comparison with other routine procedures, *Alcohol Alcohol* 43:569, 2008.

Schummer C, Appenzeller BM, Wennig R. Quantitative determination of ethylglucuronide in sweat, *Ther Drug Monit* 30:536, 2008.

Seidl S. The role of biological alcohol markers in DUI offenders appraisal for regranting of licenses, *Blutalkohol* 41:12, 2004.

Seidler L, Kaszkin M, Kinzel V. Primary alcohols and phosphatidylcholine metabolism in rat brain synaptosomal membranes via phospholipase D, *Pharmacological Toxicolog*78:249, 1996.

Selvam AP, Muthukumar S, Kamakoti V, Prasad S. A wearable biochemical sensor for monitoring alcohol consumption lifestyle through ethyl glucuronide (EtG) detection in human sweat, *Sci Rep* 6:23111, 2016.

Shi Y, Shen B, Xiang P, Yan H, Shen M. Determination of ethyl glucuronide in hair samples of Chinese people by protein precipitation (PPT) and large volume injection-gas chromatography-tandem mass spectrometry (LVI-GC/MS/MS), *J Chromatogr B* 878:3161, 2010.

Shor S, Nulman I, Kulaga V, Koren G. Heavy in utero ethanol exposure is associated with the use of other drugs of abuse in a high-risk population, *Alcohol* 44:623, 2010.

Sillanaukee P, Olsson U. Improved diagnostic classification of alcohol abusers by combining carbohydrate-deficient transferrin and gamma-glutamyltransferase, *Clin Chem* 47:681, 2001.

Sillanaukee P, Strid N, Allen JP, Litten RZ. Possible reasons why heavy drinking increases carbohydrate-deficient transferrin, *Alcohol Clin Exp Res* 25:34, 2001.

Skipper GE, Weinmann W, Thierauf A, Schaefer P, Wiesbeck G, Allen JP, Miller M, Wurst FM. Ethyl glucuronide: A biomarker to identify alcohol use by health professionals recovering from substance use disorders, *Alcohol Alcohol* 39:445, 2004.

Skipworth JR, Pereira SP. Acute pancreatitis, *Curr Opin Crit Care* 14:172, 2008.

Skopp G, Schmitt G, Pötsch L, Drönner P, Aderjan R, Mattern R. Ethylglucuronide in human hair, *Alcohol Alcohol* 35:283, 2000.

Society of Hair Testing. 2016. 2016 consensus for the use of alcohol markers in hair for assessment of both abstinence and chronic excessive alcohol consumption. https://www.soht.org/images/pdf/Revision%202016_Alcoholmarkers.pdf (Accessed July 31, 2019).

Soderberg BL, Salem RO, Best CA. Fatty acid ethyl esters. Ethanol metabolites that reflect ethanol intake, *Am J Clin Pathol* 119:S94, 2003.

Sorio D, De Palo EF, Bertaso A, Bortolotti F, Tagliaro F. Fluorescent adduct formation with terbium: a novel strategy for transferrin glycoform identification in human body fluids and carbohydrate-deficient transferrin HPLC method validation, *Anal Bioanal Che* 409:1369, 2017.

Spies CD, Emadi A, Neumann T, Hannemann L, Rieger A, Schaffartzik W, Rahmanzadeh R, Berger G, Funk T, Blum S, et al. Relevance of carbohydrate-deficient transferrin as a predictor of alcoholism in intensive care patients following trauma, *J Trauma* 39:742, 1995.

Spies CD, Kissner M, Neumann T Blum S, Voigt C, Funk T, Runkel N, Pragst F. Elevated carbohydrate-deficient transferrin predicts prolonged intensive care unit stay in traumatized men, *Alcohol Alcohol* 33:661, 1998.

Stewart SH, Comte-Walters S, Bowen E, Anton RF. Liver disease and HPLC quantification of disialotransferrin for heavy alcohol use: A case series, *Alcohol Clin Exp Res* 34:1956, 2010a.

Stewart SH, Doscher A, Miles S, Borg KT. Identification and risk-stratification of problem alcohol drinkers with minor trauma in the emergency department, *West J Emerg Med* 11:133, 2010b.

Stewart SH, Law TL, Randall PK, Newman R. Phosphatidylethanol and alcohol consumption in reproductive age women, *Alcohol Clin Exp Res* 34:488, 2010c.

Stewart SH, Reuben A, Anton RF. Relationship of abnormal chromatographic pattern for carbohydrate-deficient transferrin with severe liver disease, *Alcohol Alcohol* 52:24, 2017.

Stibler H, Allgulander C, Borg S, Kjellin KG. Abnormal micro-heterogeneity of transferrin in serum and cerebrospinal fluid in alcoholism, *Acta Med Scand* 204:49, 1978.

Stibler H, Borg S. Glycoprotein glycosyltransferase activities in serum in alcohol-abusing patients and healthy controls, *Scand J Clin Lab Invest* 51:43, 1991.

Süsse S, Selavka CM, Mieczkowski T, Pragst F. Fatty acid ethyl ester concentrations in hair and self-reported alcohol consumption in 644 cases from different origin, *Forensic Sci Int* 196:111, 2010.

Takahashi N, Kameoka J, Takahashi N, Tamai Y, Murai K, Honma R, Noji H, Yokoyama H, Tomiya Y, Kato Y, et al. Causes of macrocytic anemia among 628 patients: Mean corpuscular volumes of 114 and 130 fL as critical markers for categorization, *Int J Hematol* 104:344, 2016.

Tarcomnicu I, van Nuijs AL, Aerts K, De Doncker M, Covaci A, Neels H. Ethyl glucuronide determination in meconium and hair by hydrophilic interaction liquid chromatography-tandem mass spectrometry, *Forensic Sci Int* 196:121, 2010.

Thierauf A, Gnann H, Wohlfarth A, Auwärter V, Perdekamp MG, Buttler KJ, Wurst FM, Weinmann W. Urine tested positive for ethyl glucuronide and ethyl sulphate after the consumption of "non-alcoholic" beer, *Forensic Sci Int* 202:82, 2010a.

Thierauf A, Halter CC, Rana S, Auwaerter V, Wohlfarth A, Wurst FM, Weinmann W. Urine tested positive for ethyl glucuronide after trace amounts of ethanol, *Addiction* 104:2007, 2009.

Thierauf A, Kempf J, Perdekamp MG, Auwärter V, Gnann H, Wohlfarth A, Weinmann W. Ethyl sulphate and ethyl glucuronide in vitreous humor as postmortem evidence marker for ethanol consumption prior to death, *Forensic Sci Int* 210:63, 2011.

Thierauf A, Wohlfarth A, Auwärter V, Perdekamp MG, Wurst FM, Weinmann W. Urine tested positive for ethyl glucuronide and ethyl sulfate after the consumption of yeast and sugar, *Forensic Sci Int* 202:e45, 2010b.

Topic A, Djukic M. Diagnostic characteristics and application of alcohol biomarkers, *Clin Lab* 59:233, 2013.

Varga A, Alling C. Formation of phosphatidylethanol in vitro in red blood cells from healthy volunteers and chronic alcoholics, *J Lab Clin Med* 140:79, 2002.

Varga A, Hansson P, Johnson G, Alling C. Normalization rate and cellular localization of phosphatidylethanol in whole blood from chronic alcoholics, *Clin Chim Acta* 299:141, 2000.

Varga A, Hansson P, Lundqvist C, Alling C. Phosphatidylethanol in blood as a marker of ethanol consumption in healthy volunteers: Comparison with other markers, *Alcohol Clin Exp Res* 22:1832, 1998.

Verbeek J, Crunelle CL, Leurquin-Sterk G, Michielsen PP, De Doncker M, Monbaliu D, Pirenne J, Roskams T, van der Merwe S, Cassiman D, et al. Ethyl glucuronide in hair Is an accurate biomarker of chronic excessive alcohol use in patients with alcoholic cirrhosis, *Clin Gastroenterol Hepatol* 16:454, 2018b.

Verbeek J, Neels H, Nevens F. Carbohydrate deficient transferrin in patients with cirrhosis: A Tale of bridges, *Alcohol Alcohol* 53:350, 2018a.

Vignali C, Ortu S, Stramesi C, Freni F, Moretti M, Tajana L, Osculati AMM, Groppi A, Morini L. Variability on ethyl glucuronide concentrations in hair depending on sample pretreatment, using a new developed GC-MS/MS method, *J Pharm Biomed Anal* 159:18, 2018.

Vonlaufen A, Wilson JS, Pirola RC, Apte MV. Role of alcohol metabolism in chronic pancreatitis, *Alcohol Research Health* 30:48, 2007.

Walsham NE, Sherwood RA. Ethyl glucuronide and ethyl sulfate, *Adv Clin Chem* 67:47, 2014.

Walter H, Hertling I, Benda N, König B, Ramskogler K, Riegler A, Semler B, Zoghlami A, Lesch OM. Sensitivity and specificity of carbohydrate-deficient transferrin in drinking experiments and different patients, *Alcohol* 25:189, 2001.

Wang S, Yang R, Ji F, Li H, Dong J, Chen W. Sensitive and precise monitoring of phosphatidylethanol in human blood as a biomarker for alcohol intake by ultrasound-assisted dispersive liquid-liquid microextraction combined with liquid chromatography tandem mass spectrometry, *Talanta* 166:315, 2017.

Werner J, Saghir M, Fernandez-del Castillo C, Warshaw AL, Laposata M. Linkage of oxidative and nonoxidative ethanol metabolism in the pancreas and toxicity of nonoxidative ethanol metabolites for pancreatic acinar cells, *Surgery* 129:736, 2001.

Weykamp C, Wielders JP, Helander A, Anton RF, Bianchi V, Jeppsson JO, Siebelder C, Whitfield JB, Schellenberg F, IFCC Working Group on Standardization of Carbohydrate-Deficient Transferrin (WG-CDT). Toward standardization of carbohydrate-deficient transferrin (CDT) measurements: III. Performance of native serum and serum spiked with disialotransferrin proves that harmonization of CDT assays is possible, *Clin Chem Lab Med* 51:991, 2013.

Whitfield JB, Dy V, Madden PA, Heath AC, Martin NG, Montgomery GW. Measuring carbohydrate-deficient transferrin by direct immunoassay: Factors affecting diagnostic sensitivity for excessive alcohol intake, *Clin Chem* 54:1158, 2008.

Wiegand S, Thamm M, Kiess W, Körner A, Reinehr T, Krude H, Hoffmeister U, Holl RW (on behalf of the APV Study Group and the German Competence Network Adipositas). Gamma-glutamyl transferase is strongly associated with degree of overweight and sex, *J Pediatr Gastroenterol Nutr.* 52:635, 2011.

Wu PH, Coultrap S, Browning MD, Proctor WR. Correlated changes in NMDA receptor phosphorylation, functional activity, and sedation by chronic ethanol consumption, *J Neurochem* 115:1112, 2010.

Wurst FM, Alexson S, Wolfersdorf M, Bechtel G, Forster S, Alling C, Aradóttir S, Jachau K, Huber P, Allen JP, et al. Concentration of fatty acid ethyl esters in hair of alcoholics: Comparison to other biological state markers and self reported-ethanol intake, *Alcohol Alcohol* 39:33, 2004.

Wurst FM, Dürsteler-MacFarland KM, Auwaerter V, Ergovic S, Thon N, Yegles M, Halter C, Weinmann W, Wiesbeck GA. Assessment of alcohol use among methadone maintenance patients by direct ethanol metabolites and self-reports, *Alcohol Clin Exp Res* 32:1552, 2008b.

Wurst FM, Kelso E, Weinmann W, Pragst F, Yegles M, Sundström Poromaa I. Measurement of direct ethanol metabolites suggests higher rate of alcohol use among pregnant women than found with the AUDIT—A pilot study in a population-based sample of Swedish women, *Am J Obstet Gynecol* 198:407, 2008c.

Wurst FM, Thon N, Aradottir S, Hartmann S, Wiesbeck GA, Lesch O, Skala K, Wolfersdorf M, Weinmann W, Alling C. Phosphatidylethanol: normalization during detoxification, gender aspects and correlation with other biomarkers and self-reports, *Addict Biol* 15:88, 2010.

Wurst FM, Yegles M, Alling C, Aradottir S, Dierkes J, Wiesbeck GA, Halter CC, Pragst F, Auwaerter V. Measurement of direct ethanol metabolites in a case of a former driving under the influence (DUI) of alcohol offender, now claiming abstinence, *Int J Legal Med* 122:235, 2008a.

Xin Y, Lasker JM, Lieber CS. Serum carbohydrate-deficient transferrin: Mechanism of increase after chronic alcohol intake, *Hepatology* 22:1462, 1995.

Yamazaki K, Gilg T, Kauert G, von Meyer L, Eisenmenger W. Nonoxidative ethanol and methanol changes in the heart and brain tissue of alcohol abusers, *Nihon Hoigaku Zasshi* 51:380, 1997.

Yegles M, Labarthe A, Auwärter V, Hartwig S, Vater H, Wennig R, Pragst F. Comparison of ethyl glucuronide and fatty acid ethyl ester concentrations in hair of alcoholics, social drinkers and teetotalers, *Forensic Sci Int* 145:167, 2004.

Zimmermann CM, Jackson GP. Gas chromatography tandem mass spectrometry for biomarkers of alcohol abuse in human hair, *Ther Drug Monit* 32:216, 2010.

Use of Non-alcohol Drugs and Impaired Driving

IV

Driving Under the Influence of Non-alcohol Drugs

Review of Earlier Studies*

10

JØRG G. MØRLAND

Contents

* This chapter is in essence an unchanged version of a review article previously published in *Forensic Science Review*: Mørland JG: Driving under the influence of non-alcohol drugs; *Forensic Sci Rev* 12 (1/2):79; 2000. This chapter covers the status of the DUID-field at that time as well as results from experimental and epidemiological studies published up to 1999. In Chapters 11 and 12 results from more recent experimental and epidemiological studied are reviewed. In general, the findings from the period before 2000 have been confirmed, but also expanded, strengthening our knowledge base.

10.1 Introduction

The negative role of alcohol in vehicular traffic has been recognized for a long time, as documented by epidemiological and experimental research in several countries (Borkenstein et al. 1974; Simpson 1986; Kerr and Hindmarch 1998). In spite of legal and other countermeasures to combat drunken driving, it still persists at an almost unacceptable level as demonstrated, for example, by a high recidivism rate for convicted drunken drivers in many countries (Brewer et al. 1994; Wells-Parker et al. 1995), and by high percentages of alcohol involvement in fatal crashes. In fact, the US National Highway Traffic Safety Administration estimated that 44% of fatal crashes in 1993 involved alcohol use (US National Highway Traffic Safety Administration 1994). The risk of causing a fatal car accident for a driver with a high blood alcohol level has been demonstrated to be greatly increased (Perrine et al. 1971; Borkenstein et al. 1974; Klebelsberg 1988; Sleet et al. 1989; Robertson and Drummer 1994).

During recent years, the problem of drugged driving (i.e., driving under the influence of non-alcohol drugs) has received considerable attention. In many countries the first studies in this field dealt with possible dangerous side effects which could occur during treatment with medicinal drugs in therapeutic doses (Seppala et al. 1979). As drug abuse and drug dependence problems developed in the United States and Europe, interest on illicit drug and abuse of medicinal drugs and traffic safety has increased. The Pompidou group of the European Council this year (1999) arranged a seminar on "Road traffic and illicit drugs." In this seminar as well as from several reviews of the literature published in recent years (Hindmarch et al. 1991; Ferrara 1987; Albery et al. 1998; Moskowitz 1976; Seppala et al. 1979), it has been stated that our knowledge about drugged driving is less comprehensive than about drunken driving. Two main questions have frequently been discussed as the most important ones for any non-alcohol drug:

- To what extent will the use of a particular drug constitute a risk to traffic safety?
- To what extent do drivers on the roads use a particular drug which might constitute a traffic hazard?

In the following review I will first briefly discuss the methods available to answer these questions in Section 10.2. Then some results will be presented for the groups of drugs which have been studied, to an extent allowing some answers to the two main questions, in Section 10.3. This will be followed by sections briefly discussing assessment of drug impairment in practice, problems connected with the detection of potentially dangerous drugged driving and some legal issues. Finally, a short description of the situation in Norway, which has a very high detection rate of drugged drivers, will be given in addition to a discussion of prevention and future research issues in this field.

10.2 Methodological Issues

The information obtained with relevance to the first of the two main questions, "To what extent will the use of a particular drug constitute a risk to traffic safety?," has originated from two major sources (Simpson and Vingilis 1992): (a) Controlled experimental studies and (b) Analytical epidemiological investigations.

10.2.1 Controlled Experimental Studies

This type of study comprises a series of different performance tests thought to be of importance for various aspects of the process of operating a car, as well as simulated driving and real driving under controlled conditions (Table 10.1). The idea behind the performance tests

Table 10.1 Tests That Have Been Used in Controlled Experimental Studies on Drugs with Relevance to Driving

Test	Observation
Performance test	Psychophysical, perceptual, psychological
	Simple motor performance, reaction time
	Information processing
	Sustained attention
	Speed estimation
	Short-term memory
	Learning comprehension
Simulated Driving	Complex psychomotor performance
	Decision-making
	Response to multiple stimuli
Driving	Closed circuit
	"Real" traffic

Based on information (modified) provided in Zacny, J.P., *Exp. Clin. Psychopharmacol.*, 3, 432, 1995.

is that they should represent important mental and behavioral functions relevant to driving. Particular emphasis has been put on tests that measure sedation and drowsiness, divided attention, continuous perceptual-motor co-ordination, speed and accuracy of decision making, vigilance and short-term memory, to mention a few (de Gier and Vermeeren 1995; Vermeeren et al. 1993). It has also been pointed out that a battery of tests which are mutually independent should be used to characterize the effects of the drugs tested (Zacny 1995). Many drugs have so far been tested in experiments with single or combinations of various performance tests. Simulated driving experiments have not been conducted to the same extent. Simulators can be of two major types, interactive (wherein the driver has control of the speed and the path of the vehicle) and non-interactive (wherein the driver is only capable of making decisions, but cannot actually control the vehicle) (Irving 1988). Various levels of sophistication with respect to computer interface, robotics, and virtual reality applications also exist. The real driving experiments have mostly been conducted in closed circuits, but some studies on open roads and in city traffic have been performed in special cars equipped with double control systems; allowing an experienced co-driver to make the necessary corrections.

The main advantages of all these controlled experimental set-ups are that they can unequivocally demonstrate a causal relationship between the taking of a certain drug and a certain effect. This can be achieved by well-controlled experiments, good randomization protocols for participating subjects, or balanced cross-over designs, the use of placebo, the use of reference drugs (often referred to as "verum," one of which is usually alcohol at certain dosages) influencing performance, as well as the testing of different doses of the drug in question with accompanying determination of blood or plasma concentrations over time within the study period. In this way possible drug dose, or better, drug concentration effect relationships can be established if existing. If the studies are conducted over a certain period of time, usually more than 2–4 hours, changing relationships between effects and plasma/blood drug concentrations can be demonstrated, usually being a consequence of changed blood/brain drug distribution over time, the development of acute drug tolerance within hours, or a combination of both phenomena.

The controlled experiments also give the possibility of repeating the experiments at placebo and drug conditions, testing the robustness of the effects and making registration of inter- and intra-subject variation with respect to any possible test available. It is also possible to test the effect of drug-alcohol combinations, which has sometimes been done (Mørland et al. 1974; Sellers and Busto 1982) as well as non-alcohol drug combinations, which is seldom performed. Another important feature, which is well suited for controlled experimental testing, is the combination of sleep deprivation and drug use.

The main objection to the performance tests is lack of demonstration of their ability to predict real-life driving skills. As concluded by (Hindmarch and Gudgeon 1980) the results of a great number of laboratory psychomotor tests could not justifiably be generalized to the driving act. A recent report (European Monitoring Centre for Drugs and Drug Addiction 1999) states that a solid, reliable, and valid battery of powerfully predictive performance tests remains as much of a priority as it has ever done. That report also cites other papers indicating the difficulties in making assumptions that the driver would be generally impaired from tests where single or few behaviors are compromised disregarding possible interactions between task components that might occur to reduce such separate effects. Laboratory performance tests can be criticized also for so far only to a limited extent testing single components of the mental and behavioral state that could be critical to real driving as risk willingness, risk avoidance and aggression.

The objections so far discussed for laboratory performance tests would also apply to at least some extent for the two other types of controlled experimental approaches, simulated and "real" driving. One might argue against this by saying that driving experiments are fair representations of real driving, but there are several objections to this view. First, simulator studies usually only represent part of the real driving situation (Moskowitz 1985) and in addition the driver under study will all the time know that the conditions are artificial, no panic will arise to the same extent as in real life when a critical situation is created. In closed circuit driving and other "real" driving experiments, it is also for ethical reasons impossible to create situations that would include the potential of an accident. Instead, more operational skills such as tracking, adjustment of speed, braking, lane positioning, and vehicle maneuvering are studied during simulated and controlled experimental driving. It should also be mentioned that simulated and real driving studies are complicated to perform, are time consuming and costly compared to laboratory testing.

Furthermore, all controlled experimental studies have been criticized for sometimes being performed before the test subjects are fully trained on the task, giving rise to learning during the study sessions obscuring correct conclusions to be drawn. Another critical point is that the subjects might artificially improve their performance during test sessions due to increased vigilance as a psychological consequence of being monitored (Sanders 1986). Criticisms have also been forwarded on the study protocol often using young healthy volunteers (being unrepresentative of the driving population), only testing acute drug effects (usually those taking place during the first hours after drug intake, the period in which most side-effects are most prominent), and the restrictions imposed for ethical reasons only to use therapeutic drugs (and not illicit ones) and to use moderate drug doses. Thus, real-life doses of drugs of abuse are usually not tested nor are the effects of drug tolerance in the chronic user of licit or illicit drugs. The interactions of disease and drug treatment with the possibility of improvements of function brought about by drugs have thus not been systematically looked at, and the effects of drugs in certain subgroups, for example elderly drivers are seldom reported from controlled experiments.

In spite of the shortcomings discussed above, most researchers agree that one might gain valuable information from controlled experimental studies. The comparison with the effects of alcohol (which might act as some kind of gold standard) appears to be particularly important. Sometimes marked sedative effects are observed, for example the test subjects fall asleep during a test session, a sign according to this author, should be regarded as having a high degree of relevance with respect to real-life traffic risk increase.

If the controlled experiments show a clear dose or concentration-effect relationship, with marked effect on, a psychomotor function tested at the highest dose, and one knows that drug abusers might attain 10–20 times the tested concentration in real life, it would be allowable to suspect such use to increase real life risk of accident. The development of chronic tolerance in real life, possibly reducing drug influence, has been mentioned as a factor, which makes it difficult to interpret results from acute drug experiments in a meaningful way in comparison with the real-life situation. However, the effect of acute doses in tolerant subjects can be tested to some extent in experimental set ups (Ingum et al. 1993; Linnoila et al. 1983). Subgroups of drivers (such as the elderly) can be tested and compared to other groups (such as young people) with and without drugs under controlled conditions. Also, problems linked to the possible interactions between disease and drug therapy can be subject to controlled studies by using the patients' baseline performance (drug free) before treatment, and possibly after end of treatment as a control for drug-induced influence on performance tests or driving capability under controlled conditions (van Laar et al.1992).

In summary, the results of controlled experimental studies appear to be important, and to constitute a relevant basis for the determination of any drug's impact on traffic safety. The results should, however, be interpreted with great caution, and their external validity should be critically examined. The development of new tests and better study designs appears highly desirable.

Two major concerns appear to remain for experimental studies at the present stage. First, even the best test discussed so far would have limitations in testing all aspects of the driving process. According to one model of the theoretical framework of the driving process (Jansen 1979; Rothengatter 1997; Sanders 1986), it is composed of three different levels: the operational level (tracking, braking, and adjustment of speed), the tactical level (vehicle maneuvering, overtaking decisions, distance between vehicles, avoidance of objects/situations), and the strategic level (trip planning, route selection, risk assessment). For performance on all levels, mental and perceptual functions are critical, but most controlled experimental studies appear to test mainly the operational level.

Second, even when we assume that a series of different tests can be applied, theoretically covering all aspects of driving behavior, the experimental testing of all performances critical to the occurrence and seriousness of a traffic accident could be still more difficult. Traffic accidents are in most cases the result of multifactorial complex processes, which are very difficult to analyze in sufficient detail to reveal all cause-effect relationships that might be involved and which might have caused the accident (Klebelsberg 1988).

At the present stage, the evaluation of risk connected to the use of any drug to traffic safety can hardly rely on experimental data alone. Risk assessment will also depend on results from real-life epidemiological studies allowing at least some estimation of risk for accidents to occur when the drug is used. This situation is similar to the situation for alcohol, where our perception of the magnitude of traffic risk is based upon studies from controlled experiments supported by real-life epidemiological investigations (Borkenstein et al. 1974; Seppala et al. 1979; Kerr and Hindmarch 1998).

10.2.2 Analytical Epidemiological Studies (Allowing Traffic Accident Risk Evaluation)

Any registration of the frequency of the occurrence of a phenomenon (e.g., presence of drug in a body fluid, etc.) in the total population of part of it (e.g., in fatally injured drivers) can be considered to represent some form of epidemiological knowledge. The finding of drugs in the blood of, for example, fatally injured drivers, might give valuable information with respect to the size of the phenomenon, but no information on the causality of drugs in such cases. Such studies are usually named descriptive or survey studies. Under certain conditions, however, when the study design meets some requirements and contains control groups, the observations might allow estimation of relative risks for the phenomenon under study to be calculated. In such cases the study would be regarded as an analytical epidemiological study which might indicate causal relationships although not prove them. The most important types of analytical epidemiological studies in the field of drugged driving are: case-control studies and cohort studies.

In the case-control design, the case is the person one wants to study, such as a driver who causes a traffic accident, or a driver who is involved in a traffic accident. The control is a person who is as similar to the case as possible, i.e., is a driver (of same age, sex, driving experience, driving in the same place, same time on the same weekday, etc.), but who has not caused or been involved in an accident. When the cases are known, the controls are drawn according to the principles mentioned from the material available. The cases and the controls are then analyzed with respect to presence of the factor thought to be of importance to the accident, in this case the presence of drugs, for example, by questionnaire or by drug analysis. If drug use or positive analytical drug findings or higher drug concentrations are present more frequently among the cases than the controls, a relative risk increase can be calculated.

In the cohort design, a defined group, such as drivers on a certain medication, is followed for a certain period of time, and traffic accidents occurring in this group are registered. Over the same period another group, such as drivers not on medication, is followed with respect to accidents. If relatively more accidents occur in the drug cohort compared to the non-drug cohort, a relative risk increase will be demonstrated. The two groups should be as similar as possible except for the drug use. This is often difficult to achieve. In such cases one tries to correct for the known differences between the groups, for example with respect to age, driving experience, distance travelled per year, but such corrections might be difficult to estimate correctly. A variant of this design is to allow people to serve as their own controls during periods when they are not on drugs.

It should also be mentioned that there are other designs of similar types combining elements from both case-control and cohort studies. Some of these mixed designs have been applied to study the impact of drugs on risk of traffic accidents; for references see (Neutel 1998).

The main advantage of analytical epidemiological studies compared to controlled experimental studies is that they provide evidence based on practical real-life experience, and thus make evaluation of relative risk feasible. As will be discussed in Section 10.3, there are rather few analytical epidemiological studies within the field of drugged driving. It should also be stressed that increased relative risk ratios (or no demonstration of changed risk ratios) should be interpreted with caution, because causal relationships in the strictest sense cannot be deduced even from the best designed epidemiological studies of these two types.

The main reason for this is the presence of confounding variables in the groups that are being studied, i.e., variables that are making the study group and the control group different in more respects than the object of the study (the use of drug). A patient using a drug to treat an illness will be different from a control person at least with respect to both the use of drug and illness, if the design is not such that untreated patients constitute the control group. If increased risk ratios are seen in a drug-treated group compared to a healthy control population, it is difficult to know whether this increase is a consequence of drug, disease, or some drug-disease interaction. There will often exist other differences between study and control groups, that cannot be corrected for by study design (such as somatic illness accompanying drug abuse) and unknown confounders. One of the most important confounders in studies on alcohol or drugs on traffic accident risk is the presence of somatic and mental changes in the drug using group, changes that are consequences of long-time use or abuse. It appears that this factor is surprisingly seldom taken into account when such studies are discussed. It is known that a large proportion of drunken drivers are heavy drinkers (Gjerde et al. 1986, 1988b; Gjerde 1987). Heavy drinking is especially abundant among drivers arrested with high blood alcohol concentrations (BAC) (Gjerde et al. 1986). Nevertheless, the increased risk seen at high BAC is usually considered the sole consequence of the acute alcohol intake at that occasion and is not connected to the coexisting changes caused by long-term heavy drinking. The same would apply to chronic drug users where somatic illness (e.g., brain damage) and mental changes (such as dependence) might be present. In general, any risk increase observed in a population using drugs should therefore be regarded as a consequence of both the acute use (the actual drug concentrations) and the previous drug history. Another important confounder is the presence of alcohol in people who use drugs, and vice versa (and not so often taken into account) i.e., the presence of drugs in people with measurable BAC. The detection of these confounders will depend critically on the analytical repertoire and the sensitivity of the analytical methods applied.

These factors will obviously also be of critical importance to the catchment of cases. If the methods used are not sensitive enough, drug use might escape detection. Problems might also arise when "too sensitive" methods are applied, in the sense that urine analyses for drugs are used, with the possibility of detecting drug use over the last days (weeks) before sampling and not a high blood concentration most likely related to increased risk of an accident. Case-control studies might also be flawed, because drug use is remembered or detected more easily by the "cases" when questioned, or subjected to toxicological analysis, than in control populations. In prospective cohort studies, the assessment of medication compliance is often difficult, as is the use of alcohol or other drugs. A further constraint on prospective cohort studies is that they can hardly be applied to users of illicit drugs, although retrospective studies have been performed on this user group (Smart 1974; Elliott 1987).

As we see, several difficulties are encountered in analytical epidemiological studies, and relative risk rates calculated from such studies must accordingly be interpreted with caution.

The importance of non-alcohol drug use to traffic safety will, in addition to the risk connected to the use of the drug, depend on the answers to the second main question, "To what extent do drivers on the roads use a drug which might constitute a traffic hazard?" The relevant information in this respect comes from various types of survey studies.

10.2.3 Survey Studies (Descriptive Epidemiological Studies)

Descriptive epidemiological studies simply measure the frequency of drug use in certain groups of drivers, by means of questionnaires, interviews or analysis of drugs in body fluids. Such studies appear to have focused on four different groups of drivers:

- The general driving population (roadside survey);
- Drivers suspected of impaired driving;
- Drivers involved in accidents with non-fatal injuries; and
- Fatally injured drivers.

It should be noted that the primary intention in such studies is not to calculate the increased risk connected to drug use, but to get an indication of the magnitude of a possible problem. The data can of course constitute a basis for traffic safety risk evaluation by showing an obvious over-representation of a drug among fatally injured drivers. As discussed above it is first when the control groups have been added to the study, that stronger indications of a causal role can be obtained. The data from surveys are usually collected together to gain more information that is general and to serve as a basis to estimate the overall magnitude of a possible traffic safety problem linked to a particular drug. Such studies have often demonstrated obvious limitations for many reasons. Some of the reasons for lack of representativeness for the non-fatal and fatal cases studied are:

- Not analyzing all cases within a certain geographical region occurring within a certain period;
- Not analyzing quantitatively the relevant matrixes for recent drug use (i.e., blood, serum, plasma, saliva); and
- Not looking for all relevant drugs, alcohol included.

For the roadside survey studies, information is usually collected through self-reports and toxicological analyses of body fluids. In these studies, drop-out rates at interviews and refusal to give blood samples constitute major deficiencies. For the selected group of drivers suspected of impaired driving, variation in attention to this problem by the police and the relative interest in the role of alcohol in relation to non-alcohol drugs might give rise to problems of interpretation.

For all groups, however, the quality of information can be largely increased if repeated studies over time are performed, if the selection of cases is considered to be constant over time, if the methods used stay the same, if the same drugs are looked for and quantitated with the same analytical methods, and if comparison with alcohol findings in the same material is done. It is, however, obvious that before comparisons can be made across district, state or country borders, substantial standardizations of data collection (analytical methods) and sample collection (criteria for case selection) (Simpson and Vingilis 1992) must be undertaken.

In concluding the discussion on methodological issues, one could end up with a standpoint that the methodological fundament for our knowledge on non-alcohol drugs and traffic safety is too heavily burdened with information gaps, uncertainties and presumptions, making almost any conclusion debatable. In the mind of the present author, this would be going too far. The criticism is important, but it should not keep us away from forming a qualified opinion on the risk connected to certain drugs in relation to traffic safety. We should not forget that certain actions against drunken driving were instituted at a stage when the prevailing background knowledge about alcohol and traffic safety could have been attacked even more seriously than is the case for non-alcohol drugs today. Even today it is possible to find weak points within the methodological field of alcohol and traffic safety, without allowing this to reduce our attention, or reducing the intensity of finding countermeasures against drunken driving.

With these points in mind, the status of knowledge for some groups of non-alcohol drugs and traffic safety will be presented in the next section.

10.3 What Do We Know about Different Groups of Drugs and Traffic Safety?

From the literature, it appears that six groups of non-alcohol drugs have been studied by experimental and epidemiological methods to a degree that allows some conclusion with respect to their traffic safety hazard to be drawn. These groups are: benzodiazepines (BZDs) and related drugs, cannabis (tetrahydrocannabinol, THC, as the main psychoactive component), opioids, amphetamines and related drugs, antihistamines, and antidepressants. More than 1000 original scientific papers have been published covering various aspects of the actions of these drugs with relevance to traffic safety. To keep the number of citations at a reasonable level, the author has chosen to cite review and overview articles as often as possible, although including some references to original papers when this might illustrate certain points in an appropriate manner. This has the consequence that a large number of very important papers have not received the credit they deserve by being omitted from the citation list. The present author would like to stress that inclusion or exclusion in many instances has occurred more by chance than based on any strict criteria. Nevertheless, it is the present author's opinion that the findings presented will have support in the majority of the published literature.

10.3.1 Benzodiazepines and Related Drugs

Benzodiazepines and related drugs are used as sedatives (tranquilizers) and to induce sleep, as hypnotics.

10.3.1.1 Controlled Experimental Studies

One of the first papers to show effects of BZDs on performance tests of possible importance to driving was the demonstration (Jäättelä et al. 1971) that diazepam reduced memory and impaired digit symbol substitution test (DSST) task performance. Recently (Berghaus and Grass 1997) summarized the results of more than 500 different experimental studies involving one or more BZDs. This study took advantage of a database on drugs and driving-related performance established by a research project sponsored by the Federal Highway Research Institute of Germany (Berghaus 1997). All experimental studies with documentation of driving-related performance under the influence of a BZD were subjected to certain exclusion and inclusion criteria and information on dose-size, dose timing in relation to testing, type of performance tested (Krüger et al. 1990). Results in relation to control and verum were extracted and accumulated. Based on the dose given in the studies where no blood or serum concentration data were available, serum concentrations were calculated by means of available pharmacokinetic data from other studies. In this way plots of accumulated reduced performance could be plotted versus drug serum concentrations for a series of different BZDs, in each case based on several hundred to more than a thousand experimental test results. An almost linear correlation between serum BZD concentration and performance deficit was found for diazepam, nitrazepam, triazolam, temazepam, flunitrazepam, flurazepam, alprazolam, bromazepam, oxazepam, and lorazepam.

In simulated car driving, use of BZD caused impairment (Willumeit et al. 1984). In "real" driving tests it was shown that certain BZDs and zopiclon had effects on the standard deviation of lateral position (SDLP) (O'Hanlon et al. 1986), during long-distance driving on a four-lane primary highway in normal traffic. This measure was obtained from continuous electro-optical recording of the distance between the vehicle and the painted road delineation, followed by computer analysis of the data. The test was calibrated with respect to various BACs. It was found that some BZDs the morning after being used as hypnotics caused impairment comparable to that observed at BAC of 0.05%–0.1%.

Homogeneity: The results from several hundred studies demonstrate large similarities. Some minor differences can be observed between studies, but the overall picture is that all BZDs have the ability to cause impairment in controlled experiments, with respect to most measures tested.

Dose/Serum Concentration-Effect Relationship: As demonstrated from the results accumulated by Berghaus and Grass (1997) there exists clear dose/serum concentration-effect relationships for most BZDs investigated. More detailed single-dose studies have revealed, however, that there are significant interindividual variations in response to a given serum concentration, but that relationships exist between dose, blood drug concentration and effect in many performance tests when results from groups are presented; see (O'Hanlon et al. 1986; Ingum et al. 1992).

Acute Tolerance: Acute tolerance, defined as a decreasing drug effect relative to drug-plasma levels over a period of minutes to a few hours after drug administration, has been demonstrated following single doses of diazepam (Ellinwood et al. 1983). This effect might depend on the tasks investigated because no such effects have also been reported after diazepam administration (Ingum et al. 1994). However, in the latter study in contrast to diazepam, flunitrazepam demonstrated acute tolerance. Another report (Berghaus and Friedel 1997) found possible differences between various BZDs with respect to the duration of impairment, probably related to different degrees of development of acute tolerance. At the present time it seems appropriate to conclude that the relation between plasma concentration and effect might show considerable variation depending on the time after drug administration in studies of the acute effects of single BZD doses.

Tolerance after Repeated Dosing: Tolerance to the acute effects of 1 mg flunitrazepam did not develop when this dose was given daily for 8 days (Ingum et al. 1994). Chronic administration of diazepam (5 mg three times daily) for 9 days demonstrated extensive impairment in contrast to placebo or chronic buspirone treatment (20 mg daily, 9 days), when tested in a driving simulator (Moskowitz and Smiley 1982). Diazepam, 10 mg three times daily for 3 weeks, gave rise to the same acute psychomotor effects with no tolerance development (Linnoila et al. 1983). Diazepam, 5 mg three times daily, impaired performance measured in the first, second, and third weeks by SDLP during driving, with some tolerance developing in the fourth week (van Laar et al. 1992). In a study on subjects taking BZDs for several months it was found that tolerance developed to the sedating and psychomotor-impairing effects, but not to the impairment of short-term memory, reduction of critical flicker frequency (CFF) test and antianxiety effects caused by BZDs (Lucki et al. 1986). Taken together, studies of this type show some tolerance development after long-term drug intake; but it appears that even after chronic use the acute dose might have at least some impairing effects.

Differences between Benzodiazepines: Comparative studies of the acute impairing effects of different BZDs tested in therapeutic or higher doses, reported from the Institute for Drugs, Safety and Behavior in the Netherlands (Wolschrijn et al. 1991), presented as in the EMCDDA-report (European Monitoring Centre for Drugs and Drug Addiction 1999) showed (Table 10.2) some drugs to be more impairing than others at equivalent doses. The table, however, also shows that at high doses almost any BZD can cause severe impairment.

Table 10.2 Rating of Benzodiazepines for Acute Effects

Drug	Dosage (mg)	Impairment Rating
Alprazolam	0.25/0.5	Minor
	1.0	Moderate/not severe
Bromazepam	1.5	Minor
	3.0/6.0	Moderate/not severe
	12.0	Severe
Brotizolam	0.125/0.25	Not severe
Chlordiazepoxide	5.0/10.0/20.0–25.0	Moderate/not severe
Diazepam	2.0/5.0	Moderate
	10.0/20.0	Not severe/severe
Flunitrazepam	0.5/2.0	Severe
Flurazepam	15.0/30.0	Severe
Lorazepam	0.5/1.0	Not severe
	2.5/5.0	Severe
Lormetazepam	0.5/1.0	Moderate/not severe
	2.0	Severe
Medazepam	5.0/10.0	Minor/moderate
	15.0	Severe
Nitrazepam	2.5/5.0	Moderate/not severe
	10.0	Severe
Oxazepam	10.0/20.0	Moderate/not severe
	30.0/50.0	Severe
Temazepam	5.0/10.0	Moderate
	20.0/30.0	Severe
Triazolam	0.125/0.25	Moderate/not severe
	0.5	Severe

Using the format of (European Monitoring Centre for Drugs and Drug Addiction 1999) with data from Wolschrijn, H. et al., *Drugs and Driving: A New Categorization System for Drugs Affecting Psychomotor Performance*, Maastricht Institute for Drugs, Safety and Behaviour, University of Limburg, Maastricht, the Netherlands, 1991.

Interaction with Alcohol: Several studies have indicated pharmacodynamic interactions between different BZDs and ethanol leading to increased psychomotor impairment (Linnoila et al. 1990; Mørland et al. 1974; Taberner et al. 1983). According to (Sellers and Busto 1982), the sedative and psychomotor effects of the combination appear to be enhanced, compared to the effects of the drugs given alone. These investigators are further of the opinion that it is difficult to assess the proportion of the observed effects that is due to BZDs as opposed to ethanol, which appears to be the dominant partner in this combination.

Benzodiazepines in Patients: It has been suggested that anxious patients, who probably were unsafe drivers because of their disease, could improve their driving ability when treated with BZDs. At least three different studies have shown that this is not necessarily so. In a study (Linnoila et al. 1983) showed that treatment with 10 mg diazepam three times daily of 30 highly anxious nonpsychotic outpatients for 3–4 weeks, reduced the scores of the self-rated visual analogue scale for anxiety compared to placebo. The administration of 10 mg diazepam, however, impaired psychomotor tests such as tracking and divided attention tasks in patients and volunteers alike. Another study (O'Hanlon et al. 1995), using patients receiving therapeutic doses of lorazepam in a driving experiment on the road, found that SLDL was high despite reported decreases in anxiety. Also (Van Laar et al. 1992) reported that treatment with diazepam 5 mg three times daily for 3–4 weeks reduced anxiety symptoms significantly, while the drug treatment significantly impaired the control of lateral position during driving for the first 3 weeks of treatment.

Other Sedatives and Hypnotics: As shown above, there exists a vast literature on BZDs and impairment based on experimental studies. There are far fewer publications on meprobamate and the newer hypnotics zopiclone and zolpidem. The results reported so far for the latter two do not indicate that they are acting principally different from BZDs in performance testing (Griffiths et al. 1986; Saano et al. 1992: Salvà and Costa 1995).

10.3.1.2 Analytical Epidemiological Studies

There are numerous epidemiological publications addressing the question whether use of BZDs might be associated with increased relative risks of accidents. Four of these studies have used a case-control design.

The first (Skegg et al. 1979) investigated 57 people injured or killed while driving cars, motorcycles, or bicycles in comparison with 1452 matched controls, with respect to medicines that had been dispensed in the 3 months before the accident. There was a highly significant association between use of minor tranquilizers (BZDs, meprobamate) and the risk of a serious road accident (relative risk (RR) estimate 4.9).

In the second (Honkanen et al. 1980) analyzed serum samples from 201 drivers who presented at emergency departments within 6 hours after being injured in a road accident and 325 control drivers selected randomly at petrol stations. BZDs, in most cases diazepam, were found in 10 patients (5%) and 7 controls (2.2%). Alcohol was detected in 15% of the patients and in 1% of the controls.

The third study (Leveille et al. 1994) conducted a matched case-control study of older drivers (above 65 years) who were involved in injurious crashes and who sought medical treatment within the subsequent 7 days. Information on drug use was obtained from prescription databases for 234 cases and 447 controls. Current use of BZDs was found to have little association with increased risk for injurious collisions.

Finally (Hemmelgarn et al. 1997) also studied older drivers (aged 67–84 years) with a nested case-control design, with 5579 cases (all of whom were involved in a motor vehicle crash in which at least 1 person sustained bodily injury) and a random sample of 10 controls per case. The RR of crash involvement within the first week of taking a long-half-life BZD use was 1.45; within the first year of use, it was 1.26. In contrast, there was no increased risk after the initiation of treatment with short-half-life BZDs.

Three studies have used a design close to a case-control study by making the person thought to be responsible for the accident the case, and other persons involved, the controls.

In a study (Jick et al. 1981) examined the use of central nervous depressant drugs, from prescriptions, among 244 people hospitalized for injuries suffered in an automobile accident. This group was divided into drivers presumed at fault for the accident ($n = 93$), passengers ($n = 66$) and other drivers ($n = 85$). No significant differences were found between the groups with respect to BZD use.

Drummer studied 1045 fatally injured drivers, for whom the responsibility of the underlying accident was determined after review of 8 mitigating factors without knowing the results of drugs analysis (Drummer 1994). Based on drug findings in groups of fatally injured drivers considered culpable, contributory, and not culpable, relative risks could be calculated, and the RR for BZDs was 1.9. When BZDs and alcohol were present together, the RR increased to 9.5, while the RR for alcohol alone was 6.0. The calculated risks increased further when only drivers with drug concentrations in blood higher than those likely to reflect therapeutic use were included.

Currie et al. studied people responsible for an accident in comparison with those not responsible for an accident, who presented themselves at two hospitals with accident injuries sufficiently serious to require the taking of blood as part of routine medical procedure (Currie et al. 1995). The accidents comprised road accidents as well as other types of accidents. Drugs were present in blood samples from 63 of a total of 229 subjects. Benzodiazepines were found in 16 cases among 163 judged to be responsible, in contrast to one case among 66 not responsible, indicating a significant, greater likelihood of being involved in an accident of your own making than being a passive victim after taking a BZD.

Five studies have applied the cohort design in the investigation of BZDs and accidents. Oster et al. studied accident-related medical care (not only traffic accidents) among persons who had been prescribed BZDs and a control cohort who had been prescribed drugs other than BZDs (Oster et al. 1990). In the BZD cohort accidents occurring before and after the first prescription for BZDs were noted. Accident-related care was found more likely among persons who had been prescribed BZDs. Among these persons, the probability of an accident-related medical encounter was higher during the months in which a prescription for a BZD had recently been filled compared to other months. Persons who had filled three or more prescription for these agents in the 6 months following initiation of therapy had a significantly higher risk of an accident-related medical event than those who had only one such prescription. After controlling for age, sex, and need for prior medical treatment, a two-fold risk of accidents was found.

Ray et al. conducted a retrospective cohort study on the risk of involvement in motor vehicle crashes for drivers aged 65–84 years enrolled in the Tennessee Medicaid program. Based on 495 crashes in a cohort with 38,701 person-years to follow up, BZD treatment constituted a risk increase, RR 1.5. The relative risk increased to 2.4 when daily dosage was 20 mg or more of diazepam equivalents (Ray et al. 1993).

Neutel assessed the risk of hospitalization for injuries received in traffic accidents after a first prescription for BZDs was filled in cohorts of adults who received BZD hypnotics ($n = 78{,}000$), BZD anxiolytics ($n = 148{,}000$) and controls ($n = 98{,}000$). After the first week after the prescription was filled, the odds ratio (OR) for injury was 9.1 for hypnotics and 13.5 for anxiolytics, after 2 weeks the odds ratios were 6.5 and 5.6, respectively, and within the total first 4-week period 3.9 and 2.5, respectively. The highest risk group was males aged 20–39 years (Neutel 1995).

In another study of similar design by the same author (Neutel 1998) it was found that new BZDs users increased their risk of injurious traffic accidents within the first 4 weeks at an OR of 3.1, persons under 60 years had an OR of 3.2, older people an OR of 2.8. For individual BZDs, flurazepam showed the largest increase in risk (OR 5.1), followed by triazolam (OR 3.2), diazepam (OR 3.1), and lorazepam (OR 2.4).

Barbone et al. used a within-person case crossover study design on drivers who experienced a first road-traffic accident within a three-year period and had used a psychoactive drug within the same period prior to the accident. For each driver, the risk of having a road traffic accident while exposed and not exposed to a drug were compared. Based on 19,386 accident-involved drivers, the following odds ratios were calculated for exposure to anxiolytics and hypnotics: for anxiolytics with an intermediate half-life no increased OR was reported, but use of BZDs with a long half-life was associated with an increased risk of traffic accidents (OR 2.22). The only hypnotic, which was associated with increased risk, was zopiclone (OR 4.0). A dose–response relation was evident with BZDs, and the BZD-use associated risk decreased with increasing drivers' age (Barbone et al. 1998).

The 12 above-mentioned analytical epidemiological studies were well designed and performed, although some of the drawbacks discussed previously could not be circumvented. In 10 of the 12 studies, increased risks were observed associated with BZD use. The overall risk increase was not always large, but in several studies increased risks accompanied increased BZD doses. In addition, the following observations were made in two or more studies: younger BZD users were at greater risk than older, the risk was highest when BZD treatment started, there was a greater risk associated with the use of BZDs with long half-life, and the risk increased with concomitant alcohol use. The impact of these observations from all the analytical epidemiological studies taken together is, according to the present author, strong evidence in favor of a causative role for BZDs in traffic accidents.

10.3.1.3 Descriptive Epidemiological Studies

Data from Germany indicate that 3%–4% of the general driving population might drive after taking BZDs (Krüger et al. 1995, 1996).

In a Norwegian study (Mørland et al. 1995) BZDs were found in 17% of all blood samples taken in Norway on the suspicion of drunken or drugged driving during a period of 2 months. A Danish study from 1985 (Worm et al. 1985) demonstrated the presence of diazepam in 5%–6% of samples, taken for alcohol analysis from suspected drunken drivers. A study from Finland also demonstrated that the prevalence of BZD detection in blood samples collected on the suspicion of impaired driving (mostly because of alcohol) increased from 6% in 1979 to 23% in 1993; for discussion see (Christophersen and Mørland 1997). A similar study from Switzerland found a much lower prevalence of BZDs and related drugs, in 4% of the samples taken for alcohol testing (Ulrich 1994).

In a study of all traffic accidents which occurred in Norway during 5 months in 1993 including all cases (7%) where the police suspected drunken or drugged driving, BZDs were found in 14% of cases from which blood samples were taken, representing 1% of the total number of accidents with personal injury (Bjørneboe et al. 1996). In investigations performed on more than 7000 collision-involved drivers from Belgium (Meulmans et al. 1997) and Italy (Ferrara et al. 1990), BZDs were present in 8%–9% of the plasma samples collected. In Norway (Christophersen et al. 1993) BZDs were more often related to traffic accidents than tetrahydrocannabinol and amphetamines.

In fatally injured drivers from single-vehicle accidents representing the majority of all cases occurring during one year (1989–1990) in Norway, BZDs were found in 41% of the blood samples (Gjerde et al. 1993).

Common to some of the survey studies in this field is the frequent detection of high concentrations of BZDs in the blood samples from accident-involved subjects compared to what would be assumed the case among people using the drugs as prescribed (Bjørneboe et al. 1996). This suggests overdose or abuse of this kind of medication among people involved in traffic accidents.

10.3.1.4 Conclusions

Based on present knowledge, it can be stated that:

- The use of BZDs and related drugs constitutes a considerable risk to traffic safety when used therapeutically, and probably a much higher risk when misused in high doses.
- The prevalence of BZD use found in the general driving population, drivers suspected of impaired driving and drivers involved in non-fatal and fatal accidents indicates that BZD use might represent a major quantitative traffic safety problem in many countries.

10.3.2 Cannabis

The most common compounds are marijuana and hashish, both derived from *Cannabis sativa*. The main psychoactive compound is Δ^9-tetrahydrocannabinol (THC), which is extensively metabolized. The main metabolite in urine is the inactive compound 11-nor-9-carboxy-Δ^9-tetrahydrocannabinol (THC-COOH).

10.3.2.1 Controlled Experimental Studies

One of the first papers to report reduced attention and ability to concentrate after cannabis intake in an experimental setup was published by (Kielholz et al. 1972). A study (Manno et al. 1971) reported negative effects of THC on pursuit tracking. In a simulator study, THC was found to exert detrimental effects (stopping on red light) (Rafaelsen et al. 1973). In 1974 Klonoff was able to demonstrate detrimental effects of cannabis smoking in real-life driving (Klonoff 1974). Berghaus et al. published in 1995 a meta-analysis of 120–150 experimental studies, including laboratory, driving simulator, and on-road experiments. They performed a systematic extraction of data from the papers they reviewed, as described in their publication (Berghaus et al. 1995). To correlate effects to blood concentrations of THC they also had to calculate the THC concentrations present at the time of testing based on information about cannabis administration and a calculated THC concentration-time pharmacokinetic profile. Sixty studies fulfilled their inclusion criteria and a total of 1344 findings of effects were recorded. They plotted their results as accumulated impairment of total and separate performance functions and found in general good correlations between THC-blood concentration and effect size.

In a comprehensive series of "real" driving tests Robbe and O'Hanlon (US National Highway Traffic Safety Administration 1993) demonstrated a dose response for car lateral position variability. It was found that THC in single doses up to 300 micrograms per kg body weight impaired performance in the same way as a BAC of 0.07%. THC had fewer effects on a car following task and on driving in urban traffic.

Homogeneity: The results from a large number of quite different experimental tests show overall similarities. Some differences are found, but in many instances, they appear to reflect different sensitivities of the tests used. Tests of high complexity, such as operating a flight simulator, appear to be very sensitive to the effects of cannabis (Leirer et al. 1991; Pope et al. 1999). An additional problem compared to studies on medicinal drugs is the lack of standardization of the THC dose in some cases.

Dose/Serum-Concentration-Effect Relationship: As demonstrated from the meta-analysis performed by (Berghaus et al. 1995), there are clear dose/serum concentration-effect relationships when results from many studies are accumulated to constitute a large population. More detailed studies have shown, on the other hand, that there are significant interindividual variations in response to a given serum concentration (US National Highway Traffic Safety Administration 1993). For some THC effects, there has been reported good correlations between effects and THC concentrations at the intraindividual level.

Acute Tolerance: This phenomenon has seldom been addressed in experimental studies on THC because the THC concentration changes rapidly and markedly during the first hours after cannabis smoking.

Tolerance after Repeated Dosing: In some of the experimental studies performed, it is clearly stated that the test subjects were former occasional cannabis smokers. Systematically controlled traffic-relevant experimental studies on cannabis users with defined different patterns of previous cannabis use do not appear to have been performed.

Interaction with Alcohol: Several studies have indicated pharmacodynamic interactions between THC and ethanol causing increased impairment (Chesher et al. 1986, 1976; Moskowitz 1985; Sutton 1983). The interaction was considered to result in impairments that were greater than the effects caused by cannabis smoking or alcohol intake alone.

10.3.2.2 Analytical Epidemiological Studies

No studies using a case-control design appear to have been published on cannabis smoking and traffic accidents.

Two studies conducted responsibility analyses on fatally injured drivers. A study (Terhune et al. 1992) reported that the responsibility rate increased for drivers with BAC above 0.1%. Compared to this "positive reference" no increase was found in drivers who had taken cannabis.

In a study (Drummer 1994) a lower culpability ratio was found for the cannabis group although not statistically significant, compared to the drug-free group.

It should be added that the detection of THC was seldom done in the study of Drummer and the positive analysis for THC-COOH was used as an indicator of cannabis use, and that THC-COOH can be found for a long period after the psychoactive substance THC has disappeared from blood. There is reason to believe that concentration of THC in postmortem blood might not reflect the immediate premortal condition (Hilberg et al. 1999), making the studies of Terhune et al. and possibly Drummer somewhat difficult to interpret.

No prospective cohort studies on cannabis use and traffic accidents appear to have been published. A retrospective study on cannabis and accident probability was performed using self-report questionnaires (Smart 1974). It found that cannabis users had almost as many accidents after cannabis smoking as they had when under the influence of alcohol.

10.3.2.3 Descriptive Epidemiological Studies

Data from Germany indicate that at least 0.6% of the general driving population might drive after cannabis intake (Krüger et al. 1995, 1996).

In a Norwegian study (Mørland et al. 1995) THC was found in 12% of all blood samples taken in Norway on suspicion of drunken or drugged driving during a period of 2 months. In a paper from Finland on samples collected on the suspicion of impaired driving the same year as the Norwegian material, THC was found in 2.4% of the samples. From 1993 to 1998, the detection of THC in blood samples from drivers apprehended on the suspicion of drugged driving has increased in Norway (Christophersen and Mørland 1997) and THC was present in 17% of samples from all cases suspected of either drunken or drugged driving in 1998.

In a study on all traffic accidents that occurred in Norway during a 5-month period in 1993 including all cases where the police suspected drunken or drugged driving, THC was found in 7.6% of cases from which blood samples were taken, representing 0.5% of the total amount of accidents with personal injury (Bjørneboe et al. 1996). In studies on more than 7000 collision-involved drivers from Belgium (Meulmans et al. 1997) and Italy (Ferrara et al. 1990), 5%–6% of the urine samples collected contained cannabinoids.

In fatally injured drivers from single-vehicle accidents representing the majority of all cases in Norway during one year (1989–1990), THC was found in 35% of the blood samples (Gjerde et al. 1993). In several studies from various countries on killed drivers THC or cannabinoids have been found in body fluids with frequencies ranging from a few percent to about 49% (for review, see Albery et al. 1998; Christophersen and Mørland 1997; European Monitoring Centre for Drugs and Drug Addiction 1999).

A comparison of frequency of THC occurrence in blood samples from killed Norwegian drivers and the calculated prevalence of the presence of THC in blood samples (THC usually being present up to 4–8 hours after cannabis smoking) in the general driving population (0.04%) might indicate a considerable risk increase due to cannabis use (Bjørneboe et al. 1996).

10.3.2.4 Conclusions

Based on present knowledge, it can be stated that:

- The use of cannabis constitutes a risk to traffic safety at least for the first few hours after cannabis intake.
- The prevalence of cannabis use among the general driving population, drivers suspected of impaired driving and drivers involved in non-fatal and fatal accidents indicates a substantial quantitative traffic safety problem—at least in some countries.

10.3.3 Opioids

The term "opioids" refers to all compounds with morphine-like activity. In therapeutic medicine, they are mainly used to reduce pain.

The most common opioids studied in relation to traffic safety are morphine, codeine, heroin and similar agonists, and other opioids like methadone, buprenorphine, fentanyl, etc.

10.3.3.1 Controlled Experimental Studies

Among the earliest controlled experimental studies to demonstrate effects of opioids were the studies by Hill and collaborators (Hill et al. 1952, 1955, 1956) that demonstrated that morphine, 15 mg given intramuscularly, could increase the reaction time, although depending on environmental conditions. Zacny published in 1995 a review on relevant papers published on the effects of opioids on psychomotor and cognitive functioning in humans. In that review which contains results from more than 200 previous papers in the field, one of the main conclusions was that opioids can impair performance, but also that the impairment would depend on the particular opioid and the dose involved, the population studied and the duration of opioid use. The effects observed in healthy volunteers were primarily impairments of psychomotor performance to a larger extent than impairments of cognitive performance; behavior tended to "slow down," but did not tend to become more erratic (Zacny 1995).

Homogeneity: The results reported from different experimental studies show great variation with respect to the responses obtained. This variation appears partly to be a consequence of different sensitivities of the tests applied, but factors related to the background of the subjects themselves seem to constitute a more important basis for variation for opioids than for other drugs.

Dose/Serum Concentration-Effects Relationship: Overall dose-effect relationships have been observed across different studies for various opioids when effects obtained in standardized populations (healthy volunteers) are compared. In single studies where different doses have been tested on the same subjects in different sessions, dose-effect relationships have been found (Bradley and Nicholson 1986; Zacny et al. 1994). Most studies have tested doses of opioids within the therapeutic range. Some studies, however, have applied higher doses as used by the abusing population (Fraser et al. 1964; Isbell et al. 1948), but there are generally few controlled data resulting from high-dose experiments with opioids. Little is known with respect to the relations between opioid serum concentrations and effects in performance tests as opioid concentration have not been measured in most of the studies published, although recent papers in the field have included such data (Walker and Zacny 1998).

Acute Tolerance: Data on acute tolerance, defined as a decreasing drug effect relative to drug-plasma concentrations during the period of the first hours after opioid administration, are few, mainly because opioid plasma levels have not been measured in the majority of the experimental studies. At the present stage, accordingly, no firm conclusions about acute tolerance can be drawn.

Tolerance After Repeated Dosing: Repeated chronic use of morphine at a fixed dose to cancer patients, for example, has in several studies been demonstrated to be accompanied by disappearance of the deleterious acute effects on motor performance, indicating the development of tolerance. Similar results have been reported for other opioids including methadone (Berghaus and Friedel 1994). However, even in chronic opioid users some negative effects have been reported, also in methadone treated patients (Berghaus et al. 1993; Zacny 1995), especially after dose escalations. Less information is available on the development of chronic tolerance in drug abusers, often using much higher doses of opioids at irregular intervals. Some studies support the notion that also in these individuals considerable tolerance can build up (Zacny 1995). On the other hand, one would assume the period shortly after injection of heroin in high doses, a situation which has not been subjected to experimental testing due to ethical restriction, to demonstrate deleterious effects on performance. Withdrawal after cessation of chronic opioid treatment or abuse as well as naloxone-precipitated withdrawal seemed only to be accompanied by negligible psychomotor impairment (Zacny 1995).

Differences between Opioids: In studies comparing the acute psychomotor effects in healthy volunteers of equianalgetic doses, both buprenorphine (Zacny et al. 1997) and pentazocine (Zacny et al. 1998) caused more pronounced impairment than morphine. In general, impairment by opioids appeared to be more apparent with partial or weak agonists like buprenorphine, pentazocine, dextropropoxyphene, and codeine than with the full agonists, such as morphine (Zacny 1995).

Interaction with Alcohol: In one study on simulated driving, alcohol was not found to significantly increase the negative effects of codeine (Linnoila and Hakkinen 1974).

Opioids in Pain Treatment: It has been discussed whether pain could counteract any impairing effects that opioids might exert on psychomotor and cognitive functioning. At present, there are no clear answers to this question. The studies by Hill et al. (1952, 1955, 1956) indicated that stress might antagonize the negative effects of morphine on motor performance to some extent.

10.3.3.2 Analytical Epidemiological Studies

In a matched case-control study of older drivers (above 65 years) who were involved in injurious crashes, 234 cases and 447 controls were investigated and information on drug use was obtained from prescription databases. Use of opioid analgesics was associated with increased risk for injurious motor vehicle collisions, relative risk 1.8. The most frequently prescribed opioid was codeine (Leveille et al. 1994).

In a responsibility analysis (Drummer 1994) on fatally injured drivers, a relative risk for opioids of 2.3 was calculated. The figure was not statistically significantly different from the drug-free group.

One retrospective cohort study examined the involvement of enrollees in the Tennessee Medicaid program in injury-producing automobile accidents (Ray et al. 1993). The relative risks were not greater than unity with oral opioid analgesics.

10.3.3.3 Descriptive Epidemiological Studies

Data from Germany indicated that approximately 1% of the general driving population had used opioids in relation to driving (Krüger et al. 1965, 1996).

In a study on all blood samples taken in Norway based on the suspicion of drunken or drugged driving during 2 months in 1993, opioids were found in 58 of 1197 samples, i.e., in about 5% of the cases (Mørland et al. 1995). From 1993 to 1998, the detection of opioids in samples from drivers apprehended on the suspicion of drugged driving has almost doubled, and opioids were detected in about 9% of all cases suspected of either drunken or drugged driving in 1998.

In a study of all traffic accidents which occurred in Norway during a 5-month period in 1993, including all cases (7%) where the police suspected the driver of being influenced by either alcohol or drugs, opioids were detected in 4.3% of the blood samples, representing 0.3% of the total number of drivers involved in accidents with person injury occurring during that period (Bjørneboe et al. 1996).

In investigations performed on more than 7000 drivers involved in collisions, from Belgium (Meulmans et al. 1997) and Italy (Ferrara et al. 1990) opioids were present in 3.5–7.5% of the urine samples collected and in 0.5% of the plasma samples. Similar percentages have been reported from a smaller Canadian material on drivers injured in motor vehicle accidents (Stoduto et al. 1993).

In fatally injured drivers from single-vehicle accidents in Norway, the blood samples collected over 1 year (1989–1990) contained opioids in approximately 1% of the cases (Gjerde et al. 1993).

10.3.3.4 Conclusions

Based on present knowledge, it can be stated that:

1. The use of opioids represents a risk to traffic safety at least for people who are inexperienced with their use and/or who take the drugs in high doses.
2. The prevalence of opioid use among the general population, drivers suspected of impaired driving, and drivers involved in non-fatal and fatal accidents indicates a traffic safety problem in several countries.

10.3.4 Amphetamine and Related Drugs

The most important drugs in this group are amphetamine, methamphetamine, and the methylendioxy-substituted derivatives (MDMA, "Ecstasy"). Cocaine also belongs to this group of central nervous stimulants. These drugs are seldom used for therapeutic purposes.

10.3.4.1 Controlled Experimental Studies

Hurst and coworkers demonstrated in the 1960s that amphetamine could increase risk taking without affecting performance in complex mathematical tasks (Hurst 1962; Hurst et al. 1967). The general impression from studies of amphetamine on psychomotor functioning and performance tests has been that usually no detrimental effects have been observed or that vigilance performance in some instances has been improved (Koelega 1993; Pickworth et al. 1997). Similar results have been reported for MDMA (Ecstasy) (European Monitoring Centre for Drugs and Drug Addiction):

Homogeneity: The lack of negative effects on traditional performance tests have been reported in the majority of studies in this field (Koelega 1993).

Dose/Serum Concentration Effect Relationship: The general lack of effect on performance tests has been achieved after administration of amphetamine doses, per orally ranging from 5 to 15 mg, representing therapeutic dosing, or by using equivalent doses of other psychostimulants. It should be noted that similar doses were reported to increase risk taking (Hurst 1962). Among drug abusers amphetamines are taken at a dosage of 50–100 mg or more at a time, often intravenously to achieve the desired effect. Such doses have not been subjected to controlled experimental study. Few studies have measured the serum-concentrations of the central nervous stimulant present during controlled experiments.

Tolerance: Little is known about tolerance to the increased risk taking during amphetamine test sessions of some duration (acute tolerance), or after long-term amphetamine use. Reduced performance has been suggested during central nervous stimulant drug withdrawal (Logan 1996).

Different Amphetamines: Methamphetamine is generally thought to be somewhat more pharmacologically active than amphetamine, when similar doses are compared, but this has not been studied systematically in performance tests. The few results reported for MDMA so far appear consistent with the controlled experimental studies performed on amphetamine (European Monitoring Centre for Drugs and Drug Addiction 1999).

10.3.4.2 Analytical Epidemiological Studies

In a study on 1882 fatally injured drivers, Terhune et al. (1992) carried out a responsibility analysis to assess the contribution of drugs to accidents. They found a responsibility rate higher than unity (representing drug-free drivers) in the amphetamine positive drivers.

In a responsibility analysis (Drummer 1994) on 1045 fatally injured drivers, a relative risk for central nervous stimulants of 1.6 was calculated.

10.3.4.3 Descriptive Epidemiological Studies

Data from Germany indicate that somewhat less than 0.1% of the general driving population had taken amphetamines or cocaine in relation to driving (Krüger et al. 1995, 1996). A study on drug use in truck drivers on a major US transcontinental highway reported methamphetamine in 2% of those drivers voluntarily tested (Lund et al. 1988).

In a study on all blood samples taken in Norway because of suspicion of drunken or drugged driving during 2 months in 1993, amphetamines were found in 81 of 1197 samples, i.e., in about 7% of the cases (Mørland et al. 1995). From 1993 to 1998 the detection of amphetamines in samples from drivers apprehended on the suspicion of drugged driving has approximately doubled, and amphetamines were detected in about 14% of all cases suspected of either drunken or drugged driving in 1998, or in 28% of the suspected DUID (driving under the influence of drugs) cases in Norway. The corresponding figure for suspected DUID cases in Canton de Vaud (Switzerland) was 4% (Augsburger and Rivier 1997). On the other hand, the prevalence of cocaine use was 10.5% in that material compared to less than 1% in Norway.

In a study on all traffic accidents which occurred in Norway during a 5-month period in 1993 including all cases (7%) where the police suspected that the involved driver was influenced by either alcohol or drugs, amphetamines were present in 4.1% of the blood samples, representing about 0.3% of the total amount of drivers involved in accidents with person injury occurring during that period (Bjørneboe et al. 1996). In investigations performed on more than 7000 collision-involved drivers from Belgium (Meulmans et al. 1997) and Italy (Ferrara et al. 1990), central nervous stimulants were present in 2.7–3.7% of the urine samples collected and in 0.5% of the plasma samples.

In fatally injured drivers from single vehicle accidents in Norway, the blood samples collected over one year (1989–1990) contained amphetamine in approximately 1% of the cases (Gjerde et al. 1993). Studies performed in the United States have reported higher prevalence of stimulant use, in some reports with cocaine as the most prevalent; for review, see (Christophersen and Mørland 1997). A study reported on the prevalence of drug use in fatally injured truck drivers, and found amphetamine or methamphetamine in 7% of the cases (Crouch et al. 1993). By comparison with data reported 5 years earlier (Lund et al. 1988), there is some reason to suggest that findings of amphetamines are over-represented in fatally injured truck drivers.

Finally, it should be mentioned that the blood concentrations of amphetamine in suspected drugged drivers, most of whom were considered impaired by clinical examination, were higher than expected after taking the drug in therapeutic doses (Gjerde et al. 1992).

Investigation of 146 accident reports in which methamphetamine was found in the drivers revealed rather high blood levels (Logan et al. 1998). Postmortem concentration changes, however, add some uncertainty to the interpretation of the latter results (Hillberg et al. 1999).

10.3.4.4 Conclusions

Based on present knowledge, it can be stated that:

1. The use of amphetamine and related drugs, at least in high doses, appears to constitute a risk to traffic safety.
2. The prevalence of central stimulant use among the general driving population, drivers suspected of impaired driving and drivers involved in non-fatal and fatal accidents indicates a quantitatively important traffic safety problem—at least in some countries.

10.3.5 Antihistamines

Antihistamines are used in the treatment of allergic diseases like hay fever and in the prevention of motion sickness. This drug group can roughly be divided into two classes, the "older" antihistamines like brompheniramine, triprolidine, etc., and the "newer" antihistamines like terfenadine, loratadine, cetirizine, and similar.

10.3.5.1 Controlled Experimental Studies

The results from these studies will only be briefly reviewed and the reader is referred to the EMCDDA-report (European Monitoring Centre for Drugs and Drug Addiction 1999) for more detailed information. Several experiments have demonstrated that "older" antihistamines cause impairment, generally in a dose-dependent manner. "Newer" antihistamines do not have such effects with a few exceptions for high dosages.

10.3.5.2 Analytical Epidemiological Studies

In a case-controlled study (Skegg et al. 1979) on 57 people injured or killed while driving cars, motorcycles or bikes in comparison with 1452 matched controls a relative risk of 1.8 was found for antihistamine use. The risk increase was, however, not statistically significant.

In a matched case-control study of older drivers who were involved in injurious crashes (Leveille et al. 1994), it was found that current use of sedating antihistamines had little association with increased risk for injurious collisions.

A study examined the use of antihistamines among 244 people hospitalized for injuries suffered in automobile accidents (Jick et al. 1981). No significant differences in antihistamine use was found between faulty drivers and other drivers.

In a retrospective cohort study on the risk of involvement in motor vehicle crashes, no risk increase was found to be associated with antihistamine use (Ray et al. 1993).

Thus, none of the cited analytical epidemiological studies reported significant risk increases for antihistamine users.

10.3.5.3 Descriptive Epidemiological Studies

Antihistamines do not appear to have been detected to any significant extent in samples collected from the general driving population, from drivers suspected of impaired driving or collision-involved drivers. In a material on fatally injured drivers from Norway

(Gjerde et al. 1993), antihistamines were not detected, while antihistamines were found in 2.1% of samples taken from fatally injured Ontario drivers (Cimbura et al. 1982).

The general lack of detection of antihistamines in most materials could be related both to drivers exerting care when taking the drugs and the almost non-existing potential for abuse of antihistamine drugs.

10.3.5.4 Conclusions

1. The use of "old" antihistamines might constitute a risk to traffic safety, which does not appear to be shared by "new" antihistamines.
2. The prevalence of antihistamine use found in different types of drivers indicates that antihistamine use does not represent an important traffic safety problem.

10.3.6 Antidepressants

These drugs are mainly used in the treatment of various depressive disorders. This drug class has several members; two important types are represented by tri- and tetracyclic antidepressants such as amitriptyline, mianserin, doxepin, and similar drugs on the one hand, and paroxetine, fluvoxamine, fluoxetine (serotonin-reuptake inhibitors), and other "modern" drugs on the other.

10.3.6.1 Controlled Experimental Studies

The results from these studies can be briefly reviewed as follows (see European Monitoring Centre for Drugs and Drug Addictions 1999 for further details): The cyclic antidepressants have in a series of controlled experimental studies been shown to impair performance. Generally, cyclic antidepressants which are most sedative, such as amitriptyline, demonstrated the most pronounced effects in acute experiments. After repeated use in volunteers and in patients, impairment was reduced and for some depressed patients the impairing effects of depression on performance could be reduced by treatment with cyclic antidepressants. The modern antidepressants do not seem to interfere with performance, except in some cases when high doses resulted in minor impairment.

10.3.6.2 Analytical Epidemiological Studies

A matched case-controlled study of older drivers who were involved in injurious crashes (Leveille et al. 1994) demonstrated that use of antidepressants was associated with increased risk of motor vehicle collisions compared with non-users; current users of cyclic antidepressants had an adjusted relative risk of 2.3.

A study (Currie et al. 1995) analyzed 229 blood samples from responsible-for-accident and non-responsible drivers. They found that there was a higher incidence of tricyclic antidepressants among the responsible group compared with the non-responsible group.

In a retrospective cohort study on the risk of involvement in motor vehicle crashes, an increased risk was found for current users of cyclic antidepressants, RR 2.2 (Ray et al. 1993).

In another study (Barbone et al. 1998) no increased association between use of tricyclic antidepressants or serotonin-reuptake inhibitors and traffic accidents was found.

10.3.6.3 Descriptive Epidemiological Studies

Cyclic antidepressants have not appeared in any substantial fraction of samples collected from the general driving population or from drivers suspected of impairment.

In a material of 5000 collision-involved drivers from Italy (Ferrara et al. 1990), tricyclic antidepressants were found in 1.5% of the plasma samples.

Antidepressants were not detected in blood samples from fatally injured Norwegian drivers (Gjerde et al. 1993), and these drugs were not greatly represented in biological samples from fatally injured drivers in Washington State (Logan and Schwilke 1996). On the other hand, in a material from fatally injured drivers and pedestrians from France, antidepressants were found with a high frequency (Deveaux et al. 1996).

In general, it appears, however, fair to conclude that the infrequent detection of antidepressants in most materials could be related both to drivers exerting care when treated with the drugs and the almost nonexistent potential for abuse of antidepressants.

10.3.6.4 Conclusion

- The use of cyclic antidepressants might constitute a risk to traffic safety, especially in patients who have used the drug for a short time only. "Modern" antidepressants do not appear to represent a substantial traffic risk.
- The prevalence of use of cyclic antidepressant found in different materials from drivers does not appear to be of an order of magnitude, which should constitute a major quantitative traffic safety problem—with the possible exception of some countries.

10.3.7 Summary

In concluding section 10.3 it should first be mentioned that there are few data available on other drugs than the six groups discussed above with regard to performance tests and epidemiological studies. It appears that the main problem with respect to therapeutic drugs is experienced with BZDs and related drugs. A much smaller problem, although not negligible, exists for the therapeutic use of opioids and antidepressants. The major problem within the field of drugged driving as it appears today in the United States and Europe is related to the high dose use (abuse) of BZDs and related drugs, opioids and illicit drugs as cannabis, amphetamines, cocaine, and other central nervous stimulants. In these cases often more than one drug is found in the samples analyzed (Mørland et al. 1995). Combinations with alcohol are also frequently found. There are few controlled studies on the effects of drug combinations on performance tests. The frequent finding of such combinations in samples from accident-involved drivers indicates potentiation of traffic hazards due to drug combinations (Bjørneboe et al. 1996; Christophersen and Mørland 1997; Drummer 1994; Gjerde et al. 1993). It seems fair to conclude that the presence of abused drugs at high blood concentrations likely to be accompanied by intoxication, too high to be tested in controlled experiments for ethical reasons, can be regarded to represent a substantial traffic hazard. This conclusion has also been supported by results of accident culpability analysis (Drummer 1994).

10.4 The Assessment of Drug Impairment

In many countries, there are road traffic acts prohibiting a person unfit because of drug use from driving a motor vehicle. Being under the influence of an agent or being impaired by drugs are other expressions used. Further definitions of how actually the expression "unfit," "influenced," or "impaired" by drugs should be understood and determined are, however, generally missing from the traffic acts.

For alcohol this problem has in most countries been solved by introducing a certain BAC (or corresponding concentration in expired air) as the legal limit, defining higher BACs as illegal. It has been demonstrated in several studies that subjects with the same BAC might behave quite differently and also show wide variations of performance impairment; such variations will, however, have little practical importance for alcohol where BAC *per se* laws are operating. Since no countries so far have enacted *per se* laws for drug concentrations corresponding to the legal alcohol concentrations limits, the measurement of drug impairment constitutes a point of critical importance.

To prove the presence of impairment, most countries require some kind of assessment of the individual in question. Ideally impairment should be established by a battery of tests that would reflect driving ability and which could also measure the accident risk. As discussed in section 10.3, such tests are presently unavailable.

One way to evaluate impairment, which is often used, is performance of a more general examination of the suspect by the police officer or a police physician. This examination can be more or less causal, or according to a fixed protocol. Various protocols have been tested. In the United States, one originally developed by the Los Angeles Police Department during the 1970s has founded the basis for drug recognition examiners or experts (DREs). Modifications have obtained acceptance in other countries, such as in Germany where the Institute of Legal Medicine at the University of Saarland has developed a training program for police officers (M. Möller, Personal Communication). Various types of clinical examinations originally developed for the clinical testing of neurological patients have also found broad application (Table 10.3). In most cases, drug analyses are performed in urine or blood samples taken at the time of impairment testing. The combination of impairment signs in the test and positive drug findings may thus constitute the basis for a statement about drug impairment, as has been done in the United States by the development of the Drug Evaluation and Classification (DEC) program (US National Highway Traffic Safety

Table 10.3 Clinical Tests Used in Norway to Assess Drug-Impaired Drivers

Test	Observation
General	Consciousness
	Orientation in time and space
	General behavior
	Backward counting
	Articulation
	Ability to participate in normal conversation
Heart rate	
Neurological signs	Pupillary diameter, reaction to light
	Nystagmus
	Gait performances
	Romberg's test
	Coordination tests
	Tremor
Mental state	Mood
	Psychotic symptoms
Cognitive performance	

Administration 1990). The drug detection by the DEC program has been validated with regard to positive drug analyses (Heishman et al. 1996, 1998; Kunsman et al. 1997).

For many performance tests of relevance to driving, some drug blood concentration-effect relationship has been established (Berghaus et al. 1995; Berghaus and Grass 1997). Since the blood concentration of a drug will, when distribution equilibrium is reached, reflect the drug concentration present at critical receptors on brain neurons, this concentration-effect relationship would be expected. Similar relations would accordingly not be assumed to exist for urine drug concentrations, which are not in equilibrium with drug concentrations in the brain. The measurement of the blood concentration of any drug with an impairing potential would give important information on the likelihood of impairment, generally increasing at increasing drug concentrations. On the other hand, marked individual differences in impairment at a certain blood concentration have been demonstrated for all impairing drugs, alcohol included (Goldberg 1943; Perper et al. 1986; Iten 1994). Furthermore, differences between different observers' ability to assess impairment constitute a problem.

The best approach presently appears to be to integrate the results of an examination testing several independent measures of possible traffic-relevant impairment and the measurement(s) of blood concentration(s) of the drug(s), which is (are) present (Iten 1994). By relating these findings to available studies on drug concentration-effect relationships, and knowledge about the drug use pattern of the suspect, a picture of the impairment of the individual under investigation can be made by trained specialists in pharmacology and toxicology. In this way several factors indicating impairment can be evaluated in an integrated fashion and observer differences can to some extent be corrected for. The approach is not perfect, in that the subject's baseline performance is unknown, that the relevance of the applied tests to driving ability can be disputed, and that the procedure is time and personnel demanding.

10.5 Roadside Detection of Non-alcohol Drugged Driving

The roadside detection of a driver influenced by non-alcohol drugs can be difficult. There will be no smell of alcohol, which can raise the suspicion of an investigating police officer.

Presently two main sets of observations can lead to the detection of drugged driving.

10.5.1 Observation of Behavior

This will in some form always constitute the starting point. Some peculiarity in the driving behavior or in the behavior of the driver when in contact with police or witnesses is in general the first cause for suspicion. Further interview and conducting of simple roadside performance tests might increase or decrease a primary suspicion. In the United States as well as in other countries the police often at this stage in the investigation perform more systematic testing of the suspect by means of test batteries (see section 10.4). Such testing might, depending on outcome, be followed by collection of a blood sample. In some countries a breath alcohol screening test will be performed at the roadside. The combination of positive behavioral symptoms with a negative breath test should direct the suspicion toward influence by non-alcohol drugs.

10.5.2 Drug Screening

Systems for rapid drug screening, mostly by means of immunological techniques, have been developed for urine, saliva, and sweat.

Urine test kits have been on the market for several years, and new improved tests appear frequently. It should be noted that the specificity of such drug tests is not sufficient for forensic purposes, and that positive results have to be confirmed by alternative techniques. One main problem with urine testing and drugged driving is that drugs or metabolites may be present in urine for a long time after impairment has disappeared, thus giving rise to false positive results. Another problem is that urine testing might be impractical to perform at the roadside.

Saliva testing appears to be an interesting alternative. Many drugs are transported into saliva where they can be found at concentrations somewhat lower than in plasma, although saliva/plasma concentration ratios higher than unity have been reported (Samyn et al. 1999). Furthermore, for some drugs, the concentration-time profile in saliva after drug intake is quite similar to the profile in blood (Cone et al. 1988; Samyn et al. 1999). Saliva testing can conveniently be performed at the roadside. Devices using immunological techniques for rapid roadside screening are presently being tested in several countries in Europe, with the purpose of acting as a screening procedure to be followed by subsequent collection of a blood sample for confirmatory analysis and determination of drug concentrations, as well as other procedures.

Drug measurement in sweat appears to be less suitable, since the drug-concentration time profile of sweat is different from the profile in blood for some drugs (Kintz et al. 1996). Furthermore, it might be difficult to collect a sample which has a sufficient volume for analysis. Usually a patch has to be worn for several hours in order to collect a sufficient quantity of sweat.

10.6 Legislation

There are several legal regulations of interest to drugged driving concerning police activities connected to the detection of drugged driving as well as post-arrest processing of the cases and regranting of suspended driving licenses. There are also different legal regulations in various countries concerning drugs in general, for example with respect to possession and personal use. These points, however, will fall outside the scope of this paper.

Impairment or Zero Tolerance? Many countries have specific laws dealing with the problem of drugged driving, and have then pursued an "impairment approach" that imposes sanctions against drivers who are under the influence of substances and have impaired ability to drive a vehicle. Since impairment might be considered difficult to demonstrate, some countries have in addition introduced so-called zero-tolerance laws concerning various illicit substances and in some cases including medicinal drugs, making it illegal to drive with blood drug concentrations above the analytical cut-off limits. Germany was the first country to introduce the zero-tolerance principle in 1998. The introduction was accompanied by sanctions so that violation of the analytical zero-tolerance limit led to an administrative sanction (fine) while violation of the impairment "limit" resulted in a criminal sanction.

The zero-tolerance laws have been introduced in some countries (Germany, Sweden, Belgium) to fill a gap in law enforcement, considered troublesome in these countries where it was found difficult to obtain convictions according to impairment-law principles.

The experience with zero-tolerance laws is at the present stage very limited, but the principle is interesting and deserves some discussion. Most countries, which have implemented zero-tolerance limits, have done so only for illicit drugs. However, some patients will legally use illicit drugs, and if, for example, BZDs are included among illegal drugs as in Sweden, many patients will be affected by the zero-tolerance principle. It has been suggested that potential problems in this respect could be solved by exempting from sanctions patients who could document a physician's prescription for the drug in question. On the other hand, high dose abuse of a prescribed drug by a driver could in this way pass unpunished. It seems therefore wise that zero-tolerance laws should be coupled to "impairment" laws preventing high dose use, as has been done in countries like Germany and Sweden.

Most countries have restricted the zero-tolerance approach to illicit drugs. This obviously makes it easier for the public to accept this type of law. On the other hand, the rationale behind this can be questioned from a traffic safety point of view. A drug which is illicit is not necessarily more impairing than a medicinal drug. It appears from section 10.3 that most documentation of traffic safety risks has been collected on BZDs. No country other than Sweden has so far included BZDs among "zero limit drugs." However, use of these drugs according to ordination by a physician is not a punishable offense in Sweden. It might be, however, difficult to decide whether this is the case or not, based on toxicological analysis.

From this discussion, a more fundamental question emerges: Is it correct to implement a law that infers that the mere detection of a drug at a blood concentration, which is not impairing, can be considered illegal for a driver? It can be argued in favor of the zero-tolerance principle, by stating that the drug at higher concentrations will have the ability to impair, and that the borderline between impairing and non-impairing concentrations is difficult to draw. On the other hand, by saying this one should consequently consider the implementation of zero-tolerance laws for alcohol as well as for all medicinal drugs that are impairing at high concentrations. A consequent practice of the zero-tolerance principle would thus have large implications for laws on drunken driving and on the possibilities for many patients on drugs to drive at all.

10.7 Non-alcohol Drugged Driving in Norway

The reason to include this chapter is the following. It has been argued that "impairment" legislation may lead to too few sanctions against drugged driving, and accordingly little interest in the problem by the police because no sentences or other reactions would follow the apprehension of drugged drivers. As mentioned in section 10.6, this has led to the implementation of zero-tolerance laws in some countries. Some problems connected to the implementation of *per se* zero-tolerance laws were discussed, and it was suggested that zero-tolerance legislation should be supplemented by an "impairment based" legislation. Norway has only "impairment-based" legislation, and it might therefore be interesting to observe what can be achieved with that type of background.

The first point to mention is that Norway probably has the highest detection rate of drugged driving reported from any country around the world.

The drug detection rate among drivers was approximately 750 cases per million inhabitants per year in 1998. The corresponding figures in, Finland, Sweden, Denmark, and the UK, for example, are 190, 90, 40, and 30, respectively, and are markedly lower than the Norwegian detection rate.

A drugged driving case starts in Norway as in most other countries, by the police being called to a scene of a car accident, by the police or witness observing reckless or dangerous driving, by the police performing speed controls or sobriety roadblock checks. There are no data indicating that such encounters between drivers and police occur much more frequently in Norway than in other countries. The point seems, however, to be that a request for a blood sample for drug analysis is a much more frequent result of such encounters in Norway than elsewhere.

The Norwegian Road Traffic Act dealing with drugged driving seems at first glance not to represent a system that would lead to frequent blood sampling on the suspicion of drugged driving. The Road Traffic Act in practice requires proof for impaired driving in each individual case based on blood drug concentration results, the outcome of a clinical examination performed by a police physician or another "neutral" physician shortly after the incident, witness reports and other evidence, often supported by expert witness evaluation of the results of drug analysis and the clinical tests.

Some standard routines have developed during the last 10–20 years. The blood samples have always been analyzed by the same national institute, the National Institute of Forensic Toxicology (NIFT) by a rather broad analytical program, encompassing most drugs of abuse as well as some medicinal drugs, which might lead to impairment. As elsewhere in forensic toxicology, all positive screening results are confirmed by gas chromatography – mass spectrometry (GC/MS) or other alternative methods, and the amount of drug is quantified. The results of the analysis evaluated together with the results from clinical examination (which accompany the blood samples to NIFT) are reported back to the police with a recommendation with respect to which cases should probably be dropped and which could be followed up. The police might then request an expert witness statement on the probability of impairment in that particular case after supplying NIFT with further information on the case. The written expert statement concludes on the probability of impairment from "not impaired," "impairment cannot be excluded," "possibly impaired," "likely impaired," to "impaired." The police can then decide to bring the case to court. The experience so far has shown that the driver is very often sentenced when the expert witness statement concludes on "likely impaired" or "impaired." More than 90% of cases with these conclusions end with a court sentence.

In 1998 drugs were detected in 2951 blood samples (68%) of a total of 4336 samples taken from suspected drunken drivers and submitted for analysis that year. The average number of different drugs detected in drug positive samples was 2.6. The most frequently occurring drugs were tetrahydrocannabinol, amphetamines, and BZDs (mainly diazepam and flunitrazepam). In very few cases, the BZD findings appeared to reflect therapeutic prescription doses as judged from the drug concentration measured and coexistence of other drugs in the sample. The blood samples from suspected drugged drivers in general seldom contained therapeutic drugs in therapeutic concentrations.

The typical drugged drivers in Norway are young men (median age about 30 years). Approximately 60% of these drivers are apprehended for the same type of crime within a period of three years from the first apprehension (Gjerde et al. 1988a; Christophersen et al. 1996). A majority of the Norwegian drugged drivers appear to be drug abusers with dependency problems.

Statistics on drug abuse in general do not place Norway in a special position among European countries. There appears to be no reason to believe that drug users drive more frequently in Norway than in other countries, although this possibly cannot be ruled out completely due to lack of information on this particular subject. If we assume that there are no substantial differences between Norway and other countries in this respect, there is reason to believe that many other countries have a large undetected problem of drugged driving.

Which clues exist to explain the frequent and correct suspicion of drugged driving by the police? The following factors might be of importance. First, the Norwegian police force is organized in rather small units, which in general have obtained a high level of knowledge about the local population. These local police often know the suspects as people with previous drug problems. As drugged drivers have a high rate of criminal recidivism, they might be known to the police as previous and potential drugged drivers when they are observed behind the wheel. In such cases the police suspicion will be present by the mere observation of the former drugged driver driving a motor vehicle. Another factor is a routine, which the police have developed during the later years. Any time tablets, cannabis, other drugs, needles or syringes are found in a car or on people in a car, the driver is suspected of drugged driving regardless of signs of impairment. This procedure has led to a series of drug detections in blood samples from this group of drivers. A third factor that has recently been added is more systematic training of Norwegian police officers in recognition of symptoms and signs of drug impairment.

The attention of the police toward the phenomenon of drugged driving was markedly increased when NIFT could demonstrate a very high prevalence of drugs in blood samples that were submitted on the suspicion of drunken driving only. Such studies that were carried out in the late 1980s led the police to focus on drugs as well as alcohol as the reason for impaired driving. The studies were feasible since at that time alcohol analysis in blood samples was the only accepted way of detecting drunken driving. Later, in 1996 evidential breath testing of drunken driving was introduced and approximately 50% of the drunken driving cases in Norway are presently covered by this method. We have observed that in some police districts the introduction of evidential breath test instruments has meant a setback for the detection of drugged driving. By focusing on the question on whether alcohol was present at the time of testing or not, it appeared that some police officers forgot to think of other possibilities underlying impairment, although it was stressed that they should consider the involvement of other drugs in such cases. This problem seems to be under better control now, but it shows that too much focus on alcohol can in fact be counterproductive to the detection of drugged driving. The importance of how police officers are trained on the use of evidential breath alcohol instruments thus appears to be critical.

The role of the police physicians in the Norwegian system should also be mentioned. By performing the clinical examination and taking a drug history shortly after the apprehension, they often add important information to the case by indicating additional analyses which should be performed at NIFT. It should also be stressed that these physicians have no possibility of rejecting a case where, for example, the driver shows a prescription of a certain drug or make other claims that possible drug findings might be referred to treatment for disease. The physician is operating as a consultant for the police, and makes observations and notes, but has no right to interfere with the further handling of the case.

In conclusion, it is not easy to find a single factor within the Norwegian system that explains why this country has a high rate of detection of drugged driving. The most important point might be what can be summarized as the experience factor. Through its operation on the existing legal background, the system has given the police the experience that people apprehended under the suspicion of drugged driving very often have drugs in their blood samples, and that they often are impaired by these drugs. Furthermore, the courts appear to react to the cases brought to the courtrooms to the general satisfaction of the police.

10.8 Prevention

There are numerous preventive measures, which can be considered in the process of preventing non-alcohol drugged driving. It will fall outside the scope of the present article to give a full presentation of these measures. Here only one topic will be briefly discussed, namely the choice of preventive strategy in relation to driver category.

The prevention of drugged driving can be looked at as directed toward two main groups of drivers; on the one hand those using medicinal drugs for treatment of an illness and on the other hand those using psychotropic drugs for recreational purposes, and drug abusers or those who are drug dependent to various extents. The prevention strategies for the two groups will be different.

For the former group information from physicians and pharmacies will be important, as well as drug package inserts, and package labeling (as has been conducted in some countries). Information to physicians encouraging prescribing less traffic-hazardous drugs in cases where various options of drugs are available can also be valuable. In cases of long-term drug treatment with potentially unsafe drugs such as methadone, the patient should be closely examined by the physician after drug treatment for a substantial period of time before driving is allowed. The same procedure should be encouraged after drug dose adjustments are made. In any case, driving during the first 2–4 hours after taking a drug dose should be avoided if possible. O'Hanlon has presented a summary of guidelines for the prevention of therapeutic drugged driving (O'Hanlon 1995).

For the second group, the drug abusers, information on the risk would also be important, but probably have less impact. The group would also be less accessible for information. Secondary prevention therefore appears to be the keystone in such cases. This means that when a drugged driving case is detected, some preventive reaction should be instituted. The experience from Norway where the individual preventive measure so far has been imprisonment and/or fines is not too encouraging with high rates of recidivism to drugged driving offenses. Other approaches should therefore be considered aiming more directly at the main problem in most of these cases, drug abuse. So far, however, no major experience has been gained for drugged drivers in this respect. In the field of drunken driving several types of rehabilitation have been studied, some of which appear to reduce drinking/driving recidivism and alcohol-related crashes by 10%, as reviewed by (Wells-Parker et al. 1995).

10.9 Further Research

There are obvious gaps in our knowledge with respect to the effects of certain drugs, drug combinations and traffic safety. This would also be the case for new drugs that will appear on the market. There is accordingly a need to develop experimental techniques and undertaking of experimental studies which can be documented to be of importance to critical parts of the planning and performance of the act of driving and which can disclose behaviors critical to the occurrence of traffic accidents. The necessary development of new methods in this field would require collaboration between researchers with a wide range of different experiences. Future studies in the field should carefully consider the guidelines published by the Institute for Human Psychopharmacology in the Netherlands (Vermeeren et al. 1993; de Gier and Vermeeren 1995) and strategies discussed (Klebelsberg 1988).

Within the field of epidemiology, among several needs, two types of studies would be particularly rewarding. More knowledge about the traffic safety of therapeutic use of medicinal drugs is needed. Randomized controlled trials on patients treated with different drugs with similar therapeutic effect, but with uncertain and possibly different effects on risk of traffic accidents, could be performed within an acceptable ethical framework. In such epidemiological studies on patients treated with drugs, accident cases should if possible be screened for drugs and blood concentrations determined, to exclude effects of other drugs or misuse of the prescribed drug. The other type of studies which one would like to see published more often are studies where the cause or the culpability of the accident is related to drug findings (Terhune 1983; Robertson and Drummer 1994).

With respect to the testing of drug impairment, the comparison of simpler, easy-to-perform tests with more complex established tests or test batteries would be of great importance. This would apply to simple field test procedures, more advanced drug testing and clinical examinations. To some extent, such comparisons have been performed (Kuitunen 1994; Heishman et al. 1996, 1998; Kunsman et al. 1997). The development of new simple instrumental tests would be welcomed, but problems with respect to lack of individual baseline performance should be borne in mind. Field sobriety testing of all kinds should also be applied (evaluated) on apprehended drugged drivers where results from drivers involved in accidents could be compared to those not involved.

For the detection of drugged driving at the roadside the development of simple instruments for impairment evaluation would be welcomed. The newly introduced salivary drug screening tests should be further developed and probably also analysis of other biomatrixes could be valuable.

International collaboration between countries with different drugged driving legislation combined with studies on the populations in these countries with respect to drugged driving frequencies, accident involvement and relapses, could give valuable hints to which types of legislative measures would be most effective.

Within the field of prevention, countermeasures versus recidivism among apprehended drug drivers should have a major focus. Individual educational and treatment strategies coupled to regranting of drivers' licenses should be evaluated as well as the effects of tough measures such as car confiscations. The development of a system where a valid driver's license also functioned as necessary equipment (such as ignition-key) for the driving of a car has been proposed as an interesting idea in this field (Goldberg 1995). In general, elements from a public health approach should be evaluated in comparison with elements from a criminal justice approach to the problem, for the prevention of drugged driving recidivism as for the prevention of other drug-related criminal relapses.

10.10 Conclusions

The basis for our insight into the field of drug use and driving has certain restrictions and shortcomings and accordingly our knowledge is limited and there are several uncertainties.

So far, on the existing basis it may be stated that the main problem with therapeutic use of medicinal drugs is seen for BZDs and related sedatives or hypnotics, and to a lesser extent for opioids and cyclic antidepressants. For the use of antidepressants of the serotonin-uptake inhibitor type and antihistamines, the traffic safety problem does not appear to be serious. Our knowledge about therapeutic use of other drugs is very limited, but there are few signs that such use should constitute a serious problem.

The major problem within the field of drugged driving as it emerges today from the United States and Europe is high-dose use (abuse) of BZDs and related drugs, opioids and illicit drugs, in particular cannabis, amphetamines, cocaine, and other central nervous stimulants. Furthermore, evidence indicates that these drugs often are mutually combined or are taken together with alcohol, in all cases with the possibility of increasing traffic hazard.

One main challenge in the field is to implement ways to increase the detection rate of drugged driving. Another is to prevent dangerous drugged driving as well as its recidivism.

Future research should therefore be conducted to strengthen our knowledge base, to find new measures which can increase detection of potentially harmful drugged driving, and to create strategies for effective primary and secondary prevention of deleterious non-alcohol drugged driving.

Acknowledgments

The collaboration of my colleagues at the National Institute of Forensic Toxicology, Norway, is highly appreciated. Their work has been essential to the preparation of this review. In particular I would like to thank doctors Anders Bjørneboe, Asbjørg Christophersen, Hallvard Gjerde, John Ingum, and Svetlana Skurtveit for their contributions and discussions during many years. Finally, the comments and assistance by Dr. Wayne Jones, Linköping, Sweden, in preparing this manuscript are gratefully acknowledged.

References

Albery IP, Gossop M, Strang J. Illicit drugs and driving: A review of epidemiological, behavioural and psychological correlates. *J Subst Misuse* 3:140, 1998.

Augsburger M, Rivier L. Drugs and alcohol among suspected impaired drivers in Canton de Vaud. *Forensic Sci Int* 85:95, 1997.

Barbone F, McMahon AD, Davey PG, Morris AD, Reid IC, McDevitt DG, MacDonald TM. Association of road-traffic accidents with BZD use. *Lancet* 352:1331, 1998.

Berghaus G, Friedel B. Aspects of time for the assessment of driver fitness under therapy with BZDs. In Mercier-Guyon C (Ed): *Proceedings—14th International Conference on Alcohol, Drugs and Traffic Safety.* Centre d'Etudes et de Recherches en Médecine du Trafic: Annecy, France. p. 711, 1997.

Berghaus G, Friedel B. Methadone-substitution und Fahreignung (Methadone substitution and driving aptitude). *Neue Z Wehrr* 7:377, 1994.

Berghaus G, Grass H. Concentration-effect relationship with BZD therapy. In Mercier-Guyon C (Ed), *Proceedings—14th International Conference on Alcohol, Drugs and Traffic Safety.* Centre d'Etudes et de Recherches en Médecine du Trafic: Annecy, France. p 705, 1997.

Berghaus G, Scheer N, Scmidt P. Effects of cannabis on psychomotor skills and driving performance —A metaanalysis of experimental studies. In Kloeden CN, McLean AJ (Eds): *Proceedings —13th International Conference on Alcohol, Drugs and Traffic Safety.* NHMRC Road Accident Research Unit, The University of Adelaide: Adelaide, Australia. p 403, 1995.

Berghaus G, Staak M, Glazinski R, Höher K, Joo S, Friedel B. Complementary empirical study on the driver fitness of methadone substitution patients. In Utzelmann HD, Berghaus G, Kroj G (Eds): *Proceedings—12th International Conference on Alcohol, Drugs and Traffic Safety.* Verl TÜV Rheinland: Cologne, Germany. p 120, 1993.

Berghaus G. *Arzneimittel und Fahrtüchtigkeit. Metaanalyse Eexperimenteller Studien.* Bundesanstalt für Strassenwesen: Bergisch Gladbach, Germany, 1997.

Bjørneboe A, Beylich KM, Christophersen AS, Fosser S, Glad A, Mørland J. Prevalence of alcohol and other intoxicants in blood samples from drivers involved in road traffic accidents. *Norsk Epi* 6:49, 1996.

Borkenstein RF, Crowther RF, Shumate RP, Ziel WB, Zylman R. The role of the drinking driver in traffic accidents (The Grand Rapids Study). *Blutalkohol* 11:1, 1974.

Bradley CM, Nicholson AN. Effects of a mu opioid receptor agonist (codeine phosphate) on visuo-motor coordination and dynamic visual acuity in man. *Br J Clin Pharmacol* 22:507, 1986.

Brewer RD, Morris PD, Cole TB, Watkins S, Patetta MJ, Popkin C. The risk of dying in alcohol-related automobile crashes among habitual drunk drivers. *N Engl J Med* 331:513, 1994.

Chesher GB, Dauncey H, Crawford J, Horn K. *The Interaction between Alcohol and Marijuana.* Psychopharmacology Research Unit, Department of Pharmacology, Sidney University: Sidney, Australia, 1986.

Chesher GB, Franks HM, Hensley VR, Hensley WJ, Jackson DM, Starmer GA, Teo RKC: The interaction of ethanol and delta-9-tetrahydrocannabinol in man: Effects on perceptual, cognitive and motor functions. *Medical J Aust* 2:159, 1976.

Christophersen AS, Beylich KM, Skurtveit S, Bjørneboe A, Mørland J. Recidivism among drunken and drugged drivers in Norway. *Alcohol* 31:609, 1996.

Christophersen AS, Gjerde H, Mørland J. BZDs, tetrahydrocannabinol and drugged driving in Norway. In Utzelman HD, Berghaus G, Kroj G (Eds): *Proceedings—12th International Conference on Alcohol, Drugs and Traffic Safety.* Verl TÜV Rheinland: Cologne, Germany. p 1082, 1993.

Christophersen AS, Mørland J. Drugged driving, a review based on the experience in Norway. *Drug Alcohol Depend* 47:125, 1997.

Cimbura G, Lucas DM, Bennet RC, Warren RA, Simpson HM. Incidence and toxicological aspects of drugs detected in 484 fatally injured drivers and pedestrians in Ontario. *J Forensic Sci* 27:855, 1982.

Cone EJ, Kumor K, Thompson LK, Sherer M. Correlation of saliva cocaine levels with plasma levels and with pharmacologic effects after intravenous cocaine administration in human subjects. *J Anal Toxicol* 12:200, 1988.

Crouch DJ, Birky MM, Gust SW, Rollins DE, Walsh JM, Moulden JV, Quinlan KE, Beckel RW. The prevalence of drugs and alcohol in fatally injured truck drivers. *J Forensic Sci* 38:1342, 1993.

Currie D, Hashemi K, Fothergill J, Findlay A, Harris A, Hindmarch I. The use of anti-depressants and benzodiazepines in the perpetrators and victims of accidents. *Occup Med* (London) 45:323, 1995.

de Gier JJ, Vermeeren A. Methodological guidelines for experimental research on medicinal drugs affecting driving performance: What happened after Padua and Cologne? In Kloeden CN, McLean AJ (Eds): *Proceedings—12th International Conference on Alcohol, Drugs and Traffic Safety.* NHMRC Road Accident Research Unit, The University of Adelaide: Adelaide, Australia. p 653, 1995.

Deveaux M, Prangere R, Marson J, Goldstein P, Gosset D. The incidence of psychotropic drugs, opiates, and alcohol in fatally injured drivers: A prospective study in northern France. *J Anal Toxicol* 20:74, 1996.

Drummer OH. *Drugs in Drivers Killed in Australian Road Traffic Accidents*, Report of the Victorian Institute of Forensic Pathology (No. 0594). The Victorian Institute of Forensic Pathology: Melbourne, Australia, 1994.

Ellinwood EH Jr, Linnoila M, Easler ME, Molter DW. Profile of acute tolerance to three sedative anxiolytics. *PSCHO* 79:137, 1983.

Elliott D. Self-reported driving while under the influence of alcohol/drugs and the risk of alcohol/drugs-related accidents. *Alcohol Drugs Driv* 3(3/4):31, 1987.

European Monitoring Centre for Drugs and Drug Addiction: *Literature Review on the Relation between Drug Use, Impaired Driving and Traffic Accidents* (CT.97.EP.14). European Monitoring Centre for Drugs and Drug Addiction: Lisbon, Portuguese, 1999.

Ferrara SD, Zancaner S, Snenghi R, Berto F. Psychoactive drugs involvement in traffic accidents in Italy. In Perrine MW (Ed): *Proceedings—7th International Conference on Alcohol, Drugs and Traffic Safety.* National Safety Council: Chicago, IL. p 260, 1990.

Ferrara SD. Alcohol, drugs and traffic safety. *Br J Addict* 82:871, 1987.

Fraser HF, Jones BE, Rosenberg DE, Thompson AK. Effect of a cycle addiction to intravenous heroin on certain physiological measurements. *Bull Narc* 16(3):17, 1964.

Gjerde H, Beylich KM, Mørland J. Incidence of alcohol and drugs in fatally injured car drivers in Norway. *Accid Anal Prev* 25:479, 1993.

Gjerde H, Bjorneboe A, Bjorneboe GE, Bugge A, Drevon CA, Mørland J. A three-year prospective study of rearrests for driving under influence of alcohol or drugs. *Accid Anal Prev* 20:53, 1988a.

Gjerde H, Johnsen J, Bjorneboe A, Bjorneboe GE, Mørland J. A comparison of serum carbohydrate-deficient transferrin with other biological markers of excessive drinking. *Scand J Clin Lab Invest* 48:1, 1988b.

Gjerde H, Christophersen AS, Mørland J. Amphetamine and drugged driving. *J Traffic Med* 20:21, 1992.

Gjerde H, Sakshaug J, Mørland J. Heavy drinking among Norwegian male drunken drivers: A study of gamma-glutamyltransferase. *Alcohol Clin Exp Res* 10:209, 1986.

Gjerde H. Daily drinking and drunken driving. *Scand J Soc Med* 15:73, 1987.

Goldberg F. Electronic driving licences: Key to a new traffic safety system. In Kloeden CN, McLean AJ (Eds): *Proceedings—12th International Conference on Alcohol, Drugs and Traffic Safety.* NHMRC Road Accident Research Unit, The University of Adelaide: Adelaide, Australia. p 683, 1995.

Goldberg L. Quantitative studies on alcohol tolerance in man. The influence of ethyl alcohol on sensory, motor and psychological functions referred to blood alcohol in normal and habituated individuals. *Acta Psysh Scand* 5(Suppl):16, 1943.

Griffiths AN, Jones DM, Richens A. Zopiclone produces effects on human performance similar to flurazepam, lormetazepam and triazolam. *Br J Clin Pharmacol* 21:647, 1986.

Heishman SJ, Singleton EG, Crouch DJ. Laboratory validation study of drug evaluation and classification program: Ethanol, cocaine, and marijuana. *J Anal Toxicol* 20:468, 1996.

Heishman SJ, Singleton EG, Crouch, DJ. Laboratory validation study of drug evaluation and classification program: Alprazolam, *d*-amphetamine, codeine, and marijuana. *J Anal Toxicol* 22:503, 1998.

Hemmelgarn B, Suissa S, Huang A, Boivin JF, Pinard G. Benzodiazepine use and the risk of motor vehicle crash in the elderly. *JAMA* 278:27, 1997.

Hilberg T, Rogde S, Mørland J. Postmortem drug redistribution—Human cases related to results in experimental animals. *J Forensic Sci* 44:3, 1999.

Hill HE, Belleville RE, Wikler A. Motivational determinants in modification of behaviour by morphine and pentobarbital. *AMA Arch Neurol Psychiatry* 67:28, 1956.

Hill HE, Belleville RE, Wikler A. Studies on anxiety associated with anticipation of pain: Comparative effects of pentobarbital and morphine. *AMA Arch Neurol Psychiatry* 73:602, 1955.

Hill HE, Kornetsky CH, Flanary HG, Wikler A. Studies on anxiety associated with anticipation of pain: Effects of morphine. *AMA Arch Neurol Psychiatry* 67:612, 1952.

Hindmarch I, Gudgeon AC. The effects of clobazam and lorazepam on aspects of psychomotor performance and car handling ability. *Br J Clin Pharmacol* 10:145, 1980.

Hindmarch I, Kerr JS, Sherwood N. The effects of alcohol and other drugs on psychomotor performance and cognitive function. *Alcohol* 26:71, 1991.

Honkanen R, Ertama L, Linnoila M, Alha A, Lukkari I, Karlsson M, Kiviluoto O, Puro M. Role of drugs in traffic accidents. *Br Med J* 281:1309, 1980.

Hurst PM, Weidner MF, Radlow R. The effects of amphetamines upon judgments and decisions. *PSCHO* 11:397, 1967.

Hurst PM. The effects of *d*-ampehtamine on risk-taking. *PSCHO* 3:283, 1962.

Ingum J, Beylich KM, Mørland J. Amnesic effects and subjective ratings during repeated dosing of flunitrazepam to healthy volunteers. *Eur J Clin Pharmacol* 45:235, 1993.

Ingum J, Bjorklund R, Bjorneboe A, Christophersen AS, Dahlin E, Mørland J. Relationship between drug plasma concentrations and psychomotor performance after single doses of ethanol and benzodiazepines. *PSCHO* 107:11, 1992.

Ingum J, Bjorklund R, Volden R, Mørland J. Development of acute tolerance after oral doses of diazepam and flunitrazepam. *PSCHO* 113:304, 1994.

Irving A. A proposed investigation into drug impairment testing methodology. *Int Clin Psychopharmacol* 3(Suppl 1):99, 1988.

Isbell H, Wickler A, Eisenman AJ, Daingerfield M, Frank K. Liability of addiction to 6-dimethyl-amino-4-4-diphenyl-3-deptanone (methadone, "Amidone" or "10820") in man. *Arch Int Med* 82:362, 1948.

Iten P. *Fahren unter Drogen-oder Medikamenteinfluss.* Institut für Rechtsmedizin Forensische Toxicologie, Universität Zürich: Zürich, Switzerland, 1994.

Jäättelä A, Mannisto P, Paatero H, Tuomisto J. The effects of diazepam or diphenhydramine on healthy human subjects. *PSCHO* 21:202, 1971.

Jansen WH. *Routeplanning en geleiding: Een Literatuur-studie*, Rapport IZF 1979-C13. Institute for Perception TNO: Soesterberg, the Netherlands, 1979.

Jick H, Hunter JR, Dinan BJ, Madsen S, Stergachis A. Sedating drugs and automobile accidents leading to hospitalization. *Am J Pub Health* 71:1399, 1981.

Kerr JS, Hindmarch I. The effects of alcohol alone or in combination with other drugs on information processing, task performance and subjective responses. *Hum Psychopharmacol* 13:1, 1998.

Kielholz P, Goldberg L, Hobi V, Ladewig D, Reggiani G, Richter R. Hashish and driving behavior. An experimental study. *Dtsch Med Wochenschr* 97:789, 1972.

Kintz P, Tracqui A, Jamey C, Mangin P. Detection of codeine and phenobarbital in sweat collected with a sweat patch. *J Anal Toxicol* 20:197, 1996.

Klebelsberg D. Drugs and Traffic Safety, some basic reflections. *IATSS Research* 12:24, 1988.

Klonoff H. Marijuana and driving in real-life situations. *Science* 186:317, 1974.

Koelega HS. Stimulant drugs and vigilance performance: A review. *PSCHO* 111:1, 1993.

Krüger H, Kohnen R, Diehl M, Hüppe A. *Auswirkungen geringer Alkoholmengden auf Fahrverhalten und Verrkehrssicherheit*, Bericht Nr 213. der Bundesanstalt für Strassenwesen: Bergish Gladbach, Germany, 1990.

Krüger H, Schulz E, Magerl H, Hein PM, Hilsenbeck T, Vollrath M. *Medikamenten- und Droggennachweis bei Verkehrsunauffälligen Fahrern.* Berichte der Bundesanstalt für Strassenwesen: Bast, Germany. Heft M60, 1996.

Krüger H, Schulz E, Magerl H. Saliva analyses from an unselected driver population: Licit and illicit drugs. In Kloeden CN, McLean A (Eds): *Proceedings—12th International Conference on Alcohol, Drugs and Traffic Safety.* NHMRC Road Accident Research Unit, The University of Adelaide: Adelaide, Australia. p 55, 1995.

Kuitunen T. Drug and ethanol effects on the clinical test for drunkenness: Single doses of ethanol, hypnotic drugs and antidepressant drugs. *Pharmacol Toxicol* (Copenhagen) 75:91, 1994.

Kunsman GW, Levine B, Costantino A, Smith ML. Phencyclidine blood concentrations in DRE cases. *J Anal Toxicol* 21:498, 1997.

Leirer VO, Yesavage J, Morrow DG. Marijuana carry-over effects on aircraft pilot performance. *Aviat Space Eviron Med* 62:221, 1991.

Leveille SG, Buchner DM, Koepsell TD, McCloskey LW, Wolf ME, Wagner EH. Psychoactive medications and injurious motor vehicle collisions involving older drivers. *Epidemiology* 5:591, 1994.

Linnoila M, Erwin CW, Brendle A, Simpson D. Psychomotor effects of diazepam in anxious patients and healthy volunteers. *J Clin Psychopharmacol* 3:88, 1983.

Linnoila M, Hakkinen S. Effects of diazepam and codeine, alone and in combination with alcohol, on simulated driving. *Clin Pharmacol Ther* 15:368, 1974.

Linnoila M, Stapleton JM, Lister R, Moss H, Lane E, Granger A, Eckardt MJ. Effects of single doses of alprazolam and diazepam, alone and in combination with ethanol, on psychomotor and cognitive performance and on autonomic nervous system reactivity in healthy volunteers. *Eur J Clin Pharmacol* 39:21, 1990.

Logan BK, Fligner CL, Haddix T. Cause and manner of death in fatalities involving methamphetamine. *J Forensic Sci* 43:28, 1998.

Logan BK, Schwilke EW. Drug and alcohol use in fatally injured drivers in Washington State. *J Forensic Sci* 41:505, 1996.

Logan BK. Methamphetamine and driving impairment. *J Forensic Sci* 40:457, 1996.

Lucki I, Rickels K, Geller AM. Chronic use of benzodiazepines and psychomotor and cognitive test performance. *PSCHO* 88:426, 1986.

Lund AK, Preusser DF, Blomberg RD, Williams AF. Drug use by tractor-trailer drivers. *J Forensic Sci* 33:648, 1988.

Manno JE, Kiplinger GF, Scholz N, Forney RB. The influence of alcohol and marihuana on motor and mental performance. *Clin Pharmacol Ther* 12:202, 1971.

Meulmans A, Hooft P, Van Camp L, DeVrieze N, Buylaert W, Verstrate A, Vansnick M. *Belgian Toxicology and Trauma Study*, 1, 1997.

Mørland J, Beylich KM, Bjørneboe A, Christophersen AS. Driving under the influence of drugs: An increasing problem. In Kloeden CN, McLean AJ (Eds): *Proceedings—12th International Conference on Alcohol, Drugs and Traffic Safety*. NHMRC Road Accident Research Unit, The University of Adelaide: Adelaide, Australia. p 780, 1995.

Mørland J, Setekleiv J, Haffner JF, Stromsaether CE, Danielsen A, Wethe GH. Combined effects of diazepam and ethanol on mental and psychomotor functions. *Acta Pharmacol Toxicol* (Copenhagen) 34:5, 1974.

Moskowitz H, Smiley A. Effects of chronically administered buspirone and diazepam on driving-related skills performance. *J Clin Psychiatry* 43:45, 1982.

Moskowitz H. Drugs and driving: Introduction. *Accid Anal Prev* 8:1, 1976.

Moskowitz H. Marihuana and driving. *Accid Anal Prev* 17:323, 1985.

Neutel CI. Risk of traffic accident injury after a prescription for a benzodiazepine. *Ann Epidemiol* 5:239, 1995.

Neutel I. Benzodiazepine-related traffic accidents in young and elderly drivers. *Hum Psychopharmacol* 13:S115, 1998.

O'Hanlon JF, Brookhuis KA, Louwerens JW, Volkerts ER. Performance testing as part of drug registration. In O'Hanlon JF, deGrier JJ (Eds): *Drugs and Driving*. Taylor & Francis Group: London, UK. p 311, 1986.

O'Hanlon JF, Vermeeren A, Uiterwijk MM, van Veggel LM, Swijgman HF. Anxiolytics' effects on the actual driving performance of patients and healthy volunteers in a standardized test. An integration of three studies. *Neuropsychobiology* 31:81, 1995.

O'Hanlon JF. Ten ways for physicians to minimize the risk of patients causing traffic accidents while under the influence of prescribed psychoactive drugs. *Primary Care Psychiatry* 1:77, 1995.

Oster G, Huse DM, Adams SF, Imbimbo J, Russell MW. Benzodiazepine tranquilizers and the risk of accidental injury. *Am J Public Health* 80:1467, 1990.

Perper JA, Twerski A, Wienand JW. Tolerance at high blood alcohol concentrations: A study of 110 cases and review of the literature. *J Forensic Sci* 31:212, 1986.

Perrine MV, Waller JA, Harris LS. *Alcohol and Highway Safety: Behavioral and Medical Aspects* (US Department of Transportation, NHTSA Technical Report DOT HS-800-599). US Department of Transportation: Washington, DC, 1971.

Pickworth WB, Rohrer MS, Fant RV. Effects of abused drugs on psychomotor performance. *Exp Clin Psychopharmacol* 5:235, 1997.

Pope H, Gruber AJ, Yurgeluntodd D. The residual neuropsychological effects of cannabis- the current status of research. *Drug Alcohol Depend* 38:25, 1999.

Rafaelsen OJ, Bech P, Christiansen J, Christrup H, Nyboe J, Rafaelsen L. Cannabis and alcohol: Effects on simulated car driving. *Science* 179:920, 1973.

Ray WA, Thapa PB, Shorr RI. Medications and the older driver. *Clin Geriatr Med* 9:413, 1993.

Robertson MD, Drummer OH. Responsibility analysis: A methodology to study the effects of drugs in driving. *Accid Anal Prev* 26:243, 1994.

Rothengatter T. Psychological aspects of road user behaviour. *Applied Psychology: An International Review* (London) 46:223, 1997.

Saano V, Hansen PP, Paronen P. Interactions and comparative effects of zopiclone, diazepam and lorazepam on psychomotor performance and on elimination pharmacokinetics in healthy volunteers. *Pharmacol Toxicol* (Copenhagen) 70:135, 1992.

Salvà P, Costa J. Clinical pharmacokinetics and pharmacodynamics of zolpidem. *Clin Pharmacokin* 29:142, 1995.

Samyn N, Verstraete A, van Haeren C, Kintz P. Analysis of drugs of abuse in saliva. *Forensic Sci Rev* 11:2, 1999.

Sanders AF. Drugs, driving and the measurement of human performance. In O'Hanlon JF, de Grier JJ (Eds): *Drugs and Driving*. Taylor and Francis: London, UK. p 3, 1986.

Sellers EM, Busto U. Benzodiazepines and ethanol: Assessment of the effects and consequences of psychotropic drug interactions. *J Clin Psychopharmacol* 2:249, 1982.

Seppala T, Linnoila M, Mattila MJ. Drugs, alcohol and driving. *Drugs* 17:389, 1979.

Simpson HM, Vingilis E. Epidemiology and special population surveys. In Ferrara SD, Giorgetti R (Eds): *Methodology in Man-Machine Interaction and Epidemiology on Drugs and Traffic Safety*, Monograph Series Research. The Addiction Research Foundation of Italy: Padova, Italy. p 51, 1992.

Simpson HM. Epidemiological and laboratory studies on alcohol, drugs and traffic safety. In Noordizj PC, Roszenbach R, De Gier JJ, Neuteboom W, Zweipfenning P (Eds): *Alcohol, Drugs and Traffic Safety*. Elsevier Publications: Amsterdam, The Netherland. p 86, 1986.

Skegg DC, Richards SM, Doll R. Minor tranquillisers and road accidents. *Br Med J* 1:917, 1979.

Sleet D, Wagenaar A, Waller P. Drinking, driving, and health promotion. *Health Educ Q* 16:329, 1989.

Smart RB. Marihuana and driving risk among college students. *J Safe Res* 6:155, 1974.

Stoduto G, Vingilis E, Kapur BM, Sheu WJ, Mclellan BA, Liban CB. Alcohol and drug use among vehicle collision victims admitted to a regional trauma unit: Demographic, injury, and crash characteristics. *Accid Anal Prev* 25:411, 1993.

Sutton LR. The effects of alcohol, marihuana and their combination on driving ability. *J Stud Alcohol* 44:438, 1983.

Taberner PV, Roberts CJ, Shrosbree E, Pycock CJ, English L. An investigation into the interaction between ethanol at low doses and the benzodiazepines nitrazepam and temazepam on psychomotor performance in normal subjects. *PSCHO* 81:321, 1983.

Terhune KW, Ippolito CA, Hendrics DL, Michalovic JG, Bogema SC, Santinga P, Blomberg R, Preusser DF. *The Incidence and Role of Drugs in Fatally Injured Drivers*, DOT HS-808 065. US National Highway Traffic Safety Administration. Washington, DC, 1992.

Terhune KW. An evaluation of responsibility analysis for assessing alcohol and drug crash effects. *Accid Anal Prev* 15:237, 1983.

Ulrich L. Benzodiazepines in blood samples of alcohol intoxicated drivers. *Blutalkohol* 31:165, 1994.

US National Highway Traffic Safety Administration. *Drug Evaluation and Classification Program*. US Department of Transportation: Washington, DC, 1990.

US National Highway Traffic Safety Administration. *Marijuana and Actual Driving Performance*. US Department of Transportation: Washington, DC, 1993.

US National Highway Traffic Safety Administration. *Traffic Safety Facts 1993: Alcohol*. US Department of Transportation, National Center for Statistics and Analysis: Washington, DC, 1994.

van Laar MW, Volkerts ER, van Willigenburg AP. Therapeutic effects and effects on actual driving performance of chronically administered buspirone and diazepam in anxious outpatients. *J Clin Psychopharmacol* 12:86, 1992.

Vermeeren A, de Grier JJ, O'Hanlon JF. *Methodological Guidelines for Experimental Research on Medicinal Drugs Affecting Driving Performance An International Expert Survey.* Institute for Human Psychopharmacology: Maastricht, the Netherlands, 1993.

Walker DJ, Zacny JP. Subjective, psychomotor, and analgesic effects of oral codeine and morphine in healthy volunteers. *PSCHO* 140:191, 1998.

Wells-Parker E, Bangert-Drowns R, McMillen R, Williams M. Final results from a meta-analysis of remedial interventions with drink/drive offenders. *Addiction* 90:907, 1995.

Willumeit HP, Ott H, Neubert W. Simulated car driving as a useful technique for the determination of residual effects and alcohol interaction after short- and long-acting benzodiazepines. *Psychopharmacol Suppl* 1:182, 1984.

Wolschrijn H, de Grier JJ, de Smet PAGM: *Drugs and Driving: A New Categorization System for Drugs Affecting Psychomotor Performance.* Maastricht Institute for Drugs, Safety and Behaviour, University of Limburg: Maastricht, the Netherlands, 1991.

Worm K, Christensen H, Steentoft A. Diazepam in blood of Danish drivers: Occurrence as shown by gas-liquid chromatographic assay following radio receptor screening. *J Forensic Sci Soc* 23:407, 1985.

Zacny JP, Conley K, Galinkin J. Comparing the subjective, psychomotor and physiological effects of intravenous buprenorphine and morphine in healthy volunteers. *J Pharmacol Exp Ther* 282:1187, 1997.

Zacny JP, Hill JL, Black ML, Sadeghi P. Comparing the subjective, psychomotor and physiological effects of intravenous pentazocine and morphine in normal volunteers. *J Pharmacol Exp Ther* 286:1197, 1998.

Zacny JP, Lichtor JL, Flemming D, Coalson DW, Thompson WK. A dose-response analysis of the subjective, psychomotor, and physiological effects of intravenous morphine in healthy volunteers. *J Pharmacol Exp Ther* 268:1, 1994.

Zacny JP. A review of the effects of opioids on psychomotor and cognitive functioning in humans. *Exp Clin Psychopharmacol* 3:432, 1995.

Driving Under the Influence of Non-alcohol Drugs Experimental Studies*

11

MAREN C. STRAND, HALLVARD GJERDE, AND JØRG G. MØRLAND

Contents

* This chapter is an updated version of a review article previously published in *Forensic Science Review*: Strand MC, Gjerde H, Mørland JG: Driving under the influence of non-alcohol drugs —An update. Part II: Experimental studies; *Forensic Sci Rev* 28:79; 2016.

11.1 Introduction

A review on the effect of drug use on road traffic safety is presented in Chapter 10. The chapter covers experimental and epidemiological studies published before 1998 for the following drug groups: benzodiazepines and related drugs, cannabis, opioids, amphetamine and related drugs, antihistamines, and antidepressants. Many investigations have been performed since then. An update of epidemiological studies is presented in Chapter 12. In this chapter, experimental studies on the acute effect of drugs on psychomotor and cognitive performance as well as actual and simulated driving performance published after 1998 are reviewed.

Experimental studies are most commonly performed for medicinal drugs using healthy individuals taking relatively small drug doses and can be used to determine whether a drug may impair several driving-related functions. In many countries it is impossible to perform experimental studies on illicit drugs in humans for ethical reasons. In countries where such studies are allowed, the doses given and drug exposure times are often lower than those used by problem-drug users and may therefore not reflect the actual risks posed by illicit drug users in regular road traffic.

There are, however, a number of advantages with experimental investigations compared with epidemiological studies. First, several factors that may interfere with drug-related effects can be controlled for or excluded, such as age, gender, driving experience, health, exhaustion or sleepiness, the concomitant use of other psychoactive substances, previous or current drug abuse problems, risk-taking personality, criminal behavior, etc.; second, several types of cognitive and psychomotor functions that are relevant for safe driving may be studied, such as automative behavior (i.e., well-learned, automatic action patterns), control behavior (controlled action patterns), and executive planning behavior (interaction with ongoing traffic); third, well-documented, validated standardized tests may be used so that findings can be compared with other similar studies (Roth et al. 2014). Recommendations for experimental research on drugs and driving have been published (Walsh et al. 2008).

Another type of study, which may be regarded as "semi-experimental," is the study of psychomotor performance by drug users who have been taking a psychoactive drug *ad libitum*, either for therapeutic or recreational purposes, usually after previous drug use for an uncontrolled length of time, and therefore have varying experience and degrees of tolerance to the drug in question. Such studies are, for example, those where drivers suspected of impaired driving are subjected to an examination by a neutral observer (e.g., a physician) at the time when a blood sample is drawn for drug analysis. In some countries this is a standard procedure, and some publications have emerged on the relation between blood drug concentration and observed impairment. These types of studies have been included as they have some similarities to experimental studies of acute drug effects.

This review is an update of a previous review of studies performed before 1998 (Chapter 10). We have therefore included experimental studies published during 1998–2015 for different psychoactive drugs. In addition, a recent publication by the authors on the acute effects of methadone and buprenorphine on actual driving was included (Strand et al. 2019).

11.2 Methodological Issues—Data Sources and Search Strategy

A broad search of the English-language literature was performed incorporating both electronic and manual components. The electronic search was performed using PubMed.

The principal inclusion criteria for experimental studies on the impairing effects of drugs of relevance to driving were:

- Laboratory tests of traffic relevance (i.e., measuring sedation, drowsiness, divided attention, continuous perceptual-motor coordination, speed and accuracy of decision making, vigilance, and short-term memory) or on-the-road driving or driving simulator tests
- Alcohol as reference drug
- Pharmacokinetic data
- More than eight participants
- Published in 1998 or later.

For some drugs we were not able to retrieve any studies complying with the above criteria, and in such cases, additional studies were included according to the following criteria:

- Studies without a reference drug, but testing "standard deviation of lateral position" (SDLP) in real life or in a driving simulator, and some studies with simulated driving without SDLP
- Studies using other drugs than alcohol as "reference" drug where indirect comparison of impairment can be made
- Studies without pharmacokinetic data, but where the blood drug concentrations can be estimated from the information given (drug dose and time).

The search included the following drugs: alprazolam; amphetamine; antidepressants; antihistamines; buprenorphine; clonazepam; cocaine; codeine; diazepam; fentanyl; flunitrazepam; gamma-hydroxybutyrate (GHB); ketamine; 3,4-methylenedioxymethamphetamine (MDMA) (ecstasy); methadone; methamphetamine; methylphenidate; morphine; nitrazepam; oxazepam; oxycodone; phenazepam; THC (tetrahydrocannabinol); tramadol; zolpidem; and zopiclone. The drugs were selected based on a previous review article on the effect of drug use on traffic safety (Chapter 10). The studies included in this review are presented in Table 11.1.

In addition to the experimental studies, this review also includes a number of studies of clinical signs of impairment after *ad libitum* intake (semi-experimental studies).

Table 11.1 Experimental Studies

Drug, Administration, and Dose[a]	Time of Testing After Given Drug	Subjects (n, m/f, age)[b]	Pharmacokinetics[c]	Methodology[d]	Test(s)	Effects[e]	Control[f]	Analysis of Biol. Samples[g]	References
Alprazolam po IR/XR 1 mg	1–5.5 h (tasks) 4–5 h (driving)	n = 18 (9/9) HV 20–45 years	Mean serum concentration 4.9 ng/mL (IR) 1.7 ng/mL (XR) (55 min)	Co Db Pc Rd	Actual driving Cognitive/ psychomotor performance	Y	P	N	Leufkens et al. (2007)
Alprazolam po 1 mg	1 h (driving) 2.5 h (tasks)	n = 20 (8/12) HV 25.1 ± 2.0 years	N	Co Db Pc Rd	Actual driving Cognitive/ psychomotor performance	Y	P	Br U	Verster et al. (2002b)
Amphetamines (d,l-MA) 0.42 mg/kg	2.5 h	n = 20 (10/10) Healthy recreational illicit stimulant users 21–34 years	Mean blood concentration 90 ng/mL (120 min) 95 ng/mL (170 min) 105 ng/mL (240 min)	Db Pc	Simulated driving	N	P	N	Silber et al. (2012a)
Amphetamines (d,l-MA) po 0.42 mg/kg	3–4 h	n = 20 (10/10) HV 21–34 years	Mean blood concentration 90 ng/mL (120 min) 95 ng/mL (170 min) 105 ng/mL (240 min)	Db Pc	Cognitive/ psychomotor performance	Y/N/↑	P	N	Silber et al. (2006)
Amphetamines (d-A) 10 mg (LD) 40 mg (HD)	1.5–11.5 h	n = 18 (18/0) HV 23–40 years	Plasma Cmax 40 ng/mL (LD 140 ng/mL (HD)	Co Db Pc	Simulated driving	↑	P	Br U	Hjälmdahl et al. (2012)

(*Continued*)

Table 11.1 (*Continued*) Experimental Studies

Drug, Administration, and Dose[a]	Time of Testing After Given Drug	Subjects (n, m/f, age)[b]	Pharmacokinetics[c]	Methodology[d]	Test(s)	Effects[e]	Control[f]	Analysis of Biol. Samples[g]	References
Amphetamines (d-A) po 0.42 mg/kg	120 min	n = 20 (10/10) HV 21–32 years	Mean blood concentration 83 ng/mL (120 min) 98 ng/mL (170 min)	Rd Db Pc	Simulated driving	Y	P	N	Silber et al. (2005a)
Amphetamines (d–A) po 0.42 mg/kg	3–4 h	n = 20 (10/10) HV 21–32 years	Mean blood concentration 83 ng/mL (120 min) 98 ng/mL (170 min) 96 ng/mL (240 min)	Db Pc	Cognitive/ psychomotor performance	Y/N/↑	P	N	Silber et al. (2006)
Amphetamines (d-A) po 10 mg	120–170 min	n = 18 (12/4) Infrequent users of alcohol and amphetamine-like substances 21–37 years	Blood concentration 20.8 ng/mL (range 11.9–39.1) (120 min)	Co Db Pc Rd	Simulated driving Cognitive/ psychomotor performance	N	Alc P	Br U	Simons et al. (2012)
Amphetamines (d-MA) po 0.42 mg/kg	3–4 h	n = 20 (10/10) HV 21–32 years	Mean blood concentration 72 ng/mL (120 min) 67 ng/mL (170 min) 59 ng/mL (240 min)	Db Pc	Cognitive/ psychomotor Performance	Y/N/↑	P	N	Silber et al. (2006)

(*Continued*)

Table 11.1 (*Continued*) Experimental Studies

Drug, Administration, and Dose[a]	Time of Testing After Given Drug	Subjects (n, m/f, age)[b]	Pharmacokinetics[c]	Methodology[d]	Test(s)	Effects[e]	Control[f]	Analysis of Biol. Samples[g]	References
Amphetamines (d-MA) po 0.42 mg/kg	2.5 h	n = 20 Healthy recreational illicit stimulant users 21–32 years	Mean blood concentration 72 ng/mL (120 min) 67 ng/mL (170 min) 59 ng/mL (240 min)	Db Pc	Simulated driving	N	P	N	Silber et al. (2012b)
Amphetamines (d-MA) po 0.42 mg/kg	3 h 24 h	n = 61 (28/33) Abstinent recreational users of illicit drugs 21–34 years	Peak blood concentration 91.65 ng/mL (3 h)	Db Pc	Cognitive/psychomotor performance	Y/N/↑	P	B	Stough et al. (2012b)
Amphetamines (MA) po 10 mg	1.75–8.25 h	n = 9 (9/0) Stimulant and alcohol users 34–47 years	N	Db Pc	Cognitive/psychomotor performance	N	Alc P	N	Kirkpatrick et al. (2012a)
Amphetamines (MA) po 20 mg (LD) 40 mg (HD)	1–6.75 h	n = 11 (9/2) Previous experience with MA and MDMA 29.3 ± 5.0 years	Peak plasma concentration 50 ng/mL (LD) 120 ng/mL (HD) (3 h)	Co Pc	Cognitive/psychomotor performance	N/↑ (dd)	P	N	Kirkpatrick et al. (2012b)
Amphetamines (MA) po 0.42 mg/kg	3 h 24 h	n = 61 (28/33) Abstinent recreational users 21–34 years	Peak blood concentration 91.65 ng/mL (3 h)	Db Pc	Simulated driving	Y	P	B	Stough et al. (2012a)

(*Continued*)

Table 11.1 (*Continued*) Experimental Studies

Drug, Administration, and Dose[a]	Time of Testing After Given Drug	Subjects (n, m/f, age)[b]	Pharmacokinetics[c]	Methodology[d]	Test(s)	Effects[e]	Control[f]	Analysis of Biol. Samples[g]	References
Buprenorphine sl 0.2 mg (LD) 0.4 mg (HD)	2–3 h 5.5–6.5 h (tasks) 4–5 h (driving)	n = 22 (11/11) HV 23–49 years	Mean (SD) blood concentration 0.07 (0.04) ng/mL (LD) 0.13 (0.05) ng/mL (HD) (3.5 h)	Co Db Pc Rd	Actual driving Cognitive/ psychomotor performance	Y/N	P	Br U	Strand et al. (2019)
Cocaine po 300 mg	15–60 min	n = 61 (48/13) Heavy cannabis users with history of cocaine use 18–32 years	Mean serum concentration 284 ± 198 ng/mL (50 min)	Co Db Pc	Cognitive/ psychomotor performance	Y/N/↑	P	Br U	Van Wel et al. (2013)
Codeine po 20 mg (LD) 40 mg (MD) 60 mg (HD)	1–4 h	n = 16 (8/8) HV 22.4 ± 2.7 years	Mean serum concentration 18.26 ± 14.01/26.12 ± 16.46 ng/mL (LD) 31.85 ± 21.28/43.62 ± 13.07 ng/mL (MD) 40.33 ± 34.37/57.12 ± 19.41 ng/mL (HD) (1 h/4 h)	Co Db Pc Rd	Simulated driving Cognitive/ psychomotor performance	Y/N	P		Amato et al. (2013)
Codeine po 30 mg	1–4 h	n = 24 (24/0) HV 24 ± 3 years	N	Co Db Rd	Cognitive/ psychomotor performance	Y/N	B	N	Pickering et al. (2005)
Diazepam po 15 mg	1–5 h	n = 12 (7/5) HV 21–28 years	Mean plasma concentration 342 ng/mL (1.5 h)	Co Db Pc Rd	Simulated driving Cognitive/ psychomotor performance	Y/N	Alc B P	N	Mattila et al. (1998)

(*Continued*)

Table 11.1 (*Continued*) Experimental Studies

Drug, Administration, and Dose[a]	Time of Testing After Given Drug	Subjects (n, m/f, age)[b]	Pharmacokinetics[c]	Methodology[d]	Test(s)	Effects[e]	Control[f]	Analysis of Biol. Samples[g]	References
Diazepam po 15 mg	1.5 4 h	n = 9 (6/3) HV 22–24 years	Mean plasma concentration 0.27 ng/mL (2 h)	Co Db Pc	Simulated driving Cognitive/ psychomotor performance	Y	Alc B P	N	Vanakoski et al. (2000)
Diazepam po 10 mg	1.5 h 4 h	n = 9 (5/4) HV 55–77 years	Mean plasma concentration 0.21 ng/ L (2 h)	Co Db Pc	Simulated driving Cognitive/ psychomotor performance	Y/N	Alc B P	N	Vanakoski et al. (2000)
Fentanyl inj 0.2 μg/kg	15 min	n = 24 (24/0) HV 27.3 ± 4.92 years	Plasma concentration 1.91 27.3 ± 1.17 ng/mL (15 min)	Co Pc Rd	Cognitive/ psychomotor performance	Y/N	Alc P	N	Schneider et al. (1999)
Flunitrazepam po 1.25 mg	0.25–6 h	n = 12 (12/0) Recreational users of GHB 22–33 years	Cmax mean 14.5 ng/mL Concentrations peaked between 15–90 min	Co Db Pc Rd	Cognitive/ psychomotor performance	Y	Alc B P	Br U	Abanades et al. (2007)
Flunitrazepam po 1 mg	10 h	n = 16 (8/8) HV 55–65 years	Mean concentration 1.6 ng/mL (range: 1.0–2.4) (9.5 h) 1.3 ng/mL (range: 1.5–2.8) (14.5 h)	Co Db Pc Rd	Simulated driving	N	P	U	Bocca et al. (2011)
GHB po 40 mg/kg (LD) 60 mg/kg (HD)	0.25–6 h	n = 12 (12/0) Recreational users of GHB 22–33 years	Cmax mean 111 ± 37.4 μg/mL (LD) 166.9 ± 48.4 μg/mL (HD) Concentrations peaked between 30–90 min	Co Db Pc Rd	Cognitive/ psychomotor performance	Y (dd)	Alc B P	Br U	Abanades et al. (2007)

(*Continued*)

Table 11.1 (*Continued*) Experimental Studies

Drug, Administration, and Dose[a]	Time of Testing After Given Drug	Subjects (n, m/f, age)[b]	Pharmacokinetics[c]	Methodology[d]	Test(s)	Effects[e]	Control[f]	Analysis of Biol. Samples[g]	References
GHB po 12.5 mg/kg (LD) 25 mg/kg (HD)	15–180 min	n = 12 (6/6) HV 22–36 years	N	Co Db Pc Rd	Cognitive/ psychomotor performance	N	B P	N	Ferrara et al. (1999)
GHB po 1–10 g/70 kg	0.5–24 h	n = 14 (11/3) Previous history of sedative abuse 21–50 years	N	Db Pc	Cognitive/ psychomotor performance	Y(dd)/N	Alc B P	N	Johnson and Griffiths (2013)
Ketamine im 0.2 mg/kg 0.4 mg/kg	5–10 min 125 min	n = 20 (10/10) HV 19–42 years	N	Co Db Pc	Cognitive/ psychomotor Performance	Y/N	B P	Br U	Carter et al. (2013)
Ketamine iv 0.26 mg/kg bolus + 0.65 mg/kg per hour	5–180 min	n = 23 HV 31.3 ± 2.9 years	Plasma concentration 200 ng/mL	Db Pc Rd	Cognitive/ psychomotor performance	Y (dd) / N	B P	U	Krystal et al. (1998)
Lorazepam po 0.03 mg/kg	15–180 min	n = 12 (6/6) HV 22–36 years	N	Co Db Pc Rd	Cognitive/ psychomotor performance	Y	B P	N	Ferrara et al. (1999)
Lorazepam po 2 mg	5–180 min	n = 23 HV 31.3 ± 2.9 years	Peak plasma concentration 19 ng/mL (15 min)	Db Pc Rd	Cognitive/ psychomotor performance	Y/N	B P	U	Krystal et al. (1998)

(*Continued*)

Table 11.1 (*Continued*) Experimental Studies

Drug, Administration, and Dose[a]	Time of Testing After Given Drug	Subjects (n, m/f, age)[b]	Pharmacokinetics[c]	Methodology[d]	Test(s)	Effects[e]	Control[f]	Analysis of Biol. Samples[g]	References
Lorazepam po 2 mg	15–300 min	n = 18 (9/9) HV 24.1 ± 2.6 years	N	Co Db Pc Rd	Cognitive/ psychomotor performance	Y	B P	Br U	Zacny and Gutierrez (2003)
MDMA po 25 mg (LD) 50 mg (MD) 100 mg (HD)	2–4 h 12–14 h (no sleep)	n = 16 (8/8) Recreational MDMA users 22 years (mean age)	Mean serum concentration 25.8 ± 3.3 ng/mL (LD) 64 ± 6.4 ng/mL (MD) 157 ± 9.5 ng/mL (HD) (1.5 h)	Co Db Pc Rd	Actual driving	N	P	Br U	Bosker et al. (2012)
MDMA po 100 mg	30–360 min	n = 16 (9/7) Regular users of ecstasy 18–29 years	Cmax 202.5 ± 74.1 ng/mL (150 min)	Co Db Pc Rd	Cognitive/ psychomotor performance	N/↑	Alc B P	U	Dumont et al. (2010)
MDMA po 100 mg	15–300 min	n = 16 (12/4) Regular users of ecstasy 18–27 years	Mean Cmax 213 ng/mL (105 min)	Co Db Pc Rd	Cognitive/ psychomotor performance	Y/N	B P	U	Dumont et al. (2011)
MDMA po 100 mg	1–6.75 h	n = 11 (9/2) Previous experience with MA and MDMA 29.3 ± 5.0 years	Peak plasma concentration 220 ng/ mL (3 h)	Co Pc	Cognitive/ psychomotor performance	N	P	N	Kirkpatrick et al. (2012b)
MDMA po 75 mg (LD) 100 mg (HD)	1.5–2 h (tasks) 3–5 h (driving)	n = 18 (9/9) Recreational MDMA users 26.6 ± 5.4 years	137.4 ± 31.9 ng/mL (LD) 191.8 ± 49.1 ng/mL (HD) (1.5 h)	Co Db Pc Rd	Actual driving Cognitive/ psychomotor performance	N/↑	Alc P	Br U	Kuypers et al. (2006)

(*Continued*)

Table 11.1 (*Continued*) Experimental Studies

Drug, Administration, and Dose[a]	Time of Testing After Given Drug	Subjects (n, m/f, age)[b]	Pharmacokinetics[c]	Methodology[d]	Test(s)	Effects[e]	Control[f]	Analysis of Biol. Samples[g]	References
MDMA po 75 mg	3–5 h	n = 18 (9/9) Recreational MDMA users 21–39 years	Mean plasma concentration 113.4 ± 37.4 ng/mL (3 h)	Co Db Pc Rd	Actual driving	Y/↑	P	Br U	Ramaekers et al. (2006)
MDMA po 100 mg	3 h 24 h	n = 61 (28/33) Abstinent recreational users 21–34 years	Peak blood concentration 203.11 ng/mL (3 h)	Db Pc	Simulated driving	Y	P	B	Stough et al. (2012a)
MDMA po 100 mg	3 h 24 h	n = 61 (28/33) Abstinent recreational users of illicit drugs 21–34 years	Peak blood concentration 203.11 ng/mL (3 h)	Db Pc	Cognitive/ psychomotor performance	Y/N	P	B	Stough et al. (2012b)
MDMA po 100 mg	1.5–3.5 h	n = 19 (10/9) HV Experience with MDMA and alcohol use 21–40 years	Average (SD) blood concentration 170.41 (160.22) ng/mL (1.5 h)	Co Db Pc Rd	Simulated driving	↑	Alc P	Br U	Veldstra et al. (2012)
Methadone po 5 mg (LD) 10 mg (HD)	2–3 h 5.5–6.5 h (tasks) 4–5 h (driving)	n = 22 (11/11) HV 23–49 years	Mean (SD) blood Concentration 11.23 (2.89) ng/mL (LD) 20.16 (4.73) ng/mL (HD) (3.5 h)	Co Db Pc Rd	Actual driving Cognitive/ psychomotor performance	Y/N	P	Br U	Strand et al. (2019)

(*Continued*)

Table 11.1 (*Continued*) Experimental Studies

Drug, Administration, and Dose[a]	Time of Testing After Given Drug	Subjects (n, m/f, age)[b]	Pharmacokinetics[c]	Methodology[d]	Test(s)	Effects[e]	Control[f]	Analysis of Biol. Samples[g]	References
Morphine po 40 mg	15–300 min	n = 18 (9/9) HV 24.1 ± 2.6 years	N	Co Db Pc Rd	Cognitive/ psychomotor performance	N	B P	Br U	Zacny and Gutierrez (2003)
MPH po 20 mg	3–5 h	n = 18 (9/9) Recreational MDMA users 21–39 years	Mean plasma concentration 95.9 ± 78.4 ng/mL (ritalinic acid) (3 h)	Co Db Pc Rd	Actual driving	N/↑	P	Br U	Ramaekers et al. (2006)
Oxazepam po 30 mg	1–5 h	n = 12 (7/5) HV 21–28 years	Mean plasma concentration 190 ng/mL (1.5 h)	Co Db Pc Rd	Simulated driving Cognitive/ psychomotor performance	Y/N	Alc B P	N	Mattila et al. (1998)
Oxycodone po 5 mg (LD) 10 mg (HD)	1 h 2.5 h (tasks)	n = 18 (6/12) (driving) 24.0 ± 1.6 years	N HV	Co Db Pc Rd	Actual driving Cognitive/ psychomotor performance	Y (dd)/ N	P	Br U	Verster et al. (2006)
Oxycodone po 10 mg (LD) 20 mg (MD) 30 mg (HD)	15–300 min	n = 18 (9/9) HV 24.1 ± 2.6 years	N	Co Db Pc Rd	Cognitive/ psychomotor performance	Y (dd)/ N	B P	Br U	Zacny and Gutierrez (2003)
Oxycodone po 10 mg	60–360 min	n = 14 (8/6) HV 26.7 ± 4.7 years	N	Co Db Pc Rd	Cognitive/ psychomotor performance	N	B P	Br U	Zacny and Gutierrez (2011)

(*Continued*)

Table 11.1 (*Continued*) Experimental Studies

Drug, Administration, and Dose[a]	Time of Testing After Given Drug	Subjects (n, m/f, age)[b]	Pharmacokinetics[c]	Methodology[d]	Test(s)	Effects[e]	Control[f]	Analysis of Biol. Samples[g]	References
Temazepam po 20 mg	8.75–9.5 h (tasks) 10–11 h (driving)	n = 18 (8/10) HV 55–75 years	N	Co Db Pc Rd	Actual driving Cognitive/ psychomotor performance	Y/N	P	N	Leufkens and Vermeeren (2009)
THC inh 1.8% (LD) 3% (HD)	25 min	n = 80 (49/31) Recreational users of cannabis and alcohol (both regular and non-regular cannabis users) 21–35 years	Mean ± SD Plasma concentration Pre-drive 73.46 ± 37.36 ng/mL (LD) 90.06 ± 38.65 ng/mL (HD) Post-drive 38.20 ± 15.86 ng/mL (LD) 44.90 ± 17.90 ng/mL (HD)	Db Pc	Simulated driving	Y	Alc P	B	Downey et al. (2013)
THC inh 4 + 6 + 6 mg Interval of 90 min	15–300 min	n = 16 (12/4) Regular users of ecstasy 18–27 years	Mean plasma concentration 4 mg: 59.7 ± 5.6 ng/mL 6 mg (1st): 84.5 ± 9.0 ng/mL 6 mg (2nd): 74.8 ± 6.9 ng/mL (5 min)	Co Db Pc Rd	Cognitive/ psychomotor performance	Y/N	B P	U	Dumont et al. (2011)

(*Continued*)

Table 11.1 (*Continued*) Experimental Studies

Drug, Administration, and Dose[a]	Time of Testing After Given Drug	Subjects (n, m/f, age)[b]	Pharmacokinetics[c]	Methodology[d]	Test(s)	Effects[e]	Control[f]	Analysis of Biol. Samples[g]	References
THC inh 19 mg (LD) 38 mg (HD)	5 min	n = 25 Experienced drivers 25–40 years n = 22 Inexperienced drivers 18–21 years	7.4 ± 3.87 ng/mL (LD) 12.01 ± 5.53 ng/mL (HD) (25 min)	Co Db Pc	Simulated driving	Y (dd)	Alc P	N	Lenne et al. (2010)
THC inh 100 µg/kg 200 µg/kg	30 min	n = 18 (9/9) Current users of marijuana and alcohol 20–28 years	N	Co Db Pc	Actual driving	Y/N	Alc P	Br U	Ramaekers et al. (2000)
THC inh 400 µg/kg	20–200 min	n = 21 (15/6) Heavy cannabis users 19–38 years	Mean serum concentration 112.1 ± 47.5 ng/mL (15 min)	Co Db Pc	Cognitive/ psychomotor performance	Y/N	Alc B P	U	Ramaekers et al. (2011)
THC inh 13 mg (LD) 17 mg (HD)	30–58 min	n = 14 (10/4) Recreational users of alcohol and marihuana 26.1 ± 1.3 years	N	Co Db Pc	Simulated driving	Y (dd)/ N	Alc B P	N	Ronen et al. (2008)
THC inh 13 mg	15–80 min	n = 12 (7/5) Recreational users of alcohol and marihuana 24–29 years	N	Co Db Pc	Simulated driving Cognitive/ psychomotor performance	Y	Alc B P	N	Ronen et al. (2010)

(*Continued*)

Table 11.1 (*Continued*) Experimental Studies

Drug, Administration, and Dose[a]	Time of Testing After Given Drug	Subjects (n, m/f, age)[b]	Pharmacokinetics[c]	Methodology[d]	Test(s)	Effects[e]	Control[f]	Analysis of Biol. Samples[g]	References
THC inh 300 µg/kg	15–60 min	n = 61 (48/13) Heavy cannabis users with history of cocaine use 18–32 years	Mean serum concentration 55.3 ± 29.5 ng/mL (5 min)	Co Db Pc	Cognitive/psychomotor performance	Y	Coc P	Br U	Van Wel et al. (2013)
Tramadol po 37.5 mg	60–240 min	n = 24 (24/0) HV 24 ± 3 years	N	Co Db Rd	Cognitive/psychomotor performance	N	B	N	Pickering et al. (2005)
Triazolam po 0.2 mg/70 kg 0.4 mg/70 kg	80–200 min	n = 20 (10/10) HV 19–42 years	N	Co Db Pc	Cognitive/psychomotor performance	Y	B P	Br U	Carter et al. (2013)
Zolpidem po 10 mg	10 h	n = 16 (8/8) HV 55–65 years	Mean concentration 95.4 ng/mL (range: 15–240) (9.5 h) 54.7 ng/mL (range: 15–115) (14.5 h)	Co Db Pc Rd	Simulated driving	Y	P	U	Bocca et al. (2011)
Zolpidem po 15 mg	1–5 h	n = 12 (7/5) HV 21–28 years	Mean plasma concentration 196 ng/mL (1.5 h)	Co Db Pc Rd	Simulated driving Cognitive/psychomotor performance	Y	Alc B P	N	Mattila et al. (1998)

(*Continued*)

Table 11.1 (*Continued*) Experimental Studies

Drug, Administration, and Dose[a]	Time of Testing After Given Drug	Subjects (n, m/f, age)[b]	Pharmacokinetics[c]	Methodology[d]	Test(s)	Effects[e]	Control[f]	Analysis of Biol. Samples[g]	References
Zolpidem po 10 mg (LD) 20 mg (HD)	4 h	n = 30 (15/15) HV 24 ± 2.4 years	N	Co Db Pc	Actual driving Cognitive/ psychomotor performance	Y (dd)	Alc P	Br U	Verster et al. (2002a)
Zopiclone po 7.5 mg	1–5 h	n = 12 (7/5) HV 21–28 years	Mean plasma concentration 93 ng/mL (1.5 h)	Co Db Pc Rd	Simulated driving Cognitive/ psychomotor Performance	Y/N	Alc B P	N	Mattila et al. (1998)
Zopiclone Po 7.5 mg	10 h	n = 16 (8/8) HV 55–65 years	Mean concentration 25.4 ng/mL (range: 18–33) (9.5 h) 11.7 (range: 2–23) (14.5 h)	Co Db Pc Rd	Simulated driving	Y	P	U	Bocca et al. (2011)
Zopiclone po 5 mg (LD) 10 mg (HD)	1–6.5 h	n = 16 (16/0) HV 20–28 years	Mean Cmax 26 ± 2 ng/mL (LD) 50 ±3 ng/mL (HD) (1.7 h)	Co Db Pc Rd	Cognitive/ psychomotor performance	Y	Alc B P	U	Gustavsen et al. (2011)
Zopiclone po 5 mg 10 mg	1–6.5 h	n = 16 (16/0) HV 20–28 years	Estimated Cmax 74 ng/mL	Co Db Pc Rd	Cognitive/ psychomotor performance	Y(cd)	Alc B P	U	Gustavsen et al. (2012)

(*Continued*)

Table 11.1 (*Continued*) Experimental Studies

Drug, Administration, and Dose[a]	Time of Testing After Given Drug	Subjects (n, m/f, age)[b]	Pharmacokinetics[c]	Methodology[d]	Test(s)	Effects[e]	Control[f]	Analysis of Biol. Samples[g]	References
Zopiclone po 7.5 mg	8.75–9.5 h (tasks) 10–11 h (driving)	n = 18 (8/10) HV 55–75 years	N	Co Db Pc Rd	Actual driving Cognitive/ psychomotor performance	Y/N	P	N	Leufkens and Vermeeren (2009)
Zopiclone po 7.5 mg	10 h	n = 30 (15/15) HV 21–45 years	N	Co Db Pc Rd	Actual driving Cognitive/ psychomotor performance	Y/N	Alc P	U	Vermeeren et al. (2002)

[a] Abbreviations for drug, dose, and administration: d-A = dexamphetamine; d,l-MA = dextro, levo-methamphetamine; d-MA = dexmetphamphetamine; HD = high dose; im = intramuscular; inh = inhalation; inj = injection; IR = immediate release; iv = intravenous injection; LD = low dose; MA = methamphetamine; MD = medium dose; MDMA = 3,4-methylenedioxymethamphetamine; MPH = methylphenidate; po = per os (through the mouth); sl = sublingual (under the tongue); THC = tetrahydrocannabinol; XR = extended release.

[b] Abbreviations for subjects: f = number of females; HV = healthy volunteers; m = number of males; n = total number.

[c] Abbreviations for pharmacokinetics: Cmax = maximum concentration, h = hours; min = minutes.

[d] Abbreviations for methodology: Bl = blinded; Co = crossover; Db = double blind; Pc = placebo controlled; Rd = randomized.

[e] Abbreviations for effects: ↑ = improvement; cd = concentration dependent; dd = dose dependent; N = no impairment; Y = impairment.

[f] Abbreviations for control group: Alc = alcohol; B = baseline; P = placebo.

[g] Abbreviations for biological samples: B = blood; Br = breath (testing for alcohol); N = none; U = urine.

An electronic search for published studies describing the relationship between drug concentrations in blood and the outcome of a clinical test of impairment (CTI) was also performed using PubMed. The principal inclusion criteria were:

- Drug was used *ad libitum*
- Analysis of alcohol and a wide range of psychoactive drugs in blood samples
- Only one drug detected in the blood sample
- Performance of a CTI when collecting blood sample
- Published in 1998 or later.

The included semi-experimental studies are presented in Table 11.2.

Table 11.2 Semi-experimental Studies

Substance	Subjects (n)[a]	Methodology[b]	Concentration-Dependent Association (Y/N)	Reference Group	References
Amphetamine Methamphetamine	n = 878	CTI	Y	None	Gustavsen et al. (2006)
Amphetamine	n = 70	CTI	N	None	Jones (2007)
Benzodiazepines	n = 818	CTI	Y	Alcohol only; n = 10,759	Bramness et al. (2002)
Benzodiazepines	n = 818	CTI	Y	None	Bramness et al. (2003)
Codeine	n = 43	CTI	Y	None	Bachs et al. (2003)
Flunitrazepam	n = 415	CTI	Y	None	Bramness et al. (2006)
GHB	n = 25	CTI	Y	GHB negative; n = 32	Al-Samarraie et al. (2010)
Heroin	n = 70	CTI	Y	Negative; n = 79	Bachs et al. (2006)
Methadone	Methadone; n = 635 Methadone only; n = 10	CTI	N	None	Bernard et al. (2009)
THC	n = 589	CTI	Y	Alcohol only; n = 3,480 Negative; n = 79 THC and alcohol; n = 894	Bramness et al. (2010)
THC	n = 456	CTI	Y	None	Khiabani et al. (2006)
Zolpidem Zopiclone	Zopiclone only; n = 79 Zolpidem only; n = 43	CTI	N	Alcohol only; n = 3,480	Gustavsen et al. (2009)

[a] Abbreviation for subjects: n = total number.
[b] Abbreviation for methodology: CTI = clinical test of impairment.

11.2.1 On-the-Road Driving

The on-road driving-test methodology was developed in The Netherlands (O'Hanlon et al. 1982) and resulted in a highly standardized test (Verster and Roth 2011) that is performed on a public highway in normal traffic. The test driver operates a specially instrumented vehicle over a 100-km distance on a highway. Drivers are instructed to drive with a steady lateral position within the right traffic lane while maintaining a constant speed of 95 km/h. The speed and mean lateral position are continuously recorded, and the weaving of the car is calculated as the SDLP, and in addition a broad range of driving tasks at operational and tactical levels may also be assessed (Ramaekers et al. 2006) allowing all behavioral levels to be tested.

In a road-tracking test (Ramaekers et al. 2006), instruments are continuously measuring the distance between the vehicle and the left lane-line. The data are used to calculate means and variances for speed and position, such as the SDLP.

In a car-following test (Ramaekers et al. 2006), two motor vehicles are driving in tandem with a distance of 15–30 m between the cars. The first vehicle is under an investigator's control, and the following vehicle is under the test driver's control. During the experiment, speed changes of the leading car are controlled by a computer, which also activates the brake lights by random. The test driver in the following car is instructed to react to brake lights by removing his/her foot from the speed pedal as quickly as possible. The speed, distance between cars, and reaction times are recorded.

11.2.2 Driving Simulator

In a driving simulator, the subjects perform a computer simulation of a driving task. Tests in a driving simulator are used to evaluate driving performance. However, even very sophisticated driving simulators cannot fully replicate real driving conditions (Helland et al. 2016).

The main advantages of driving simulation are that driving tasks can be standardized and data can be obtained safely.

The risk of simulator sickness may be a problem when using driving simulators (Barkley et al. 2005). This is a form of motion sickness in which participants experience slight cognitive disorientation or dizziness and often nausea. In some cases, this sickness can occur to a degree that participants cannot complete the driving course.

It is necessary to practice on the simulator situation, both to reduce dropout as a result of nausea and to ensure familiarization to the driving environment of the simulator.

11.2.3 Psychomotor and Cognitive Testing

Driving is an example of complex behavior (Verster et al. 2004), where simultaneous use of multiple skills is required. Laboratory tests are used to measure specific driving-related skills (Verstraete et al. 2014). They can be useful in examining functions that are essential to safe driving even though they can never fully reproduce the complexity of real driving (Helland et al. 2013). Examples of performance tasks are reaction time, attention, divided attention, psychomotor skills, visual functions, tracking, and en-/decoding (Krüger et al. 2008). Some experimental studies also include physiological measurements, such as blood pressure, pulse and eye movements, as well as subjective evaluations, mainly using visual analogue scales to report effects such as drug liking, sedation, or pain. The results of subjective evaluations have not been included in our review.

11.2.4 Studies of Clinical Signs of Impairment after *Ad Libitum* Intake

In cases of suspected drugged driving, a CTI can be performed when collecting the blood sample from the apprehended driver. The observations retrieved from the CTI can be evaluated in relation to the drug findings. This type of study does not obtain objective information regarding time and the amount of drug intake. However, an individual evaluation of impairment can be made.

11.3 Results

11.3.1 Benzodiazepines and Related Drugs

Benzodiazepines are classified as anxiolytic and hypnotic drugs and act selectively on $GABA_A$ receptors (Rang et al. 2007). All benzodiazepines have common pharmacodynamic properties (Drummer 2002). We have included 17 studies on acute effects of benzodiazepines that met our inclusion criteria in this review (see also Table 11.1).

Abanades et al. found that 1.25 mg flunitrazepam impaired psychomotor performance (digit symbol substitution test, Maddox Wing and balance task) up to 5 hours after administration (Abanades et al. 2007).

Bocca et al. administered 1 mg flunitrazepam to subjects aged 55–65 years and found that driving parameters measured in a driving simulator were not affected by flunitrazepam (Bocca et al. 2011). They also administered 10 mg zolpidem and 7.5 mg zopiclone to subjects at nighttime and tested simulated driving the next morning. The study showed that both drugs had residual effects on driving performance 10 hours after the drugs were administered.

Bramness et al. studied the relationship between drug concentrations in benzodiazepine users and performance in a CTI in persons suspected of driving under the influence (Bramness et al. 2002). Only drivers found positive for one single drug were included in this study. The probability of being assessed as impaired rose with increasing blood levels of diazepam, oxazepam, and flunitrazepam.

Bramness et al. studied the relationship between benzodiazepine concentration and simple CTI in apprehended drivers suspected of driving under the influence of benzodiazepines (Bramness et al. 2003). Thirteen of 25 subtests and observations were significantly related to blood benzodiazepine concentrations.

Carter et al. studied psychomotor and cognitive effects and found that triazolam (0.2 and 0.4 mg/kg) impaired all tests examined (Carter et al. 2013). Triazolam also produced an underestimation of cognitive impairment as measured with subjective ratings of the drug effects.

Ferrara et al. found that lorazepam (approximately 2 mg) worsened performance on all psychomotor tests (critical fusion frequency, critical tracking test, response competition task, choice reaction time, and visual vigilance task) as compared to placebo (Ferrara et al. 1999).

Gustavsen et al. studied psychomotor effects at three levels of behavior (i.e., automative behavior, control behavior, and executive planning behavior) and found that 10 mg zopiclone caused impairment at all levels 1 hour after intake (Gustavsen et al. 2011). Blood zopiclone concentrations at approximately 39 ng/mL, achieved 1 hour after intake of 10 mg zopiclone, were accompanied by comparable or more impairment than blood alcohol concentration (BAC) of 0.74 g/L. No test components were impaired at 6.5 hours after administration, in spite of the fact that the same concentration in blood was associated with impairment about 1 hour after intake. The group also found a clear positive concentration–effect relationship above 16 ng/mL (up to 74 ng/mL) for zopiclone (5 and 10 mg) for both automotive and control behaviors as well as a modest relationship for executive planning behavior (Gustavsen et al. 2012).

Gustavsen et al. investigated the relationship between zopiclone and zolpidem blood concentrations and driving impairment as judged by a CTI (Gustavsen et al. 2009). No significant relationship was found, although there was a tendency toward an increased proportion of drivers judged as impaired with higher blood zopiclone concentrations. For alcohol-positive drivers, the proportion of impaired drivers was significantly related to blood BACs.

Leufkens et al. found that the acute impairing effects of 1 mg alprazolam extended-release (XR) on driving and psychomotor functions were generally less, as compared to its immediate-release (IR) equivalent, but still of sufficient magnitude to increase the risk of impairment (Leufkens et al. 2007). Both formulations impaired driving performance severely between 4 and 5 hours after administration. The magnitude of driving impairment with XR formulation was about half of that observed with IR.

Leufkens and Vermeeren found that 7.5 mg of zopiclone impaired a highway driving test as well as cognitive and psychomotor tests in healthy elderly subjects aged 55–75 years at least until 11 hours after intake (Leufkens and Vermeeren 2009). The magnitude of impairing effects was comparable with those found previously in younger volunteers. They also concluded that 20 mg temazepam was unlikely to impair driving 10 hours or more after bedtime administration in healthy elderly subjects.

Mattila et al. studied the effects of 15 mg diazepam, 30 mg oxazepam, 15 mg zolpidem, and 7.5 mg zopiclone on performance (symbol digit substitution, simulated driving, flicker fusion, and body sway) and memory (Mattila et al. 1998). The data indicate that zolpidem produces more decrements on psychomotor performance and immediate memory and learning than the comparator drugs. All drugs impaired three or more out of the five psychomotor tests performed.

Vanakoski et al. tested driving after intake of diazepam in subjects aged 22–24 years (15 mg) and 55–77 years (10 mg), under light and dark conditions, and found that simulated driving was impaired in both groups compared to baseline and placebo (Vanakoski et al. 2000). It was concluded that young subjects made good baseline scores but were sensitive to diazepam and alcohol, whereas older subjects showed poorer baseline scores but were less sensitive to both drugs.

Vermeeren et al. studied effects of 7.5 mg zopiclone on actual driving and concluded that zopiclone caused marked residual impairment 10 hours after intake and that patients should be advised to avoid driving the morning after zopiclone administration (Vermeeren et al. 2002). The subjects did not feel significantly less alert in the morning after zopiclone than after placebo. The magnitude of impairment in the driving test (SDLP) after zopiclone was twice that observed after alcohol with an average BAC of 0.3 g/L.

Verster et al. found a dose–response relationship between 10 and 20 mg of zolpidem as well as an impaired performance of actual driving, memory and psychomotor performance after 20 mg zolpidem (Verster et al. 2002a). Driving ability was measured 4 hours after administration, and memory and psychomotor performance (word learning test, critical tracking test, divided attention test, digit substitution test) 6 hours after administration.

Relative to placebo, SDLP after both doses of zolpidem was of a greater magnitude than SDLP observed at BACs up to 0.5 g/L. On the other hand, the SDLP after the recommended dose of zolpidem (10 mg) was comparable to SDLP observed in placebo conditions in previous investigations.

Verster et al. administered 1 mg alprazolam to healthy volunteers and test subjects who then performed a standardized driving test as well as a laboratory test battery (Verster et al. 2002b). Alprazolam caused serious driving impairment and significantly impaired performance on the laboratory tests compared to placebo. The increment of SDLP caused by alprazolam was comparable to a BAC of 1.5 g/L as shown in a previous study (Louwerens et al. 1986).

Zacny et al. tested psychomotor and cognitive performance in healthy volunteers after 2 mg lorazepam and found significant impairment on all tests performed (Zacny and Gutierrez 2003).

11.3.2 Cannabis

The most commonly used cannabis products are marijuana and hashish, both derived from the plant *Cannabis sativa* (Huestis 2002). The main psychoactive compound is Δ^9-tetrahydrocannabinol (THC). We have included nine studies on acute effects of cannabis that met the inclusion criteria in this review (see also Table 11.1).

A driving simulator study, performed by Downey et al., illustrated how THC negatively affects driving ability in both regular and nonregular THC users after administration of cannabis cigarettes containing 1.8% THC (0.8 g cigarette) and 3% THC (1.8 g cigarette), which represents about 14 and 53 mg THC, respectively (Downey et al. 2013). Generally, experienced cannabis users displayed more driving errors than nonregular cannabis users. The mean level of THC in plasma was higher in the regular cannabis users (approximately 100 ng/mL) than nonregular users (approximately 80 ng/mL). Driving was tested 25 minutes after smoking cannabis. The mean THC blood concentrations after low and high dose were 73 and 90 ng/mL, respectively, before driving and 38 and 45 ng/mL, respectively, after driving.

Dumont et al. found that THC (4 + 6 + 6 mg) induced cognitive impairment but did not affect eye movements compared to placebo (Dumont et al. 2011).

Khiabani et al. studied the relationship between THC concentration in blood and impairment in apprehended drivers suspected of driving under the influence of drugs (Khiabani et al. 2006). The time between apprehension and completing the CTI with simultaneous collection of blood samples was about 2 hours. Drivers with blood THC concentrations above 3 ng/mL had an increased risk for being judged impaired by CTI compared to drivers with lower concentration ranges. The relationship between concentration and impairment at the time of CTI and blood sampling does not necessarily reflect the degree of impairment at the time of driving.

Lenné et al. tested simulated driving performance in experienced and inexperienced drivers and found dose-related impairment (Lenne et al. 2010). Cannabis was associated with increases in speed and lateral position variability; a high dose of THC was associated with decreased mean speed, increased mean and greater variability in headways (distance between cars in car-following task), and longer reaction time.

Actual driving performance was tested by Ramaekers et al. after administration of two doses of THC (100 and 200 μg/kg, i.e., about 7 and 14 mg) (Ramaekers et al. 2000). Both doses of THC significantly impaired the subjects' performances in the driving tests, and both doses increased SDLP more than a BAC of approximately 0.4 g/L.

Ramaekers et al. measured perceptual motor control, dual task processing, motor inhibition and cognition in heavy cannabis users, and found that THC (400 μg/kg, i.e., about 28 mg) generally did not affect task performance (Ramaekers et al. 2011). THC did not affect performance of the critical tracking task, the stop-signal task, and the Tower of London Test, tasks that have previously been shown to be very sensitive to the impairing effects of THC when administered to infrequent cannabis users. It was concluded that heavy cannabis users develop tolerance to the impairing effects of THC on neurocognitive task performance, but no cross-tolerance to the impairing effects of alcohol.

A moderate dose of alcohol (BAC 0.5 g/L) and a THC dose of 13 mg were equally detrimental to some of the driving abilities (reaction time and steering wheel variability), with some differences between the drugs, as measured in simulated driving (Ronen et al. 2008). After THC administration, subjects drove significantly slower than in the control condition, whereas alcohol caused subjects to drive significantly faster. The effects on driving ability were dose-dependent at dosages of 13 and 17 mg THC. No THC-related effects were measured 24 hours after smoking the high dose of THC.

Ronen et al. studied the effect of THC (13 mg, smoked) on performance of simulated driving and nondriving tasks (e.g., reaction time) and found that THC impaired both driving and nondriving performance (Ronen et al. 2010).

Van Wel et al. demonstrated that heavy cannabis users showed impairment in a broad range of neuropsychological domains during THC intoxication (Van Wel et al. 2013). The tests used measured impulse control and psychomotor function (critical tracking test, divided attention test, matching familiar figures test, stop signal test, and Tower of London test). Single doses of cannabis (300 μg/kg, i.e., about 21 mg, smoked) impaired psychomotor performance and increased response errors during impulsivity tasks.

11.3.3 Opioids

The term opioid refers to substances with morphine-like effects (Rang et al. 2007). Opioids, acting through the μ-opioid receptor, are widely used as analgesics. The opioid drug class includes numerous compounds that are structurally related to morphine and many other compounds that are pharmacologically related, but structurally unrelated (Stout and Farrell 2003). The drugs included in our review were buprenorphine, codeine, fentanyl, methadone, morphine, and oxycodone. Nine studies on acute effects of opioids met the inclusion criteria (see also Table 11.1).

Amato et al. tested driving performance in healthy volunteers using a driving simulator and found that driving and psychomotor performance were not affected by any of three codeine doses administered (20, 40, and 60 mg) (Amato et al. 2013).

Bachs et al. studied the relationship between codeine blood concentration and the conclusions from the corresponding individual CTI in apprehended drivers suspected of drugged driving (Bachs et al. 2003). Only cases with detected codeine but not morphine were included. The odds ratios (ORs) for being judged as impaired were 6 and 19 for the "medium high" and "high" codeine blood concentration group, respectively. Codeine appeared to have some concentration-dependent effect on the central nervous system, independent of measurable morphine blood concentration, supporting the view that some codeine effects are not mediated by its conversion to morphine.

Bachs et al. found no relationship between the concentration of morphine, as the main metabolite of heroin, and the results from a CTI (Bachs et al. 2006). However, concentration-dependent effects were observed for the pharmacologically active metabolite morphine-6-glucuronide (M6G) and the sum of morphine and M6G.

Bernard et al. found no correlation between methadone blood concentration and impairment as judged by a CTI neither when detected alone or in combination with other drugs (Bernard et al. 2009).

Pickering et al. found that 30 mg codeine caused a longer choice reaction time than did 37.5 mg tramadol in young healthy volunteers; none of the drugs affected a memorization test and no difference was seen between the two treatments (Pickering et al. 2005).

Schneider et al. administered 0.2 µg/kg fentanyl by injection to healthy volunteers and compared the results of the cognitive testing to placebo and BAC 0.3 g/L (Schneider et al. 1999). In contrast to the alcohol data, fentanyl (as compared to placebo) produced a significant impairment of auditory reaction time, signal detection, sustained attention, and a subtest of the memory test. The fentanyl plasma concentrations measured in relation to the testing were comparable to patient plasma levels when fentanyl is used as an analgesic during anesthesia in outpatient surgical procedures.

Strand et al. found that 0.4 mg of buprenorphine significantly increased SDLP as compared to placebo (Strand et al. 2019). Both methadone (5 and 10 mg) and buprenorphine (0.2 and 0.4 mg) produced impairments of cognitive task performance (e.g., divided attention, reaction time, and tracking) and increased sleepiness particularly at the highest dose.

Verster et al. found no significant treatment effects of oxycodone (5 and 10 mg) on driving ability relative to placebo, although a significant dose–response effect was found for SDLP (Verster et al. 2006). The increment of SDLP was, however, found to be less than that observed with BAC of 0.5 g/L.

Zacny et al. tested psychomotor and cognitive performance in healthy volunteers after 10, 20, and 30 mg of oral oxycodone, and found impairment in some of the tests after the higher doses, indicating that psychomotor impairment may occur with clinically prescribed doses of oxycodone (Zacny and Gutierrez 2003).

Zacny et al. found no evidence of impairment of psychomotor and cognitive performance after 10 mg of oral oxycodone compared to placebo (Zacny and Gutierrez 2011).

11.3.4 Stimulants

Among the drugs with stimulating CNS effects are amphetamine, methamphetamine, MDMA, cocaine, and methylphenidate. These drugs are widely used as recreational drugs and sometimes for therapeutic purposes. We have included 19 studies on the acute effects of stimulants that met the inclusion criteria in this review (see also Table 11.1).

Bosker et al. tested three acute doses of MDMA (25, 50, and 100 mg) in recreational MDMA users (Bosker et al. 2012). In general, MDMA did not affect any of the driving measures of actual driving nor did it change the impairing effects due to sleep loss.

Dumont et al. found an increase in psychomotor speed, but not accuracy, after administration of 100 mg MDMA (Dumont et al. 2010). In another study, it was found that saccadic eye movements (a measure for psychomotor speed and sedation), immediate recall, and body sway were impaired after administration of single acute doses of 100 mg MDMA in regular users of ecstasy (Dumont et al. 2011).

Gustavsen et al. found a positive concentration–effect relationship between blood concentrations of amphetamine and/or methamphetamine and clinical impairment as assessed by CTI in drivers suspected of driving under the influence of nonalcoholic drugs (Gustavsen et al. 2006). The relationship reached a ceiling at blood amphetamines concentrations of 270–530 ng/mL. The concentration–effect relationship was apparently less pronounced than previously found in studies regarding benzodiazepines, carisoprodol, codeine, and alcohol. Younger drivers were more often judged impaired than older drivers at similar concentrations.

Hjälmdal et al. studied simulated driving performance and found few significant results, showing both improved and worsened driving performance, after administering 10 or 40 mg of *d*-amphetamine to healthy volunteers (Hjälmdahl et al. 2012). The low dose led to improved driving performance for three out of the five primary indicators measured. The positive effects of the low dose were not further improved or even sustained by increasing the dose, which might indicate that at still higher doses there are few or no positive effects of *d*-amphetamine. The data did not show any evidence that taking *d*-amphetamine prevented the subjects from becoming successively sleepier during the night, suggesting that the drug does not compensate for impairment of driving due to fatigue.

Jones did not find any correlation between blood amphetamine concentration and results of clinical tests of impairment in apprehended drivers (Jones 2007).

Kirkpatrick et al. administered 20 and 40 mg methamphetamine and found that performance on tasks measuring response time and vigilance were improved by the 40 mg methamphetamine dose (Kirkpatrick et al. 2012b). They also found that 100 mg MDMA had no effect on performance.

Kirkpatrick et al. found in another study that 10 mg methamphetamine did not have acute nor residual cognitive or psychomotor effects (Kirkpatrick et al. 2012a).

Kuypers et al. found that MDMA (75 and 100 mg) reduced SDLP and standard deviation of speed in actual driving (Kuypers et al. 2006).

Ramaekers et al. tested actual driving and concluded that 75 mg MDMA may improve performance in certain aspects of the driving task, such as road-tracking performance (SDLP), but cause impairment in other aspects, such as accuracy and speed adaption during car-following performance (Ramaekers et al. 2006). In the same study it was found that 20 mg methylphenidate improved tracking performance as indicated by a significant decrease in SDLP.

Silber et al. have studied simulated driving performance following amphetamine or methamphetamine administration in several studies (Silber et al. 2005a, 2006, 2012a, 2012b). The studies provide evidence of low-level amphetamine-related enhancement of function (Silber et al. 2006), but no significant (overall) effect on simulated driving performance (Silber et al. 2012a, 2012b) and a decrease in overall simulated driving ability following amphetamine administration (Silber et al. 2005a) at the same dosages (0.42 mg/kg). The authors concluded that the results shed little light as to how amphetamine may contribute to driving fatalities as there were no direct demonstrations of amphetamine-related impairments (Silber et al. 2006). It is worth mentioning that the studies performed by Silber et al. are all describing the acute effects of amphetamine and methamphetamine after intake of single and relatively low (therapeutic) doses, in contrast to a realistic setting with binge or intensive use and higher doses.

Another simulated driving study, performed by Simons et al., showed that 10 mg dexamphetamine alone caused the least number of collisions and less passing of red traffic lights, and the best performance on divided attention and vigilance tasks, as compared to alcohol (BAC 0.64–0.91 g/L) or a combination of the two substances (Simons et al. 2012).

A simulator study by Stough et al. showed that overall impairment scores for driving and signaling were worse in the methamphetamine condition (0.42 mg/kg) compared to placebo, but this difference was not significant (Stough et al. 2012a). They also found that the overall impairment scores for driving and signaling were worse in the MDMA condition compared to both the placebo and methamphetamine conditions.

Stough et al. found more accurate performance on a choice reaction task in the methamphetamine condition (0.42 mg/kg) compared to placebo, whereas impairment of working memory was observed (Stough et al. 2012b). They also found poorer performance in the MDMA condition at peak concentration for the trail-making measures, and a trend level of working memory, as compared to the placebo condition.

Van Wel et al. found that single doses of cocaine improved psychomotor function and decreased response time in impulsivity tasks, but increased errors, in heavy cannabis users (Van Wel et al. 2013).

Veldstra et al. tested driving performance and traffic safety by means of a driving simulator after administration of 100 mg MDMA (Veldstra et al. 2012). The study showed that simulated driving, including SDLP, improved under the MDMA condition compared to both placebo and alcohol.

11.3.5 GHB

GHB is a potent sedative and anxiolytic drug with additional euphoric effects. In addition to being prescribed to patients with narcolepsy and its previous use as an anesthetic, GHB is a popular recreational drug of abuse (Drasbek et al. 2006; Nicholson and Balster 2001). It has a substantial risk of acute toxicity after overdose (Gable 2004; King and Nutt 2007). Drivers apprehended by the police for suspicion of DUI testing positive for GHB show signs of sedation as well as agitation, impaired balance, nystagmus, and irrational behavior (Al-Samarraie et al. 2010; Bosman and Lusthof 2003; Jones et al. 2008). We have included four studies on acute effects of GHB that met the inclusion criteria in this review (see also Table 11.1).

Abanades et al. tested a psychomotor performance battery. Two different doses of GHB were administered (40 and 60 mg/kg), and the negative effects of GHB were dose-dependent and peaked 1 hour after its administration (Abanades et al. 2007).

Al-Samarraie et al. investigated the possible relationship between GHB blood concentrations and clinical effects in car drivers (Al-Samarraie et al. 2010). During an 8-year period, 25 car drivers who had tested positive for only GHB in their blood were identified among drivers suspected of drugged driving. The median blood GHB concentration was 131 μg/mL, which is quite high, and CTI results indicated impairment that depressed central nervous system activity. The effect of GHB on the degree of impairment and consciousness tended to be concentration-dependent, and the number of drivers who were impaired or had reduced consciousness was highly increased in GHB drivers compared to controls.

Ferrara et al. administered two therapeutic doses of GHB (12.5 and 25 mg/kg) and found that performance after both doses was not different from placebo (Ferrara et al. 1999). Psychomotor performance was measured using tests of attention, vigilance, alertness, short-term memory, and psychomotor coordination.

Johnson and Griffiths reported that GHB (1–10 g/70 kg) caused significant decreases in performance on all cognitive and motor tasks tested, with peak effects at 60 minutes (Johnson and Griffiths 2013). Dose-related effects were observed.

11.3.6 Ketamine

Ketamine is used therapeutically to induce anesthesia prior to the administration of a general anesthetic or for brief surgical procedures (Carter et al. 2013). Ketamine is also used recreationally for its mood-altering properties. The misuse of ketamine as a recreational drug has increased remarkably over the last decade (Giorgetti et al. 2015). We have included two studies on acute effects of ketamine that met the inclusion criteria in this review (see also Table 11.1).

Carter et al. found that 0.2 and 0.4 mg ketamine administered intramuscular impaired several of the psychomotor and cognitive tasks measured (i.e., balance, circular lights, digit symbol substitution task, divided attention task, and episodic and working memory), and the results suggest that the impairing effects of ketamine are more closely related to its dissociative effects as opposed to its sedative effects (Carter et al. 2013).

Krystal et al. assessed a spectrum of behaviors associated with frontal cortex functionality (e.g., vigilance to visual stimuli, distractibility, verbal fluency, abstraction, and the Wisconsin Card Sorting Test) as well as memory and psychomotor function after administration of a bolus of 0.26 mg/kg followed by a 1-hour infusion of 0.65 mg/kg ketamine (Krystal et al. 1998). Ketamine impaired six out of seven functions measured; one of the tests also showed dose-dependent impairment.

11.3.7 Antihistamines and Antidepressants

We did not find any studies that complied with our inclusion criteria.

11.4 Discussion

A large number of experimental studies have been performed. We have made literature searches with rather limiting inclusion criteria; therefore, a number of studies that did not comply with our criteria have not been taken into consideration in this review. Making limitations based on a judgment of quality in the way we have done in this review makes it easier to select the most relevant studies, but also implies a risk of leaving out studies of importance.

Publication bias is a well-known problem with regard to experimental studies. Researchers and journals might not want to publish null results; consequently, it is more likely that positive findings are published. This would further influence the results of systematic literature reviews and meta-analysis.

Only publications in English have been included. Relevant studies might have been lost due to this limitation. Experimental studies published before 1998 were also not included in this review since they have been discussed in a previous review on publications published before 1998 (see Chapter 10).

11.4.1 Benzodiazepines and Related Drugs

11.4.1.1 Impairing Effects of a Single Dose

All of the studies on acute effects, except one, found that the different benzodiazepines and benzodiazepine-like drugs cause some degree of impairment (Abanades et al. 2007; Bocca et al. 2011; Carter et al. 2013; Ferrara et al. 1999; Gustavsen et al. 2011, 2012;

Leufkens and Vermeeren 2009; Leufkens et al. 2007; Mattila et al. 1998; Vanakoski et al. 2000; Vermeeren et al. 2002; Verster et al. 2002a, 2002b; Zacny and Gutierrez 2003). Only one study on acute effects reported that a benzodiazepine (flunitrazepam, 1 mg) did not cause impairment, as assessed by a driving simulator test performed 10 hours after drug administration (Bocca et al. 2011). The explanation for this could be that the dose administered was not sufficient to impair performance at the time of testing. Also, previous reviews (Couper and Logan 2014; Drummer 2002; Verster et al. 2004; Verstraete et al. 2014) and meta-analysis (Roth et al. 2014) have concluded that benzodiazepines can impair skills relevant to safe driving. In general, these papers reported that therapeutic doses of long-acting benzodiazepines, such as diazepam and flunitrazepam, can impair skills relevant to safe driving, whereas shorter-acting benzodiazepines, such as oxazepam, show little or no significant adverse effects on psychomotor performance. Benzodiazepine-like drugs, such as zopiclone, zolpidem, and zaleplon, can also cause significant effects on driving. The duration of action of benzodiazepines is largely dependent on their pharmacokinetic half-lives. Data demonstrating impairing effects on driving-related skills will therefore depend critically on the time of testing in relation to time of administration (Drummer 2002).

11.4.1.2 Dose/Blood Concentration–Effect Relationship

A positive concentration–effect relationship was found for zopiclone with respect to automotive and control behaviors (Gustavsen et al. 2012).

Semi-experimental studies demonstrated a concentration–effect relationship for benzodiazepines among persons suspected of drugged driving (Bramness et al. 2002, 2003), but no such effect was found for zopiclone and zolpidem (Gustavsen et al. 2009).

Dose-dependent performance impairment has been described for hypnotics (Verster et al. 2004). A meta-analysis concentration of several benzodiazepines that produced impairment equivalent to a BAC of 0.5 g/L has been determined (Berghaus et al. 2011). Berghaus et al. performed, as part of the European DRUID (Driving Under the Influence of Drugs, Alcohol and Medicines) project, a meta-analysis of studies measuring acute effects after intake of several benzodiazepines as well as z-hypnotics. For example, experimental studies with single administration of diazepam doses between 5 and 40 mg to healthy volunteers were included. Curves showing time- and concentration-dependent impairment were calculated. It was established that a BAC of 0.5 g/L caused impairment in 30% of the tests, and the same percentage of impaired tests was seen at a diazepam concentration of 320 ng/mL in plasma (i.e., about 179 ng/mL blood). A dose/concentration–effect relationship was found for diazepam. The equivalents to a BAC of 0.5 g/L for the other benzodiazepines and z-hypnotics were, in plasma (blood), as follows: alprazolam 9(7.3) ng/mL, checked doses 0.25–2.0 mg; flunitrazepam 5.4(4) ng/mL, checked doses 0.5–4.0 mg; lorazepam 9 ng/mL, checked doses 0.5–9.0 mg; nitrazepam not calculable due to different impairment profiles dependent on time of administration; oxazepam 330 (300) ng/mL, checked doses 10–90 mg; triazolam 1.6 (1) ng/mL, checked doses 0.125–3.0 mg; zopiclone 26 (23) ng/mL, checked doses 2.5–10 mg; zolpidem 71 (50) ng/mL, checked doses 5–20 mg. Furthermore, an expert panel proposed concentrations for several benzodiazepines in blood that were equivalent to a BAC of 0.5 g/L with respect to psychomotor impairment: alprazolam 6 ng/mL; diazepam 143 ng/mL; flunitrazepam 3 ng/mL; nitrazepam 42 ng/mL; oxazepam 430 ng/mL; zolpidem 77 ng/mL; and zopiclone 23 ng/mL (Vindenes et al. 2012).

11.4.1.3 Tolerance

Acute tolerance to the effects of zopiclone was demonstrated as blood concentrations measured less than 1 hour after intake were more often accompanied by impairment than the same blood drug concentration at a later point of time (Gustavsen et al. 2011).

It has been postulated that the phenomenon of acute tolerance can be predicted at a population level, but not for individuals (dos Santos et al. 2009). Previous studies have shown that regular users will develop tolerance to most of the adverse effects of benzodiazepines (Drummer 2002). A meta-analysis concluded that moderate-to-large weighted effect sizes were found for all cognitive domains suggesting that long-term benzodiazepine users were significantly impaired in all of the areas that were assessed as compared to controls (Barker et al. 2004a). Results of meta-analyses also indicated that long-term benzodiazepine users showed recovery of function in many areas after withdrawal, although there may have been some permanent deficits or deficits that took longer than six months to completely recover (Barker et al. 2004b). It has been described that impairment was most pronounced after treatment initiation, typically after one or two nights of administration (Verster et al. 2004).

11.4.1.4 Interaction with Alcohol

None of the studies included in this review evaluated interaction with alcohol.

In general, an increased impairment of psychomotor and other driving skills has been observed when alcohol was administered to subjects who already had consumed benzodiazepines, especially during the first days to weeks of treatment with these drugs (Drummer 2002). It has been described that the combination of alcohol and temazepam, lorazepam, or triazolam caused clear impairment (Verstraete et al. 2014).

11.4.1.5 Comparison with Findings in Epidemiological Studies

Most epidemiological studies found an association between the use of benzodiazepines or z-hypnotics and increased crash risk (see Chapter 12). The reviewed experimental studies are on line with the epidemiological studies indicating that a significant risk of road traffic crash (RTC) involvement is present among users of benzodiazepines/z-hypnotics.

11.4.2 Cannabis

11.4.2.1 Impairing Effect of a Single Dose

Most of the studies included in this review found that cannabis affected driving ability in regular (Downey et al. 2013; Lenne et al. 2010; Ramaekers et al. 2000; Ronen et al. 2008, 2010; Van Wel et al. 2013) and nonregular (Downey et al. 2013; Lenne et al. 2010) users. All of these studies, but one (Van Wel et al. 2013), investigated the effects of THC on actual driving or simulated driving. Dumont et al. found that THC induced cognitive impairment but had no significant effect on eye movements (Dumont et al. 2011). Ramaekers et al. found that a high dose of THC of about 28 mg generally did not affect performance tests (i.e., the critical tracking test, the stop-signal task, and the Tower of London test) in heavy cannabis users (Ramaekers et al. 2011). The divided attention task was, however, affected by THC, indicating that the sensitivity to different tests can vary.

It has been stated that results from experimental studies clearly indicated that cannabis use can have a detrimental impact on driving ability, as it impaired some cognitive and psychomotor skills that are necessary for driving (Verstraete et al. 2014). A review of experimental studies concluded that performance of complex tasks deteriorates after smoking cannabis (Hartman and Huestis 2013). Another review concluded that there was strong evidence from performance studies that THC had significant effects on the cognitive and psychomotor tasks associated with driving, but that it could still be debated whether these effects increased RTC risk (Huestis 2002).

11.4.2.2 Dose/Blood Concentration–Effect Relationship

Dose-related impairment was observed in both inexperienced (Lenne et al. 2010) and experienced drivers (Lenne et al. 2010; Ramaekers et al. 2000; Ronen et al. 2008), as tested in simulated driving (Lenne et al. 2010; Ronen et al. 2008) and actual driving (Ramaekers et al. 2000).

Semi-experimental studies revealed a positive relationship between the blood THC concentration and the number of persons classified as impaired by a CTI (Khiabani et al. 2006). Similarly, Papafotiou et al. found a positive correlation between the dose of THC administered and the impairment found when using standardized field sobriety tests (Papafotiou et al. 2005). It is worth mentioning that a time lag between intake of cannabis and blood sampling would not obscure the relationship between blood THC concentration and clinical outcome as long as the blood sample is collected at the same time as CTI is performed.

The US National Highway Traffic Safety Administration (NHTSA) expert panel (Couper and Logan 2014) assessed the driving risks after use of cannabis and stated that the use of low doses caused moderate impairment, whereas severe impairment was seen after high doses and chronic use. Previously, it has been found that blood concentrations of THC were not closely related to the degree of impairment (Robbe 1998). An international working group of experts evaluated possible approaches to developing *per se* limits for driving under the influence of cannabis (Grotenhermen et al. 2007) and concluded that epidemiological studies indicated that serum concentrations of THC below 10 ng/mL (i.e., about 5 ng/mL blood) were not associated with an elevated RTC risk, and experimental studies on driving-related skills suggested that a THC concentration of 7–10 ng/mL in serum (i.e., about 3.5–5 ng/mL blood) was associated with impairment equivalent to a BAC of 0.5 g/L. A meta-analysis calculated that a 0.5 g/L alcohol equivalent was around 3.8 ng/mL THC in plasma (i.e., about 2 ng/mL blood) with respect to impairment, but it was stated that there was a considerable variation (Berghaus et al. 2011). An expert panel proposed that a THC concentration in blood of 3.0 ng/mL is equivalent to a BAC of 0.5 g/L with respect to impairment (Vindenes et al. 2012).

11.4.2.3 Tolerance

A study on neurocognitive task performance generally demonstrated that heavy cannabis users developed tolerance to the impairing effects of THC, but not cross-tolerance to the impairing effects of alcohol (Ramaekers et al. 2011). The study describes that tolerance was not apparent in all performance tasks, which could explain that some studies, on the other hand, have reported that heavy users showed impaired psychomotor performance (Van Wel et al. 2013), and experienced cannabis users made more driving errors than nonregular users (Downey et al. 2013). It has also been suggested that drivers might be able to compensate for the effects of cannabis by, for example, driving at slower speeds (Lenne et al. 2010).

Neurocognitive performance has been tested in occasional and heavy users, and it was observed that THC affected performance in more tasks in occasional users than in heavy users (Ramaekers et al. 2009). Cannabis smoking impaired psychomotor function significantly more in occasional users than in frequent users (Desrosiers et al. 2015).

11.4.2.4 Interaction with Alcohol

Some studies found that the combination of THC and alcohol produced synergistic effects (Downey et al. 2013; Ramaekers et al. 2000; Ronen et al. 2010), whereas one study found that alcohol did not produce synergistic effects when combined with cannabis (Lenne et al. 2010). The latter study also described that alcohol alone, at the doses used (0.4 and 0.6 g/kg), had few effects on simulated driving, indicating rather low sensitivity of the test, at least to the acute effects of alcohol, which could explain the lack of synergistic effects. Additive and synergistic effects of alcohol and THC were shown in heavy cannabis users (Ramaekers et al. 2011).

Additive effects of THC and alcohol on driving performance have been observed by others (Lamers and Ramaekers 2001; Robbe 1998; Sexton et al. 2002). Additive effects were reported in occasional cannabis users (Ramaekers et al. 2004). Verstraete et al. concluded that combining alcohol and marijuana would eliminate the ability that marijuana users may have to effectively compensate for some impairing effects while driving by using different behavioral strategies (Verstraete et al. 2014). On the other hand, some studies found that the combination of cannabis and alcohol did not produce different effects on performance than when each drug was tested individually (Lamers and Ramaekers 2001; Liguori et al. 2002).

It has been shown that co-administration of alcohol and cannabis gave significantly increased blood THC concentrations compared to cannabis alone (Downey et al. 2013; Hartman et al. 2015). This might explain increased performance impairment observed from cannabis-alcohol combinations.

11.4.2.5 Comparison with Findings in Epidemiological Studies

Epidemiological studies have reported a significant association between cannabis use and RTCs and injuries (see Chapter 12). Cohort, case-control, and responsibility/case-crossover studies have found a significant association, but some studies also report lack of such association. The reviewed experimental studies are on line with the epidemiological studies indicating that there is an increased risk of RTC in both experienced and inexperienced users of cannabis.

11.4.3 Opioids

11.4.3.1 Impairing Effect of a Single Dose

The studies included in this review found variable results for opioids with respect to impairment. The reason for this could be the sensitivity of the different tests used and/or the sensitivity of the participants to drug-induced effects. Pickering et al. found that 30 mg codeine affected choice reaction time (Pickering et al. 2005), and Amato et al. found that 20 mg codeine impaired SDS (standard deviation of speed) but did not find any effect on SDLP or reaction time after administration of up to 60 mg (Amato et al. 2013). Also, for oxycodone, some studies found that some tests were affected while others were not (Verster et al. 2006; Zacny and Gutierrez 2003), and one study found no effect at all after 10 mg

(Zacny and Gutierrez 2011). Schneider et al. (1999) found significant effects for fentanyl at a dose of 0.2 μg/kg. Strand et al. found significant effects of 0.4 mg buprenorphine on SDLP, and both methadone (5 and 10 mg) and buprenorphine (0.2 and 0.4 mg) produced impairment of neurocognitive tasks (Strand et al. 2019).

The NHTSA expert panel concluded that morphine can severely impair driving skills if used in acute situations or taken illicitly (Couper and Logan 2014). A review of the literature on acute effects after administration of single doses of morphine to healthy, opioid-naïve subjects concluded that blood morphine concentrations below 14.3 ng/mL were probably accompanied by few effects in traffic-relevant performance tasks (Strand et al. 2011). Verstraete et al. summarized the acute effects of morphine, fentanyl, methadone, buprenorphine, and codeine as investigated in experimental studies, and concluded that opioids may cause some cognitive and psychomotor impairment (Verstraete et al. 2014). These effects are highly dependent on the type of opioid at issue and the dose administered, and are mostly moderate. Stout and Farrell summarized the literature relating selected opioids to performance, specifically driving (Stout and Farrell 2003). They concluded that opioids appeared to impair psychomotor functioning in such a way that is likely to be important for the performance of complex, divided-attention tasks such as driving, and the impairment was notably more prevalent in individuals with no history of opioid use than individuals with long-term use. A systematic review found that both methadone and buprenorphine were confirmed as having impairing potentials of cognitive and psychomotor functions in opioid-naïve subjects, but not in compliant stable users with tolerance (Strand et al. 2013).

11.4.3.2 Dose/Blood Concentration–Effect Relationship

A dose–response study of codeine found no correlation between concentration and effects (Amato et al. 2013). Dose-dependent effect was observed for SDLP after administration of oxycodone (Verster et al. 2006). Both methadone and buprenorphine produced dose-dependent impairment of neurocognitive tasks (Strand et al. 2019).

A semi-experimental study found that codeine appeared to have some dose-dependent effect on the central nervous system in drivers suspected of drugged driving (Bachs et al. 2003). No correlation was found between methadone blood concentration and impairment as judged by the CTI, neither when detected alone nor in combination with other drugs (Bernard et al. 2009). Concentration-dependent effects for the combination of the heroin metabolites morphine and morphine-6-glucuronide in blood in semi-experimental studies have been observed (Bachs et al. 2006).

11.4.3.3 Tolerance

None of the studies included in this review evaluated tolerance.

A structured evidence-based review has included studies on psychomotor abilities, cognitive function, effect of opioid dosing on psychomotor abilities, motor vehicle driving violations and RTCs, and driving impairment as measured in driving simulators and off/on-road driving (Fishbain et al. 2003). The majority of the reviewed studies appeared to indicate that opioids do not impair driving-related skills in opioid-dependent/tolerant patients. However, impairments of psychomotor and cognitive functions have been observed among both methadone-maintained patients and buprenorphine-maintained patients when compared to control groups (Strand et al.

2013), and a systematic review concluded that it cannot be generalized that patients on stable opioid doses are safe to drive (Mailis-Gagnon et al. 2012). Studies have found that tolerance develops early to the duration and intensity of euphoria after use of morphine (Couper and Logan 2014).

11.4.3.4 Interaction with Alcohol

Oxycodone (10 mg, oral) combined with alcohol (0.3 and 0.6 g/kg) did not affect psychomotor and cognitive performance, possibly due to insensitivity to the tests used or dosages being unable to produce impairment. Oxycodone combined with alcohol did not affect psychomotor and cognitive performance (Zacny and Gutierrez 2011). It was observed that oxycodone decreased the absorption of alcohol (Zacny and Gutierrez 2011). No synergistic effects between alcohol and methadone or buprenorphine as used by maintenance participants were observed in a study of simulated driving (Lenne et al. 2003).

11.4.3.5 Comparison with Findings in Epidemiological Studies

Most epidemiological studies also found statistically significant associations between use of opioids and RTC (see Chapter 12). The reviewed experimental studies, on the other hand, indicate that opioids cause only moderate effects on driving-related performance.

11.4.4 Stimulants

11.4.4.1 Impairing Effect of a Single Dose

Most experimental studies of amphetamine, methamphetamine, and MDMA in doses of up to 40 mg amphetamine, 40 mg methamphetamine, and 100 mg MDMA found no major detrimental effect on psychomotor tests or actual driving (Bosker et al. 2012; Kirkpatrick et al. 2012a, 2012b; Silber et al. 2012a, 2012b); some studies found minor improvements (Dumont et al. 2010; Hjälmdahl et al. 2012; Kirkpatrick et al. 2012b; Kuypers et al. 2006; Ramaekers et al. 2006; Silber et al. 2006; Simons et al. 2012; Stough et al. 2012b; Van Wel et al. 2013; Veldstra et al. 2012), and some studies found some negative effects (Dumont et al. 2011; Hjälmdahl et al. 2012; Ramaekers et al. 2006; Silber et al. 2005a; Stough et al. 2012a, 2012b; Van Wel et al. 2013).

As part of the European DRUID project, a meta-analysis of studies measuring effects after intake of amphetamine and cocaine, and a review of results from studies on MDMA, was performed (Berghaus et al. 2011). Doses up to 36 mg *d*-amphetamine were administered, and while some improvement was observed, none of the effects measured were impaired. The same results were found for the effects after cocaine administration in doses up to 210 mg. MDMA had primarily no risk potential on driver fitness, as tested with doses up to 125 mg of MDMA in experimental studies. Verstraete et al. concluded that acute use of amphetamine and methamphetamine can have positive effects, as well as negative effects, on cognitive and psychomotor skills (Verstraete et al. 2014). Especially in sleep-deprived or fatigued subjects, stimulants can improve performance. Experimental studies of acute use of MDMA have also found both negative and positive effects on performance. A review of the effects of methamphetamine on human performance and behavior concluded that anything other than therapeutic administration of low-dose methamphetamine was likely to cause some impairment of performance in complex psychomotor tasks such as driving (Logan 2002). A PET scan study found that relatively high doses of amphetamine, presumably at least 1 mg/kg, increased cerebral glucose metabolism and caused signs of mania and thought disorder (Vollenweider et al. 1998).

It can further be noted that amphetamine is administered in daily doses of 5–60 mg for therapeutic use in adults (Baselt 2009), in some cases probably somewhat higher, and doses up to 1 mg/kg body weight are given to voluntary participants in experimental studies (Vollenweider et al. 1998). However, commonly abused doses are reported to be 100–1,000 mg/day, and up to 5,000 mg/day in chronic binge use (Couper and Logan 2014). Controlled experimental studies of these high doses cannot be performed for ethical reasons, and therefore higher concentrations of amphetamines are not studied. Large doses of amphetamines may have harmful effects on self-perception, critical judgment, and risk taking, whereas the stimulating effects are disappearing, followed by a period associated with fatigue, anxiety, and irritability (see Chapters 12 and 15). The single, therapeutic doses administered in these experimental studies do not reflect the realistic setting of binging or intensive use of amphetamines.

11.4.4.2 Dose/Blood Concentration–Effect Relationship

Experimental studies have not found any dose–effect relationship. This is probably related to the fact that the doses used in experimental studies are small compared to the doses used by problem amphetamine users (Gustavsen et al. 2006).

Semi-experimental studies have reported divergent results. A positive concentration–effect relationship between blood amphetamines concentrations and clinical impairment as assessed by CTI in drivers suspected of driving under the influence of nonalcoholic drugs was found (Gustavsen et al. 2006). The relationship reached a ceiling at blood amphetamines concentrations of 270–530 ng/mL. On the other hand, no relationship was observed between blood amphetamine concentration and impairment in another study of apprehended drivers (Jones 2007). It was reported that doses of approximately 30 mg amphetamine or methamphetamine did not impair performance on the SFSTs (Silber et al. 2005b). It can be noted that an oral dose of approximately 30 mg amphetamine has been shown to lead to blood concentrations up to approximately 100 ng/mL (Silber et al. 2006). Current methamphetamine users were more likely to speed and weave from side to side, as measured by SDLP, when simulator performance was studied (Bosanquet et al. 2013). The main measures of risky driving were not associated with current methamphetamine, or its main metabolite amphetamine, levels in blood.

The NHTSA expert panel (Couper and Logan 2014) described that lower doses of amphetamines could cause improvement of some psychomotor tasks and otherwise had few effects on cognitive functioning, whereas at higher doses risk-taking increased and responses became inappropriate.

11.4.4.3 Tolerance

The development of tolerance was not investigated in the studies included in this review.

It has been stated that tolerance to the effects of amphetamines may develop (Couper and Logan 2014; Verstraete et al. 2014). Habituation to certain effects can occur within an intake (acute tolerance) so that the sense of intoxication decreases while the substance is still present in the body (Logan 2002). Significant subjective effects have been observed after administering methamphetamine, effects that subsided rapidly and before the concentrations in blood decreased markedly, suggesting development of acute tolerance (Cook et al. 1993). A case series of drivers apprehended for driving under the influence of drugs reported abnormally high concentrations of amphetamine in blood, ranging from 5,000 ng/mL to 17,000 ng/mL (Jones and Holmgren 2005). The authors speculated that these very high concentrations were tolerated without any fatalities due to a pronounced adaption to the pharmacological effects of this drug.

Chronic tolerance to Ecstasy/MDMA in humans has been observed, and many recreational users reported reduced subjective efficacy with repeated drug use, together with dosage escalation, and bingeing (Parrott 2005).

11.4.4.4 Interaction with Alcohol

It was stated that oral methamphetamine combined with alcohol produced a profile of effects that was different from either drug alone (Kirkpatrick et al. 2012a). Methamphetamine attenuated alcohol-related performance decrements as participants performed worse on measures of divided attention and vigilance following administration of alcohol alone. The combination of dexamphetamine and alcohol was associated with a higher frequency of red-light running and collisions than the dexamphetamine or placebo conditions in simulated driving (Simons et al. 2012). The risk scenarios and measures employed in the study were very sensitive to both alcohol and the combination treatment. The impairing effects of alcohol on skills related to driving were not improved by the stimulatory effects of co-administration of 10 mg dexamphetamine.

A driving study found that MDMA moderated alcohol-induced impairment of road tracking performance (SDLP), but did not affect alcohol impairments of car-following and laboratory task performance (Kuypers et al. 2006), whereas another study did not find a significant effect on driving performance (e.g., SDLP) when combining the two drugs (Veldstra et al. 2012). Equivalence testing in the latter showed that combined use may lead to impaired driving for some, but not all, drivers. Co-administration of MDMA and alcohol improved psychomotor speed, but impaired psychomotor accuracy, compared with placebo and also reversed alcohol-induced sedation (Dumont et al. 2010).

The combination of MDMA and alcohol has been shown to cause subjects to feel euphoric and less sedated and might have the feeling of doing better, but actual performance ability continued to be impaired by the effect of alcohol (Hernandez-Lopez et al. 2002).

Plasma concentrations of MDMA have shown a 13% increase after the use of alcohol, whereas plasma concentrations of alcohol have shown a 9%–15% decrease after MDMA administration (Hernandez-Lopez et al. 2002).

11.4.4.5 Comparison with Findings in Epidemiological Studies

Epidemiological studies reported a clear association between use of amphetamines and cocaine and increased RTC risk (see Chapter 12). After alcohol, amphetamines were found to be the substances associated with the highest RTC risk. It is likely that problematic amphetamine users and addicts constitute a larger traffic safety problem than drivers that occasionally are taking small doses of amphetamines to stay awake and alert during long journeys. The general lack of findings in controlled experimental studies reviewed in this review is not at odds with epidemiological findings that the use of amphetamines and cocaine, at least in higher doses, is associated with a significant RTC risk.

11.4.5 GHB

Abanades et al. and Johnson and Griffiths found dose-dependent effects on cognitive and psychomotor performance (Abanades et al. 2007; Johnson and Griffiths 2013), whereas Ferrara et al., who administered markedly lower doses of GHB than did the other two studies, found that psychomotor performance did not differ from placebo (Ferrara et al. 1999). On the other hand, Ferrara et al. tested performance in healthy volunteers, whereas Abanades et al. and Johnson and Griffiths tested subjects who were recreational users of GHB or had a history of sedative abuse, respectively.

A semi-experimental study found that the effect of GHB on the degree of impairment and consciousness tended to be concentration-dependent and the number of drivers who were impaired or had reduced consciousness was highly increased in GHB drivers compared to controls (Al-Samarraie et al. 2010).

The NHTSA expert panel concluded that recreational use of GHB has the potential to produce moderate to severe driving impairment due to its ability to induce sleep and unconsciousness (Couper and Logan 2014). It was reported that tolerance can develop to GHB with chronic abuse, although tolerance does not develop to all effects of GHB, like enhanced sleep. Cross-tolerance exists between GHB and alcohol. Dose-dependent cognitive and psychomotor impairment after acute use of GHB after doses typically consumed by users has been described (Verstraete et al. 2014). Furthermore, it was found that there were additive, but not synergetic, effects of GHB and alcohol on cognitive impairment.

11.4.6 Ketamine

Both studies included in this review found that ketamine impaired cognitive and psychomotor tasks related to driving (Carter et al. 2013; Krystal et al. 1998); one test showed dose-dependent impairment (Krystal et al. 1998).

A systematic review on the effects of ketamine on psychomotor, cognitive, visual, and perceptual functions related to safe driving using wider inclusion criteria has been published (Giorgetti et al. 2015). The authors concluded that significant impairment in multiple functional domains essential to driving has been described and could reasonably warrant an increased risk of dangerous driving under the influence of ketamine.

The NHTSA expert panel concluded that ketamine can cause moderate to severe psychomotor, cognitive, and residual effects on driving skills (Couper and Logan 2014). The expert panel stated that the use of ketamine therefore was not compatible with safe driving. As to tolerance, high tolerance was described after long-term exposure.

11.4.7 Antihistamines and Antidepressants

We did not find any studies that complied with our inclusion criteria, but some recent review articles have dealt with this topic (Berghaus et al. 2011; Ramaekers 2003; Veldhuijzen et al. 2006; Verster et al. 2002; Verster and Volkerts 2004).

11.5 Conclusions

Benzodiazepines and Related Drugs: The evidence from the experimental studies reviewed, as well as other reviews and meta-analyses, indicate that all benzodiazepines studied have impairing effects that are dose-related. Tolerance to these effects has only to a limited extent been studied in the experimental reports reviewed. Moderate but incomplete tolerance was suggested in a meta-analysis. Synergistic interaction with alcohol was shown in some studies, in accordance with several review articles.

Cannabis: The reviewed studies revealed that cannabis can cause dose-dependent impairment of driving skills in both experienced and inexperienced users. Tolerance may develop to many of the effects of cannabis. Additive effects of THC and alcohol have been reported, while other studies found that the combination did not produce such effects.

Opioids: The studies showed that opioids can have some impairing effects on cognitive and psychomotor performance, but the effects seem moderate with dose relation only for some opioids. Tolerance to these effects can develop in chronic opioid users. Synergistic effects between opioids and alcohol have not been shown.

Stimulants: In experimental studies where doses up to 40 mg of amphetamine were administered, both improvement and impairment on performance have been observed, as well as no effects. However, there are indications that higher doses may impair traffic-related skills. Tolerance has been reported for amphetamines and MDMA. The effects of combining amphetamines and alcohol in experimental studies are variable.

GHB: Experimental studies have reported dose-dependent cognitive and psychomotor impairment after use of GHB.

Ketamine: Experimental studies reported cognitive and psychomotor impairment after use of ketamine, and dose-dependent impairment was described.

References

Abanades S, Farre M, Barral D, Torrens M, Closas N, Langohr K, Pastor A, de la Torre R: Relative abuse liability of gamma-hydroxybutyric acid, flunitrazepam, and ethanol in club drug users; *J Clin Psychopharmacol* 27: 625; 2007.

Al-Samarraie MS, Karinen R, Mørland J, Stokke Opdal M: Blood GHB concentrations and results of medical examinations in 25 car drivers in Norway; *Eur J Clin Pharmacol* 66:987; 2010.

Amato JN, Marie S, Lelong-Boulouard V, Paillet-Loilier M, Berthelon C, Coquerel A, Denise P, Bocca ML: Effects of three therapeutic doses of codeine/paracetamol on driving performance, a psychomotor vigilance test, and subjective feelings; *Psychopharmacology (Berl)* 228:309; 2013.

Bachs L, Hoiseth G, Skurtveit S, Mørland J: Heroin-using drivers: Importance of morphine and morphine-6-glucuronide on late clinical impairment; *Eur J Clin Pharmacol* 62:905; 2006.

Bachs L, Skurtveit S, Mørland J: Codeine and clinical impairment in samples in which morphine is not detected; *Eur J Clin Pharmacol* 58:785; 2003.

Barker MJ, Greenwood KM, Jackson M, Crowe SF: Cognitive effects of long-term benzodiazepine use: A meta-analysis; *CNS Drugs* 18:37; 2004a.

Barker MJ, Greenwood KM, Jackson M, Crowe SF: Persistence of cognitive effects after withdrawal from long-term benzodiazepine use: A meta-analysis; *Arch Clin Neuropsychol* 19:437; 2004b.

Barkley RA, Murphy KR, O'Connell T, Connor DF: Effects of two doses of methylphenidate on simulator driving performance in adults with attention deficit hyperactivity disorder; *J Safety Res* 36:121; 2005.

Baselt RC: *Disposition of Toxic Drugs and Chemicals in Man*, 8th ed; Biomedical Publications: Foster City, CA; 2009.

Berghaus G, Sticht G, Grellner W, Lenz D, Naumann T, Wiesenmüller S: *Meta-analysis of Empirical Studies Concerning the Effects of Medicines and Illegal Drugs Including Pharmacokinetics on Safe Driving* (DRUID Deliverable 1.1.2b); University of Würzburg: Würzburg, Germany; 2011.

Bernard JP, Mørland J, Krogh M, Khiabani HZ: Methadone and impairment in apprehended drivers; *Addiction* 104:457; 2009.

Bocca ML, Marie S, Lelong-Boulouard V, Bertran F, Couque C, Desfemmes T, Berthelon C, Amato JN, Moessinger M, Paillet-Loilier M, et al.: Zolpidem and zopiclone impair similarly monotonous driving performance after a single nighttime intake in aged subjects; *Psychopharmacology* (Berl) 214:699; 2011.

Bosanquet D, Macdougall HG, Rogers SJ, Starmer GA, McKetin R, Blaszczynski A, McGregor IS: Driving on ice: Impaired driving skills in current methamphetamine users; *Psychopharmacology* (Berl) 225:161; 2013.

Bosker WM, Kuypers KP, Conen S, Kauert GF, Toennes SW, Skopp G, Ramaekers JG: MDMA (ecstasy) effects on actual driving performance before and after sleep deprivation, as function of dose and concentration in blood and oral fluid; *Psychopharmacology (Berl)* 222:367; 2012.

Bosman IJ, Lusthof KJ: Forensic cases involving the use of GHB in The Netherlands; *Forensic Sci Int* 133:17; 2003.

Bramness JG, Khiabani HZ, Mørland J: Impairment due to cannabis and ethanol: Clinical signs and additive effects; *Addiction* 105:1080; 2010.

Bramness JG, Skurtveit S, Mørland J: Clinical impairment of benzodiazepines—Relation between benzodiazepine concentrations and impairment in apprehended drivers; *Drug Alcohol Depend* 68:131; 2002.

Bramness JG, Skurtveit S, Mørland J: Testing for benzodiazepine inebriation—Relationship between benzodiazepine concentration and simple clinical tests for impairment in a sample of drugged drivers; *Eur J Clin Pharmacol* 59:593; 2003.

Bramness JG, Skurtveit S, Mørland J: Flunitrazepam: Psychomotor impairment, agitation and paradoxical reactions; *Forensic Sci Int* 159:83; 2006.

Carter LP, Kleykamp BA, Griffiths RR, Mintzer MZ: Cognitive effects of intramuscular ketamine and oral triazolam in healthy volunteers; *Psychopharmacology* (Berl) 226:53; 2013.

Cook CE, Jeffcoat AR, Hill JM, Pugh DE, Patetta PK, Sadler BM, White WR, Perez-Reyes M: Pharmacokinetics of methamphetamine self-administered to human subjects by smoking S-(+)-methamphetamine hydrochloride; *Drug Metab Dispos* 21:717; 1993.

Couper FJ, Logan BK: *Drugs and Human Performance Fact Sheets* (DOT HS 809 725); US National Highway Traffic Safety Administration: Washington, DC; 2014.

Desrosiers NA, Ramaekers JG, Chauchard E, Gorelick DA, Huestis MA: Smoked cannabis' psychomotor and neurocognitive effects in occasional and frequent smokers; *J Anal Toxicol* 39:251; 2015.

Dos Santos FM, Goncalves JC, Caminha R, da Silveira GE, Neves CS, Gram KR, Ferreira CT, Jacqmin P, Noel F: Pharmacokinetic/pharmacodynamic modeling of psychomotor impairment induced by oral clonazepam in healthy volunteers; *Ther Drug Monit* 31:566; 2009.

Downey LA, King R, Papafotiou K, Swann P, Ogden E, Boorman M, Stough C: The effects of cannabis and alcohol on simulated driving: Influences of dose and experience; *Accid Anal Prev* 50:879; 2013.

Drasbek KR, Christensen J, Jensen K: Gamma-hydroxybutyrate—A drug of abuse; *Acta Neurol Scand* 114:145; 2006.

Drummer OH: Benzodiazepines—Effects on human performance and behavior; *Forensic Sci Rev* 14:14; 2002.

Dumont GJ, Schoemaker RC, Touw DJ, Sweep FC, Buitelaar JK, van Gerven JM, Verkes RJ: Acute psychomotor effects of MDMA and ethanol (co-) administration over time in healthy volunteers; *J Psychopharmacol* 24:155; 2010.

Dumont GJH, van Hasselt JGC, de Kam M, van Gerven JMA, Touw DJ, Buitelaar JK, Verkes RJ: Acute psychomotor, memory and subjective effects of MDMA and THC co-administration over time in healthy volunteers; *J Psychopharmacol* 25: 478; 2011.

Ferrara SD, Giorgetti R, Zancaner S, Orlando R, Tagliabracci A, Cavarzeran F, Palatini P: Effects of single dose of gamma-hydroxybutyric acid and lorazepam on psychomotor performance and subjective feelings in healthy volunteers; *Eur J Clin Pharmacol* 54:821; 1999.

Fishbain DA, Cutler RB, Rosomoff HL, Rosomoff RS: Are opioid-dependent/tolerant patients impaired in driving-related skills? A structured evidence-based review; *J Pain Symptom Manage* 25:559; 2003.

Gable RS: Comparison of acute lethal toxicity of commonly abused psychoactive substances; *Addiction* 99:686; 2004.

Giorgetti R, Marcotulli D, Tagliabracci A, Schifano F: Effects of ketamine on psychomotor, sensory and cognitive functions relevant for driving ability; *Forensic Sci Int* 252:127; 2015.

Grotenhermen F, Leson G, Berghaus G, Drummer OH, Kruger HP, Longo M, Moskowitz H, Perrine B, Ramaekers JG, Smiley A, Tunbridge R: Developing limits for driving under cannabis; *Addiction* 102:1910; 2007.

Gustavsen I, Al-Sammurraie M, Mørland J, Bramness JG: Impairment related to blood drug concentrations of zopiclone and zolpidem compared to alcohol in apprehended drivers; *Accid Anal Prev* 41:462; 2009.

Gustavsen I, Hjelmeland K, Bernard JP, Mørland J: Psychomotor performance after intake of zopiclone compared with intake of ethanol: A randomized, controlled, double-blinded trial; *J Clin Psychopharmacol* 31:481; 2011.

Gustavsen I, Hjelmeland K, Bernard JP, Mørland J: Individual psychomotor impairment in relation to zopiclone and ethanol concentrations in blood—A randomized controlled double-blinded trial; *Addiction* 107:925; 2012.

Gustavsen I, Mørland J, Bramness JG: Impairment related to blood amphetamine and/or methamphetamine concentrations in suspected drugged drivers; *Accid Anal Prev* 38:490; 2006.

Hartman RL, Brown TL, Milavetz G, Spurgin A, Gorelick DA, Gaffney G, Huestis MA: Controlled cannabis vaporizer administration: Blood and plasma cannabinoids with and without alcohol; *Clin Chem* 61:850; 2015.

Hartman RL, Huestis MA: Cannabis effects on driving skills; *Clin Chem* 59:478; 2013.

Helland A, Jenssen GD, Lervag LE, Moen T, Engen T, Lydersen S, Mørland J, Slørdal L: Evaluation of measures of impairment in real and simulated driving: Results from a randomized, placebo-controlled study; *Traffic Inj Prev* 17:245; 2016.

Helland A, Jenssen GD, Lervåg L-E, Westin AA, Moen T, Sakshaug K, Lydersen S, Mørland J, Slørdal L: Comparison of driving simulator performance with real driving after alcohol intake: A randomised, single blind, placebo-controlled, cross-over trial; *Accid Anal Prev* 53:9; 2013.

Hernandez-Lopez C, Farre M, Roset PN, Menoyo E, Pizarro N, Ortuno J, Torrens M, Cami J, de La Torre R: 3,4-Methylenedioxymethamphetamine (ecstasy) and alcohol interactions in humans: Psychomotor performance, subjective effects, and pharmacokinetics; *J Pharmacol Exp Ther* 300:236; 2002.

Hjälmdahl M, Vadeby A, Forsman A, Fors C, Ceder G, Woxler P, Kronstrand R: Effects of *d*-amphetamine on simulated driving performance before and after sleep deprivation; *Psychopharmacology* (Berl) 222:401; 2012.

Huestis MA: Cannabis (Marijuana)—Effects on human behavior and performance; *Forensic Sci Rev* 14:46; 2002.

Johnson MW, Griffiths RR: Comparative abuse liability of GHB and ethanol in humans; *Exp Clin Psychopharmacol* 21:112; 2013.

Jones AW, Holmgren A, Kugelberg FC: Driving under the influence of gamma-hydroxybutyrate (GHB); *Forensic Sci Med Pathol* 4:205; 2008.

Jones AW, Holmgren A: Abnormally high concentrations of amphetamine in blood of impaired drivers; *J Forensic Sci* 50:1215; 2005.

Jones AW: Age- and gender-related differences in blood amphetamine concentrations in apprehended drivers: Lack of association with clinical evidence of impairment; *Addiction* 102:1085; 2007.

Khiabani HZ, Bramness JG, Bjørneboe A, Mørland J: Relationship between THC concentration in blood and impairment in apprehended drivers; *Traffic Inj Prev* 7:111; 2006.

King LA, Nutt D: Seizures in a night club; *Lancet* 370:220; 2007.

Kirkpatrick MG, Gunderson EW, Levin FR, Foltin RW, Hart CL: Acute and residual interactive effects of repeated administrations of oral methamphetamine and alcohol in humans; *Psychopharmacology (Berl)* 219:191; 2012a.

Kirkpatrick MG, Gunderson EW, Perez AY, Haney M, Foltin RW, Hart CL: A direct comparison of the behavioral and physiological effects of methamphetamine and 3,4-methylenedioxymethamphetamine (MDMA) in humans; *Psychopharmacology* (Berl) 219:109; 2012b.

Krüger H, Hargutt V, Schnabel E, Brookhuis K: *Theoretical Framework for Substance Effects on Safe Driving* (DRUID Deliverable 1.1.1); University of Würzburg: Würzburg, Germany; 2008.

Krystal JH, Karper LP, Bennett A, D'Souza DC, Abi-Dargham A, Morrissey K, Abi-Saab D, Bremner JD, Bowers MB Jr, Suckow RF, et al.: Interactive effects of subanesthetic ketamine and subhypnotic lorazepam in humans; *Psychopharmacology* (Berl) 135:213; 1998.

Kuypers KP, Samyn N, Ramaekers JG: MDMA and alcohol effects, combined and alone, on objective and subjective measures of actual driving performance and psychomotor function; *Psychopharmacology* (Berl) 187:467; 2006.

Lamers CTJ, Ramaekers JG: Visual search and urban city driving under the influence of marijuana and alcohol; *Hum Psychopharm Clin* 16:393; 2001.

Lenne MG, Dietze P, Rumbold GR, Redman JR, Triggs TJ: The effects of the opioid pharmacotherapies methadone, LAAM and buprenorphine, alone and in combination with alcohol, on simulated driving; *Drug Alcohol Depend* 72:271; 2003.

Lenne MG, Dietze PM, Triggs TJ, Walmsley S, Murphy B, Redman JR: The effects of cannabis and alcohol on simulated arterial driving: Influences of driving experience and task demand; *Accid Anal Prev* 42:859; 2010.

Leufkens TRM, Vermeeren A, Smink BE, van Ruitenbeek P, Ramaekers JG: Cognitive, psychomotor and actual driving performance in healthy volunteers after immediate and extended release formulations of alprazolam 1 mg; *Psychopharmacology* (Berl) 191:951; 2007.

Leufkens TRM, Vermeeren A: Highway driving in the elderly the morning after bedtime use of hypnotics—A comparison between temazepam 20 mg, zopiclone 7.5 mg, and placebo; *J Clin Psychopharmacol* 29:432; 2009.

Liguori A, Gatto CP, Jarrett DB: Separate and combined effects of marijuana and alcohol on mood, equilibrium and simulated driving; *Psychopharmacology* (Berl) 163:399; 2002.

Logan B: Methamphetamine—Effects on human performance and behavior; *Forensic Sci Rev* 14:133; 2002.

Louwerens J, Gloerich A, de Vries G, Brookhuis KA, O'Hanlon J: The relationship between drivers' blood alcohol concentration (BAC) and actual driving performance during high speed travel; In: Noordzij PC, Roszbach R (Eds), *Proceedings—10th International Conference on Alcohol, Drugs and Traffic Safety*; Excerpta Medica: Amsterdam, the Netherlands; pp 183–192; 1986.

Mailis-Gagnon A, Lakha SF, Furlan A, Nicholson K, Yegneswaran B, Sabatowski R: Systematic review of the quality and generalizability of studies on the effects of opioids on driving and cognitive/psychomotor performance; *Clin J Pain* 28:542; 2012.

Mattila MJ, Vanakoski J, Kalska H, Seppälä T: Effects of alcohol, zolpidem, and some other sedatives and hypnotics on human performance and memory; *Pharmacol Biochem Behav* 59:917; 1998.

Nicholson KL, Balster RL: GHB: A new and novel drug of abuse; *Drug Alcohol Depend* 63:1; 2001.

O'Hanlon JF, Haak TW, Blaauw GJ, Riemersma JB: Diazepam impairs lateral position control in highway driving; *Science* 217:79; 1982.

Papafotiou K, Carter JD, Stough C: An evaluation of the sensitivity of the standardised field sobriety tests (SFSTs) to detect impairment due to marijuana intoxication; *Psychopharmacology* (Berl) 180:107; 2005.

Parrott AC: Chronic tolerance to recreational MDMA (3,4-methylenedioxymethamphetamine) or ecstasy; *J Psychopharmacol* 19:71; 2005.

Pickering G, Estrade M, Dubray C: Comparative trial of tramadol/paracetamol and codeine/paracetamol combination tablets on the vigilance of healthy volunteers; *Fundam Clin Pharmacol* 19:707; 2005.

Ramaekers JG, Berghaus G, van Laar M, Drummer OH: Dose related risk of motor vehicle crashes after cannabis use; *Drug Alcohol Depend* 73:109; 2004.

Ramaekers JG, Kauert G, Theunissen EL, Toennes SW, Moeller MR: Neurocognitive performance during acute THC intoxication in heavy and occasional cannabis users; *J Psychopharmacol* 23:266; 2009.

Ramaekers JG, Kuypers KP, Samyn N: Stimulant effects of 3,4-methylenedioxymethamphetamine (MDMA) 75 mg and methylphenidate 20 mg on actual driving during intoxication and withdrawal; *Addiction* 101:1614; 2006.

Ramaekers JG, Robbe HWJ, O'Hanlon JF: Marijuana, alcohol and actual driving performance; *Hum Psychopharm Clin* 15:551; 2000.

Ramaekers JG, Theunissen EL, de Brouwer M, Toennes SW, Moeller MR, Kauert G: Tolerance and cross-tolerance to neurocognitive effects of THC and alcohol in heavy cannabis users; *Psychopharmacology* (Berl) 214:391; 2011.

Ramaekers JG: Antidepressants and driver impairment: Empirical evidence from a standard on-the-road test; *J Clin Psychiatr* 64:20; 2003.

Rang HP, Dale MM, Ritter JM, Flower RJ: *Rang and Dale's Pharmacology, 6th edition;* Elsevier Churchill Livingstone: London, UK; 2007.

Robbe H: Marijuana's impairing effects on driving are moderate when taken alone but severe when combined with alcohol; *Hum Psychopharm Clin* 13: S70; 1998.

Ronen A, Chassidim HS, Gershon P, Parmet Y, Rabinovich A, Bar-Hamburger R, Cassuto Y, Shinar D: The effect of alcohol, THC and their combination on perceived effects, willingness to drive and performance of driving and non-driving tasks; *Accid Anal Prev* 42:1855; 2010.

Ronen A, Gershon P, Drobiner H, Rabinovich A, Bar-Hamburger R, Mechoulam R, Cassuto Y, Shinar D: Effects of THC on driving performance, physiological state and subjective feelings relative to alcohol; *Accid Anal Prev* 40:926; 2008.

Roth T, Eklov SD, Drake CL, Verster JC: Meta-analysis of on-the-road experimental studies of hypnotics: Effects of time after intake, dose, and half-life; *Traffic Inj Prev* 15:439; 2014.

Schneider U, Bevilacqua C, Jacobs R, Karst M, Dietrich DE, Becker H, Muller-Vahl KR, Seeland I, Gielsdorf D, Schedlowski M, et al.: Effects of fentanyl and low doses of alcohol on neuropsychological performance in healthy subjects; *Neuropsychobiology* 39:38; 1999.

Sexton B, Tunbridge R, Board A, Jackson P, Wright K, Stark M, Engelhard K: *The Influence of Cannabis and Alcohol on Driving;* Transport Research Laboratory: Crowthorne, UK: 2002.

Silber BY, Croft RJ, Downey LA, Camfield DA, Papafotiou K, Swann P, Stough C: The effect of *d*, *l*-methamphetamine on simulated driving performance; *Psychopharmacology* (Berl) 219:1081; 2012a.

Silber BY, Croft RJ, Downey LA, Papafotiou K, Camfield DA, Stough C: The effect of *d*-methamphetamine on simulated driving performance; *Hum Psychopharm Clin* 27:139; 2012b.

Silber BY, Croft RJ, Papafotiou K, Stough C: The acute effects of *d*-amphetamine and methamphetamine on attention and psychomotor performance; *Psychopharmacology* (Berl) 187:154; 2006.

Silber BY, Papafotiou K, Croft RJ, Ogden E, Swann P, Stough C: The effects of dexamphetamine on simulated driving performance; *Psychopharmacology* (Berl) 179:536; 2005a.

Silber BY, Papafotiou K, Croft RJ, Stough CKK: An evaluation of the sensitivity of the standardised field sobriety tests to detect the presence of amphetamine; *Psychopharmacology* (Berl) 182:153; 2005b.

Simons R, Martens M, Ramaekers J, Krul A, Klopping-Ketelaars I, Skopp G: Effects of dexamphetamine with and without alcohol on simulated driving; *Psychopharmacology* (Berl) 222:391; 2012.

Stough C, Downey LA, King R, Papafotiou K, Swann P, Ogden E: The acute effects of 3,4-methylenedioxymethamphetamine and methamphetamine on driving: A simulator study; *Accid Anal Prev* 45:493; 2012a.

Stough C, King R, Papafotiou K, Swann P, Ogden E, Wesnes K, Downey LA: The acute effects of 3,4-methylenedioxymethamphetamine and *d*-methamphetamine on human cognitive functioning; *Psychopharmacology* (Berl) 220:799; 2012b.

Stout PR, Farrell LJ: Opioids—Effects on human performance and behavior; *Forensic Sci Rev* 15:29; 2003.

Strand MC, Fjeld B, Arnestad M, Mørland J: Can patients receiving opioid maintenance therapy safely drive? A systematic review of epidemiological and experimental studies on driving ability with a focus on concomitant methadone or buprenorphine administration; *Traffic Inj Prev* 14:26; 2013.

Strand MC, Fjeld B, Arnestad M, Mørland J: *Psychomotor Relevant Performance after Administration of Opioids, Narcoanalgesics and Hallucinogens* (DRUID Deliverable 1.1.2c); Norwegian Institute of Public Health: Oslo, Norway; 2011.

Strand MC, Vindenes V, Gjerde H, Mørland JG, Ramaekers JG: A clinical trial on the acute effects of methadone and buprenorphine on actual driving and cognitive function of healthy volunteers; *Br J Clin Pharmacol* 85:442; 2019.

Van Wel JHP, Kuypers KPC, Theunissen EL, Toennes SW, Spronk DB, Verkes RJ, Ramaekers JG: Single doses of THC and cocaine decrease proficiency of impulse control in heavy cannabis users; *Br J Pharmacol* 170:1410; 2013.

Vanakoski J, Mattila MJ, Seppala T: Driving under light and dark conditions: Effects of alcohol and diazepam in young and older subjects; *Eur J Clin Pharmacol* 56:453; 2000.

Veldhuijzen DS, van Wijck AJ, Verster JC, Kenemans JL, Kalkman CJ, Olivier B, Volkerts ER: Acute and subchronic effects of amitriptyline 25 mg on actual driving in chronic neuropathic pain patients; *J Psychopharmacol* 20:782; 2006.

Veldstra JL, Brookhuis KA, de Waard D, Molmans BH, Verstraete AG, Skopp G, Jantos R: Effects of alcohol (BAC 0.5 per thousand) and ecstasy (MDMA 100 mg) on simulated driving performance and traffic safety; *Psychopharmacology* (Berl) 222:377; 2012.

Vermeeren A, Riedel WJ, van Boxtel MPJ, Darwish M, Paty I, Patat A: Differential residual effects of zaleplon and zopiclone on actual driving: A comparison with a low dose of alcohol; *Sleep* 25:224; 2002.

Verster JC, Roth T: Standard operation procedures for conducting the on-the-road driving test, and measurement of the standard deviation of lateral position (SDLP); *Int J Gen Med* 4:359; 2011.

Verster JC, Veldhuijzen DS, Volkerts ER: Effects of an opioid (oxycodone/paracetamol) and an NSAID (bromfenac) on driving ability, memory functioning, psychomotor performance, pupil size, and mood; *Clin J Pain* 22:499; 2006.

Verster JC, Veldhuijzen DS, Volkerts ER: Residual effects of sleep medication on driving ability; *Sleep Med Rev* 8:309; 2004.

Verster JC, Volkerts ER, Schreuder AHCML, Eijken EJE, van Heuckelum JHG, Veldhuijzen DS, Verbaten MN, Paty I, Darwish M, Danjou P, et al. Residual effects of middle-of-the-night administration of zaleplon and zolpidem on driving ability, memory functions, and psychomotor performance; *J Clin Psychopharmacol* 22:576; 2002a.

Verster JC, Volkerts ER, Verbaten MN: Effects of Alprazolam on driving ability memory functioning and psychomotor performance: A randomized, placebo-controlled study; *Neuropsychopharmacol* 27:260; 2002b.

Verster JC, Volkerts ER: Antihistamines and driving ability: Evidence from on-the-road driving studies during normal traffic; *Ann Allergy Asthma Immunol* 92:294; 2004.

Verstraete AG, Legrand S-A, Vandam L, Hughes B, Griffiths P, Drugs EMCf, Addiction D, Portugal: *Drug Use, Impaired Driving and Traffic Accidents;* Publications Office of the European Union: Luxembourg; 2014.

Vindenes V, Jordbru D, Knapskog AB, Kvan E, Mathisrud G, Slørdal L, Mørland J: Impairment based legislative limits for driving under the influence of non-alcohol drugs in Norway; *Forensic Sci Int* 219:1; 2012.

Vollenweider FX, Maguire RP, Leenders KL, Mathys K, Angst J: Effects of high amphetamine dose on mood and cerebral glucose metabolism in normal volunteers using positron emission tomography (PET); *Psychiatry Res Neuroimaging* 83:149; 1998.

Walsh JM, Verstraete AG, Huestis MA, Mørland J: Guidelines for research on drugged driving; *Addiction* 103:1258; 2008.

Zacny JP, Gutierrez S: Characterizing the subjective, psychomotor, and physiological effects of oral oxycodone in non-drug-abusing volunteers; *Psychopharmacology* (Berl) 170:242; 2003.

Zacny JP, Gutierrez S: Subjective, psychomotor, and physiological effects of oxycodone alone and in combination with ethanol in healthy volunteers; *Psychopharmacology* (Berl) 218:471; 2011.

Driving Under the Influence of Non-alcohol Drugs
Epidemiological Studies*

12

HALLVARD GJERDE, MAREN C. STRAND, AND JØRG G. MØRLAND

Contents

* This chapter is an updated version of a review article previously published in *Forensic Science Review*: Gjerde H, Strand MC; Mørland JG: Driving under the influence of non-alcohol drugs—An update. Part I: Epidemiological studies; *Forensic Sci Rev* 27:89, 2015.

12.1 Introduction

A review on the effect of drug use on road traffic safety is presented in Chapter 10. The review covers experimental and epidemiological studies published before 1998 for the following drug groups: benzodiazepines and related drugs, cannabis, opioids, amphetamine and related drugs, antihistamines, and antidepressants. Many investigations have been performed since then. In this chapter, epidemiological studies on drugs and traffic safety published 1998 are reviewed. An update of experimental studies is presented in Chapter 11.

Experimental studies can be used to determine whether a drug may impair driving-related functions and are most commonly performed for medicinal drugs using healthy individuals taking relatively small drug doses (see Chapters 11 and 15). In many countries it is impossible to perform experimental studies of illicit drugs in humans for ethical reasons. In countries where such studies are allowed, the doses given and drug exposure times are often lower than those used by problematic drug users and may therefore not reflect the actual risks in road traffic.

The resulting effects of drug use on traffic safety are a function of the degree to which the drugs are used, the levels and manners in which they are used, and the populations that are using them (Moskowitz 2005). Therefore, epidemiological studies are needed to determine the actual consequences of drug use on road traffic safety.

An important advantage with epidemiological studies is that they may be used to determine the impact of drug use in the general population of drivers, which includes users of illicit drugs, patients taking medicinal drugs for treatment of illness or relief from symptoms, and drivers using the same type of drugs for recreational purposes or because of drug addiction. In the latter case, the taken dose may be substantially higher than doses taken by patients for therapeutic purposes. Medicinal drugs that are used for the treatment of severe pain, anxiety, insomnia, narcolepsy, or hyperactivity are among those most frequently used for nontherapeutic purposes.

This review is primarily based on articles found by searching the major scientific literature databases. We have only included studies published in English. We have only assessed risk estimates adjusted for covariables, if available. If crude estimates are presented, this has been specified.

12.2 Methodological Issues

Challenges and Difficulties. There are four main types of epidemiological studies on the incidence and consequences of drug-impaired driving in various driving populations, primarily those involved in road traffic crashes (RTCs): (a) cross-sectional, descriptive studies on the prevalence of drug use; (b) cohort and population studies on RTC involvement among drug users compared to nondrug users; (c) case-control studies comparing drug use among RTC-involved and non-RTC-involved drivers; and (d) studies on RTC-involved drivers only, such as responsibility studies and case-crossover studies. Results from cross-sectional studies may be used to propose hypotheses on RTC risk related to the use of individual medicinal or illicit drugs, whereas cohort studies, case-control studies, responsibility studies, and case-crossover studies are analytical studies that may be used to estimate the actual RTC risks associated with the use of individual drugs.

A general difficulty in all types of epidemiological studies of RTCs is a possible selection bias in the inclusion of RTC-involved drivers (Kim and Mooney 2016). It is only possible to include drivers involved in RTCs that are recorded in databases or registries, self-reported RTC-involved drivers, injured drivers receiving treatment, drivers involved in RTCs that are subject to blood sampling for toxicological testing, or fatally injured drivers subject to legal autopsy. If including a control population, a selection bias may occur as well.

Knowledge about alcohol and drug use may be incomplete for both those involved in accidents and for a control population of drivers who are not crash-involved. If data is based on self-reports, underreporting might be a significant problem (af Wåhlberg et al. 2010; Fendrich et al. 2004; Harrison and Hughes 1997; Musshoff et al. 2006; Tourangeau and Yan 2007). If basing the study on drug testing of biological samples, only cases where sampling is performed are included, and a limited number of psychoactive substances are looked for in most studies. Thus, the use of some drugs or drug combinations that can affect the results may not be detected.

If information is obtained from prescription registries, the data just tells us that the medicinal drug has been dispensed at a pharmacy, not that it is actually taken and if so, taken in recommended doses. Another difficulty is related to the fact that the patient has received the prescription for a medicinal drug due to illness or disease, which itself may affect the RTC risk. In fact, the patient might be a more dangerous driver in some cases of nonmedicated disease than when medication is taken. In studies using data from prescription registries, the use of alcohol and illicit drugs is not taken into consideration, as well as nonrecorded use of medicinal drugs.

RTC involvement does not mean responsibility. In RTCs between a drug-impaired driver and a sober driver, the driver who is injured and therefore included in the study as RTC-involved might not be the one who was responsible for the RTC. This will cause a "dilution" of the calculated RTC risk, as previously described for alcohol in case-control studies (Gjerde et al. 2014a). Studies of only responsible drivers would eliminate this error. In some studies, drivers injured or killed in single-vehicle RTCs are investigated separately because they are almost always responsible in such cases.

A low participation rate may give a significant sampling bias. The refusal rate may be related to study design and/or to cultural issues. It might be suggested that a large proportion of those who voluntarily participate in studies are conscientious individuals without significant social or behavioral problems, whereas some of those who refuse to participate might be careless or might not want to reveal any less acceptable behavior.

Covariates (confounding or interacting variables) that are usually included in matching cases and controls or in data analysis are: age, gender, time of day/week, and geographical region. Some other possibly important covariates are: driving experience, personality characteristics, state of physical and mental health, sleep deprivation, state of alertness, exhaustion, distractions, use of caffeine, hunger, thirst, socioeconomic factors, driving alone or with passengers, speed limit, weather conditions, visibility, traffic density, the condition of the road, and the condition of the motor vehicle.

Covariates related to personality are often not included. If cases and controls are different in relation to impulsivity, sensation-seeking and risk-taking behavior, the calculated risk for RTC involvement will not reflect the risk posed by the drug alone, but a combination of substance use with personality factors. A particular problem is the association between the use of illicit drugs and risk-taking personality (Beirness and Simpson 1988; Bingham and Shope 2005; Dunlop and Romer 2010; Karjalainen et al. 2012; Walter et al. 2012), which in itself may be associated with high RTC risk also in the absence of drug use. In addition, risk-taking behavior might again be increased after using some types of drugs.

It is often difficult to relate any increased RTC risk to drug doses or blood drug concentrations in epidemiological studies due to lack of statistical power; therefore, assessments are in most studies performed using dichotomous data (drug used: yes/no).

It is important to remember that the types of epidemiological studies included in this review cannot be used to prove causality; the studies can merely be used to document an association between drug use and involvement in RTCs. Any observed association may also, at least partly, be related to confounding factors that are not controlled for.

Guidelines for research on drugged driving were published in 2008 (Walsh et al. 2008). They include recommendations for roadside surveys, studies of drivers injured in RTCs (hospital studies), fatal RTC studies, and the collection and analysis of biological samples. Similar recommendations for cohort studies or research using registries or self-reported data have, to our knowledge, not been published. However, general guidelines on observational studies in epidemiology (STROBE Statement) have been developed (von Elm et al. 2008), and guidelines for assessing the quality of non-randomized studies in meta-analyses (Newcastle-Ottawa Scale) are valuable tools when assessing the quality of epidemiological studies (Wells et al. 2011).

12.2.1 Cross-Sectional Studies

The use of drugs by drivers who are involved in RTCs is investigated in descriptive cross-sectional studies. After alcohol, the most frequently found drugs are cannabis, benzodiazepines, stimulants, and opioids (Drummer et al. 2012; Gonzalez-Wilhelm 2007; Legrand et al. 2013, 2014; Mørland et al. 2011; Romano and Pollini 2013). Combinations of alcohol and drugs or multiple drugs are also commonly found. We have not reviewed cross-sectional studies in this article.

12.2.2 Cohort and Population Studies

RTC involvement among drivers who are using a specified drug may be compared with RTC involvement among drivers who are not using the drug. The use of medicinal drugs can be studied by using data from prescription registries, and data on RTC involvement or injury may be obtained from accident registries or health databases. The date for dispensing from a pharmacy is regarded as the starting date for drug use. RTCs during the first 7 or 14 days after dispensing date are often measured and compared with RTCs among drivers who have not purchased the same type of drug. The drug-using driver may be his own control; the number of RTCs during periods of drug use is then compared with RTCs during periods without using the drug in question. This type of study is called "case-crossover study."

The selection of the drivers in the drug-exposed and nondrug-exposed cohorts is independent of any RTC involvement; this is in contrast to case-control studies, where RTC-involved drivers are selected as cases, as well as in responsibility studies, where only RTC-involved drivers are studied.

Studies of the association between self-reported use of medication or illicit drugs and RTCs are also performed. In those surveys, participants are selected by random within geographical areas and sometimes within specified age groups by using population registries of different types, such as driver license, health, social insurance, or resident registries. Information is gathered by using questionnaires or telephone interviews. The frequency of drug use is recorded as well as involvements in RTCs under the influence of the drug in question and RTCs when not using the substance in question. A list of cohort and population studies published after 1998 is presented in Table 12.1.

Table 12.1 Cohort and Population Studies of Road Traffic Crash (RTC) Involvement among Drug Users and Nondrug Users

Methodology	Size of Population, Survey, or Cohort	Data Source[a]	Substances Assessed[b]	Covariates[c]	References Country of Study
Student survey	6,087 senior students	Q	can[d]	edu, exp, fak, sex, urb	Asbridge et al. (2005) Canada
Population study	3.1 million, age 18–70	Prescription DB, RTC DB	cod[d], tra	age, sex	Bachs et al. (2009) Norway
Population study	3.1 million, age 18–69	Prescription DB, RTC DB	car[d], dia[d], sal	–	Bramness et al. (2007) Norway
Population study	3.1 million, age 18–70	Prescription DB, RTC DB	and[d]	–	Bramness et al. (2008) Norway
Population study	3.1 million, age 18–70	Prescription DB, RTC DB	lit, val	age, sex	Bramness et al. (2009) Norway
Population study	3.1 million, age 18–70	Prescription DB, RTC DB	met[e]	age, sex	Bramness et al. (2012) Norway
Population study	3.1 million, age 18–69	Prescription DB, RTC DB	ben[d], bet, cra, nsa[d], opi[d], pen[e]	age, sex, sea	Engeland et al. (2007) Norway
Birth cohort study	907, age 18–21	Q	can[d]	age, att, beh, ddb, exp, sex	Fergusson and Horwood (2001) New Zealand
Birth cohort study	936, age 18–21	Q	can	beh, dui, exp	Fergusson et al. (2008) New Zealand
Healthcare cohort study	64, 657	Q	can[e]	age, bmi, dis, dri, mar, som	Gerberich et al. (2003) US
Population study	3.1 million, age 18–69	Prescription DB, RTC DB	hyp[d]	age, sex	Gustavsen et al. (2008) Norway
Exposed & non-exposed cohorts	Exposed: 8,188, Non-exp.: 32,752	Health Insurance DB	zol[d]	age, dis, dru, sex	Lai et al. (2014) Taiwan
Population survey	2,676	Q	can[d]	age, edu, inc, mar, sex	Mann et al. (2007) Canada
Population survey	8,481	Q	can[d]	age, dri, edu, exp, inc, mar, sex	Mann et al. (2010) Canada
Population study	1 million	Prescription DB, Health Insurance DB, Hospital DB	ben[d]	age, alc, dru, sex	Neutel (1998) Canada
Population survey	17,484	Q	can[d], coc[d]	age, alc, dru, edu, eth, occ, exp, sex	Pulido et al. (2011) Spain
Population study	3.1 million, age 18–69	Prescription DB, RTC DB	adb[e]	age, sex	Skurtveit et al. (2009) Norway

(Continued)

Table 12.1 (*Continued*) Cohort and Population Studies of Road Traffic Crash (RTC) Involvement among Drug Users and Nondrug Users

Methodology	Size of Population, Survey, or Cohort	Data Source[a]	Substances Assessed[b]	Covariates[c]	References Country of Study
Population survey	8,107	Q	coc[d]	age, dui, exp, inc, sex	Stoduto et al. (2012) Canada
Population survey	4,754	Q	can[d]	age, dis, dri, edu, inc, occ, per, sex, smo	Wadsworth et al. (2006) UK
Population survey	3,428	Q	opi[d]	age, dri, edu, exp, geo, mar, sex	Wickens et al. (2017) Canada
Population survey	7,857	Q	opi[d]	age, ddb, dis, dri, edu, exp, geo, inc, mar, sex	Wickens et al. (2018) Canada

[a] Abbreviations for data sources: DB = database or registry; Q = questionnaire or interview.

[b] Abbreviations for substances: adb = antidiabetics; and = antidepressants; ben = benzodiazepines; bet = beta blockers; can = cannabis; car = carisoprodol; coc = cocaine; cod = codeine; cra = calcium receptor antagonists; dia = diazepam; hyp = hypnotics; lit = litium; met = methadone; nsa = nonsteroidal anti-inflammatory drugs; opi = opioids; pen = pencillins; sal = salbutamol; tra = tramadol; val = valproate; zol = zolpidem.

[c] Abbreviations for covariates: age = age of driver; alc = alcohol used; att = attitudes to risky driving; beh = driving behavior; bmi = body mass index; ddb = drink driving behavior; dis = disease or health status; dri = drinking habits; dui = previous driving under the influence; dru = drug(s) used; edu = education grade; eth = ethnicity; exp = driver experience or milage; fak = used fake ID to get alcohol; geo = geographical region; inc = income; mar = marital status; occ = occupational status; per = personality; sea = season of the year; smo = smoking; urb: urbanity.

[d] Statistically significant association between drug use and RTC was reported.

[e] Statistically significant association was reported for some groups of drivers.

12.2.3 Case-Control Studies

Case-control studies are in general used to study the association between a defined exposure and an outcome of active exposure and are sometimes regarded as the optimal methodological approach for studying the RTC risk when driving after using alcohol or drugs (Berghaus et al. 2007; Houwing et al. 2009). This statement might be questionable due to a number of difficulties (Gjerde et al. 2018; Kim and Mooney 2016); we have discussed some of them below. However, there is no doubt that a well-performed case-control study of drug use and RTC involvement provides important information on the association between drugs and RTC risks among drivers in actual road traffic.

Cases are drivers involved in RTCs. They may be selected from police records, insurance records, hospital records, postmortem autopsy records, other databases or registries on RTC-involved drivers, or by self-reported RTC involvement.

Controls are drivers who are not involved in RTCs and may be selected from random traffic, from driver's-license databases, or by self-reported noninvolvement in RTCs.

The exposure to drugs may be determined in different ways: by analyzing drugs in biological samples (blood, oral fluid, urine, or sweat), by self-reporting, or by using data from prescription registries.

If using biological samples, blood or oral fluid may be used to study real-time drug exposure (i.e., at the time of sample collection), whereas samples of sweat or urine may be used to detect drug use once or more during the last days or weeks, to study drug-using drivers (i.e., not only drug exposure at the time of sample collection).

Normally, the odds ratios (ORs) for involvement in RTCs are calculated in case-control studies using logistic regression analysis. The reference group in the regression analysis may either be (a) drivers who have not used alcohol or any psychoactive drugs before driving; or (b) drivers who have not used the substance in question (but they may have used alcohol or other drugs). Those two calculation options give different ORs.

Most often the OR is calculated for single drug use (i.e., not combined with alcohol or other drugs), but sometimes the OR is calculated for any use of that particular drug (i.e., either alone or in combination with alcohol or drugs). Previous studies have shown that those calculation methods may give very different ORs (Gjerde et al. 2011, 2013). The chosen method is in some studies not properly described.

An important requirement for case-control studies is that cases and controls must be selected by random from the same population; i.e., controls should be selected in an unbiased manner from those individuals who would have been included in the case series, had they been involved in an RTC (Miettinen 1985). To enable this, cases and controls should be matched regarding important covariates, or more commonly, covariates should be included in the data analysis. It is very difficult to control for all significant factors. Therefore, the outcome of case-control studies seldom determines the increase in RTC risk due to only the drug *per se*, but instead the RTC risk posed by the drug user, which also includes behavioral and personality factors in addition to physical and mental health. Long-term drug abuse may also cause somatic and mental changes that may increase the RTC risk. Case-crossover studies may be used to overcome this problem, at least partly, because important covariates such as age, gender, and behavioral and personality factors are the same.

If using biological samples, blood samples should ideally be collected from both cases and controls because blood samples reflect recent intake and exposure to drugs. Blood samples should be taken from cases immediately after RTCs to eliminate concentration changes due to metabolism or postmortem redistribution (Ferner 2008; Han et al. 2012; Rodda and Drummer 2006). Blood samples are the best type of biological matrix for drug analysis that can be used for evaluation of RTC risk related to the drug concentration, which is expected to reflect the drug concentration in the central nervous system and therefore most likely the degree of drug influence.

The controls are drivers who are not involved in RTCs and who have the option of refusing to participate. Some drivers may refuse because of fear of detection and prosecution, whereas others may refuse because of the invasiveness or intrusiveness of the sampling or because they do not want to spend the amount of time required. The refusal rate is often particularly high when collecting blood samples; in recent roadside surveys of alcohol, drugs, and driving, the refusal rate was 24% in Lithuania; it was 52% when collecting blood or oral fluid in Belgium, and 25% refused to give a blood sample but 20% were willing to give a sample of oral fluid instead of blood in the Netherlands (Houwing et al. 2011). In American roadside surveys, 50%–60% refused to give blood samples (Lacey et al. 2007, 2009).

Oral fluid has sometimes been collected from controls in case-control studies because it reflects drug presence in blood (Samyn et al. 1999; Verstraete 2004). When collecting oral fluid, the refusal rate was less than 10% in roadside surveys in Denmark, Norway, Poland, Portugal, and Spain; however, it was higher in Sweden, Finland, the Czech Republic, and Hungary (Houwing et al. 2011). The refusal rates were about 20%–30% in North American roadside surveys (Beirness and Beasley 2010; Johnson et al. 2012; Lacey et al. 2009). It has thus been possible to obtain high participation rates if collecting oral fluid when using a good study design. However, other factors, such as cultural issues, may also have affected the participation rate.

Because of different drug concentration in oral fluid and blood, it can be difficult to compare the prevalence of drugs. However, the prevalence of a drug in paired samples of oral fluid and blood from the same cohort are equal if using equivalent (not equal) cutoff concentrations (Gjerde et al. 2014b; Gjerde and Verstraete 2011), then the average drug detection time in oral fluid will be the same as in blood. Equivalent cutoff concentrations for oral fluid and blood have been used in a few previous studies (Bernhoft et al. 2012; Gjerde et al. 2011, 2013; Hels et al. 2013). If equivalent cutoff concentrations are not used, the OR for RTC involvement will either be overestimated or underestimated, depending on differences in drug detection times in oral fluid and blood after intake of a single drug dose. Drug concentrations in oral fluid cannot be used to accurately estimate concentrations in blood because of large inter- and intraindividual variations in drug-concentration ratios between oral fluid and blood (Langel et al. 2014; Wille et al. 2009).

Some studies have compared results for blood samples from cases with urine samples from controls or used a mixture of data from blood and urine samples (Dussault et al. 2000; Movig et al. 2004; Woratanarat et al. 2009). That type of case-control design makes interpretation of results difficult, because a drug finding in urine does not indicate active drug exposure while driving. Urine samples may be positive for a drug and/or metabolite for a number of days longer than a blood sample, with very large variation between individuals, and it is therefore impossible to define equivalent cutoff concentrations in blood and urine, and the calculated OR for RTC involvement may be very much underestimated. If using urine samples, urine should be collected from all cases and all controls. This type of study will determine any association between drug users and RTCs and not between active drug exposure and RTCs.

Biological samples should be analyzed for a broad range of psychoactive substances. Multidrug use and combinations of alcohol and drugs is commonly observed among drivers injured or killed in RTCs (Legrand et al. 2013; 2014; Romano and Pollini 2013) because it may increase impairment and thus also the RTC risk. If only analyzing for a small number of substances, multidrug use may not be detected and the calculated ORs may be incorrectly high, while risks related to drugs that are not analyzed will not be detected at all.

Some studies have compared results for blood samples from cases with self-reported drug use among controls (Blows et al. 2005; Haworth et al. 1997). It is well known that underreporting of drug use is common and it may vary for different drugs and between different cohorts or cultures (af Wåhlberg et al. 2010; Fendrich et al. 2004; Harrison and Hughes 1997; Musshoff et al. 2006; Tourangeau and Yan 2007). However, results of studies of this type may be used to propose hypotheses on increased RTC risk after using certain drugs.

Random and systematic errors and weaknesses in case-control studies of drugs and RTC involvement have been discussed in detail elsewhere (Gjerde et al. 2018; Houwing et al. 2013).

It is practically impossible to fulfill the requirements for optimal case-control studies of drugs and RTCs. It is easy to handle some confounding factors, such as age, gender, time of day, day of week, and type of road or crash site, but more difficult to handle selection bias, low participation rate, and lack of control of important confounding factors. The calculated OR for involvement in an RTC will not only be related to risks posed by the substance *per se*, but very much affected by the study design, participation rate, confounding factors that are not adjusted for during matching or data analysis, and often an uncertainty introduced because of using different biological fluids from cases and controls. Lists of case-control studies published in English after 1998 are presented in Tables 12.2 and 12.3.

12.2.4 Responsibility and Case-Crossover Studies

Responsibility studies are case-case studies performed without any non-RTC control group. Judgments about responsibility for causing the RTC are made by examining the circumstances leading up to the RTC without having information about alcohol or drug use by the drivers, who are classified according to their degree of responsibility for the RTC. Then drug use is compared for each category, and ORs for RTC responsibility are calculated for drug users. Blood samples should be used for all categories of RTC responsibility and the samples should be taken immediately after the RTC.

Table 12.2 Case-Control Studies Using Biological Samples (Cases Were Killed or Injured in RTCs, Controls Were Not Involved in RTCs)

Cases	Participation Rate (%)[a]	Controls	Participation Rate (%)[a]	Samples[b]	Equivalent Cutoffs[c]	Substances Analyzed[d]	Substances Assessed[d]	Covariates[e]	References Country of study
87 killed or injured car/van/minibus drivers	Unknown	410 drivers in normal traffic	87	Alcohol: B or BR; Drugs: B (cases); OF (controls)	No	alc, amp, ben, can, coc, ecs, opi	amp[f], ben[f], can, mul[f], opi	–	Assum et al. (2005) Norway
902 killed drivers	Unknown	4,711	68.4	Alcohol: B or BR; Drugs: B (cases); OF (controls)	No	alc, amp, ben, can, opi	can[f]	–	Beirness et al. (2013) Canada
1,112 killed car/van drivers	FI 94.3, NO 59, PT 79, SE 94	21,917 drivers in normal traffic	FI 52, NO 94, PT 97, SE 62	Alcohol: B or BR; Drugs: B (cases), OF (controls)	Yes	alc, amp, ben, can, coc, ecs, opi, zhy	amp[f], ben/zhy[f], can, coc[f], mul[f], opi[f]	age, geo, sex	Bernhoft et al. 2012) Hels et al. (2011) Europe (4 countries)
2,490 injured car/van drivers	BE 94.6, DK 95, FI 91.5, IT 100, LT 100, NL unknown	15,832 drivers in normal traffic	BE 48, DK 95, FI 52, IT 100, LT 76, NL 95	Alcohol: B or BR; Drugs: B (cases), B or OF (controls)	Yes	alc, amp, ben, can, coc, ecs, opi, zhy	amp[f], ben/zhy[f], can[f], coc, mul[f], opi[f]	age, geo, sex	Bernhoft et al. 2012) Hels et al. 2011) Hels et al. (2013) Europe (6 countries)
96 injured car/van drivers	93	5,305 drivers in normal traffic	93.8	Cases: B; Controls: OF coc, ecs, opi, zhy	Yes	alc, amp, ben, can,	mul[f]	age, sex, tim	Bogstrand et al. (2012) Norway

(Continued)

Table 12.2 (*Continued*) Case-Control Studies Using Biological Samples (Cases Were Killed or Injured in RTCs, Controls Were Not Involved in RTCs)

Cases	Participation Rate (%)[a]	Controls	Participation Rate (%)[a]	Samples[b]	Equivalent Cutoffs[c]	Substances Analyzed[d]	Substances Assessed[d]	Covariates[e]	References Country of study
2,738 drivers arrested for DUI with BAC <0.2 g/L (794 RTC-involved)	Unknown	9,375 drivers in normal traffic with BAC <0.2 g/L	94	Cases: B; Controls: OF	Yes	alc, amp, ben, can, coc, ecs, opi, zhy	amp[g], ben[g], can[g], coc[g], ecs[g], mul[g], opi[g], zop[g]	age, geo, sea, sex, tim	Bogstrand and Gjerde (2014) Norway
512 killed drivers of passenger vehicles	38.3	5,931 drivers in normal traffic	49.6	Alcohol: B or BR Drugs: U	Yes	alc, amp, bar, ben, can, coc, opi, pcp	amp[f], bar, ben[f], can[f], coc[f], opi[f], pcp[f]	age, sex, tim	Brault et al. (2004) Canada
1,944 killed drivers	Unknown	7,719 drivers in normal traffic	70.7	Alcohol: B or BR; Drugs: B or U (cases); OF (controls)	No	alc, can, opi, sed, sti, ill	can[f]	age, geo, sex	Chihuri et al. (2017) US
3,095 drivers involved in RTC	79.6	6,190 drivers in normal traffic	83.7	OF	Yes	alc, and, can, opi, sed, sti	and, can, opi, sed, sti	age, alc, sex	Compton and Berning (2015); Lacey et al. (2016) US
1,406 RTC- involved	Unknown	1,953 professional drivers undergoing mandatory drug testing	Unknown	U	Yes	alc, amp, can, coc, opi	can[f]		Del Balzo et al. (2018) Italy

(*Continued*)

Table 12.2 (*Continued*) Case-Control Studies Using Biological Samples (Cases Were Killed or Injured in RTCs, Controls Were Not Involved in RTCs)

Cases	Participation Rate (%)[a]	Controls	Participation Rate (%)[a]	Samples[b]	Equivalent Cutoffs[c]	Substances Analyzed[d]	Substances Assessed[d]	Covariates[e]	References Country of study
204 killed car/van drivers	61	10,540 drivers in normal traffic	88	Cases: B; Controls: OF	Yes	alc, amp, ben, can, car, coc, ecs, opi, zhy	amp[f], ben, can, mul[f], zop	age, sea, sex tim	Gjerde et al. (2011) Norway
508 killed car/van drivers	61	9,210 drivers in normal traffic	94	Cases: B; Controls: OF	Yes	alc, amp, ben, can, coc, ecs, opi, zhy	amp[f], ben[f], can, mûl[f], zop	age, geo, sea, sex, tim, urb	Gjerde et al. (2013) Norway
254 injured drivers	93	254	76	Alcohol: B or BR; Drugs: B or U	No	alc, amp, and, bar, ben, can, coc, opi, pcp	and, bar, ben[f]	age, geo, mar, sex, tim	Hou et al. (2012) Taiwan
612 arrested RTC-involved	Unknown	3,027 drivers in normal traffic	93.8	Cases: B; Controls OF	Yes	alc, amp, sed, can, coc, ecs, opi, zhy	amp[f], sed[f], can[f], mul[f], zop[f]	age, alc, sex, tim	Jamt et al. (2019) Norway
337 injured car/van drivers	27.0	2,726 drivers in normal traffic	44.8	Alcohol: BR; Drugs: B	Yes	alc, amp, ben, can, coc, ecs, opi, zhy	amp[f], ben, can[f], coc, mul[f], opi, zhy[f]	age, sex, tim	Kuypers et al. (2012) Belgium
737 killed drivers[i]	35.6	7,719 drivers in normal traffic	70.7	Alcohol: B or BR; Drugs: B or U (cases); OF (controls)	No	alc, amp, and, anh, ben, can, car, coc, ecs, ket, opi, php, zhy	can[f], opi[f], mul[f], sti[f]	age, geo, sex, tim	Li et al. (2013) US
3,606 killed drivers[i]	53.2	15,600 drivers in normal traffic	71	Alcohol: B or BR; Drugs: B or U (cases); OF or B (controls)	No	alc, and, can, opi, sed, sti	opi[f]	age, alc, geo, sex, tim	Li and Chihuri (2019) US
296 age 18–35 injured drivers	Unknown	278 age 18–35 other patients	Unknown	Cases: U; Controls: U	Yes	amp, can, coc, ecs, opi	can[h], opi	age, geo, sex	Marquet et al. (1998) France
184 injured drivers	88.9	3,374 drivers in normal traffic	87.6	Alcohol: B or BR; Drugs: B (cases); B, U or Q (controls)	No	alc, amp, and, ben, can, coc, opi	ben[f], can, cod, mor[f], mul[f]	–	Mathijssen and Houwing (2005) Netherlands

(*Continued*)

Table 12.2 (*Continued*) Case-Control Studies Using Biological Samples (Cases Were Killed or Injured in RTCs, Controls Were Not Involved in RTCs)

Cases	Participation Rate (%)[a]	Controls	Participation Rate (%)[a]	Samples[b]	Equivalent Cutoffs[c]	Substances Analyzed[d]	Substances Assessed[d]	Covariates[e]	References Country of study
110 injured drivers	Unknown	816 drivers in normal traffic	79.3	Alcohol: B or BR; Drugs: B or U	No	alc, amp, and, bar, ben, opi	amp, ben[f], can, coc, mul[f], opi	age, sea, sex, tim	Movig et al. (2004) Netherlands
900 injured drivers	96	900 non-trauma Patients	96	B and either U or SW	Yes	alc, amp, and, bar, ben, can, coc, opi	ben[f], can[f], mor[f]	age, sex	Mura et al. (2003) France
427 killed drivers	Unknown	687 drivers at petrol station	63.4	Cases: B; Controls: B, Q	Yes	anh	anh	age	Perttula et al. (2014) Finland
1,766 killed drivers[i]	Unknown	3,424 drivers in normal traffic	71	Alcohol: B or BR; Drugs: B or U (cases) and OF (controls)	No	alc, amp, and, anh, ben, can, car, coc, ecs, ket, opi, php, zhy	can[f], opi, sti[f]	age, eth, sex	Romano et al. (2014) US
200 injured drivers	Unknown	849 drivers at petrol stations	Unknown	Alcohol: B or BR; Drugs: U, Q	Yes	alc, amp, and, ane, anh, bar, ben, can, coc, mit, mus, opi	amp[f], and, anh, can, mor[f], mul	–	Woratanarat et al. (2009) Thailand

[a] Abbreviations for countries: BE = Belgium; DK = Denmark; FI = Finland; IT = Italy; LT = Lithuania; NL = The Netherlands; NO = Norway; PT = Portugal; SE = Sweden.

[b] Abbreviations for samples: B = blood; BR = breath; OF = oral fluid; Q = questionnaire or interview; SW = sweat; U = urine.

[c] Equivalent cutoffs for cases and controls.

[d] Abbreviations for substances: alc = alcohol; amp = amphetamines; and = antidepressants; ane = antiepileptics; anh = antihistamines; bar = barbiturates; ben = benzodiazepines; can = cannabinoids; car = carisoprodol; cod = codeine; coc = cocaine/metabolites; ecs = ecstacy (MDMA); ket = ketamine; ill=illicit drugs; mit = mitragynine; mor = morphine/heroin; mul = multiple drug use; mus = muscle relaxants; opi = opioids; sed = sedatives; sti = stimulants; zhy = z-hypnotics (zolpidem, zopiclone); zop = zopiclone.

[e] Abbreviations for covariates: age = age of driver; eth = ethnicity; geo = geographical area; mar = marital status; sea = season of the year; tim = time of day or week; urb = urbanity.

[f] Statistically significant association between drug use and road traffic crash (RTC) was reported.

[g] Calculated ORs were not relative to sober drivers; ranks between ORs for arrest after using single or multiple drugs were calculated.

[h] Statistically significant association was reported for some groups of drivers.

[i] Data from the Fatality Analysis Reporting System (FARS), an US database operated by the National Highway Traffic Safety Administration.

Table 12.3 Case-Control Studies Using Questionnaires or Registries (Cases Were Drivers Injured or Involved in RTCs)

No. of Cases; Crash Outcome	Participation Rate (%)[a]	No. of Controls	Participation Rate (%)[a]	Data Sources[b]	Substances Assessed[c]	Covariates[d]	References Country of Study
571 involved in injurious or fatal RTC	92.8	588 random	78.8	Alcohol: B or BR Cannabis: Q	can[e]	age, alc, bel, edu, eth, exp, pas, sex, spe, tim, veh	Blows et al. (2005) New Zealand
5,183 injured	n/a	31,093 matched by age, sex, year	n/a	National Health Ins. Research DB	and[f], anp, ben[f], zhy[f]	com, nop, psy, urb	Chang et al. (2013) Taiwan
5,579 age 67–84 involved in injurious RTC	n/a	12,911 age 67–84 not involved in injurious RTC	n/a	Driver Insurance DB Health Insurance DB	War	age, dis, dru, rec, sex, urb	Delaney et al. (2006) Canada
5,579 age 67–84 involved in injurious RTC	n/a	13,300 age 67–84 drivers	n/a	Driver Insurance DB Health Insurance DB	lit[f], caa	age, dru, exp, geo, rec, sex	Etminan et al. (2004) Canada
74,503 age 67–84 involved in RTC	n/a	744,663 matched by age, geo, follow-up duration	n/a	Driver Insurance DB Health Insurance DB	ben[f], and[g], com[g]	age, dru, fup, ppv, rec, sex	Fournier et al. (2015) Canada
5,300 injured	n/a	5,300 matched	n/a	Prescription DB Health DB	opi[f]	age, dru, pat, ppv, sex	Gomes et al. (2013) Canada
5,579 age 67–84 involved in injurious RTC	n/a	13,300 age 67–84	n/a	Driver Insurance DB Health Insurance DB	adb[f]	age, geo, ins, rec, sex	Hemmelgarn et al. (2006) Canada
30,845 age 50–80 involved in non-alcohol injurious RTC	n/a	123,380 matched by age, sex, geo	n/a	RTC DB Prescription DB	ben[f]	alc, age, dru, mar, occ, sex	Johnell et al. (2014) Sweden
447 age 65 + involved in RTC	79.8	454 matched by age, sex	74.1	Q	ace[f], adb, anc[f], and, bet, ben, nsa[f]	exp, age, eth, sex	McGwin et al. (2000) US

(Continued)

Table 12.3 (*Continued*) Case-Control Studies Using Questionnaires or Registries (Cases Were Drivers Injured or Involved in RTCs)

No. of Cases; Crash Outcome	Participation Rate (%)[a]	No. of Controls	Participation Rate (%)[a]	Data Sources[b]	Substances Assessed[c]	Covariates[d]	References Country of Study
27,096 age 50–80 involved in injurious RTC	n/a	108,384 matched by age, sex, geo	n/a	RTC DB Patient DB	zhy[f] Socioeconomic DB	age, com, geo, dru, mar, occ, sex	Nevriana et al. (2017)[i] Sweden
3,963 injured	n/a	18,828 matched	n/a	RTC DB Prescription DB	and[f], anp, anx[f], hyp[f], sed	dru	Ravera et al. (2011) Netherlands
140 involved in injurious RTC	90.3	752 random	84.3	Q	kav[f]	age, alc, eth, hou, kha, roa, spe, tim	Wainiqolo et al. (2016) Fiji

[a] n/a = not applicable or not known.

[b] Abbreviations for data sources: B = blood; BR = breath; DB = database or registry; Q = questionnaire or interview.

[c] Abbreviations for substances: ace = angiotensin converting enzyme inhibitors; adb = antidiabetics; anc = anticoagulants; and = antidepressants; anp = antipsychotics; anx = anxiolytics; ben = benzodiazepines; bet = beta blockers; caa = carbamazepine; can = cannabinoids; com = combined drug use; hyp = hypnotics; kav = kava; kha = cava use habits; lit = litium; nsa = nonsteroidal anti-inflammatory drugs; opi = opioids; sed = sedatives; war = warfarin; zhy = z-hypnotics (zolpidem, zopiclone).

[d] Abbreviations for covariates: age = age of driver; alc = alcohol used; bel = seatbelt use; com = comorbidity score; dis = disease or health status; dru = drug(s) used; edu = education grade; eth = ethnicity; exp = driver experience or milage; fup = follow-up time; geo = geographical area; hou = household income; ins = insulin use; mar = marital status; nop = nonpsychiatric outpatient visits; occ = occupational status; pas = passengers in car; pat = previous alcoholism treatment; ppv = previous physician visits; psy = psychiatric outpatient visits; roa = road condition; rec = previous driving records; spe = speed; tim = time of day or week; urb = urbanity; veh = vehicle age.

[e] Statistically significant association was reported for some groups of drivers.

[f] Statistically significant association between drug use and RTC was reported.

[g] Statistically significant association between use of some drugs and RTC was reported.

[i] Also case-crossover study.

The second-best alternative is to collect samples of oral fluid. If collecting urine samples, drug intake during the last days or weeks is detected, not only active drug exposure at the time of the RTC. Some responsibility studies are using self-reported use of drugs, which may introduce difficulties due to underreporting of drug intake, incorrect categorization of active drug exposure, or incorrect reporting of RTCs and RTC responsibilities.

As with case-control studies, a large number of psychoactive substances should be included in the analysis of blood samples to eliminate cases with additive effects due to multidrug use or combinations of alcohol or drugs. Ideally, drug concentrations in blood at the time of the RTC should be included in data analysis. However, this is difficult because of few cases within each relevant drug-concentration interval.

The judgment of responsibility, including any police judgments, may easily be biased, for example by suspicion or knowledge about current or previous alcohol or drug use, previous RTC involvement, traffic violations, or criminal records. It is therefore important that this judgment is done in accordance with predefined criteria (Drummer 2009; Robertson and Drummer 1994; Salmi et al. 2014).

A potential difficulty is that RTC-involved drivers who are judged to have little or no responsibility for the RTC might not represent randomly selected drivers because they fail to avoid an RTC. This may be related to differences in significant confounding factors regarding personality, sleep deprivation, alertness, health, alcohol or drug use, etc., and may introduce an error in risk estimates.

Another problem is the inclusion of drivers involved in single-vehicle RTCs, who are virtually all responsible for their RTCs. It may not be relevant to compare those drivers with nonresponsible drivers, who are almost exclusively included in multiple-vehicle RTCs.

A review of previous responsibility studies and difficulties and faults has recently been published (Salmi et al. 2014). Difficulties were often related to selection procedures, the definition of responsibility, the use of undocumented factors when assessing responsibility, lack of blinded exposure assessment, varying or missing data on the proportion of responsible drivers, and lacking discussion of confounding and mitigating factors.

Case-crossover studies are comparing the number of RTCs for each individual during periods of drug use with periods without drug use. Each person in the study is both a case and his own self-matched control. This study design eliminates the need for matching cases and controls regarding a number of confounding factors that may affect the RTC risk. Periods of drug exposure may be based on either self-reported use or data recorded in prescription registries, whereas data on RTCs may be based on self-reports or RTC registries. An important difficulty with this study design is that nontreated illness during periods with no drug use may bias the risk calculations.

A list of responsibility and case-crossover studies published in English after 1998 is presented in Table 12.4.

Table 12.4 Studies of Only RTC-Involved Drivers

Methodology	Drivers	Data Source[a]	Substances Analyzed[b]	Substances Assessed[b]	Covariates[c]	References Country of Study
Case-crossover	860 injured in RTC	B, Q	alc	can[d]	ben, coc	Asbridge et al. (2014) Canada
Case-crossover	19,386 RTC-involved	Prescription DB RTC DB	n/a	and, ben[d]	–	Barbone et al. (1998) UK
Recorded unsafe driving action[e]	32,543 killed in RTC	B or U; FARS DB	alc, amp, ben, can, coc, opi, opd	can[f]	age, alc, sex, rec	Bedard et al. (2007) US
Recorded unsafe driving action[e]	36,642 killed drivers	B or U; FARS DB	alc, amp, ben, can, coc, opd, opi	opi[f]	age, alc, rec, sex, sur	Chihuri and Li (2019) US
Responsibility	72,685 involved in injurious RTC	Police DB Health Insurance DB	n/a	bup[d], met[d]	age, alc, dis, opd, geo, inj, occ, sex, tim, vet	Corsenac et al. (2012) France
Responsibility	3,398 killed in RTC	B; Police Crash Reports	alc, amp, ben, can, coc, ecs, opi	ben, can[d], opi, sti[g]	age, alc, geo, sex, sin, yea	Drummer et al. (2004) Australia
Responsibility	2,638 killed drivers	B; Coroner records	alc, amp, and, anh, anp, ben, can, coc, opi	amp[d], and, anh anp, ben, can[d], opi	–	Drummer and Yap (2016) Australia
Recorded unsafe driving action[e]	72,026 involved in non-alcohol fatal RTC	B or U; FARS DB	alc, amp, ben, can, coc, opi, opd	ben[f,h]	age, opd, rec, sex	Dubois et al. (2008) US
Recorded unsafe driving action[e]	72,026 involved in non-alcohol fatal RTC	B or U; FARS DB	alc, amp, ben, can, coc, opi, opd	opi[f,g]	age, opd, rec, sex	Dubois et al. (2010) US
Responsibility	6,932 involved in fatal RTC	Alcohol: B if BR+ Drugs: B if U+ RTC DB	alc, amp, can, coc, opi	amp, can[d], coc, opi	age, sex	Gadegbeku et al. (2011) France
Recorded unsafe driving action[e]	8,325 male truck drivers involved in non-alcohol fatal RTC	B or U; FARS DB	alc, amp, ben, can, coc, opi, opd	can, opi[f], sti[f]	age, dru, rec	Gates et al. (2013) US
Case-crossover Case-series	49,821 involved in RTC	Health DB	n/a	and[h,i], anh[i], ben[d], bet, hyp[h,i], opi[d]	–	Gibson et al. (2009) UK
Responsibility	10,748 killed in RTC	Alcohol: B if BR+ Drugs: B if U+ RTC DB	alc, amp, can coc, opi	can[d]	age, alc, tim, vet	Laumon et al. (2005) France

(Continued)

Table 12.4 (*Continued*) Studies of Only RTC-Involved Drivers

Methodology	Drivers	Data Source[a]	Substances Analyzed[b]	Substances Assessed[b]	Covariates[c]	References Country of Study
Recorded unsafe driving action[e]	36,642 killed drivers	B or U; FARS DB	alc, amp, ben, can, coc, opd, opi	can[f]	age, alc, rec, sex	Li et al. (2017) US
Responsibility	2,500 injured in RTC	B; Police Crash Reports	alc, ben, can, sti	can, sti	–	Longo et al. (2000) Australia
Responsibility	2,500 injured in RTC	B; Police Crash Reports	alc, ben, can, sti	ben[d]	–	Longo et al. (2001) Australia
Responsibility	414 injured in RTC	U RTC DB	alc, amp, bar, ben, can, coc, lsd, mep, opi, pcp, xyl	can	age, bel, sex, tim	Lowenstein and Koziol-McLain (2001) US
Responsibility	4,059 killed drivers	B; Traffic Crash DB	alc, amp, can, coc, opi	can[d]	age, sex, tim, vet	Martin et al. (2017) France
Case-crossover	616 age 60 + injured in RTC	Prescription DB Hospital DB	n/a	and[d], ben[d], opi[d]	age, dis, eth, geo, mar, sex	Meuleners et al. (2011) Australia
Case-crossover	26,586 drivers age 50–80 involved in injurious RTC	RTC DB Patient DB Socioeconomic DB	n/a	zhy[d]	dru	Nevriana et al. (2017) Sweden
Case-crossover Responsibility	72,685 drivers involved in injurious RTC	Health Insurance DB Police DB Police Reports	n/a	hyp[h]	age, alc, dis, dru, geo, occ, sev, sex, tim, vet	Orriols et al. (2011) France
Case-crossover Responsibility	72,685 drivers involved in injurious RTC	Health Insurance DB Police DB Police Reports	n/a	and[d]	age, alc, dis, dru, geo, occ, sev, sex, tim, vet	Orriols et al. (2012) France
Case-crossover Responsibility	72,685 drivers involved in injurious RTC	Health Insurance DB Police DB Police Reports	n/a	ane[d]	age, alc, dis, dru, geo, occ, sev, sex, tim, vet	Orriols et al. (2013a) France
Case-crossover	2,919 age 66–84 Antidepressants used at day of RTC	Car Insurance DB Health Insurance DB	n/a	and[d]	–	Orriols et al. (2013b) Canada

(*Continued*)

Table 12.4 (*Continued*) Studies of Only RTC-Involved Drivers

Methodology	Drivers	Data Source[a]	Substances Analyzed[b]	Substances Assessed[b]	Covariates[c]	References Country of Study
Responsibility	142,763 drivers involved in injurious RTC	Health Insurance DB RTC DB Police Reports	n/a	ben[d], zhy[d]	age, alc, dis, dru, geo, sev, sex, soc, tim, vet	Orriols et al. (2016) France
Responsibility	142,771 drivers involved	Health Insurance DB RTC DB Police Reports	n/a	anh, hyx[d]	age, alc, dis, geo, sev, sex, soc, tim, vet	Orriols et al. (2017) France
Responsibility	1,046 killed in RTC	B; Police Crash Reports	alc, amp, ben, can, ecs, opd, opi	can	age, lic, sex, sin, urb, vet	Poulsen et al. (2014) New Zealand
Case time-to-event	159,678 drivers age 65+	Health Insurance DB RTC DB	n/a	and[g], anf, anp[d], ben[d], mul[d], ppi	dru, lic, sex	Rapoport et al. (2011) Canada
Recorded unsafe driving action[e]	8,325 male truck drivers killed in non-alcohol RTC	B or U; FARS DB	alc, amp, ben, can, coc, opd, opi	opi[f]	age, dru, rec, sex	Reguly et al. (2014) US
Responsibility	4,294 killed drivers	B or U; FARS DP; SWITRS DB	alc, amp, ben, can, coc, opd, opi	can[d]	alc, dru	Romano et al. (2017b) US
Case-crossover	611 RTC-involved drivers ≥65 years	Medical records	n/a	and, hyd, oxy, tra[d], zol, + 14 other pre	nom	Rudisill et al. (2016) US
Responsibility	4,448 RTC-involved	Q	n/a	and[d]	age, dis, exp	Sagberg (2006) Norway
Responsibility	2,537 injured in RTC	Alcohol: B; Drugs: U Hospital DB; RTC DB	Not specified	can, coc[d]	age, sex	Soderstrom et al. (2005) US

(*Continued*)

Table 12.4 (*Continued*) Studies of Only RTC-Involved Drivers

Methodology	Drivers	Data Source[a]	Substances Analyzed[b]	Substances Assessed[b]	Covariates[c]	References Country of Study
Recorded unsafe driving action[e]	174 THC-positive and 174 matched killed drivers (no alcohol or drugs detected)	B; RTC DB	alc, can, opd	can[f]	age, sex	Van Elslande et al. (2012) France
Case-crossover	12,929 injured in RTC	Health Insurance Research DB	n/a	ben[d], zhy[d]	–	Yang et al. (2011) Taiwan
Case-crossover	1,250 antidepressant-using killed drivers	RTC DB Health Insurance DB	n/a	and[d]	cha, dru, dis	Yang et al. (2019) South Korea
Case-crossover	714 zolpidem-using killed drivers	RTC DB Health Insurance DB	n/a	zol[d]	age, dis, dru, res	Yang et al. (2018) South Korea

[a] Abbreviations for data sources: B = blood; BR = breath; DB = database or registry; Q = questionnaire or interview; FARS = Fatality Analysis Reporting System, an US database operated by the National Highway Traffic Safety Administration; SWITRS = California Statewide Integrated Traffic Records System.

[b] Abbreviations for substances: alc = alcohol; amp = amphetamines; and = antidepressants; ane = antiepileptics; anf = antifungal drugs; anh = antihistamines; anp = antipsychotics; bar = barbiturates; ben = benzodiazepines; bet = beta blockers; bup = pubrenorphine; cad = change in antidepressant use; can = cannabinoids; coc = cocaine/metabolites; ecs = ecstacy (MDMA); hyd = hydrocodone; hyp = hypnotics; hyx = hydroxyzine; mep = meprobamate; met = methadone; mul = multiple drug use; opd = other psychoactive drugs; opi = opioids; oxy = oxycodone; ppi = proton pump inhibitors; pre = prescription medication; sti = stimulants; tra = tramadol; xyl = xylene; zhy = z-hypnotics (zolpidem, zopiclone); zol = zolpidem; n/a = not applicable.

[c] Abbreviations for covariates: age = age of driver; alc = alcohol used; bel = seatbelt use; dis = disease; dru = drug(s) used; eth = ethnicity; exp = driver experience or milage; geo = geographical area; inj = previous injuries; lic = driver license status; mar = marital status; nom = number of medications; occ = occupational status; rec = previous driving records; res = responsibility score; sev = injury severity; sin = single vehicle crash; soc = socioeconomy; sur = survival status; tim = time of day or week; urb: urbanity; vet = vehicle type; yea = year of crash.

[d] Statistically significant association between drug use and RTC involvement or responsibility.

[e] Proxy measure for RTC responsibility.

[f] Statistically significant association between drug use and unsafe driving action.

[g] Statistically significant association for some groups of drivers.

[h] Statistically significant association for some drugs.

[i] For long-term use.

12.3 Results

Study Quality. Many large studies based on registry data have been performed. The quality of those studies depends primarily on the quality and completeness of the registries, both regarding RTCs and drug use. The individual use of alcohol, illicit drugs, and medicinal drugs obtained on the illicit market is not included in those registries and may cause a study bias.

Many large population surveys have also been performed. It is well known that both the use of drugs and involvement in RTCs is often underreported, particularly the use of illicit drugs (af Wåhlberg et al. 2010; Fendrich et al. 2004; Harrison and Hughes 1997; Musshoff et al. 2006; Tourangeau and Yan 2007). In many studies, the participants have not been asked about the use of alcohol or important drug groups, only selected drugs (e.g., only cannabis). Most surveys have not included factors related to alcohol or drug behavior, other behavioral factors, or personality factors, which may be important confounders.

We have previously assessed the quality of 17 case-control studies of drug use and crash involvement (Gjerde et al. 2018). We found problems in all of them; the major difficulties were related to likely selection bias, information bias, and confounding. Other weaknesses included lacking explanation of the assessment of drug exposure, missing covariates, lacking description of statistical methods, and lack of discussion of bias and confounding. The conclusions of this study type may therefore not always be accurate.

The largest and best-performed case-control studies on drugs and RTC involvement were part of the European Project DRUID (Driving Under the Influence of Drugs, Alcohol and Medicines) (Bernhoft et al. 2012; Hels et al. 2011, 2013) and complied with most of the recommendations published by Walsh and co-workers (Walsh et al. 2008). Some small studies were also well performed; however, the statistical power was weaker in those studies due to small numbers of cases and controls.

Four large case-control studies have also been performed in the United States. However, for three of them (Li et al. 2013; Li and Chihuri 2019; Romano et al. 2014), the cases were selected from the US Fatality Analysis Reporting System (FARS) database, whereas the controls were selected from roadside surveys (Lacey et al. 2009; Kelley-Baker et al. 2016a,b). The FARS database has limitations that do not allow calculation of reliable estimates of the risk of RTC involvement resulting from drug use (Berning and Smither 2014; Compton and Berning 2015; Romano et al. 2017a). This is due to many factors, including inconsistent drug testing between states, a bias in selecting cases for drug testing (only about half of fatal-RTC drivers are tested for drugs), failure to record all drug findings in the database, and data on drug findings were based on either blood or urine testing with cutoff concentrations not specified. In addition, the cutoff concentrations in blood from cases and oral fluid from controls were not equivalent; for some drugs the cutoffs for oral fluid testing were therefore too low and for others too high compared to those used for blood. Thus, drug exposure was defined differently for cases and controls. Those issues introduced unpredictable errors in the studies. The calculated ORs would certainly have been different if only blood samples had been collected for cases and controls.

The third large US case-control study was performed in Virginia Beach, VA (Compton and Berning 2015; Lacey et al. 2016). More than 3,000 RTC-involved drivers and 6,000 drivers in normal road traffic. Oral fluid samples were collected and analyzed for a large number of drugs to estimate the odds ratio for crash involvement. After adjusting for age and gender, no drug gave statistically significant odds ratio for RTC involvement, contrary to most other studies. This might have been caused by weaknesses in the used methodology.

Some other studies used partly blood and partly urine samples and in one study only sweat samples were collected from some participants; this makes interpretation of data difficult.

Problems mentioned above pertaining to study quality are referred to for only some of the studies that are presented in this chapter.

We have primarily included peer-reviewed articles in this review. We have only included studies that accurately specified drugs or drug groups; studies on the association between RTCs and the use of "prescribed drugs," "psychoactive drugs," or "CNS drugs" without specifying which groups were excluded. Studies published until 1998 discussed in Chapter 10 have not been included.

12.3.1 Benzodiazepines and z-Hypnotics

A population study using Norwegian prescription and RTC databases (see Table 12.1) found an increased RTC risk during the first seven days after patients started using benzodiazepines (standardized incidence ratio, SIR, of 2.9, 95% CI 2.5–3.5 for tranquillizers and SIR 3.3, 95% CI 2.1–4.7 for hypnotics) (Engeland et al. 2007). A similar increased risk was found for patients starting to use diazepam (SIR 2.8, 95% CI 2.2–3.6) (Bramness et al. 2007).

A similar study using Norwegian databases investigated RTCs during the first week after a hypnotic drug was dispensed (Gustavsen et al. 2008). The largest risk increase was observed for flunitrazepam (SIR 4.0, 95% CI 2.4–6.4), followed by nitrazepam (SIR 2.7, 95% CI 1.8–3.9), and lowest for z-hypnotics (zopiclone and zolpidem; SIR 2.3, 95% CI 2.0–2.7). A study of patients using zolpidem in Taiwan found increased risk for major injury (hazard ratio (HR) 1.67, 95% CI 1.19–2.34); the risk increased with increasing dosage (Lai et al. 2014).

The two DRUID case-control studies (Bernhoft et al. 2012; Hels et al. 2011, 2013) (see Table 12.2) found significant associations between the use of benzodiazepines or z-hypnotics and being injured (OR 1.77, 95% CI 1.16–2.69) or killed (OR 4.59, 95% CI 3.28–6.43) in RTCs. The Belgian part of the DRUID case-control studies found a significant association between the use of z-hypnotics and being injured (crude OR 6.45, 95% CI 1.63–25.52) but no significant association for benzodiazepines (Kuypers et al. 2012).

Gjerde and co-workers found significant association between the use of only one benzodiazepine drug and being killed in an RTC (OR 8.8, 95% CI 4.7–16.5), and similar results for using only diazepam (OR 6.4, 95% CI 2.5–16.7) (Gjerde et al. 2013). No significant association was found for the use of only zopiclone and fatal injury among drivers. A case-control study comparing crash-involved drivers arrested for DUI with drivers in random road traffic found an OR of 21.0 (95% CI 9.9–44.4) for crash-related arrest associated with testing positive for benzodiazepines and similar substances (excluding clonazepam and zopiclone) (Jamt et al. 2019). The OR was 41.5 (95% CI 3.7–464.4) for clonazepam and 10.6 (95% CI 2.5–45.3) for zopiclone. It is, however, likely that there was a significant selection bias because of the study design.

Significant associations between benzodiazepine use and being injured or killed in RTCs were found in other case-control studies: OR 12.6 (95% CI 1.3–122.8) (Assum et al. 2005); OR 3.9, (95% CI 2.5–6.1) (Brault et al. 2004); OR 3.41 (95% CI 1.76–6.70) (Hou et al. 2012); OR 2.98 (95% CI 1.31–6.75) (Mathijssen and Houwing 2005); OR 5.05 (95% CI 1.82–14.04) (Movig et al. 2004); and OR 1.7 (95% CI 1.2–2.4) (Mura et al. 2003).

A population-based case-control study in Taiwan (see Table 12.3) found an adjusted OR of 1.64 (95% CI 1.43–1.88) for an RTC after one week's use of benzodiazepines and an OR of 1.37 (95% CI 1.06–1.75) for z-hypnotics (Chang et al. 2013). A Swedish study found an OR of 1.26 (95% CI 1.17–1.36) for involvement in an injurious RTC after using benzodiazepines without combination with other drugs (Johnell et al. 2014).

A case-control study performed in the Netherlands used prescription data linked with police RTC data and driving license data (Ravera et al. 2011). A significant association was found between the use of hypnotic benzodiazepines with intermediate half-life and involvement in an RTC (OR 6.44, 95% CI 1.44–28.78), but no significant associations were found for other hypnotics or sedatives.

A Canadian nested case-control study of drivers aged 67–84 years using registry data found that the risk for RTC involvement was higher in current users of long-acting benzodiazepines (OR 1.23, 95% CI 1.16–1.29) than among users of short-acting benzodiazepines (OR 1.05, 95% CI 1.02–1.08) (Fournier et al. 2015). A similar study was performed in Sweden for users of zolpidem and zopiclone aged 50–80 years (Nevriana et al. 2017). The highest OR was found for newly initiated zolpidem use (OR 2.27, 95% CI 1.21–4.24 for involvement in single vehicle crash), followed by frequent combined zolpidem and zopiclone users (OR 2.20, 95% CI 1.21–4.00). Also, case-crossover calculations were performed, showing that newly initiated treatment with zolpidem or zopiclone gave an OR of 2.66 (95% 1.04–6.81) for RTC involvement within two weeks after start of the treatment.

A case-series study in the UK found an incidence rate ratio (IRR) of 1.94 (99% CI 1.62–2.32) for benzodiazepines in the first four weeks of treatment and increased with extended exposure (Gibson et al. 2009) (see Table 12.4). Short-term use of z-hypnotics was not associated with an increased RTC risk, but longer-term use was associated with a modest increased risk (IRR 1.37, 95% CI 1.05–1.79).

Longo and coworkers (Longo et al. 2001) found in a responsibility study that drivers who tested positive for benzodiazepines had a higher culpability rate than drug-free drivers. They also found a significant linear relationship between benzodiazepine concentration and culpability for drivers who tested positive for benzodiazepines alone.

Orriols and co-workers performed a responsibility study using registry data. Exposure to benzodiazepine anxiolytics was associated with an increased risk of being responsible for RTC (OR 1.42, 95% CI 1.24–1.62) (Orriols et al. 2016). The risk decreased immediately after introduction of a color-graded warning pictogram, but increased again over time.

A population-based case-crossover study of older drivers based on data from registries found that benzodiazepine users had an OR of 5.3 (95% CI 3.6–7.8) for hospitalization due to RTC (Meuleners et al. 2011).

Rapoport and co-workers found a significant association between benzodiazepine use and RTC involvement among elderly drivers (HR 1.05, 95% CI 1.03–1.07) in a case-only, time-to-event study (Rapoport et al. 2011).

A case-crossover study based on data from the Taiwanese health insurance research database found an OR for RTCs of 1.74 (95% CI 1.25–2.43) after taking one defined daily dose of zolpidem, OR 1.55 (95% CI 0.98–2.45) for zopiclone, OR 1.74 (95% CI 1.26–2.40) for long half-life benzodiazepines, and OR 1.13 (1.04–1.23) for short half-life benzodiazepines (Yang et al. 2011). A Korean case-crossover study based on registry data found an OR of 1.48 (95% CI 1.06–2.07) for fatal RTC associated with prescription for zolpidem the previous day (Yang et al. 2018).

Dubois and co-workers used the FARS database to study unsafe driving actions among drivers killed in RTCs (Dubois et al. 2008). Compared with drivers not using benzodiazepines, drivers taking intermediate or long-half-life benzodiazepines demonstrated increased odds for an unsafe driving action from ages 25 to 55. Drivers taking short-half-life benzodiazepines did not demonstrate increased odds.

Orriols' research team in France performed a registry-based responsibility study, and found that the risk for being responsible for an RTC was higher in users of benzodiazepine hypnotics (OR 1.39, 95% CI 1.08–1.79) and among drivers to whom a dosage of more than one pill of zolpidem a day had been dispensed during the five months before an RTC (OR 2.46, 95% CI 1.70–3.56); no association was found for zopiclone and risk of an RTC (Orriols et al. 2011).

In the Virginia Beach study, RTC-involved drivers were found to be significantly more likely to test positive for sedatives. However, if adjusting for age, gender, ethnicity, and presence of alcohol, the OR for RTC involvement was not statistically significant (Compton and Berning 2015; Lacey et al. 2016). Drummer and co-workers (2004) found no significant association between benzodiazepine use and RTC responsibility; however, the number of cases was small, so the study had low statistical power.

A small study in Norway found no significant associations between single use of diazepam, any benzodiazepine, or zopiclone with involvement in fatal RTC, probably because of lower statistical power (Gjerde et al. 2011). However, significant associations were found for any use of those substances (alone or in combination with other drugs or alcohol). An American case-crossover study of drivers ≥65 years found no significant crash risk among older drivers related to use of zolpidem (Rudisill et al. 2016).

McGwin and co-workers found, in an American case-control study based on registry data, a weak although not statistically significant association; OR of 5.2 (95% CI 0.9–30.0) (McGwin et al. 2000). Drummer and Yap did not find any significant association between benzodiazepine use and crash responsibility (Drummer and Yap 2016).

12.3.2 Cannabis

Asbridge et al. (Table 12.1) studied the association between self-reported driving under the influence of cannabis with RTCs among senior students. A statistically significant association was found; the adjusted OR was 2.39 ($p < 0.001$) (Asbridge et al. 2005).

A study in New Zealand investigated the association between cannabis use and RTC involvement in a young birth cohort (Fergusson and Horwood 2001). They found a statistically significant relationship between reported annual cannabis use and RTC rates ($p < 0.001$). They concluded that the risk appeared to reflect the characteristics of the cannabis users rather than the effect of cannabis use on driver performance. In a second study of the same cohort published seven years later (Fergusson et al. 2008), the investigators found a marginally significant association ($p = 0.064$) between driving under the influence of cannabis and RTCs after adjustment for annual distance driven and self-reported risky behaviors.

Gerberich and co-workers found a significant association between current marijuana use and hospitalization due to RTCs among men (IRR 1.96, 95% CI 1.23–3.14) but no statistically significant association for women (IRR 1.23, 95% CI 0.71–2.05) (Gerberich et al. 2003). However, the total number of RTCs was only 188 (100 for men and 88 for women), so the statistical power of this study was not very high.

A significant association between self-reported cannabis use more than once a week and self-reported RTC involvement (OR 2.76, 95% CI 1.50–5.08) was found in a Canadian population survey (Mann et al. 2007). They also found a significant association between self-reported driving within an hour after cannabis use and RTC (OR 2.61, 95% CI 1.45–4.68). They found similar results in a study performed three years later using a larger dataset (Mann et al. 2010); the OR for self-reported collision after cannabis use was 1.84 (95% CI 1.23–2.76).

A Spanish national survey found a significant association between self-reported cannabis use more than four days per week and self-reported RTC injury (OR 1.6, 95% CI 1.0–2.6), but no significant association for less frequent use (Pulido et al. 2011).

A study in Wales using postal questionnaires found that cannabis use during the previous year was associated with involvement in RTCs (OR 1.92, 95% CI 1.04–3.54) (Wadsworth et al. 2006).

The DRUID case-control studies (Table 12.2) found a significant association between THC and RTC injury (OR 1.91, 95% CI 1.15–3.17), but no statistically significant association with fatal RTCs (OR 1.25, 95% CI 0.45–3.51) (Bernhoft et al. 2012; Hels et al. 2011, 2013). The Belgian part of the DRUID study found a very high OR of 13.40 (95% CI 3.95–45.42) for involvement in injurious RTCs using blood samples from cases and controls (Kuypers et al. 2012).

American case-control studies (Chihuri et al. 2017; Li et al. 2013; Romano et al. 2014) found significant crude ORs of 1.54 (95% CI 1.16–2.03), 1.83 (95% CI 1.39–2.39) and 1.55 (95% CI 1.42–1.94), respectively. In the Virginia Beach study, crude data indicated an elevated risk of RTCs. However, when adjusting for age, gender, ethnicity, and presence of alcohol, the OR was not statistically significant (Compton and Berning 2015; Lacey et al. 2016).

A case-control study using data from British Columbia, Canada, found an OR of 4.95 (95% CI 3.70–6.62). The study is not very well described and the cutoff concentrations in oral fluid for controls and blood for cases were most likely not equivalent (Beirness et al. 2013). Another Canadian case-control study using urine samples an OR for fatal RTCs associated with cannabis alone of 1.6 (96% CI 1.1–2.4); for all cannabis cases (with or without other substances) the OR was 4.5 (95% CI 3.3–6.0) (Brault et al. 2004).

In a French case-control study, a significant association between cannabis and RTC injury was found for THC (OR 2.5, 95% CI 1.5–4.2) when analyzing blood, urine, or sweat samples (Mura et al. 2003). Another study found significant difference in cannabis findings in urine samples from female drivers involved in RTCs in France compared to non-trauma patients ($p = 0.02$), but not for male drivers; however, the number of cases ($n = 296$) and controls ($n = 278$) were low, giving low statistical power, and the study was flawed as alcohol and sedative therapeutic drugs were not analyzed (Marquet et al. 1998).

An Italian study compared urine test results for drivers injured in RTCs with test results for professional drivers undergoing mandatory urine testing as control population. An OR of 10.88 ($p < 0.0001$) was estimated (Del Balzo et al. 2018).

A case-control study comparing crash-involved drivers arrested for DUI in with drivers in random road traffic found an OR of 15.3 (95% CI 6.0–39.0) for arrest associated with testing positive for THC (Jamt et al. 2019).

Blows and co-workers (Table 12.3) found in a population-based case-control study in New Zealand based on self-reported data that there was no significant association between acute marijuana intake and RTC injury (OR 0.8, 95% CI 0.2–3.3), whereas there was a strong association between habitual use and RTC injury (OR 9.5, 95% CI 2.8–32.3). The authors concluded that the nature of this relationship was unclear (Blows et al. 2005).

A Canadian case-crossover study using blood sample analysis and self-reported data that cannabis used was associated with a fourfold increased odds of an RTC (OR 4.11, 95% CI 1.98–8.52), whereas a regression relying on self-reports measures found no significant association (Asbridge et al. 2014) (Table 12.4).

Using data from the American FARS database to study fatally injured drivers, the presence of cannabis in biological samples was associated with significantly increased odds for potentially unsafe driving actions (OR 1.29, 95% CI 1.11–1.50) (Bedard et al. 2007). Another study based on FARS data compared culpable drivers (RTC initiators) with non-culpable drivers (non-initiators) and found an OR of 1.62 (95% CI 1.43–1.84) for crash-initiation among cannabis-positive drivers (Li et al. 2017). A responsibility study combining FARS records from California with SWITRS data found that cannabis was associated with an OR of 1.89 (95% CI 1.34–2.66) for crash responsibility (Romano et al. 2017b).

An Australian responsibility study found that drivers with THC in their blood had a significantly higher likelihood of being culpable for an RTC than drug-free drivers (OR 2.7, 95% CI 1.02–7.0); for drivers with THC concentrations of 5 ng/mL or higher the OR was 6.6 (95% CI 1.5–28.0) (Drummer et al. 2004). A later study found an OR of 3.0 ($p < 0.05$) (Drummer and Yap 2016). Responsibility studies in France found OR of 1.89 (95% CI 1.43–2.51) (Gadegbeku et al. 2011), OR of 3.32 (95% CI 2.63–4.18) (Laumon et al. 2005), and OR 1.65 (95% CI 1.16–2.34) (Martin et al. 2017); ORs in relation to THC concentration intervals were presented in all studies. Another French study found that drivers who were killed in RTCs with THC in blood (and no detection of other drugs or alcohol) had significantly higher rates of driving failures than matched controls (i.e., fatally injured drivers without any alcohol or drugs detected in their blood test). The THC-positive drivers had significantly lower levels of attention ($p < 0.01$) and significantly higher level of risky driving ($p < 0.01$) as well as significantly higher frequencies of other failures (Van Elslande et al. 2012).

No significant association between cannabis use and RTC involvement was found in the first Norwegian case-control study (Assum et al. 2005). However, the number of cases ($n = 87$) and controls ($n = 410$) were far too low to give sufficient statistical power; in addition, the cutoff concentrations in oral fluid and blood were not equivalent. Two larger studies did neither find significant associations between THC and fatal RTCs after using only cannabis (OR 0.9, 95% CI 0.1–7.3; and OR 1.9, 95% CI 0.8–4.6), probably due to low statistical power, but significant associations if also including cases and controls with THC in combination with other drugs (OR 8.6, 95% CI 3.9–19.3; and OR 8.9, 95% CI 5.2–15.4) (Gjerde et al. 2011, 2013).

A study of data on truck drivers involved in fatal RTCs based using the American FARS database found an OR of 1.14 (95% CI 0.84–1.53) for performing an unsafe driving action associated with cannabinoids, which was detected by either blood or urine testing (Gates et al. 2013).

A Dutch study using blood samples from cases and urine or blood samples from controls found no statistically significant association with RTCs (Mathijssen and Houwing 2005). Urine samples may be positive for cannabinoids for weeks after use. Thus, urine samples are particularly unsuitable for case-control studies on the association between cannabis use and RTCs, except if only urine samples are collected from both cases and controls. Therefore, this study design gave incorrect risk estimates. The number of included cases was also low (n = 184). Another Dutch study found neither any significant association between cannabis use and RTC involvement using the case-control design (Movig et al. 2004). They collected either blood or urine from cases and controls. The fraction giving urine samples was significantly higher among controls (85%) than cases (39%), thereby underestimating the calculated ORs because urine samples are positive for drugs for a significantly longer time period than blood samples after drug use. In addition, the number of cases was low (n = 110), giving poor statistical power.

In a Thai study, urine samples were collected from both cases and controls (Woratanarat et al. 2009). Very few samples from cases and controls were positive for cannabis, and no significant association between cannabis use and RTCs was found. As only urine samples were used, the study did not determine cannabis use immediately prior to the RTC but rather cannabis use during the last week(s).

No significant association between THC and responsibility for an RTC in an Australian study (Longo et al. 2000). Neither two American studies found any significant association between cannabis in urine and RTC responsibility (Lowenstein and Koziol-McLain 2001; Soderstrom et al. 2005).

Poulsen and co-workers found only a weak association, although not statistically significant, between THC alone in blood and culpability for fatal RTCs in New Zealand (OR 1.3, 95% CI 0.8–2.3) when studying 1,046 fatally injured drivers (Poulsen et al. 2014).

12.3.3 Opioids

A Norwegian population study linking data from prescription registries with RTC databases found increased risk for involvement in RTCs among patients using natural opium alkaloids (SIR 2.0, 95% CI 1.7–2.4) (Engeland et al. 2007) (Table 12.1). Another Norwegian study (Bachs et al. 2009) found significant increased RTC risk among patients using codeine (SIR 1.9, 95% CI 1.6–2.2) but no significant accident risk associated with the use of tramadol (SIR 1.5, 95% CI 0.9–2.3). Bramness and co-workers found that male opioid maintenance treatment patients using methadone had increased RTC risk (SIR 2.4, 95% CI 1.5–3.6) but no significantly increased risk was observed for female patients (Bramness et al. 2012).

Two Canadian studies based on self-reported data found ORs of 1.97 (95% CI 1.08–3.60) and 1.60 (95% CI 1.06–2.40) for RTC involvement related to use of prescription opioids (Wickens et al. 2018; Wickens et al. 2017).

Bernhoft, Hels, and coworkers (Table 12.2) (Bernhoft et al. 2012; Hels et al. 2011, 2013) found in the European DRUID case-control studies an OR for being injured after using medicinal opioids of 7.37 (95% CI 4.99–10.88) and for being killed an OR of 4.07 (95% CI 2.14–7.72). For illicit opiates, the OR was not statistically significant for injured drivers, whereas for killed drivers, the OR was 10.04 (95% CI 2.04–19.32). The Belgian part of the DRUID study calculated an OR for being injured of 3.91 (95% CI 0.97–8.68) after analyzing blood samples from cases and controls (Kuypers et al. 2012).

Significantly increased risks for RTCs were also found in case-control studies for all opiate cases (OR 3.1, 95% CI 1.5–6.5) (Brault et al. 2004), for morphine: OR 8.2 (95% CI 2.5–27.3) (Mura et al. 2003); OR 27.97 (95% CI 9.77–80.08) (Woratanarat et al. 2009); for morphine/heroin OR 32.4 (95% CI 1.78–592) (Mathijssen and Houwing 2005); for narcotic analgesics a crude OR of 3.03 (95% CI 2.00–4.48) (Li et al. 2013), and for prescription opioids OR 1.72/95% CI 1.37–2.17) (Li and Chihuri 2019).

A Canadian population-based nested case-control study found a statistically significant association between opioid dose and risk for RTC trauma among drivers; the OR was 1.29 (95% CI 1.06–1.57) for moderate doses and 1.42 (95% CI 1.15–1.76) for high doses (Gomes et al. 2013) (Table 12.3).

An Australian case-crossover study based on prescription and hospital databases found a significant risk for injurious RTCs among older patients using opioid analgesics (OR 1.5, 95% CI 1.0–2.3) (Meuleners et al. 2011) (Table 12.4). A study using data from the American FARS database found that male truck drivers using opioid analgesics involved in fatal RTCs had greater odds of committing unsafe driver actions (OR 2.80, 95% CI 1.64–4.81) (Reguly et al. 2014).

Corsenac and co-workers used data from three French national databases and performed responsibility and case-crossover analyses. Drivers who had been exposed to methadone and/or buprenorphine on the same day as an RTC had significantly higher odds for being responsible for the crash (OR 2.02, 95% CI 1.40–2.91) (Corsenac et al. 2012) (Table 12.4).

A study based on data from the American FARS database found that female drivers who tested positive for opioid analgesics demonstrated increased odds for performing an unsafe driving action from age groups 25–34 years (OR 1.35, 95% CI 1.05–1.74) to 55–64 years (OR 1.30, 95% CI 1.07–1.58); for male drivers this was true from age groups 25–34 years (OR 1.66, 95% CI 1.32–2.09) to 65–74 years (OR 1.39, 95% CI 1.17–1.67) (Dubois et al. 2010). Another study, which used pair-matched data from FARS, found that the OR for crash initiation associated with use of medicinal opioids was 2.18 (95% CI 1.91–2.48) (Chihuri and Li 2019).

A case-series study using a British health database found that initiation of opioid treatment was associated with an increased risk of RTCs (IRR 1.70; 99% CI 1.39–2.08) (Gibson et al. 2009).

A study of truck drivers involved in fatal RTCs showed that those who were positive for opioid analgesics had higher odds for committing an unsafe driving action (OR 1.63, 95% CI 1.12–2.35) (Gates et al. 2013).

Rudisill and coworkers found in an American case-crossover study of older drivers a statistically significant association with RTC related to use of tramadol (OR 11.41, 95% CI 1.27–102.15), but not for hydrocodone and oxycodone (Rudisill et al. 2016). A French responsibility study found OR of 2.21 (95% CI 1.02–4.78) for involvement in fatal RTC related to opioid concentrations ≥20 ng/mL in blood (Martin et al. 2017) but with low prevalence, requiring caution in interpreting these findings.

Other studies did not find any statistically significant association between opiate use and RTC involvement (Assum et al. 2005; Compton and Berning 2015; Movig et al. 2004; Romano et al. 2014) (Drummer et al. 2004; Gadegbeku et al. 2011); the statistical power of some of those studies was very low. Marquet and co-workers found no significant association, but the study was flawed because analysis of alcohol and sedative therapeutic drugs was not performed (Marquet et al. 1998). Drummer and Yap found no statistical association in a responsibility study (Drummer and Yap 2016).

12.3.4 Stimulants

12.3.4.1 Amphetamines

Bernhoft, Hels, and coworkers (Table 12.2) found in the European DRUID case-control studies that the use of amphetamines alone was associated with adjusted ORs of 14.15 (95%

CI 5.82–34.42) for being injured (Bernhoft et al. 2012; Hels et al. 2011, 2013) and 34.34 (95% CI 13.18–89.49) for being killed. Blood samples were collected and analyzed from cases and oral fluid or blood samples from controls using equivalent cutoff concentrations for blood and oral fluid. Two similar studies in Norway found adjusted ORs of 20.9 (95% CI 7.3–60.0) (Gjerde et al. 2011) and 41.6 (95% CI 12.6–137.1) (Gjerde et al. 2013) after using only amphetamine or methamphetamine, while the ORs were 57.1 (95% CI 27.3–119.5) and 76.9 (95% CI 38.7–152.9) for use of amphetamines in total (i.e., with or without other substances). Blood and oral fluid were analyzed with equivalent cutoff concentrations. The latest study included practically the same control material as used in the Norwegian contribution to the DRUID Project and samples from killed drivers for several more years. Results from the Belgian part of the DRUID case-control study using blood samples from cases and controls found a crude OR of 54.82 (95% CI 6.09–493.12) for being injured in an RTC associated with amphetamines (single use); an adjusted OR was not calculated (Kuypers et al. 2012).

A case-control study comparing crash-involved drivers arrested for DUI with drivers in random road traffic found an OR of 171.3 (95% CI 29.7–990.1) for crash-related arrest associated with testing positive for amphetamine or methamphetamine (Jamt et al. 2019); however, there was a large selection bias which artificially amplified the estimated OR.

A Canadian case-control study found an OR of 11.0 (95% CI 2.9–41.3) for being killed in an RTC after use of amphetamines when analyzing urine samples; this included also amphetamines in combination with other substances (Brault et al. 2004). OR of 8.88 (95% CI 4.54–17.39), also based on analysis of urine samples from cases and controls, was found in Thai study (Woratanarat et al. 2009).

Assum and co-workers found amphetamines in blood samples from eight cases and none of the controls in a small Norwegian study (Assum et al. 2005). In order to calculate the OR, 0.5 unit was added to negatives and positives among cases and controls and 37 negative cases were added to correct for sampling bias. The calculated OR for RTC involvement was then 29.5 (95% CI 1.5–575.6). The statistical power of this study was poor.

Three other studies did not find any significant association between amphetamines and RTC involvement (Gadegbeku et al. 2011; Martin et al. 2017; Movig et al. 2004); however, problems were low statistical powers, and in one study the use of either blood or urine from cases and controls, with higher fraction of urine samples from controls (85%) than cases (39%) (Movig et al. 2004), thereby underestimating the calculated ORs because urine samples are positive for drugs for a significantly longer time period than blood samples after drug use.

12.3.4.2 Cocaine

A Spanish population study using questionnaires found a significant association between weekly cocaine use and involvement in nonfatal RTC injury (OR 2.8, 95% CI 1.1–7.1) but not for less frequent use (Pulido et al. 2011) (Table 12.1). A similar Canadian study found a significant association between self-reported cocaine use last year and involvement in an RTC (OR 2.11, 95% CI 1.06–4.18) (Stoduto et al. 2012).

The DRUID case-control studies (Table 12.2) found no significant association between the use of cocaine and injuries; the adjusted OR was 1.65 (95% CI 0.66–4.16) (Bernhoft et al. 2012; Hels et al. 2011, 2013). For fatal RTCs the adjusted OR could not be calculated; the crude OR was 22.34 (95% CI 3.66–36.53) (Bernhoft et al. 2012; Hels et al. 2011). Brault and co-workers found OR of 4.5 (95% CI 1.2–16.3) for the association with fatal RTCs for cocaine alone and 17.2 (95% CI 10.8–27.2) for all cocaine cases altogether based on urine testing (Brault et al. 2004).

An American responsibility study found significant associations between cocaine and RTC injury for male drivers (OR 2.17, 95% CI 1.14–4.13); for female drivers a positive association was also found, although not statistically significant (OR 2.34, 95% CI 0.86–6.35) (Soderstrom et al. 2005) (Table 12.4).

No significant association was found in French studies based on the calculations of only 34 cocaine-positive drivers (Gadegbeku et al. 2011) or 12 cocaine-positive drivers (Martin et al. 2017). No significant associations were found in two other studies with poor statistical power (Kuypers et al. 2012; Movig et al. 2004).

12.3.4.3 Stimulants in Total Rather Than Specified Substances

Two studies used data recorded in the FARS database combined with data from a roadside survey of drugs and driving (Li et al. 2013; Romano et al. 2014) (Table 12.2). The two studies reported crude OR for stimulants of 3.57 (95% CI 2.63–4.76) and 1.87 (95% CI 1.45–2.43), respectively, for association with fatal RTCs based on case-control calculations without specifying the cutoff concentrations used. Analytical findings in urine or blood samples from cases and samples of oral fluid from controls were used to calculate the risk. The Virginia Beach study found no significant association between the use of stimulants and RTC involvement (Compton and Berning 2015; Lacey et al. 2016).

The FARS database was also used to study unsafe driving actions associated with stimulant use. An OR of 1.78 (95% CI 1.41–2.26) was found (Gates et al. 2013) (Table 12.4).

An Australian responsibility study found that a higher proportion of drivers who tested positive for stimulants in blood were culpable compared to those who were drug-free although not statistically significant (Longo et al. 2000). Another Australian responsibility study found a nonsignificant OR of 2.27 (95% CI 0.9–5.6) between stimulant findings and culpability; for truck drivers the calculated OR was 8.83 (95% CI 1.00–78) (Drummer et al. 2004). A later study found an OR of 4.1 ($p < 0.05$) (Drummer and Yap 2016).

12.3.5 Antidepressants

A minor risk increase was observed for sedating antidepressants (SIR 1.4, 95% CI 1.2–1.6) and nonsedating antidepressants (SIR 1.6, 95% CI 1.5–1.7) in a Norwegian population study using data from prescription and RTC registries (Bramness et al. 2008) (Table 12.1).

A Taiwanese registry-based case-control study found an increased risk for RTC after one week's use of antidepressants (OR 1.71, 95% CI 1.29–2.26) (Chang et al. 2013) (Table 12.3). Also, a similar Dutch study found significant association between the use of SSRIs and involvement in RTCs (OR 2.03, 95% CI 1.31–3.14) (Ravera et al. 2011).

A Canadian nested case-control study of drivers aged 67–84 years used registry data. The risk for RTC involvement was increased for current users of SSRIs (OR 1.13, 95% CI 1.04–1.22), while it was not for users of tricyclic antidepressants (Fournier et al. 2015).

A population-based case-crossover study found greater risk for RTC involvement among drivers aged 60 or older (OR 1.8, 95% CI 1.0–3.3), highest among patients with a chronic condition (OR 3.4, 95% CI 1.3–8.5) (Meuleners et al. 2011) (Table 12.4).

A French study used data from the national healthcare insurance database, the national police database, and police reports to perform responsibility and case-crossover studies (Orriols et al. 2012). They found a significant association between the risk of being responsible for an RTC and prescription of antidepressants (OR 1.34, 95% CI 1.22–1.47); the case-crossover analysis showed no association with treatment prescription, but the risk of RTCs increased after an initiation of antidepressant treatment (OR 1.49, 95% CI 1.24–1.79) and after a change in antidepressant treatment (OR 1.32, 95% CI 1.09–1.60); the exposure was considered to start on the day following dispensing.

A case-crossover study of elderly drivers (Orriols et al. 2013b) found an increased risk of RTCs in drivers with a prescription of antidepressants before their RTC when compared with a prescription of antidepressants four to eight months before the RTC; OR of 1.19 (95% CI 1.08–1.30) to OR of 1.42 (95% CI 1.30–1.55).

A Canadian study found a significant association between antidepressant use and RTCs among elderly drivers (HR 1.07, 95% CI 1.05–1.10) (Rapoport et al. 2011). A prescription of a benzodiazepine along with the antidepressant was associated with a higher risk (HR 1.23, 95% CI 1.17–1.28), whereas the lack of concomitant benzodiazepine yielded no increase in RTC risk associated with antidepressant use. Similarly, concomitant use of some anticholinergic drugs was associated with significantly higher risk.

Significant risk associated with the use of antidepressants was also found in a Norwegian responsibility study using questionnaires (OR 1.70, $p < 0.04$) (Sagberg 2006).

Gibson and co-workers did not find any elevated risk for RTC involvement when using tricyclic antidepressants in a case-series study; however, extended use of SSRIs was associated with a small increased risk (IRR 1.16, 99% CI 1.06–1.28) (Gibson et al. 2009).

A Korean case-crossover study using registry data found an OR of 1.30 (95% CI 1.03–1.63) for involvement in a fatal RTC during a 30-day hazard period (Yang et al. 2019).

No significant associations were found in case-control studies in Taiwan (Hou et al. 2012), USA (Compton and Berning 2015; Rudisill et al. 2016), and Thailand (Woratanarat et al. 2009); and no association was found in an American study based on interviews and RTC registry data (McGwin et al. 2000) and in an Australian responsibility study (Drummer and Yap 2016), but the statistical power was poor.

12.3.6 Other Drugs

Increased RTC risk was found during the first week after patients started using carisoprodol (SIR 3.7, 95% CI 2.9–4.8) when linking the Norwegian prescription registry with the RTC registry, and no risk increase for salbutamol (Bramness et al. 2007) (Table 12.1). In a similar study, no significant risk increase was observed for lithium or valproate, except for young female drivers on lithium (OR 3.2, 95% CI 1.3–6.6) (Bramness et al. 2009). An increased risk for RTCs among elderly drivers in Canada using lithium (OR 1.80, 95% CI 1.00–3.24) (Etminan et al. 2004).

A Canadian case-control study based on analysis of biological samples found significant association between any use of PCP (alone or in combination) and being killed in an RTC (OR 31.4, 95% CI 9.2–107.4) (Brault et al. 2004) (Table 12.2).

A Norwegian study found a significant association between NSAIDs and RTC involvement (for men: OR 1.6, 95% CI 1.2–2.1; for women: OR 1.5 (95% CI 1.0–2.0) (Engeland et al. 2007) (Table 12.1). A significant association was also found for penicillins for men: OR 1.4 (95% CI 1.0–2.0); no significant association was found for women. No significant associations were found for the use of beta-blockers and calcium receptor antagonists.

A Canadian case-control study on antidiabetic drugs based on registry data found elevated risk for injurious RTC involvement among elderly patients using insulin (relative risk (RR) 1.4, 95% CI 1.0–2.0) and combined use of sulfonylurea and metformin (RR 1.3, 95% 1.0–1.7) (Hemmelgarn et al. 2006) (Table 12.3).

Significant association have been found between the use of antipsychotic drugs and RTC involvement among elderly drivers (HR 1.17, 95% CI 1.07–1.27) (Rapoport et al. 2011). The use of proton pump inhibitors or antifungal drugs was not associated with RTCs.

A Norwegian registry study found a significant association between RTCs and the use of insulin (SIR 1.4, 95% CI 1.2–1.6); however, the association was not statistically significant for drivers above 35 years of age (Skurtveit et al. 2009) (Table 12.1).

A case-control study in the US based on questionnaires found significant associations between the use of NSAIDs (OR 1.7, 95% CI 1.0–2.6), angiotensin-converting enzyme inhibitors (OR 1.6, 95% CI 1.0–2.7), or anticoagulants (OR 2.6, 95% CI 1.0–73) with RTCs among the elderly (McGwin et al. 2000) (Table 12.3). The reasons for these associations are unclear and might be related to the diseases rather than the medication. No significant association was found for other hypertension or heart medication or for the use of insulin, oral hypoglycemics, diuretics, hormones, or arthritis glaucoma medication.

Drivers exposed to prescribed antiepileptic medicines had increased risk of being responsible for an RTC (OR 1.74, 95% CI 1.29–2.34); the association was also significant for the most severe epileptic patients (OR 2.20, 95% CI 1.31–3.69) (Orriols et al. 2013a) (Table 12.4). However, case-crossover analysis found no association between RTC risk and treatment prescription, suggesting that the RTC risk was more likely to be related to the disease with seizures than to the effect of antiepileptic medicines.

No effect was found for receiving a prescription for antihistamines on short-term risk for RTCs, but extended use was associated with increased risk (IRR 1.21; 99% CI 1.04–1.41) (Gibson et al. 2009). They found no significant association for the use of beta-blockers.

Orriols and co-workers also performed a combined responsibility and case-crossover study on sedating antihistamines using registry data (Orriols et al. 2017). The responsibility study found an increased risk of being responsible for an injurious RTC among hydroxyzine users with long-term chronic disease (OR 1.67, 95% CI 1.22–2.30), higher for those with highest exposure levels. The case-crossover analysis showed no impact of antihistamine treatment initiation on the RTC risk. Drummer and Yap found no significant association in a responsibility study, but the statistical power was poor (Drummer and Yap 2016).

A study in Fiji found a significant association between use of kava with RTC injury (OR 4.70, 95% CI 1.90–11.63) in a population-based case-control study (Wainiqolo et al. 2016). Kava is a popular intoxicating beverage extracted from the roots of a plant in most Pacific islands.

Other studies found no significantly increased RTC involvement for barbiturates (Brault et al. 2004; Hou et al. 2012) and antihistamines (Perttula et al. 2014; Woratanarat et al. 2009) and for elderly patients using warfarin (Delaney et al. 2006), carbamazepine (Etminan et al. 2004) or antipsychotics (Chang et al. 2013).

12.3.7 Multiple Drug Use

The DRUID case-control studies (Bernhoft et al. 2012; Hels et al. 2011, 2013) (Table 12.2) found that the OR associated with multiple drug use was larger than for single drug use except for amphetamines. When using DRUID data from Belgium based on analysis of blood samples from cases and controls, OR of 210.97 (95% CI 4.90–9088.71) was found for combination of stimulants and sedatives and OR of 13.70 (95% CI 2.95–63.66) for multiple sedatives (Kuypers et al. 2012).

The first case-control study in Norway found an OR for RTC involvement of 63.2 (95% CI 3.6–1115.3) after using two drugs and 29.5 (95% CI 1.5–575.6) when using three drugs (Assum et al. 2005). A more recent study found that the OR for being injured in an RTC after using two drugs was 13.3 (95% CI 4.2–41.3) and after using three or more drugs 38.9 (95% CI 8.2–185.0) (Bogstrand et al. 2012). A study of drivers arrested for drugged driving (both those arrested after involvement in an RTC and those arrested for other reasons) found that multiple drug use was associated with very high risk for arrest, particularly the combination of amphetamines and benzodiazepines. Arrests for drugged driving based on dangerous driving behavior was in this study regarded as a proxy for RTC responsibility (Bogstrand and Gjerde 2014). Gjerde and coworkers found significantly higher OR after using two or more drugs than after using only one drug in case-control studies; after using two or more medicinal drugs the calculated OR was 17.1 (95% CI 5.7–51.9) (Gjerde et al. 2011) and OR 28.8 (95% CI 7.3–113.6) (Gjerde et al. 2013); for two or more illegal drugs the OR was 49.7 (95% CI 4.4–561.6) (Gjerde et al. 2011). Highest ORs were found for the combination of amphetamines and benzodiazepines: 98.2 (95% CI 24.9–386.9) (Gjerde et al. 2013).

A case-control study comparing crash-involved drivers arrested for DUI with drivers in random road traffic found, however, that the OR for combinations of different psychoactive substances did not increase the OR more than the single drug with highest OR (Jamt et al. 2019).

Dutch studies found OR of 24.0 (95% CI 11.5–49.7) (Mathijssen and Houwing 2005) and OR of 6.05 (95% CI 2.60–14.10) (Movig et al. 2004) for becoming injured in an RTC after using combinations of drugs. In the United States, Li and co-workers found an OR of 3.41 (95% CI 2.43–4.73) (Li et al. 2013). A study in Thailand did not find significantly different ORs for multiple and single drug use (Woratanarat et al. 2009).

12.4 Discussion

The present review includes only studies published in the English language, primarily in peer-reviewed journals, from January 1998 to March 2019. The results of a large number of investigations have been published during this period, and in general the findings confirm the conclusions made in Chapter 10.

The European DRUID Project has so far been the most comprehensive study of alcohol, drugs, and RTC risk. The project included large case-control studies (Bernhoft et al. 2012; Hels et al. 2011, 2013; Kuypers et al. 2012; Ravera et al. 2011), a responsibility study (Gadegbeku et al. 2011), and other epidemiological and experimental studies that are not reviewed in this article (for an overview, see project deliverables at https://www.bast.de/Druid/EN/Home/home_node.html).

The DRUID Project and other investigations documented that alcohol constitutes larger RTC risk than the use of any single drug when disregarding the concentrations in blood samples of the substances used. However, the largest increase in RTC risk has been observed for combined use of alcohol and drugs, a combination that has not been discussed in this article.

As mentioned above, a large case-control study was performed recently in Virginia Beach, VA (Compton and Berning 2015; Lacey et al. 2016). The prevalence of drugs was found to be 16.0% among RTC-involved drivers and 14.4% among matched drivers in normal traffic. The calculated risks for RTC involvement in that study was significantly lower for both alcohol and drugs than the risks reported in many other studies and not statistically significant for any drug. The OR for RTC involvement was calculated based on drug testing of oral fluid samples from cases and controls in order to avoid using different biological matrices from cases than from controls. However, the use of oral fluid testing will cause random misclassification of drug exposure from both cases and controls; this may obscure the effect of drug use on the RTC risk. Extremely low cut-offs were used, which made it impossible to distinguish between drug-impaired drivers and non-impaired drivers who had used the drug within the past couple of days. In contrast to most other studies, only a small proportion of the included drivers had been involved in serious crashes; 66% were involved in crashes with property damage only. The participation rates for suspected DUI offenders, injured drivers and hit-and-run drivers were also fairly low. Drivers who were too impaired to give informed consent were excluded. It is likely that those issues may have contributed to the unexpected low risk estimates.

The prevalence of drugs in fatally injured drivers in the US (28.3% in 2010) (Brady and Li 2014) was significantly higher than that reported in the Virginia Beach study (16.0%). This could be related to the inclusion of all types of RTCs, even quite trivial ones, in the study (Compton and Berning 2015; Lacey et al. 2016), in addition to the factors mentioned above.

12.4.1 Benzodiazepines and z-Hypnotics

A total of 36 different analytical epidemiological studies dealt with effects of benzodiazepines and/or z-hypnotics or sedatives in general. In 29 of these studies there was a statistically significant association between benzodiazepines/z-hypnotics (or use of unspecified sedatives) and RTCs. Seven studies did not report a significant association, most of these had low statistical power. Thus, in sum, analytical epidemiological studies published since 1998 in general found a clear association between use of benzodiazepines and/or z-hypnotics and increased RTC risk.

12.4.2 Cannabis

A total of 43 different analytical epidemiological studies have presented data for the effects of cannabis, and 30 found a statistically significant association between cannabis use and RTCs and injuries. The calculated OR was typically in the range 1–4, and was thus similar to the risk observed after starting therapeutic use of a benzodiazepine. Thirteen studies did not report significant associations, but seven of these had either low statistical power or questionable study design. Significant associations as well as lack of significant associations were reported in all three types of study design (i.e., in cohort, case-control, and responsibility/case-crossover).

12.4.3 Opioids

A total of 31 different analytical epidemiological studies dealing with the effects of opioids were identified. In 22 of these studies a statistically significant association between opioid use and RTCs was found; in eight studies the association was not statistically significant. However, nine of those studies had either low statistical power and/or questionable design. Significant as well as nonsignificant associations were found in case-control and responsibility/case-crossover studies. The three cohort studies performed found significant associations between prescribed opioids (with the exception of tramadol) and RTC risk. Thus, in sum, analytical epidemiological studies performed after 1998 found in most cases an association between opioid use and RTCs.

12.4.4 Stimulants

12.4.4.1 Amphetamines

Twelve different analytical epidemiological studies have included amphetamines: eight case-control studies and four responsibility studies. Ten of these found statistically significant associations between amphetamine use and RTC risk. The two studies that reported no significant associations still reported a trend. One of these studies most probably underestimated the calculated risk due to different distribution of blood and urine samples among control and cases. Thus in sum, the epidemiological studies performed since 1998 report a clear association between amphetamine use and increased RTC risk. Several of these studies found that amphetamine and methamphetamine were associated with higher RTC risk than any other drug, also when not combined with other psychoactive substances.

High concentrations of amphetamines may have harmful effects on self-perception, critical judgment, and risk taking, whereas when the stimulating effects are disappearing, a period associated with fatigue, anxiety, and irritability may occur even if the drug is still present in the body. The risk for involvement in RTCs might be increased both during the stimulated and fatigue periods when taking high doses (Logan 1996). It is likely that problematic amphetamine users and addicts constitute a larger traffic safety problem than drivers that occasionally are taking small doses of amphetamines to stay awake and alert during long journeys with little time for resting.

12.4.4.2 Cocaine

Nine different analytical epidemiological investigations studied the effect of cocaine. Five found an association between cocaine use and crashes, whereas four studies did not conclude with a significant association. Three of the latter had, however, low statistical power. The ORs reported in all studies were in general lower than those reported for amphetamines. Six of the studies included both amphetamines and cocaine. In all of these, regardless of whether an association between stimulant use and accidents was found or not, the OR-values were always higher for amphetamines. Thus in sum analytical epidemiological studies performed since 1998 found in most cases an association between cocaine use and crash risk. This association appeared, however, to be somewhat weaker than for amphetamines.

12.4.5 Antidepressants

Seventeen different analytical epidemiological studies dealing with the effects of antidepressants were identified. In eleven of these there was a statistically significant association between use of antidepressants and RTCs; one additional study reported a small risk increase for SSRIs, but not for tricyclic antidepressants. No significant association was observed in six studies, some had low statistical power. Significant as well as nonsignificant associations were found in case-control and responsibility/case-crossover studies. The only cohort study performed found a statistically significant association. One crossover study indicated that the condition itself (depression) was associated with increased risk, but also that the initial period after start of drug treatment represented a similar association. In sum, the analytical epidemiological studies published since 1998 indicate that there is some association between the use of antidepressants, both tricyclic and SSRIs, and increased RTC risk. The calculated statistically significant ORs were, however, around two or lower.

12.4.6 Other Drugs

In general, there were few studies on the associations between other drugs and RTCs. Antihistamines were studied in five reports; four of them did not find an association with RTCs, while one found a modest increased risk. The most marked risk increase (OR 31.4) was found for the association between RTCs and any use of PCP, and the risk increases after using kava (OR 4.70) or carisoprodol (SIR 3.8) were higher than for many benzodiazepines.

12.4.7 Multiple Drug Use

Twelve different analytical epidemiological studies published since 1998 all found that drug combinations increased the ORs for the association with RTCs compared to single drug use. In some studies, the calculated increases in OR were very marked.

12.5 Conclusions

Approximately 15 analytical epidemiological studies published as of 1998 were included in the review presented in Chapter 10. In the present chapter we have identified 91 analytical epidemiological studies published after those included in the former review. The scientific basis has thus increased substantially within this field of research, and thus constitutes a broader background for the following conclusions.

Epidemiological studies have found that after alcohol, amphetamines are the single substances with highest risk for RTC involvement. Increased RTC risk has also been well documented for cocaine, cannabis, benzodiazepines, z-hypnotics, opioids, and for some antidepressants. Increased RTC risk has also been found for carisoprodol and PCP, although few epidemiological studies have been performed on those substances. Associations with RTCs have been found for some other drugs as well, but it is unclear whether this association was more dependent on the underlying disease than the drug use *per se*.

The combination of two or more psychoactive drugs has been found to be more risky than single use. However, the combination of psychoactive drugs with alcohol is associated with the highest RTC risk.

The calculated risks for involvement in RTCs associated with the use of different drugs, particularly nontherapeutic use, are closely related to behavioral factors such as risk-taking behavior and impulsivity. The attitudes toward driving after drug use may also vary between countries and between groups within countries. Therefore, the calculated risks associated with drug use may vary between different studies. In addition, abuse of drugs for longer periods can cause somatic and mental changes that may increase the RTC risk as well. Therapeutic drug use may also constitute a lower risk for RTC involvement than non-treated illness. For those reasons it is difficult to determine quantitatively the risk posed by the use of a single drug dose *per se* in epidemiological studies. The risk depends on who is taking the drug, why, when, how much, how often, and under which circumstances.

Disclaimer

This chapter is an update of a review article published in *Forensic Science Review* in 2015 covering results from epidemiological studies on the association between use of non-alcohol drugs and RTC involvement for the period 1998–2015. This update is based on searching PubMed and similar databases for additional studies published between 2015 and March 2019. Our searches might not have identified all relevant studies published during this period.

References

af Wåhlberg AE, Dorn L, Kline T: The effect of social desirability on self reported and recorded road traffic accidents; *Transp Res Part F Traffic Psychol Behav* 13:106; 2010.

Asbridge M, Mann R, Cusimano MD, Trayling C, Roerecke M, Tallon JM, Whipp A, Rehm J: Cannabis and traffic collision risk: Findings from a case-crossover study of injured drivers presenting to emergency departments; *Int J Public Health* 59:395; 2014.

Asbridge M, Poulin C, Donato A: Motor vehicle collision risk and driving under the influence of cannabis: Evidence from adolescents in Atlantic Canada; *Accid Anal Prev* 37:1025; 2005.

Assum T, Mathijssen MPM, Houwing S, Buttress SC, Sexton B, Tunbridge RJ, Oliver J: *The Prevalence of Drug Driving and Relative Risk Estimations. A Study Conducted in The Netherlands, Norway and the United Kingdom*; Kuratorium für Verkehrssicherheit: Vienna, Austria; 2005.

Bachs LC, Engeland A, Mørland JG, Skurtveit S: The risk of motor vehicle accidents involving drivers with prescriptions for codeine or tramadol; *Clin Pharmacol Ther* 85:596; 2009.

Barbone F, McMahon AD, Davey PG, Morris AD, Reid IC, McDevitt DG, MacDonald TM: Association of road-traffic accidents with benzodiazepine use; *Lancet* 352:1331; 1998.

Bedard M, Dubois S, Weaver B: The impact of cannabis on driving; *Can J Public Health* 98:6; 2007.

Beirness DJ, Beasley EE, Boase P: A comparison of drug use by fatally injured drivers and drivers at risk; In Watson B (Ed): *Proceedings—20th International Council on Alcohol, Drugs and Traffic Safety Conference*; Center for Accident Research and Road Safety Queensland: Brisbane, Australia; pp 96; 2013.

Beirness DJ, Beasley EE: A roadside survey of alcohol and drug use among drivers in British Columbia; *Traffic Inj Prev* 11:215; 2010.

Beirness DJ, Simpson HM: Lifestyle correlates of risky driving and accident involvement among youth; *Alcohol Drugs Driving* 4:193; 1988.

Berghaus G, Ramaekers JG, Drummer OH: Demands on scientific studies in different fields of forensic medicine and forensic sciences. Traffic medicine—Impaired driver: Alcohol, drugs, diseases; *Forensic Sci Int* 165:233; 2007.

Bernhoft IM, Hels T, Lyckegaard A, Houwing S, Verstraete AG: Prevalence and risk of injury in Europe by driving with alcohol, illicit drugs and medicines; *Procedia Soc Behav Sci* 48:2907; 2012.

Berning A, Smither DD: *Understanding the Limitations of Drug Test Information, Reporting, and Testing Practices in Fatal Crashes* (Research Note DOT HS 812 072); US National Highway Traffic Safety Administration: Washington, DC; 2014; https://crashstats.nhtsa.dot.gov/Api/Public/ViewPublication/812072 (Accessed April 9, 2019).

Bingham CR, Shope JT: Adolescent predictors of traffic crash patterns from licensure into early young adulthood; *Annu Proc Assoc Adv Automot Med* 49:245; 2005.

Blows S, Ivers RQ, Connor J, Ameratunga S, Woodward M, Norton R: Marijuana use and car crash injury; *Addiction* 100:605; 2005.

Bogstrand ST, Gjerde H, Normann PT, Rossow I, Ekeberg O: Alcohol, psychoactive substances and non-fatal road traffic accidents—A case-control study; *BMC Public Health* 12:734; 2012.

Bogstrand ST, Gjerde H: Which drugs are associated with highest risk for being arrested for driving under the influence? A case-control study; *Forensic Sci Int* 240:21; 2014.

Brady JE, Li G: Trends in alcohol and other drugs detected in fatally injured drivers in the United States, 1999–2010; *Am J Epidemiol* 179:692; 2014.

Bramness JG, Skurtveit S, Mørland J, Engeland A: An increased risk of motor vehicle accidents after prescription of methadone; *Addiction* 107:967; 2012.

Bramness JG, Skurtveit S, Mørland J, Engeland A: The risk of traffic accidents after prescriptions of carisoprodol; *Accid Anal Prev* 39:1050; 2007.

Bramness JG, Skurtveit S, Neutel CI, Mørland J, Engeland A: An increased risk of road traffic accidents after prescriptions of lithium or valproate? *Pharmacoepidemiol Drug Saf* 18:492; 2009.

Bramness JG, Skurtveit S, Neutel CI, Mørland J, Engeland A: Minor increase in risk of road traffic accidents after prescriptions of antidepressants: A study of population registry data in Norway; *J Clin Psychiatry* 69:1099; 2008.

Brault M, Dussault C, Bouchard J, Lemire AM: The contribution of alcohol and other drugs among fatally injured drivers in Quebec: Final results; In Oliver J, Williams P, Clayton A (Eds): *Proceedings—17th International Conference on Alcohol, Drugs and Traffic Safety* (CD-ROM); International Council on Alcohol, Drugs and Traffic Safety: Glasgow, Scotland; 2004.

Chang CM, Wu EC, Chen CY, Wu KY, Liang HY, Chau YL, Wu CS, Lin KM, Tsai HJ: Psychotropic drugs and risk of motor vehicle accidents: a population-based case-control study; *Br J Clin Pharmacol* 75:1125; 2013.

Chihuri S, Li G, Chen Q: Interaction of marijuana and alcohol on fatal motor vehicle crash risk: A case-control study; *Injury Epidemiol* 4:8; 2017.

Chihuri S, Li G: Use of prescription opioids and initiation of fatal 2-vehicle crashes; *JAMA Netw Open* 2:e188081; 2019.

Compton RP, Berning A: *Drug and Alcohol Crash Risk* (Research Note DOT HS 812 117); US National Highway Safety Administration: Washington, DC; 2015; http://www.nhtsa.gov/staticfiles/nti/pdf/812117-Drug_and_Alcohol_Crash_Risk.pdf (Accessed April 9, 2019).

Corsenac P, Lagarde E, Gadegbeku B, Delorme B, Tricotel A, Castot A, Moore N, Philip P, Laumon B, Orriols L: Road traffic crashes and prescribed methadone and buprenorphine: A French registry-based case-control study; *Drug Alcohol Depend* 123:91; 2012.

Del Balzo G, Gottardo R, Mengozzi S, Dorizzi RM, Bortolotti F, Appolonova S, Tagliaro F: "Positive" urine testing for Cannabis is associated with increased risk of traffic crashes; *J Pharm Biomed Anal* 151:71; 2018.

Delaney JA, Opatrny L, Suissa S: Warfarin use and the risk of motor vehicle crash in older drivers; *Br J Clin Pharmacol* 61:229; 2006.

Drummer OH, Gerostamoulos J, Batziris H, Chu M, Caplehorn J, Robertson MD, Swann P: The involvement of drugs in drivers of motor vehicles killed in Australian road traffic crashes; *Accid Anal Prev* 36:239; 2004.

Drummer OH, Kourtis I, Beyer J, Tayler P, Boorman M, Gerostamoulos D: The prevalence of drugs in injured drivers; *Forensic Sci Int* 215:14; 2012.

Drummer OH, Yap S: The involvement of prescribed drugs in road trauma; *Forensic Sci Int* 265:17; 2016.

Drummer OH: Epidemiology and traffic safety: Culpability studies; In Verster JC, Pandi-Lerumal SR, Ramaekers JG, de Gier JJ (Eds): *Drugs, Driving and Traffic Safety*; Birkhäuser Verlag: Basel, Switzerland; p. 93; 2009.

Dubois S, Bedard M, Weaver B: The association between opioid analgesics and unsafe driving actions preceding fatal crashes; *Accid Anal Prev* 42:30; 2010.

Dubois S, Bedard M, Weaver B: The impact of benzodiazepines on safe driving; *Traffic Inj Prev* 9:404; 2008.

Dunlop SM, Romer D: Adolescent and young adult crash risk: Sensation seeking, substance use propensity and substance use behaviors; *J Adolesc Health* 46:90; 2010.

Dussault C, Lemire AM, Bouchard J, Brault M: Drug use among Quebec drivers: The 1999 roadside survey; In Laurell H, Schlyter F (Eds): *Proceedings—15th Conference on Alcohol, Drugs and Traffic Safety; 21–26 May 2000, Stockholm* (CD ROM); Swedish National Road Administration: Borlänge; Paper 309; 2000.

Engeland A, Skurtveit S, Mørland J: Risk of road traffic accidents associated with the prescription of drugs: A registry-based cohort study; *Ann Epidemiol* 17:597; 2007.

Etminan M, Hemmelgarn B, Delaney JA, Suissa S: Use of lithium and the risk of injurious motor vehicle crash in elderly adults: Case-control study nested within a cohort; *Br Med J* 328:558; 2004.

Fendrich M, Johnson TP, Wislar JS, Hubbell A, Spiehler V: The utility of drug testing in epidemiological research: Results from a general population survey; *Addiction* 99:197; 2004.

Fergusson DM, Horwood LJ, Boden JM: Is driving under the influence of cannabis becoming a greater risk to driver safety than drink driving? Findings from a longitudinal study; *Accid Anal Prev* 40:1345; 2008.

Fergusson DM, Horwood LJ: Cannabis use and traffic accidents in a birth cohort of young adults; *Accid Anal Prev* 33:703; 2001.

Ferner RE: Post-mortem clinical pharmacology; *Br J Clin Pharmacol* 66:430; 2008.

Fournier JP, Wilchesky M, Patenaude V, Suissa S: Concurrent use of benzodiazepines and antidepressants and the risk of motor vehicle accident in older drivers: A nested case-control study; *Neurol Ther* 4:39; 2015.

Gadegbeku B, Amoros E, Laumon B: Responsibility study: Main illicit psychoactive substances among car drivers involved in fatal road crashes; *Ann Adv Automot Med* 55:293; 2011.

Gates J, Dubois S, Mullen N, Weaver B, Bedard M: The influence of stimulants on truck driver crash responsibility in fatal crashes; *Forensic Sci Int* 228:15; 2013.

Gerberich SG, Sidney S, Braun BL, Tekawa IS, Tolan KK, Quesenberry CP: Marijuana use and injury events resulting in hospitalization; *Ann Epidemiol* 13:230; 2003.

Gibson JE, Hubbard RB, Smith CJ, Tata LJ, Britton JR, Fogarty AW: Use of self-controlled analytical techniques to assess the association between use of prescription medications and the risk of motor vehicle crashes; *Am J Epidemiol* 169:761; 2009.

Gjerde H, Bogstrand ST, Lillsunde P: Why is the odds ratio for involvement in serious road traffic accident among drunk drivers in Norway and Finland higher than in other countries? *Traffic Inj Prev* 15:1; 2014a.

Gjerde H, Langel K, Favretto D, Verstraete AG: Estimation of equivalent cutoff thresholds in blood and oral fluid for drug prevalence studies; *J Anal Toxicol* 38:92; 2014b.

Gjerde H, Christophersen AS, Normann PT, Mørland J: Associations between substance use and fatal road traffic accidents among car and van drivers in Norway: A case-control study; *Transp Res Part F Traffic Psychol Behav* 17:134; 2013.

Gjerde H, Normann PT, Christophersen AS, Samuelsen SO, Mørland J: Alcohol, psychoactive drugs and fatal road traffic accidents in Norway: A case-control study; *Accid Anal Prev* 43:1197; 2011.

Gjerde H, Romeo G, Mørland J: Challenges and common weaknesses in case-control studies on drug use and road traffic injury based on drug testing of biological samples; *Ann Epidemiol* 28:812; 2018.

Gjerde H, Verstraete AG: Estimating equivalent cutoff thresholds for drugs in blood and oral fluid using prevalence regression: A study of tetrahydrocannabinol and amphetamine; *Forensic Sci Int* 212:e26; 2011.

Gomes T, Redelmeier DA, Juurlink DN, Dhalla IA, Camacho X, Mamdani MM: Opioid dose and risk of road trauma in Canada: A population-based study; *JAMA Intern Med* 173:196; 2013.

Gonzalez-Wilhelm L: Prevalence of alcohol and illicit drugs in blood specimens from drivers involved in traffic law offenses. Systematic review of cross-sectional studies; *Traffic Inj Prev* 8:189; 2007.

Gustavsen I, Bramness JG, Skurtveit S, Engeland A, Neutel I, Mørland J: Road traffic accident risk related to prescriptions of the hypnotics zopiclone, zolpidem, flunitrazepam and nitrazepam; *Sleep Med* 9:818; 2008.

Han E, Kim E, Hong H, Jeong S, Kim J, In S, Chung H, Lee S: Evaluation of postmortem redistribution phenomena for commonly encountered drugs; *Forensic Sci Int* 219:265; 2012.

Harrison L, Hughes A: *The Validity of Self-Reported Drug Use: Improving the Accuracy of Survey Estimates* (NIDA Research Monograph no. 167); National Institute on Drug Abuse: Rockville, MD; 1997; https://archives.drugabuse.gov/sites/default/files/monograph167_0.pdf (Accessed April 9, 2019).

Haworth N, Vulcan P, Bowland L, Pronk N: *Estimation of Risk Factors for Fatal Single Vehicle Crashes*; Monash University Accident Research Centre: Victoria, Australia; 1997; http://www.monash.edu.au/miri/research/reports/muarc121.pdf (Accessed April 9, 2019).

Hels T, Bernhoft IM, Lyckegaard A, Houwing S, Hagenzieker M, Legrand SA, Isalberti C, van der Linden T, Verstraete A: *Risk of Injury by Driving with Alcohol and Other Drugs* (DRUID Deliverable D 2.3.5); Technical University of Denmark: Copenhagen, Denmark; 2011; http://hdl.handle.net/1854/LU-1988746 (Accessed April 9, 2019).

Hels T, Lyckegaard A, Simonsen KW, Steentoft A, Bernhoft IM: Risk of severe driver injury by driving with psychoactive substances; *Accid Anal Prev* 59:346; 2013.

Hemmelgarn B, Levesque LE, Suissa S: Anti-diabetic drug use and the risk of motor vehicle crash in the elderly; *Can J Clin Pharmacol* 13:e112; 2006.

Hou CC, Chen SC, Tan LB, Chu WY, Huang CM, Liu SY, Chen KT: Psychoactive substance use and the risk of motor vehicle crash injuries in southern Taiwan; *Prev Sci* 13:36; 2012.

Houwing S, Hagenzieker M, Mathijssen R, Bernhoft IM, Hels T, Janstrup K, van der Linden T, Legrand SA, Verstraete A: *Prevalence of Alcohol and Other Psychoactive Substance in Drivers in General Traffic. Part I: General Results* (DRUID Deliverable D 2.2.3); SWOV Institute for Road Safety Research: Leidschendam, The Netherlands; 2011; http://orbit.dtu.dk/fedora/objects/orbit:89486/datastreams/file_6341069/content (Accessed April 9, 2019).

Houwing S, Hagenzieker M, Mathijssen RP, Legrand SA, Verstraete AG, Hels T, Bernhoft IM, Simonsen KW, Lillsunde P, Favretto D, et al.: Random and systematic errors in case-control studies calculating the injury risk of driving under the influence of psychoactive substances; *Accid Anal Prev* 52:144; 2013.

Houwing S, Mathijssen R, Brookhuis KA: Case-control studies; In Verster J, Pandi-Perumal SR, Ramaekers JG, de Gier JJ (Eds): *Drugs, Driving and Traffic Safety*; Birkhäuser Verlag AG: Basel, Switzerland; p. 107; 2009.

Jamt REG, Gjerde H, Romeo G, Bogstrand ST: Association between alcohol and drug use and arrest for driving under the influence after crash involvement in a rural area of Norway: A case-control study; *BMJ Open* 9:e023563; 2019.

Johnell K, Laflamme L, Moller J, Monarrez-Espino J: The role of marital status in the association between benzodiazepines, psychotropics and injurious road traffic crashes: A register-based nationwide study of senior drivers in Sweden; *PLoS One* 9:e86742; 2014.

Johnson MB, Kelley-Baker T, Voas RB, Lacey JH: The prevalence of cannabis-involved driving in California; *Drug Alcohol Depend* 123:105; 2012.

Karjalainen K, Blencowe T, Lillsunde P: Substance use and social, health and safety-related factors among fatally injured drivers; *Accid Anal Prev* 45:731; 2012.

Kelley-Baker T, Berning A, Ramirez A, Lacey JH, Carr K, Waehrer G, Moore C, Pell K, Yao J, Compton R: *2013–2014 National Roadside Study of Alcohol and Drug Use by Drivers: Drug Results* (DOT HS 812 411); US National HIghway Traffic Safety Administration: Washington, DC; 2016a; https://www.nhtsa.gov/document/2013-2014-national-roadside-study-alcohol-and-drug-use-drivers-drug-results (Accessed April 9, 2019).

Kelley-Baker T, Lacey JH, Berning A, Ramirez A, Moore C, Brainard K, Yao J, Tippetts AS, Romano E, Carr K, Pell K: *2013–2014 National Roadside Study of Alcohol and Drug Use by Drivers: Methodology* (DOT HS 812 294); US National Highway Traffic Safety Administration: Washington, DC; 2016b; https://www.nhtsa.gov/sites/nhtsa.dot.gov/files/812294-national-roadside-study-methodology-report-2013-2014.pdf (Accessed April 9, 2019).

Kim JH, Mooney SJ: The epidemiologic principles underlying traffic safety study designs; *Int J Epidemiol* 45:1668; 2016.

Kuypers KP, Legrand SA, Ramaekers JG, Verstraete AG: A case-control study estimating accident risk for alcohol, medicines and illegal drugs; *PLoS One* 7:e43496; 2012.

Lacey JH, Kelley-Baker T, Berning A, Romano E, Ramirez A, Yao J, Moore C, Brainard K, Carr K, Pell K, Compton R: *Drug and Alcohol Crash Risk: A Case-Control Study* (DOT HS 812 355); US National Highway Traffic Safety Administration: Washington, DC; 2016; https://www.nhtsa.gov/sites/nhtsa.dot.gov/files/documents/812355_drugalcoholcrashrisk.pdf (Accessed April 9, 2019).

Lacey JH, Kelley-Baker T, Furr-Holden D, Brainard K, Moore C: *Pilot Test of New Roadside Survey Methodology for Impaired Driving* (DOT HS 810 704); US National Highway Traffic Safety Administration: Washington, DC; 2007; http://www.nhtsa.gov/DOT/NHTSA/Traffic%20Injury%20Control/Articles/Associated%20Files/PilotTest_NRSM.pdf (Accessed April 9, 2019).

Lacey JH, Kelley-Baker T, Furr-Holden D, Voas RB, Romano E, Ramirez A, Brainard K, Moore C, Torres P, Berning A: *2007 National Roadside Survey of Alcohol and Drug Use by Drivers—Drug Results* (DOT HS 811 249); US National Highway Safety Administration: Washington, DC; 2009; www.nhtsa.gov/DOT/NHTSA/Traffic%20Injury%20Control/Articles/Associated%20Files/811249.pdf (Accessed April 9, 2019).

Lai MM, Lin CC, Lin CC, Liu CS, Li TC, Kao CH: Long-term use of zolpidem increases the risk of major injury: A population-based cohort study; *Mayo Clin Proc* 89:589; 2014.

Langel K, Gjerde H, Favretto D, Lillsunde P, Øiestad EL, Ferrara SD, Verstraete AG: Comparison of drug concentrations between whole blood and oral fluid; *Drug Test Anal* 6:461; 2014.

Laumon B, Gadegbeku B, Martin JL, Biecheler MB: Cannabis intoxication and fatal road crashes in France: Population based case-control study; *Br Med J* 331:1371; 2005.

Legrand SA, Gjerde H, Isalberti C, van der Linden T, Lillsunde P, Dias MJ, Gustafsson S, Ceder G, Verstraete AG: Prevalence of alcohol, illicit drugs and psychoactive medicines in killed drivers in four European countries; *Int J Inj Contr Saf Promot* 21:17; 2014.

Legrand SA, Isalberti C, der Linden TV, Bernhoft IM, Hels T, Simonsen KW, Favretto D, Ferrara SD, Caplinskiene M, Minkuviene Z, et al.: Alcohol and drugs in seriously injured drivers in six European countries; *Drug Test Anal* 5:156; 2013.

Li G, Brady JE, Chen Q: Drug use and fatal motor vehicle crashes: A case-control study; *Accid Anal Prev* 60:205; 2013.

Li G, Chihuri S, Brady JE: Role of alcohol and marijuana use in the initiation of fatal two-vehicle crashes; *Ann Epidemiol* 27:342; 2017.

Li G, Chihuri S: Prescription opioids, alcohol and fatal motor vehicle crashes: A population-based case-control study; *Inj Epidemiol* 6:11; 2019.

Logan BK: Methamphetamine and driving impairment; *J Forensic Sci* 41:457; 1996.

Longo MC, Hunter CE, Lokan RJ, White JM, White MA: The prevalence of alcohol, cannabinoids, benzodiazepines and stimulants amongst injured drivers and their role in driver culpability: Part II: The relationship between drug prevalence and drug concentration, and driver culpability; *Accid Anal Prev* 32:623; 2000.

Longo MC, Lokan RJ, White JM: The relationship between benzodiazepine concentration and vehicle crash culpability; *J Traffic Med* 29:36; 2001.

Lowenstein SR, Koziol-McLain J: Drugs and traffic crash responsibility: A study of injured motorists in Colorado; *J Trauma* 50:313; 2001.

Mann RE, Adlaf E, Zhao J, Stoduto G, Ialomiteanu A, Smart RG, Asbridge M: Cannabis use and self-reported collisions in a representative sample of adult drivers; *J Safety Res* 38:669; 2007.

Mann RE, Stoduto G, Ialomiteanu A, Asbridge M, Smart RG, Wickens CM: Self-reported collision risk associated with cannabis use and driving after cannabis use among Ontario adults; *Traffic Inj Prev* 11:115; 2010.

Marquet P, Delpla PA, Kerguelen S, Bremond J, Facy F, Garnier M, Guery B, Lhermitte M, Mathe D, Pelissier AL, Renaudeau C, Vest P, Seguela JP: Prevalence of drugs of abuse in urine of drivers involved in road accidents in France: A collaborative study; *J Forensic Sci* 43:806; 1998.

Martin JL, Gadegbeku B, Wu D, Viallon V, Laumon B: Cannabis, alcohol and fatal road accidents; *PLoS One* 12:e0187320; 2017.

Mathijssen MPM, Houwing S: European Union research Project IMMORTAL: The risk of drink and drug driving—Results of a case-control study conducted in the Netherlands; In *Drugs and Traffic: Transportation Research Circular E-C096*; Transportation Research Board: Washington, DC; p. 22; 2005; http://onlinepubs.trb.org/onlinepubs/circulars/ec096.pdf (Accessed April 9, 2019).

McGwin G, Jr., Sims RV, Pulley L, Roseman JM: Relations among chronic medical conditions, medications, and automobile crashes in the elderly: A population-based case-control study; *Am J Epidemiol* 152:424; 2000.

Meuleners LB, Duke J, Lee AH, Palamara P, Hildebrand J, Ng JQ: Psychoactive medications and crash involvement requiring hospitalization for older drivers: A population-based study; *J Am Geriatr Soc* 59:1575; 2011.

Miettinen OS: The "case-control" study: Valid selection of subjects; *J Chronic Dis* 38:543; 1985.

Mørland J, Steentoft A, Simonsen KW, Ojanperä I, Vuori E, Magnusdottir K, Kristinsson J, Ceder G, Kronstrand R, Christophersen A: Drugs related to motor vehicle crashes in northern European countries: A study of fatally injured drivers; *Accid Anal Prev* 43:1920; 2011.

Moskowitz H: Commentary on variability among epidemiological studies of drugs and driving; In *Drugs and Traffic: A Symposium Transportation Research Circular E-C096*; Transportation Research Board: Washington, DC; p. 36; 2005; http://onlinepubs.trb.org/onlinepubs/circulars/ec096.pdf (Accessed April 9, 2019).

Movig KL, Mathijssen MP, Nagel PH, van Egmond T, de Gier JJ, Leufkens HG, Egberts AC: Psychoactive substance use and the risk of motor vehicle accidents; *Accid Anal Prev* 36:631; 2004.

Mura P, Kintz P, Ludes B, Gaulier JM, Marquet P, Martin-Dupont S, Vincent F, Kaddour A, Goulle JP, Nouveau J et al.: Comparison of the prevalence of alcohol, cannabis and other drugs between 900 injured drivers and 900 control subjects: Results of a French collaborative study; *Forensic Sci Int* 133:79; 2003.

Musshoff F, Driever F, Lachenmeier K, Lachenmeier DW, Banger M, Madea B: Results of hair analyses for drugs of abuse and comparison with self-reports and urine tests; *Forensic Sci Int* 156:118; 2006.

Neutel I: Benzodiazepine-related traffic accidents in young and elderly drivers; *Hum Psychopharmacol Clin Exp* 13: S115; 1998.

Nevriana A, Moller J, Laflamme L, Monarrez-Espino J: New, occasional, and frequent use of zolpidem or zopiclone (zlone and in combination) and the risk of injurious road traffic crashes in older adult drivers: A population-based case-control and case-crossover study; *CNS Drugs* 31:711; 2017.

Orriols L, Foubert-Samier A, Gadegbeku B, Delorme B, Tricotel A, Philip P, Moore N, Lagarde E: Prescription of antiepileptics and the risk of road traffic crash; *J Clin Pharmacol* 53:339; 2013a.

Orriols L, Wilchesky M, Lagarde E, Suissa S: Prescription of antidepressants and the risk of road traffic crash in the elderly: A case-crossover study; *Br J Clin Pharmacol* 76:810; 2013b.

Orriols L, Luxcey A, Contrand B, Benard-Laribiere A, Pariente A, Gadegbeku B, Lagarde E: Road traffic crash risk associated with prescription of hydroxyzine and other sedating H1-antihistamines: A responsibility and case-crossover study; *Accid Anal Prev* 106:115; 2017.

Orriols L, Luxcey A, Contrand B, Gadegbeku B, Delorme B, Tricotel A, Moore N, Salmi LR, Lagarde E: Road traffic crash risk associated with benzodiazepine and z-hypnotic use after implementation of a colour-graded pictogram: A responsibility study; *Br J Clin Pharmacol* 82:1625; 2016.

Orriols L, Philip P, Moore N, Castot A, Gadegbeku B, Delorme B, Mallaret M, Lagarde E: Benzodiazepine-like hypnotics and the associated risk of road traffic accidents; *Clin Pharmacol Ther* 89:595; 2011.

Orriols L, Queinec R, Philip P, Gadegbeku B, Delorme B, Moore N, Suissa S, Lagarde E: Risk of injurious road traffic crash after prescription of antidepressants; *J Clin Psychiatry* 73:1088; 2012.

Perttula A, Pitkaniemi J, Heinonen OP, Finkle WD, Triche T Jr, Gergov M, Vuori E: Second-generation antihistamines exhibit a protective effect on drivers in traffic—A preliminary population-based case-control study; *Traffic Inj Prev* 15:551; 2014.

Poulsen H, Moar R, Pirie R: The culpability of drivers killed in New Zealand road crashes and their use of alcohol and other drugs; *Accid Anal Prev* 67:119; 2014.

Pulido J, Barrio G, Lardelli P, Bravo MJ, Regidor E, de la Fuente L: Association between cannabis and cocaine use, traffic injuries and use of protective devices; *Eur J Public Health* 21:753; 2011.

Rapoport MJ, Zagorski B, Seitz D, Herrmann N, Molnar F, Redelmeier DA: At-fault motor vehicle crash risk in elderly patients treated with antidepressants; *Am J Geriatr Psychiatry* 19:998; 2011.

Ravera S, van RN, de Gier JJ, de Jong-van den Berg LT: Road traffic accidents and psychotropic medication use in The Netherlands: A case-control study; *Br J Clin Pharmacol* 72:505; 2011.

Reguly P, Dubois S, Bedard M: Examining the impact of opioid analgesics on crash responsibility in truck drivers involved in fatal crashes; *Forensic Sci Int* 234:154; 2014.

Robertson MD, Drummer OH: Responsibility analysis: A methodology to study the effects of drugs in driving; *Accid Anal Prev* 26:243; 1994.

Rodda KE, Drummer OH: The redistribution of selected psychiatric drugs in post-mortem cases; *Forensic Sci Int* 164:235; 2006.

Romano E, Pollini RA: Patterns of drug use in fatal crashes; *Addiction* 108:1428; 2013.

Romano E, Torres-Saavedra P, Voas RB, Lacey JH: Drugs and alcohol: Their relative crash risk; *J Stud Alcohol Drugs* 75:56; 2014.

Romano E, Torres-Saavedra P, Voas RB, Lacey JH: Marijuana and the risk of fatal car crashes: What can we learn from FARS and NRS data? *J Prim Prev* 38:315; 2017a.

Romano E, Voas RB, Camp B: Cannabis and crash responsibility while driving below the alcohol per se legal limit; *Accid Anal Prev* 108:37; 2017b.

Rudisill TM, Zhu M, Davidov D, Long DL, Sambamoorthi U, Abate M, Delagarza V: Medication use and the risk of motor vehicle collision in West Virginia drivers 65 years of age and older: A case-crossover study; *BMC Res Notes* 9:166; 2016.

Sagberg F: Driver health and crash involvement: A case-control study; *Accid Anal Prev* 38:28; 2006.

Salmi LR, Orriols L, Lagarde E: Comparing responsible and non-responsible drivers to assess determinants of road traffic collisions: Time to standardise and revisit; *Inj Prev* 20:380; 2014.

Samyn N, Verstraete A, van Haeren C, Kintz P: Analysis of drugs of abuse in saliva; *Forensic Sci Rev* 11:2; 1999.

Skurtveit S, Strom H, Skrivarhaug T, Mørland J, Bramness JG, Engeland A: Road traffic accident risk in patients with diabetes mellitus receiving blood glucose-lowering drugs. Prospective follow-up study; *Diabet Med* 26:404; 2009.

Soderstrom CA, Dischinger PC, Kufera JA, Ho SM, Shepard A: Crash culpability relative to age and sex for injured drivers using alcohol, marijuana or cocaine; *Annu Proc Assoc Adv Automot Med* 49:327; 2005.

Stoduto G, Mann RE, Ialomiteanu A, Wickens CM, Brands B: Examining the link between collision involvement and cocaine use; *Drug Alcohol Depend* 123:260; 2012.

Tourangeau R, Yan T: Sensitive questions in surveys; *Psychol Bull* 133:859; 2007.

Van Elslande P, Fournier JY, Jaffard M: Influence of cannabis on fatal traffic crash: A detailed analysis; *Transp Res Rec* 2281:2012.

Verstraete AG: Detection times of drugs of abuse in blood, urine, and oral fluid; *Ther Drug Monit* 26:200; 2004.

von Elm E, Altman DG, Egger M, Pocock SJ, Gotzsche PC, Vandenbroucke JP: The strengthening the reporting of observational studies in epidemiology (STROBE) statement: Guidelines for reporting observational studies; *J Clin Epidemiol* 61:344; 2008.

Wadsworth EJ, Moss SC, Simpson SA, Smith AP: A community based investigation of the association between cannabis use, injuries and accidents; *J Psychopharmacol* 20:5; 2006.

Walsh JM, Verstraete AG, Huestis MA, Mørland J: Guidelines for research on drugged driving; *Addiction* 103:1258; 2008.

Walter M, Hargutt V, Krüger HP: *German Smartphone Survey Part II: Person-Related Characteristics of Drug Users and Drug Drivers Compared to Controls* (DRUID Deliverable 2.2.2); University of Würzburg: Würzburg, Germany; 2012; http://www.psychologie.uni-wuerzburg.de/izvw//texte/2011_walter_hargutt_DRUID_Deliverable_2_2_2_Part2.pdf (Accessed April 9, 2019).

Wainiqolo I, Kafoa B, Kool B, Robinson E, Herman J, McCaig E, Ameratunga S: Driving following kava use and road traffic injuries: A population-based case-control study in Fiji (TRIP 14); *PLoS One* 11:e0149719; 2016.

Wells GA, Shea B, O'Connel D, Peterson J, Welsh V, Losos M, Tugwell P: *The Newcastle-Ottawa Scale (NOS) for Assessing the Quality of Nonrandomised Studies in Meta-Analyses*; Ottawa Hospital Research Institute: Ottawa, Canada; 2011; http://www.ohri.ca/programs/clinical_epidemiology/oxford.asp (Accessed March 21, 2019).

Wickens CM, Mann RE, Brands B, Ialomiteanu AR, Fischer B, Watson TM, Matheson J, Stoduto G, Rehm J: Driving under the influence of prescription opioids: Self-reported prevalence and association with collision risk in a large Canadian jurisdiction; *Accid Anal Prev* 121:14; 2018.

Wickens CM, Mann RE, Ialomiteanu AR, Rehm J, Fischer B, Stoduto G, Callaghan RC, Sayer G, Brands B: The impact of medical and non-medical prescription opioid use on motor vehicle collision risk; *Transp Res Part F Traffic Psychol Behav* 47:155; 2017.

Wille SMR, Raes E, Lillsunde P, Gunnar T, Laloup M, Samyn N, Christophersen AS, Moeller MR, Hammer KP, Verstraete A: Relationship between oral fluid and blood concentrations of drugs of abuse in drivers suspected of DUID; *Ther Drug Monit* 31:511; 2009.

Woratanarat P, Ingsathit A, Suriyawongpaisal P, Rattanasiri S, Chatchaipun P, Wattayakorn K, Anukarahanonta T: Alcohol, illicit and non-illicit psychoactive drug use and road traffic injury in Thailand: A case-control study; *Accid Anal Prev* 41:651; 2009.

Yang BR, Kim YJ, Kim MS, Jung SY, Choi NK, Hwang B, Park BJ, Lee J: Prescription of zolpidem and the risk of fatal motor vehicle collisions: A population-based, case-crossover study from South Korea; *CNS Drugs* 32:593; 2018.

Yang BR, Kwon KE, Kim YJ, Choi NK, Kim MS, Jung SY, Shin JY, Ahn YM, Park BJ, Lee J: The association between antidepressant use and deaths from road traffic accidents: A case-crossover study; *Soc Psychiatry Psychiatr Epidemiol* 54:485; 2019.

Yang YH, Lai JN, Lee CH, Wang JD, Chen PC: Increased risk of hospitalization related to motor vehicle accidents among people taking zolpidem: A case-crossover study; *J Epidemiol* 21:37; 2011.

International Trends in Alcohol and Drug Use Among Motor Vehicle Drivers*

13

ASBJØRG S. CHRISTOPHERSEN,
JØRG G. MØRLAND, KATHRYN STEWART,
AND HALLVARD GJERDE

Contents

* This chapter is an updated version of a review article previously published in *Forensic Science Review*: Christophersen AS, Mørland JG, Stewart K, Gjerde H: International trends in alcohol and drug use among motor vehicle drivers; *Forensic Sci Rev* 28:37; 2016.

13.1 Introduction

13.1.1 Alcohol and Drug Use as Traffic Safety Risks

The number of road traffic deaths worldwide continues to rise steadily reaching 1.35 million persons in 2016, up to about 50 million people are injured in road traffic crashes (RTCs) (WHO 2018a). RTCs is the eighth leading cause of death for people of all ages and the number-one cause of death for children and young adults 5–29 years of age. With an average rate of 27.5 deaths per 100,000 population; the risk is more than three times higher in low-income countries than in high-income countries where the average rate is 8.3 deaths 100,000 population. RTCs in low- and middle-income countries (LMCs) accounted for about 93% of the world's RTC fatalities, while those countries had 85% of the world's population and 60% of the world's motor vehicles (WHO 2018a). The number of RTC fatalities is decreasing in high-income countries but significantly increasing in LMCs (Ameratunga et al. 2006; WHO 2018a). If no effective measures are taken, the estimated annual worldwide number of RTC deaths may nearly double to 2.4 million by 2030 (WHO 2009), mainly due to increases in motorization and RTCs in LMCs caused by economic growth in those countries, enabling more people to buy motor vehicles. In the Sustainable Development Goals, world leaders have committed to halve the number of deaths from road crashes by 2020 (WHO 2018b). The WHO report from 2018 shows that far too little progress has been made to reach the goal. There is an urgent need to scale up evidence-based interventions and investment.

Driving under the influence (DUI) of alcohol has for many years been well known as a risk for road traffic safety (Borkenstein et al. 1974; Moskowitz and Burns 1990). Despite extensive focus in the scientific literature on the negative effects caused by alcohol, general warnings in mass media, and improving law enforcement, alcohol is still one of the main contributing factors for RTCs (NHTSA 2018b; WHO 2018a).

The negative effects caused by use of illicit drugs and psychoactive medicines on the ability to drive safely gained little attention until the 1970s, when the first studies on drugs relevant to traffic safety were published (see Chapter 10). Later, traffic safety related to drug use received steadily increasing attention at international conferences organized by the International Council on Alcohol, Drugs and Traffic Safety (ICADTS), and many studies have been performed to document the effects of drugs on traffic safety. Numerous review articles have been published (Gjerde et al. 2015; OECD 2010; Ogden and Moskowitz 2004; Penning et al. 2010; Raes et al. 2008; Verster and Mets 2009; Verstraete et al. 2014), see also Chapters 10–12.

The majority of the world's countries do not have robust data on the involvement of alcohol and drugs in nonfatal RTC injuries (WHO 2018a), and almost half of all countries lack data on alcohol-related RTC deaths. Only 94 countries, mostly high- and middle-income countries, have data on road traffic deaths that involve alcohol consumption amongst drivers; only 72 countries carry out alcohol testing of fatally injured drivers routinely for all cases. In a review of available data from low-income countries in Africa, Southeast Asia, Latin America, and the Caribbean, it was reported that 8%–29% of drivers in nonfatal crashes had alcohol in their systems, whereas alcohol was present in 33%–69% of fatally injured drivers (Davis et al. 2003). Since alcohol use is increasing in many (LMCs) (Davis et al. 2003; Gururaj 2004; Ingsathit et al. 2009; Mokolobate 2017), it is also expected that the number of alcohol-related accidents will increase if efficient actions are not taken to prevent driving after drinking.

13.1.2 Historical Background

The first described arrest for drunk driving was in 1897 when a London taxi driver slammed his car into a building after drinking alcohol (Editorial 1897). In 1904, the first study on alcohol involvement in RTCs was published; the study included RTCs where 24 persons were killed and several seriously injured. The investigation found that most of the drivers had used alcohol shortly before the accidents (Editorial 1904). At that time, the knowledge of the risks associated with alcohol use before driving was sparse, and no suitable analytical methods for alcohol in blood samples had been developed.

The Swedish scientist Eric Widmark developed a method for analysis of alcohol in blood samples in 1922 (Widmark 1932). This method was used for several decades, but has been replaced by an enzymatic technique (based on alcohol dehydrogenase) and gas chromatography to determine BACs in most countries (Jones and Pounder 2007). Modifications of the Widmark method are still in use in some countries, e.g., in Chile (Congress of Chile 2010).

Another great analytical achievement was the development of a "Drunkometer" in 1938 (Harger et al. 1938), an instrument to measure the alcohol content of exhaled breath, which was used in a US case-control study of alcohol and RTC that was published in 1938 (Holcomb 1938). A "breathalyzer" was presented in 1961 (Borkenstein and Smith 1961), and improvements in breathalyzer technology made large scale screening for alcohol among drivers possible (Jones et al. 1975).

The first large scientific study that documented a relationship between BAC levels and risk of RTCs was performed by Borkenstein and co-workers in a study carried out in Grand Rapids, Michigan, at the beginning of 1960s (Borkenstein et al. 1974). More studies have been performed later using more modern techniques showing an exponential increase of crash risk beginning at a BAC of about 0.5 g/L (Blomberg et al. 2009; Voas et al. 2012; Zador et al. 2000).

Chromatographic methods for analysis of drugs in blood and urine were developed from the 1950s (Curry 1960); the first methods were based on paper and thin layer chromatography. A number of gas chromatography (GC) and liquid chromatography (LC) methods where developed in the 1970s and 1980s, which made systematic drug screening of blood samples from suspected drug-impaired drivers possible. Later, gas chromatography-mass spectrometry (GC-MS) and liquid chromatography-mass spectrometry (LC-MS) methods were implemented for systematic drug analysis (Logan et al. 2013; Maurer 1992; Polettini 1999).

Immunological tests for drugs were developed in the 1970s (Cleeland et al. 1976; Wisdom 1976), first for urine and blood, later for oral fluid. This enabled mass screening for drug use among drivers. Immunological screening combined with GC, LC, GC-MS or LC-MS confirmation has been commonly used since the 1990s (Council on Scientific Affairs 1987; Logan et al. 2013). At present, cost-efficient LC-MS/MS methods that may eliminate the need for immunological drug screening are available (Badawi et al. 2009; Eichhorst et al. 2012; Maurer 2007; Montenarh et al. 2015; Sergi et al. 2009; Øiestad et al. 2007, 2011). These methods can be used to simultaneously analyze large numbers of different drugs in a small sample volume (0.5 mL or less).

Systematic studies of drug use among suspected drug-impaired drivers and drivers killed in RTCs have been performed since the late 1980s (Christophersen and Mørland 1997; Gonzalez-Wilhelm 2007). The first studies on the prevalence of drugs among random drivers were performed in Australia and Germany in the 1990s (Krüger et al. 1995; Starmer et al. 1994). Many similar studies have been performed since then. The RTC risk associated with drug use have been investigated in some studies, mainly during the last 15 years (Gjerde et al. 2015; Raes et al. 2008; Verstraete et al. 2014).

13.1.3 Legislation

13.1.3.1 Alcohol

Norway was the first country to introduce a legal limit for DUI of alcohol; in 1936 the chosen legal limit was 0.5 g/kg blood (about 0.5 g/L). Sweden introduced a legal limit of 0.8 g/kg in 1941. It took some years before other European countries followed; most of them established a limit of 0.8 g/L. During the 1970s, Finland and Sweden reduced the legal limit to 0.5 g/kg; most of the other European countries did the same during the 1990s, whereas Scotland changed to 0.5 g/L in December 2014. Sweden and Norway lowered the BAC limit to 0.2 g/kg in 1990 and 2001, respectively. The BAC limits in Eastern Europe range from zero to 0.5 g/L (WHO 2013). Several countries have lower BAC limits for professional and young drivers (WHO 2013).

The majority of the US states implemented their first legislative BAC limit of 1.0 g/L in the period of 1975–1984; the limits in some states were reduced to 0.8 g/L during the 1980s (Mann et al. 2001). By 2005, all states had changed the BAC limit to 0.8 g/L (Berning et al. 2015). Utah changed to 0.5 g/L December 30, 2018 (Fiorentino and Martin 2018). Canada implemented 0.8 g/L in 1969 (Chambers et al. 1974), which has later been changed to 0.5g/L. Australia also first implemented BAC limit of 0.8 g/L in all states and territories except Victoria, but the limit was later reduced to 0.5 g/L (Haworth and Johnston 2004).

Brazil first implemented a BAC limit of 0.8 g/L in 1989, which was reduced to 0.6 g/L in 1997, further to 0.2 g/L in 2008, and to zero in 2012 (more correctly a BAC limit of 0.1 g/L) (Gjerde et al. 2014b). Most other South American countries have BAC limits of 0.5 g/L or lower (WHO 2013).

Different legal BAC limits have been implemented in other parts of the world varying from zero to 0.8 g/L; about 30 countries have no defined BAC limits (WHO 2013).

13.1.3.2 Non-alcohol Drugs

Legal regulations for DUI of illicit drugs, psychoactive medicines and other substances have been implemented in many countries. However, the scientific documentation of accident risk became available much later than for alcohol. Still, DUI of non-alcohol drugs often does not result in prosecution. Testing for drugs other than alcohol is more expensive, and interpretation of drug findings may be difficult. Most countries seem to focus less on drugs during police controls, and police officers are often not adequately trained to detect possible drug-related impairment. The police in some countries have introduced on-site drug screening of drugs in oral fluid to detect drug-using drivers more easily (Pil and Verstraete 2008; Strano-Rossi et al. 2012; Vanstechelman et al. 2012; Verstraete 2005).

Three different types of law regulations have been implemented: (a) impairment-based laws, (b) *per se* laws, and (c) zero-tolerance laws (sometimes zero-tolerance laws are regarded as *per se* laws).

The first type of law to be implemented was impairment based. In order to be convicted for DUI of drugs, signs and symptoms of performance impairment must be documented using a standardized protocol, in addition to finding drug concentrations in the blood sample that may be associated with impairment. The process from DUI arrest to conviction is long and time consuming: primary investigation of impairment on the road-side, in some cases using standardized field sobriety tests (Anderson and Burns 1997; Burns and Moskowitz 1977) or Drug Recognition Tests (Smith et al. 2002). In case of maintained suspicion, the driver is brought to a physician or nurse for blood sampling and clinical examination of impairment. The samples are analyzed at a forensic laboratory and positive results are interpreted for the court to assess possible impairment. As an example, the routines from Norway have been described in a previous article (Christophersen and Mørland 1997). Despite the fact that such laws entail a rather resource-demanding routine, the impairment law has worked rather well in some countries, e.g., in Norway. One important reason has been well trained police officers with high focus on the problem.

Information from some other countries indicated that the impairment-based law did not work according to the intention and few cases came to the court (Jones 2005; Steentoft et al. 2010). Some of these countries have therefore changed the law (see below). Impairment-based laws are used as supplement to *per se* and zero-tolerance laws in several countries.

Per se limits (legislative blood concentration limits) have been implemented for alcohol in most countries. With *per se* limits, no other proof of impairment is required to sentence a driver for DUI if the drug concentration in blood is above the set limit. *Per se* blood concentration limits for several non-alcohol drugs were implemented in Denmark in 2007 (Steentoft et al. 2010) and for 20 illicit drugs and psychoactive medicines in Norway in 2012 (Vindenes et al. 2012). The concentrations limits in Norway were primarily based on experimental data, and were set to correspond to the BACs of 0.2 g/L (the legal limit for alcohol), of 0.5 g/L and 1.2 g/L, which are limits for graded sanctions. Apprehended drivers with blood concentrations above the legislative limits for medicinal drugs who have valid drug prescriptions are assessed individually to determine whether concentrations are according to recommended therapeutic doses and further in relation to the impairment law. Cases with detection of relevant drugs that are not among those with defined limits are also handled according to the impairment law. The list of drugs with legislative limits will be extended when relevant data from scientific studies become available; limits for some other drugs have already been suggested (Vindenes et al. 2015). Legislative *per se* limits were implemented in England and Wales in 2015 (UK Secretary of State 2014) and *per se* limits were implemented in the Netherlands in 2017 (Government of the Netherlands 2016). In December 2009, Walsh reported that a three US states had implemented *per se* limits (i.e., other than zero: Nevada, Ohio, and Virginia), whereas

14 states had zero-tolerance laws (see below) (Walsh 2009); by July 2015, 19 states had implemented *per se* or zero-tolerance limits (GHSA 2019b). Since then, more US states have implemented legislative limits.

There is limited documentation of the actual RTC risks associated with different drug concentrations in blood, in contrast to the documentation for alcohol. Therefore, zero-tolerance laws were established in many countries and states (EMCDDA 2019; Lacey et al. 2010; Walsh 2009; Walsh et al. 2004). Zero-tolerance laws can be regarded as a special case of *per se* laws whereby the legal limit is set to an analytical zero limit in the biological matrix (Walsh et al. 2004). Essentially, driving with any measurable amount of the specified substance in the blood constitutes an offence. The laws have been well accepted for illicit drugs, but more problematic for psychoactive medicines prescribed for medical treatment. Some countries therefore implemented a zero-tolerance law for illicit drugs and impairment law for medicines (EMCDDA 2009; Lillsunde and Gunnar 2005; Senna et al. 2010). The laws are in most countries or states related to any drug present in blood or serum (i.e., low concentration limits related to the quantitation limits for the analytical methods used); however, some countries or states allow the testing of urine instead of blood. Belgium, France, Spain, and some Australian states have also implemented zero-tolerance concentration limits in oral fluid (Parliament of Belgium 2009; Parliament of France 2003; Parliament of Spain 2014; Parliament of Victoria 2003).

13.1.4 Aims of This Article

The aim of this article is to give an overview of trends in DUI of alcohol, illicit drugs and psychoactive medication in general traffic and among those involved in fatal RTCs. Few countries have performed studies that may document trends in the use of drugs among drivers; most of the studies have been performed in North America, Europe, and Australia. We have selected countries with relevant data for both alcohol and drugs from different part of the world, including Australia, Brazil, Norway, Spain, and the United States. The trends in driving under the influence of alcohol in selected countries has been described and discussed previously (Stewart 2001; Stewart and Sweedler 2008; Sweedler 2007; Sweedler et al. 2004), but very little information has been summarized regarding trends in driving under the influence of drugs.

13.2 Methodological Issues and Limitations

13.2.1 Alcohol and Drugs in the General Driving Population

Data on the prevalence of DUI among drivers in general road traffic is important information for legal regulations, law enforcement, as well as preventive measures. Two methods have been used to obtain data on DUI prevalence: (a) surveys on self-reported DUI using questionnaires or interviews, and (b) road-side surveys or testing at enforcement road-blocks (sobriety checkpoints).

Surveys based on self-reported DUI (Aguilera et al. 2015; Alvarez et al. 1995; Chou et al. 2006; Watson and Freeman 2007) may be associated with measurement problems, e.g., the respondents may remember incorrectly, or deliberately underreport (Davis et al. 2010;

Tourangeau and Yan 2007; Van de Mortel 2008). The extent of under-reporting may depend on the attitudes toward driving after drinking or after using psychoactive drugs in the studied cohort, and may vary between countries or cohorts. A difficulty in some investigations is that only the use of one drug is studied, without asking for any simultaneous use of alcohol or other drugs.

Roadside surveys are performed by stopping random drivers at roads and time intervals selected at random or systematically. Breathalyzer tests for alcohol may be performed, and biological samples, such as oral fluid, blood or sweat, may be collected for analyses of alcohol and drugs. Data on self-reported alcohol and drug use, attitude toward DUI and previous DUI episodes may also be collected using questionnaires or interviews. This type of roadside survey is resource intensive and requires detailed planning to obtain representative sampling and prevalence estimates for alcohol and drug use in the general population. Roadside surveys may cover selected geographical areas and time periods or cover all days and time periods of the week.

An important challenge in studies with voluntary participation is to obtain high participation rate in order to get as correct data as possible. The proportion of refusers may be high, particularly if blood samples are collected; usually, the participation rate is higher if collecting oral fluid samples (Gjerde et al. 2011). However, many drivers may refuse to participate if they are not absolutely assured that the results will be anonymous.

Roadside surveys on alcohol using breathalyzers have been conducted in many countries for a number of years to study DUI of alcohol. Surveys that also included drug testing were previously more complicated due to lack of techniques for analysis many drugs simultaneously in small volumes of biological samples. However, during the last 15 years, roadside surveys using oral fluid for drugs analyses have become more feasible due to appropriate collection devices available on the marked, and improved analytical technique for detecting large number of substances simultaneously in very small volumes (Badawi et al. 2009; Bosker and Huestis 2009; Sergi et al. 2009; Øiestad et al. 2007). In roadblock studies and at sobriety checkpoints, breathalyzer tests or on-site drug tests are performed only for drivers who have been judged by police to appear to have been drinking or to be under the influence of drugs, unless the country's law allows testing without prior suspicion. This may generate a serious sampling bias because some drivers who are impaired by alcohol or drugs are not detected.

Recommendation on how to perform roadside surveys have been published (Walsh et al. 2008). The main difficulties when comparing results from various studies are that drugs included and cut-off concentrations may be different, different sampling devices may have been used if collecting oral fluid, and it may be difficult to compare prevalence data for oral fluid and blood if not using equivalent cut-off concentrations (Gjerde et al. 2014a; Gjerde and Verstraete 2011; Verstraete et al. 2011). Another problem is the refusal rate in voluntary studies. It is likely that a large proportion of those who had been driving under the influence of alcohol or drugs do not want to participate in such a study, particularly if it is part of a sobriety check organized by the police, as observed in Brazilian and American investigations (Pechansky et al. 2010; Wells et al. 1997). Prevalence rates measured at roadside surveys may not be comparable to prevalence rates at enforcement roadblocks.

Results from roadside and roadblock studies in five countries are presented in Table 13.1 and summarized in Section 13.3. Results from three countries are also presented in Figure 13.1.

Table 13.1 Roadside Surveys and Random Tests of Alcohol and Drugs among Drivers

Country (study area)[a]	Year of Study	Cohort[b]	N	Participation Rate	Samples & Data Source[c]	Main Findings[d]	References
Australia (Adelaide, SA)	1979–1994	Drivers in random traffic (10 pm–3 am)[e]	Unk	Unk	BR	BAC ≥ 0.8 g/L: 1979 ca. 12%; 1982 ca. 3.5%; 1983 ca. 5%; 1987 ca. 4%; 1993 ca. 2%	McLean et al. (1995)
Australia (Adelaide, SA)	1989	Drivers in random traffic (10 pm–3 am)[e]	5,751	90%	BR	Before easter: BAC ≥ 0.5 g/L 8.2%, ≥0.8 g/L 4.2% After easter: BAC ≥ 0.5 g/L 5.8%, ≥0.8 g/L 2.5%	McLean et al. (1991)
Australia (Adelaide, SA)	1991–1993	Drivers in random traffic (10 pm–3 am)[e]	20,734	95%	BR	1991 pre 0.5 g/L limit: BAC ≥ 0.5 g/L 5.1%, ≥0.8 g/L 2.5% 1991 post 0.5 g/L limit: BAC ≥ 0.5 g/L 4.6%, ≥0.8 g/L 2.1% 1993: BAC ≥ 0.5 g/L 3.5%, ≥0.8 g/L 1.5%	Kloeden and McLean (1994)
Australia (Vic)	2004–2006	Drivers in random traffic[e]	25,317	99.93%	OF; if pos B or OF	Drugs: 2.1% (ecs 1.1%, met 1.8%, mul 0.5% thc 0.6%)	Boorman and Owens (2009)
Australia (Melbourne, Vic)	2004–2005	Drivers in random traffic[e]	13,176	Unk	Alcohol: BR. Drugs: OF; if pos: B or OF	Alcohol: 1.0%. Drugs: 2.4% (ecs 1.3%, met 2.1%, thc 0.7%, thc+amps 0.6%)	Drummer et al. (2007)
Australia (Vic)	2001–2010	Drivers in random traffic[e]	Unk	Unk	BR	BAC ≥ 0.5 g/L decreased from 0.57% to 0.37% from 2002 to 2010 (estimated)	McIntyre et al. (2011)
Australia (Vic)	2009–2010	Drivers in random traffic[e]	Unk	Unk	OF	Drugs: 853 samples (coc 68, cod 78, ecs 141, mam 41, met 661, mor 66, thc 355)	Chu et al. (2012)
Australia (Vic)	2005–2013	Drivers in random traffic[e]	Unk	Unk	OF	Drugs: 2.3% in 2005; 1.1% in 2009; 5.0% in 2012, 6.3% in 2013	Chu (2014); Swann (2014)

(Continued)

Table 13.1 (*Continued*) Roadside Surveys and Random Tests of Alcohol and Drugs among Drivers

Country (study area)[a]	Year of Study	Cohort[b]	N	Participation Rate	Samples & Data Source[c]	Main Findings[d]	References
Australia (Qld)	2006–2007	Drivers in random traffic (5 pm–1 am)[e]	2,657	Unk; 74.1% in sub–sample	OF	Drugs: 3.8% (amps 0.9%, coc 0.2%, ecs 2.0%, thc 1.7%)	Davey et al. (2009)
Australia (Brisbane, Qld)[f]	2006–2007	Drivers in random traffic (5 pm–1 am)[e]	1,587	Unk; 74.1% in sub-sample	OF	Drugs: 3.7% (amps 1.1%, coc 0.1%, ecs 2.2%, thc 1.3)	Davey and Freeman (2009)
Australia (Townsville, Qld)[f]	2006–2007	Drivers in random traffic (5 pm–1 am)[e]	781	Unk; 74.1% in sub-sample	Alcohol: BR Drugs: OF	Alcohol: 0.8%. Drugs: 3.5% (amps 1.4%, can 1.7%)	Davey et al. (2007)
Australia (Qld)	2007–2012	Drivers in random traffic[e]	80,624	Unk	OF	Drugs: 2.7% (ecs 0.2%, met 1.8%; thc 1.5%). Increasing from 2% in 2007 to 4% in 2012.	Davey et al. (2014)
Australia (SA)	2006–2012	Drivers in random traffic[e]	Unk	Unk	OF	met: 2006–7 ca. 2%, 2011–12 ca. 5%; thc: 2006–7 ca. 1.5%, 2011–12 ca. 3.3%	Thompson (2013)
Brazil (Diadema, SP)[g]	2005–2006	Drivers at sobriety checkpoints Fri–Sat nights and Sun afternoons[e]	655 (active breath-alyzer)	66%	BR	BAC ≥ 0.6 g/L: 17.1%	Duailibi et al. (2007)
Brazil (Belo Horizonte, MG)[g]	2005–2006	Drivers at sobriety checkpoints Fri–Sat (10 pm–3 am)[e]	913	67%	BR	BAC ≥0.6 g/L: 19.6%	Campos et al. (2008)
Brazil (South-East)	2005–2007	Drivers at sobriety checkpoint, mostly Fri–Sat (10 pm–3 or 4 am); some Sun (3–7 pm), some Thu (10 pm–4 am)[e]	3,488	83%	BR	BAC ≥ 0.6 g/L: 15.9%	Campos et al. (2013a)

(*Continued*)

Table 13.1 (*Continued*) Roadside Surveys and Random Tests of Alcohol and Drugs among Drivers

Country (study area)[a]	Year of Study	Cohort[b]	N	Participation Rate	Samples & Data Source[c]	Main Findings[d]	References
Brazil (SP)	2007–2009	Drivers at sobriety checkpoints Fri–Sat (11 pm–3 am)[e]	3,229	76%	BR	BAC > 0.2 g/L: 27% in 2007; 11% in 2009	Campos et al. (2013c)
Brazil (Belo Horizonte, MG)	2009	Drivers at sobriety checkpoints Fri–Sat (11 pm–3 am)[e]	1,254	73%	BR	BAC > 0.2 g/L: 13.6%, BAC > 0.6 g/L: 6.4%	Campos et al. (2013b)
Brazil (27 state capitals)	2008–2009	Drivers in random traffic Fri–Sat (12 am–12 pm)	3,326	97%	Alcohol: BR Drugs: OF	BAC > 0.2 g/L: 2.7%, BAC > 0.1 g/L: 4.8% Drugs: ben: 1.0%, sti 1.0%, thc 0.5%	Gjerde et al. (2014b)
Brazil (Palmas, TO; Teresina, PI)	2011–2012	Drivers at sobriety checkpoints Wed–Sat (7 pm–2 am), Sun (4 pm to 2 am)[e]	492	48%	BR	BAC > 0.0 g/L: 8.8% in Palmas, 5.0% in Teresina	Sousa et al. (2013)
Brazil (Curitiba, PR)	2012	Drivers at sobriety checkpoints Wed–Sat (8 pm–1 am)[e]	183	36%	BR	BAC > 0.1 g/L: 2.7%	Aguilera et al. (2015)
Brazil (3 of 4 regions)	1996	Truck drivers in random traffic[e]	728	Unk	U	Drugs: amp 4.8%, can 0.27%, coc 0.27%, met 0.00%	Silva et al. (2003)
Brazil (SP)	2002–2008	Truck drivers in random traffic[e]	1,250	98.4%	OF	Alcohol: 1.44% Drugs: amp 0.64%, coc 0.56%, mul 0.08%, thc 0.40%	Yonamine et al. (2013)
Brazil (SP)	2008–2011	Truck drivers in random traffic[e]	993	94%	U	Drugs: amps 5.4%, coc 2.6%, can 1.0% Significant association between amp use and travel length	Sinagawa et al. (2015)

(*Continued*)

Table 13.1 (*Continued*) Roadside Surveys and Random Tests of Alcohol and Drugs among Drivers

Country (study area)[a]	Year of Study	Cohort[b]	N	Participation Rate	Samples & Data Source[c]	Main Findings[d]	References
Brazil (SP)	2009	Truck drivers in random traffic[e]	456	93.4%	U	Drugs: amp 5.8% (mainly fenproporex), can 1.1%, coc 2.2%, mul 0.2%	Leyton et al. (2012)
Brazil (SP)	2009–2012	Truck drivers in random traffic[e]	1,370	97%	U	amp: 5.4% in 2009, 1.7% in 2012 coc: 2.5% in 2009, 3.9% in 2012	Sinagawa et al. (2013)
Brazil (SP)	2010	Truck drivers in random traffic[e]	134	Unk	U	amp 10.8%	Takitane et al. (2013)
Brazil (SP)	2012	Truck drivers in random traffic[e]	427	Unk	U	amp 2.7%	Oliveira et al. (2013)
Brazil (Paranagua, PR)	2012	Truck drivers in at terminal port	62	28%	U	amp 1.6%, can 0.0%, coc 4.8%, mul 1.6%	Peixe et al. (2014)
Brazil (SP)	2014–2015	Truck drivers in random traffic[e]	762	99.7%	OF	dru 5.2% (coc 2.8%, amp 2.1%, thc 1.1%)	Bombana et al. (2017)
Brazil (SP)	2009–2016	Truck drivers in random traffic[e]	4,125	99%	U	dru 7.8% (bze 3.6%, amp 3.4%, can 1.6%)	Leyton et al. (2019)
Norway (Oslo)	1970–1971	Random drivers (10 pm–2 am)	1,927	Unk	BR	BAC > 0.5 g/L: 2.0%	Bø (1972)
Norway (Oslo)	1977	Random drivers (10 pm–2 am)	1,152	98%	BR	BAC > 0.5 g/L: 1.0%	Christensen et al. (1978)
Norway (Nationwide)	1981–1982	Random drivers	71,999	100%	BR	BAC > 0.5 g/L: 0.27% 10 pm–2 am: BAC > 0.5 g/L: 0.2%	Glad (1985)
Norway (Oslo & Bergen)	2003–2004	Random drivers	410	94%	BR	BAC > 0.5 g/L: 0.0%, drugs: 1.0%	Assum et al. (2005)

(*Continued*)

Table 13.1 (*Continued*) Roadside Surveys and Random Tests of Alcohol and Drugs among Drivers

Country (study area)[a]	Year of Study	Cohort[b]	N	Participation Rate	Samples & Data Source[c]	Main Findings[d]	References
Norway (South-East)	2005–2006	Random drivers	10,816	88%	OF	Alcohol: 0.4% (BAC > 0.2 g/L 0.3%) 10 pm–2 am: BAC > 0.5 g/L <0.1% Drugs: med 3.4% (ben 1.4%, coc/bze 0.1%, cod 0.8%, zop 1.4%); ill 1.0% (amps 0.3%, thc 0.6%)	Gjerde et al. (2008)
Norway (4 regions)	2008–2009	Random drivers	9,410	94%	OF	Alcohol: 0.3% (BAC > 0.2 g/L: 0.2%) 10 pm–2 am: BAC > 0.5 g/L: <0.1% Drugs: med 3.2% (ben 1.6%, cod 0.4%, zop 1.4%); ill 1.5% (amp 0.3%, coc/bze 0.4%, thc 1.1%)	Gjerde et al. (2013a)
Norway (Nationwide)	2011	Random drivers[e]	30,441	Unk	BR	BAC > 0.2 g/L: 0.16%	TISPOL (2011)
Norway (North)	2014–2015	Random drivers	3,027	94%	OF	BAC > 0.5 g/L: 0.1%. Drugs: 3.9% (med 2.5%, ill 1.6%)	Jamt et al. (2017)
Norway (South-east)	2016–2017	Random drivers	5,034	91%	OF	BAC > 0.2 g/L: 0.2%; >0.5 g/L: 0.1% Drugs: 4.6% (med 3.0%, ill 1.7%)	Furuhaugen et al. (2018)
Spain	1989–1998	Random drivers[e]	>1 mill. per year	Unk	BR	Alcohol: increase from about 1% in 1989 to 3.5% in 1998.	Alvarez et al. (2000)
Spain (Catalonia)	2013	Random drivers	7,596	100%	BR	BAC > 0.5 g/L: 1.29% (Sat 1.90%, Sun 4.21%).	Alcañiz et al. (2014)

(*Continued*)

Table 13.1 (*Continued*) Roadside Surveys and Random Tests of Alcohol and Drugs among Drivers

Country (study area)[a]	Year of Study	Cohort[b]	N	Participation Rate	Samples & Data Source[c]	Main Findings[d]	References
Spain (4 regions)	2008–2009	Random drivers	3,302	98%	Alcohol: BR Drugs: OF	BAC > 0.1 g/L: 6.6% (including alc+dru). Drugs 6.93% (amps 0.06%, ben 0.17%, thc 5.28%, coc 1.28%, opi 0.14%, mul 0.55%); alc+dru: 1.69%	Fierro et al. (2015)
Spain (4 regions)	2012	Random drivers	2,932	100%	Alcohol: BR Drugs: OF	BAC > 0.1 g/L: 4.1% (including alc+dru) Drugs: 4.87% (amps 0.12%, ben 0.09%, coc 0.87%, mul 0.90%, opi 0.03%, thc 3.13%); alc+dru: 0.72%.	Fierro et al. (2015)
Spain (Catalonia)	2014	Random drivers	521	100%	OF	Drugs 16.4% (thc 12.4%, met 3.4%, amp 2.2%, coc 1.8%, opi 0.7%, ben 0.4%)	Alcañiz et al. (2018)
Spain (Nationwide)	2005	Random drivers	2,744	100%	Alcohol: BR Drugs: OF	BAC > 0.1 g/L: 2.6%. Drugs: 9.8% (thc 7.5%, coc 4.7%, amf 1.3%, ben 0.7%, opi 0.4%, ket 0.2%)	Domingo-Salvany et al. (2017)
US (18 states)	1973	Random drivers Fri, Sat (10–12 pm) Sat, Sun (1–3 am)	3,192	86%	BR	BAC ≥ 0.2 g/L: 22.6%, BAC ≥ 0.5 g/L:13.5%, BAC ≥ 1.0 g/L:5.0%	Wolfe (1974)
US (24 areas)	1986	Random drivers Fri, Sat (10–12 pm) Sat, Sun (1–3 am)	2,850	92 %	BR	BAC ≥ 0.2 g/L:19.5, BAC ≥ 0.5 g/L:8.4%, BAC ≥ 1.0 g/L: 3.2%	Lund and Wolfe (1991)
US (24 areas)	1996	Random drivers Fri, Sat (10–12 pm) Sat, Sun (1–3 am)	6,028	96%	BR	BAC ≥ 0.05 g/L :17.0%, BAC ≥ 0.5 g/L: 7.8%, BAC ≥ 1.0 g/L: 2.8%	Voas et al. (1998)

(*Continued*)

Table 13.1 (*Continued*) Roadside Surveys and Random Tests of Alcohol and Drugs among Drivers

Country (study area)[a]	Year of Study	Cohort[b]	N	Participation Rate	Samples & Data Source[c]	Main Findings[d]	References
US (24 areas)	2005	Random drivers Fri, Sat (10–12 pm) Sat, Sun (1–3 am)	761 BR 642 OF 406 B	79% 67% 42%	Alcohol: BR Drugs: OF and/or B	BAC ≥0.05 g/L :14.5%, BAC ≥ 0.5 g/L: 5.6%, BAC ≥ 1.0 g/L: 2.1%. Drugs only:13.3%; alc+dru: 1.7%. amp 2.2%, ben 1.6%, can 7.4%, coc 2.2%	Lacey et al. (2007)
US (300 locations)	2007	Random drivers Fri, Sat (10–12 pm) Sat, Sun (1–3 am)	9,413 BR 7,719 OF 3,276 B	87% 71% 39%	Alcohol: BR Drugs: OF and/or B	Weekend nights: BAC ≥ 0.05 g/L:12.4.%,; BAC > 0.5 g/L: 4.5%, BAC > 0.8 g/L: 2.2%; Drugs: ill11.4% (amp 0.45%, can 8.7%, coc 3.9%; met 0.84%); med 3.9% (alp 0.64%, hyd 0.68%, oxy 0.82%)	Lacey et al. (2009a, 2009b)
US (300 locations)	2013–2014	Random drivers Fri, Sat (10–12 pm) Sat, Sun (1–3 am)	9,455 BR 7,881 OF 4,686 B	85% 71% 42%	Alcohol: BR Drugs: OF and/or B	Weekend nights: BAC > 0.05 g/L 8.3%; BAC > 0.5 g/L 3.1%, BAC > 0.8 g/L 1.5%; Drugs: ill 15.1% (can 12.6%); only med 4.9%	Berning et al. (2015)

[a] Abbreviations for study area: MG = Minas Gerais; PI = Piauí; PR = Paraná; Qld = Queensland; SA = South Australia; SP = São Paulo; TO = Tocantins; Vic = Victoria.
[b] The term "driver" may include different categories of motor vehicle drivers and motorcycle riders if not specified.
[c] Abbreviations for samples and data sources: B = blood; BR = breath; OF = oral fluid.
[d] Abbreviations for main findings: alc = alcohol; alp = alprazolam; amp = amphetamine; amps = amphetamines; BAC = blood alcohol concentration; ben = benzodiazepines; bze = benzoylecgonine (cocaine metabolite); coc = cocaine; cod = codeine; dru = drugs; ecs = ecstasy; hyd = hydrocodone; ill = illicit drugs; med = psychoactive medicinal drugs; met = methamphetamine; mul = multiple drug use; opi = opioids; oxy = oxycodone; sti = stimulants; thc = tetrahydrocannabinol; zop = zopiclone.
[e] Based on data from police operations, which may introduce a selection bias because the choice of time periods and roads is not by random.
[f] Data also included in the article by Davey and Freeman (2009).
[g] Data also included in the article by Campos et al. (2013a).

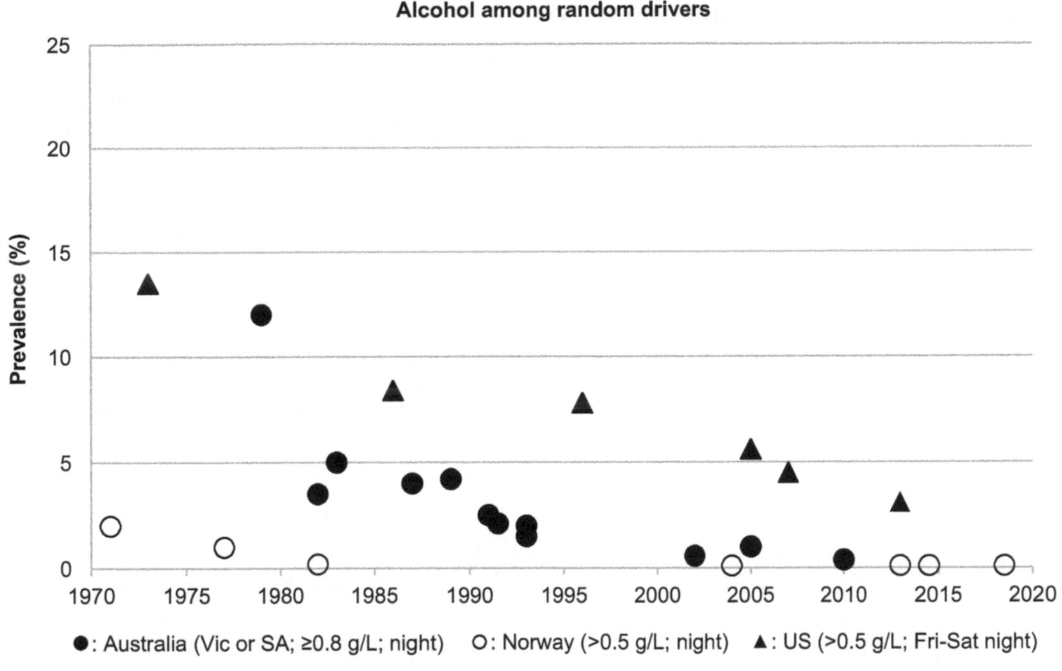

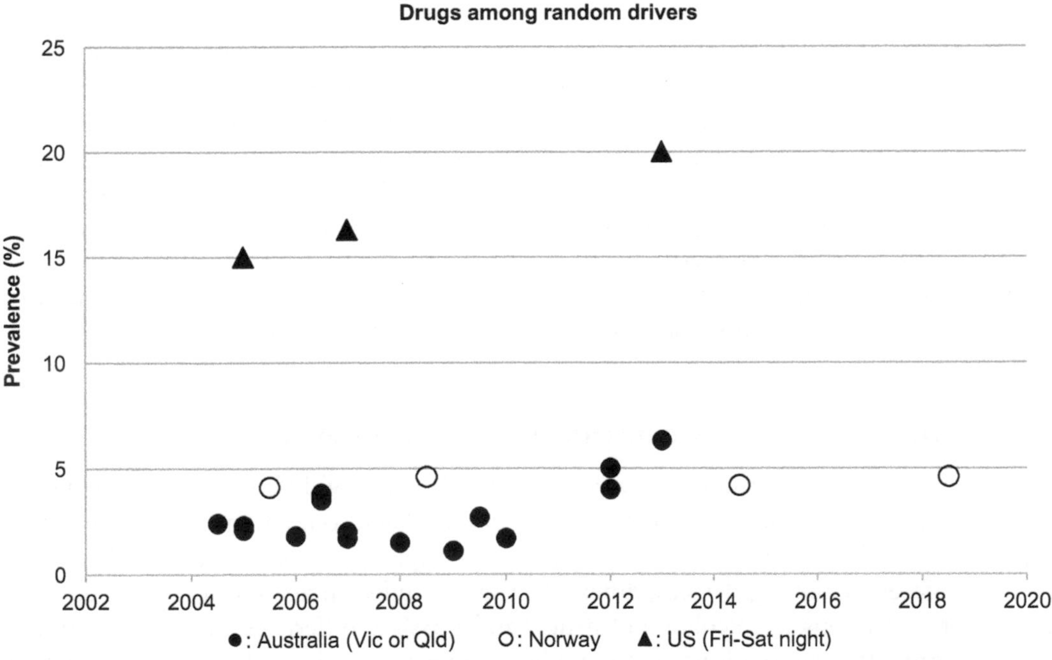

Figure 13.1 Trends in alcohol and drug findings among random drivers in Australia, Norway, and the US. Some of the time points represent averages for periods of several years.

13.2.2 Studies of RTC-Involved Drivers

The prevalence of alcohol and other substances among drivers involved in RTCs gives valuable information of the association between DUI and RTC, and data on alcohol and drug trends among drivers and possible effects after changes in law and enforcement. It is then important that the studies are performed using a standardized protocol. Recommendations for studies on RTC-involved drivers (Walsh et al. 2008) and for toxicological investigations of drug-impaired driving and RTC (Logan et al. 2013) have been published.

In studies of drivers injured in RTCs, there is always a selection bias: only those who are treated for injuries or those who are apprehended by the police due to RTC-involvement are included in the studies. Thus, large proportions of drivers with minor injuries or non-injurious RTCs are often not included. If the study requires voluntary participation, a high refusal rate may also be a problem. Another difficulty is related to the time of blood sampling after the RTC occurred. The concentration of alcohol and drugs may decline before the sample is taken. This is especially a problem for drugs with short elimination times, such as THC (in the distribution phase) (Wood et al. 2016) and cocaine (Cone 1995), which may have declined to insignificant levels before a sample is collected. To avoid the problems due to the selection bias based on severity of crash or injury and decline in alcohol and drug concentrations before blood samples were taken from injured drivers, we have in this review only included drivers (and motorcycle riders) who were killed in RTCs.

In studies of fatal RTCs, there may also be a selection bias as the proportion of drivers who are subject to legal autopsy and/or drug testing may be low. This may be due to lack of suspicion of DUI by the police, and may bias the findings significantly. Another difficulty is that a decrease or increase in alcohol and drug concentrations may have occurred after the accident or death; decrease due to metabolism or degradation; and increase due to absorption or re-distribution (Drummer 2004; Skopp 2010). The findings also depend on the analytical program employed.

Results from studies of fatally injured drivers are presented in Table 13.2 and summarized in Section 13.3. Results from three countries are also presented in Figure 13.2.

13.2.3 Difficulties When Comparing Results of Different Studies

It is difficult to compare findings in various studies because of differences in study design. For roadside surveys, the differences are most often related to different time periods during the day, week or year for the studies, different sample types (oral fluid, blood, urine or sweat), different sampling devices, different drugs included in analytical testing, different cutoff concentrations for alcohol and drugs, and possibly difference between urban and rural areas and types of roads where the studies were performed. In addition, low participation rates may bias the findings.

For studies of RTC fatalities, the magnitude of the selection bias (see above) may be different. In some studies, data for drivers, passengers, pedestrians and other road users are not separated. This may be due to lack of access to important crash data, or because the aim is to study RTC victims in total, not drivers. If studying only drivers, most studies do not distinguish between drivers who are culpable or non-culpable for the crash.

Table 13.2 Studies and Statistics on Drivers Fatally Injured in Road Crashes

Country (Study Area)[a]	Year of Study	Cohort[b]	N	Participation Rate	Samples & Data Data Source[c]	Main Findings[d]	References
Australia	1981–1998	Fatally injured drivers autopsied	Unk	Unk	B	BAC ≥ 0.5 g/L declined from 44% in 1981 to 26% in 1998	Australian Transportation Safety Bureau (2001)
Australia	2000–2008	Fatally injured drivers autopsied	Unk	Unk	B	BAC > 0.5 g/L increased from 24% in 2000 to about 34% in 2007 and 28% in 2008	Australian Transport Council (2011)
Australia	2005–2008	Road fatalities	Unk	Unk	B	Prevalence of alcohol and drugs varied across states and territories; alcohol from 11% in TAS to 48% in NT; drugs from 6% in TAS to 32% in Vic	Owens and Boorman (2011)
Australia (Except Vic)	2013	Fatally injured drivers autopsied	Unk	Unk	B	BAC > 0.5 g/L: 22.4%	BITRE (2015)
Australia (Except Vic, WA)	2016	Fatally injured drivers autopsied	Unk	Unk	B	BAC > 0.5 g/L: 17.8%	BITRE (2018)
Australia (SA)	1979–1993	Fatally injured drivers autopsied	Unk	Unk	B	BAC ≥ 0.8 g/L: 1979 ca. 55%, 1982 ca. 40%, 1987 ca. 45%, 1993 ca. 22%	McLean et al. (1995)
Australia (Vic)	1987–2012	Fatally injured drivers and riders	Unk	Unk	B	BAC ≥ 0.5 g/L: decreased from 38% in 1987 to 24% in 2012	TAC (2013)
Australia (Vic)	2001–2013	Fatally injured drivers and riders	Unk	Unk	B	BAC > 0.5 g/L (total) decreased from 22% in 2001 to 20% in 2013; alcohol + drugs increased from 10% to 17%, and drugs (total) increased from 20% to 41%	Swann (2014)

(Continued)

Table 13.2 (*Continued*) Studies and Statistics on Drivers Fatally Injured in Road Crashes

Country (Study Area)[a]	Year of Study	Cohort[b]	N	Participation Rate	Samples & Data Data Source[c]	Main Findings[d]	References
Australia (WA)	1985–1995	Fatally injured drivers autopsied	2,388	Unk	B, U	CNS-acting drugs: increase from 6% (1985) to 32% (1995)	Swensen and Jones (1996)
Australia (WA)	2000–2012	Fatally injured drivers autopsied	1,375	90%	B	BAC ≥ 0.5 g/L: 34.2%. Drugs: ill 22.7% (thc 18.0%, met 7.4%, ecs 1.6%); med: opi 11.9%, and 7.3%, ben 5.7%, sti 2.0%	Palamara et al. (2014)
Australia (Vic, NSW, WA)	1990–1992	Fatally injured drivers autopsied	1,045	Unk	B	BAC ≥ 0.1 g/L: 36%. Drugs: 22% (can 11%, sti 3.7%, opi 2.7%, ben 3.1%, opd 5.6%)	Gerostamoulos et al. (2000)
Australia (Vic, NSW, WA)	1995–1996	Fatally injured drivers autopsied	Vic 590 NSW 143 WA 188	94% 27% 94%	B	BAC ≥ 0.1 g/L: 32%. Drugs: 27% (can 13%, sti 3.2%, ben 3.8%, opi 4.0%, opd 10%)	Gerostamoulos et al. (2000)
Australia (Vic, NSW, WA)	1990–1999	Fatally injured drivers autopsied	3,398	Unk	B	BAC ≥ 0.5 g/L: 29.1%. Psychotropic drugs: 23.5%; can 13.5%; opi 4.9%; sti 4.1%; ben 4.1%	Drummer et al. (2003)
Australia (Qld)	2000–2013	Fatally injured drivers autopsied	2,638	97%	B	BAC > 0.5 g/L: 24.8%, alc + dru 11.0%, med 21.2%, ill 18.4%	Drummer and Yap (2016)
Australia (SA)	2012–2016	Fatally injured drivers autopsied	281	93%	B	Alcohol or drugs: 37%. Alc 12%; ill 24%	Government of South Australia (2017)
Brazil (São Paulo, SP)	1999	Fatally injured traffic crash victims autopsied	2,360	Unk	B	44.9% of victims killed in collisions had BAC ≥ 0.1 g/L	Leyton et al. (2005)

(*Continued*)

Table 13.2 (*Continued*) Studies and Statistics on Drivers Fatally Injured in Road Crashes

Country (Study Area)[a]	Year of Study	Cohort[b]	N	Participation Rate	Samples & Data Data Source[c]	Main Findings[d]	References
Brazil (São Paulo, SP)	2005	Fatally injured traffic crash victims autopsied	907 (309 drivers)	Unk	B	43.4% of car drivers and motorcyclists had BAC ≥ 0.6 g/L	De Carvalho Ponce et al. (2011)
Brazil (Brasilia, DF)	2005	Fatally injured traffic crash victims autopsied	158	Unk	B	48% of victims of collisions and overturns had BAC > 0.6 g/L.	Dos Santos Modelli et al. (2008)
Brazil (São Paulo, SP)	2007–2008	Fatally injured traffic crash victims autopsied	1,095	Unk	B	44.4% (2007) and 38.4% (2008) of car drivers, passengers, cyclists and motorcyclists had BAC ≥ 0.2 g/L. For 2nd half of 2008: 36.1%	Koizumi et al. (2010)
Brazil (São Paulo, SP)	2014–2015	Fatallly injured traffic crash victims autopsied	56	Unk	B	Alcohol: 42.9%	Andreuccetti et al. (2017)
Norway (South-East)	1959–1969 1973–1975	Fatally injured traffic crash victims autopsied	134	Unk	B	BAC > 0.5 g/L: 25% (1959–1969); 45% (1973–1975)	Lundevall and Olaisen (1976)
Norway (Nationwide)	1976–1977	Fatally injured traffic crash victims autopsied	133	82%	B	32% of killed drivers had BAC > 0.5 g/L	Andenæs and Sørensen (1979)
Norway (16 of 19 counties)	1989–1990	Fatally injured drivers autopsied	159	57%	B	Alcohol 28.3% (BAC > 0.5 g/L: 27.0%). Drugs: 16.4% (amp 0.6%, cod 1.3%, dia 6.3%, thc 5.0%)	Gjerde et al. (1993)
Norway (10 of 19 counties)	1994–1999	Fatally injured drivers autopsied	163	34%	B	BAC > 0.5 g/L: 17%. Drugs 27.1%.	Brevig et al. (2004)

(*Continued*)

Table 13.2 (*Continued*) Studies and Statistics on Drivers Fatally Injured in Road Crashes

Country (Study Area)[a]	Year of Study	Cohort[b]	N	Participation Rate	Samples & Data Data Source[c]	Main Findings[d]	References
Norway (16 of 19 counties)	2001–2010	Fatally injured car and van drivers autopsied or investigated for alcohol or drug use	676	63%	B	BAC > 0.2 g/L: 25.3% (BAC > 0.5 g/L: 24.0%) Drugs: 21.9%; med 14.4% (dia 5.5%, oxa 2.7%, zop 2.5%); ill 14.1% (amp 8.0%, met 3.8%, thc 7.2%)	Christophersen and Gjerde (2014)
Norway (16 of 19 counties)	2001–2010	Fatally injured motorcycle riders autopsied or investigated for alcohol or drug use	207	63%	B	BAC > 0.2 g/L: 17.4%. Drugs: med 7.2% (clo 1.0%, dia 3.4%, flu 1.0%, zop 1.0%); ill 9.2% (amp 5.3%, thc 4.3%)	Christophersen and Gjerde (2015)
Norway (Nationwide)	2011–2015	Fatally injured car and van drivers autopsied or investigated for alcohol or drug use	337	69%	B	BAC > 0.5 g/L: 14.2%. Drugs: 15.9% (above graded sanction limits corresponding to BAC 0.5 g/L)	Valen et al. (2019)
Spain (North-West)	1980s	Fatally injured drivers autopsied	113	Unk	B	BAC > 0.1 g/L: 77%, BAC > 0.5 g/L: 71%	Bermejo et al. (1993)
Spain (North-West)	1996–1998	Fatally injured drivers autopsied	338	Unk	B, U	BAC detected: 58.9%; BAC > 0.8 g/L: 33%; ben 19%; can 4%	Lopez-Rivadulla and Cruz (2000)
Spain	1991–1998	Fatally injured drivers autopsied	3,191	Unk	B	Alcohol 47.3%, BAC > 0.8 g/L: 35.1% (42.2% in 1991, 30.4% in 1998). Drugs: med 4.8% (6.6% in 1991,4.5% in 1998); ill 8.9% (7.7% in 1991, 9.4% in 1998)	Alvarez et al. (2000)
Spain	1994–1996	Fatally injured drivers autopsied	285	Unk	B	Alcohol 50.5% (BAC ≥ 0.8 g/L 35.4%); med 9.1%; ill 10.2% (amps 1.4%, can 1.4%, coc 7.4%, ecs 1.1%, opi 4.9%)	Del Rio and Alvarez (1999, 2000)

(*Continued*)

Table 13.2 (*Continued*) Studies and Statistics on Drivers Fatally Injured in Road Crashes

Country (Study Area)[a]	Year of Study	Cohort[b]	N	Participation Rate	Samples & Data Data Source[c]	Main Findings[d]	References
Spain	1991–2000	Fatally injured drivers autopsied	5,745	9.7%[e]	B	Alcohol 43.8% (BAC > 0.8 g/L 32.0%); ill 8.8% (amp 1.2%, can 2.2%, coc 5.2%, opi 3.2%); med 4.7% (ana 0.4%, and 0.6%, ben 3.4%)	Del Rio et al. (2002)
Spain	2012	Fatally injured drivers autopsied	615	53%	B	Alcohol 35.1%; med 13.5%; ill 12.7%	Alvarez and Gonzalez-Luque (2014)
Spain	2014	Fatally injured drivers autopsied	614	71%	B	Alcohol 26.2%; med 10.7%; ill 13.3%	Arroyo et al. (2016)
US	1982–2011	Fatally injured drivers autopsied	Unk	Unk	B, U (FARS)	1982: BAC ≥ 0.5 g/L 52%, BAC ≥ 0.8 g/L: 33%. 2011: BAC ≥ 0.5 g/L: 49%, BAC ≥ 0.8 g/L: 31%. Drugs: 27%, can 8% (increase from 4% in 2000 to 11% in 2010), sti 7%	Fell and Romano (2013)
US (24 states)	1999–2010	Fatally injured drivers autopsied	95,654	Unk	B, U (FARS)	BAC ≥ 0.8 g/L: 33%. Drugs: 24.6%, increased by 49% from 1999–2000 to 2009–2010, particularly for ben, can, opi	Rudisill et al. (2014)
US	2005–2009	Fatally injured drivers autopsied	Unk	Unk	B, U (FARS)	Drugs: Increase from 28% (2005, 2006 and 2007) to 30% in 2008 and 33% in 2009	CESAR (2010)
US (14 states)	2005–2009	Fatally injured drivers autopsied	20,150	Unk	B, U (FARS)	Alcohol 40.2%. Drugs 31.8% (can 10.5%, sti 9.0%, opi 5.7%, dep 4.0%)	Brady and Li (2013)
US (6 states)	1999–2010	Fatally injured drivers autopsied	23,591	Unk	B, U (FARS)	Alcohol 39.7%. Drugs 24.8% (increase from 16.6% in 1999 to 28.3% in 2010; can increase from 4.2% in 1999 to 12.2% in 2010)	Brady and Li (2014)

(*Continued*)

Table 13.2 (*Continued*) Studies and Statistics on Drivers Fatally Injured in Road Crashes

Country (Study Area)[a]	Year of Study	Cohort[b]	N	Participation Rate	Samples & Data Data Source[c]	Main Findings[d]	References
US (20 states)	1998–2010	Fatally injured drivers autopsied, single vehicle crashes only	16,942	Unk	B, U (FARS)	BAC ≥ 0.8 g/L: 39.9%. Drugs: 25.9% (can 7.1%, dep 1.5%, mul 4.1%, opi 2.1%, sti 7.2%	Romano and Pollini (2013)
US	1982–2016	Fatally injured drivers autopsied	818,718	Unk	B (FARS)	BAC ≥ 0.8 g/L: 20%–48%	NHTSA (2018)
US	2017	Fatally injured drivers/MC riders	23,611	Unk	B (FARS)	BAC ≥ 0.8 g/L: 20%	NHTSA (2019)

[a] Abbreviations for study area: DF = Distrito Federal; NSW = New South Wales; NT = Northern Territory; Qld = Queensland; SA = South Australia; SP = São Paulo; TAS = Tasmania; Vic = Victoria; WA = Western Australia.

[b] The term "drivers" may include different categories of motor vehicle drivers and motorcycle riders if not specified.

[c] Abbreviations for samples and data sources: B = blood; BR = breath; OF = oral fluid; FARS = Fatality Analysis Reporting System, a US database operated by the National Highway Traffic Safety Administration.

[d] Abbreviations for main findings: amp = amphetamine; amps = amphetamines; ana = analgesics; and = antidepressants; BAC = blood alcohol concentration; can = cannabis; clo = clonazepam; coc = cocaine; dep = depressants; dia = diazepam; ecs = ecstasy; flu = flunitrazepam; ill = illicit drugs; med = psychoactive medicinal drugs; mul = multiple drugs; opd = other psychoactive substances; opi = opioids (called "narcotics" in some American studies); oxa = oxazepam; sti = stimulants; thc = tetrahydrocannabinol; zop = zopiclone.

[e] From 2.8% in 1991 to 23.8% in 2000.

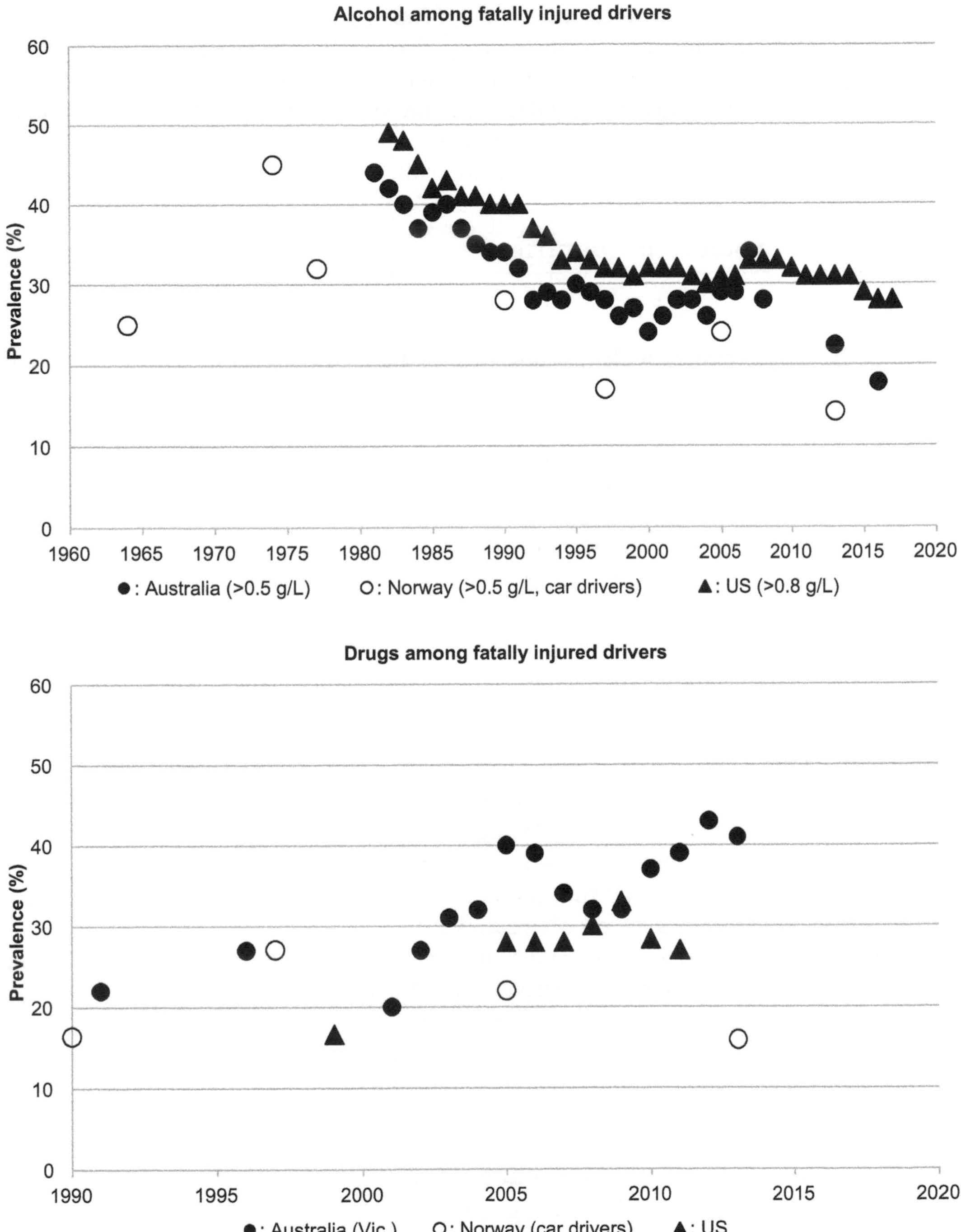

Figure 13.2 Trends in alcohol and drug findings among fatally injured drivers in Australia, Norway, and the US. Some of the time points represent averages for periods of several years.

Another difficulty is that a small selection of substances may be included in the alcohol and drug testing program. Sometimes only alcohol is tested for, in other cases only illicit drugs in addition to alcohol. To obtain optimal data, a wide selection of psychoactive drugs and metabolites should be included. In many studies, non-psychoactive drugs are also included when calculating the total prevalence of drugs. This makes comparison of the total drug prevalence in different studies difficult.

13.3 Trends in Selected Countries

13.3.1 Australia

Australia is a large country with vast distances and large differences between states and territories regarding RTC fatalities. The overall number of RTC fatalities decreased from 17.5 per 100,000 population in 1988 to 9.5 in 2000 and 5.1 in 2018 (BITRE 2018), ranging from 3.8 in the Australian Capital Territory to 20.0 in Northern Territory in 2015. The vision of the government for the future is that none should be killed or seriously injured on Australian roads; the target for 2020 is a reduction in the number of RTC fatalities by at least 30% and the number of serious injuries by at least 30% as compared with the number in 2010 (Australian Transportation Council 2011).

13.3.1.1 Law and Enforcement

The nine Australian states and territories have different DUI laws. BAC limits were implemented by in the late 1960s and 1970s; all states and territories except Victoria chose 0.8 g/L as limit. The BAC limits were reduced to 0.5 g/L in all states by 1994 (Haworth and Johnston 2004). Random breath testing was first introduced in Victoria in 1976 and was implemented in all other states and territories by 1988 (Owens and Boorman 2011). Some states have implemented zero limits for learners and professional drivers, and alcohol ignition interlocks were introduced for repeat-offenders in some states. Australia has a strong community support for drink driving countermeasures, with nearly universal agreement for random breath testing of drivers (Petroulias 2013).

From December 2004, a new drug driving legislation framework was implemented in Victoria as the first Australian state (Parliament of Victoria 2003); the law opened for random roadside drug testing in oral fluid performed by the police. Other states and territories followed with zero-tolerance laws for methamphetamine, ecstasy and cannabis and roadside surveys collecting oral fluid for drug analysis among randomly stopped or suspected drivers (Davey et al. 2014). Some areas may also test for other drugs (Owens and Boorman 2011).

13.3.1.2 Roadside Surveys and Random Testing

Results from studies on alcohol and drugs among random drivers in normal road traffic are presented in Table 13.1 and Figure 13.1. Random breath testing studies in South Australia documented a decline of alcohol related driving from 1979 to 1994; the proportion with BAC $\geq$ 0.8 g/L between 10 pm and 3 am declined from 12% to 2% (Kloeden and McLean 1994; McLean et al. 1991, 1995). Reduced incidence of drink driving was observed after a marked increase in the level of publicity of police random breath testing operations (McLean et al. 1991). A study in Victoria found a decrease in the prevalence of BAC $\geq$ 0.5 g/L from 0.57% in 2002 to 0.37% in 2010 (McIntyre et al. 2011).

Random testing in Victoria and Queensland during 2004–2006 found drugs (i.e., methamphetamine, THC or ecstasy) in 2.3%–3.8% of the samples (Boorman and Owens 2009; Davey et al. 2014; Davey and Freeman 2009; Davey et al. 2009; Davey et al. 2007; Drummer et al. 2007). The proportion of drug positive oral fluid samples increased from about 2% in 2007 to about 4% in 2012 (Davey et al. 2014). The rate of drug detection in Victoria decreased from 1:43 (2.3%) in 2005 to 1:94 (1.1%) in 2009, but has later increased to 1:16 (6.3%) in 2013 (Chu 2014; Swann 2014). Analysis of a broader selection of drugs found significantly lower prevalence of cocaine, codeine, morphine and monoacetylmorphine (6-MAM) than ecstasy, THC and methamphetamine in oral fluid samples from random drivers (Chu et al. 2012). Also, random testing in South Australia from 2006 to 2012 found a large increase in drug detections (Thompson 2013). However, if the study is part of police enforcement operations, the drug testing sites may be strategically chosen to be near locations where and when drug use is expected. So, data from such studies do not represent the true prevalence of drug use in random road traffic.

13.3.1.3 Drivers Killed in RTCs

Results from studies on alcohol and drugs among fatally injured drivers and riders are presented in Table 13.2 and Figure 13.2. Analysis of alcohol among drivers and motorcycle riders killed in RTCs showed a declining prevalence from 44% in 1981 to 24% in 2000, followed by an increase during 2001–2007 and a decline in 2008 (Australian Transport Council 2011; Australian Transportation Safety Bureau 2001); 34% had BAC above the legal limit in 2007 (Australian Transport Council 2011). Out of 608 fatally injured drivers and riders who died in all Australian states and territories except Victoria in 2013, 22.4% were reported to have BAC above the legal limit (BITRE 2015), whereas out of 527 fatally injured drivers in 2016 (except Victoria and Western Australia), 17.8% had BAC above the legal limit, indicating a further reduction in alcohol-related deaths (BITRE 2018).

Data from Victoria show that the percentage of alcohol related fatalities declined from 38% in 1987 to 18%–28% in 2006–2012 (TAC 2013). From 2001 to 2013, the prevalence of alcohol (total) in samples from killed drivers in Victoria was practically unchanged (decrease from 22% to 20%); the combination of alcohol plus drugs increased from 10% to 17%, and drugs (total) increased from 20% to 41% (Swann 2014). In Adelaide Metropolitan Area, South Australia, the prevalence of BAC ≥ 0.8 g/L among fatally injured drivers declined from about 55% in 1979 to about 22% in 1993 (McLean et al. 1995).

For fatally injured drivers in three Australian states (Victoria, New South Wales, Western Australia), the prevalence of BAC ≥ 0.1 g/L was 36% and drugs 22% in 1990–1992 (Gerostamoulos et al. 2000). For the period 1995–1995, the prevalence of BAC ≥ 0.1 g/L was 32% and a prevalence of drugs 27% (Gerostamoulos et al. 2000). A study covering 1999–2002 found prevalence of BAC ≥ 0.5 g/L of 29.1% and psychotropic drugs of 23.5%, respectively. The authors concluded that the prevalence of drugs increased from 1990 to 1999 particularly cannabis and opioids, while alcohol decreased (Drummer et al. 2003).

The prevalence of central nervous system (CNS)-acting drugs in samples from drivers and riders killed in RTCs in Western Australia found an increase from 6% in 1985 to 32% in 1995 (Swensen and Jones 1996). A study for the period 2000–2012 found that the prevalence of BAC ≥ 0.5 g/L was 34.2%, illicit drugs 22.7% (cannabis 18.0%); for medicinal drugs the most frequently found group was opioids (11.9%) followed by antidepressants (7.3%) and benzodiazepines (3.1) (Palamara et al. 2014).

The prevalence of alcohol and drugs in RTC fatalities varied between states and territories; the prevalence of alcohol was from 11% in Tasmania to 48% in Northern Territory in 2006/2008, while the prevalence of drugs varied from 6% in Tasmania to 32% in Victoria (Owens and Boorman 2011). A study of fatally injured motor vehicle drivers in South Australia found that 37% tested positive for alcohol or drugs during 2011–2016. The prevalence of alcohol declined, but drugs remained fairly steady compared to earlier five-year periods (Government of South Australia 2017). In a study on fatally injured drivers ($n = 2638$) in Victoria covering the period from 2000 to 2013, representing 97% of the fatalities, alcohol ≥0.5 g/L, alcohol plus drugs, medicinal and illicit drug were found among 24.8%, 11.9%, 21.2% and 18.4%, respectively, of the drivers. Increased crash risks were documented for use of alcohol, amphetamines and cannabis (Drummer and Yap 2016).

13.3.1.4 Trends

After the implementation of random breath testing, the incidence of drink driving and the proportion of alcohol-related RTCs declined significantly. Australia has therefore been deemed to have the most successful random breath testing program in the world, measured in terms of alcohol-related RTCs (Erke et al. 2009). This reduction was assumed to be related to the widespread use of random breath testing, formal and informal publicity about drink driving, a reduction in alcohol consumption, and other vehicle safety measures (Sweedler 2007). The number of random breath testing related to number of licensed drivers is 1:1 or greater in five states and territories (Ferris et al. 2015).

However, the proportion of the population who considered that drink driving was the factor that most often lead to RTCs fell from 23% in 1993 to 11% in 2012 (Petroulias 2013); the change was most significant during the first three years. The percentage reporting they never drink and drive was 34% in 1993 and 38% in 2012.

The proportion of drivers in random traffic with illicit drugs present in their system has been increasing. Similarly, the proportion of drug-related fatal crashes has increased during the last decades. The proportion of killed drivers and riders with BAC above the legal limit also increased during 2000–2007, but decreased significantly during recent years.

13.3.2 Brazil

Many studies on DUI have been performed in Brazil as compared with other middle-income countries. The country has deep regional differences; the Human Development Index (HDI) in the south and southeast is similar to that of Portugal, whereas the HDI in the north and northeast is similar to Botswana and Indonesia (Ribeiro et al. 2014). It might therefore be difficult to assess trends over time based on results from studies in different regions. The number of RTC fatalities decreased from 36.9 to 24.8 per 100,000 population from 2000 to 2015. Large variations between different states have been recorded (Ladeira et al. 2017). Trucks were involved in about 28% of all RTCs on federal highways in 2004 (Istituto de Pesquisa Econômica Aplicada, Departamento Nacional de Trânsito 2006). The number of RTC fatalities per 100,000 inhabitants (2000–2008 average) varied between regions: 17.8 in northeast, 19.5 in north, 19.4 in southeast, 26.0 in south and 29.7 in central-west of Brazil (Chandran et al. 2013).

13.3.2.1 Law and Enforcement

Brazil introduced a legal BAC limit of 0.8 g/L in 1989, which was reduced to 0.6 g/L in 1997 (Law 9.503/97) (Congress of Brazil 1997), and a "zero limit" was introduced in 2008 with suspension of driving privileges for a BAC above 0.2 g/L or a breath alcohol concentration (BrAC) of 0.1 mg/L (Law 11.705/8 "Dry Law") (Congress of Brazil 2008). The new law was followed by media campaigns and more active enforcement. The law was amended in 2012 (Law 12.760/12) (Congress of Brazil 2012); a concentration of alcohol in expired breath of 0.05 mg/L or more but less than 0.34 mg/L (corresponding to a BAC of 0.10–0.59 g/L) is regarded as an "administrative violation" resulting in a fine and suspension of the driving license, whereas a BrAC ≥ 0.34 mg/L (BAC ≥ 0.6 g/L) is regarded as a crime and may lead to imprisonment for 6 to 36 months in addition to suspension or prohibition of obtaining driving license. Signs of psychomotor impairment (without alcohol testing) may also lead to conviction ("administrative violation").

A survey among young adults aged 18–25 years living in São Paulo (in the southeast region of Brazil) was performed in 1998. The study found that many participants had low level of knowledge about the DUI law (Pinsky et al. 2001). A study performed in the city of Belo Horizonte (in the southeast region) in 2005–2006 found that 13.1% knew the BAC limit that would result to arrest (Campos et al. 2008). A study of drivers in 27 metropolitan areas performed in 2008–2009 found that 8.1% of the drivers knew the BAC limit that would result in arrest (Da Conceicao et al. 2012). Thus, only a small proportion of the drivers were aware of the law.

The enforcement of the DUI law has not been as strong as in many developed countries, such as Australia, Canada, United States, and many European countries. Drivers can refuse to give a breath or blood sample in accordance with the American Convention on Human Rights "Pact of San Jose, Costa Rica" (OAS 1978). As a large number of DUI suspects refused to provide a breath test or blood sample (Sousa et al. 2013), stricter legal sanctions were introduced in 2014, including sanctions for refusing to provide a breath or blood sample, which is an "administrative violation" (National Department of Traffic of Brazil 2014).

13.3.2.2 Roadside Surveys

Roadside surveys performed in southeast Brazil in 2005–2007 found that about 16%–20% of the drivers on Friday and Saturday nights had BAC above 0.6 g/L (Campos et al. 2008, 2013a; Duailibi et al. 2007) (Table 13.1). In Belo Horizonte, the proportion of drivers with BAC ≥ 0.6 g/L during those time periods declined from 19.6% in 2005–2006 (Campos et al. 2008) to 6.4% in 2009 (Campos et al. 2013b). The proportions of drivers with BAC > 0.2 g/L in 27 state capitals during Fridays and Saturdays between noon and midnight was 2.7% in 2008–9 (Gjerde et al. 2014b). When studying Wednesday to Saturday nights (7 pm–2 am), the prevalence of BAC > 0.0 g/L was 5.0%–8.8% in Palmas and Teresina in 2012 (Sousa et al. 2013), and the prevalence of BAC > 0.1 g/L Wednesday to Saturday nights (8 pm–1 am) in Curitiba was 2.7% in 2012 (Aguilera et al. 2015). It must be emphasized that the participation rates in the two last mentioned studies was less than 50%, so the figures are probably very much under-estimated.

Only one of the studies (performed in the state capitals) included analysis of drugs (Gjerde et al. 2014b). The most prevalent drugs were stimulants (4.8%, which included amphetamines and cocaine), benzodiazepines (1.0%) and THC (0.5%). Use of stimulants was most prevalent among truck drivers.

A study performed in 2011–2012 at police sobriety checkpoints in the southeast found that the prevalence of recent alcohol drinking was very high among those who refused to give a breathalyzer test or who fled the roadblock (Sousa et al. 2013); for example, 51% of drivers in the city of Palmas who reported that they had consumed alcohol within 6 hours before a breath sample was requested by the police refused to give a sample. Therefore, the official results of roadblock studies were under-estimating the actual prevalence of DUI significantly.

Many studies of truck drivers have been performed; all studied have found high prevalence of stimulant use. The reason is that many trucks drive long distances, often during the night, with little rest or sleep, in order to obtain a good monthly income. The reported prevalence of amphetamines in urine samples from truck drivers ranged from 3% to 10% with an average around 5% (Leyton et al. 2012; Oliveira et al. 2013; Peixe et al. 2014; Silva et al. 2003; Sinagawa et al. 2015; Sinagawa et al. 2013; Takitane et al. 2013). One study reported a decline in amphetamine detections from 5.4% in 2009 to 1.7% in 2012 and an increase in cocaine detections from 2.5% to 3.9% during the same period (Sinagawa et al. 2013). A study of drugs in oral fluid from truck drivers found, as expected, lower prevalence than in those studies that used urine samples (Yonamine et al. 2013). A study of drugs in oral fluid from truck drivers in the highways of Sao Paulo during 2014–2015 found that 5.2% tested positive for drugs. The most frequently detected substances were cocaine (2.8%), amphetamines (2.1%) and THC (1.1%) (Bombana et al. 2017). A study based on analysis of urine samples from truck drivers found a total prevalence of illicit drugs of 7.8%. The cocaine-metabolite benzoylecgonine was the most prevalent substance (3.6%), followed by amphetamine (3.4%) and the cannabis-marker THC-COOH (1.6%) (Leyton et al. 2019).

13.3.2.3 Drivers Killed in RTCs

Most studies have not differentiated between different types of killed road users; the studies found that 43%–48% of RTC victims were positive for alcohol (Andreuccetti et al. 2017; De Carvalho Ponce et al. 2011; Dos Santos Modelli et al. 2008; Koizumi et al. 2010; Leyton et al. 2005). One study reported the prevalence of alcohol among fatally injured drivers and motorcycle riders: 43% had BAC $\geq$ 0.6 g/L (De Carvalho Ponce et al. 2011) (Table 13.2).

13.3.2.4 Trends

After reducing the legal BAC limit in 2008, Campos et al. (2013c) found that there was a 45% reduction in the number of alcohol-positive drivers in São Paulo when using a passive alcohol sensor. Also, a smaller proportion of the drivers reported drinking earlier during the study day. A similar reduction was found in Belo Horizonte (De Souza Salgado et al. 2012). A study of drivers who had drunk at alcohol outlets in Porto Alegre found that only 40% had changed their drinking behavior before driving after the law change (De Boni et al. 2014). Of those who had changed behavior, 50% reported that they were drinking less than before, 31% reported using public transportation, 17% reported using a designated driver, and 14% reported not driving after drinking. A study in Brasilia found a reduction in binge drinking before driving after the law was implemented, but this seemed not to be a permanent change in behavior (Moura et al. 2009).

Studies have found that after reducing the BAC limit from 0.6 to 0.2 g/L in 2008, the number of RTC injuries and fatalities declined in São Paulo municipal district and São Paulo state (Andreuccetti et al. 2011; Koizumi et al. 2010), and the number of killed alcohol-positive RTC victims decreased (Koizumi et al. 2010). According to Madruga et al. (2011), the reduction in RTC fatalities was sustained in cities where enforcement was steadily maintained during the two years following the change in legislation. De Mello Jorge and Koizumi (2009) found that there was a drop of 28.3% in hospitalizations due to

RTC injuries after the law was implemented. On the other hand, Nunes and Nascimento (2012) found a reduction of RTC fatalities of only 2.67%.

If the proportion of alcohol and drug related fatal RTCs is unchanged and if the number of RTC fatalities will still increase, the total number of fatalities related to DUI will also increase.

The use of amphetamines among truck drivers may have declined, however, the use of cocaine might have increased. More research data are needed to confirm this trend.

13.3.3 Norway

The Norwegian government has a vision of a transport system in which no one is killed or severely injured ("Vision Zero"); a preliminary goal is to reduce the number of killed or seriously injured road users from 1593 in year 2000 to 350 (for a population of 5.3 million) in 2030 (Ministry of Transport and Communications 2017). The total number of road users killed in RTCs has decreased significantly during the last decades, from 14.5 per 100,000 in 1970 to 7.6 in 2000, 2.3 in 2015 and 2.0 in 2017 (Statistics Norway 2018).

13.3.3.1 Law and Enforcement

A legal BAC limit of 0.5 g/kg blood (about 0.5 g/L) was introduced in 1936; the legal limit was reduced to 0.2 g/kg or 0.1 mg/L expired breath in 2001 (Ministry of Justice 2012). The Norwegian Road Traffic Act was extended to include an impairment law for other drugs in 1959 (Christophersen and Mørland 1997). From 1981 the police were allowed to perform random breath testing without any suspicion of DUI. Legislative blood concentration limits were implemented for 20 illicit drug and psychoactive medicines in 2012 in addition to limits for graded sanctions for drug concentration in blood corresponding to impairment comparable to BACs of 0.5 and 1.2 g/L for 13 substances (Ministry of Transport and Communications 2016; Vindenes et al. 2012). DUI offenders with BAC of 0.21–0.50 g/L or equivalent drug concentrations are sentenced to a fine, which normally is 1.5 times the driver's monthly gross income. For BAC > 0.50 g/L, the driver is also sentenced to conditional (for BAC of 0.50–1.20 g/L) or unconditional (for BAC > 1.20 g/L) prison (Ministry of Justice 2012). For BAC > 0.50 g/L, the driving license is suspended for 1–5 years depending on BAC, accident involvement, repeated offence, etc.

Random breath testing campaigns are frequently performed. In 2008, 0.34 breath tests were performed per inhabitant (Jost et al. 2010). In 2008, about 2,100 drivers per million inhabitants were suspected for DUI of alcohol or drugs and subject to evidential breath testing for alcohol or blood sampling for alcohol or drug testing (Edland-Gryt 2012).

13.3.3.2 Roadside Surveys

Nine roadside surveys on alcohol or drug use among motor vehicle drivers were conducted in the period 1970–2017 (Table 13.1 and Figure 13.1). During the first years, only drivers between 10 pm and 2 am were studied. From 1970 to 1982 the prevalence of BAC > 0.5 g/L during this time period decreased from 2.0% to 0.3%, and has later decreased even further (Bø 1972; Christensen et al. 1978; Furuhaugen et al. 2018; Gjerde et al. 2013a, 2008; Glad 1985; Jamt et al. 2017). In the studies performed in 2008–2009 and 2016–2017, only 0.2% of random drivers had BAC > 0.2 g/L (Furuhaugen et al. 2018; Gjerde et al. 2013a). This is similar to findings from random police controls, where 0.16% were found to have breath alcohol concentrations above the legal limit (TISPOL 2011).

Drugs were also analyzed in samples of oral fluid in the five latest roadside surveys. Assum et al. (2005) found a prevalence of drugs of only 1% in 2003–2004; however, this study included only 410 drivers. In the study by Gjerde et al. (2008) in 2005–2006, when about 10,800 drivers were included, medicinal drugs were found in 3.4% and illicit drugs in 1.0% of the samples; whereas in their study in 2008–2009, which included about 9,400 drivers, medicinal drugs were found in 3.2% and illicit drugs in 1.5% (Gjerde et al. 2013a). Slightly higher prevalence of drugs was found in a smaller study in northern Norway in 2014–2015 (Jamt et al. 2017). A study performed in south-eastern Norway in 2016–2017 found medicinal drugs in 3.0% and illicit drugs in 1.7% of the collected oral fluid samples (Furuhaugen et al. 2018). The most prevalent medicinal drugs were benzodiazepines and z-hypnotics, and the most prevalent illicit drugs were cannabis and amphetamines (see Table 13.1).

13.3.3.3 Drivers Killed in RTCs

The first study of drivers killed in RTCs found that 25% of drivers killed in 1959–1969 ($n = 56$) and 45% of drivers killed during 1973–1975 ($n = 69$) had BAC > 0.5 g/L (Lundevall and Olaisen 1976) (Table 13.2 and Figure 13.2). A nation-wide study in 1976–1977 found that 32% of killed drivers had BAC > 0.5 g/L (Andenæs and Sørensen 1979).

A study of 159 fatally injured drivers during 1989–1990 found that 27% had BAC > 0.5 g/L and drugs were found in 16% of the samples (Gjerde et al. 1993); diazepam was detected in 6%, THC in 5%, amphetamine in 0.6%. In addition, about 4% were positive for other drugs.

BAC > 0.5 g/L was found in 17% of 163 fatally injured drivers in 1994–1999; psychoactive medicinal or illicit drugs were found in blood samples from 27% (Brevig et al. 2004).

A larger study of 676 fatally injured car and van drives during 2001–2010 found that 25% had BAC > 0.2 g/L (24% had BAC > 0.5 g/L); the prevalence of alcohol was 22%–25% during 2001–2006 and 27%–28% during 2007–2010. Psychoactive medication was found in 14%, and illicit drugs in 14% of the samples (Christophersen and Gjerde 2014). The most prevalent drugs were amphetamine 8%, THC 7%, diazepam 5%, methamphetamine 4% and oxazepam 3%. No changes in the total prevalence of alcohol or drugs were observed during the study period, but the proportion of methamphetamine findings increased and amphetamine decreased, and the proportion of flunitrazepam findings decreased while clonazepam increased. A study of 207 motorcycle riders who were fatally injured during the same period found lower prevalence of alcohol (17%), psychoactive medication (7%) and illicit drugs (9%) (Christophersen and Gjerde 2015). The latest data from killed car and van drivers (for 2011–2015) showed that 14.2% had BAC > 0.5 g/kg and 15.9% had drugs in concentrations above the Norwegian graded sanction limits corresponding to BAC of 0.5 g/kg (Valen et al. 2019). There was a significant decline in the prevalence of alcohol compared to the period 2005–2010, but no significant change for drugs.

13.3.3.4 Trends

The incidence of DUI of alcohol in general road traffic has decreased significantly during the last decades. For DUI of drugs, two comprehensive studies have been performed fairly close in time (2005–2006 and 2008–2009) in addition to two minor ones (2003–2004 and 2014–2015). Different sampling devices for oral fluid and different cut-off concentrations were used, so it is difficult to study any change in drug use among random drivers.

The prevalence of drugs in blood samples from fatally injured drivers seems to have increased over time, particularly amphetamines. However, cut-off concentrations for drugs were not equal in the different studies, so exact comparisons are difficult.

The total number of road users killed in RTCs has decreased significantly during the last decades. The number of alcohol and drug related deaths have also decreased, particularly for alcohol during the latest years.

13.3.4 Spain

The relative number of RTC fatalities has declined from 12.4 in 2000 to 3.6 per 100,000 population in 2015 (European Commission 2018). The government's strategy for 2020 is to keep the relative number of fatalities lower than 3.7 and reduce the number of serious injuries by 35% as compared with the base figure for 2009 (General Directorate for Traffic 2014).

13.3.4.1 Law and Enforcement

A legal BAC limit of 0.8 g/L was introduced in 1973 (Government of Spain 1973). The general legal limit was lowered to 0.5 g/L in 1998 and became effective in 1999, and the BAC limit for commercial and novice drivers was lowered to 0.3 g/L (Spanish Ministry of the Interiors 1998). Drug testing of oral fluid was introduced in 2010 (Parliament of Spain 2010), and a zero-tolerance law for DUI of drugs was introduced in 2014 (Parliament of Spain 2014). A driver can be sentenced based on a positive drug finding in oral fluid. Random breath testing for alcohol and oral fluid testing for drugs is allowed. DUI is regulated as an "administrative violation" if the BAC is between 0.5 and 1.2 g/L (or BrAC between 0.25 and 0.60 mg/L) and as a crime if the BAC is above 1.2 g/L (or BrAC above 0.60 mg/L) (Alcañiz et al. 2014). DUI of drugs is regulated similarly; the law differentiates between "presence of drugs," which is an "administrative violation" based on the zero-tolerance criterion, and "influence of drugs," which is a crime (Alvarez and Gonzalez-Luque 2014; Alvarez et al. 2015). The fine for driving with BAC between 0.5 and 1.2 g/L or driving with the presence of drugs in the driver's system, or for refusing to undergo the detection tests, is established at €500–1,000, along with the loss of 6 driver's license points. The legal sanction for driving with BAC above 1.2 g/L or under the impairment of drugs is either a fine, community work, or imprisonment in addition to suspension of the driving license (Alvarez and Gonzalez-Luque 2014; Alvarez et al. 2015).

13.3.4.2 Roadside Surveys

The results of breathalyzer testing of random drivers showed an increase in positive alcohol tests from about 1% in 1989 to about 3.5% in 1998 (Alvarez et al. 2000). The first roadside survey that included drug use among random drivers in Spain was performed as a part of the DRUID project in 2008–2009 (Fierro et al. 2015; Gomez-Talegon et al. 2012). A follow-up was performed in 2013, and findings were compared with the first study (Fierro et al. 2015) (Table 13.1). The prevalence of alcohol decreased from 6.6% to 4.1%, and the prevalence of drug positive cases decreased from 6.9% to 4.9%, mainly due to less use of cannabis combined with driving.

A road-side study on the use of alcohol was conducted in the Catalonia region during 2012. The prevalence of BAC > 0.5 g/L was found to be 1.29%, with the highest prevalence on Sundays (4.29%) (Alcañiz et al. 2014).

A new study from the same region was performed during the autumn of 2014. The study included THC, amphetamines, cocaine, opiates and benzodiazepines, showing an overall prevalence of 16.4% and THC as the most frequently found substance (12.4%) (Alcañiz et al. 2018).

A nationwide road-side study using 128 police check points included 2,744 drivers in 2015. Overall, 11.6% drivers tested positive for alcohol or drugs. The most frequently detected compounds were cannabis (7.5%), cocaine (4.7%), and alcohol (2.6%). A comparison of the results with an earlier study from 2012 showed a similar proportion of drivers who tested positive (12.3%); the prevalence of alcohol decreased (from 3.4%), while other substances increased (8% to 10.7%) (Domingo-Salvany et al. 2017).

13.3.4.3 Drivers Killed in RTCs

Several studies on alcohol and drugs among fatally injured drivers in Spain have been conducted (Table 13.2). In a study from the 1980s, alcohol was found in samples from 77% of the drivers; 71% had BAC above 0.5 g/L (Bermejo et al. 1993). In a study covering 1994–1996, alcohol, illicit drugs, and medicines were found in blood samples from 50.5%, 10.2% and 9.1%, respectively, of the drivers (Del Rio and Alvarez 1999, 2000). A study in Northern Spain for 1996–1998 found that 58.9% had alcohol present in the blood, 33% had BAC > 0.8 g/L, while 19% were positive for benzodiazepines and 4% for cannabis (Lopez-Rivadulla and Cruz 2000).

In a larger study covering 1991–1998, alcohol was found in 47.3% (BAC > 0.8 g/L: 35.1%), and less frequently illicit (8.9%) and medicinal drugs (4.8%) (Alvarez et al. 2000). The prevalence of alcohol decreased during the study period, while the prevalence of illicit drugs increased slightly.

In a study covering 1991–2000, BAC > 0.8 g/L was found in 32.0% of the blood samples from fatally injured drivers, medicinal drugs in 4.7% and illicit drugs in 8.8%, mainly cocaine (5.2%) and cannabis (2.2%) (Del Rio et al. 2002). The proportion of included fatally injured drivers increased from 3.8% in 1991 to 23.8% in 2000 (Del Rio et al. 2002), suggesting that a variation in the selection bias might have affected the observed trend. In 2012, alcohol was found in 35.1%, medicinal drugs in 13.5% and illicit drugs in 12.7% of autopsied fatally injured drivers; the inclusion rate was 53% (Alvarez and Gonzalez-Luque 2014).

A study on drivers ($n = 614$) killed in road traffic accidents during 2014 showed a prevalence of 39% for one or more substances. Alcohol, illicit drugs and psychoactive medicines were found among 26.2%, 13.3% and 10.7%, respectively, of the killed drivers. Substances most often detected in the group of illicit drugs findings were cocaine (50%) and cannabis (46.3%). Compared to earlier studies, the prevalence of alcohol had decreased while illicit and medicinal drugs had increased (Arroyo et al. 2016).

13.3.4.4 Trends

The results of the roadside surveys suggest that there was an increase in the presence of alcohol among random drivers from 1989 to 1998, and a reduction from 2008 to 2013. The results also suggest that there was a reduction in the presence of illicit drugs from 2008 to 2013. The reduced prevalence may be related to changes in the road traffic law with lower limits for alcohol and introduction of random drug testing.

It is more difficult to assess the prevalence of alcohol and drugs in samples from fatally injured drivers because the proportion of the killed drivers that was tested for alcohol and drugs increased. When comparing data for blood samples from fatal RTCs in 2012 with earlier years, the prevalence of alcohol has decreased while the prevalence of medicinal drugs and illicit drugs has increased. It is likely that the police requested analysis of alcohol and drugs more often if they suspected alcohol or drug use, which caused a selection bias. The extent of bias may have changed over time.

The prevalence of alcohol in breath samples taken by the police in non-fatal crashes showed an increase from 1979 to 1999 from about 5% to about 7% (Alvarez and Del Rio 2000). Those data are thus not in line with the data from fatal accidents. Trends from both recent roadside and fatal RTC studies indicate a decrease in the prevalence of alcohol but increase for other substances.

13.3.5 United States of America

There has been a significant reduction of fatal RTCs during the last 35 years. In 1982, the death rate was 19.0 per 100,000 inhabitants, it declined to 14.9 in 2000 and 10.9 in 2015 (IIHS 2018b). There was large variation in fatal RTCs between the states, varying from 3.4 (District of Columbia) to 24.7 (Wyoming) per 100,000 inhabitants in 2015 (IIHS 2016).

13.3.5.1 Law and Enforcement

When US Department of Transportation was established in 1969, there was a growing recognition of the traffic safety risks associated with DUI of alcohol. A report on highway traffic safety prepared in 1968 for the congress recommended the establishment of a system for improved data registration on drinking, driving and accidents (Voas et al. 1998). The report was the background for the decision of BAC testing of all fatally injured drivers and pedestrians, and the establishment of the Fatality Analysis Reporting System (FARS) in 1975.

The majority of US states implemented their first legislative BAC limit of 1.0 g/L during the period from 1975 to 1984 (Mann et al. 2001); several states reduced the limit to 0.8 g/L during the 1980s and 1990s. In 2005, all 50 states and the District of Colombia had implemented a BAC limit of 0.8 g/L (Berning et al. 2015). In 2018, Utah was the first state in US to adopt 0.5 g/L as the BAC limit (Fiorentino and Martin 2018).

US law does not allow random alcohol breath testing of drivers. The majority of the states are using "sobriety checkpoints" as enforcement tools (Elder et al. 2002). Unlike with random breath testing, this enforcement technique requires that the driver shows signs of impairment before a test can be performed. The laws and practices regulating the use and frequencies of such controls vary between the states (GHSA 2019c). In cases of suspected alcohol use, a law enforcement officer may submit drivers to breath testing. However, the drivers may refuse to participate with reference to the "American Convention on Human Rights" (OAS 1978; Voas and Fell 2011). Those who refuse are penalized in various ways, depending on the state where the incident occurs (Voas and Fell 2011).

The majority of US states have implemented impairment laws for drugs other than alcohol. By March 2019, 16 states have zero-tolerance legislation that forbids the presence of a prohibited substance or drug in the driver's body while in control of the vehicle, without any other evidence of impairment, while seven states have *per se* limits for particular drugs (GHSA 2019a).

13.3.5.2 Roadside Surveys

National roadside studies on alcohol use among night-time drivers have been performed in 1973, 1986, 1996, 2005 (pilot study), 2007 and 2013–2014 (Berning et al. 2015; Kelley-Baker et al. 2013; Lacey et al. 2007; Lacey et al. 2009a, 2009b; Lund and Wolfe 1991; Voas et al. 1998; Wolfe 1974). The surveys performed in 1973, 1986 and 1996 studied alcohol use among drivers during weekend nights. In the 2005, 2007 and 2013–2014 surveys, oral fluid and blood samples were also collected for drug analysis (Table 13.1 and Figure 13.1).

The proportion of drivers with BAC of at least 0.5 g/L decreased from 14% in 1973 to 8.1% in 1986, but was not significantly different in the 1996 survey (7.8%). However, a significant decrease was recorded for night time drivers below 20 years of age (Lund and Wolfe 1991; Voas et al. 1998; Wolfe 1974); this was in the period during which all states raised the minimum drinking age to 21. The proportion of drivers with BAC ≥ 0.5 g/L had decreased further to 5.6% in 2005 (a pilot study) (Lacey et al. 2007), 4.5% in 2007 (Lacey et al. 2009b) and 3.1% in 2013–2014 (Berning et al. 2015).

The pilot study conducted in 2005 included drugs for the first time in a US roadside survey by collecting and analyzing oral fluid and/or blood samples. The total prevalence of drugs in the 2005 study was 15%. However, the data are not quite comparable to the two next surveys, due some protocol variations and drugs analyzed (Lacey et al. 2007). When comparing the 2007 and 2013–2014 surveys, the prevalence of illicit drugs in oral fluid and/or blood among night-time drivers increased from 11.4% to 15.1%. The drug representing the largest increase was THC (an increase from 8.7% to 12.6%). For medicines, a minor increase was found, from 3.9% to 4.9% (Berning et al. 2015).

13.3.5.3 Drivers Killed in RTCs

Results from testing of alcohol and drugs in biological samples from drivers killed in RTCs in all states are recorded in the FARS database. Alcohol registration started in 1975 and drugs were included from 1998.

A large number of articles and overviews have been published on fatal RTCs from different states, in particular on alcohol, but during the last years drugs have also been included. However, the procedures and protocols used in the different states for inclusion of cases and the program for drug analyses do not represent a consistent policy (Berning and Smither 2014). To get a total overview on the situation in the United States, we will mainly include data from the FARS database (Table 13.2 and Figure 13.2).

In 1982, BACs of at least 0.8 g/L were found among 48% of the killed drivers; the prevalence declined steadily, and was 28%–32% during the period 1996–2016 (Fell and Romano 2013; IIHS 2018a; NHTSA 2018b). The data also show large variation of alcohol among fatally injured drivers in the different states; the prevalence of cases with BAC ≥ 0.8 g/L in 2015 varied from 21% (New Jersey and West Virginia) to 48% (Arizona), with a national mean of 30% (IIHS 2016).

When it comes to illicit drugs and medicines that may affect road traffic safety, it has been recommended that the data available from FARS should be interpreted with caution (Berning and Smither 2014). The inclusion of cases, type of biological matrix used for testing, drugs included in the analytical program and their cut-off limits for reporting positive results vary between the states. Overall, drugs were found in 25%–27% of the drivers during the period from 1998/1999/2000 to 2010 (Fell and Romano 2013; Romano and Pollini 2013; Rudisill et al. 2014) and increased from 28% to 33% in the period from 2005 to 2009 (CESAR 2010). The drugs most frequently detected were cannabis (7%–8%) and stimulants (7%) (Fell and Romano 2013; Romano and Pollini 2013). Nearly 60% of the drivers who were positive for cannabis and 42% of those were positive for stimulants also had BACs ≥ 0.8 g/L (Fell and Romano 2013). The prevalence of alcohol and drugs was higher in samples from men than women (Brady and Li 2014).

A study based on data from six states (California, Hawaii, Illinois, New Hampshire, Rhode Island and West Virginia) documented an increase in drug findings among drivers who died in RTCs from 16.6% in 1999 to 28.3% in 2010. Results were based on 90.9% of the drivers who died within 1 hour after the accident. The prevalence of cannabis increased from 4.2% to 12.2% during the study period (Brady and Li 2014); a similar increase was found by Fell and Romano (2013).

Another study from the same period (1999–2010) that included 24 states focused mainly on the changes in drugs among fatal RTC drivers (Rudisill et al. 2014) (some of the states were also included in the study by Brady and Li [2013, 2014]). A total of 95,654 drivers were included in the study and 25.6% ($n = 23{,}500$) of these drivers tested positive for at least one drug (Rudisill et al. 2014). During the study period, the prevalence of drugs among the tested fatally injured drivers increased by 49%. The largest increase of individual drugs was found for illicit compounds, depressants, cannabinoids, and benzodiazepines.

13.3.5.4 Trends

A significant decline of alcohol among drivers in normal traffic has been documented when comparing results from roadside survey from 1973 to the 2013–2014 survey. The decrease may be due to implementing legal BAC limits and lowering the limit to 0.8 g/L for all states. Public information about the crash risk when combining use of alcohol with driving may also have contributed to the positive development. The organization MADD (Mothers Against Drunk Driving) has received important credit for changing the attitudes against drunk driving during more than 30 years' work. It has been documented that MADD is recognized by more than 90% of US citizens (Fell and Voas 2006).

However, the prevalence of BAC above the legal limit among drivers in regular US road traffic is still higher than in many European countries and Australia (Davey et al. 2007; Houwing et al. 2011). The legal BAC limit is also higher in United States compared to Australia and most EU countries, where a legislative limit of 0.5 g/L and even lower have been implemented. As noted before, in 2018, Utah became the first state in the United States to adopt a limit of 0.5 g/L. An additional factor may be that random alcohol roadside testing is not allowed in the United States, in contrast to Australia and several European countries (Voas and Fell 2011).

It is more difficult to come to conclusions about the changes in drug use among drivers in regular traffic as these compounds have been included only in the last surveys from the last years. However, the data indicate an increasing use of drugs among drivers when comparing the 2007 and 2013–2014 surveys. The increase may be partly be due to the legalization of medical and recreational use of cannabis in some states, which showed an increased from 4.2% to 12.2% during the study period.

Similar trend of reduction in the detection of alcohol has also been found for fatal RTCs (Fell and Romano 2013; Williams 2006); however, the proportion of positive drug findings has increased significantly (Brady and Li 2013; Rudisill et al. 2014). A frequent combination of cannabis or stimulants with alcohol contributes to a negative trend as well (Fell and Romano 2013).

Several states have implemented changes in cannabis law: medical legalization, decriminalization, or legalization. The consequences of legalization on the number of cannabis-related RTCs are still somewhat unclear. Increased prevalence of cannabis detections after decriminalization was found among fatally injured drivers in some states, while no changes were detected in other states (Masten and Guenzburger 2014; Pollini et al. 2015; RMHIDTA 2014; Salomonsen-Sautel et al. 2014; Sevigny 2018). Lee and co-workers found that the prevalence of THC in fatally injured drivers increased after decriminalization or legalization, but not after legalization of cannabis for medical use (Lee et al. 2018). The Highway Loss Data Institute reported in 2018 that legalization of cannabis sales was associated with a 6.0% increase in collision claim frequency (HLDI 2018).

13.4 Discussion

13.4.1 High-Income Countries

The increasing focus on the effects of alcohol use on driving safety caused an implementation of legal limits for alcohol in blood in practically all high-income countries over some decades. The law was most often combined with strong enforcement and information campaigns. The proportion of drink drivers in random traffic decreased significantly in Australia, Norway, Spain, the United States, and other high-income countries (Sweedler et al. 2004). The prevalence of DUI of alcohol among random drivers is at present very low in Australia, Norway, and other Scandinavian countries, mainly because of widespread use of random breath testing, information campaigns for many decades, and a deterrent effect caused by fairly strong legal actions against DUI offenders. This has caused a shift in the public attitudes over some decades; now, DUI of alcohol is regarded as unacceptable by the vast majority of the citizens in those countries, and random breath testing is widely accepted (Assum 2010; Petroulias 2013).

The number of RTC fatalities has decreased significantly in high-income countries during the last decades. The proportion of drink drivers among those who were fatally injured in RTCs also declined, as shown for Australia, Norway, Spain, and United States (see Section 13.3), and also for other countries (see previously published reviews [Stewart and Sweedler 2008; Sweedler 2007; Sweedler et al. 2004]). For Norway, there has been a slight increase in the proportion of drink drivers, but a reduction in the absolute number of drivers killed in alcohol-related RTCs per year. Thus, the number of alcohol-related fatalities has not always decreased by the same extent as the decline in RTC fatalities in total.

As more information on the effects of psychoactive drugs on traffic safety became available, an increasing number of countries changed their laws to also include impairment by drugs. During the period from the 1950s to 1990s, many countries implemented impairment laws, which required that the presence of drugs in blood alone was not sufficient to sentence a driver for drug impaired driving; other indications on impairment were needed. To simplify the legal issues and to clearly state that the use of illicit drugs should not be combined with driving, several countries and states implemented zero-tolerance laws. A few countries instead implemented legal limits for drugs similar to legal limits for alcohol. The prevalence of illicit drugs among random drivers seems, however, to have increased, in spite of implementing drug driving laws. The prevalence of illicit drugs in blood samples from fatally injured drivers has also increased during the last decades.

The number of drivers arrested on suspicion of drug impaired driving depends on law regulation, enforcement and police prioritization, public attitudes, media focus, as well as analytical capabilities. In Norway, blood samples from 426 drivers suspected of drug impaired driving were analyzed for drugs in 1978 (Bjørneboe et al. 1987), 1,223 in 1989 (Gjerde et al. 1990), and after implementing legal limits in 2012, 5,850 samples were analyzed in 2014 (NIPH 2015). When Sweden introduced a zero-tolerance limit in 1999, the number of samples from drivers suspected for drug-impaired driving increased more than ten-fold within five years (Jones 2005), with a prevalence of drugs of approximately 85%. Similarly, when Denmark implemented legal limits for drugs in 2007, the number of investigated cases increased from 237 in 2006 to 1,176 in 2008 (Steentoft et al. 2010). The prevalence of drug findings in blood samples before and after the change was 87% and 73%, respectively. Similar tendency has also been registered in Finland (Ojaniemi et al. 2009). When France changed the legislation in 2008 to allow drug screening of oral fluid, the number of samples for drug testing increased by more than five-fold (Roussel et al. 2014). Thus, improving the law and enforcement caused the apprehension and probably conviction of significantly larger numbers of DUI offenders. This might have had a deterring effect.

Studies from some countries have documented a tendency of decreased prevalence of alcohol among drivers included in roadside studies and also among fatally injured drivers. However, the prevalence of other drugs seems to have increased during the same time period.

Another change that is worth following is decriminalization of cannabis, not only in US states, but also in Uruguay and Canada. Discussions of liberalization or decriminalization of cannabis is ongoing in other counties. At present, the impact on road traffic safety is unknown.

13.4.2 Low- and Middle-Income Countries

While RTCs have decreased in high-income countries during the last decades, the problem is increasing in low- and middle-income countries (Ameratunga et al. 2006; Gururaj 2004; Sharma 2008; WHO 2018a). According to the latest WHO report, the RTC fatality rate per 100,000 inhabitants is about 26.6 in the African region, about 20.7 in South-East Asia and the Western Pacific regions, and about 9.3 in the European region, varying from about 2 in some European countries to more than 30 in some African, Asian, Central American and South American countries (WHO 2018a). If comparing the number of RTC fatalities per 10,000 motor vehicles, the differences are much larger (Wikipedia.org 2019). The exact numbers of RTCs that are related to alcohol or drug use are unknown. However, since alcohol use is increasing in many low- and middle-income countries (Davis et al. 2003; Gururaj 2004; WHO 2014), it is also expected that alcohol related accidents will increase. There are few roadside studies performed in low- and middle-income countries on alcohol and drugs use in traffic, including alcohol and drug related accidents.

The number of fatalities per 100,000 inhabitants and the incidence of drink driving seem to have decreased in Brazil, but can still be further reduced. In some other middle-income countries, such as Thailand, the prevalence of drink driving is similar to the situation in Brazil (Ingsathit et al. 2009), whereas a study in Kenya found that the prevalence of BACs above 0.5 g/L among drives in random traffic was 8.4% (Odero and Zwi 1997), and similar studies in Ghana found prevalence of BAC above 0.8 g/L of 5.5%–7.3% (Damsere-Derry et al. 2014; Damsere-Derry et al. 2015; Mock et al. 2001). Thus, the incidence of drink driving is very high in some countries.

Pedestrians are a special vulnerable group in many African countries. A study form South Africa, which included more 4,000 pedestrian fatalities, found that 58% tested positive for alcohol (Mabunda et al. 2008).

Work to improve road traffic safety is in not prioritized in many low- and middle-income countries. Knowledge about the risks associated with DUI of alcohol is also less widespread than in high-income countries. The police in many LMCs have no or few breathalyzers, and the police often prioritize other criminal acts. As the economic situation in some middle-income countries is improving, more people can afford to buy a motorcycle or car, which in itself will increase the number of RTCs, if the countries do not implement significant road safety improvements.

Studies have been done in China (Bhalla et al. 2013; Wang et al. 2015) and Vietnam (Bachani et al. 2013) in addition to Brazil (see Section 13.3.2) to monitor changes in DUI after implementing changes in law, enforcement or public information campaigns. Some of the studies found significant reductions in DUI.

13.4.3 The Future

An increasing use of alcohol in a population may also affect drinking among drivers. However, this may not always be associated with more drink driving. If the attitude among drivers is that drinking and driving shall not be combined, and if it is not socially accepted to drink and drive, the prevalence of alcohol among drivers might not be affected. In Norway, the alcohol consumption per adult increased by 35% from 1990 to 2010, while the number of DUI cases with BAC $\geq$ 0.5 g/L decreased by 42% (Gjerde et al. 2013b), and the prevalence of BAC $\geq$ 0.5 g/L among drivers in random traffic decreased from 0.3% in the 1980s (Glad 1985) to 0.1% in 2008–2009 (Gjerde et al. 2013a).

The pattern of illicit drug use among drivers may also be related to drug use in the general population. However, most individuals refrain from driving while impaired by drugs. Therefore, the pattern of drugs found in blood samples from arrested drug-impaired drivers may not exactly mirror drug use in the general, adult population. Studies in Norway found that drivers arrested by the police for DUI of drugs most often had used amphetamines, benzodiazepines, and combinations of several drugs, often in very high doses, whereas guests at nightclubs had primarily used cocaine or cannabis without combining with other drugs (Gjerde et al. 2016). Thus, the pattern of drug use among drug impaired drivers may not reflect the recreational drug use pattern.

If the use of cannabis in the society is increasing, the number of THC-positive blood samples may also be expected to increase. However, the DUI law and enforcement combined with public information may affect the number who actually drive within the first few hours after smoking cannabis, which is the period when cannabis may affect the ability to drive safely most significantly. The combined use of alcohol in addition to cannabis will constitute a larger threat to road safety than using cannabis alone.

If drivers use cannabis instead of alcohol, the number of alcohol-related RTCs might be reduced while the number of cannabis-related RTCs might increase. In general, the crash risk associated with cannabis use is lower than for binge drinking of alcohol (Bernhoft et al. 2012). If combined, the crash risk is high (Hartman and Huestis 2013). At present, it is too early to assess the consequences of legalization of cannabis as far as RTCs are concerned. This has to be monitored closely both in US and other countries in order to obtain better data for discussions on cannabis legalization elsewhere.

The use of new psychoactive substances, sometimes called "designer drugs" is increasing. The analysis of these newly created substances in blood samples from suspected DUI offenders is challenging because of the vast number of drugs that have been synthesized and the constantly changing illicit market for these drugs.

Any discussion of future trends in impaired driving must take into account the rapid changes in LMCs. The dramatic progress we have seen in recent decades in higher income countries has been gratifying, but increased motorization combined with increased alcohol consumption in some countries can result in greater crash risk—especially when these countries have less developed infrastructure, less safe vehicles, and a high number of vulnerable road users. The lessons learned in higher income countries can have applicability in low- and middle-income countries, but the lack of legal structure, enforcement resources, and public awareness present challenges (Stewart et al. 2012).

Another important trend is advances in vehicle technology. Much of the overall progress in improving traffic safety, including impaired driving, in higher income countries has resulted from safer vehicles and safer roadways. Further improvements based on advanced technologies are likely to bring benefits—especially for impaired drivers. Recently developed features, such as collision avoidance systems, lane deviation warnings, and the like, can help prevent crashes when the driver is impaired—whether by drugs and alcohol, or by fatigue, distractions, or other problems (Highway Loss Data Institute 2014).

Technological advances specific to impaired driving are also in development. For example, less expensive and easier to use oral fluid tests may make it easier to detect drug using drivers and thus make drug impaired driving enforcement less costly and more effective (Logan et al. 2013). In the United States, a program to develop in-vehicle alcohol detection systems is underway with the intent of preventing any driver over the legal alcohol limit from starting a car (NHTSA 2016).

While these technologies show promise for further reducing impaired driving and related crashes, LMCs are likely to lag far behind in the implementation of these new technologies.

Acknowledgments

Thanks to Professor Dr. Dimitri Gerostamoulos and Dr. Mark Chu (Victorian Institute of Forensic Medicine: Melbourne, Victoria, Australia), Professor Dr. Vilma Leyton and Dr. Gabriel Andreuccetti (University of São Paulo: São Paulo, Brazil) and to Professor Dr. Javier Alvarez (University of Valladolid: Valladolid, Spain) for reviewing the sections about Australia, Brazil, and Spain, respectively.

Disclaimer

This chapter is an update of a review article published in Forensic Science Review in 2016. This update is based on searching PubMed and similar electronic databases for studies published between 2015 and March 2019. Our searches might not have identified all relevant studies published during this period.

References

Aguilera SL, Sripad P, Lunnen JC, Moyses ST, Chandran A, Moyses SJ: Alcohol consumption among drivers in Curitiba, Brazil; *Traffic Inj Prev* 16:219; 2015.

Alcañiz M, Guillen M, Santolino M: Prevalence of drug use among drivers based on mandatory, random tests in a roadside survey; *PLoS One* 13:e0199302; 2018.

Alcañiz M, Guillen M, Santolino M, Sanchez-Moscona D, Llatje O, Ramon L: Prevalence of alcohol-impaired drivers based on random breath tests in a roadside survey in Catalonia (Spain); *Accid Anal Prev* 65:131; 2014.

Alvarez FJ, del Rio MC: Alcohol y accidentes de tráfico: ¿Hemos progresado en estos últimos 25 años? (Alcohol and traffic accidents: Have we progressed in the last 25 years?); *Rev Esp Drogodepend* 25:377; 2000.

Alvarez FJ, del Rio MC, Prada R: Drinking and driving in Spain; *J Stud Alcohol* 56:403; 1995.

Alvarez FJ, del Rio MC, Sancho M, Rams MA, Gonzalez-Luque JC: Alcohol and illicit drugs among Spanish drivers; In Laurell H, Schlyter F (Eds): *Alcohol, Drugs and Traffic Safety. Proceedings—15th International Conference on Alcohol, Drugs and Traffic Safety*; ICADTS: Stockholm, Sweden; 2000.

Alvarez FJ, Gonzalez-Luque JC: *Drogas, Adicciones y Aptitud para Conducir, Ed. 2 (Drugs, Addiction, and Fitness to Drive*, 2nd ed); University of Valladolid: Valladolid, Spain; 2014; http://www.drogasyconduccion.com/download.php?folder=materiales&file=materiales_1.pdf (Accesssed April 5, 2019).

Alvarez FJ, Gonzalez-Luque JC, Segui-Gomez M: Drugs, substance use disorder and driving: Intervention of health professionals in the treatment of addictions; *Adicciones* 27:159; 2015.

Ameratunga S, Hijar M, Norton R: Road-traffic injuries: Confronting disparities to address a global-health problem; *Lancet* 367:1533; 2006.

Andenæs J, Sørensen RK: Alkohol og Dødsulykker i Trafikken (Alcohol and Fatal Traffic Accidents); *Lov og Rett* (Oslo) 18:83; 1979.

Anderson EW, Burns M: Standardized field sobriety tests: A field study; In Mercier-Guyon C (Ed): *Alcohol, Drugs and Traffic Safety. Proceedings—14th International Conference on Alcohol, Drugs and Traffic Safety T'97*; Centre d'Etudes et de Recherches en Médicin du Traffic: Annecy, France; p. 635; 1997.

Andreuccetti G, Carvalho HB, Cherpitel CJ, Ye Y, Ponce JC, Kahn T, Leyton V: Reducing the legal blood alcohol concentration limit for driving in developing countries: A time for change? Results and implications derived from a time-series analysis (2001–2010) conducted in Brazil; *Addiction* 106:2124; 2011.

Andreuccetti G, Leyton V, Lemos NP, Miziara ID, Ye Y, Takitane J, Munoz DR, Reingold AL, Cherpitel CJ, de Carvalho HB: Alcohol use among fatally injured victims in Sao Paulo, Brazil: Bridging the gap between research and health services in developing countries; *Addiction* 112:596; 2017.

Arroyo A, Marrón MT, Leal MJ, Vidal C: Fatal road accidents in Spain: Psychoactive substances in killed drivers in 2014; *J Forensic Sci Criminol* 4:502; 2016.

Assum T: Reduction of the blood alcohol concentration limit in Norway—Effects on knowledge, behavior and accidents; *Accid Anal Prev* 42:1523; 2010.

Assum T, Mathijsen MPM, Houwing S, Buttress SC, Sexton B, Tunbridge RJ, Oliver J: *The Prevalence of Drug Driving and Relative Risk Estimations. A Study Conducted in The Netherlands, Norway and the United Kingdom*; Kuratorium für Verkehrssicherheit: Vienna, Austria; 2005.

Australian Transport Council: *National Road Safety Strategy 2011–2020*; Australian Transport Council: Canberra, Australia; 2011; https://roadsafety.gov.au/nrss/files/NRSS_2011_2020.pdf (Accessed April 5, 2019).

Australian Transportation Safety Bureau: *Alcohol and Road Fatalities. Monograph 5*; Australian Transport Safety Bureau: Canberra, Australia; 2001; https://www.infrastructure.gov.au/roads/safety/publications/2001/pdf/Alc_fat_4.pdf (Accessed April 5, 2019).

Bachani AM, Jessani NS, Pham VC, Quang LN, Nguyen PN, Passmore J, Hyder AA: Drinking & driving in Viet Nam: Prevalence, knowledge, attitudes, and practices in two provinces; *Injury* 44(Suppl 4):S38; 2013.

Badawi N, Simonsen KW, Steentoft A, Bernhoft IM, Linnet K: Simultaneous screening and quantification of 29 drugs of abuse in oral fluid by solid-phase extraction and ultraperformance LC-MS/MS; *Clin Chem* 55:2004; 2009.

Bermejo A, Lopez B, Garcia R, Fernandez P, Sanches I, Cruz A, Lopez-Rivadulla M: Alcohol and drugs involved in fatal accident in the North West of Spain; In Utzelmann H-D, Berghaus G, Kroj G (Eds): *Alcohol, Drugs and Traffic Safety Proceedings—12th International Conference on Alcohol, Drugs and Traffic Safety*; Cologne, Germany; Verlag TÜV Rheinland: Cologne, Germany; p. 981; 1993.

Bernhoft IM, Hels T, Lyckegaard A, Houwing S, Verstraete AG: Prevalence and risk of injury in Europe by driving with alcohol, illicit drugs and medicines; *Procedia Soc Behav Sci* 48:2907; 2012.

Berning A, Compton R, Wochinger K: *Traffic Safety Facts. Results of the 2013–2014 National Roadside Survey of Alcohol and Drugs Use by Drivers* (DOT HS 812 118); US National Highway Traffic Safety Administration: Washington, DC; 2015; www.nhtsa.gov/staticfiles/nti/pdf/812118-Roadside_Survey_2014.pdf (Accessed April 5, 2019).

Berning A, Smither DD: *Traffic Safety Facts. Understanding the Limitations of Drug Test Information, Reporting, and Testing Practices in Fatal Crashes* (DOT HS 812 072); US National Highway Traffic Safety Administration: Washington, DC; 2014; http://www-nrd.nhtsa.dot.gov/Pubs/812072.pdf (Accessed April 5, 2019).

Bhalla K, Li Q, Duan L, Wang Y, Bishai D, Hyder AA: The prevalence of speeding and drunk driving in two cities in China: A mid project evaluation of ongoing road safety interventions; *Injury* 44(Suppl 4):S49; 2013.

BITRE: *Road Trauma Australia—2014 Statistical Summary*; Department of Infrastructure and Regional Development: Canberra, Australia; 2015; https://bitre.gov.au/publications/ongoing/files/Road_trauma_Australia_2014_statistical_summary_N_ISSN.pdf (Accessed April 5, 2019).

BITRE: *Road Trauma Australia—2017 Statistical Summary*; Bureau of Infrastructure, Transport and Regional Economics: Canberra, Australia; 2018; https://bitre.gov.au/publications/ongoing/files/Road_Trauma_Australia_2017.pdf (Accessed April 5, 2019).

Bjørneboe A, Bjørneboe GEA, Bugge A, Christophersen A, Drevon CA, Gadeholt G, Gjerde H, Mørland J: Drugged driving in Norway 1978–1986; In Jones GR, Singer PP (Eds): *Proceedings—24th International Meeting of The International Association of Forensic Toxicologists*; Banff, Canada; Alberta Society of Clinical and Forensic Toxicologists: Edmonton, Canada; p. 258; 1987.

Blomberg RD, Peck RC, Moskowitz H, Burns M, Fiorentino D: The Long Beach/Fort Lauderdale relative risk study; *J Safety Res* 40:285; 2009.

Bombana HS, Gjerde H, Dos Santos MF, Jamt REG, Yonamine M, Rohlfs WJC, Munoz DR, Leyton V: Prevalence of drugs in oral fluid from truck drivers in Brazilian highways; *Forensic Sci Int* 273:140; 2017.

Boorman M, Owens K: The Victorian legislative framework for the random testing drivers at the roadside for the presence of illicit drugs: An evaluation of the characteristics of drivers detected from 2004 to 2006; *Traffic Inj Prev* 10:16; 2009.

Borkenstein RF, Crowther RF, Shumate RF, Ziel WB, Zylman R: The role of the drinking driver in traffic accidents (The Grand Rapids Study); *Blutalkohol* 11:1; 1974.

Borkenstein RF, Smith HW: The breathalyzer and its application; *Med Sci Law* 4:13; 1961.

Bosker WM, Huestis MA: Oral fluid testing for drugs of abuse; *Clin Chem* 55:1910; 2009.

Brady JE, Li G: Prevalence of alcohol and other drugs in fatally injured drivers; *Addiction* 108:104; 2013.

Brady JE, Li G: Trends in alcohol and other drugs detected in fatally injured drivers in the United States, 1999–2010; *Am J Epidemiol* 179:692; 2014.

Brevig T, Arnestad M, Mørland J, Skullerud K, Rognum TO: Hvilken betydning har sykdom, ruspåvirkning og selvmord ved dødsfall blant bilførere? (Of what significance are diseases, intoxication and suicide in fatal traffic accidents?) *Tidsskr Nor Laegeforen* 124:916; 2004.

Burns M, Moskowitz H: *Psychophysical Tests for DWI Arrest (DOT HS 802 424);* US National Highway Traffic Safety Administration: Washington, DC; 1977; https://rosap.ntl.bts.gov/view/dot/1186 (Accessed April 5, 2019).

Bø O: *Screening av Alkoholbelastningen blant Bilførere i Normal Trafikk. En Undersøkelse fra Oslo Våren 1970 og 1971 (Screening of Alcohol Use among Car Drivers in Normal Traffic. A Study from Oslo during the Spring of 1970 and 1971)*; Institute for Transport Economics: Oslo, Norway; 1972.

Campos VR, de Souza ESR, Duailibi S, Laranjeira R, Palacios EN, Grube JW, Pinsky I: Drinking and driving in southeastern Brazil: Results from a roadside survey study; *Addict Behav* 38:1442; 2013a.

Campos VR, Salgado Rde S, Rocha MC: Bafômetro positivo: Correlatos do comportamento de beber e dirigir na cidade de Belo Horizonte, Minas Gerais, Brasil (Positive breathalyzer test: Factors associated with drinking and driving in the city of Belo Horizonte, Minas Gerais State, Brazil); *Cad Saude Publica* 29:51; 2013b.

Campos VR, Salgado Rde S, Rocha MC, Duailibi S, Laranjeira R: Prevalência do beber e dirigir em Belo Horisonte, Minas Gerais, Brasil (Drinking-and-driving prevalence in Belo Horizonte, Minas Gerais State, Brazil); *Cad Saude Publica* 24:829; 2008.

Campos VR, Silva dSe, Duailibi S, dos Santos JF, Laranjeira R, Pinsky I: The effect of the new traffic law on drinking and driving in Sao Paulo, Brazil; *Accid Anal Prev* 50:622; 2013c.

CESAR: One-third of fatally injured drivers with known test results tested positive for at least one drug in 2009; *Cesar Fax* 19:1; 2010.

Chambers LW, Roberts RS, Voelker CC: The epidemiology of traffic accidents and the effect of the 1969 breathalyzer law in Canada; In Israelstam S, Lambert S (Eds): *Alcohol, Drugs and Traffic Safety. Proceedings—6th International Conference on Alcohol, Drugs and Traffic Safety, Toront*; Addiction Research Foundation: Toronto, Canada; p. 689; 1974.

Chandran A, Khan G, Sousa T, Pechansky F, Bishai DM, Hyder AA: Impact of road traffic deaths on expected years of life lost and reduction in life expectancy in Brazil; *Demography* 50:229; 2013.

Chou SP, Dawson DA, Stinson FS, Huang B, Pickering RP, Zhou Y, Grant BF: The prevalence of drinking and driving in the United States, 2001–2002: Results from the national epidemiological survey on alcohol and related conditions; *Drug Alcohol Depend* 83:137; 2006.

Christensen P, Fosser S, Glad A: *Drunken Driving in Norway*; Institute for Transport Economics: Oslo, Norway; 1978.

Christophersen AS, Gjerde H: Prevalence of alcohol and drugs among car and van drivers killed in road accidents in Norway: An overview from 2001–2010; *Traffic Inj Prev* 15:523; 2014.

Christophersen AS, Gjerde H: Prevalence of alcohol and drugs among motorcycle riders killed in road crashes in Norway during 2001–2010; *Accid Anal Prev* 80:236; 2015.

Christophersen AS, Mørland J: Drugged driving, a review based on the experience in Norway; *Drug Alcohol Depend* 47:125; 1997.

Chu M: Random oral fluid drug testing of Victorians: A 10-year perspective; *The 52nd International Meeting of The International Association of Forensic Toxicologists, Young Scientist's Meeting*; Buenos Aires, Argentina; 2014.

Chu M, Gerostamoulos D, Beyer J, Rodda L, Boorman M, Drummer OH: The incidence of drugs of impairment in oral fluid from random roadside testing; *Forensic Sci Int* 215:28; 2012.

Cleeland R, Christenson J, Usategui-Gomez M, Heveran J, Davis R, Grunberg E: Detection of drugs of abuse by radioimmunoassay: A summary of published data and some new information; *Clin Chem* 22:712; 1976.

Cone EJ: Pharmacokinetics and pharmacodynamics of cocaine; *J Anal Toxicol* 19:459; 1995.

Congress of Brazil: Lei N° 9.503, de 23 de setembro de 1997—O código de trânsito brasileiro; http://www.planalto.gov.br/ccivil_03/LEIS/L9503.htm (Accessed April 3, 2019).

Congress of Brazil: Lei N° 11.705, de 19 de junho de 2008; http://www.planalto.gov.br/ccivil_03/_ato2007-2010/2008/lei/l11705.htm (Accessed April 3, 2019).

Congress of Brazil: Lei N° 12.760, de 20 de dezembro de 2012; http://www.planalto.gov.br/ccivil_03/_Ato2011-2014/2012/Lei/L12760.htm (Accessed April 3, 2019).

Congress of Chile: Resolución exenta N° 8.833 de 3 de septiembre de 2010. Aprueba instrucciones y normativa técnica sobre exámenes de alcoholemia (Decision on instructions and technical regulations for alcohol testing); http://www.leychile.cl/Navegar?idNorma=1017485&idVersion=2010-09-30 (Accessed April 3, 2019).

Council on Scientific Affairs: Scientific issues in drug testing; *JAMA* 257:3110; 1987.

Curry AS: Toxicological analysis; *J Pharm Pharmacol* 12:321; 1960.

Da Conceicao TV, De Boni R, Duarte PCAV, Pechansky F: Awareness of legal blood alcohol concentration limits amongst respondents of a national roadside survey for alcohol and traffic behaviours in Brazil; *Int J Drug Policy* 23:166; 2012.

Damsere-Derry J, Afukaar F, Palk G, King M: Determinants of drink-driving and association between drink-driving and road traffic fatalities in Ghana; *Int J Alcohol Drug Res* 3:135; 2014.

Damsere-Derry J, Palk G, King M: Prevalence of alcohol-impaired driving and riding in northern Ghana; *Traffic Inj Prev* 17:226; 2015.

Davey J, Armstrong K, Martin P: Results of the Queensland 2007–2012 roadside drug testing program: The prevalence of three illicit drugs; *Accid Anal Prev* 65:11; 2014.

Davey J, Freeman J: Screening for drugs in oral fluid: Drug driving and illicit drug use in a sample of Queensland motorists; *Traffic Inj Prev* 10:231; 2009.

Davey J, Freeman J, Lavelle A: Screening for drugs in oral fluid: Illicit drug use and drug driving in a sample of urban and regional Queensland motorists; *Transp Res Part F Traffic Psychol Behav* 12:311; 2009.

Davey J, Leal N, Freeman J: Screening for drugs in oral fluid: Illicit drug use and drug driving in a sample of Queensland motorists; *Drug Alcohol Rev* 26:301; 2007.

Davis A, Quimby A, Odero W, Gururaj G, Hijar H: *Improving Road Safety by Reducing Impaired Driving in Developing Countries: A Scoping Study*; Road research laboratory: Crowthorne, England; 2003; http://legacy.grsproadsafety.org/sites/default/files/Impaired%20driving%20full%20report.pdf (Accessed April 5, 2019).

Davis CG, Thake J, Vilhena N: Social desirability biases in self-reported alcohol consumption and harms; *Addict Behav* 35:302; 2010.

De Boni RB, Pechansky F, Vasconcellos MT, Bastos FI: Have drivers at alcohol outlets changed their behavior after the new traffic law? *Rev Bras Psiquiatr* 36:11; 2014.

De Carvalho Ponce J, Munoz DR, Andreuccetti G, de Carvalho DG, Leyton V: Alcohol-related traffic accidents with fatal outcomes in the city of Sao Paulo; *Accid Anal Prev* 43:782; 2011.

De Mello Jorge MHP, Koizumi MS: Acidentes de trânsito causando vítimas: Possível reflexo da lei seca nas internações hospitalares (Traffic accidents that cause victims: A probable reflection of the "dry law" in hospital admittances); *Rev ABRAMET* 27:16; 2009.

De Souza Salgado R, Campos VR, Duailibi S, Laranjeira RR: O impacto da "Lei Seca" sobre o beber e dirigir em Belo Horizonte/MG (The Impact of Prohibition on drinking and driving in Belo Horizonte in the State of Minas Gerais); *Cien Saude Colet* 17:971; 2012.

Del Rio MC, Alvarez FJ: Alcohol use among fatally injured drivers in Spain; *Forensic Sci Int* 104:117; 1999.

Del Rio MC, Alvarez FJ: Presence of illegal drugs in drivers involved in fatal road traffic accidents in Spain; *Drug Alcohol Depend* 57:177; 2000.

Del Rio MC, Gomez J, Sancho M, Alvarez FJ: Alcohol, illicit drugs and medicinal drugs in fatally injured drivers in Spain between 1991 and 2000; *Forensic Sci Int* 127:63; 2002.

Domingo-Salvany A, Herrero MJ, Fernandez B, Perez J, Del Real P, Gonzalez-Luque JC, de la Torre R: Prevalence of psychoactive substances, alcohol and illicit drugs, in Spanish drivers: A roadside study in 2015; *Forensic Sci Int* 278:253; 2017.

Dos Santos Modelli ME, Pratesi R, Tauil PL: Blood alcohol concentration in fatal traffic accidents in the Federal District, Brazil; *Rev Saude Publica* 42:350; 2008.

Drummer OH: Postmortem toxicology of drugs of abuse; *Forensic Sci Int* 142:101; 2004.

Drummer OH, Gerostamoulos D, Chu M, Swann P, Boorman M, Cairns I: Drugs in oral fluid in randomly selected drivers; *Forensic Sci Int* 170:105; 2007.

Drummer OH, Gerostamoulos J, Batziris H, Chu M, Caplehorn JR, Robertson MD, Swann P: The incidence of drugs in drivers killed in Australian road traffic crashes; *Forensic Sci Int* 134:154; 2003.

Drummer OH, Yap S: The involvement of prescribed drugs in road trauma; *Forensic Sci Int* 265:17; 2016.

Duailibi S, Pinsky I, Laranjeira R: Prevalência do beber e dirigir em Diadema, estado de São Paulo (Prevalence of drinking and driving in a city of Southeastern Brazil); *Rev Saude Publica* 41:1058; 2007.

Editorial: Drunken motor car driver; *The Morning Post* September 11, 1897.

Editorial: *Q J Inebriety* 26:308; 1904.

Edland-Gryt M, Skretting A, Lund M, Bye EK: *Rusmidler i Norge 2012 (Alcohol and Drugs in Norway)*; Norwegian Institute for Alcohol and Drug Research: Oslo, Norway; 2012; https://www.fhi.no/publ/2012/rusmidler-i-norge-2012/ (Accessed April 5, 2019).

Eichhorst JC, Etter ML, Hall PL, Lehotay DC: LC-MS/MS techniques for high-volume screening of drugs of abuse and target drug quantitation in urine/blood matrices; *Methods Mol Biol* 902:29; 2012.

Elder RW, Shults RA, Sleet DA: Effectiveness of sobriety checkpoints for reducing alcohol-involved crashes; *Traffic Inj Prev* 3:266; 2002.

EMCDDA: *Legal Approaches to Drugs and Driving.* Lisbon, Portugal: European Monitoring Centre for Drugs and Drug Addiction; 2019; http://www.emcdda.europa.eu/html.cfm/index19034EN.html (Accessed April 4, 2019).

EMCDDA: *Responding to Drug Driving in Europe;* Office for Official Publications of the European Communities: Luxembourg; 2009; http://www.emcdda.europa.eu/publications/drugs-in-focus/driving (Accessed April 5, 2019).

Erke A, Goldenbeld C, Vaa T: The effects of drink-driving checkpoints on crashes—A meta-analysis; *Accid Anal Prev* 41:914; 2009.

European Commission: *Fatalities as Reported by Road User Type in EU Countries*; European Commission: Brussels, Belgium; 2018; https://ec.europa.eu/transport/road_safety/sites/roadsafety/files/pdf/statistics/historical_country_person_class.pdf (Accessed April 4, 2019).

Fell JC, Romano E: Alcohol and other drugs involvement in fatally injured drivers in the United States; In Watson B (Ed): *Proceedings—20th International Council on Alcohol, Drugs and Traffic Safety Conference*; Brisbane, Australia; Center for Accident Research and Road Safety Queensland: Brisbane, Australia; p. 232; 2013.

Fell JC, Voas RB: Mothers Against Drunk Driving (MADD): The first 25 years; *Traffic Inj Prev* 7:195; 2006.

Ferris J, Devaney M, Sparkes-Carroll M, Davis G: *A National Examination of Random Breath Testing and Alcohol-Related Traffic Crash Rates (2000–2012)*; Foundation for Alcohol Research & Education: Canberra, Australia; 2015; http://fare.org.au/a-national-examination-of-random-breath-testing-and-alcohol-related-traffic-crash-rates-2000-2012/ (Accessed April 5, 2019).

Fierro I, Gonzalez-Luque JC, Segui-Gomez M, Alvarez FJ: Alcohol and drug use by Spanish drivers: Comparison of two cross-sectional road-side surveys (2008–9/2013); *Int J Drug Policy* 26:794; 2015.

Fiorentino DD, Martin BD: Survey regarding the 0.05 blood alcohol concentration limit for driving in the United States; *Traffic Inj Prev* 19:345; 2018.

Furuhaugen H, Jamt REG, Nilsson G, Vindenes V, Gjerde H: Roadside survey of alcohol and drug use among Norwegian drivers in 2016–2017: A follow-up of the 2008–2009 survey; *Traffic Inj Prev* 19:555; 2018.

General Directorate for Traffic: *Main Figures on Road Safety Data, Spain 2013*; General Directorate for Traffic: Madrid, Spain; 2014; http://www.dgt.es/Galerias/seguridad-vial/estadisticas-e-indicadores/publicaciones/principales-cifras-siniestralidad/Main-figures-on-Road-Safety-Data.-Spain-2013.pdf (Accessed April 5, 2019).

Gerostamoulos J, Batziris H, Drummer OH: Involvement of drugs in accident causation; *Probl Forensic Sci* 43:79; 2000.

GHSA: *Drug Impaired Driving*; Governors Highway Safety Association: Washington, DC; 2019a; https://www.ghsa.org/state-laws/issues/drug%20impaired%20driving (Accessed April 4, 2019).

GHSA: *Drug Impaired Driving Laws*; Governors Highway Safety Association: Washington, DC; 2019b; http://www.ghsa.org/html/stateinfo/laws/dre_perse_laws.html (Accessed April 5, 2019).

GHSA: *Sobriety Checkpoints*; Governors Highway Safety Association: Washington, DC; 2019c; https://www.ghsa.org/state-laws/issues/sobriety%20checkpoints (Accessed April 5, 2019).

Gjerde H, Beylich KM, Mørland J: Incidence of alcohol and drugs in fatally injured car drivers in Norway; *Accid Anal Prev* 25:479; 1993.

Gjerde H, Christophersen AS, Bjørneboe A, Sakshaug J, Mørland J: Driving under the influence of other drugs than alcohol in Norway; *Acta Med Leg Soc* (Liege) 40:71; 1990.

Gjerde H, Christophersen AS, Normann PT, Assum T, Øiestad EL, Mørland J: Norwegian roadside survey of alcohol and drug use by drivers (2008–2009); *Traffic Inj Prev* 14:443; 2013a.

Gjerde H, Christophersen AS, Normann PT, Mørland J: Increased population drinking is not always associated with increased number of drink driving convictions; *Addiction* 108:2221; 2013b.

Gjerde H, Langel K, Favretto D, Verstraete AG: Estimation of equivalent cutoff thresholds in blood and oral fluid for drug prevalence studies; *J Anal Toxicol* 38:92; 2014a.

Gjerde H, Nordfjærn T, Bretteville-Jensen AL, Edland-Gryt M, Furuhaugen H, Karinen R, Øiestad EL: Comparison of drugs used by nightclub patrons and criminal offenders in Oslo, Norway; *Forensic Sci Int* 265:1; 2016.

Gjerde H, Normann PT, Pettersen BS, Assum T, Aldrin M, Johansen U, Kristoffersen L, Øiestad EL, Christophersen AS, Mørland J: Prevalence of alcohol and drugs among Norwegian motor vehicle drivers: A roadside survey; *Accid Anal Prev* 40:1765; 2008.

Gjerde H, Sousa TR, De Boni R, Christophersen AS, Limberger RP, Zancanaro I, Øiestad EL, Normann PT, Mørland J, Pechansky F: A comparison of alcohol and drug use by random motor vehicle drivers in Brazil and Norway; *Int J Drug Policy* 25:393; 2014b.

Gjerde H, Strand MC, Mørland J: Driving under the influence of non-alcohol drugs—An update. Part I: Epidemiological studies; *Forensic Sci Rev* 27:89; 2015.

Gjerde H, Verstraete AG: Estimating equivalent cutoff thresholds for drugs in blood and oral fluid using prevalence regression: A study of tetrahydrocannabinol and amphetamine; *Forensic Sci Int* 212:e26; 2011.

Gjerde H, Øiestad EL, Christophersen AS: Using biological samples in epidemiological research on drugs of abuse; *Nor Epidemiol* 21:5; 2011; https://www.ntnu.no/ojs/index.php/norepid/article/view/1420 (Accessed April 5, 2019).

Glad A: *Omfanget av og Variasjonen i Promillekjøringen* (*Prevalence and Variation in Drunk Drivin*); Institute of Transport Economics: Oslo, Norway; 1985.

Gomez-Talegon T, Fierro I, Gonzalez-Luque JC, Colas M, Lopez-Rivadulla M, Javier Alvarez F: Prevalence of psychoactive substances, alcohol, illicit drugs, and medicines, in Spanish drivers: A roadside study; *Forensic Sci Int* 223:106; 2012.

Gonzalez-Wilhelm L: Prevalence of alcohol and illicit drugs in blood specimens from drivers involved in traffic law offenses. Systematic review of cross-sectional studies; *Traffic Inj Prev* 8:189; 2007.

Government of South Australia: *Alcohol and Drugs in Road Crashes in South Australia—Fact Sheet*; Safety Policy Unit, Department of Planning, Transport and Infrastructure: Adelaide, Australia; 2017.

Government of Spain: Decreto 1890/1973, de 26 de julio, por el que se modifican determinados articulos del Código de la Circulación; *Bol Oficial Estado* 15972; 1973; http://www.boe.es/boe/dias/1973/08/06/pdfs/A15972-15972.pdf (Accessed April 5, 2019).

Government of the Netherlands: Besluit van 14 december 2016, houdende regels over de voorlopige onderzoeken en de vervolgonderzoeken die ter vaststelling van het gebruik van alcohol, drugs en geneesmiddelen in het verkeer; *Staatsblad* 529:1; 2016; https://zoek.officielebekendmakingen.nl/stb-2016-529.pdf (Accessed April 5, 2019).

Gururaj G: Alcohol and road traffic injuries in South Asia: Challenges for prevention; *J Coll Physicians Surg Pak* 14:713; 2004.

Harger RN, Lamb EB, Hulpieu HR: A rapid chemical test for intoxication employing breath; *JAMA* 110:1076; 1938.

Hartman RL, Huestis MA: Cannabis effects on driving skills; *Clin Chem* 59:478; 2013.

Haworth NL, Johnston IR: Why isn't the involvement of alcohol in road crashes in Australia lower? In Oliver J, Williams P, Clayton A (Eds): *Proceedings—17th International Conference on Alcohol, Drugs and Traffic Safety*, T2004 (CD ROM); X-CD Technologies: Glasgow, UK; 2004.

Highway Loss Data Institute: Honda Accord collision avoidance features: Initial results; *HLDI Bulletin* 31(2):1; 2014; http://www.iihs.org/media/a4bf654e-6a8a-4e2c-81f4-3b437c095dc0/-1220194404/HLDI%20Research/Bulletins/hldi_bulletin_31.2.pdf (Accessed April 5, 2019).

HLDI: Recreational marijuana and collision claim frequencies; *HLDI Bulletin* 35(8):1; 2018; https://www.iihs.org/media/e0028841-76ee-4315-a628-32a704258980/gmJeDw/HLDI%20Research/Bulletins/hldi_bulletin_35-08.pdf (Accessed April 5, 2019)

Holcomb RL: Alcohol in relation to traffic accidents; *JAMA* 111:1076; 1938.

Houwing S, Hagenzieker M, Mathijssen R, Bernhoft IM, Hels T, Janstrup K, van der Linden T, Legrand SA, Verstraete A: *Prevalence of Alcohol and Other Psychoactive Substance in Drivers in General Traffic. Part I: General Results* (DRUID Deliverable D 2.2.3); SWOV Institute for Road Safety Research: Leidschendam, The Netherlands; 2011; http://orbit.dtu.dk/fedora/objects/orbit:89486/datastreams/file_6341069/content (Accessed April 5, 2019).

IIHS: *Fatality Facts—Alcohol 2017*; Insurance Institute of Highway Safety: Arlington, VA; 2018a; https://www.iihs.org/iihs/topics/t/alcohol-and-drugs/fatalityfacts/alcohol-and-drugs (Accessed April 4, 2019).

IIHS: *Fatality Facts—General Statistics*; Insurance Institute for Highway Safety: Arlington, VA; 2018b; https://www.iihs.org/iihs/topics/t/general-statistics/fatalityfacts/overview-of-fatality-facts (Accessed April 5, 2019).

IIHS: *Fatality Facts—State by State 2015*; Insurance Institute for Highway Safety: Arlington, VA; 2016; https://www.iihs.org/iihs/topics/t/general-statistics/fatalityfacts/state-by-state-overview (Accessed April 5, 2019).

Ingsathit A, Woratanarat P, Anukarahanonta T, Rattanasiri S, Chatchaipun P, Wattayakorn K, Lim S, Suriyawongpaisal P: Prevalence of psychoactive drug use among drivers in Thailand: A roadside survey; *Accid Anal Prev* 41:474; 2009.

Istituto de Pesquisa Econômica Aplicada, Departamento Nacional de Trânsito: *Impactos Sociais e Econômicos dos Acidentes de Trânsito nas Rodovias Brasileiras* (*Social and Economical Impacts of Road Traffic Accidents in Brazil*); Departamento Nacional de Trânsito: Brasilia, Brazil; 2006; http://www.denatran.gov.br/images/Educacao/Publicacoes/custos_acidentes_transito.pdf (Accessed April 5, 2019).

Jamt REG, Gjerde H, Normann PT, Bogstrand ST: Roadside survey on alcohol and drug use among drivers in the Arctic county of Finnmark (Norway); *Traffic Inj Prev* 18:681; 2017.

Jones AW: Driving under the influence of drugs in Sweden with zero concentration limits in blood for controlled substances; *Traffic Inj Prev* 6:317; 2005.

Jones AW, Pounder DJ: Update on clinical and forensic analysis of alcohol; In Karch SB (Ed): *Drug Abuse Handbook*, 2nd ed; CRC Press: Boca Raton, FL; p. 333; 2007.

Jones AW, Wright BM, Jones TP: A historical and experimental study of the breath/blood alcohol ratio; In Israelstam S, Lambert S (Eds): *Proceedings—6th International Conference on Alcohol, Drugs and Traffic Safety*; Toronto, September 8–13, 1974; Addiction Research Foundation of Ontario: Toronto, Canada; p. 509; 1975.

Jost G, Popolizio M, Allsop R, Eksler V: *Road Safety Target in Sight: Making Up for Lost Time. 4th Road Safety PIN Report;* European Transport Safety Council: Brussels, Belgium; 2010; http://archive.etsc.eu/documents/ETSC%20PIN%20Report%202010.pdf (Accessed April 5, 2019).

Kelley-Baker T, Lacey JH, Voas RB, Romano E, Yao J, Berning A: Drinking and driving in the United States: Comparing results from the 2007 and 1996 National Roadside Surveys; *Traffic Inj Prev* 14:117; 2013.

Kloeden CN, McLean AJ: *Late Night Drink Driving in Adelaide Two Years after the Introduction of the 0.05 limit*; South Australian Department of Transport, The Office of Road Safety: Adelaide, Australia; 1994; http://casr.adelaide.edu.au/casrpubfile/769/CASRlatenightdrinkdriving264.pdf (Accessed April 5, 2019).

Koizumi MS, Leyton V, de Carvalho DG, Coelho CA, de Mello Jorge MHP, Gianvecchio V, Gawryszewski VP, de Godoy CD, Sinagawa DM, Araujo GL, Munoz DR: Alcoolemia e mortalidade por acidentes de trânsito no município de São Paulo, 2007/2008 (Alcohol use and mortality by traffic accidents in the municipal district of São Paulo, 2007/2008); *Rev ABRAMET* 28:25; 2010.

Krüger HP, Schultz E, Magerl H: The German roadside survey 1992–1994: Saliva analyses from an unselected driver population: Licit and illicit drugs; In Cloeden CN, McLean AJ (Eds): *Proceedings—13th International Conference on Alcohol, Drugs and Traffic Safety*, T'95; University of Adelaide: Adelaide, Australia; p. 55; 1995.

Lacey JH, Brainard K, Snitow S: *Drug Per Se Laws: A Review of Their Use in States* (DOT HS 811 317); US National Highway Traffic Safety Administration: Washington, DC; 2010; http://www.nhtsa.gov/staticfiles/nti/impaired_driving/pdf/811317.pdf (Accessed April 5, 2019).

Lacey JH, Kelley-Baker T, Furr-Holden D, Brainard K, Moore C: *Pilot Test of New Roadside Survey Methodology for Impaired Driving* (DOT HS 810 704); US National Highway Traffic Safety Administration: Washington, DC; 2007; http://www.nhtsa.gov/DOT/NHTSA/Traffic%20 Injury%20Control/Articles/Associated%20Files/PilotTest_NRSM.pdf (Accessed April 5, 2019).

Lacey JH, Kelley-Baker T, Furr-Holden D, Voas RB, Romano E, Ramirez A, Brainard K, Moore C, Torres P, Berning A: *2007 National Roadside Survey of Alcohol and Drug Use by Drivers—Drug Results* (DOT HS 811 249); National Highway Safety Administration: Washington, DC; 2009a; www.nhtsa.gov/DOT/NHTSA/Traffic%20Injury%20Control/Articles/Associated%20 Files/811249.pdf (Accessed April 5, 2019).

Lacey JH, Kelley-Baker T, Furr-Holden D, Voas RB, Romano E, Torres P, Tippetts AS, Ramirez A, Brainard K, Berning A: *2007 National Roadside Survey of Alcohol and Drug Use by Drivers—Alcohol Results* (DOT HS 811 248); US National Highway Safety Administration: Washington, DC; 2009b; http://www.nhtsa.gov/DOT/NHTSA/Traffic%20Injury%20Control/Articles/ Associated%20Files/811248.pdf (Accessed April 5, 2019).

Ladeira RM, Malta DC, Morais OLN, Montenegro MMS, Soares AMF, Vasconcelos CH, Mooney M, Naghavi M: Road traffic accidents: Global burden of disease study, Brazil and federated units, 1990 and 2015; *Rev Bras Epidemiol* 20(Suppl 01):157; 2017.

Lee J, Abdel-Aty A, Park J: Investigation of associations between marijuana law changes and marijuana-involved fatal traffic crashes: A state-level analysis; *J Transp Health* 10:194; 2018.

Leyton V, Bombana HS, Magalhães JG, Panizza HN, Sinagawa DM, Takitane J, de Carvalho HB, Andreuccetti G, Yonamine M, Gjerde H, et al.: Trends in the use of psychoactive substances by truck drivers in São Paulo State, Brazil: A time-series cross sectional roadside survey (2009–2016); *Traffic Inj Prev* 20:122; 2019.

Leyton V, Greve JM, de Carvalho DG, Muñoz DR: Perfil epidemiológico das vítimas fatais por acidente de trânsito e a relação com o uso do álcool (Epidemiological profile of fatally injured victims in motor vehicles accidents and the relation with alcohol use); *Saude Etica Just* 10:12; 2005.

Leyton V, Sinagawa DM, Oliveira KC, Schmitz W, Andreuccetti G, De Martinis BS, Yonamine M, Munoz DR: Amphetamine, cocaine and cannabinoids use among truck drivers on the roads in the State of Sao Paulo, Brazil; *Forensic Sci Int* 215:25; 2012.

Lillsunde P, Gunnar T: Drugs and driving: The finnish perspective; *Bull Narc* 57:213; 2005.

Logan BK, Lowrie KJ, Turri JL, Yeakel JK, Limoges JF, Miles AK, Scarneo CE, Kerrigan S, Farrell LJ: Recommendations for toxicological investigation of drug-impaired driving and motor vehicle fatalities; *J Anal Toxicol* 37:552; 2013.

Lopez-Rivadulla M, Cruz A: Drugs and driving in Spain; *Blutalkohol* 37:28; 2000.

Lund AK, Wolfe AC: Changes in the incidence of alcohol-impaired driving in the United States, 1973–1986; *J Stud Alcohol* 52:293; 1991.

Lundevall J, Olaisen B: Alkoholpåvirkning hos motorvognførere drept i trafikkulykker (Alcohol impairment among motor vehicle drivers killed in traffic accidents); *Lov og Rett* (Oslo) 271; 1976.

Mabunda MM, Swart LA, Seedat M: Magnitude and categories of pedestrian fatalities in South Africa; *Accid Anal Prev* 40:586; 2008.

Madruga C, Pinsky I, Laranjeira R: Commentary on Andreuccetti et al. (2011): The gap between stricter blood alcohol concentration legislation and enforcement in Brazil; *Addiction* 106:2132; 2011.

Mann RE, Macdonald S, Stoduto LG, Bondy S, Jonah B, Shaikh A: The effects of introducing or lowering legal per se blood alcohol limits for driving: An international review; *Accid Anal Prev* 33:569; 2001.

Masten SV, Guenzburger GV: Changes in driver cannabinoid prevalence in 12 U.S. States after implementing medical marijuana laws; *J Safety Res* 50:35; 2014.

Maurer HH: Current role of liquid chromatography-mass spectrometry in clinical and forensic toxicology; *Anal Bioanal Chem* 388:1315; 2007.

Maurer HH: Systematic toxicological analysis of drugs and their metabolites by gas chromatography-mass spectrometry; *J Chromatogr* 580:3; 1992.

McIntyre A, Cockfield S, Niewesteeg M: Drink and drug driving in Victoria: Lessons from 10 years of TAC research; *A Safe System: Making It Happen; Proceedings—Australasian College of Road Safety Conference*; Melbourne; Australasian; College of Road Safety: Melbourne, Australia; 2011.

McLean AJ, Kloeden CN, McCaul KA: Drink-driving in the general night-time driving population, Adelaide 1989; *Aust J Public Health* 15:190; 1991.

McLean AJ, Kloeden CN, McRoll RA, Laslett R: Reduction in the legal blood alcohol limit from 0.08 to 0.05: Effects on drink driving and alcohol-related crashes in Adelaide; In Kloeden CN, McLean AJ (Eds): *Alcohol, Drugs and Traffic Safety. Proceedings—13th International Conference on Alcohol, Drugs and Traffic Safety*, T'95; National Health and Medical Research Council: Adelaide, Australia; p. 373; 1995.

Ministry of Justice: Lov om vegtrafikk (LOV-1965-06-18-4) (Road Traffic Act); 2012; https://lovdata.no/dokument/NL/lov/1965-06-18-4 (Accessed April 3, 2019).

Ministry of Transport and Communications: Forskrift om faste grenser for påvirkning av andre berusende eller bedøvende middel enn alkohol m.m. (FOR-2016-01-12-19) (Regulations on Fixed Legal Limits for Impairment by Intoxicating Substances Other than Alcohol); 2016; https://lovdata.no/dokument/SF/forskrift/2012-01-20-85 (Accessed April 5, 2019).

Ministry of Transport and Communications: *National Transport Plan 2018–2029. Meld. St. 33 (2016–2017) Report to the Storting* (white paper); Ministry of Transport and Communications: Oslo, Norway; 2017; https://www.regjeringen.no/contentassets/7c52fd2938ca42209e4286fe86bb28bd/en-gb/pdfs/stm201620170033000engpdfs.pdf (Accessed April 5, 2019).

Mock C, Asiamah G, Amegashie J: A random, roadside breathalyzer survey of alcohol impaired driving in Ghana; *J Crash Prevent Inj Contr* 2:193; 2001.

Mokolobate K: Effects of alcohol consumption in South Africa: From the cradle to the grave; In *Mail & Guardian*, October 27, 2017; Johannesburg, South Africa; 2017; https://mg.co.za/article/2017-10-27-00-effects-of-alcohol-consumption-in-south-africa-from-the-cradle-to-the-grave (Accessed April 5, 2019).

Montenarh D, Hopf M, Warth S, Maurer HH, Schmidt P, Ewald AH: A simple extraction and LC-MS/MS approach for the screening and identification of over 100 analytes in eight different matrices; *Drug Test Anal* 7:214; 2015.

Moskowitz H, Burns M: Effects of alcohol on driving performance; *Alcohol Health Res World* 14:12; 1990.

Moura EC, Malta DC, Morais Neto OL, Penna GO, Temporao JG: Motor vehicle driving after binge drinking, Brazil, 2006 to 2009; *Rev Saude Publica* 43:891; 2009.

National Department of Traffic of Brazil: Portaria N° 219, de 19 de novembro de 2014; Departamento Nacional de Trânsito: Brasilia, Brazil; 2014; http://www.denatran.gov.br/download/Portarias/2014/Portaria2192014.pdf (Accessed April 5, 2019).

NHTSA: *Driver Alcohol Detection System for Safety*; US National Highway Traffic Safety Administration: Washington, DC; 2016; https://one.nhtsa.gov/Vehicle-Safety/DADSS (Accessed April 3, 2019).

NHTSA: *Traffic Safety Facts 2016. Compilation of Motor Vehicle Crash Data from the Fatality Analysis Reporting System and the General Estimates Sys*tem (DOT HS 812 554); US National Highway Traffic Safety Administration: Washington, DC; 2018; https://crashstats.nhtsa.dot.gov/Api/Public/ViewPublication/812554 (Accessed April 5, 2019).

NHTSA: *Traffic Safety Facts 2017. A Compilation of Motor Vehicle Crash Data* (DOT HS 812 806); US National Highway Traffic Safety Administration: Washington, DC; 2019; https://crashstats.nhtsa.dot.gov/Api/Public/Publication/812806 (Accessed February 18, 2020).

NIPH: *Rusmiddelstatistikk—Funn i blodprøver hos bilførere mistenkt for påvirket kjøring 2014 (Drug Statistics—Findings in Blood Samples from Drivers Suspected for Drugged Driving in 2014)*; Norwegian Institute of Public Health: Oslo, Norway; 2015; https://www.fhi.no/globalassets/dokumenterfiler/rapporter/2015/2015-rusmiddelstatistikk-pdf.pdf (Accessed April 5, 2019).

Nunes MN, Nascimento LF: Spatial analysis of deaths due to traffic accidents, before and after the Brazilian Drinking and Driving Law, in micro-regions of the state of Sao Paulo, Brazil; *Rev Assoc Med Bras* 58:685; 2012.

OAS: *American Convention on Human Rights "Pact of San Jose, Costa Rica"* (B-32); Organization of American States: Washington, DC; 1978; http://www.oas.org/dil/treaties_B-32_American_Convention_on_Human_Rights.pdf (Accessed April 5, 2019).

Odero W, Zwi AB: Drinking and driving in an urban setting in Kenya; *East Afr Med J* 74:675; 1997.

OECD: *Drugs and Driving: Detection and Deterrence*; OECD Publishing: Paris, France; 2010; doi:10.1787/9789282102763-en (Accessed April 5, 2019).

Ogden EJ, Moskowitz H: Effects of alcohol and other drugs on driver performance; *Traffic Inj Prev* 5:185; 2004.

Øiestad EL, Johansen U, Christophersen AS: Drug screening of preserved oral fluid by liquid chromatography-tandem mass spectrometry; *Clin Chem* 53:300; 2007.

Øiestad EL, Johansen U, Øiestad ÅML, Christophersen AS: Drug screening of whole blood by ultra-performance liquid chromatography-tandem mass spectrometry; *J Anal Toxicol* 35:280; 2011.

Ojaniemi KK, Lintonen TP, Impinen AO, Lillsunde PM, Ostamo AI: Trends in driving under the influence of drugs: A register-based study of DUID suspects during 1977–2007; *Accid Anal Prev* 41:191; 2009.

Oliveira LG, Endo LG, Sinagawa DM, Yonamine M, Munoz DR, Leyton V: A continuidade do uso de anfetaminas por motoristas de caminhão no Estado de São Paulo, Brasil, a despeito da proibição de sua produção, prescrição e uso (Persistent amphetamine consumption by truck drivers in Sao Paulo State, Brazil, despite the ban on production, prescription, and use); *Cad Saude Publica* 29:1903; 2013.

Owens KP, Boorman M: *Evaluating the Deterrent Effect of Random Breath Testing (RBT) and Random Drug testing (RDT)—The Driver's Perspective. Research Findings* (Monograph Series No. 41); National Drug Law Enforcement Research Fund: Canberra, Australia; 2011; http://www.ndlerf.gov.au/pub/Monograph_41.pdf (Accessed April 5, 2019).

Palamara P, Broughton M, Chambers F: *Illicit Drugs and Driving: An Investigation of Fatalities and Traffic Offences in Western Australia* (Report no. RR 13-001); Curtin-Monash Accident Research Centre: Bentley, Australia; 2014; http://c-marc.curtin.edu.au/local/docs/final-drugs-and-driving-november-2014_upload.pdf (Accessed April 5, 2019).

Parliament of Belgium: Loi relative à l'introduction des tests salivaires en matière de drogues dans la circulation—Wet tot invoering van speekseltesten op drugs in het verkeer; *Moniteur Belge* 179:62185; 2009; http://reflex.raadvst-consetat.be/reflex/pdf/Mbbs/2009/09/15/114286.pdf (Accessed April 5, 2019).

Parliament of France: Loi n° 2003-87 du 3 février 2003 relative à la conduite sous l'influence de substances ou plantes classées comme stupéfiants; *J Off Rep France* 2103; 2003; *http://legifrance.gouv.fr/eli/loi/2003/2/3/2003-87/jo/texte* (Accessed April 5, 2019).

Parliament of Spain: Ley 6/2014, de 7 de abril, por la que se modifica el texto articulado de la Ley sobre Tráfico, Circulación de Vehículos a Motor y Seguridad Vial, aprobado por el Real Decreto Legislativo 339/1990, de 2 de marzo; *Bol Oficial Estado* Sec. I:29508; 2014; https://www.boe.es/boe/dias/2014/04/08/pdfs/BOE-A-2014-3715.pdf (Accessed April 5, 2019).

Parliament of Spain: Ley Orgánica 5/2010, de 22 de junio, por la que se modifica la Ley Orgánica 10/1995, de 23 de noviembre, del Código Penal; *Bol Oficial Estado* 54811; 2010; http://www.boe.es/boe/dias/2010/06/23/pdfs/BOE-A-2010-9953.pdf (Accessed April 5, 2019).

Parliament of Victoria: *Road Safety (Drug Driving) Bill 2003*; Parliament of Victoria: Melbourne, Australina; 2003; http://www.austlii.edu.au/au/legis/vic/bill/rsdb2003257/ (Accessed April 2, 2019).

Pechansky F, Von Diemen L, Soibelman M, de Boni R, Bumaguin DB, Fürst MC: Clinical signs of alcohol intoxication as markers of refusal to provide blood alcohol readings in emergency rooms: An exploratory study; *Clinics* (Sao Paulo) 65:1391; 2010.

Peixe TS, de Almeida RM, Girotto E, de Andrade SM, Mesas AE: Use of illicit drugs by truck drivers arriving at Paranaguá port terminal, Brazil; *Traffic Inj Prev* 15:673; 2014.

Penning R, Veldstra JL, Daamen AP, Olivier B, Verster JC: Drugs of abuse, driving and traffic safety; *Curr Drug Abuse Rev* 3:23; 2010.

Petroulias T: *Community Attitudes to Road Safety—2013 Survey Report;* Australian Government Department of Infrastructure and Transport: Canberra, Australia; 2013.

Pil K, Verstraete A: Current developments in drug testing in oral fluid; *Ther Drug Monit* 30:196; 2008.

Pinsky I, Labouvie E, Pandina R, Laranjeira R: Drinking and driving: Pre-driving attitudes and perceptions among Brazilian youth; *Drug Alcohol Depend* 62:231; 2001.

Polettini A: Systematic toxicological analysis of drugs and poisons in biosamples by hyphenated chromatographic and spectroscopic techniques; *J Chromatogr B Biomed Sci Appl* 733:47; 1999.

Pollini RA, Romano E, Johnson MB, Lacey JH: The impact of marijuana decriminalization on California drivers; *Drug Alcohol Depend* 150:135; 2015.

Raes E, Van den Neste T, Verstraete AG, Lopez D, Hughes B, Griffiths P: *Drug Use, Impaired Driving and Traffic Accidents*; Office for Official Publications of the European Communities: Luxembourg; 2008; http://www.emcdda.europa.eu/attachements.cfm/att_65871_EN_Insight8.pdf (Accessed April 5, 2019).

Ribeiro M, Perrenoud LO, Duailibi S, Duailibi LB, Madruga C, Marques ACPR, Laranjeira R: The Brazilian drug policy situation: The public health approach based on research undertaken in a developing country; *Public Health Rev* 35:143; 2014.

RMHIDTA: *The Legalization of Marijuana in Colorado—The Impact*, Vol. 2; August 2014; Rocky Mountain High Intensity Drug Trafficking Area: Denver, CO; 2014; https://www.rmhidta.org/html/August%202014%20Legalization%20of%20MJ%20in%20Colorado%20the%20Impact.pdf (Accessed April 5, 2019).

Romano E, Pollini RA: Patterns of drug use in fatal crashes; *Addiction* 108:1428; 2013.

Roussel O, Perrin-Rosset M, Fuché C, Carlin M: The French experience of establishing an oral fluid roadside drug test; *Toxicol Anal Clin* 26:S2; 2014.

Rudisill TM, Zhao S, Abate MA, Coben JH, Zhu M: Trends in drug use among drivers killed in U.S. traffic crashes, 1999–2010; *Accid Anal Prev* 70:178; 2014.

Salomonsen-Sautel S, Min SJ, Sakai JT, Thurstone C, Hopfer C: Trends in fatal motor vehicle crashes before and after marijuana commercialization in Colorado; *Drug Alcohol Depend* 140:137; 2014.

Senna MC, Augsburger M, Aebi B, Briellmann TA, Donze N, Dubugnon JL, Iten PX, Staub C, Sturm W, Sutter K: First nationwide study on driving under the influence of drugs in Switzerland; *Forensic Sci Int* 198:11; 2010.

Sergi M, Bafile E, Compagnone D, Curini R, D'Ascenzo G, Romolo FS: Multiclass analysis of illicit drugs in plasma and oral fluids by LC-MS/MS; *Anal Bioanal Chem* 393:709; 2009.

Sevigny EL: The effects of medical marijuana laws on cannabis-involved driving; *Accid Anal Prev* 118:57; 2018.

Sharma BR: Road traffic injuries: A major global public health crisis; *Public Health* 122:1399; 2008.

Silva OA, Greve JMD, Yonamine M, Leyton V: Drug use by truck drivers in Brazil; *Drugs Educat Prev Pol* 10:135; 2003.

Sinagawa DM, De Carvalho HB, Andreuccetti G, Do Prado NV, De Oliveira KC, Yonamine M, Munoz DR, Gjerde H, Leyton V: Association between travel length and drug use among Brazilian truck drivers; *Traffic Inj Prev* 16:5; 2015.

Sinagawa DM, Takitane J, Endo LG, Carvalho HB, Andreuccetti G, Yonamine M, Rohlfs WJC, Novo GC, Santos AJ, Leyton V: Drug use by truck drivers in Brazil: A historical analysis during 2009–2012; *Abstracts—51st Annual Meeting of the International Association of Forensic Toxicologists* (TIAFT 2013); Madeira, Portugal; Instituto Nacional de Medicina Legal e Ciencias Forenses: Coimbra, Portugal; p. 88; 2013.

Skopp G: Postmortem toxicology; *Forensic Sci Med Pathol* 6:314; 2010.

Smith JA, Hayes CE, Yolton RL, Rutledge DA, Citek K: Drug recognition expert evaluations made using limited data; *Forensic Sci Int* 130:167; 2002.

Sousa T, Lunnen JC, Goncalves V, Schmitz A, Pasa G, Bastos T, Sripad P, Chandran A, Pechansky F: Challenges associated with drunk driving measurement: Combining police and self-reported data to estimate an accurate prevalence in Brazil; *Injury* 44(Suppl 4):S11; 2013.

Spanish Ministry of the Interiors: Real Decreto 2282/1998, de 23 de octubre, por el que se modifican los artículos 20 y 23del Reglamento General de Circulación, aprobado por Real Decreto 13/1992, de 17 de enero; *Bol Oficial Estado* 36202; 1998; http://www.boe.es/boe/dias/1998/11/06/pdfs/A36202-36202.pdf (Accessed April 5, 2019).

Starmer GA, Mascord D, Tattam B, Zeleny R: *Analysis for Drugs in Saliva;* Australian Government Publishing Service: Canberra, Australia; 1994.

Statistics Norway: *Veitrafikkulykker med personskade 2017* (*Injurious Road Traffic Crashes 2017*); Statistics Norway: Kongsvinger, Norway; 2018; https://www.ssb.no/transport-og-reiseliv/statistikker/vtu/aar/2018-05-29 (Accessed April 3, 2019).

Steentoft A, Simonsen KW, Linnet K: The frequency of drugs among Danish drivers before and after the introduction of fixed concentration limits; *Traffic Inj Prev* 11:329; 2010.

Stewart K: *Alcohol Involvement in Fatal Crashes. Comparison among Countries* (DOT HS 809 355); US National Highway Traffic Safety Administration: Washington, DC; 2001; https://rosap.ntl.bts.gov/view/dot/1709 (Accessed April 5, 2019).

Stewart K, Silcock D, Wegman F: Reducing drink driving in low- and middle-income countries: Challenges and opportunities; *Traffic Inj Prev* 13:93; 2012.

Stewart K, Sweedler BM: Worldwide trends in impaired driving: Past experience and future progress; In Nickel WR, Koran M (Eds): *Proceedings—3rd International Traffic Expert Congress*; Prague, Czech Republic; June 2008; Kirschbaum Berlag: Bonn, Germany; 2008.

Strano-Rossi S, Castrignano E, Anzillotti L, Serpelloni G, Mollica R, Tagliaro F, Pascali JP, di Stefano D, Sgalla R, Chiarotti M: Evaluation of four oral fluid devices (DDS®, Drugtest 5000®, Drugwipe 5+® and RapidSTAT® for on-site monitoring drugged driving in comparison with UHPLC-MS/MS analysis; *Forensic Sci Int* 221:70; 2012.

Swann P: Drugs and driving Victoria Australia update; *2nd International Symposium on Drugs and Driving;* Wellington, November 12–13, 2014; Wellington, New Zealand; 2014; https://www.youtube.com/watch?v=z_Uv8NdwedE (Accessed April 5, 2019).

Sweedler BM: Worldwide trends in alcohol and drug impaired driving; In Logan BK, Isenschmid DS, Walsh JM, Beimess D, Mørland J (Eds): *Proceedings of the 18th International Council on Alcohol, Drugs and Traffic Accident Conference*, T2007; Seattle WA; ICADTS: Seattle, WA; 2007.

Sweedler BM, Biecheler MB, Laurell H, Kroj G, Lerner M, Mathijssen MP, Mayhew D, Tunbridge RJ: Worldwide trends in alcohol and drug impaired driving; *Traffic Inj Prev* 5:175; 2004.

Swensen G, Jones S: *Drug-Related Traffic Fatalities in Western Australia*; Task Force on Drug Abuse: Perth, Australia; 1996.

TAC: *Drink Driving Statistics*; Transport Accident Commission: Melbourne, Australia; 2013; http:// www.tac.vic.gov.au/road-safety/statistics/summaries/drink-driving-statistics (Accessed April 4, 2019).

Takitane J, de Oliveira LG, Endo LG, de Oliveira KC, Munoz DR, Yonamine M, Leyton V: Uso de anfetaminas por motoristas de caminhão em rodovias do Estado de São Paulo: um risco à ocorrência de acidentes de trânsito? (Amphetamine use by truck drivers on highways of Sao Paulo State: A risk for the occurrence of traffic accidents?); *Cien Saude Colet* 18:1247; 2013.

Thompson P: Changing trend of drug driving detections in South Australia; In Watson B (Ed): *Proceedings—20th International Council on Alcohol, Drugs and Traffic Safety Conference*; August 22–25, 2013; Center for Accident Research and Road Safety Queensland: Brisbane, Australia; 2013.

TISPOL: Almost one million drivers tested for alcohol in summer operation; *TISPOL Bull* 4; 2011.

Tourangeau R, Yan T: Sensitive questions in surveys; *Psychol Bull* 133:859; 2007.

UK Secretary of State: *The Drug Driving Specified Limits Regulations 2014 (England and Wales)*; Secretary of State: London, UK; 2014; http://www.legislation.gov.uk/id/uksi/2014/2868 (Accessed April 4, 2019).

Valen A, Bogstrand ST, Vindenes V, Frost J, Larsson M, Holtan A, Gjerde H: Alcohol and drug use and crash characteristics for fatally injured drivers in Norway 2005–2015; *Traffic Inj Prev* (in press); 2019.

Van de Mortel TF: Faking it: Social desirability response bias in self-report research; *Aust J Adv Nurs* 25:40; 2008.

Vanstechelman S, Isalberti C, Van der Linden T, Pil K, Legrand SA, Verstraete AG: Analytical evaluation of four on-site oral fluid drug testing devices; *J Anal Toxicol* 36:136; 2012.

Verster JC, Mets MA: Psychoactive medication and traffic safety; *Int J Environ Res Public Health* 6:1041; 2009.

Verstraete A, Knoche A, Jantos R, Skopp G, Gjerde H, Vindenes V, Mørland J, Langel K, Lillsunde P: *Per Se Limits—Methods of Defining Cut-off Values for Zero Tolerance. DRUID* (Deliverable D1.4.2); Ghent University: Ghent, Belgium; 2011; https://biblio.ugent.be/publication/1988464/file/1988490.pdf (Accessed April 5, 2019).

Verstraete AG: Oral fluid testing for driving under the influence of drugs: History, recent progress and remaining challenges; *Forensic Sci Int* 150:143; 2005.

Verstraete AG, Legrand SA, Vandam L, Hughes B, Griffiths B: *Drug Use, Impaired Driving, and Traffic Accidents, Second Edition;* Publications Office of the European Union: Luxembourg; 2014; http://www.emcdda.europa.eu/publications/insights/2014/drugs-and-driving (Accessed April 5, 2019).

Vindenes V, Aamo T, Innerdal C, Mathisrud G, Mørland J, Riedel B, Slørdal L, Strand MC: *Revidering av "forskrift om faste grenser for påvirkning av andre berusende eller bedøvende middel enn alkohol m.m."—Vurdering av eksisterende faste grenser og forslag til faste grenser for flere stoffer* (*Revision of "Regulations on Fixed Limits for Impairment by Other Intoxicating or Anaesthetic/Sedative Substances than Alcohol etc."—Assessment of Existing Fixed Limits and Proposed Fixed Limits for Additional Substances*); Ministry of Transport and Communications: Oslo, Norway; 2015; https://www.regjeringen.no/contentassets/21dac5b787734d7b80f45d30c88e8632/hbrev2304rapport.pdf (Accessed April 5, 2019).

Vindenes V, Jordbru D, Knapskog AB, Kvan E, Mathisrud G, Slørdal L, Mørland J: Impairment based legislative limits for driving under the influence of non-alcohol drugs in Norway; *Forensic Sci Int* 219:1; 2012.

Voas RB, Fell JC: Preventing impaired driving opportunities and problems; *Alcohol Res Health* 34:225; 2011.

Voas RB, Torres P, Romano E, Lacey JH: Alcohol-related risk of driver fatalities: An update using 2007 data; *J Stud Alcohol Drugs* 73:341; 2012.

Voas RB, Wells J, Lestina D, Williams A, Greene M: Drinking and driving in the United States: The 1996 national roadside survey; *Accid Anal Prev* 30:267; 1998.

Walsh JM: *A State-by-State Analysis of Laws Dealing with Driving Under the Influence of Drugs* (DOT HS 811 236): US National Highway Traffic Safety Administration: Washington, DC; 2009; http://www.nhtsa.gov/staticfiles/nti/pdf/811236.pdf (Accessed April 5, 2019).

Walsh JM, de Gier JJ, Christophersen AS, Verstraete AG: Drugs and driving; *Traffic Inj Prev* 5:241; 2004.

Walsh JM, Verstraete AG, Huestis MA, Mørland J: Guidelines for research on drugged driving; *Addiction* 103:1258; 2008.

Wang Z, Zhang Y, Zhou P, Shi J, Wang Y, Liu R, Jiang C: The underestimated drink driving situation and the effects of zero tolerance laws in China; *Traffic Inj Prev* 16:429; 2015.

Watson B, Freeman J: Perceptions and experiences of random breath testing in Queensland and the self-reported deterrent impact on drunk driving; *Traffic Inj Prev* 8:11; 2007.

Wells JK, Greene MA, Foss RD, Ferguson SA, Williams AF: Drinking drivers missed at sobriety checkpoints; *J Stud Alcohol* 58:513; 1997.

WHO: *Global Status Report on Alcohol and Health 2014*; World Health Organization: Geneva, Switzerland; 2014; http://www.who.int/substance_abuse/publications/global_alcohol_report/msb_gsr_2014_1.pdf (Accessed April 5, 2019).

WHO: *Global Status Report on Road Safety 2013 Supporting a Decade of Action*; World Health Organization: Geneva, Switzerland; 2013; http://www.who.int/violence_injury_prevention/road_safety_status/2013/en/ (Accessed April 5, 2019).

WHO: *Global Status Report on Road Safety 2018;* World Health Organization: Geneva, Switzerland; 2018a; https://www.who.int/violence_injury_prevention/road_safety_status/2018/en/ (Accessed April 5, 2019).

WHO: *Global Status Report on Road Safety—Time for Action*; World Health Organization: Geneva, Switzerland; 2009; http://www.who.int/violence_injury_prevention/road_safety_status/2009/en/index.html (Accessed April 5, 2019).

WHO: *World Health Statistics 2018: Monitoring Health for the Sustainable Development Goals*; World Health Organization: Geneva, Switzerland; 2018b; https://www.who.int/healthinfo/en/ (Accessed April 5, 2019).

Widmark EMP: *Theoretischen Grundlagen und die praktische Verwendbarkeit der gerichtlich-medizinischen Alkoholbestimmung* (*The Theoretical Basis and Applications of Medicolegal Alcohol Determination*); Urban & Schwarzenberg: Berlin, Germany; 1932.

Wikipedia.org: *List of Countries by Traffic-Related Death Rate* http://en.wikipedia.org/wiki/List_of_countries_by_traffic-related_death_rate (Accessed March 25, 2019).

Williams AF: Alcohol-impaired driving and its consequences in the United States: The past 25 years; *J Safety Res* 37:123; 2006.

Wisdom GB: Enzyme-immunoassay; *Clin Chem* 22:1243; 1976.

Wolfe AC: *1973 U.S. National Roadside Breath Testing Survey: Procedures and Results* (DOT HS 801 241); University of Michigan Safety Research Institute: Ann Arbor, MI; 1974; *https://rosap.ntl.bts.gov/view/dot/1118* (Accessed April 5, 2019).

Wood E, Brooks-Russell A, Drum P: Delays in DUI blood testing: Impact on cannabis DUI assessments; *Traffic Inj Prev* 17:105; 2016.

Yonamine M, Sanches LR, Paranhos BA, de Almeida RM, Andreuccetti G, Leyton V: Detecting alcohol and illicit drugs in oral fluid samples collected from truck drivers in the state of Sao Paulo, Brazil; *Traffic Inj Prev* 14:127; 2013.

Zador PL, Krawchuk SA, Voas RB: Alcohol-related relative risk of driver fatalities and driver involvement in fatal crashes in relation to driver age and gender: an update using 1996 data; *J Stud Alcohol* 61:387; 2000.

V

Epidemiology, Enforcement, and Countermeasures

Alcohol Limits and Public Safety*,†

14

DENNIS V. CANFIELD, KURT M. DUBOWSKI, MACK COWAN, AND PATRICK M. HARDING

Contents

14.1 Introduction

Recently the National Transportation Safety Board (NTSB) recommended lowering the legal blood-alcohol limit to 0.05 g/dL for motor vehicle operators in the United States (NTSB/SR-13/01 2013). This recommendation has prompted other organizations, including the National Safety Council (NSC), to consider this proposed action. The authors were asked to evaluate the NTSB recommendation and to submit a scientific report on the feasibility of lowering the blood-alcohol limit to 0.05 g/dL for drivers. The authors have conducted this study based on the available published scientific literature and herein provide

* This chapter is an updated version of a review article previously published in *Forensic Science Review*: Canfield DV, Dubowski KM, Cowan M, Harding PM: Alcohol limits and public safety; *Forensic Sci Rev* 26:9; 2014.

† The views and opinions expressed by the authors do not necessarily reflect those of the agencies or institutions with which they were or are affiliated.

an overview of alcohol limits and public safety. Alcohol concentrations in this article are expressed in g/dL in blood and g/210 L in breath.

Approximately 133 million (51.8%) Americans aged 12 or older reported being current users of alcohol in 2012; approximately 58.3 million (22.6%) reported participating in binge drinking and approximately 15.9 million (6.2%) reported being heavy drinkers (NSDUH, (SMA) 12-4713 2012). The direct and indirect economic costs of alcohol abuse have been estimated at $223.5 billion for 2006 (Bouchery et al. 2011). This does not include the psychological toll associated with loss of human life and recovery from serious injuries.

Robert F. Borkenstein, in his groundbreaking study correlating accident rates with breath-alcohol concentrations, provided the first clear and convincing scientific evidence that individuals who drink and drive are at greater risk of being involved in a traffic crash (Borkenstein et al. 1964). His study has been repeated several times using more modern techniques by research scientists with similar results (Figure 14.1) (Blomberg et al. 2009; Krüger et al. 1995, 2004; Zador 1991). It has been proved that the relative risk of having a motor vehicle crash increases as a function of alcohol concentration with, for example, an

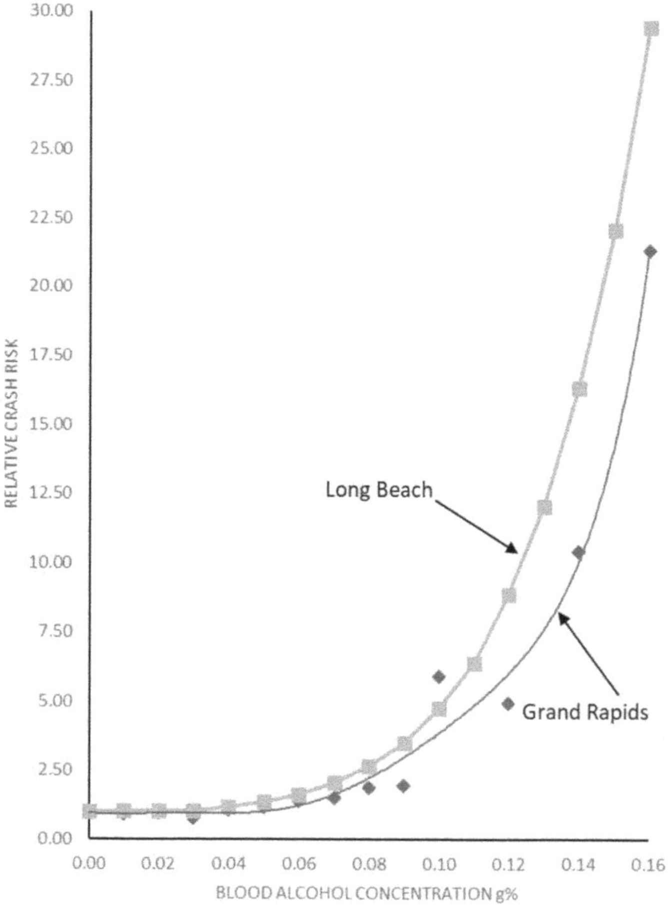

Figure 14.1 Comparison of Long Beach crash data (gray squares) with Grand Rapids data (black diamonds). (Figure is constructed based on data appearing in Blomberg, R.D. et al., *J. Safety Res.*, 40, 2, 2009; Borkenstein, R.F. et al., *The Role of the Drinking Driver in Traffic Accidents*, Department of Police Administration, Indiana University, Bloomington, IN, 1964.)

18% increased crash risk at 0.04. It took many years after Professor Borkenstein's original work was published for the documented dangers associated with drinking and driving to be recognized in the form of *per se* driving laws. Professor Borkenstein's original research is also supported by human-subject impairment studies that demonstrate increased impairment with increasing blood-alcohol concentrations (Landauer and Howat 1982; Moskowitz et al. [DOT HS 809 075] 2000).

In 1995 the US Department of Transportation (DOT) established a mandatory *per se* blood-alcohol testing limit of 0.04 for commercial drivers and other individuals in safety-related positions (Dubowski et al. 2008). The effectiveness of this program in reducing alcohol-related fatal motor-carrier crashes was evaluated by examining accidents involving 69,295 motor-carrier drivers and 83,436 non–motor-carrier drivers involved in 66,138 fatal multivehicle accidents (Brady et al. 2009). Overall, alcohol-related fatal motor-vehicle crashes declined by 80% after the introduction of the DOT regulation and by 41% for non-motor-carrier drivers not covered by the regulation. After the removal of confounding factors such as age and gender, the mandatory 0.04 rule for motor-carrier drivers showed a 23% reduction in alcohol-related fatal accidents (Brady et al. 2009). The above-mentioned research clearly demonstrates that the DOT mandatory 0.04 alcohol testing program significantly reduced the number of alcohol-related fatal motor-carrier accidents.

Many state laws already provided a 0.04 limit for individuals flying an aircraft and/or driving a commercial vehicle. So, this lower alcohol limit is not a totally new concept for states. The limits are not always applied equally across all modes of transportation. Oklahoma law states it is unlawful to operate an aircraft with a breath- or blood-alcohol concentration at or above 0.04 within 2 hours after the arrest of such person concentration has been associated with driving (Oklahoma Code Title 3—Aircraft and Airports 2006).

There have been numerous studies that examined the effects of low alcohol concentrations on driving ability and crash risk. After a review of the vast scientific literature on the subject of the increased risks associated with alcohol use and accidents, it is clear there is a loss of driving ability at 0.05 concentration and even lower concentration with more severe impairment occurring at increasing concentrations (AMA Council on Scientific Affairs 1986). It has been understood for many years that alcohol present in the body at any concentration causes an increased crash risk (Kuypers et al. 2012). Cognitive functions for a range of alcohol concentrations showed more changes in cognitive function between placebo and 0.05 than was found between 0.05 and 0.10 (Kennedy et al. 1993). Alcohol at any concentration has been associated with driving impairment (AMA Council on Scientific Affairs CSA Rep 14: A-97 1997). Gross and persistent impairment has been demonstrated between 0.04 and 0.05 and increases with subsequent increases of alcohol concentration (AMA Council on Scientific Affairs CSA Rep 14: A-97 1997). Current published reviews of the literature support the conclusion that a 0.05 alcohol concentration impairs drivers and causes increased numbers of accidents (Martin et al. 2013).

The American Medical Association (AMA) in 1997 gathered information from other countries with a legal limit of 0.02 or less and based on this information proposed a national *per se* 0.02 alcohol driving limit at any age in the United States (AMA Council on Scientific Affairs CSA Rep 14: A-97 1997). The AMA for many years has supported legal limits of 0.05 for adults and 0.02 for individuals under 21 (AMA Council on Scientific Affairs CSA Rep 14: A-97 1997). Even though alcohol-abuse intervention has proved very effective, emergency room doctors often cannot detect or intervene when treating alcohol-related crash victims, leading to the underreporting of alcohol related accidents (Miller et al. 2012).

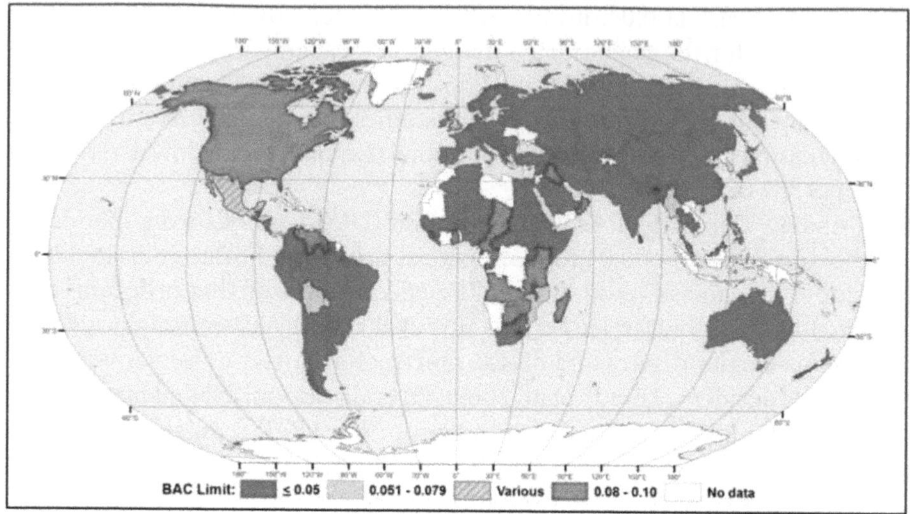

Figure 14.2 A comparison of the United States' breath-alcohol concentration (BrAC) limit with those of other countries [NSC Policy #130 2016].

Other nations discovered long ago that they could save lives and prevent injuries by lowering the alcohol limit for driving. Out of all the countries listed in the National Safety Council's "Position/Policy Statement, Low Alcohol Concentration National Culture Change," available online, only a few highlighted countries have a higher breath-alcohol limit than the United States (Figure 14.2) (NSC Policy #130 2016). The majority of the countries (60%) have alcohol limits at or below the 0.05 recommended by the NTSB.

14.2 Risks Associated with Alcohol Limits

14.2.1 Crash Data

Research has proved that drinking drivers are at high risk of suffering injury or death when compared with nondrinking drivers (Waller et al. 1986). With single-vehicle accidents involving fatalities, it has been estimated that approximately twice the number of drivers will be involved in an accident for every 0.02 increase in the alcohol concentration in the body compared with 0-alcohol drivers. Increased crash risk was associated with an increasing alcohol concentration for all the age and gender groups studied at alcohol concentrations from 0.05 to 0.09, with the odds of a crash being nine times greater than individuals at 0-alcohol concentrations (Zador 1991).

Many studies have shown that alcohol concentrations of less than 0.04 cause impairment and crash risk to increase. Using a control group with an alcohol concentration of 0, the estimated relative risk of death increased even with an alcohol concentration of 0.01 by 30% with a 95% confidence interval between 20% and 40% (Smith et al. 2001). There was a threefold increase in crash risk associated with crash injuries even with blood-alcohol concentrations below 0.05 (Connor et al. 2004). When concentrations were at or above 0.05, there was a 23-fold increase in crash risk (Connor et al. 2004).

Other studies have found the risk associated with fatal accidents increases drastically between 0.04 and 0.05, with an even greater risk at 0.10 (AMA Council on Scientific Affairs CSA Rep 14: A-97 1997).

Each single drink of alcohol consumed increases the risk of roadside traffic crashes (Di Bartolomeo et al. 2009). Associations between alcohol intake and traffic risk behaviors were compared with abstainers: individuals who consumed only one alcohol unit were found more likely to be a passenger in a car driven by a drunk driver, increasing their risk of being in an accident by almost four times (Goncalves et al. 2012). Individuals consuming five or more alcoholic drinks increased their risk of being in a car crash by almost five times (Goncalves et al. 2012). Individuals drinking three alcoholic beverages were four times more likely to be involved in a crash than someone who consumed one alcoholic beverage (Goncalves et al. 2012).

14.2.2 Experimental Data

Alcohol impairment begins at very low alcohol concentrations and rapidly increases as a function of alcohol concentration. Laboratory experiments with low concentration of blood alcohol clearly demonstrate that impairment begins at 0.015 and increases with rising alcohol concentration (Moskowitz et al. 1985). A study of blood-alcohol concentration at 0.00, 0.021, 0.05, and 0.073 found increased decision and reaction times as a function of increasing alcohol concentration (Landauer and Howat 1982). Performance impairment by alcohol occurred with all concentrations from 0.02 to 0.10, with a magnitude of increased impairment with increasing alcohol concentrations (Moskowitz et al. [DOT HS 809 075] 2000). The relative change in the measured performance from 0 to 0.10 alcohol concentration based on data from table 2 of the DOT HS 809 075 report using the equation (Performance Index–Performance Index^0)/Performance Index^0 (Figure 14.3) showed a twofold decrease in performance from 0.02 alcohol concentration to 0.04.

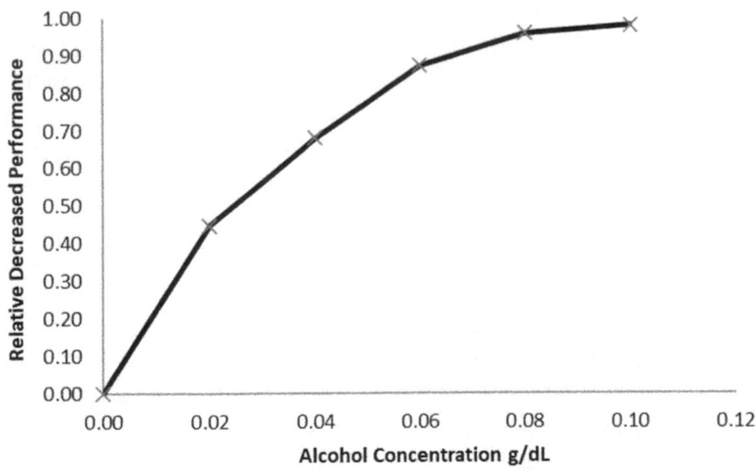

Figure 14.3 Relative decreased performance at different concentrations of alcohol versus no alcohol. (Figure is constructed by the authors based on data appearing in Moskowitz, H. et al., *Driver Characteristics and Impairment at Various BACs*, (DOT HS 809 075), National Highway Traffic Safety, Washington, DC, 2000.)

14.2.3 Medical Data

Hospital studies (Fabbri et al. 2001) have demonstrated that positive alcohol trauma patients have a:

- 89% greater chance of suffering from critical injuries when examined;
- 67% increased risk of being killed or permanently disabled;
- 87% greater chance of needing intensive care;
- 91% greater chance of needing surgery; and
- 94% increased probability of blood transfusions and acute medical complications.

Additional emergency room studies have shown a direct correlation to injuries and alcohol-positive patients (Cherpitel 1989). Certain medical conditions have been associated with an increased risk for alcohol impairment, as can be seen with patients suffering from obstructive sleep apnea being more impaired at a given concentration of alcohol than would be found in healthy individuals (Vakulin et al. 2009). Fatigue has also been found to increase alcohol impairment. A Utah study on crash risks associated with alcohol and fatigue compared drivers in motor vehicle crashes with hospital discharge records. This study found that alcohol intoxication and fatigue together increased the likelihood of hospitalization or death (Smith et al. 2004). Others studies have also shown increased impairment at low alcohol concentration with partially sleep-deprived subjects (Banks et al. 2004).

14.3 Instrument Reliability

14.3.1 Instrument Data

14.3.1.1 Breath

A study published in 1999 found that the coefficient of variation for evidential federally approved breath-testing devices never exceeded 2% for repeated tests at four different concentrations (0.02, 0.04, 0.06, and 0.10) (Dubowski and Essary 1999). The probability of a breath-test result being at the extreme positive or negative ends of the variability accepted by federal regulations for evidential breath-testing devices for a 0.08 of ±0.005 (6%) are less than 0.1%, whereas there is more than a 99.9% probability that the result will fall within this very narrow 6% legally accepted instrument variability of the actual breath concentration. This has been confirmed in another study that found "nine subjects had linear regression coefficients for the end-expiratory results that were not significantly different from zero ($P > 0.05$)" (Gullberg 1995). Only minor variations were observed using simulator solutions in the third decimal place, showing that the instrumentation is very precise (Gullberg 1989).

Simulator devices containing alcohol used to calibrate and evaluate the performance of breath-testing instruments have been examined for reliability and found to be accurate in the delivery of a known concentration of alcohol (Dubowski and Essary 1991, 1992; Silverman et al. 1997). Even when studies were conducted using less or more than the 500 mL of solution used in simulators, the variability remained within a coefficient of variation (CV) of 1% regardless of the volume used. Variations of ±20% "from the 500-mL volume in a simulator do not result in a statistically significant difference where between-day measurements are evaluated" (Speck et al. 1991). Simulator tests at six different concentrations, ranging from 0.060 to 0.120, with a total of 779 repeated tests showed consistent and satisfactory results with laboratory tests that conformed with established testing protocols "as an effective quality assurance measure in evidential breath-alcohol analysis" (Dubowski and Essary 1992).

Some individuals have claimed gastroesophageal reflux disease (GERD) as the cause for their failure to pass a breath-alcohol test. However, experiments with individuals suffering from this illness did not show any "risk of alcohol erupting from the stomach into the mouth owing to gastric reflux and falsely increasing the result of an evidential breath-alcohol test" (Kechagias et al. 1999). Another claim is that mouth alcohol causes the elevated reading. Research has demonstrated that mouth alcohol levels drop below significant values within 15 minutes after alcohol exposure (Dubowski 1975; Gullberg 1992; Logan and Distefano 1998; Logan et al. 1998; Logan and Gullberg 1998; Watterson and Ellefsen 2009). Following standard breath-testing procedures of waiting 15 minutes and conducting duplicate tests will prevent interference from mouth alcohol with breath-testing devices (Gullberg 2001).

Alcohol concentrations reported by breath-alcohol instruments in the United States typically are lower than those found in the blood (Currier et al. 2006; Fransson et al. 2005; Gullberg 1990; Harding et al. 1990). A Wisconsin study using "404 pairs of breath- and blood-alcohol results from specimens collected within 1 hour of each other" were examined and 94% of the breath tests were lower than or equal to the blood-alcohol concentration (Harding and Field 1987). Breathalyzers used in the United States are programmed with a breath/blood-alcohol conversion factor of 1/2100 but the general population has a mean breath/blood-alcohol ratio of approximately 1/2300 (Jones 1985a), causing the breath-alcohol results from an instrument programmed at 1/2100 to be typically lower than the actual blood-alcohol concentration (Jones 1985b). This means the majority of the drivers convicted of violating alcohol laws in the United States actually had a higher blood-alcohol concentration than the reported breathalyzer results. Blood-alcohol concentrations vary even within the body, with venous blood differing from the concentration found in arterial blood. It is interesting that the arterial blood-alcohol concentration correlates better with breath-alcohol than it does with venous blood (Martin et al. 1984). Medical studies comparing breath- and blood-alcohol concentrations have found a high diagnostic reliability with the use of breath-alcohol testing (Heifer et al. 1995).

The specificity of breath testing has been evaluated with regard to the presence of acetone, a naturally occurring substance in the body of individuals suffering from ketoacidosis. Studies have shown the presence of acetone in the body did not interfere with the accuracy of breath-alcohol testing devices. A review of the literature of ambulatory patients and other information regarding acetone production in the human body, considering the low acetone cross reactivity of the breath-alcohol testing devices, it "is not considered to be a significant problem in breath-alcohol analysis for traffic law enforcement purposes" (Dubowski and Essary 1983, 1984; Jones 1987). Other investigations have proven that inhalation of nasal sprays and other vapors do not interfere with the breath-alcohol test (Gomm et al. 1990, 1991).

Breath- and blood-alcohol concentrations involving patients with pulmonary dysfunctions were studied to determine what, if any, difference could be found with healthy individuals. The analysis did not find any "significant difference between directly and indirectly established blood-alcohol concentration with regard to pulmonary disorders" (Heifer et al. 1995).

14.3.1.2 Blood

There are many different types of blood-alcohol instruments and procedures, which need not be discussed in detail. At the present time the accepted forensic practice is to use an internal standard, two different types of gas chromatography columns, and flame ionization detectors (FIDs) to quantitate and confirm alcohol in blood (Harding and Field 1987; Jaffe et al. 2013). This procedure has been accepted in all courts of law as a scientifically acceptable procedure for the analysis of alcohol in blood. Repeated in-house analysis of a blind blood-ethanol control using an internal standard, two column headspace gas chromatography, and an FID method for a period of over 2 years gave a CV of 0.02, a standard deviation (SD) of 0.002, and a mean of 0.081 with no outliers. An open control run for 2 years had a CV of 0.02, an SD of 0.001, and a mean of 0.050 with no outliers. An open control run for 1 year had a CV of 0.03, an SD of 0.001, and a mean of 0.024 mg/dL. This demonstrates the high reliability of blood-alcohol analysis using a legally accepted forensic procedure.

14.3.1.3 Saliva

Enzymatic saliva-testing devices have proved very reliable in the detection of alcohol. This test is easy to administer and does not require invasive procedures in the collection of specimens. Observed specimen collection can be used to avoid problems associated with the validity of the specimen collected. Acetone, methanol, 2-butanone, and ethylene glycol did not react with the QED when tested in vitro. Control solutions at 0.050, 0.100, and 0.140 were tested using saliva and gave readings of 0.050 ± 0.002 (SD), 0.102 ± 0.003, and 0.136 ± 0.005, corresponding to recoveries of 100%, 102%, and 97%, respectively (Jones 1995). Good correlation was found between the enzymatic procedure and venous blood-alcohol concentrations. Saliva analysis has proved very successful in the analysis of alcohol, with the results comparing well with venous blood concentrations and breath testing (Jones 1995). Saliva can also be collected and confirmed using other procedures such as gas chromatography, providing a more specific and strong correlation between saliva and blood-alcohol concentrations (Gubala and Zuba 2002). Saliva-testing devices approved on the NHTSA's conforming products lists (CPL) can be used as a screening device for DOT workplace alcohol testing.

14.3.1.4 Urine

Urine-alcohol concentrations are not well correlated with blood-alcohol concentrations or with driver impairment due to the elimination characteristics of alcohol into the bladder as well as other causes. It is possible that all blood alcohol has been eliminated from the body into the bladder and therefore not available to impair the individual. Voiding the urine and waiting 20 minutes before the collection of the test specimen can provide a more reliable ratio of urine to blood of approximately 1.3 to 1.4 (Jones 2006). All alcohol found in the urine specimen collected after waiting 20 minutes will be from the bloodstream, assuming all urine was voided from the bladder in the sample collected 20 minutes prior to the test specimen. The analysis of bladder urine is not recommended in traffic law enforcement (Dubowski 1985; Jones 2006).

14.3.2 Arrest Data

Even with repeated measurements on individuals arrested for DUI within several different jurisdictions, the variations in the breath instruments were found to be minimal. When sample conditions were maximized to cause the largest variance, the duplicate test differences were found to be 0.008 or less from all participating jurisdictions, demonstrating that subject manipulation of exhalation time and volume had very little effect on breath-alcohol testing results (Gullberg and Polissar 2011).

A study was conducted using 30,224 duplicate breath-alcohol tests collected from eight different age groups to determine what, if any, differences occurred as a result of age. Based on a statistical analysis of this data, it was determined that the breath-alcohol test provided acceptable agreement at all ages, even in elderly subjects where the risk of respiratory difficulty increases (Gullberg 1993).

14.4 Law Enforcement and Adjudication

14.4.1 Probable Cause

Establishing probable cause at a 0.05 or lower limit using today's standards of impairment detection may prove difficult without some new standard for establishing probable cause to test. Standardized field sobriety tests (SFST) were developed to assist law enforcement personnel in identifying alcohol-impaired drivers and were originally validated at an alcohol concentration of 0.10 (Tharp et al. 1981). SFST consists of the one-leg stand, the walk and turn, and an assessment of the person's horizontal gage nystagmus. Findings from the 1998 NHTSA study of SFST "results strongly suggest that the SFSTs also accurately discriminate even at 0.04 percent BAC" (Stuster and Burns 1998).

When the *per se* definition for impairment was lowered to 0.08, the SFST criteria were reassessed and validated at the lower alcohol concentration. Lowering the SFST criteria from 0.10 to 0.08 required no changes to the SFST procedure. The 0.08 SFST validation study established that, when using the same scoring criteria, properly trained officers correctly identified a person with a 0.08 alcohol concentration 91% of the time (Stuster and Burns 1998) while in the original validation study police officers correctly identified a person with a 0.10 alcohol concentration only 81% of the time (Tharp et al. 1981). NHTSA concludes that the greater component and overall accuracies found during the 1998 study are attributable to 17 years of law enforcement experience with the SFSTs since the original study. The change to 0.05 will likely not be so simple. Lowering the alcohol concentration to 0.05 will likely require changes to the scoring of the SFST procedure, such as lowering the number of visible horizontal gaze nystagmus (HGN) clues from six to four. Additional tests, yet to be determined, may also be required to produce a reliable 0.05 SFST (Stuster 2001). By moving away from observed impairment, which may or may not identify impaired drivers, to a limit, the new law will rely heavily on test results. Research has shown measured alcohol at all concentrations does not necessarily correlate with the outward physical signs of impairment and expected signs of intoxication, especially in those individuals who abuse alcohol on a regular basis (Olson et al. 2013). Law enforcement and the general public need to be made aware of the fact that individuals who have developed a tolerance to alcohol will mask the signs of intoxication and go undetected using standard physical impairment criteria (Olson et al. 2013). Even at today's legal limit of 0.08, some chronic drinkers are missed by all but the most highly trained police officers using today's standards of determining observed impairment.

In the United States, commercial motor vehicle (CMV) guidelines for drivers do not allow CMV drivers to have any measurable or detectable amount of alcohol in their bodies when in control of the vehicles (Federal Motor Carrier Safety Administration 2019). If a police officer smells the odor of an alcoholic beverage on the breath of a CMV driver, the driver is placed out of service for 24 hour. If the driver has a blood- or breath-alcohol concentration of 0.04 or more, his or her CMV license will be revoked for a year. Establishing zero tolerance for alcohol in CMV drivers simplified the probable-cause element necessary to require the testing of CMV drivers. Probable cause for the arrest is greatly simplified if the smell of an alcoholic beverage on a person's breath is sufficient to make an arrest. Unless new laws are similarly worded or contain some other mechanism to allow for the testing of persons suspected of having an alcohol concentration of 0.05 or greater, the identification of drivers with a high tolerance for alcohol, based solely on visible signs of impairment, may prove to be difficult.

With the lowering of the legal limit to 0.05 there will be a commensurate lowering in the visible signs and symptoms of alcohol impairment in many people who are at or near the limit. This will result in a greater reliance on test results. It is important to ensure alcohol laws include sections dealing with testing procedures such as time-of-test laws for breath or blood specimens. A search of the scientific literature by the NSC's Committee on Alcohol and Other Drugs, Subcommittee on Alcohol: Technology, Pharmacology & Toxicology found time-of-test laws to be scientifically sound and supported by the scientific literature (Cowan and Dubowski 2005). Time-of-test laws define the offense as the time the blood or breath sampling occurred, usually within 2–3 hours of driving, as opposed to laws that define the offense as occurring while driving. New *per se* laws should specify the alcohol concentration at the time of sampling and not at the time of driving. This would serve the dual purpose of making any new *per se* law more enforceable and greatly reduce the need for retrograde extrapolation (Dubowski 2006).

14.4.2 Current Laws

Many states, including Wisconsin, already have 0.02 laws on the books for repeat offenders (Wisconsin Department of Transportation 2013). As expected, very few are arrested with 0.02 alcohol concentrations based on the physical indication of impaired driving. That does not mean the law is ineffective or unenforceable; drivers with low alcohol concentrations do indeed get arrested after an initial stop for an equipment violation, crash investigation, suspended license offense, etc., and an odor of intoxicants or other sign of alcohol use. In addition, many states have 0.04 rules for individuals who fly an aircraft or drive commercial vehicles.

14.4.3 Enforcement

DUI checkpoints have been and continue to be an effective tool for reducing crashes: those involving alcohol by 17% at a minimum and all crashes, independent of alcohol involvement, by about 10–15% (Erke et al. 2009). There are many ways alcohol-impaired driver accidents can be reduced using an enforcement program to screen the whole driving population to identify those individuals, primarily chronic alcohol users, who do not exhibit physical signs of impairment, but are cognitively impaired and at high risk of being involved in a crash. Screening all drivers can identify those drinking drivers who are at great risk of an accident and provide for corrective actions from punitive to therapeutic, based on the needs of the offender, and establish a deterrence to individuals considering the risk of being detected and arrested (Borkenstein 1976).

It is often difficult to determine if the postabsorptive state has been reached at any given time or if other pharmacokinetic variability caused an abnormal blood–breath ratio to occur (Simpson 1987). Pharmacokinetic factors often make it impossible or infeasible to convert the alcohol concentration of breath or urine to the simultaneous blood-alcohol concentration with forensically acceptable certainty, especially under *per se* or absolute alcohol concentration laws. Laws should include *per se* breath-alcohol concentrations in drunk-driving statutes to avoid unnecessary conversion of breath-alcohol analysis results into equivalent blood-alcohol concentrations (Dubowski 1985; Mason and Dubowski 1976).

14.4.4 Adjudication

There is debate on the appropriate actions needed to prevent recidivism after the arrest and conviction of an individual for an alcohol-related offense. Interlock devices, education, treatment, license revocation, increased penalties, or some combination of these actions have been suggested and are used in some state courts as possible sentencing options (Bjerre and Thorsson 2008; Jones and Holmgren 2009; Lahausse and Fildes 2009; McCartt et al. 2013; McDermott 1986).

Mandating the installation of interlock devices on all DUI convictions has proved successful in reducing the number of repeat offenders. Even when interlock usage rates were low, a reduced number of accidents occurred (McCartt et al. 2013). Increased use of interlock devices would most likely provide an even lower rate of recidivism (Beck et al. 1999; Coben and Larkin 1999; Voas et al. 2002). The use of interlock devices has been found to reduce health care costs (Bjerre et al. 2007). Completion of programs involving interlock devices "appears to have lasting effects (even 2.5 years later) in terms of far lower rates of DWI recidivism and maybe also lower crash rates" (Bjerre 2005). Individuals who did not participate in the interlock program or dropped out of the program returned rapidly to driving after the use of alcohol (Bjerre 2005). Given the rapid return to alcohol abuse after removal of the device, it is recommended that the device only be removed after a driver demonstrates abstinence from alcohol for an extended period of time (Raub et al. 2003). Interlock devices along with other variables have proved very successful in identifying repeat offenders. Previous DUIs and repeated interlock warnings within the first 5 months of usage identified 60% of the drivers who would become repeat offenders with an accuracy of ±10% (Marques et al. 2001).

14.5 Conclusions

The scientific data provided in this report support the NTSB recommendations, but the recommendation needs to be modified to include units for breath-alcohol concentration (BrAC) in addition to blood-alcohol concentration (BAC). Scientific research has clearly proved that impairment and increased crash risk do occur at low concentrations. Tests that are commonly used in law enforcement today are effective at detecting and analyzing alcohol limits such as 0.05 or lower and are considered forensically acceptable.

Based on a review of the literature and personal experience, it is clear that breath-alcohol testing must be included in all laws regarding *per se* alcohol-concentration limits. The majority of the states and the federal government use breath-alcohol testing to determine the concentration of alcohol, not blood testing. Blood is not readily available and involves an invasive procedure that needs specialized staff and equipment. The federal government only allows workplace alcohol testing using an instrument approved on the NHTSA's CPL for evidential and nonevidential alcohol devices. At the present time NHTSA has only approved breath and saliva testing for use in workplace alcohol testing.

The present quality assurance procedures used in the analysis of breath and blood alcohol provide highly reliable and dependable results for use in court. Quality assurance safeguards implemented by law enforcement "have withstood adversarial challenges in the judicial system for more than 30 years" (Dubowski 1994).

When asked the question at what alcohol concentration is it safe to drive, the answer must be no alcohol concentration (Moskowitz and Fiorentino 2000), and that is why many countries have adopted zero-alcohol-limit laws for drivers. Furthermore, many US states already have zero-alcohol-limit laws for teenage drivers.

The degree of impairment of an individual is an elusive and largely subjective assessment, whereas the correlation between alcohol concentration and increased crash risk has been well established in the scientific literature. The object of a legal *per se* law should not be to establish the absolute degree of impairment, but to establish a legal limit that will significantly reduce deaths and injuries known to occur above certain alcohol concentrations. The scientific literature establishes with a high degree of scientific certainty the increased crash risk associated with accidents at different concentrations of alcohol and this needs to be the final deciding factor when establishing a *per se* legal alcohol limit. The ultimate goal of a *per se* alcohol limit is public safety and the reduction of deaths and injuries known to be associated with increasing alcohol concentrations. Considering the published literature, one must conclude that a minimum of 2,000 lives will likely be saved per year in the United States if the alcohol limit is lowered to 0.05.

References

American Medical Association Council on Scientific Affairs: Alcohol and the driver; *J Am Med Assoc* 255:522; 1986.

American Medical Association Council on Scientific Affairs: Drivers impaired by alcohol; *CSA Rep* 14:A-97; 1997.

Banks S, Catcheside P, Lack L, Grunstein RR, McEvoy RD: Low levels of alcohol impair driving simulator performance and reduce perception of crash risk in partially sleep deprived subjects; *Sleep* 27:1063; 2004.

Beck KH, Rauch WJ, Baker EA, Williams AF: Effects of ignition interlock license restrictions on drivers with multiple alcohol offenses: A randomized trial in Maryland; *Am J Public Health* 89:1696; 1999.

Bjerre B: Primary and secondary prevention of drunk driving by the use of alcolock device and program: Swedish experiences; *Accident Anal Prev* 37:1145; 2005.

Bjerre B, Kostela J, Selen J: Positive health-care effects of an alcohol ignition interlock programme among driving while impaired (DWI) offenders; *Addiction* 102:1771; 2007.

Bjerre B, Thorsson U: Is an alcohol ignition interlock programme a useful tool for changing the alcohol and driving habits of drink-drivers? *Accident Anal Prev* 40:267; 2008.

Blomberg RD, Peck RC, Moskowitz H, Burns M, Fiorentino D: The long beach/Fort Lauderdale relative risk study; *J Safety Res* 40:2; 2009.

Borkenstein RF: Efficacy of law enforcement procedures concerning alcohol, drugs, and driving; *Mod Probl Pharm* 11:1; 1976.

Borkenstein RF, Crowther FR, Shumate RP, Ziel WB, Zylman R: *The Role of the Drinking Driver in Traffic Accidents*; Department of Police Administration, Indiana University: Bloomington, IN; 1964.

Bouchery EE, Harwood HJ, Sacks JJ, Simon CJ, Brewer RD: Economic costs of excessive alcohol consumption in the U.S., 2006; *Am J Prev Med* 41:516; 2011.

Brady JE, Baker SP, Dimaggio C, McCarthy ML, Rebok GW, Li G: Effectiveness of mandatory alcohol testing programs in reducing alcohol involvement in fatal motor carrier crashes; *Am J Epidemiol* 170:775; 2009.

Cherpitel CJ: Breath analysis and self-reports as measures of alcohol-related emergency room admissions; *J Stud Alcohol* 50:155; 1989.

Coben JH, Larkin GL: Effectiveness of ignition interlock devices in reducing drunk driving recidivism; *Am J Prev Med* 16:81; 1999.

Connor J, Norton R, Ameratunga S, Jackson R: The contribution of alcohol to serious car crash injuries; *Epidemiology* 15:337; 2004.

Cowan M, Dubowski KM: *Scientific Soundness of Time-of-Test Laws* (report of the Alcohol Technology, Pharmacology, and Toxicology Subcommittee, National Safety Council Committee on Alcohol and Other Drugs); 2005.

Currier GW, Trenton AJ, Walsh PG: Innovations: Emergency psychiatry: Relative accuracy of breath and serum alcohol readings in the psychiatric emergency service; *Psychiatr Serv* 57:34; 2006.

Di Bartolomeo S, Valent F, Sbrojavacca R, Marchetti R, Barbone F: A case-crossover study of alcohol consumption, meals and the risk of road traffic crashes; *BMC Public Health* 9:316; 2009.

Dubowski KM: Absorption, distribution and elimination of alcohol: Highway safety aspects; *J Stud Alcohol Suppl* 10:98; 1985.

Dubowski KM: Quality assurance in breath-alcohol analysis; *J Anal Toxicol* 18:306; 1994.

Dubowski KM: Studies in breath-alcohol analysis: Biological factors; *Z Rechtsmed* 76:93; 1975.

Dubowski KM: *Time-of-Test DUI Laws vs. BAC Extrapolation*; Borkenstein Course, Indiana University: Bloomington, IN; 2006.

Dubowski KM, Caplan YH, Canfield DV: Alcohol testing in the workplace; In Garriott JC (Ed): *Garriot's Medicolegal Aspects of Alcohol*; Lawyers & Judges Publishing: Tucson, AZ; 2008.

Dubowski KM, Essary NA: Evaluation of commercial breath-alcohol simulators: Further studies; *J Anal Toxicol* 15:272; 1991.

Dubowski KM, Essary NA: Field performance of current generation breath-alcohol simulators; *J Anal Toxicol* 16: 325; 1992.

Dubowski KM, Essary NA: Measurement of low breath alcohol concentrations: Laboratory studies and field experience; *J Anal Toxicol* 23:386; 1999.

Dubowski KM, Essary NA: Response of breath-alcohol analyzers to acetone; *J Anal Toxicol* 7:231; 1983.

Dubowski KM, Essary NA: Response of breath-alcohol analyzers to acetone: Further studies; *J Anal Toxicol* 8:205; 1984.

Erke A, Goldenbeld C, Vaa T: The effects of drink-driving checkpoints on crashes—A meta-analysis; *Accident Anal Prev* 41:914; 2009.

Fabbri A, Marchesini G, Morselli-Labate AM, Rossi F, Cicognani A, Dente M, Iervese T, Ruggeri S, Mengozzi U, Vandelli A: Blood alcohol concentration and management of road trauma patients in the emergency department; *J Trauma* 50:521; 2001.

Federal Motor Carrier Safety Administration: *49 CFR 392.5—Alcohol Prohibition*; https://www.fmcsa.dot.gov/regulations/title49/section/392.5 (Accessed May 10, 2019).

Fransson M, Jones AW, Andersson L: Laboratory evaluation of a new evidential breath-alcohol analyser designed for mobile testing—The Evidenzer; *Med Sci Law* 45:61; 2005.

Gomm PJ, Osselton MD, Broster CG, Johnson NM, Upton K: The effect of salbutamol on breath alcohol testing in asthmatics; *Med Sci Law* 31:226; 1991.

Gomm PJ, Weston SI, Osselton MD: The effect of respiratory aerosol inhalers and nasal sprays on breath alcohol testing devices used in Great Britain; *Med Sci Law* 30:203; 1990.

Goncalves PD, Cunha PJ, Malbergier A, do Amaral RA, de Oliveira LG, Yang JJ, de Andrade AG: The association between low alcohol use and traffic risk behaviors among Brazilian college students; *Alcohol* 46:673; 2012.

Gubala W, Zuba D: Saliva as an alternative specimen for alcohol determination in the human body; *Pol J Pharmacol* 54:161; 2002.

Gullberg RG: An application of probability theory to a group of breath-alcohol and blood-alcohol data; *J Forensic Sci* 35:1342; 1990.

Gullberg RG: Breath alcohol analysis in one subject with gastroesophageal reflux disease; *J Forensic Sci* 46:1498; 2001.

Gullberg RG: Breath alcohol test precision: An in vivo vs. in vitro evaluation; *Forensic Sci Int* 43:247; 1989.

Gullberg RG: Evaluating the variability of duplicate breath alcohol analyses as a function of subject age; *Med Sci Law* 33:110; 1993.

Gullberg RG: Repeatability of replicate breath alcohol measurements collected in short time intervals; *J Forensic Sci Soc* 35:5; 1995.

Gullberg RG: The elimination rate of mouth alcohol: Mathematical modeling and implications in breath alcohol analysis; *J Forensic Sci* 37:1363; 1992.

Gullberg RG, Polissar NL: Factors contributing to the variability observed in duplicate forensic breath alcohol measurement; *J Breath Res* 5:016004; 2011.

Harding P, Field PH: Breathalyzer accuracy in actual law enforcement practice: A comparison of blood- and breath alcohol results in Wisconsin drivers; *J Forensic Sci* 32:1235; 1987.

Harding PM, Laessig RH, Field PH: Field performance of the Intoxilyzer 5000: A comparison of blood- and breath alcohol results in Wisconsin drivers; *J Forensic Sci* 35:1022; 1990.

Heifer U, Loos U, Klaes D, Schyma C: Time course of breath and blood alcohol concentration in disorders of lung function; *Blutalkohol* 32:218; 1995.

Jaffe DH, Siman-Tov M, Gopher A, Peleg K: Variability in the blood/breath alcohol ratio and implications for evidentiary purposes; *J Forensic Sci* 58:1233; 2013.

Jones AW: Breath-acetone concentrations in fasting healthy men: Response of infrared breath-alcohol analyzers; *J Anal Toxicol* 11:67; 1987.

Jones AW: Electrochemical measurement of breath-alcohol concentration: Precision and accuracy in relation to blood levels; *Clin Chim Acta* 146:175; 1985a.

Jones AW: Evaluation of breath-alcohol instruments. III. Controlled field trial with Alcolmeter pocket model; *Forensic Sci Int* 28:147; 1985b.

Jones AW: Measuring ethanol in saliva with the QED enzymatic test device: Comparison of results with blood- and breath-alcohol concentrations; *J Anal Toxicol* 19:169; 1995.

Jones AW: Urine as a biological specimen for forensic analysis of alcohol and variability in the urine-to-blood relationship; *Toxicol Rev* 25:15; 2006.

Jones AW, Holmgren A: Age and gender differences in blood-alcohol concentration in apprehended drivers in relation to the amounts of alcohol consumed; *Forensic Sci Int* 188:40; 2009.

Kechagias S, Jonsson KA, Franzen T, Andersson L, Jones AW: Reliability of breath-alcohol analysis in individuals with gastroesophageal reflux disease; *J Forensic Sci* 44: 814; 1999.

Kennedy RS, Turnage JJ, Wilkes RL, Dunlap WP: Effects of graded dosages of alcohol on nine computerized repeated measures tests; *Ergonomics* 36:1195; 1993.

Krüger HP, Kazenwadel J, Vollrath M: *Grand Rapids Effects Revisited*; Accidents, Alcohol and Risk Centre for Automotive Safety Research: Adelaide, Australia; 1995.

Krüger HP, Vollrath M: The alcohol-related accident risk in Germany: Procedure, methods and results; *Accident Anal Prev* 36:125; 2004.

Kuypers KP, Legrand SA, Ramaekers JG, Verstraete AG: A case-control study estimating accident risk for alcohol, medicines and illegal drugs; *PloS One* 7:e43496; 2012.

Lahausse JA, Fildes BN: Cost-benefit analysis of an alcohol ignition interlock for installation in all newly registered vehicles; *Traffic Injury Prev* 10:528; 2009.

Landauer AA, Howat PA: Alcohol and the cognitive aspects of choice reaction time; *Psychopharmacology* (Berlin) 78:296; 1982.

Logan BK, Distefano S: Ethanol content of various foods and soft drinks and their potential for interference with a breath-alcohol test; *J Anal Toxicol* 22:181; 1998.

Logan BK, Distefano S, Case GA: Evaluation of the effect of asthma inhalers and nasal decongestant sprays on a breath alcohol test; *J Forensic Sci* 43:197; 1998.

Logan BK, Gullberg RG: Lack of effect of tongue piercing on an evidential breath alcohol test; *J Forensic Sci* 43:239; 1998.

Marques PR, Tippetts AS, Voas RB, Beirness DJ: Predicting repeat DUI offenses with the alcohol interlock recorder; *Accident Anal Prev* 33:609; 2001.

Martin E, Moll W, Schmid P, Dettli L: The pharmacokinetics of alcohol in human breath, venous and arterial blood after oral ingestion; *Eur J Clin Pharmacol* 26:619; 1984.

Martin TL, Solbeck PAM, Mayers DJ, Langille RM, Buczek Y, Pelletier MR: A review of alcohol-impaired driving: The role of blood alcohol concentration and complexity of the driving task; *J Forensic Sci* 58:1238; 2013.

Mason MF, Dubowski KM: Breath-alcohol analysis: Uses, methods, and some forensic problems—Review and opinion; *J Forensic Sci* 21:9; 1976.

McCartt AT, Leaf WA, Farmer CM, Eichelberger AH: Washington State's alcohol ignition interlock law: Effects on recidivism among first-time DUI offenders; *Traffic Injury Prev* 14:215; 2013.

McDermott FT: Alcohol on wheels; *Aust NZ J Surg* 56:19; 1986.

Miller TR, Gibson R, Zaloshnja E, Blincoe LJ, Kindelberger J, Strashny A, Thomas A, Ho S, Bauer M, Sperry S, et al.: Underreporting of driver alcohol involvement in United States police and hospital records: Capture-recapture estimates; *Ann Adv Automot Med* 56:87; 2012.

Moskowitz H, Burns M, Fiorentino D, Smiley A, Zador P: *Driver Characteristics and Impairment at Various BACs*; (DOT HS 809 075); National Highway Traffic Safety: Washington, DC; 2000.

Moskowitz H, Burns M, Williams AF: Skills performance at low blood alcohol levels; *J Stud Alcohol* 46:482; 1985.

Moskowitz H, Fiorentino D: *A Review of the Literature on the Effects of Low Doses of Alcohol on Driving-Related Skills* (DOT HS 809 028); National Highway Traffic Safety: Washington, DC; 2000.

National Safety Council: *Low Alcohol Concentration National Culture Change*; 2016 https://www.nsc.org/Portals/0/Documents/DistractedDrivingDocuments/Low-BAC-policy.pdf (Accessed May 10, 2019).

National Transportation Safety Board: *Reaching Zero: Actions to Eliminate Alcohol-Impaired Driving* (NTSB/SR13/01); National Transportation Safety Board: Washington, DC; 2013.

Oklahoma: Operation of aircraft under influence of intoxicants (Section 301); In *2006 Oklahoma Code Title 3—Aircraft and Airports;* 2006.

Olson KN, Smith SW, Kloss JS, Ho JD, Apple FS: Relationship between blood alcohol concentration and observable symptoms of intoxication in patients presenting to an emergency department; *Alcohol Alcohol* 48:386; 2013.

Raub RA, Lucke RE, Wark RI: Breath alcohol ignition interlock devices: Controlling the recidivist; *Traffic Injury Prev 4 Suppl* 1:28; 2003.

Silverman LD, Wong K, Miller S: Confirmation of ethanol compressed gas standard concentrations by an NIST traceable, absolute chemical method and comparison with wet breath alcohol simulators; *J Anal Toxicol* 21:369; 1997.

Simpson G: Accuracy and precision of breath alcohol measurements for subjects in the absorptive state; *Clin Chem* 33:753; 1987.

Smith GS, Keyl PM, Hadley JA, Bartley CL, Foss RD, Tolbert WG, McKnight J: Drinking and recreational boating fatalities: A population-based case-control study; *J Am Med Assoc* 286:2974; 2001.

Smith R, Cook LJ, Olson LM, Reading JC, Dean JM: Trends of behavioral risk factors in motor vehicle crashes in Utah, 1992–1997; *Accident Anal Prev* 36:249; 2004.

Speck PR, McElroy AJ, Gullberg RG: The effect of breath alcohol simulator solution volume on measurement results; *J Anal Toxicol* 15:332; 1991.

Stuster J: *Development of a Standardized Field Sobriety Test (SFST) Training Management System* (HS 809 400); National Highway Traffic Safety Administration: Washington, DC; 2001.

Stuster J, Burns M: *Validation of the Standardized Field Sobriety Test Battery at BACs Below 0.10 Percent* (DOT HS 808 839); US National Highway Traffic Safety Administration: Washington, DC; 1998.

Substance Abuse and Mental Health Services Administration: *Results from the 2011 National Survey on Drug Use and Health: Summary of National Findings* (NSDUH Series H-44, HHS Publication No. (SMA) 12-4713); Center for Behavioral Health Statistics and Quality, Substance Abuse and Mental Health Services Administration: Rockville, MD; 2012.

Tharp V, Burns M, Moskowitz H: *Development and Field Test of Psychophysical Tests for DWI Arrest* (DOT HS-805 864); US National Highway Traffic Safety Administration: Washington, DC; 1981.

Vakulin A, Baulk SD, Catcheside PG, Antic NA, van den Heuvel CJ, Dorrian J, McEvoy RD: Effects of alcohol and sleep restriction on simulated driving performance in untreated patients with obstructive sleep apnea; *Ann Intern Med* 151:447; 2009.

Voas RB, Blackman KO, Tippetts AS, Marques PR: Evaluation of a program to motivate impaired driving offenders to install ignition interlocks; *Accident Anal Prev* 34:449; 2002.

Waller PF, Stewart JR, Hansen AR, Stutts JC, Popkin CL, Rodgman EA: The potentiating effects of alcohol on driver injury; *J Am Med Assoc* 256:1461; 1986.

Watterson JH, Ellefsen KN: Examination of some performance characteristics of breath alcohol measurements obtained with the Intoxilyzer 8000C following social drinking conditions; *J Anal Toxicol* 33:514; 2009.

Wisconsin Department of Transportation: Prohibited alcohol concentration; In *Wis Stats Chapter 340 Vehicles—General Provisions* (Title 340.01, Section 46m); 2013.

Zador PL: Alcohol-related relative risk of fatal driver injuries in relation to driver age and sex; *J Stud Alcohol* 52:302; 1991.

Methodologies for Establishing the Relationship between Alcohol/Drug Use and Driving Impairment

15

Differences between Epidemiological, Experimental, and Real-Case Studies*

HALLVARD GJERDE, JOHANNES G. RAMAEKERS, AND JØRG G. MØRLAND

Contents

* This chapter is an updated version (format only) of a review article previously published in *Forensic Science Review*: Gjerde H, Ramaekers J, Mørland JG: Methodologies for establishing the relationship between alcohol/drug use and driving impairment—Differences between epidemiological, experimental and real-case studies; *Forensic Sci Rev* 31:141; 2019.

15.1 Introduction

A large proportion of road traffic crashes are caused by driver impairment after using alcohol or other psychoactive substances (World Health Organization 2015). Analysis of blood samples from those arrested for driving under the influence (DUI) of alcohol or drugs, or from crash-involved drivers, show variations in detected substances across countries related to regional differences in the use of alcohol, recreational drugs and psychoactive medicines, including problematic use and addiction, as well as differences in attitudes towards driving after using alcohol or drugs (Gonzalez-Wilhelm 2007; Legrand et al. 2013, 2014) (see also Chapter 13). Such differences make comparisons between studies difficult. In general, alcohol is the most commonly used psychoactive substance among drivers, followed by cannabis, central nervous stimulants, such as amphetamines and cocaine, and central nervous depressants, such as sedatives, hypnotics and narcotic analgesics. Multi-substance use is also common among arrested DUI offenders (Holmgren et al. 2007; Karjalainen et al. 2010; Valen et al. 2017b).

Most countries have implemented statutory alcohol concentration limits in blood or breath for DUI of alcohol. Many countries have also laws on driving under the influence of drugs other than alcohol, which may either be based on documented impairment, zero tolerance for psychoactive drugs, or concentration *per se* limits in blood (Walsh et al. 2004) (see also Chapter 13). Zero tolerance laws make it a criminal offense to have a drug or metabolite in the body while operating a motor vehicle, and is sometimes regarded as a type of *per se* legislation. This legal framework was constructed, at least in part, to simplify the evidence necessary for a successful prosecution (Jones 2005).

Standardized research methods are needed in order to generate accurate and reproducible data when studying the effects of alcohol and drugs on the ability to drive safely. The first recommendations and guidelines were published in the 1980s and 1990s (Donelson et al. 1980; International Council on Alcohol Drugs and Traffic

Safety 1993, 1999; Joscelyn and Donelson 1980). In 2007, an expert meeting was held in Talloires (France) where guidelines on both experimental and epidemiological research were discussed (Walsh et al. 2007). As an outcome of that meeting, more detailed guidelines and recommendations were developed (Walsh et al. 2008). The US National Highway Traffic Safety Administration published a consensus protocol for assessing the potential of drugs to impair driving in 2011, although with less details (Kay and Logan 2011), and a white paper on drugged driving research was published by the Drugged Driving Committee of the Institute for Behavior and Health in the US, also in 2011 (DuPont et al. 2011). Finally, the Food and Drug Administration published Guidance for Industry on the evaluation of drug effects on the ability to operate a motor vehicle in 2017 (Food and Drug Administration 2017), although less detailed than other guidelines.

The aim of this chapter is to describe the methodologies used to investigate the effect of alcohol and drugs on the ability to drive safely, present the main advantages and challenges, and discuss disagreements between findings for some substances.

15.2 Experimental Studies

Experimental studies on the acute effects of alcohol and/or drugs on a person's ability to drive safely are performed by giving a defined amount of substance to a number of test persons and measure the effect on performance at predefined time points.

Participants are included in accordance with predefined specifications regarding age, sex, disease, current or previous substance use, and other issues. Studies in healthy volunteers serve as a good model to demonstrate principal drug effects on human performance, whereas patient studies in addition allow estimating the net effect of drug-induced impairments and therapeutic benefits, e.g., symptom relief, on performance. Experimental studies can also take into account contributing factors that may affect drug effects on driving, such as age, gender, concomitant use of drugs and alcohol as well as duration of treatment.

Often, blood samples are taken to determine the drug concentration at the time of performing the tests to study whether there is a correlation between substance concentration and performance. Acute drug effects are often assessed around the time of maximal drug concentration (T_{max}) which is a time point when effects are most prominent (EMCDDA 1999). However, assessments should also be repeated over a prolonged period to assess whether the relationship between effect and substance concentration in blood may change over time due to changed blood/brain substance concentration ratio and/or development of acute tolerance. Sub-acute effects may also be studied, such as residual effects (hangover) of hypnotics the morning after intake as well as withdrawal effects after long-term use. Ideally, participants should also receive multiple doses during several weeks of treatment to assess their influence on performance beyond acute use.

The optimal approach is to use a randomized double-blind study, where neither the researchers nor the participants are aware of the order of treatment conditions to which participants are randomized. A crossover study design should be used, where each participant is tested with different doses of the test substance and placebo, and with a well-documented benchmark substance, such as alcohol.

When testing medicinal drugs, low to medium doses that fall within the therapeutic window are given acutely or subchronically. Ethical approval for studying large doses and chronic dosing is normally not given. It is also difficult to get ethical approval for studying illicit drugs. If approved, low to regular recreational doses are normally tested, and it is required that the test persons must have previous experience with the drug. For all substances, a risk assessment must be performed before submitting ethical committee and clinical trial applications.

The main advantage of experimental studies is that researchers have full control over substance dosing; they can compare different doses and different substances. Each study participant can perform different types of tests, and different types of subjects can be included. Well-documented tests on cognitive and psychomotor performance can be used. The studies can therefore easily be repeated in order to study the robustness of effects, study inter- and intrasubject variations, study sleep-deprived persons, or compare the effects of a drug alone with drug-alcohol or drug-drug combinations.

Experimental studies have other advantages as well. They only require small sample sizes to achieve sufficient statistical power to detect drug-induced impairment. They can be used as part of drug development programs to predict driver impairment of novel compounds before these enter the market. They also allow studying individual drugs rather than drug categories as is often the case in epidemiological studies.

The main limitations are: (a) that only low doses are tested, so the findings may not reflect real-life situations of repeated intake, perhaps of large doses; (b) effects of any hangover and withdrawal symptoms after repeated abuse of large doses cannot easily be studied; (c) the participants know they are being tested; they may therefore act differently or overachieve versus being in a normal driving setting; (d) researchers have often neglected to include assessments that may indicate whether people actually want to drive when feeling "high" or impaired by the substance, or be extra careful if they decide to drive, or whether they prefer to avoid driving situations; and (e) the performed tests may not be relevant to skills necessary for safe driving and ability to drive in the traffic flow and react to emergency situations.

A potential problem is that the participating subjects may improve their performance over time due to repeated practicing in the behavioral tests performed after drug treatment. This learning over time may interfere and obscure effects of the substance being studied if the study design is not taking this into account. So, the participants must be sufficiently trained before the study starts to achieve a steady performance level. Placebo studies may also be performed throughout the study period to control for the potential obscuring effects due to learning, and treatment orders across subjects can be counterbalanced. Another potential challenge is that acute tolerance to the drug may be developed, causing less impairment at the same blood drug concentration after some hours. This must be taken into account when designing the study.

Experimental methods cannot be used to determine crash risk, only the degree of impairment of driving performance under somewhat artificial conditions, as well as cognitive, psychomotor, and other mental functions related to driving caused by the given substance doses, or correlated with concentrations in blood at defined time points after substance intake. They can therefore only be used to determine whether a substance may reduce the ability to drive safely and whether this effect is related to drug dose or drug concentration in blood.

Many experimental studies have been performed for alcohol (see Section 15.5.1), and Strand and co-workers have summarized findings in studies of antidepressants, antihistamines, benzodiazepines and similar drugs, cannabis, GHB, ketamine, opioids, stimulants; see Chapter 11.

15.2.1 Controlled Laboratory Studies

These types of studies are utilizing neurocognitive performance tests that are important for various aspects of the process of operating a car. Many skills that are needed to drive safely are tested. This may include attention, auditory and visual skills, cognitive performance, reaction time, motor coordination skills, vigilance, sedation, wakefulness, risk-taking or risk avoidance, aggression, and psychotomimetic symptoms.

Many different functions should be tested in order to characterize the effects of the tested substance because different substances may affect different mental functions, and the tests may have different sensitivities for different substances. Testing should therefore be performed at three "Core Levels": Automative Behavior (well-learned, automatic action patterns), Control Behavior (controlled action patterns), and Executive Planning Behavior (general plans in interaction with ongoing traffic) (Owens and Ramaekers 2009; Walsh et al. 2008).

A number of validated computerized tests of basic psychomotor and cognitive functioning are available (Verstraete et al. 2014; Wetherell 1996). An assessment of the sensitivity of different test assessing driving related skills to dose-related impairment by alcohol has been published (Jongen et al. 2016).

15.2.2 Driving Simulator Studies

Driving simulators can be used to study psychomotor and cognitive functioning in a situation that is more similar to driving on the road (Liguori 2009). It is then possible to study different types of driving conditions, such as different road types, traffic densities, speed, day/night, different weather types, unexpected events, and challenging situations, including situations where crash involvement is likely to happen.

The main advantage is that driving tests can be systematically designed, presented and reproduced and that the performance is not associated with any driving risks.

A limitation is that the driving conditions are artificial, so the driver's response in a critical situation, e.g., when avoiding a crash, may be different in a simulator situation than when driving in actual road traffic. Moskowitz stated that no simulator was capable of representing every aspect of the driving act simultaneously, but only a subset of them (Moskowitz 1985). Even after technical improvements of the simulator technology, this might also be the situation at present, although to a lesser extent than in the earlier days of simulator studies.

Another challenge is that many drivers may experience simulator sickness, which may cause more careful driving (Helland et al. 2016b). It is, however, possible that simulator sickness can be reduced by repeated training sessions, as well as by drugs, complicating interpretation of the results. Simulators are also associated with higher levels of subjective and physiological sleepiness than real driving, which may hamper their comparability (Hallvig et al. 2013).

A validation study found that behavioral responses of sober drivers, as expressed by type and number of errors, were similar in a simulator and on-the-road driving (Shechtman et al. 2009). Another study comparing a simulator study on the effects of alcohol with on-the-road driving found that the standard deviation of lateral position (SDLP) was largest when using a simulator; this may reflect a lack of perceived danger in the simulator and may therefore be more sensitive (Helland et al. 2013). Others have, however, reported that the overall sensitivity of driving simulators to detect drug-induced impairment was lower than on-the-road driving tests, particularly at low doses (Jongen et al. 2016; Veldstra et al. 2015).

15.2.3 On-the-Road Driving Studies

On-the-road driving tests are often considered as a "gold standard" for assessing driving impairment after using a psychoactive substance (Ramaekers 2017; Verster and Mets 2009; Verster and Ramaekers 2009). The primary test measure is SDLP, which quantifies the weaving while driving; this measure has been found to be more sensitive than other driving-related measures (Helland et al. 2016a). Studies may be performed on highways in actual traffic or in closed circuits. Specially equipped cars are used to measure the distance to the midline of the road or to a car in front. Lateral position, speed, distance between vehicles, and the use of accelerator and brake are recorded. In addition, it may be possible to record eye movements. There is always a licensed driving instructor present.

A limitation is that driving must be performed without challenging situations with increased risk for crash involvement; thus, the ability to avoid crash involvement cannot be studied.

Examples of measured performance in basic computerized tests and driving simulators or on-the-road driving are presented in Table 15.1.

Table 15.1 Examples of Measured Performance in Experimental Studies

Core Level	Basic Computerized Tests	Simulator and On-the-Road Driving
Automative behavior	Tracking	Tracking
	Alertness and vigilance	Performance over time
		Steering, weaving
		Vision
Control behavior	Response time (too fast/slow)	Distance to car in front
	Speed estimation	Frequency of brake/accelerator use
	Visual search	Reaction to stop signs
	Divided attention	Maneuvering during overtaking
	Psychomotor function	Divided attention
Executive planning behavior	Memory	Planning of driving route
	Planning skills	Speed choice
	Risk taking	Risk taking
	Impulsivity	Hazard avoidance
		Inhibition of motor or cognitive responses
		Reaction to unexpected events

15.3 Epidemiological Studies

Analytical epidemiological studies involve comparing crash involvement among drivers who are using, versus not using, a substance that may potentially affect the ability to drive safely, or substance use among crash-involved versus non–crash-involved drivers. This may include cohort, case-crossover, case-control, and responsibility studies (Kim and Mooney 2016). It is more difficult to perform well-controlled epidemiological studies on the risk of crash involvement due to substance use than experimental studies on impairment after substance use. The main limitations are selection bias, information bias, and confounding (Grimes and Schulz 2002; Kelsey et al. 1996). Therefore, there are large variations in the risk estimates found in epidemiological studies.

Epidemiological studies are used to determine the crash risk posed by substance using drivers in real driving situations; not only the substance *per se*, as other factors than the substance itself are important, such as insight into own impairment, willingness to drive after substance use, and ability to compensate for impairment while driving.

Some large studies have also found significant associations between substances use and crash severity, or higher odds ratio for fatal crash than injurious crash, particularly for alcohol (Behnood and Mannering 2017; Bernhoft et al. 2012; Kim et al. 1995; Shyhalla 2014; Traynor 2005). This potential association should be kept in mind when comparing the findings in different studies, and when designing new studies.

15.3.1 Selection Bias

The studied drivers should constitute a random selection from the total population of drivers, but this is not always the case (Kim and Mooney 2016). If participation is voluntary, the refusal rate may be higher among those who have used a psychoactive substance if they fear that it will be detected. Then, the prevalence of alcohol and drugs will be under-estimated. If data are based on drivers selected by the police for toxicological investigation, such as crash-involved drivers, there may be a selection bias because drivers who appear unlikely to have used alcohol or drugs may less frequently be subject to alcohol and drug testing. Then, the prevalence of alcohol and drugs will be over-estimated. On the other hand, hit-and-run drivers cannot easily be included, resulting in likely under-estimation of alcohol and drug use.

It is therefore important to have very high participation rates; the best situation would be that nonparticipation is not allowed or could be excluded. High participation rates may be obtained by using data from road traffic registries combined with drug prescription data, so long as the registries contain complete information.

15.3.2 Information Bias

Information about substance exposure may be inaccurate or misinterpreted. If exposure data is based on self-reports, underreporting is common (af Wåhlberg et al. 2010; Krumpal 2013; Tourangeau and Yan 2007), but overreporting may also occur in some settings. If asked about substance use before being involved in a previous crash, the driver may incorrectly associate crash involvement with substance use due to inaccurate memory if this might be a plausible explanation for the crash.

If based on analytical testing of biological samples, the type of biological matrix and the cutoff concentration will affect the detection window after use, i.e., for how long time after last substance intake will the analytical finding be regarded as "positive" and thus indicate substance exposure. If only substance concentrations that may affect the ability to drive safely shall be studied, blood samples and appropriate cutoff concentrations must be used (Gjerde et al. 2011b, 2018; Verstraete 2004). Misinterpretation of these issues may cause information bias.

For drivers injured in road traffic crashes, the blood sample for alcohol and drug testing may be taken several hours after the crash; the analytical results may therefore not always reflect the concentrations in blood at the time of the crash. This decrease of drug concentrations may be particularly fast for cocaine, gamma-hydroxybutyric acid (GHB) and tetrahydrocannabinol (THC) (Cone 1995; Liechti et al. 2016; Wood et al. 2016). In studies of drivers injured or killed in crashes, findings of medicinal drugs may be a result of therapeutic administration after the crash during emergency care or resuscitation efforts; those findings must be excluded from the dataset. Analysis of postmortem blood samples may not reflect the alcohol and drug concentrations in blood at the time of death due to postmortem changes (Drummer et al. 2013; Han et al. 2012; Pelissier-Alicot et al. 2003).

There may also be information bias regarding crash involvement if data is based on self-reports.

15.3.3 Covariates and Confounding

Several factors may be related both to substance use and crash involvement, such as age, sex, time of day, day of the week, and driving experience. Also, impulsivity, sensation-seeking behavior, and subjective norms may predict alcohol and drug use and driving behaviors. Other factors that may modulate the risk of crash involvement after using a psychoactive substance are weekly driving distance, whether or not the driver has passengers, and whether passengers are impaired by alcohol or drugs, road traffic speed, weather conditions, exhaustion or sleepiness, and diseases. Some of the covariates may be difficult or practically impossible to include in statistical evaluation of findings.

15.3.4 Pharmacoepidemiological Cohort Studies

Cohort studies on substance use and crash involvement are studies investigating two groups with different substance exposure. In most cases, a substance-exposed cohort comprises drivers who are using a medicinal drug, while an unexposed cohort comprises drivers who are not taking the drug in question. The numbers of crashes in those two cohorts are recorded and the standardized incidence rate for crash involvement is calculated. Some studies use a case-control design instead and calculate the odds ratio for crash involvement. Significant covariates such as age, sex, driving experience, and annual driving distance may be adjusted for in the statistical evaluation of data. If relatively more crashes have occurred among drivers using the drug than among non-drug using drivers when adjusted for confounders, an association between the drug and crash involvement may be found.

Drug exposure is in most studies based on records in prescription registries, whereas crash involvements are found in road traffic crash databases, hospital or police records, or insurance databases. Information about drug use and crash involvement may also be based on self-reports.

The main strengths of cohort studies are that drivers in actual road traffic are studied, many hundred thousand drivers may be included when using large databases, and crash risk associated with prescription of medicinal drugs may be calculated.

One major limitation is that comprehensive and accurate data are required and that coupling of information for individuals can be done. Road traffic crashes are recorded only if detected and reported by the police or insurance companies, depending on regional legislation and routines, and may therefore be inaccurate. Another major limitation is that actual drug use is not recorded, only that the prescription had been given, or that the drug has been dispensed at a pharmacy, or that the participant reports use. In addition, there is no recorded information on whether the taken dose is according to the prescription and whether alcohol or other drugs are taken in addition to, or instead of, the prescribed drug. It is also difficult to distinguish between crashes related to drug use and those related to the disease that is being treated—i.e., confounding by indication bias (Signorello et al. 2002).

Another limitation is that driving patterns, including the weekly driving distance, may be different among drug users than other drivers. The drivers may choose not to drive as frequently as before when taking medication, and the need for driving may be significantly reduced if they are on sick leave.

A third limitation is that cohort studies of this type are using data on crash involvement, not crash responsibility.

Cohort studies based on prescription and road traffic crash registries have been performed for benzodiazepines and similar substances, opioids, and some other medicinal drugs, whereas studies on cannabis have been based on self-reported data; see Chapter 12.

15.3.5 Case-Crossover Studies

A special type of pharmacoepidemiological cohort studies is the case-crossover design, which examines the crash rate in a cohort of drivers who have received a prescription drug. The standardized incidence rate for crash involvement is calculated for the first weeks after the drug has been dispensed at a pharmacy and compared with periods where the drug is not used. Thus, the cases (i.e., drivers who are taking the drug) can be their own controls (i.e., when the drivers are not taking the drug). Thereby, a number of confounders can be eliminated, such as age, sex, driving experience, traffic safety attitudes, and personality. However, it may still be difficult to distinguish between increased crash risk due to disease itself or due to medication to treat the disease. Studies based on prescription and crash registries have been performed for antidepressants, benzodiazepines, opioids, and some other medicinal drugs; see Chapter 12.

Case-crossover studies may also be performed based on self-reported data (Asbridge et al. 2014).

15.3.6 Case-Control Studies

Case-control studies are often regarded as theoretically the best epidemiological method to calculate the association between an exposure and an outcome (Berghaus et al. 2007; Houwing et al. 2009; Schulz and Grimes 2002). In our setting, the exposure (independent variable) is substance use, whereas the outcome (dependent variable) is crash involvement. Cases are drivers involved in crashes, whereas controls are drivers stopped at random in road traffic. Substance use is determined by analysis of oral fluid, blood or urine samples, or by self-report. Cases are most often selected from hospital emergency rooms or autopsy databases, whereas controls are most often selected in roadside surveys, most often in collaboration with the police. The risk for crash involvement associated with substance use is calculated as odds ratio.

The main strength of case-control studies of this type is that actual drivers in normal road traffic are being studied, both therapeutic and recreational use and misuse are included, the studies require lower numbers of participants than cohort studies, and the actual crash risk associated with the use of psychoactive substances can be estimated.

It is, however, very difficult to perform good studies on substance use and crash risk using a case-control approach, mainly because it is almost impossible to avoid serious selection bias (Gjerde et al. 2018; Kim and Mooney 2016). Information bias is also a frequently encountered error, particularly misclassification of substance use, or defining substance exposure differently for cases than for controls (Gjerde et al. 2018; Grimes and Schulz 2002). Substance concentrations are mostly re-coded as positive or negative. However, the median substance concentration may be very much different among substance-positive drivers defined as cases compared to the controls, even when the same cutoff concentrations are used. This may cause a significant information bias. Case-control studies also require fairly large samples sizes to achieve sufficient statistical power because prevalence of drug use among cases and controls are generally quite low.

Also confounding factors make interpretation of findings difficult (Gjerde et al. 2018). To avoid the most serious errors related to confounders, the data should at least be adjusted for age and gender and time and day of week, as those factors are among the most important confounders. Other confounders may also significantly affect the estimation of the crash risk associated with substance use (see the section on Covariates and Confounding above).

The crash-involved drivers who are included as cases in the studies are not always responsible for the crash. It is expected that the odds ratio for crash involvement will be higher if only crash responsible drivers are included and drivers who are not responsible are excluded.

A number of case-control studies on the association between use of alcohol or drugs with crash involvement have been published; see Chapter 12.

15.3.7 Responsibility Studies

Responsibility studies (also called culpability studies) constitute a subtype of the case-control study design (Kim and Mooney 2016; Robertson and Drummer 1994; Salmi et al. 2014). Drivers identified as being partly or mainly responsible for a road traffic crash are selected as cases, and drivers who are involved in crashes but not responsible are selected as controls, assuming that they constitute a random selection from the driving population. The incidence of substance exposure among drivers who are responsible for crashes is compared to those who are not responsible. The association between being responsible for a crash (as dependent variable) and alcohol or drug exposure (as independent variables) are calculated as odds ratios.

The main strength is that blood samples are normally collected from both responsible and nonresponsible drivers; then, substance exposure can be defined equally among both cases and controls. Other strengths are that real drivers in normal road traffic are studied, and that substance concentrations reflect actual substance use in the studied population, both therapeutic and recreational use and misuse.

The main limitation is that it may be difficult to determine responsibility in an unbiased way and that a driver who is deemed not responsible may have some partial responsibility, as the driver was unable to avoid the crash. The crash risk estimates may therefore differ from "standard" case-control studies, as it is likely that the nonresponsible driver may not represent a random selection of drivers from normal road traffic, and cases are not merely crash-involved drivers, but crash-responsible. Another likely bias is that substance concentrations may not reflect the concentrations at the time of crash. They are in most studies reported as negative/positive; differences in median substance concentrations between cases and controls can then not be taken into account, which may cause a significant information bias.

Very few studies have investigated acute substance intoxication; most studies have defined substance exposure as detecting traces of the used substance in blood samples by using low concentration cutoffs that may detect substance intake several hours or days later.

A number of responsibility studies have been published, see Chapter 12; some studies were based on recorded unsafe driving actions as a proxy for crash responsibility. Salmi and co-workers have published a review on responsibility studies of use of drugs, mobile phone, distraction and diseases, including critical discussion of the methodology (Salmi et al. 2014).

15.3.8 Meta-analyses and Systematic Reviews

A number of meta-analyses on the association between substance use and road traffic crashes have been published. In those reports, data from many independent studies have been combined. The validity of the meta-analyses depends on the quality of the selected independent studies as well as the overall evaluation. The same applies to systematic reviews.

Knowledge about pharmacology, epidemiology, statistics, and traffic safety research is needed in order to prepare meta-analyses and systematic reviews of good quality. In general, some published meta-analyses and systematic reviews may suffer from lack of insight into one or more of those scientific fields, being unable to exclude studies of poor quality or misunderstand the findings (Ioannidis 2016). One example is that the authors may not understand whether substance exposure is defined as substance-induced impairment or merely detection of traces of substance in biological samples, reflecting intake during the last days, such as in a recent meta-analysis of studies on acute cannabis intoxication (Gjerde and Mørland 2016; Røgeberg and Elvik 2016). Sometimes, data from studies based on urine testing, blood sample testing, and self-reports are mixed into the same meta-analysis. Therefore, the conclusions in some meta-analyses and systematic reviews may be inaccurate.

15.4 Real-Case Studies

Real-case studies are descriptive studies of drug-impaired drivers. This may be DUI offenders apprehended by the police or involved in road traffic crashes. In contrast to analytical epidemiological studies, the drivers are normally not compared with a reference (control) group.

15.4.1 Drivers Arrested for Driving Under the Influence

Cross-sectional studies of drivers arrested by the police suspected for DUI of alcohol or drugs show which substances are most commonly used by those who are apprehended as well as substance concentrations and multi-substance use. Most DUI offenders are arrested due to dangerous or aberrant driving, such as weaving, speeding, not stopping for red light or stop sign, or crash involvement; relatively few are arrested in random roadside police controls or controls at sobriety checkpoints. There is thus a marked selection bias, where the risk for apprehension is highest for those who are most significantly impaired or intoxicated.

Repeated studies of this type may show trends in substance use among apprehended DUI offenders over time, including changes in substances used for different age groups and sex.

Data on substance type and concentrations in blood may also be compared with observations of unsafe driving actions to characterize the type of impairment that is caused by different substance types, such as alcohol, other depressants, stimulants, hallucinogens, and cannabis.

Drivers suspected for DUI are in many countries also examined using standardized clinical tests for impairment or field sobriety tests. If these tests are performed in connection with collection of a blood sample, the relationship between substance concentrations and degree of impairment may be assessed. This type of study is sometimes called "semi-experimental," as the participants are drivers who have taken substance dose(s) that are "normal" for them, but not controlled by the researchers, whereas the clinical examination comprises standardized psychomotor and cognitive tests.

The main advantage is that the substance concentrations in blood are often very much higher than those used in experimental studies. Since the researchers do not give any substance to the participants, ethical approval for such high-dose studies is not needed. The fact that the participants are actual substance users, not healthy volunteers, may also be regarded as an advantage. The results show the wide range of substance concentrations that may be associated with clinical impairment: low concentrations may be found among impaired drivers with low tolerance to the substance and high concentrations may reflect high tolerance if the clinical impairment is low to moderate. Studies of this type may also indicate whether there is an overall positive correlation between substance concentration and degree of impairment.

The main limitation is a selection bias as the included drivers are stopped by the police based on dangerous or aberrant driving. Therefore, it is not possible to determine an unbiased correlation between substance concentration in blood and results of field sobriety tests or clinical tests of impairment. Another limitation is that data on the amount of substance taken, information about the time and frequency of use, and whether it was for taken for therapeutic or recreational purposes, has in most studied not be collected because the data were based on standardized questionnaires used by the police.

Semi-experimental studies of this type have been performed for alcohol, amphetamines, benzodiazepines, and similar medicinal drugs, cannabis, and opioids; see Chapter 11.

15.4.2 Drivers Involved in Road Traffic Crashes

Cross-sectional studies of drivers involved in crashes can be used to determine the prevalence of different psychoactive substances as well as substance concentrations. These studies may be used to compare substance use among different groups, e.g., drivers arrested for DUI, drivers involved in fatal versus noninjurious crashes, or car drivers versus motorcycle riders. Substance use among sub-groups can be studied—e.g., sex, age groups, or drivers involved in single-vehicle crashes—and changes in substance use over time can be monitored.

Comparison between different countries or regions may be difficult if studies are not harmonized regarding type of biological sample, types of substances, and detection limits or cutoff concentrations if analyzing biological samples. This has so far been done in few studies (Legrand et al. 2013, 2014; Mørland et al. 2011). The same applies when monitoring changes over time in a country or region.

The risks for crash involvement cannot be calculated based on studies of this type. However, findings may be used to hypothesize which substances may cause impairment and thus increase the crash risk, and at which concentrations.

15.5 Agreements and Disagreements Between Studies

Neither experimental, epidemiological, nor real-case studies can alone provide sufficient documentation and understanding about the risks for crash involvement after using a psychoactive substance. All methods have distinct advantages and limitations. Therefore, those methodologies may in some instances apparently provide conflicting data. However, the combination of the three methods may be used to create a broader and more complete picture as they may complement each other when assessing the effects of substance use on road traffic safety.

Experimental studies indicate which substances and at which doses and concentrations the ability to drive safely may be affected. Real-case studies indicate which substances are found in drivers involved in crashes, or among arrested DUI offenders as proxy for crash involvement, and at which concentrations. Well-designed epidemiological studies (cohort-, case-crossover-, case-control- and culpability-studies) may be used to estimate the actual crash risk posed by drivers using different psychoactive substances, and compare the risks posed by users of cannabis, stimulants, hallucinogens, and depressants of different types.

To illustrate some similarities and disagreements for the three methodologies, we have presented data from a selection of representative studies of alcohol, amphetamine/methamphetamine, cannabis, and diazepam below.

15.5.1 Alcohol

15.5.1.1 Experimental Studies

The first experimental studies of alcohol-related impairment were performed in the early twentieth century. Studies included the effect of alcohol on typewriting efficiency (Heise 1934) and studies on response time between stop signaling and actual application of brakes while driving (Heise and Halporn 1932). The effect of alcohol on cognitive and psychomotor functions has later been studied in a number of computer-based studies of mental and psychomotor functioning, in driver simulators, and on-the-road driving studies, and several review articles have summarized the findings (Irwin et al. 2017; Jongen et al. 2016, 2017; Moskowitz and Robinson 1988; Schnabel et al. 2010). Due to the clear and well-documented relationship between BAC and impairment, alcohol is often used as a benchmark standard when studying other substances.

The Norwegian researcher Klaus Hansen performed a number of semi-experimental studies on the degree of impairment in relation to the BAC among drivers during 1915–1936 (Hansen 1938a, 1938b); the documentation was used to set the legal BAC limit for DUI of alcohol in Norway, as the first country in the world, to 0.05% in 1936.

15.5.1.2 Epidemiological Studies

Holocomb published the results of an analytical epidemiological study on alcohol and crash involvement in 1938, comparing the prevalence of alcohol and the BAC in random drivers and crash-involved drivers in a case-control study (Holcomb 1938). The results indicated that crash risk increased with higher BAC. The first large-scale study was performed by Borkenstein and co-workers in 1962–1963 (Borkenstein et al. 1974); they found that a BAC above 0.04% was associated with increased crash rate and that the risk increased with increasing BAC. Later studies have confirmed the findings (Blomberg et al. 2009; Krüger and Vollrath 2004; Schulze et al. 2012; Terhune 1982; Voas et al. 2012; Zador et al. 2000). However, the estimated odds ratio for crash involvement at a defined BAC has not been the same in different studies, indicating that the BAC alone cannot fully explain the crash risk (Gjerde et al. 2014). It is likely that confounders related to personality, risk perception, and social norms may also play a role. Also differences in study protocols, execution and statistical evaluations may cause variation in risk estimates.

15.5.1.3 Real-Case Studies

In the first published study of alcohol use among crash-involved drivers, which was published in 1904, found that in 19 out of 25 fatal crashes, the drivers had used alcohol during the last hour before the crash (Editorial 1904). A study of 119 crash-involved drivers published in 1934 found that the majority had been drinking (Heise 1934). Since then, many studies have confirmed the large proportion of alcohol-related crashes (Gonzalez-Wilhelm 2007).

The proportion of BAC above 0.08% among drivers killed in crashes in the United States declined from 49% in 1982 to 31% in 2011 (Fell and Romano 2013) and 28% in 2016 (National Highway Traffic Safety Administration 2018). In Sweden, 22% of drivers killed in crashes during 2008–2011 had BAC > 0.02% with a mean BAC of 0.172% (Ahlner et al. 2014). In Norway, 25.3% of drivers killed in crashes during 2001–2010 who were investigated for alcohol use had BAC > 0.02%, 20.6% had BAC > 0.1% (Christophersen and Gjerde 2014). The mean BAC of drivers killed during 2005–2015 was 0.16% (Anja Valen, Oslo University Hospital; personal communication).

15.5.1.4 Agreements between Studies

Experimental and epidemiological studies confirm the association between increasing BAC and increasing impairment and crash risk. Real-case studies show that DUI of alcohol is a contributing factor in a large proportion of crashes. There is no significant disagreement between findings in different types of studies. However, experimental methods seem more sensitive to the effects of alcohol, showing impairment of some skills at BAC of 0.02% or lower (Moskowitz and Fiorentino 2000), whereas epidemiological studies have documented increased crash risk at BAC of 0.02%–0.04% and higher (Borkenstein et al. 1974; Schnabel et al. 2010; Voas et al. 2012).

15.5.2 Amphetamine and Methamphetamine

15.5.2.1 Experimental Studies

Experimental studies of cognitive and psychomotor performance have been performed by acute administration of amphetamine or methamphetamine in doses of 10–40 mg to healthy volunteers, giving mean concentration in blood of about 50–100 ng/mL after 3–4 hours. Overall, the studies found neutral or stimulatory effects when given alone, and stimulatory effects were not strong enough to counteract the impairing effects of alcohol or sleep (Ramaekers et al. 2012). Some studies found enhancement of functions in fatigued and sleep-deprived persons, others found a small decrease in overall driving performance in a simulator after amphetamine administration at the same dosing, see also Chapter 11. Baselt has also published additional data (Baselt 2001).

A driving simulator study with 39 participants who were weekly users of methamphetamine and a control group of non-users was performed in Australia (Bosanquet et al. 2013). The methamphetamine users were significantly more likely to speed and to swerve from side to side when driving. They also left less distance between their vehicle and oncoming vehicles when making a right-hand turn. There were higher levels of impulsivity and anti-social personality disorder in the methamphetamine-using cohort.

15.5.2.2 Epidemiological Studies

In epidemiological studies, significant associations between use of amphetamine/methamphetamine and crash involvement were found in most studies, whereas a few studies did not find significant associations, see Chapter 12. Hayley and co-workers have published a more detailed systematic review of observational studies on amphetamines and RTC injury or death (Hayley et al. 2016). Most of the reviewed studies had been performed by using a classical case-control design whereas a few used responsibility design. The largest case-control study of alcohol, drugs, and crash involvement performed so far, the European DRUID Project (Driving under the Influence of Drugs, Alcohol and Medicines) (Schulze et al. 2012), included 2490 seriously injured drivers, 1112 fatally injured drivers, and more than 36,000 drivers in random road traffic as controls; the adjusted odds ratio for serious injury in road traffic crashes associated with amphetamines was 14.2 (95% CI 5.8–34.4), whereas the adjusted odds ratio for fatal injury was 34.3 (95% CI 13.2–89.5) (Bernhoft et al. 2012).

Common challenges with case-control studies are selection bias, information bias, and confounding (Gjerde et al. 2018). We therefore expect that the calculated odds ratios are inaccurate, in most studies over-estimated.

A study on the odds ratio for being arrested for DUI was higher for amphetamine/methamphetamine using drivers than for those who had used other drugs (Bogstrand and Gjerde 2014).

15.5.2.3 Real-Case Studies

The prevalence of amphetamine or methamphetamine in blood samples from drivers arrested for DUI varies a lot between different countries; the prevalence is particularly high in some northern European countries and Australia (Gonzalez-Wilhelm 2007). In Sweden, amphetamine was detected in 60% of blood samples taken from drivers suspected for DUI of drugs in the period 2000–2004 (Jones et al. 2008b). In Norway, amphetamine was detected in 27.6% and methamphetamine in 13.4% of suspected drug-impaired drivers arrested during 1990–2015 (Valen et al. 2017b), in Germany amphetamine, methamphetamine, MDMA, or MDEA was found in 21.1% of arrested drug drivers (Musshoff and Madea 2012). On the other hand, a Swiss study found methamphetamine to be present in only 3.6% of blood/urine samples from drivers suspected for DUI of drugs (Augsburger et al. 2005).

The concentrations of amphetamine in drivers arrested for DUI are often very high. The reported mean concentration in blood samples from arrested impaired drivers in Sweden with amphetamine as the only drug (n = 33,642) was 800 ng/mL (Jones and Holmgren 2013). The mean concentration among arrested drivers in Norway during 1990–2015 (n = 30,968, cutoff 40 ng/mL) was 380 ng/mL; for methamphetamine (n = 15,039, cutoff 45 ng/mL) the mean concentration was 450 ng/mL (Anja Valen, Oslo University Hospital; personal communication). A large proportion of the arrested amphetamine-impaired drivers are chronic long-term users of the drug, many take it intravenously at very high doses (Jones and Holmgren 2013). A Swedish study found that 75% of drivers killed in road traffic crashes who tested positive for amphetamines had been arrested previously for use of illicit drugs or DUI (Jones et al. 2015), confirming problematic drug use.

In a study of arrested DUI offenders in Germany where amphetamines were the only psychoactive substance found, the mean amphetamine concentration in plasma was 181 ng/mL (Musshoff and Madea 2012), which is lower than averages found in Scandinavian studies.

Among 1375 drivers/riders killed in crashes in Western Australia during 2000–2012, methamphetamine was found in 7.4% (Palamara et al. 2014). In Norway, 9.0% of 676 investigated drivers and 6.3% of 207 motorcycle riders killed in crashes during 2001–2010 tested positive for amphetamine/methamphetamine (Christophersen and Gjerde 2014, 2015). In Sweden, 3.4% of 895 drivers tested positive for amphetamines in 2008–2011 (Ahlner et al. 2014).

The mean concentration of amphetamines in killed drivers in Sweden during 2008–2011 (n = 30) was 1030 ng/mL (Ahlner et al. 2014). The mean concentration in blood samples from car drivers killed in road traffic crashes in Norway during 2005–2013 was for amphetamine 900 ng/mL (n = 29) and methamphetamine 1,070 ng/mL (n = 23) (Anja Valen, Oslo University Hospital; personal communication).

Clinical tests of impairment of arrested DUI offenders who tested positive for only amphetamine found that almost 60% of apprehended drivers with amphetamine concentrations in blood of 40–100 ng/mL were judged clinically impaired, while about 70% of those with amphetamine concentrations above 270 ng/mL were judged impaired. Younger drivers were more often judged impaired than older drivers at similar concentrations (Gustavsen et al. 2006). A Swedish study was not able to find an association between concentration and impairment; however, the statistical power was low (Jones 2007).

Case studies of arrested amphetamine impaired drivers indicated that they had been apprehended due to aberrant or dangerous driving, such as changing lane rapidly without signaling, tailgating the car ahead, speeding, and weaving (Lemos 2009; Logan 1996). Studies of arrested DUI offenders found that those who had used stimulants had difficulties when performing balance tests, walk-and-turn, and finger-nose-test (Lemos 2009; Porath-Waller and Beirness 2014).

Amphetamine and methamphetamine can be taken orally, snorted, or injected; the effects are then similar for the two substances. Methamphetamine can also be smoked as "crystal meth." The effects of amphetamine and methamphetamine on behavior and crash risk are mostly related to dose and frequency of use, but the way of administration may also have some modulating effect.

15.5.2.4 Disagreements between Studies

Experimental studies with amphetamine and methamphetamine have often showed improvement in skills related to driving or fail to find any effects at all. Most epidemiological studies, however, found that stimulant use increased the crash risk.

Experimental studies of amphetamines have mostly been performed by administration of a single, small dose to healthy volunteers, normally about 10–40 mg, giving peak plasma concentration of about 140 ng/mL (Chapter 11). Patients using amphetamine or methamphetamine for therapeutic purposes may have peak plasma concentrations of 200 ng/mL or lower (Schulz et al. 2012; Schweitzer and Holcomb 2002). It is unlikely that therapeutic use of amphetamines may significantly reduce the ability to drive safely.

The concentrations of amphetamines in most arrested or crash-involved drivers are higher, because most of them are abusers who take 50–300 mg in each dose, several times a day and for many days in a row, as described above. As a result of the large doses for extended periods of time, irrational behavior may occur, as well as fatigue, paranoia and psychotomimetic symptoms (Cruickshank and Dyer 2009; Logan 2002; Panenka et al. 2013). It is likely that the observed increase in crash risk associated with amphetamines may be related to those effects, as very high amphetamine concentrations in blood are often found in crash-involved drivers and arrested DUI offenders (Jones and Holmgren 2013; Logan 1996). However, also therapeutic amphetamine concentrations in blood are sometimes found in clinical impaired DUI offenders, suggesting that those drivers may be on a declining concentration curve after taking larger doses.

Based on the data presented above, the differences between findings in experimental studies and epidemiological studies on the association between amphetamines and the ability to drive safely are therefore most likely related to dose and frequency of use (Logan 2002).

15.5.3 Cannabis

15.5.3.1 Experimental Studies

A large number of studies have found that cannabis causes a dose-related mild to moderate impairment in neurocognitive and neurophysiological functions that may reduce the ability to drive safely, see Chapter 11. Other reviews have also been published (Bondallaz et al. 2017; Hartman and Huestis 2013; Ramaekers et al. 2004). Ramaekers and co-workers reported that the degree of performance impairment observed in experimental studies after smoking doses up to 300 μg/kg THC were equivalent to the impairing effect of an alcohol dose producing a BAC $\geq$ 0.05% (Ramaekers et al. 2004), this corresponds to an average peak THC concentration in serum of 7–10 ng/mL (Grotenhermen et al. 2007); about 3–5 ng/mL in whole blood. However, smaller performance impairments have been demonstrated to arise at THC levels >2 ng/mL in serum (Ramaekers et al. 2006).

The results of several studies indicate that highest degree of impairment appear later than the peak THC concentration in blood after smoking cannabis. A counterclockwise hysteresis relationship has been demonstrated several times (Cone and Huestis 1993; Huestis 2002; Newmeyer et al. 2017; Schwope et al. 2012). However, it has also been shown that a strong relationship between performance impairment and THC concentrations in blood can be demonstrated if the magnitude of cannabis-induced impairment is discarded. For example, Ramaekers et al. (2004) and Grotenhermen et al. (2007) determined the relationship between THC concentration in blood and a binary representation of impairment (i.e., present or absent); they found that the number of psychomotor tests showing cannabis impairment increased as a function of THC concentration in serum.

Experimental studies have demonstrated that levels of cannabis-induced impairments may differ as a function of cannabis use history. Impairment levels are maximal in occasional cannabis and less or even absent in frequent or daily users due to tolerance (Desrosiers et al. 2015; Ramaekers et al. 2009). It is unknown, at present, at which cannabis use frequency tolerance becomes complete, if ever (Ramaekers et al. 2016a, 2016b).

15.5.3.2 Epidemiological Studies

Studies on the association between cannabis use and crash risk have been performed using cohort, case-crossover, case-control, and responsibility designs. Most studies found significant association between cannabis use and crash involvement or crash responsibility. However, the odds ratios were lower than for alcohol or amphetamines, in most studies less than 3.0, see Chapter 12 and other review articles (Asbridge et al. 2012; Hartman and Huestis 2013; Li et al. 2012). Røgeberg and Elvik (Rogeberg and Elvik 2016; Røgeberg et al. 2018) attempted to recalculate the odds ratios in a meta-analysis of many previous studies to eliminate an upward bias in odds-ratio estimations. The recalculations indicated a statistically significant risk increase of low-to-moderate magnitude [random-effects model odds ratio 1.32 (95% CI 1.09–1.59), metaregression odds ratio 1.18 (95% CI 1.07–1.3)]. The included data were based on studies using low cutoff concentrations for THC in blood, or studies based on urine testing, and did therefore not specifically address the risk during acute cannabis intoxication (Gjerde and Mørland 2016). It is therefore likely that only a small proportion of those who were categorized as cannabis-exposed were actually intoxicated or "high" in the included studies, thus underestimating the risk posed by driving while intoxicated by cannabis. Røgeberg has also performed a meta-analysis of culpability studies on cannabis use and crash responsibility avoiding interpretational bias, estimating a crash risk of 1.42 (95% CI 1.16–1.40) (Røgeberg 2019).

The risk associated with likely acute cannabis intoxication, defined as a THC concentration in whole blood ≥5 ng/mL, has been studied in few investigations. Using the responsibility study design, estimated odds ratios for crash responsibility were 1.0 (95% CI 0.4–2.4), 2.1 (95% CI 1.3–3.4) and 6.6 (95% CI 1.5–28) (Drummer et al. 2004; Laumon et al. 2005; Poulsen et al. 2014), whereas a case-control study found an odds ratio for crash involvement of 14.3 (95% CI 2.0–101.1) (Kuypers et al. 2012). The main problems with those studies were low statistical power, possibly information bias as the THC concentration in the analyzed blood samples might not represent the concentration at the time of crash, and a likely selection bias for the case-control study as the participation rate was low.

15.5.3.3 Real Case Studies

Cannabis is the most common nonalcohol drug detected in blood samples from suspected drug-impaired drivers in many countries (Gonzalez-Wilhelm 2007). In Norway, THC was found in 23% of the analyzed blood samples in 2000, increasing to 34% in 2015 (Valen et al. 2017a); similarly, the proportion testing positive for THC increased from 18% in 1995 to 30% in 2003 in Sweden (Jones et al. 2008a).

In a California study, the main reasons for being apprehended for DUI of cannabis were found to be speeding, unable to maintain lane position, ran red light or stop sign, unsafe lane change, collision, going too slow, no headlights at night, no turn signals, and driving the wrong way (Declues et al. 2016). Drug recognition expert examination characteristics of cannabis-impaired drivers found that the strongest indicators were walk and turn problems, one leg stand sway, finger to nose misses, as well as eyelid tremors, blood shot eyes, and pupil rebound dilation; the speech was also often affected (Declues et al. 2016; 2018; Hartman et al. 2016).

A study of drivers arrested for drug-impaired driving in San Francisco, CA, found the mean THC concentration in blood was 4.9 ng/mL; among those who tested positive only for THC, the mean concentration was 5.8 ng/mL. Among drivers killed in crashes, the THC concentrations were higher (mean 11.7 ng/mL, 20.3 ng/mL among cannabis-only drivers) (Lemos et al. 2015).

The prevalence of THC in biological samples from drivers killed in road traffic crashes varies between different countries or states and has changed over time, see Chapter 13 and an earlier review article (Gonzalez-Wilhelm 2007). Norwegian studies found THC in blood samples from 7.2% of car and van driver killed in road traffic crashes during 2001–2010 (Christophersen and Gjerde 2014) and 4.3% among killed motorcycle riders (Christophersen and Gjerde 2015). A study of crash data from six American states found that the proportion of killed drivers who tested positive for cannabis increased from 4.2% in 1999 to 12.2% in 2010 (Brady and Li 2014). A study in Washington state estimated an increase in THC detections among killed drivers from 8.5% in 2010 to 17.0% in 2014 (Tefft et al. 2016); it is likely that this increase was related to the legalization of recreational cannabis use in December 2012. Among fatally injured drivers in Canada who were tested for drugs, the proportion who tested positive for cannabis increased from 15.9% in 2000 to 20.9% in 2015 (TIRF 2018); however, the proportion who was tested for drugs increased during this period, so the data should be interpreted with caution. The 2018 Canadian Cannabis Survey found that among those who had used cannabis during the past 12 months, 39% reported that they had ever driven within two hours of using cannabis (Government of Canada 2018). It is likely that the number of drivers testing positive for cannabis will increase further after legalization for recreational use in Canada.

15.5.3.4 Disagreements between Studies

The results from different types of studies show apparently different findings regarding the risk posed by cannabis in road traffic: experimental studies and real-case studies found significant impairment of mental and psychomotor functions, whereas epidemiological studies found a fairly low but statistically significant increase in crash risk.

There may be several reasons for the differences. First of all, it is very difficult to study the effect of acute cannabis intoxication in epidemiological studies. No study has been able to determine the THC concentration in crash-involved drivers immediately after the crash; by the time samples were taken, the THC concentrations had declined significantly. The THC concentration in blood may stay detectable but low for a very long time after use, depending on inter-individual differences as well as frequency of cannabis use. Often, THC concentrations in blood above 1 ng/mL have been regarded as proof of cannabis exposure, but cannabis use may for the vast majority of those drivers have occurred several hours ago, or perhaps more than one day ago. So, most epidemiological studies have not been able to distinguish between acute intoxication and previous cannabis use, or occasional and daily users, which may bias the study findings. Other difficulties are related to selection bias and confounding.

Investigators have reported that some cannabis users are aware of their impairment and may try to be more cautious by driving more slowly and avoid taking risks if deciding to drive while "high" (MacDonald et al. 2008; Robbe and O'Hanlon 1996). However, studies have found that drivers under the influence of cannabis were not able to compensate for weaving, had increased decision and response times, and difficulties in handling unexpected events (Hartman and Huestis 2013; Sewell et al. 2009). How much this attempted compensation reduces the crash risk is therefore not clear.

15.5.4 Diazepam

15.5.4.1 Experimental Studies

Early studies on diazepam performed in the 1960s and 1970s found that diazepam could reduce both mental and psychomotor functions that are important for safe driving (Haffner et al. 1973; Jäättelä et al. 1971; Lawton and Cahn 1963; Mørland et al. 1974). Since then, a large number of studies have been performed. A meta-analysis of 103 experimental studies of diazepam was performed by Berghaus and co-workers as part of the DRUID Project (Berghaus et al. 2011). The degree of impairment after single administration of 5–20 mg diazepam to healthy individuals was summarized, as well as studies of repeated use among patients. There was a linear correlation between drug concentrations in plasma and performance impairment. Berghaus et al. estimated that a diazepam concentration in plasma of 320 ng/mL produced the same degree of impairment as a BAC of 0.05% (Berghaus et al. 2011), whereas Vindenes et al. estimated that impairment similar to BAC of 0.05% was obtained at a diazepam concentration of 143 ng/mL in whole blood (Vindenes et al. 2012), corresponding to 260 ng/mL in plasma (the blood/plasma concentration ratio for diazepam is about 0.55 (Jones and Larsson 2004; Moffat et al. 2011).

15.5.4.2 Epidemiological Studies

Most epidemiological studies have investigated benzodiazepines as a drug group, not individual substances; see Chapter 12 and other reviews and meta-analyses (Dassanayake et al. 2011; Elvik 2013; Orriols et al. 2009; Smink et al. 2010). Statistically significant associations have been found between use of benzodiazepines, including diazepam, and crash involvement.

Among the studies that specifically addressed diazepam, investigations of crash involvement among patients using diazepam found an incidence rate ratio of 1.93 (95% CI 1.54–2.43) during the four first weeks of use (Gibson et al. 2009) and standardized incidence rates of 2.8 (95% CI 2.2–3.6) during the first week after dispensed from a pharmacy (Bramness et al. 2007), and 3.1 (95% CI 1.4–6.5) during the first four weeks in another study (Neutel 1998). A study of elderly drivers found a relative risk for injurious crash of 2.4 (95% CI 1.3–4.4) for ≥20 mg diazepam per day (Ray et al. 1992).

Case-control studies found odds ratios for crash involvement associated with diazepam of 0.9 (95% CI 0.1–7.0) (Gjerde et al. 2011a) and 6.4 (95% CI 2.5–16.7) (Gjerde et al. 2013). Similar odds ratios have been found in studies of the benzodiazepine drug group in total; see e.g., reviews by Elvik (2013) or Dassanyake et al. (Dassanayake et al. 2011). The risk for crash involvement after using benzodiazepines is lower than the average risk associated with alcohol use; the DRUID Project found for alcohol an overall adjusted odds ratio for being seriously injured of 9.8 (95% CI 8.2–11.7), and for being fatally injured of

19.0 (95% CI 14.4–25.0), whereas the odds ratios associated with the use of benzodiazepines or Z-drugs were 1.8 (95% CI 1.2–2.7) for being seriously injured and 4.6 (95% CI 3.3–6.4) for being killed (Bernhoft et al. 2012).

Other studies have found a positive correlation between daily dose of benzodiazepines and crash risk (Barbone et al. 1998; Ray et al. 1992).

15.5.4.3 Real Case Studies

The use of diazepam in Norway is fairly high compared to many other countries. During 1990–2015, on average, 15% of drivers suspected for drug impaired driving in Norway tested positive for diazepam in concentrations above 142 ng/mL in whole blood (Valen et al. 2017b), which was the maximum analytical cutoff used during the study period. About 80% of those tested also positive for one or more other drugs; the median diazepam concentration was 340 ng/mL and 7% had concentrations above 1100 ng/mL (Anja Valen, Oslo University Hospital; personal communication), corresponding to 2000 ng/mL plasma (Jones and Larsson 2004; Moffat et al. 2011); a concentration that may be regarded as the upper concentration limit of therapeutic use (Schulz et al. 2012).

Among car and van drivers killed in road traffic crashes in Norway during 2001–2010, 5.5% tested positive for diazepam (Christophersen and Gjerde 2014).

Studies of suspected DUI offenders and fatally injured drivers in several other countries also found high prevalence of benzodiazepines, but the types of benzodiazepines as well as the prevalence in blood samples differed between countries (Legrand et al. 2014; Thomas 1998).

15.5.5.4 Agreements between Studies

Results from experimental (Chapter 11) and epidemiological studies (Chapter 12) indicate that the use of diazepam may impair the ability to drive safely and increase the crash risk; see also the review by Berghaus and co-workers (Berghaus et al. 2011). The risk is related to the daily dose (Barbone et al. 1998; Ray et al. 1992), but development of tolerance may reduce the risk (Drummer 2002). Studies on the prevalence of diazepam among arrested DUI offenders and crash-involved drivers also indicate that impaired driving may be caused by diazepam, particularly when taken in large doses.

15.6 Conclusions

Experimental, epidemiological, and real-case studies have different advantages and limitations when used to study the effect of substance use on the risk for involvement in a road traffic crash. All types of studies are needed to assess the impact of the use of different psychoactive substances on road traffic safety. For some drugs, such as cannabis and stimulants, the results of experimental studies are not always in line with those of epidemiological studies. Those disagreements may be caused by limitations in study designs and in interpretation of findings. For example, many drug-impaired drivers are multi-substance users that combine high doses of illicit, prescription drugs and alcohol. Such real-life incidences cannot be mimicked in experimental studies due to ethical constraints.

References

af Wåhlberg AE, Dorn L, Kline T: The effect of social desirability on self reported and recorded road traffic accidents; *Transp Res Part F Traffic Psychol Behav* 13:106; 2010.

Ahlner J, Holmgren A, Jones AW: Prevalence of alcohol and other drugs and the concentrations in blood of drivers killed in road traffic crashes in Sweden; *Scand J Public Health* 42:177; 2014.

Asbridge M, Hayden JA, Cartwright JL: Acute cannabis consumption and motor vehicle collision risk: Systematic review of observational studies and meta-analysis; *BMJ* 344:e536; 2012.

Asbridge M, Mann R, Cusimano MD, Trayling C, Roerecke M, Tallon JM, Whipp A, Rehm J: Cannabis and traffic collision risk: Findings from a case-crossover study of injured drivers presenting to emergency departments; *Int J Public Health* 59:395; 2014.

Augsburger M, Donze N, Menetrey A, Brossard C, Sporkert F, Giroud C, Mangin P: Concentration of drugs in blood of suspected impaired drivers; *Forensic Sci Int* 153:11; 2005.

Barbone F, McMahon AD, Davey PG, Morris AD, Reid IC, McDevitt DG, MacDonald TM: Association of road-traffic accidents with benzodiazepine use; *Lancet* 352:1331; 1998.

Baselt RC: *Drug Effects on Psychomotor Performance*; Biomedical Publications: Foster City, CA; 2001.

Behnood A, Mannering FL: The effects of drug and alcohol consumption on driver injury severities in single-vehicle crashes; *Traffic Inj Prev* 18: 456; 2017.

Berghaus G, Ramaekers JG, Drummer OH: Demands on scientific studies in different fields of forensic medicine and forensic sciences. Traffic medicine-impaired driver: Alcohol, drugs, diseases; *Forensic Sci Int* 165:233; 2007.

Berghaus G, Sticht G, Grellner W, Lenz D, Naumann T, Wiesenmüller S: *Meta-Analysis of Empirical Studies Concerning the Effects of Medicines and Illegal Drugs Including Pharmacokinetics on Safe Driving*, DRUID Deliverable 1.1.2b; University of Würzburg: Würzburg, Germany; 2011.

Bernhoft IM, Hels T, Lyckegaard A, Houwing S, Verstraete AG: Prevalence and risk of injury in Europe by driving with alcohol, illicit drugs and medicines; *Procedia Soc Behav Sci* 48:2907; 2012.

Blomberg RD, Peck RC, Moskowitz H, Burns M, Fiorentino D: The Long Beach/Fort Lauderdale relative risk study; *J Safety Res* 40:285; 2009.

Bogstrand ST, Gjerde H: Which drugs are associated with highest risk for being arrested for driving under the influence? A case-control study; *Forensic Sci Int* 240:21; 2014.

Bondallaz P, Chtioui H, Favrat B, Fornari E, Giroud C, Maeder P: Assessment of cannabis acute effects on driving skills: Laboratory, simulator, and on-road studies; In Preedy VR (Ed): *Handbook of Cannabis and Related Pathologies*; Academic Press: London, UK; 2017.

Borkenstein RF, Crowther RF, Shumate RF, Ziel WB, Zylman R: The role of the drinking driver in traffic accidents (the Grand Rapids study); *Blutalkohol* 11:1; 1974.

Bosanquet D, Macdougall HG, Rogers SJ, Starmer GA, McKetin R, Blaszczynski A, McGregor IS: Driving on ice: Impaired driving skills in current methamphetamine users; *Psychopharmacology* (Berl) 225:161; 2013.

Brady JE, Li G: Trends in alcohol and other drugs detected in fatally injured drivers in the United States, 1999–2010; *Am J Epidemiol* 179:692; 2014.

Bramness JG, Skurtveit S, Mørland J, Engeland A: The risk of traffic accidents after prescriptions of carisoprodol; *Accid Anal Prev* 39:1050; 2007.

Christophersen AS, Gjerde H: Prevalence of alcohol and drugs among car and van drivers killed in road accidents in Norway: An overview from 2001–2010; *Traffic Inj Prev* 15:523; 2014.

Christophersen AS, Gjerde H: Prevalence of alcohol and drugs among motorcycle riders killed in road crashes in Norway during 2001–2010; *Accid Anal Prev* 80:236; 2015.

Cone EJ: Pharmacokinetics and pharmacodynamics of cocaine; *J Anal Toxicol* 19:459; 1995.

Cone EJ, Huestis MA: Relating blood concentrations of tetrahydrocannabinol and metabolites to pharmacologic effects and time of marijuana usage; *Ther Drug Monit* 15:527; 1993.

Cruickshank CC, Dyer KR: A review of the clinical pharmacology of methamphetamine; *Addiction* 104:1085; 2009.

Dassanayake T, Michie P, Carter G, Jones A: Effects of benzodiazepines, antidepressants and opioids on driving: A systematic review and meta-analysis of epidemiological and experimental evidence; *Drug Saf* 34:125; 2011.

Declues K, Perez S, Figueroa A: A 2-year study of delta(9)-tetrahydrocannabinol concentrations in drivers: Examining driving and field sobriety test performance; *J Forensic Sci* 61:1664; 2016.

Declues K, Perez S, Figueroa A: A two-year study of delta(9)-tetrahydrocannabinol concentrations in drivers. Part 2: Physiological signs on drug recognition expert (DRE) and non-DRE examinations; *J Forensic Sci* 63:583; 2018.

Desrosiers NA, Ramaekers JG, Chauchard E, Gorelick DA, Huestis MA: Smoked cannabis' psychomotor and neurocognitive effects in occasional and frequent smokers; *J Anal Toxicol* 39:251; 2015.

Donelson AC, Marks ME, Jones RK, Joscelyn KB: *Drug Research Methodology: Volume One—The Alcohol-Highway Safety Experience and Its Applicability to Other Drugs*, Final report (DOT HS 805 374); National Highway Traffic Safety Administration: Washington, DC; 1980.

Drummer OH: Benzodiazepines—Effects on human performance and behavior; *Forensic Sci Rev* 14:1; 2002.

Drummer OH, Gerostamoulos J, Batziris H, Chu M, Caplehorn J, Robertson MD, Swann P: The involvement of drugs in drivers of motor vehicles killed in Australian road traffic crashes; *Accid Anal Prev* 36:239; 2004.

Drummer OH, Kennedy B, Bugeja L, Ibrahim JE, Ozanne-Smith J: Interpretation of postmortem forensic toxicology results for injury prevention research; *Inj Prev* 19:284; 2013.

DuPont RL, Logan BK, Shea CL, Talpins SK, Voas RB: *Drugged Driving Research: A White Paper*; National Institute on Drug Abuse: Rockville, MD; 2011.

Editorial: *Q J Inebriety* 26:308; 1904.

Elvik R: Risk of road accident associated with the use of drugs: A systematic review and meta-analysis of evidence from epidemiological studies; *Accid Anal Prev* 60:254; 2013.

EMCDDA: *Literature Review on the Relation Between Drug Use, Impaired Driving and Traffic Accidents* (CT.97.EP.14); European Monitoring Centre for Drugs and Drug Addiction: Lisbon, Portugal; 1999.

Fell JC, Romano E: Alcohol and other drugs involvement in fatally injured drivers in the United States; In Watson B (Ed): *Proceedings—20th International Council on Alcohol, Drugs and Traffic Safety Conference*; Brisbane, Australia; August 22–25, 2013; Center for Accident Research and Road Safety Queensland: Brisbane, Australia; p. 232; 2013.

Food and Drug Administration: *Evaluating Drug Effects on the Ability to Operate a Motor Vehicle—Guidance for Industry;* Food and Drug Administration, Center for Drug Evaluation and Research: Silver Spring, MD; 2017.

Gibson JE, Hubbard RB, Smith CJ, Tata LJ, Britton JR, Fogarty AW: Use of self-controlled analytical techniques to assess the association between use of prescription medications and the risk of motor vehicle crashes; *Am J Epidemiol* 169:761; 2009.

Gjerde H, Bogstrand ST, Lillsunde P: Why is the odds ratio for involvement in serious road traffic accident among drunk drivers in Norway and Finland higher than in other countries? *Traffic Inj Prev* 15:1; 2014.

Gjerde H, Christophersen AS, Normann PT, Mørland J: Associations between substance use among car and van drivers in Norway and fatal injury in road traffic accidents: A case-control study; *Transp Res Part F Traffic Psychol Behav* 17:134; 2013.

Gjerde H, Mørland J: Risk for involvement in road traffic crash during acute cannabis intoxication; *Addiction* 111:1492; 2016.

Gjerde H, Normann PT, Christophersen AS, Samuelsen SO, Mørland J: Alcohol, psychoactive drugs and fatal road traffic accidents in Norway: A case-control study; *Accid Anal Prev* 43:1197; 2011a.

Gjerde H, Romeo G, Mørland J: Challenges and common weaknesses in case-control studies on drug use and road traffic injury based on drug testing of biological samples; *Ann Epidemiol* 28:812; 2018.

Gjerde H, Øiestad EL, Christophersen AS: Using biological samples in epidemiological research on drugs of abuse; *Nor Epidemiol* 21:5; 2011b.

Gonzalez-Wilhelm L: Prevalence of alcohol and illicit drugs in blood specimens from drivers involved in traffic law offenses. Systematic review of cross-sectional studies; *Traffic Inj Prev* 8:189; 2007.

Government of Canada: Canadian Cannabis Survey 2018 Summary; https://www.canada.ca/en/services/health/publications/drugs-health-products/canadian-cannabis-survey-2018-summary.html (Accessed March 5, 2019).

Grimes DA, Schulz KF: Bias and causal associations in observational research; *Lancet* 359:248; 2002.

Grotenhermen F, Leson G, Berghaus G, Drummer OH, Kruger HP, Longo M, Moskowitz H, Perrine B, Ramaekers JG, Smiley A, Tunbridge R: Developing limits for driving under cannabis; *Addiction* 102:1910; 2007.

Gustavsen I, Mørland J, Bramness JG: Impairment related to blood amphetamine and/or methamphetamine concentrations in suspected drugged drivers; *Accid Anal Prev* 38:490; 2006.

Haffner JF, Mørland J, Setekleiv J, Strømsæther CE, Danielsen A, Frivik PT, Dybing F: Mental and psychomotor effects of diazepam and ethanol; *Acta Pharmacol Toxicol* (Copenh) 32:161; 1973.

Hallvig D, Anund A, Fors C, Kecklund G, Karlsson JG, Wahde M, Akerstedt T: Sleepy driving on the real road and in the simulator—A comparison; *Accid Anal Prev* 50:44; 2013.

Han E, Kim E, Hong H, Jeong S, Kim J, In S, Chung H, Lee S: Evaluation of postmortem redistribution phenomena for commonly encountered drugs; *Forensic Sci Int* 219:265; 2012.

Hansen K: Alkohol und Verkehrsunfälle—Diskussionsbemerkungen [Alcohol and Traffic Accidents—Discussions]; *Forsch Alkoholfrage* (Berl) 46:130; 1938a.

Hansen K: Ueber das Verhältnis zwischen der Alkoholkonzentration im Blute und dem Grad der Alkoholbeeinflussung [Relation between the concentration of alcohol in the blood and the degree of the alcohol influence]; *Forsch Alkoholfrage* (Berl) 46:1; 1938b.

Hartman RL, Huestis MA: Cannabis effects on driving skills; *Clin Chem* 59:478; 2013.

Hartman RL, Richman JE, Hayes CE, Huestis MA: Drug Recognition Expert (DRE) examination characteristics of cannabis impairment; *Accid Anal Prev* 92:219; 2016.

Hayley AC, Downey LA, Shiferaw B, Stough C: Amphetamine-type stimulant use and the risk of injury or death as a result of a road-traffic accident: A systematic review of observational studies; *Eur Neuropsychopharmacol* 26:901; 2016.

Heise HA: Alcohol and automobile accidents; *JAMA* 103:739; 1934.

Heise HA, Halporn B: Medicolegal aspects of drunkenness; *Penn Med J* 36:190; 1932.

Helland A, Jenssen GD, Lervåg LE, Moen T, Engen T, Lydersen S, Mørland J, Slørdal L: Evaluation of measures of impairment in real and simulated driving: Results from a randomized, placebo-controlled study; *Traffic Inj Prev* 17:245; 2016a.

Helland A, Jenssen GD, Lervåg LE, Westin AA, Moen T, Sakshaug K, Lydersen S, Mørland J, Slørdal L: Comparison of driving simulator performance with real driving after alcohol intake: A randomised, single blind, placebo-controlled, cross-over trial; *Accid Anal Prev* 53:9; 2013.

Helland A, Lydersen S, Lervåg LE, Jenssen GD, Mørland J, Slørdal L: Driving simulator sickness: Impact on driving performance, influence of blood alcohol concentration, and effect of repeated simulator exposures; *Accid Anal Prev* 94:180; 2016b.

Holcomb RL: Alcohol in relation to traffic accidents; *JAMA* 111:1076; 1938.

Holmgren A, Holmgren P, Kugelberg FC, Jones AW, Ahlner J: Predominance of illicit drugs and poly-drug use among drug-impaired drivers in Sweden; *Traffic Inj Prev* 8:361; 2007.

Houwing S, Mathijssen R, Brookhuis KA: Case-control studies; In Verster JC, Pandi-Perumal SR, Ramaekers JG, de Gier JJ (Eds): *Drugs, Driving and Traffic Safety*; Birkhäuser Verlag AG: Basel, Switzerland; p. 107; 2009.

Huestis MA: Cannabis (marijuana)—Effects on human performance and behavior; *Forensic Sci Rev* 14:15; 2002.

International Council on Alcohol Drugs and Traffic Safety: *Guidelines on Experimental Studies Undertaken to Determine a Medicinal Drug's Effect on Driving or Skills Related to Driving;* Bundesanstalt für Strassenwesen: Cologne, Germany; 1999.

International Council on Alcohol Drugs and Traffic Safety: Quality assurance and standardization concerning empirical trials on drugs and driving; In Utzelmann HD, Berghaus G, Kroj G (Eds): *Alcohol, Drugs and Traffic Safety, T92*; Verlag TÜV Rheinland: Cologne, Germany; p. 804; 1993.

Ioannidis JPA: The mass production of redundant, misleading, and conflicted systematic reviews and meta-analyses; *Milbank Q* 94:485; 2016.

Irwin C, Iudakhina E, Desbrow B, McCartney D: Effects of acute alcohol consumption on measures of simulated driving: A systematic review and meta-analysis; *Accid Anal Prev* 102:248; 2017.

Jones AW: Age- and gender-related differences in blood amphetamine concentrations in apprehended drivers: Lack of association with clinical evidence of impairment; *Addiction* 102:1085; 2007.

Jones AW: Driving under the influence of drugs in Sweden with zero concentration limits in blood for controlled substances; *Traffic Inj Prev* 6:317; 2005.

Jones AW, Holmgren A: Amphetamine abuse in Sweden: Subject demographics, changes in blood concentrations over time, and the types of coingested substances; *J Clin Psychopharmacol* 33:248; 2013.

Jones AW, Holmgren A, Ahlner J: High prevalence of previous arrests for illicit drug use and/or impaired driving among drivers killed in motor vehicle crashes in Sweden with amphetamine in blood at autopsy; *Int J Drug Policy* 26:790; 2015.

Jones AW, Holmgren A, Kugelberg FC: Driving under the influence of cannabis: A 10-year study of age and gender differences in the concentrations of tetrahydrocannabinol in blood; *Addiction* 103:452; 2008a.

Jones AW, Holmgren A, Kugelberg FC: Driving under the influence of central stimulant amines: Age and gender differences in concentrations of amphetamine, methamphetamine, and ecstasy in blood; *J Stud Alcohol Drugs* 69:202; 2008b.

Jones AW, Larsson H: Distribution of diazepam and nordiazepam between plasma and whole blood and the influence of hematocrit; *Ther Drug Monit* 26:380; 2004.

Jongen S, Vermeeren A, van der Sluiszen NN, Schumacher MB, Theunissen EL, Kuypers KP, Vuurman EF, Ramaekers JG: A pooled analysis of on-the-road highway driving studies in actual traffic measuring standard deviation of lateral position (i.e., "weaving") while driving at a blood alcohol concentration of 0.5 g/L; *Psychopharmacology* (Berl) 234:837; 2017.

Jongen S, Vuurman EF, Ramaekers JG, Vermeeren A: The sensitivity of laboratory tests assessing driving related skills to dose-related impairment of alcohol: A literature review; *Accid Anal Prev* 89:31; 2016.

Joscelyn KB, Donelson AC: *Drug Research Methodology. Volume four. Epidemiology in Drugs and Highway Safety: the Study of Drug Use Among Drivers and Its Role in Traffic Crashes* (DOT HS 803 879); National Highway Traffic Aafety Administration: Washington, DC; 1980.

Jäättelä A, Mannisto P, Paatero H, Tuomisto J: The effects of diazepam or diphenhydramine on healthy human subjects; *Psychopharmacologia* 21:202; 1971.

Karjalainen KK, Lintonen TP, Impinen AO, Lillsunde PM, Ostamo AI: Poly-drug findings in drugged driving cases during 1977–2007; *J Subst Use* 15:143; 2010.

Kay GG, Logan BK: *Drugged Driving Expert Panel Report: A Consensus Protocol for Assessing the Potential of Drugs to Impair Driving* (DOT HS 811 438); National Highway Traffic Safety Administration: Washington, DC; 2011.

Kelsey JL, Whittemore AS, Evans AS, Thompson WD: *Methods in Observational Epidemiology*, 2nd ed; Oxford University Press: New York, NY; 1996.

Kim JH, Mooney SJ: The epidemiologic principles underlying traffic safety study designs; *Int J Epidemiol* 45:1668; 2016.

Kim K, Nitz L, Richardson J, Li L: Personal and behavioral predictors of automobile crash and injury severity; *Accid Anal Prev* 27:469; 1995.

Krumpal I: Determinants of social desirability bias in sensitive surveys: A literature review; *Qual Quant* 47:2025; 2013.

Krüger HP, Vollrath M: The alcohol-related accident risk in Germany: Procedure, methods and results; *Accid Anal Prev* 36:125; 2004.

Kuypers KP, Legrand SA, Ramaekers JG, Verstraete AG: A case-control study estimating accident risk for alcohol, medicines and illegal drugs; *PLoS One* 7:e43496; 2012.

Laumon B, Gadegbeku B, Martin JL, Biecheler MB: Cannabis intoxication and fatal road crashes in France: Population based case-control study; *BMJ* 331:1371; 2005.

Lawton MP, Cahn B: The effects of diazepam (Valium®) and alcohol on psychomotor performance; *J Nerv Ment Dis* 136:550; 1963.

Legrand SA, Gjerde H, Isalberti C, van der Linden T, Lillsunde P, Dias MJ, Gustafsson S, Ceder G, Verstraete AG: Prevalence of alcohol, illicit drugs and psychoactive medicines in killed drivers in four European countries; *Int J Inj Contr Saf Promot* 21:17; 2014.

Legrand SA, Isalberti C, der Linden TV, Bernhoft IM, Hels T, Simonsen KW, Favretto D, Ferrara SD, Caplinskiene M, Minkuviene Z, et al.: Alcohol and drugs in seriously injured drivers in six European countries; *Drug Test Anal* 5:156; 2013.

Lemos NP: Methamphetamine and driving; *Sci Justice* 49:247; 2009.

Lemos NP, San Nicolas AC, Volk JA, Ingle EA, Williams CM: Driving under the influence of marijuana versus driving and dying under the influence of marijuana: A comparison of blood concentrations of delta(9)-tetrahydrocannabinol, 11-hydroxy-delta9-tetrahydrocannabinol, 11-nor-9-carboxy-delta(9)-tetrahydrocannabinol and other cannabinoids in arrested drivers versus deceased drivers; *J Anal Toxicol* 39:588; 2015.

Li MC, Brady JE, DiMaggio CJ, Lusardi AR, Tzong KY, Li G: Marijuana use and motor vehicle crashes; *Epidemiol Rev* 34:65; 2012.

Liechti ME, Quednow BB, Liakoni E, Dornbierer D, von Rotz R, Gachet MS, Gertsch J, Seifritz E, Bosch OG: Pharmacokinetics and pharmacodynamics of gamma-hydroxybutyrate in healthy subjects; *Br J Clin Pharmacol* 81:980; 2016.

Liguori A: Simulator studies of drug-induced driving impairment; In Verster JC, Pandi-Perumal SR, Ramaekers JG, de Gier JJ (Eds): *Drugs, Driving and Traffic Safety*; Birkhäuser Basel: Basel, Switzerland; p. 75; 2009.

Logan BK: Methamphetamine—Effects on human performance and behavior; *Forensic Sci Rev* 14:133; 2002.

Logan BK: Methamphetamine and driving impairment; *J Forensic Sci* 41:457; 1996.

MacDonald S, Mann R, Chipman M, Pakula B, Erickson P, Hathaway A, MacIntyre P: Driving behavior under the influence of cannabis or cocaine; *Traffic Inj Prev* 9:190; 2008.

Moffat AC, Osselton MD, Widdop B: *Clarke's Analysis of Drugs and Poisons*, 4th ed; Pharmaceutical Press: London, UK; 2011.

Moskowitz H: Marihuana and driving; *Accid Anal Prev* 17:323; 1985.

Moskowitz H, Fiorentino D: *A Review of the Literature on the Effects of Low Doses of Alcohol on Driving-Related Skills*, DOT HS 809 028; National Highway Traffic Safety Administration: Washington, DC; 2000.

Moskowitz H, Robinson CD: *Effects of Low Doses of Alcohol on Driving-related Skills: A Review of the Evidence* (DOT HS 807 280); National Highway Traffic Safety Administration: Washington, DC; 1988.

Musshoff F, Madea B: Driving under the influence of amphetamine-like drugs; *J Forensic Sci* 57:413; 2012.

Mørland J, Setekleiv J, Haffner JF, Strømsæther CE, Danielsen A, Wethe GH: Combined effects of diazepam and ethanol on mental and psychomotor functions; *Acta Pharmacol Toxicol* (Copenh) 34:5; 1974.

Mørland J, Steentoft A, Simonsen KW, Ojanpera I, Vuori E, Magnusdottir K, Kristinsson J, Ceder G, Kronstrand R, Christophersen A: Drugs related to motor vehicle crashes in northern European countries: A study of fatally injured drivers; *Accid Anal Prev* 43:1920; 2011.

National Highway Traffic Safety Administration: *State Alcohol-Impaired-Driving Estimates 2016* (DOT HS 812 483); National Highway Traffic Safety Administration: Washington, DC; 2018.

Neutel I: Benzodiazepine-related traffic accidents in young and elderly drivers; *Hum Psychopharmacol Clin Exp* 13:S115; 1998.

Newmeyer MN, Swortwood MJ, Abulseoud OA, Huestis MA: Subjective and physiological effects, and expired carbon monoxide concentrations in frequent and occasional cannabis smokers following smoked, vaporized, and oral cannabis administration; *Drug Alcohol Depend* 175:67; 2017.

Orriols L, Salmi LR, Philip P, Moore N, Delorme B, Castot A, Lagarde E: The impact of medicinal drugs on traffic safety: A systematic review of epidemiological studies; *Pharmacoepidemiol Drug Saf* 18:647; 2009.

Owens K, Ramaekers JG: Drugs, driving, and models to measure driving impairment; In Verster JC, Pandi-Perumal SR, Ramaekers JD, de Gier JJ (Eds): *Drugs, Driving and Traffic Safety*; Birkhäuser Basel: Basel, Switzerland; p. 43; 2009.

Palamara P, Broughton M, Chambers F: *Illicit Drugs and Driving: An Investigation of Fatalities and Traffic Offences in Western Australia*, Report no. RR 13-001; Curtin-Monash Accident Research Centre: Bentley, Australia; 2014.

Panenka WJ, Procyshyn RM, Lecomte T, MacEwan GW, Flynn SW, Honer WG, Barr AM: Methamphetamine use: A comprehensive review of molecular, preclinical and clinical findings; *Drug Alcohol Depend* 129:167; 2013.

Pelissier-Alicot AL, Gaulier JM, Champsaur P, Marquet P: Mechanisms underlying postmortem redistribution of drugs: A review; *J Anal Toxicol* 27:533; 2003.

Porath-Waller AJ, Beirness DJ: An examination of the validity of the standardized field sobriety test in detecting drug impairment using data from the drug evaluation and classification program; *Traffic Inj Prev* 15:125; 2014.

Poulsen H, Moar R, Pirie R: The culpability of drivers killed in New Zealand road crashes and their use of alcohol and other drugs; *Accid Anal Prev* 67:119; 2014.

Ramaekers JG: Drugs and driving research in medicinal drug development; *Trends Pharmacol Sci* 38:319; 2017.

Ramaekers JG, Berghaus G, van Laar M, Drummer OH: Dose related risk of motor vehicle crashes after cannabis use; *Drug Alcohol Depend* 73:109; 2004.

Ramaekers JG, Kauert G, Theunissen EL, Toennes SW, Moeller MR: Neurocognitive performance during acute THC intoxication in heavy and occasional cannabis users; *J Psychopharmacol* 23:266; 2009.

Ramaekers JG, Kuypers KP, Bosker WM, Brookhuis KA, Veldstra JA, Simons R, Martens M, Hjalmdahl M, Forsman A, Knoche A: Effects of stimulant drugs on actual and simulated driving: Perspectives from four experimental studies conducted as part of the DRUID research consortium; *Psychopharmacology* (Berl) 222:413; 2012.

Ramaekers JG, Moeller MR, van Ruitenbeek P, Theunissen EL, Schneider E, Kauert G: Cognition and motor control as a function of delta(9)-THC concentration in serum and oral fluid: Limits of impairment; *Drug Alcohol Depend* 85:114; 2006.

Ramaekers JG, van Wel JH, Spronk DB, Toennes SW, Kuypers KP, Theunissen EL, Verkes RJ: Cannabis and tolerance: Acute drug impairment as a function of cannabis use history; *Sci Rep* 6:26843; 2016a.

Ramaekers JG, van Wel JH, Spronk DB, Toennes SW, Kuypers KP, Theunissen EL, Verkes RJ: Erratum: Cannabis and tolerance: Acute drug impairment as a function of cannabis use history; *Sci Rep* 6:31939; 2016b.

Ray WA, Fought RL, Decker MD: Psychoactive drugs and the risk of injurious motor vehicle crashes in elderly drivers; *Am J Epidemiol* 136:873; 1992.

Robbe HW, O'Hanlon JF: *Marijuana and Actual Driving Performance* (DOT HS 808 078); National Highway Traffic Safety Administration: Washington, DC; 1996.

Robertson MD, Drummer OH: Responsibility analysis: A methodology to study the effects of drugs in driving; *Accid Anal Prev* 26:243; 1994.

Røgeberg O: A meta-analysis of the crash risk of cannabis-positive drivers in culpability studies-Avoiding interpretational bias; *Accid Anal Prev* 123:69; 2019.

Røgeberg O, Elvik R: The effects of cannabis intoxication on motor vehicle collision revisited and revised; *Addiction* 111:1348; 2016.

Røgeberg O, Elvik R, White M: Correction to: The effects of cannabis intoxication on motor vehicle collision revisited and revised (2016); *Addiction* 113:967; 2018.

Salmi LR, Orriols L, Lagarde E: Comparing responsible and non-responsible drivers to assess determinants of road traffic collisions: Time to standardise and revisit; *Inj Prev* 20:380; 2014.

Schnabel E, Hargutt V, Krüger HP: *Meta-Analysis of Empirical Studies Concerning the Effects of Alcohol on Safe Driving*, DRUID Deliverable D 1.1.2a; University of Würzburg: Würzburg, Germany; 2010.

Schulz KF, Grimes DA: Case-control studies: Research in reverse; *Lancet* 359:431; 2002.

Schulz M, Iwersen-Bergmann S, Andresen H, Schmoldt A: Therapeutic and toxic blood concentrations of nearly 1,000 drugs and other xenobiotics; *Crit Care* 16:R136; 2012.

Schulze H, Schumacher M, Urmeew R, Auerbach K, Alvarez J, Bernhoft IM, de Gier H, Hagenzieker M, Houwing S, Knoche A, et al.: *Driving Under the Influence of Drugs, Alcohol and Medicines in Europe—Findings from the DRUID Project*; Publications Office of the European Union: Luxembourg; 2012.

Schweitzer JB, Holcomb HH: Drugs under investigation for attention-deficit hyperactivity disorder; *Curr Opin Investig Drugs* 3:1207; 2002.

Schwope DM, Bosker WM, Ramaekers JG, Gorelick DA, Huestis MA: Psychomotor performance, subjective and physiological effects and whole blood delta(9)-tetrahydrocannabinol concentrations in heavy, chronic cannabis smokers following acute smoked cannabis; *J Anal Toxicol* 36:405; 2012.

Sewell RA, Poling J, Sofuoglu M: The effect of cannabis compared with alcohol on driving; *Am J Addict* 18:185; 2009.

Shechtman O, Classen S, Awadzi K, Mann W: Comparison of driving errors between on-the-road and simulated driving assessment: A validation study; *Traffic Inj Prev* 10:379; 2009.

Shyhalla K: Alcohol involvement and other risky driver behaviors: Effects on crash initiation and crash severity; *Traffic Inj Prev* 15:325; 2014.

Signorello LB, McLaughlin JK, Lipworth L, Friis S, Sorensen HT, Blot WJ: Confounding by indication in epidemiologic studies of commonly used analgesics; *Am J Ther* 9:199; 2002.

Smink BE, Egberts AC, Lusthof KJ, Uges DR, de Gier JJ: The relationship between benzodiazepine use and traffic accidents: A systematic literature review; *CNS Drugs* 24:639; 2010.

Tefft BC, Arnold LS, Grabowski JG: *Prevalence of Marijuana Involvement in Fatal Crashes: Washington, 2010–2014*; AAA Foundation for Traffic Safety: Washington, DC; 2016.

Terhune KW: *The Role of Alcohol, Marijuana, and Other Drugs in the Accidents of Injured Drivers. Volume 1—Findings* (DOT HS 806 199); National Highway Traffic Safety Administration: Washington, DC; 1982.

Thomas RE: Benzodiazepine use and motor vehicle accidents. Systematic review of reported association; *Can Fam Physician* 44:799; 1998.

TIRF: *Marijuana use among drivers in Canada, 2000–2015*; Traffic Injury Research Foundation: Ottawa, ON, Canada; 2018.

Tourangeau R, Yan T: Sensitive questions in surveys; *Psychol Bull* 133:859; 2007.

Traynor TL: The impact of driver alcohol use on crash severity: A crash specific analysis; *Transp Res Part E Logist Transp Rev* 41:421; 2005.

Valen A, Bogstrand ST, Vindenes V, Gjerde H: Increasing use of cannabis among arrested drivers in Norway; *Traffic Inj Prev* 18:801; 2017a.

Valen A, Bogstrand ST, Vindenes V, Gjerde H: Toxicological findings in suspected drug-impaired drivers in Norway—Trends during 1990–2015; *Forensic Sci Int* 280:15; 2017b.

Veldstra JL, Bosker WM, de Waard D, Ramaekers JG, Brookhuis KA: Comparing treatment effects of oral THC on simulated and on-the-road driving performance: Testing the validity of driving simulator drug research; *Psychopharmacology* (Berl) 232:2911; 2015.

Verster JC, Mets MA: Psychoactive medication and traffic safety; *Int J Environ Res Public Health* 6:1041; 2009.

Verster JC, Ramaekers JG: The on-the-road driving test; In Verster JC, Pandi-Perumal SR, Ramaekers JD, de Gier JJ (Eds): *Drugs, Driving and Traffic Safety*; Birkhäuser Basel: Basel, Switzerland; p. 83; 2009.

Verstraete AG: Detection times of drugs of abuse in blood, urine, and oral fluid; *Ther Drug Monit* 26:200; 2004.

Verstraete AG, Legrand SA, Vandam L, Hughes B, Griffiths B: *Drug Use, Impaired Driving, and Traffic Accidents*, 2nd ed; Publications Office of the European Union: Luxembourg; 2014.

Vindenes V, Jordbru D, Knapskog AB, Kvan E, Mathisrud G, Slørdal L, Mørland J: Impairment based legislative limits for driving under the influence of non-alcohol drugs in Norway; *Forensic Sci Int* 219:1; 2012.

Voas RB, Torres P, Romano E, Lacey JH: Alcohol-related risk of driver fatalities: An update using 2007 data; *J Stud Alcohol Drugs* 73:341; 2012.

Walsh JM, de Gier JJ, Christophersen AS, Verstraete AG: Drugs and driving; *Traffic Inj Prev* 5:241; 2004.

Walsh JM, Huestis MA, Mørland J: *Guidelines for Drugged Driving Research. The Talloires Report*; The Walsh Group: Bethesda, MD; 2007.

Walsh JM, Verstraete AG, Huestis MA, Mørland J: Guidelines for research on drugged driving; *Addiction* 103:1258; 2008.

Wetherell A: Performance tests; *Environ Health Perspect* 104 Suppl 2:247; 1996.

Wood E, Brooks-Russell A, Drum P: Delays in DUI blood testing: Impact on cannabis DUI assessments; *Traffic Inj Prev* 17:105; 2016.

World Health Organization: *Global Status Report on Road Safety 2015*; World Health Organization: Geneva, Switzerland; 2015.

Zador PL, Krawchuk SA, Voas RB: Alcohol-related relative risk of driver fatalities and driver involvement in fatal crashes in relation to driver age and gender: An update using 1996 data; *J Stud Alcohol* 61:387; 2000.

Vehicle Safety Features Aimed at Preventing Alcohol-Related Crashes*

16

ROBERT B. VOAS

Contents

* This chapter is an updated version (format only) of a review article previously published in *Forensic Science Review*: Voas RB: Vehicle safety features aimed at preventing alcohol-related crashes; *Forensic Sci Rev* 32:55; 2020.

16.1 Introduction

16.1.1 Objectives of This Chapter

It is well understood by safety researchers and policymakers that highway crashes involve three factors: the driver, the vehicle, and the roadway. However, when it comes to the special category of alcohol-related crashes, the driver receives most of the attention. This is logical given that overconsumption of alcohol impairs both cognitive and psychomotor functioning and increases the risk of crashes and injuries on roadways. This review chronicles the substantial success that has been achieved through laws and programs focused on the drinking driver, which have included a broad range of activities such as educating the public and treating problem drinkers, as well as enacting and enforcing driving-while-impaired (DWI) laws. Progress in both roadway and automotive technology has produced substantial safety benefits, some of which are particularly relevant to reducing alcohol-related crashes. However, because of the more limited understanding of the role played by the motor vehicle and the roadway, those achievements have not been recognized as contributions to impaired driving programs. This article attempts to highlight the role of automotive technology and the public policies related to motor vehicle operation on the observed reduction in alcohol-related crashes during the twentieth century and the expected impact of vehicle factors in the twenty-first century.

16.1.2 Automobiles and Alcohol—A Deadly Relationship

The automobile is a complex vehicle that taxes key human capabilities—especially when impaired by alcohol—such as balance, attention (particularly divided attention), vision, coordination, hearing, and judgment. The appearance and rapid growth in numbers of automobiles in the twentieth century (e.g., 36 motor vehicle traffic fatalities in 1900, 36,688 in 1955) in the heavy-drinking US culture led to 1.4 million deaths in alcohol-related vehicle crashes during the twentieth century (US National Center for Statistics and Analysis 2003). These road-traffic deaths occurred despite the fact that per-capita alcohol consumption did not increase during the same period, suggesting the significance of the automobile in the epidemic of alcohol-related deaths. The private vehicles available in the nineteenth century involved slow-moving, relatively lightweight conveyances (mainly horsedrawn carriages); the twentieth century saw heavy, high-speed cars in the hands of individual owners. The combination of weight and speed in the automobile produced high acceleration loads (*g*) on a vehicle and its driver in the event of a crash.

Although there are many different types of vehicles on the road, the private vehicle became the principal source of the problem. Commercial drivers were subject to many controls not placed on the operator of a family car. In an occupational setting, employers screen applicants to select the most qualified for the job of driving heavy and potentially dangerous modes of transport. Once selected, employees are trained to operate equipment maintained by experts and work under supervisors who are empowered to terminate those who are not performing adequately. Thus, commercial transportation companies have a number of safety features that reduce the impact of an inebriated operator.

The private automobile presents a strong contrast to other industries that use vehicles. It places powerful devices in the hands of individuals who may select a vehicle for qualities such as high speed and performance rather than safety, maintain their vehicles erratically, and drive them carelessly with little or no training and no monitoring by a supervisor. This makes the driver/vehicle unit a sensitive detector of alcohol problems in a heavy-drinking society. This difference between private compared to commercial drivers is reflected in studies of fatally injured drivers, which have found that only 1% of commercial drivers in fatal crashes have illegal blood alcohol concentration (BAC) levels (≥0.08%) compared to 23% of private car drivers (Fell et al. 2009).

A fundamental feature of the private automobile that makes it such a strong national marker for potential alcohol-related crashes is its deep penetration in the US population; 87% of US citizens have driver licenses, and 85% of US households own at least one car (US Federal Bureau of Investigation 2018). Thus, while commercial transportation firms experience alcohol-related fatalities, the number of such fatalities is small relative to those involving private vehicles.

Consider, for example, what might have occurred in the twentieth century if urban Americans had relied on public transportation: trolleys, buses, subways, trains, and aircraft. Since transportation workers are trained and monitored, alcohol-related crashes would occur but be limited to a small number—not nearly enough to produce the epidemic of 1.4 million deaths. The automobile not only became the primary transportation for urban dwellers, it also revised urban lifestyle by being the prime enabler for the growth of suburban communities around urban centers.

16.1.3 Factors Related to the Effectiveness of Vehicle-Based Alcohol Safety Programs

It is well understood by safety researchers and safety activists that three factors play a role in crash causation: the driver, the vehicle, and the roadway environment. Within those three elements it is important to understand the difference between policies directed at influencing human behavior and dependent for their effectiveness on human action and policies that force conformity by changing the environment in which the behavior occurs. This framework is illustrated in Table 16.1. Impaired driving laws seek to deter impaired driving but fail to influence some drivers, while state prohibition laws seek to make drinking impossible to all drivers. Safety belts are only effective if used by the driver, whereas shatterproof windshield glass is present without any special action by the driver. Similarly, the driver may ignore speed limits, but the guardrail is always present.

The structural elements that reduce crashes and ameliorate injury are not generally viewed as "alcohol" countermeasures. They provide major safety benefits to all drivers. However, those programs that reduce crash risk and particularly those that limit crash injuries are particularly beneficial to impaired drivers, as shown in Figure 16.1. Drivers with a BAC of 0.15% are at 80 times the risk of crashing compared to a sober driver (Zador et al. 2000b). The much higher risk that drinking drivers, particularly heavy-drinking drivers, have of being in a crash shows that they clearly benefit more than the average driver from any program that lowers risk of crashing or reduces the extent of injury from crash involvement.

A third dimension on which safety programs can be arrayed is the proportion of the US population at risk that is covered by the program. Here the major difference arises from programs that affect *all* drivers, versus programs limited to the much smaller population of DWI offenders. Lund et al. (2012) calculated the relative value of a system that

Table 16.1 Safety Action Laws and Programs for Alcohol Crashes

	Programs Aimed at *Individual Behavior* Change to Prevent Harm	Programs Aimed at *Structural* Change to Prevent Harm
Drivers	DWI laws	Minimum drinking age laws
	License suspension	State alcohol control laws
	Public education programs	State responsible beverage service laws
Vehicles	Safety belts	Occupant protection system
	Turn signals	Safety belt interlocks
	Speed limit laws	Power breaks
Roadways	Speed limits	Guard rails
	Traffic lights	Freeways
	Warning signs	Breakaway signs

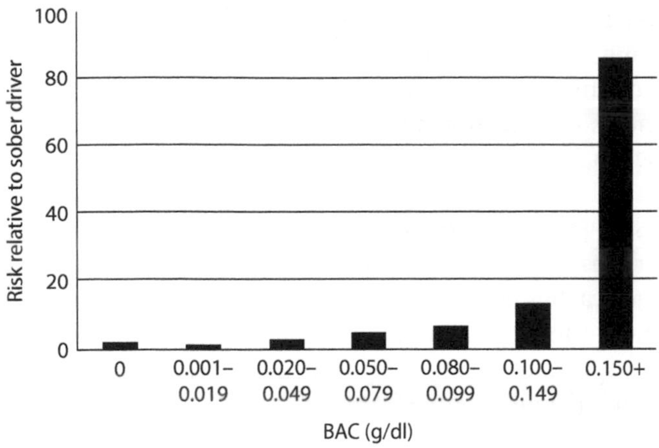

Figure 16.1 Relative risk of a driver being involved in a fatal road traffic crash in relation to BAC at autopsy compared to a sober driver. (Reproduced with permission from Lund, A.K. et al., *Contribution of Alcohol-Impaired Driving to Motor Vehicle Crash Deaths in 2010,* Insurance Institute for Highway Safety, Arlington, VA, 2012.)

prevented crashes involving *all* drivers with BACs > 0.02%, which they predicted would prevent 10,699 deaths compared to the same system applied only to DWI offenders, which would only be expected to save 785 lives.

16.1.4 Four Vehicle-Based Alcohol-Related Safety Program Areas

Automotive technology is advancing rapidly, and auto companies are competing to make driving easier and safer. Since alcohol impairs skills related to driving, any technological advance that makes operating an automobile easier or safer can be viewed as an alcohol-related safety measure. However, there are four areas in which vehicle-based programs are particularly effective in reducing alcohol-related injuries or where the program has been specifically designed to reduce alcohol-related crashes. These four areas are based on logical approaches to using the vehicle to reduce alcohol-related crashes:

- ***Reduce crash harm through occupant-protection programs:*** The first of these is the implementation of occupant-protection systems to ameliorate or prevent driver and passenger injuries in the event of a crash. Because alcohol-impaired drivers, depending on their BAC, are at much greater risk of crashing than sober drivers, they and their passengers profit substantially more than the average driver from vehicle features that protect them from injury. While vehicle crashworthiness protects all drivers and reduces injuries in all crashes, it should have its greatest impact on injury levels in alcohol-related crashes.
- ***Prevent drivers convicted of impaired driving from owning a car through vehicle registration laws:*** The attempt to prevent the driving of convicted DWI offenders

through driver license suspension has been limited by the difficulty in preventing illicit driving. Some states have adopted policies directed at separating offenders from their vehicles through cancellation of the vehicle registration or vehicle impoundment or confiscation for a DWI conviction or for unlicensed driving. Unlike the occupant-protection programs, these policies specifically target DWI offenders.

- ***Test driver sobriety and prevent starting the vehicle through an ignition interlock:*** Perhaps the most efficient and effective vehicle method for preventing alcohol-related crashes is to screen the driver for impairment. If every vehicle was fitted with an interlock, this might produce a major reduction in alcohol-related crashes. Three approaches have been taken to screening the driver: (a) measure the driver's BAC, (b) apply a performance test that measures impairment of the driver, or (c) use a feature of the vehicle operation to test the extent of driver impairment.
- ***Simplify the driving task to allow impaired drivers to operate the vehicle safely through vehicle automation:*** Making the driver's task less demanding lowers the challenge to the capability of the impaired driver and increases the possibility of avoiding a crash. The simplification of vehicle operation will progress in three steps: (a) vehicle warning systems, (b) automatic crash-avoidance systems, and (c) partially and fully automated (self-driving) vehicles. In twentieth-century cars, the driver had little assistance from crash-prevention systems, and driving presented a substantial challenge to the driver's alertness and mental condition. Current trends suggest that as we progress toward the development of self-driving vehicles in the twenty-first century, the number of automated crash-prevention systems in vehicles will increase, reducing the dependence on the competence of drivers and the significance of BAC to crash involvement. Ultimately, when/if self-driving vehicles take over the roads, alcohol-related crashes will fade away.

In this article, the opportunities and problems in implementing vehicle safety programs in each of the four areas are reviewed.

16.2 Reducing Harm from Crash Involvement

16.2.1 Occupant Protection—An Early Vehicle Safety Program

During the first half of the twentieth century, vehicle technology steadily improved, making cars easier to drive. However, much of the potential value of such safety features was reduced by customers' preference for powerful high-speed vehicles, which were promoted in sales programs by most car companies. One might assume that as cars became easier to drive and less taxing on the brain, impaired drivers could benefit more than sober drivers, but that impaired drivers could still be more dangerous in powerful high-speed vehicles. However, in the early years before the development of accurate state record systems and the establishment of the national Fatality Analysis Reporting System (FARS), adequate data to relate vehicle factors to alcohol involvement were not available. Publication of Ralph Nader's book *Unsafe at Any Speed* in 1965 (Nader 1965) changed public attitudes about vehicle safety and stimulated efforts to protect vehicle occupants in a crash. This led to two basic

Table 16.2 Examples of Vehicle Occupant Protection Programs

Protecting the Passenger Compartment	Keeping Passengers Safe and in Place
Crushable structure to absorb crash impact	Safety belts
Strengthen vehicle frame	Safety belt interlocks
Roll-over protection	Safety belt warning systems
Strengthen doors to prevent passenger ejection	Air bags
Removal of interior hazards	Child restraint seats
Installing shatterproof glass windscreen	Safety belt laws

programs that: (a) maintain the integrity of the passenger cabin to keep it from collapsing and thus injuring the occupants; and (b) prevent the passengers from being thrown against the dashboard or wall of the cabin, or being thrown outside into the roadway (Table 16.2).

16.2.2 Vehicle Crashworthiness

This effort focused on strengthening the frame of the vehicle, providing a front-end crush area to reduce the *g*-force level on impact, rollover protection, shatterproof glass, and the elimination of internal protrusions into the cabin. All of these safety features are passive, requiring no action by the driver other than purchasing vehicles equipped with these features. Since impaired drivers have a higher probability of crashing, these safety features have greater value to the drinking driver; unfortunately, however, studies have indicated that traffic offenders in alcohol-related crashes are more likely to drive older vehicles without these safety features.

16.2.3 Safety Belts

Perhaps the most important vehicle-safety regulation promulgated by the National Highway Traffic Safety Administration (NHTSA) was the requirement that manufacturers install safety belts in their vehicles. The main limit on their effectiveness has been that they require an action by the driver. Initially (1976), only 20% of American drivers fastened their belts. The passage by the states of mandatory safety belt laws in the 1980s increased the usage to about 50%. By the end of the century, enforcement of safety belt laws raised the usage rate to 80%, and by 2018, NHTSA reported that the usage rate reached 89.6%, and that safety belts had saved 14,955 lives in 2017 (Li and Pickrell 2018). However, 47% of the passengers killed in highway crashes in 2017 were not buckled up. Had they been wearing belts, 2,549 additional lives would have been saved. There is strong evidence that impaired drivers are less likely to buckle up, and nonuse of the safety belt has even been used by the police as a clue to identify impaired drivers. As a result of this relationship between belt use and drinking, mandatory safety belt laws have a greater potential benefit for impaired than for sober drivers.

16.2.4 Safety Belt Interlocks

The crashworthiness safety features described above are passive and do not require activation by the driver. This is also true of design features such as antilock brakes that function automatically when needed. But as illustrated in the case of safety belts, safety features that require activation by the driver can be substantially degraded by the failure of the operator to enable them. Given the very substantial benefits of safety belts when used and the frustrating non-use levels, in 1974 NHTSA issued a rule requiring that all vehicles be equipped with interlocks, which sensed the presence of the driver and front-seat passenger and prevented ignition of the automobile if the appropriate safety belt was not fastened. This had obvious special safety value for impaired drivers given their high non-use rate. Unfortunately, the driving public strongly objected to the inconvenience of this innovation, which, among other problems, prevented starting the vehicle when there was a heavy bag in the right-hand seat, and Congress voted to cancel the rule.

16.2.5 Safety Belt Use Laws and Warning Systems

The failure to adopt safety belt interlocks left the problem of persuading drivers to buckle up to the passage of state laws making it an infraction to be an unbelted front-seat passenger. The trend to adopt such laws was spurred by "First Ride–Safe Ride" programs providing parents with safety-reinforced baby carriers for attachment to car seats as well as promoting the use of child-safety seats and the placing of children in the rear seats of vehicles. Child-restraint programs broke ground for adult belt laws, which were implemented at two levels. At the first level, police were only allowed to issue a ticket to motorists legally stopped for other highway offenses such as speeding. The second level allowed police to stop and cite drivers who were unbelted. These laws were augmented by engineering a vehicle warning system that actuated when an unbelted occupant was sensed by the restraint system. Considerable research effort was expended in developing an on/off program with increasing frequency and volume sufficient to promote action without stimulating unacceptable annoyance.

16.2.6 Air Bags

The non-use of safety belts and the failure of belt interlocks focused attention on an emerging technology, namely use of exploding gas to inflate air bags within milliseconds in the period between the vehicle contacting a barrier and the driver's body contacting the steering wheel. Initially, this technology appeared to offer an automatic substitute for seat belts. However, when early models were placed in vehicles it turned out that air bags that deployed with enough force to stop the unbelted driver could injure children and small adults who were out of normal position (e.g., adjusting the radio). As a result, air bag technology was modified to be an adjunct to the safety belts to deal with off-center and side-impact crashes where air bags play an important role in increasing the effectiveness of seat belts but are not a replacement for them. Because they deploy automatically, they are of special benefit to impaired drivers.

16.3 Prevent DWI Offenders from Owning or Operating a Vehicle

16.3.1 Vehicle Licensing Programs

States maintain control over the traffic on their highways by licensing drivers and vehicles. State driver-licensing programs include many special features directed at reducing impaired driving, including better driver education, licensing age limits, remedial driver training, treatment programs for offenders, and license suspension/revocation, the ultimate sanction for impaired driving. But these programs are directed at drivers and fall outside the subject matter of this chapter. State vehicle licensing programs, while also primarily directed at traffic control, contain elements directed at impaired driving. These include actions to separate high-risk drivers from their vehicles through the confiscation of the vehicle plate and/or a requirement of special plates or tags on the car (see Voas and DeYoung [2002] for a general review of vehicle license cancellation and impoundment programs). Because up to two-thirds of those suspended still drive (McCartt et al. 2002; Ross and Gonzales 1988) and are difficult for police to detect unless they commit a traffic offense, the removal of the license plate or marking the license plate to indicate that the driver may be unlicensed is a powerful deterrent to impaired driving.

A national survey (Voas 1992) identified 12 states with legislation requiring the suspension of the registration of an offender-owned vehicle for the same length of time as the driver license suspension upon a DWI conviction. However, this tough sanction was frequently ameliorated by allowing registration restoration upon the demonstration that the owner had appropriate vehicle insurance (Voas and DeYoung 2002). Two states (Ohio and Minnesota) went further, requiring that convicted drivers turn in their vehicle plates and replace them with special "family plates" that the police could identify and use as a basis for stopping the vehicle to check that it was not being driven by the convicted driver. This process was implemented to allow driving by innocent family members while deterring the offender from using the vehicle. For third-time DWI offenders, Minnesota took the further step of having the police confiscate the plates when making the arrest. Rodgers found that application of this procedure reduced recidivism by 50% compared to third-time offenders who avoided having their plates confiscated (Rodgers 1994).

The states of Oregon and Washington enacted laws allowing the arresting police officer who apprehended an unlicensed driver to place a striped "zebra" tag over the issue date of the vehicle plate to alert enforcement officers to check the vehicle's driver. Non-offender owners of a vehicle driven by an unlicensed driver had to prove they had not permitted the offender to drive. Voas et al. found reductions in both states in alcohol-related offenses, but only the result in Oregon was statistically significant (Voas et al. 1997a). Both states discontinued the policy shortly after the study. The authority to confiscate license plates and to refuse to issue plates to convicted offenders gives state motor vehicle departments considerable power to limit driving by individuals convicted of a DWI offense, but few states have chosen to make extensive use of that authority.

16.3.2 Vehicle Impoundment Programs

At the time of a DWI arrest, the police generally take control of the vehicle driven by the offender and have it towed to a city impound lot where it can be picked up the following day upon payment of a towing and storage fee. This gets the vehicle out of the traffic flow and prevents the offender from recovering it while still intoxicated. Several states have implemented programs to extend the possession of the vehicle as a penalty for the DWI conviction and as a means of discouraging illegal driving by suspended offenders. In a national survey conducted in 1992 (Voas 1992), 10 states had vehicle impoundment/forfeiture laws. In most of those states, that sanction was infrequently applied, making evaluation difficult. Three states implemented programs large enough to make an evaluation possible.

In 1995 California enacted a law that allowed police to impound for 30 days the vehicle of offenders who were apprehended for driving with suspended or revoked licenses. To determine the specific deterrent impact of that law, DeYoung used propensity matching to compare the 12-month driving records of offenders whose vehicles were impounded with a similar group who did not suffer that sanction (DeYoung 1999). Offenders whose vehicles were impounded had 14% fewer DWI arrests, 18% fewer moving violations, and 25% fewer crashes. A later study of whether the impoundment law had a general deterrent effect on the general driving population produced inconclusive results (DeYoung 2000).

The impact of a state law providing for 30–60 days of impoundment for a first DWI offense and 90–180 days for a second DWI offense was evaluated by Voas in two Ohio jurisdictions: Franklin County (Voas et al. 1997b) and Hamilton County (Voas et al. 1998a). The studies produced similar results for the year in which the sanction was applied. Compared to similar offenders whose vehicles were not impounded, the recidivism rate for those who did suffer the sanction was 60% lower while their vehicles were impounded and 30% lower after their vehicles' return. The reason for the lower recidivism following the restoration of the vehicle is unclear. One factor may have been that those offenders who were driving vehicles belonging to others remained without a vehicle because they did not get access to the returned vehicle.

16.3.3 Vehicle Forfeiture Programs

In 1989, Portland, OR, enacted a law mandating that vehicles driven by suspended DWI drivers were a public nuisance and were subject to forfeiture to the city. That policy was evaluated through a comparison of the driving records of all offenders whose vehicles were seized by the city over a 5-year period (1990–1995) with a similar group of offenders whose vehicles were not forfeited (Crosby 1995). The study showed a 50% reduction in the rearrest rate for those whose vehicles were seized by the city.

A unique and interesting application of a forfeiture law was introduced in New York City in 1999 (Safir et al. 2000). The law empowered the New York Police Department to seize the vehicles of convicted DWI offenders and institute forfeiture proceedings against those owned by the offender. Between February and December of 1999, 1,458 vehicles were seized and 827 forfeiture actions were initiated. A special settlement policy allowed the vehicle to be returned to the offender on completion of a treatment program and the payment of a fee to cover administrative costs. Unfortunately, that program was never evaluated for impact on DWI arrest rates or offender recidivism.

In 1995, California augmented its 30-day impoundment program for first offenders with a forfeiture penalty for multiple offenders. However, while the impoundment penalty was widely implemented across the state only a few communities attempted to employ the forfeiture law. This was apparently the result of four factors: (a) vehicles not owned by the offender were not subject to forfeiture, (b) the cost to the locality of prosecuting the cases was substantial, (c) the value of the vehicles when sold was not adequate to reimburse the government, and (d) the forfeiture process was generally cumbersome and time-consuming. As a result of the low utilization of forfeiture programs, the impact on multiple-DWI offender recidivism could not be measured (Peck and Voas 2000, 2002).

16.4 Testing Driver Sobriety to Prevent Drinkers from Starting a Car

There are three basic approaches when the vehicle is used to detect impaired operators and prevent them from driving:

- Measure the amount of the impairing substance in the driver's body and prevent engine ignition (a blood alcohol content [BAC]-detecting interlock).

- Assess the extent of impairment produced by the substance and prevent starting the vehicle (a driver performance interlock).
- Vehicle assessment of driver capability during normal driving and taking control to prevent continued impaired driving (a vehicle safety interlock).

Early (1970s) examples of these three in-vehicle devices include the following.

16.4.1 Alcohol-Detecting Ignition Interlocks

In 1970, the Borg Warner Company brought a vehicle with a functioning BAC interlock to NHTSA headquarters (Voas 1970). While the prototype alcohol-detecting interlock demonstrated in 1970 accurately screened out drivers with measurable BACs, it required substantial further engineering development to ensure reliability and prevent circumvention, which delayed its introduction until 1990. Work was required to ensure reliability over at least a month and hardening of its sampling system against tampering and attempts to bypass the required breath sample. The current interlock (Figure 16.2) can be installed on most vehicles to prevent a drinking driver from starting a car. Typically, it consists of two units: a handheld breath-test unit accessible from the driver's-seat position in the vehicle and a box with a computer under the hood, which controls the operation of the system and maintains a time and date record (data logger) of all breath tests and engine ignitions. The threshold BAC level that prevents vehicle ignition can be varied to meet state requirements. To prevent drinking in the vehicle following a successful breath test, a rolling retest is required at random intervals following engine ignition. Security of the system is protected by temperature and flow sampling in the breath-test unit and by power connection sensors to the vehicle. Initially, DWI offenders had to bring their vehicles to the installer for monthly calibration and functional checks and download of log data. A recent major enhancement has been the development of Wi-Fi transmission of data providing for real-time reporting of performance.

16.4.2 Driver Performance Interlocks

Also, during the early 1970s, NHTSA assigned the development of a performance interlock to the NHTSA Electronics Laboratory in Boston, where it came in conflict with an ongoing

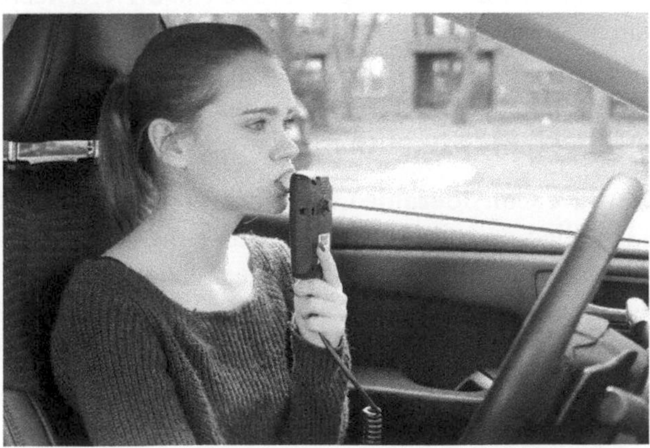

Figure 16.2 Smart start alcohol ignition interlock device (Smart Start, Inc., Grapevine, Texas).

program to develop a vehicle-borne driver cognitive performance test for a vehicle interlock (Sussman and Abernethy 1973). Such an interlock would have the significant advantage of being useful for preventing other dangerous drivers, such as drug users and medicated or drowsy drivers, from operating vehicles while cognitively impaired. Strong support for the performance interlock concept was provided by the work of Moskowitz, who conducted an important set of laboratory experiments relating BAC to the impairment of driving-related skills. He identified divided attention as being particularly sensitive to impairment by alcohol. This test became an important feature of the initial concepts for driver-performance interlocks, which generally featured a tracking task with a peripheral task involving responding to a randomly appearing signal (Sussman and Abernethy 1973). Such an interlock would have the significant advantage of being useful for preventing other types of dangerous drivers, such as drug users and medicated or drowsy drivers, from operating vehicles while cognitively impaired. Attempts to develop such a device (e.g., Klein and Jex [1975]) proved to be difficult owing to day-to-day variation in the alertness of potential drivers. There was too much variation in the subject's performance on the test to develop a reliable cutoff score that would not produce excessive numbers of (a) false positives unnecessarily preventing engine ignition and frustrating users or (b) false negatives that would allow an impaired driver to start the car.

16.4.3 Vehicle Safety Interlocks

In the 1970s, there was also a rather crude example of a vehicle safety interlock on the market called Quick Key, which tested the potential driver's reaction time as part of the engine-ignition process. The driver inserted the key and waited briefly for the sound of a buzzer and as quickly as possible turned the key. If that action was not rapid enough, the engine would not start. The number of Quick Keys installed in vehicles is unknown, but it illustrates the concept of using elements of the driving performance to determine vehicle behaviors, which are only becoming possible as vehicle automation increases.

16.4.4 Interlock Program Description

16.4.4.1 Relationship between License Suspension and the Interlock

The model of the relationship between license suspension and the interlock that has guided this review appears in Figure 16.3. The suspension of the driver's license can occur at two points in the criminal justice process: (a) at the time of arrest under administrative license revocation (ALR) laws if the driver's BAC is at or above 0.08% or under implied consent laws if the offender refuses the BAC test, or (b) at the time of conviction by the judge if the offender violates neither of those administrative laws.

16.4.4.1.1 Offenders Have Considerable Control Over Interlock Installation Because the device must be installed on a vehicle the offender owns or has permission to drive, mandatory courts and state motor vehicle departments have been forced to recognize that the lack of a vehicle is a basis for not participating in an interlock program (Voas 2007). This has allowed offenders to claim not to have a vehicle, and this (in addition to inefficiency in court probation follow-up and vehicle registration checks) has been a significant factor in the failure of most states to achieve installment rates for arrested DWI offenders above 50%. Given the offender's influence on the installation processes, the model in Figure 16.3 centers on the installation decision: whether to enroll in the interlock program

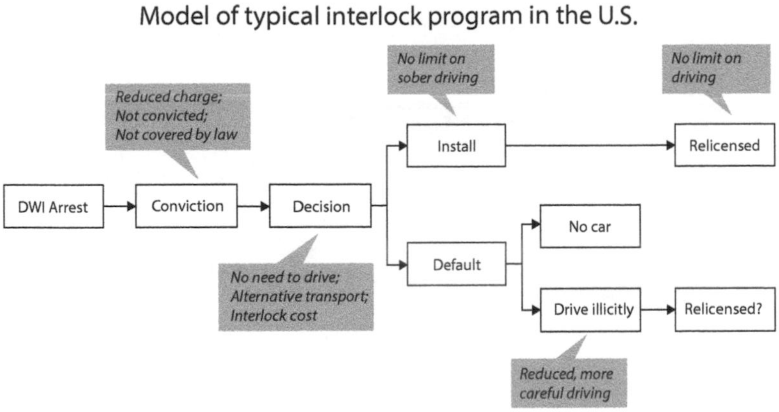

Model of typical interlock program in the U.S.

No limit on sober driving
No limit on driving
Reduced charge; Not convicted; Not covered by law
Install
Relicensed
DWI Arrest
Conviction
Decision
No car
Default
No need to drive; Alternative transport; Interlock cost
Drive illicitly
Relicensed?
Reduced, more careful driving

Figure 16.3 The interlock program model described in this chapter.

or accept the default condition of remaining on a suspended/revoked license for the period specified by the DWI charge. Courts could impose more consequential alternative penalties such as home confinement for interlock refusers but have generally declined to do so. Currently only about a third of those arrested for DWI install interlocks.

16.4.4.1.2 The Offender's Install Decision Has Received Little Study Logic suggests that the install decision is based on three major factors: the need to drive, the availability of alternate transportation opportunities, and the cost and inconvenience of operating a vehicle with an interlock. Those who opt for the interlock have no limit on their driving providing they can start their car, although some states impose a "hardship license," which can limit interlock driving to essential needs such as work and doctor appointments. Once installers complete their time on the interlock, they return to full-license status. The status of those who elect to remain suspended is less clear but can probably be divided into two groups: those who drive illicitly (but potentially with more care to avoid a new arrest) and those who do not drive but make use of other transportation sources (friends, car pools, public transport, bicycles). At what point in time these suspended offenders apply for reinstatement is less clear, particularly among those who have stopped driving.

16.4.4.1.3 Interlocks While on the Offender's Vehicle Are Effective There is persuasive evidence that interlocks while on the offender's car are an effective means of preventing or at least limiting impaired driving by DWI offenders. From early reviews (Corbin and Larkin 1999; Voas et al. 1999) to the more comprehensive meta-analyses (Elder et al. 2011; Willis et al. 2004), and the recent review (Blais et al. 2013), there is now convincing evidence that recidivism is reduced while the unit is on the offender's vehicle but rises following interlock removal.

16.4.4.2 Patterns of Attempts to Drink and Drive While on the Interlock

16.4.4.2.1 Records of Start Attempts An important feature of the interlock is that it records all attempts to start the vehicle. Thus, with the limitation that illegal driving of non-interlock vehicles is not recorded, the record reflects driving frequency and the attempts to drive that are blocked by the interlock. Studies of the patterns of those lockouts provide cues to drinking patterns and to the offender's ability to adapt to the interlock. This is clearly illustrated by the patterns of BAC tests in three different jurisdictions: two Canadian

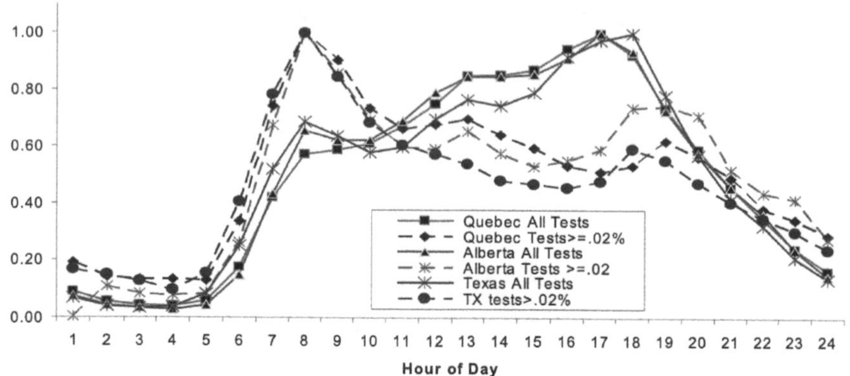

Figure 16.4 Relative rates of interlock BAC tests >0.02 g/dL (dashed lines) and all tests taken (solid lines) over 24-hour periods, Monday to Friday, in Quebec, Alberta, and Texas. Sampling base = 38 million breath tests. (Reproduced with permission from Marques, P.R. et al., *Addiction*, 98(S2),13, 2003b.)

provinces and Texas, shown in Figure 16.4 (Marques et al. 2010b). Of particular interest is the rise in lockouts in the early morning shown in the Texas data in Figure 16.4 and in more detail in data from New Mexico (Figure 16.5) apparently reflecting residual alcohol from heavy drinking the prior evening. Since these drivers could not have started their cars the night before, these cases appear to be associated with drinking at home, relying on friends to drive the night before, or using public transportation (Marques et al. 2010b). This suggests an attempt to adapt to the interlock by separating driving from the time of drinking but failure to accommodate the one-drink-per-hour clearance rate required to return to an alcohol-free condition. Interestingly, a different pattern appears on Saturdays and Sundays, when drinking apparently begins earlier in the day. Clearly the interlock record appears to provide a useful drinking-driving behavior sample for assessing crash risk.

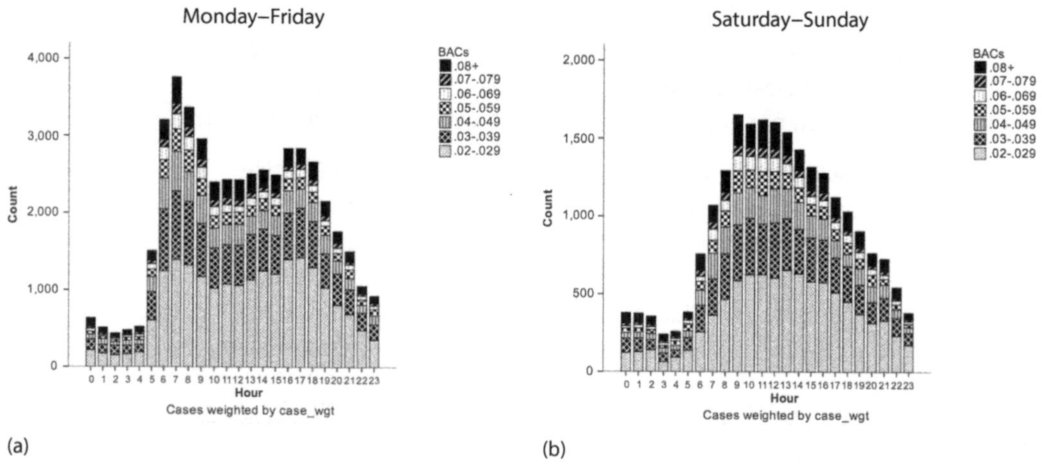

Figure 16.5 BACs of breath tests from attempt to start the vehicle by time of day and day of the week in New Mexico. (a) weekend attempts showing mid-day rise high BAC attempts and (b) week day attempt showing rise in high BAC attempts. (Reproduced from Marques, P.R. et al., *Evaluation of the New Mexico Ignition Interlock Program* (DOT HS 811 410), National Highway Traffic Safety Administration, Washington, DC, 2010b. A publication of the US government.)

16.4.4.2.2 Frequency of Lockouts Decline The frequency of lockouts decreases with time on the interlock as shown in Figure 16.6 (Marques et al. 1999; Vanlaar et al. 2010). This suggests a learning process that leads to a behavioral change that avoids the inconvenience of lockouts. To achieve this result, the offenders must reduce consumption, reduce driving, or avoid drinking in connection with driving. This demonstrates the capability of the offenders to separate drinking from their driving. Initial studies of alcohol consumption and the frequency of driving during the time on the interlock suggest that this reduction in attempts to drink and drive may be achieved without reducing either the amount of alcohol consumed or the amount of driving. As shown in Figure 16.7 (Marques et al. 2010b), alcohol biomarkers can be used to measure changes in drinking quantity from installation to removal of the interlock 8 months later. The researchers stratified the multiple offenders in their study into three groups based on the number of lockouts they experienced while on the interlock and found that whether they had a high or low number of lockouts, their volume of alcohol consumption did not change. They also measured vehicle-start attempts to determine driving frequency while on the interlock. They found no change in their alcohol consumption measures or in driving frequency despite the overall reduction in lockouts produced by the offenders' adaptation to the interlock while it was on their vehicles.

16.4.4.2.3 Failure to Adapt Predicts Recidivism The significance of this adaptation to the interlock is illustrated by its relationship to recidivism subsequent to interlock removal. Frequent lockouts provide evidence that the interlock user is not adapting to the interlock and is not separating drinking from driving. This failure to control drinking while on the interlock is associated with greater recidivism following removal as reported in several studies (Marques et al. 2003a, 2001, 2010a, 2014). This was particularly highlighted by a study tracking the recidivism of 19,959 first-DWI offenders in the Florida interlock

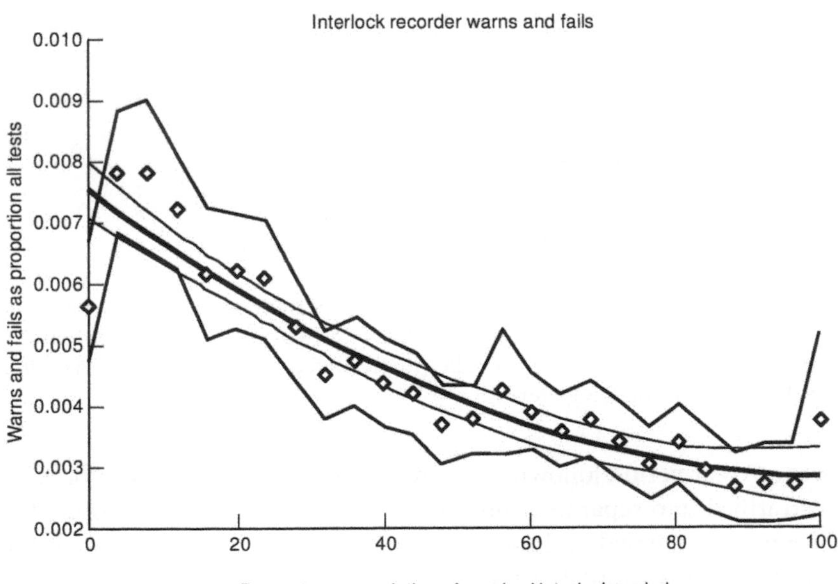

Figure 16.6 While interlocks are installed, the average rate of failed BAC tests declines by about half. (Reproduced with permission from Marques, P.R. et al., *Addiction*, 94, 1861, 1999.)

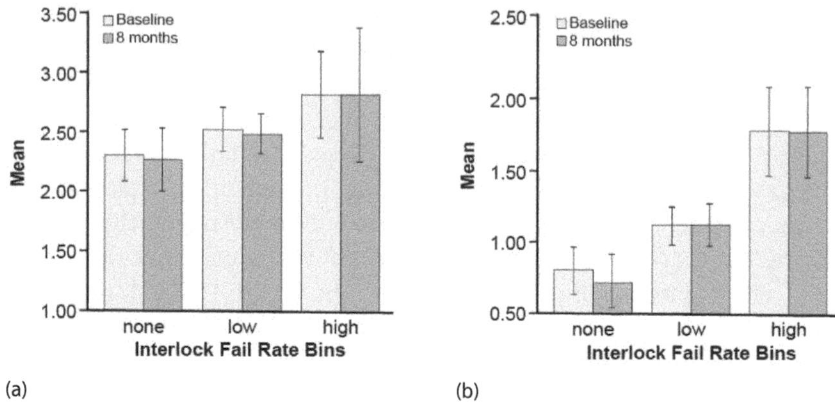

Figure 16.7 No change is shown in total alcohol consumption of interlock users over an 8-month period as determined from analysis of biomarkers %carbohydrate-deficient transferrin (CDT) and phosphatidylethanol (PEth) measured at installation and at removal of the interlock. (a) %CDT Mean +/− 2SE baseline to end and (b) PEth Mean +/− 2SE baseline to end. (Constructed based on data appearing in Marques, P.R. et al., *J. Stud. Alcohol.*, 64, 83, 2003a.)

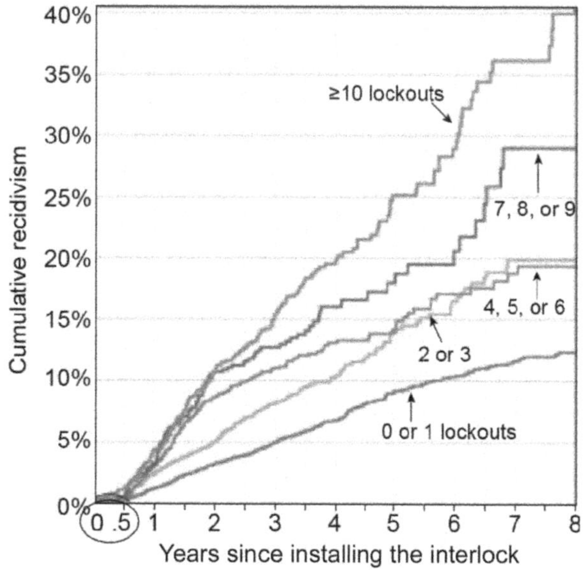

Figure 16.8 Relationship of the number of lockouts experienced by traffic offenders while the unit is on their vehicle for 6 months to their recidivism over the following 7 years. Data based on 19,959 first time DWI offenders in Florida. (Reproduced from Voas, R.B., *Alcohol. Res.*, 36, 81, 2014. A publication of the US government.)

program over a 7-year period following removal of the interlock (Figure 16.8). The participants were stratified into separate groups based on the number of lockouts they experienced in the 6 months (circled in the lower left-hand corner of the figure) that they had the device on their vehicles. Cumulative recidivism survival curves were calculated for each of the five lockout levels (Voas and Tippetts 2013).

The strong relationship between lockouts and recidivism following removal is clear. This relationship between performance on the interlock and recidivism is a long-term

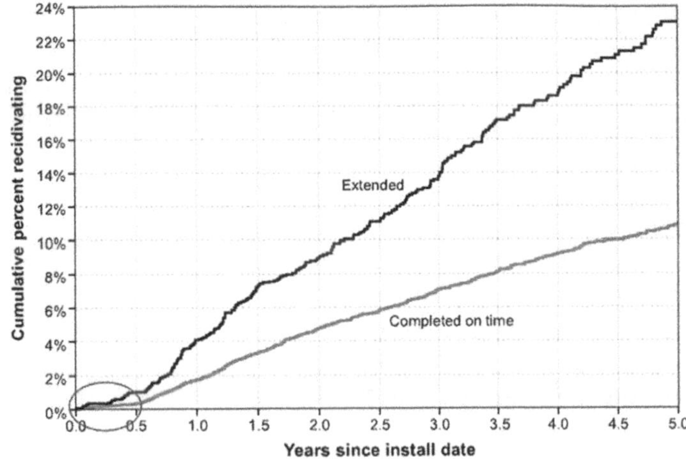

Figure 16.9 Cumulative recidivism over the 5-year period following the installation of the interlock for first DUI offenders in the Florida interlock program, comparing extended and problem cases with offenders completing normally. Based on 33,446 cases. (Reproduced from Voas, R.B., *Alcohol. Res.*, 36, 81, 2014. A publication of the US government.)

effect manifest in administrative decisions on extensions of time on the interlock and in early-withdrawal decisions of the offenders (Voas and Tippetts 2013) (Figure 16.9). An unpublished study of 33,446 first-DWI offenders in Florida convicted between July 2002 and January 2011 found that the annual recidivism rate while on the interlock was .04%; following removal, it rose to 2% for those offenders who completed the interlock period normally. In contrast, those offenders whose time was extended on the interlock because of excessive numbers of lockouts were found to have 4% postremoval recidivism rates, and offenders who dropped out of the program early had 5% annual recidivism rates.

16.4.5 Interlock Performance Provides a Method for Screening DWI Offenders for Treatment

16.4.5.1 Compliance-Based Removal

These results suggest that performance while on the interlock provides a screening method for identifying offenders with a drinking problem. One approach employed by the states is to apply a remedial program called compliance-based removal to this problem by extending the time on the interlock for those users who accumulate excessive numbers of lockouts through policies requiring zero lockouts in the final month or months on the device. The effectiveness of this type of remedial action in reducing postremoval recidivism has not been fully evaluated. However, a test of a policy in Florida banning removal of the interlock in any month in which a lockout occurred still resulted in postremoval recidivism rates markedly higher than for those who completed on time. Apparently, the poor performance on the interlock that led to the extension decision identified high-risk offenders, for which the extended time on the interlock did not fully correct their impaired-driving problem, as shown in Figure 16.9. It is clear that additional research to determine the effectiveness of compliance-based removal is needed.

16.4.5.2 Interlock Educational Interventions

This relationship between lockouts and postremoval recidivism suggests that an opportunity exists to provide intensified monitoring, treatment, and educational programs to support the behavioral adaptation that occurs while the interlock is installed, with an aim to extend the impact of the interlock after it is removed (Marques and Voas 2013). Two studies have demonstrated that intensified monitoring through more frequent contacts with the offender can reduce lockouts while the interlock is installed. An early study in Canada compared a standard interlock program in Saskatchewan with a similar program in Alberta that included a counselor who provided additional information on how the interlock functions and advised the offender on methods for avoiding lockouts. The authors found that the added support (information and counseling) resulted in a statistically significant reduction ($F = 19.79$, $p = .001$) in lockouts during the program (Marques et al. 1999). More recently in Maryland, Zador et al. (2011) demonstrated that an intensive monitoring program involving supportive messages for good behavior and additional sanctions for failures to meet program rules improved performance while on the interlock. Both of these programs involved a substantial increase in instructor resources. The rapid growth in communication technology is opening opportunities to use automation and social media to deliver educational information with more limited personnel costs. A program applying the concepts of the Zador et al. study (Zador et al. 2011)—through which prevention messages based on the user interlock records are automatically generated and transmitted to the offender's cell phone during the period the device is on the vehicle—has been developed but has yet to be evaluated.

16.4.5.3 Treatment While on the Interlock Reduces Recidivism

The Florida interlock program includes an active remedial program designed to identify and intervene with offenders experiencing high lockout rates. On the first occurrence, users receive a counseling session on methods for avoiding lockouts. A second occurrence leads to a requirement for monthly meetings with a program monitor to review their interlock records, while a third lockout results in assignment to an outpatient treatment program. Voas et al. reported on the evaluation of the treatment component of that program (Voas et al. 2016). The postremoval recidivism over a 4-year period of 640 offenders who received the treatment was compared to 806 users not mandated to treatment employing propensity matching. The ignition interlock-plus-treatment group experienced 32% lower recidivism (95% CI; 9%, 49%) following the removal of the interlock. The study estimated that this decline in recidivism would have prevented 41 rearrests, 13 crashes, and 9 injuries in crashes involving the 640 treated offenders over the period following interlock removal (Figure 16.10).

The 32% reduction in recidivism rates is impressive, but there is reason to believe that this result might be improved with a treatment protocol that makes more direct use of interlock performance data in group therapy classes (Marques et al. 2004; Timken et al. 2012). These as-yet unevaluated treatment syllabi tie the treatment program directly to the interlock data-logger reports emanating from the offender's use of the vehicle. They make use of actual instances of failure to control drinking by the users and the data loggers help get rid of denial and develop changes in behavior regarding alcohol use and driving.

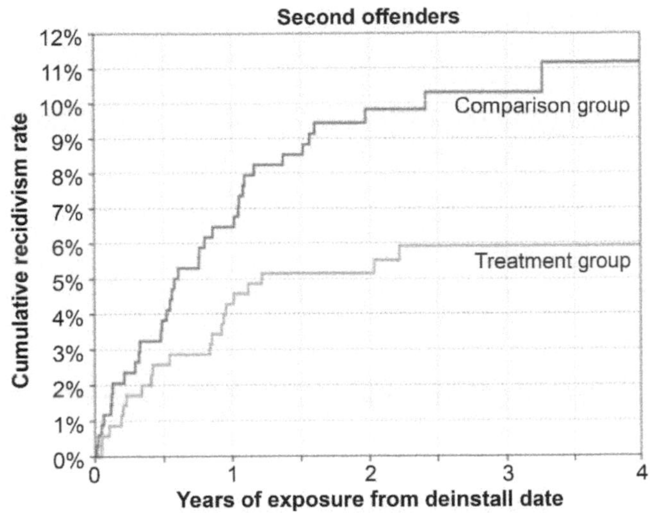

Figure 16.10 Reduction in post-interlock cumulative recidivism for 640 treated vs. 806 untreated DUI offenders in Florida. (Reproduced with permission from Voas, R.B. et al., *Alcohol. Clin. Exp. Res.*, 40, 1953, 2016.)

16.4.6 Interlock Program Implementation

This highlights the prevailing view that alcohol-involved crashes are a driver problem and outside of NHTSA's vehicle rule-making program and symptomatic of the coolness (or indifference) with which the interlock was initially received. Despite this, the interlock is by far the most widely applied of the programs directly focused on the alcohol crash problem, and if these devices had been fitted to all vehicles, they might have come close to solving the problem.

NHTSA left the major engineering effort required to ensure the development of a highly reliable sampling and measuring system and ways to protect the unit against tampering and circumvention to industry. Early models were not very robust, and it was not until a "second generation" of interlocks (Collier 1994) was introduced in the late 1980s that devices with adequate provisions for prevention of tampering and circumvention became available. These included alcohol-specific fuel cells (Collier 1995) (in place of semiconductor sensors); the requirement for special learned skills such as hum-tone recognition, which requires the operator to hum while blowing into the interlock unit, be included to prevent an untrained individual from substituting for a DWI offender; filtered-air detection (prevents blowing through a device that filters out the alcohol); blow abort (detection of too small an air sample); and significantly, the requirement for random rolling retests (i.e., take a retest once the vehicle is in motion to discourage having a person, such as a parking lot attendant, start the vehicle for the offender, or allowing a vehicle to sit idling while the owner drinks). In addition to these safeguards, a breath-alcohol test and engine operation monitor was added to the unit to (a) detect any engine starts not preceded by a breath test and (b) maintain a record of the frequency of vehicle starts that will detect any starts not preceded by a breath test and that creates a record of vehicle use through the number of engine starts each day and detects evidence the vehicle was in use and not simply stored in the driveway, while a substitute vehicle is used. These and similar measures led to devices that were more difficult to circumvent without disabling the system or, if circumvented, would result in registration of the act on a computer record and thus detected when the vehicle was brought in for routine service 1 or 2 months later (US National Highway Traffic Safety Administration 2013; Voas and Marques 1992).

The driving of an alternative non-interlock-equipped vehicle remains the one circumvention procedure that is not well controlled. Some state policies require the installing facility to record the odometer reading when the interlock-equipped vehicle comes in for service and requires that readings below a specific level be reported to the monitoring authority. In an effort to determine the extent to which offenders use alternative non-interlock-equipped vehicles, Roth (2007) conducted a study of the license plate numbers of the vehicles in which interlock program recidivist offenders in New Mexico were arrested. He found that 135 of the 178 cases (76%) were driving the interlock-equipped vehicle. That still left 24% driving a non-interlock-equipped vehicle, suggesting how big a problem use of alternative vehicles may be.

In 1992 NHTSA issued a national standard for interlocks (US National Highway Traffic Safety Administration 2015). A proposal to issue a national standard for state interlock programs (as distinct from the hardware itself) was turned down by NHTSA (Voas and Marques 1992) and as result each state was left free to design its own regulations, resulting in considerable variation in the rigor in both offender and interlock service provider monitoring across the states. NHTSA did issue a guide to state programs in 2014 (Mayer 2014).

16.4.6.1 Three-Step Introduction Process

The interlock was introduced into the criminal justice system in the 1990s, 20 years after Borg Warner displayed the first operating interlock installed in a vehicle at NHTSA as a substitute for the suspension of the driver's license. Interlocks appeared to deal with two important issues: (a) offenders who drive illicitly and become involved in alcohol-related crashes would be prevented from starting their vehicles and (b) offenders who depend on their cars to get to work or on the job would not be prevented from driving if sober. The introduction proceeded in three steps—first with individual judges establishing programs in some localities during the 1990s, which was followed by the states enacting administrative interlock laws empowering motor vehicle departments to allow the substitution of the interlock for license suspension, and finally during the early years of this century culminating in the enactment of mandatory all DWI offender laws for both motor vehicle departments and the courts.

16.4.6.2 Slow Implementation

Interlock usage was slowed initially by judges' concern with the reliability of the units and their cost, which presented a barrier for low-income offenders (Marques et al. 2010b). While these concerns were largely mitigated by the performance of the interlock, the provision of state indigent funds for interlock users and pressure to conform to all DWI laws, a more intractable problem was presented by the rejection of the interlock by the offenders themselves. The latter countered the assumption that the opportunity to drive with an interlock would be preferable to a ban on all driving, through license suspension. Instead, experience has shown that DWI offenders reject installing the device when given the opportunity to substitute the interlock for license suspension.

16.4.6.3 Programs Directed at Increasing Interlock Installations

16.4.6.3.1 License Suspension a Weak Alternative for Motivating Installation While license suspension has served moderately well as a sanction for the DWI offense, it has not proved to be a strong motivator to persuade traffic offenders to install interlocks. The limitation in the power of suspension was illustrated by studies of license-reinstatement rates. Second-DWI offenders frequently delay reinstatement for 3–5 years. It was found that in California two-thirds of first-DWI offenders and 84% of second-DWI offenders remained suspended and did not reinstate their licenses within 3 years of becoming eligible to do so (Tashima and Helander 1999). In a follow-up study covering seven large states with 40 million drivers (Voas et al. 2010), it was found that 42% of first offenders and 55% of multiple offenders delay reinstatement at least a year beyond their date of eligibility and 30% delay beyond 5 years. The reasons for the failure to reinstate the license when eligible in these studies are not clear but a number of factors such as the inability to afford a vehicle and insurance, the necessity of clearing the driver record of previous fines and assessments, and meeting court requirements for treatment appear to play a role.

16.4.6.3.2 DWI Offenders Resisted Installing Interlocks Even though interlocks offer the opportunity to drive legally, many DWI offenders reject their installation. Early state laws provided for the substitution of the interlock for a license suspension. The offender had the option of installing the unit for part or all of the suspension sanction period. However, initial studies (DeYoung 2002; Voas and Marques 2003; Voas et al. 1999) found that only a small portion (10% to 20%) of eligible DWI offenders took advantage of the interlock opportunity (Voas 2001). One example of such low rates was that of 3% among second offenders in West Virginia (Tippetts and Voas 1998). Among the 13 states in a meta-analysis (Elder et al. 2011) for which data on the eligibility to install an interlock were available, nine states reported participation rates of less than 20%. When California enacted a law allowing second-DWI offenders to substitute the interlock for the second year of their 2-year license suspension, only 1 in 10 took advantage of that opportunity (DeYoung et al. 2004). When New Mexico provided multiple-DWI offenders who had received 5- to 10-year suspensions the option of installing interlocks, only 10% opted to do so (Marquest et al. 2010b).

16.4.6.4 Alternative Sanctions More Punitive Than Suspension

16.4.6.4.1 The Alternative of Home Detention To overcome the barrier to interlock installation by offenders claiming not to have a car, an alternative sanction more punitive than license suspension is needed. One alternative implemented in two states was electronically monitored home confinement. The implementation of house arrest as an alternative to installing the interlock resulted in a 62% installation rate in Hamilton County, Indiana (Voas et al. 2002). Similarly, in Santa Fe County, New Mexico, when the judges adopted the house-arrest alternative, installations increased over other courts in the state (Figure 16.11) and recidivism was reduced (Marques et al. 2010b; Voas et al. 2002). While these studies indicate the value of providing a more severe consequence for not installing an interlock, traditional license suspension/revocation remains the principal default condition for non-installation.

16.4.6.4.2 All DWI Laws The evidence that only a relatively small (10% to 20%) segment of the DWI population was installing the interlock led to the development of mandatory all DWI laws, which, aside from extending the interlock requirement to first-DWI offenders,

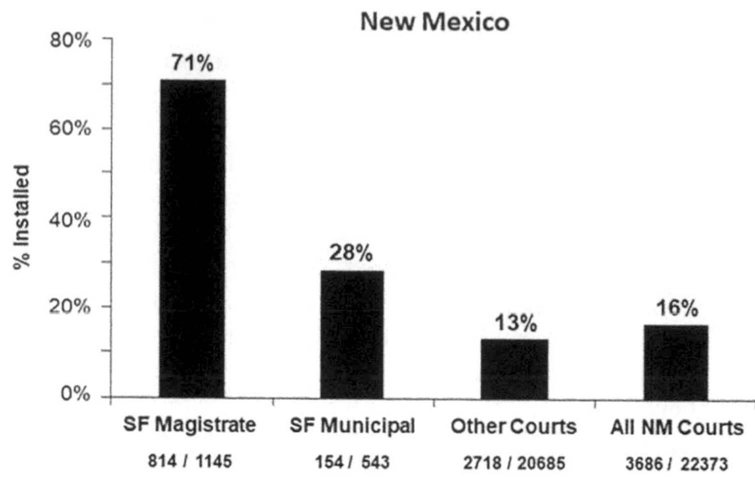

Figure 16.11 Example of the use of home detention (SF Magestraits) rather than license suspension (other New Mexico courts) as an alternative to installing an interlock). (Reproduced from Marques, P.R. et al., *Evaluation of the New Mexico Ignition Interlock Program* (DOT HS 811 410), National Highway Traffic Safety Administration, Washington, DC, 2010b. A publication of the US government.)

provided for the possibility of increased sanctions for failure to install an interlock. In court-based interlock programs, the DWI offender was placed on probation, and refusal to install an interlock could be treated as a breach of probation and subject to the sanctions for that offense. Thus, while the no-car exception remained in place, states and courts were empowered to apply less desirable alternatives than license suspension to non-installers. DWI criminal laws also resulted in the tightening of administrative interlock laws to include offenders with high arrest BACs and ultimately all first offenders. A national effort was mounted involving Mothers Against Drunk Driving (MADD 2018), NHTSA, the Centers for Disease Control and Prevention (CDC), and Congress to motivate states to pass all DWI laws, which mandate interlocks for both first- and multiple-DWI offenders. This national campaign generally succeeded as shown by a national survey of laws conducted by MADD in 2018 (Figure 16.12). Most of the states enacted all DWI laws, with only a few retaining laws that applied only to second offenders or high-BAC first offenders.

16.4.6.4.3 Interlock Installation Rates As a result of growth in all DWI laws, interlock installations increased steadily from 2014 to 2017, as shown in Figure 16.13. When existing users are added to the annual installations, the current total number of interlocks in use approaches 600,000 (Robertson et al. 2018). When the annual installation rates are related to the number of DWI offenders apprehended and convicted each year (Figure 16.14), it appears that current programs in the United States are covering a third of the arrested and half of the convicted DWIs. The discrepancy between the two figures is produced by (1) arrests of offenders not covered by the law (first and low-BAC offenders), (2) offenders receiving plea bargains, and of course (3) arrestees judged innocent.

16.4.6.4.4 Opportunity for Increasing Installation Rate Typically, state administrative interlock laws allow offenders to "wait out" the suspension period and reinstate their licenses once they have served that time with a suspended license. However, a number of

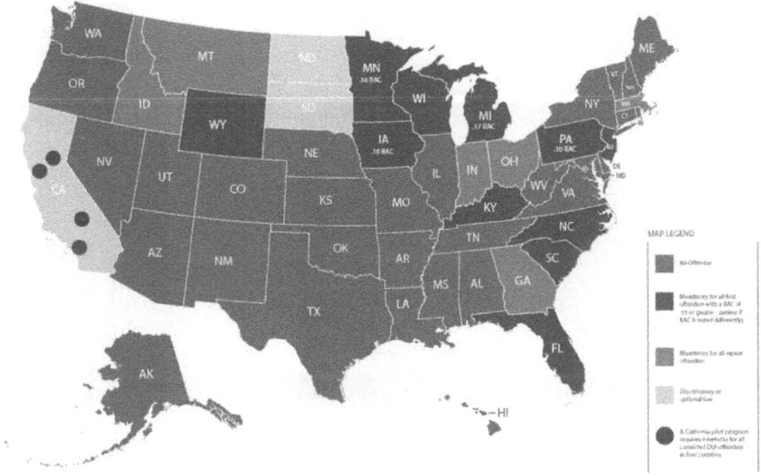

Figure 16.12 The extent to which state laws mandate that DWI offenders use an interlock varies substantially from state to state. However, the majority have all-offender laws. (Reproduced with permission from MADD: Ignition interlock laws in the United States of America; 2018; https://madd.org/wp-content/uploads/2018/06/State-IID-overview.6-18-18.pdf, Accessed December 12, 2019.)

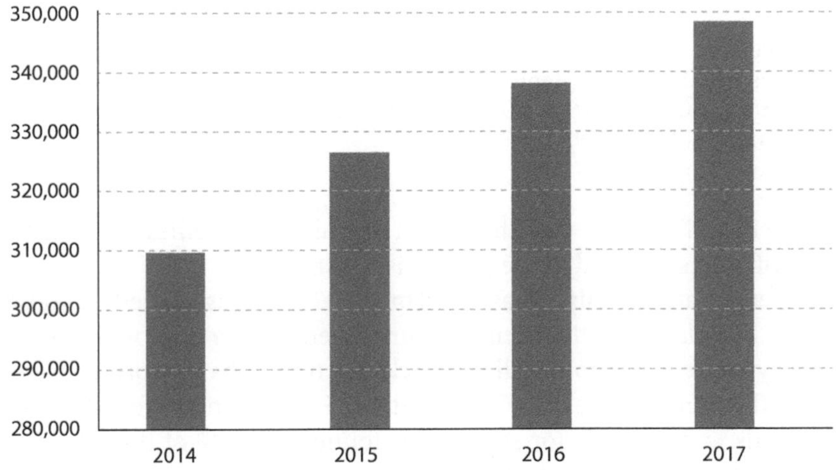

Figure 16.13 National active installations of interlocks on December 31st of each year as reported by manufacturers. (Reproduced (with modification) from Robertson, R.D. et al., Annual Ignition IID Survey 2016 & 2017, United States, Traffic Injury Research Foundation USA, Inc., Washington, DC, 2018.)

states (Florida, New Mexico, Illinois, California) with administrative interlock laws have responded to the national all DWI-law campaign by passing legislation making driving with the interlock for a specific period a prerequisite for reinstatement of the driver's license with the apparent consequence that refusal to install leaves the non-installer permanently unlicensed. This would appear to substantially increase the alternative sanction for those

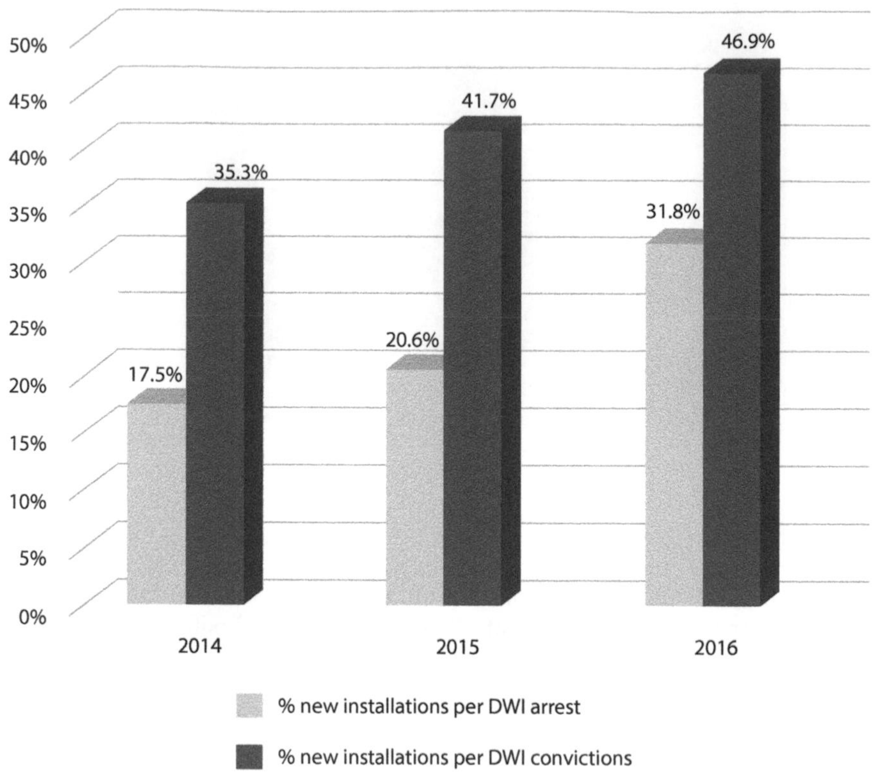

Figure 16.14 Percentage of interlock devices installed per arrests and per convictions in the United States in 2014–2020. (Reproduced (with modification) from Robertson, R.D. et al., Annual Ignition IID Survey 2016 & 2017, United States, Traffic Injury Research Foundation USA, Inc., Washington, DC, 2018.)

choosing not to install. To date, there have been no published studies of the install rate and recidivism of offenders exposed to the prerequisite sanction.

A limited, exploratory study (Voas and Tippetts 2014) was carried out on the impact of the policy in Florida where the licenses of first offenders arrested with 0.15% BACs are voided and they are required to install interlocks for 6 months as a prerequisite to license reinstatement. The retrospective study identified 8,135 first offenders for whom a full 5 years of driving records was available for study. They found that 55% of the offenders installed interlocks and were reinstated, while the driving records of the non-installers indicated they remained unlicensed through the 5-year period. The recidivism rates of installers and non-installers are shown in Figure 16.15. The recidivism rate of the installers between arrest and installing the interlock when they were suspended was high but decreased on installation and then almost doubled on removal (a pattern similar to that of most interlock studies).

The low recidivism rate for the refusers is not surprising, because based on their interlock record they remained with revoked licenses throughout the 5-year period, suggesting that they were not driving or greatly limiting their driving. However, it is difficult to determine whether those offenders continued to drive in Florida. Driving activity only appears on the driving record if offenses are recorded. Voas and Tippetts (2014) attempted to determine the driving status of the refusers by examining both driving infractions and administrative entries (e.g., address changes, etc.). They found that 23% left the state. Of the

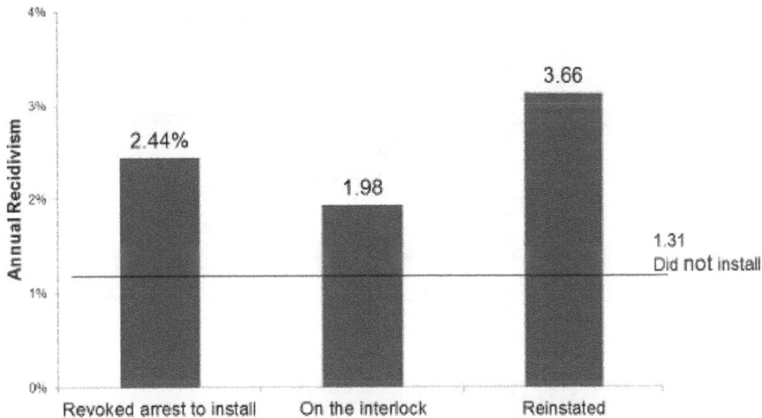

Figure 16.15 Recidivism of installers compared to non-installers under three conditions over 5 years in Florida (Total recidivism for all phases; Installers = 3.13 compared to Non-installers = 1.31; $z = 4.75$; $p < 0.001$). (Figure is reproduced from Voas, R.B. and Tippetts, A.S., Impact on recidivism of requiring time on the interlock as a pre-requisite for license reinstatement, Unpublished working paper, 2014, co-authored by the author of this review.)

remaining drivers still apparently in the state, 30% had moving violations, indicating they continued to drive. For the remainder, it was not possible to determine whether they were driving. Clearly, a large proportion of the refusers were limiting their driving or not driving at all, resulting in little or no exposure to recidivism. Meanwhile, the installers were fully licensed following their period on the interlock, continuing to drive in the state and exposed to rearrest for DWI. This study clearly suggests that when faced with the requirement to install in order to reinstate, DWI offenders who plan to continue to drive install, while those who plan to leave the state, or to stop driving and depend on others or public transportation, do not install, resulting in a lower overall recidivism rate—in this case, 1.31% compared to the overall 5-year recidivism rate of 3.13% for the installers.

It is important to note the limitations in this exploratory study. It was conducted in only one state, and while it involved a sizeable number of cases, it was conducted entirely based on license record data with no contact with the participants and no interlock record data. Instead, it used only administrative data, which does not fully reflect actual driving. However, pending confirming studies, it supports a number of logical consequences of the implementation of a regulation requiring a period on the interlock making installation the only road to reinstatement: Offenders who install are those who (a) most need to drive based on vocational or family requirements; (b) have the fewest family or public transportation alternatives; and (c) will drive more during their time on the interlock when compared with suspended drivers because they are free to drive at any time they are alcohol-free, while suspended drivers are prohibited from all driving.

16.4.7 Impact of Interlocks on Recidivism and Alcohol-Related Crashes

16.4.7.1 Impact on Recidivism

There is persuasive evidence that interlocks while on offenders' cars are an effective incapacitation system for limiting impaired driving by DWI offenders. From early reviews (Corbin and Larkin 1999; Voas et al. 1999) to the more comprehensive meta-analyses

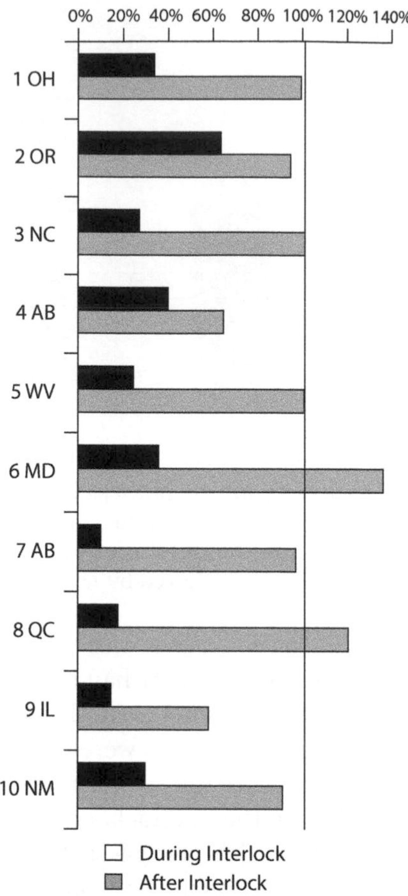

Figure 16.16 Recidivism in 10 studies: While the interlocks are on the vehicle (dark bars) and after removal (light bars). Rates are expressed relative to non-interlock license-suspended DWI offenders (vertical line) in each study. (Reproduced (with modification) from Marques, P.R. et al., *Accid. Anal. Prev.*, 33, 609, 2001.)

(Elder et al. 2011; Willis et al. 2004) and the recent review (Blais et al. 2013), studies have shown that recidivism is reduced while the unit is on the offender's vehicle but rises following interlock removal. Recidivism is a convenience measure that is recorded on the driver's record and provides a validity indicator with strong specificity since arrests are based on BAC data and sobriety tests but limited sensitivity since research indicates that there are 76–200 impaired driving trips for each DWI arrest (Zador et al. 2000a, 2000b). A compelling example of the use of the within-group technique was provided by the early studies comparing the recidivism of interlock users while the device was on their vehicle with their recidivism following interlock removal. Figure 16.16 shows this contrast for separate studies of 10 different localities (Marques et al. 2010b). These studies avoided the problem of attempting to equate non-installers with non-users in assessing the interlock.

16.4.7.2 Impact on Crashes

Crash severity may serve as a significant criterion for measuring the effectiveness of interlocks. The role of alcohol as a causal factor has been shown to vary with crash severity.

Based on data from FARS (US National Center for Statistics and Analysis 2003), 32% of all fatal crashes involve alcohol. In comparison, only approximately 10% of crashes involving lesser injuries involve alcohol, and alcohol plays a role in only 5% of the much more numerous property-damage-only crashes. Since interlocks do not limit sober driving, total crashes, wherein alcohol plays a role only 5% to 10% of the time, is not a very sensitive measure. To provide a strong criterion, fatal crashes or crashes determined to have involved a drinking driver are required.

An important challenge to the effectiveness of interlocks was raised by DeYoung, who found that first-DWI offenders were involved in more total crashes than suspended non-interlock controls but noted that their crash rate was essentially equal to that of the average driver (DeYoung et al. 2004). Vezina (2002) documented a higher *total* crash rate for drivers on interlocks. A later, more extensive study (DeYoung et al. 2004) found that interlocks reduced recidivism but increased crash involvements of interlock users relative to suspended controls. It was noted (Blais et al. 2013) that, "No studies have been able to measure miles of driving on an individual basis, so it has not been possible to determine whether interlock users drive more than suspended drivers. However, there is good reason to believe that some suspended offenders are not driving and that the total driving of many may be constrained by fear of apprehension." In contrast, the driving of interlock users is limited only by the relatively few occasions when they are unable to start their vehicles. The frequency of non–alcohol-related crashes is strongly related to driving exposure. Since the interlock does not prevent sober driving, it presumably has no effect on non–alcohol-related crash involvement. Therefore, it is likely that offenders with interlocks will experience more non–alcohol-related crashes than similar suspended drivers for whom *any driving* is illegal.

16.4.7.3 Research Methods for Assessing Interlocks

Three research designs have been employed in interlock studies:

- *Within-subject* analyses comparing recidivism rates while on the interlock with pre- and post-driving,
- *Group comparisons* of offenders on the interlock with similar offenders with suspended licenses, and
- *Before vs. after* enactment of an interlock law comparison of alcohol-related crash rates.

Within-subject designs appear to provide the strongest method since all participants experience both the interlock and control condition and avoid the potential bias problem presented in the install/no-install decision. Further the criterion measure—recidivism—minimizes the threat to validity presented by illicit use of a non-interlock car since the recidivism measure covers all driving. This methodology also has the value that outcome groups based on interlock performance can be stratified for special study. Among the significant limitations of this methodology are that it does not cover non-interlock offenders and most are limited to relatively short time periods, with small numbers of cases that preclude the use of the key criterion measure—alcohol-related crashes.

Group studies have the advantage that they can generally involve all DWI offenders creating larger *N*s for study but face the difficult problem of equating potentially quite different groups. The state before-after interlock laws appear to provide the best opportunity to study large groups of offenders over longer periods of time using the most significant outcome measure. Their main problem is to account for changes in the policy environment. They also have a problem in identifying the mechanism by which the interlock produced any benefit demonstrated; was it primary deterrence of all motorists resulting from the increased severity of the penalty for DWI, or was it secondary deterrence resulting from the interlock experience? They also have the complication that interlock users may drive more and be more exposed to crash involvement.

16.4.7.4 Impact of Interlock Laws on Alcohol-Related Crashes

The strongest studies of interlock effectiveness appear to be those that evaluate alcohol-related crash indicators before compared to after the implementation of an interlock law. Such studies can focus on the key outcome measure, the proportion of all crashes that are alcohol-related based on the presence compared to the absence of an interlock law. They are particularly convincing provided that adequate covariates have been employed to account for other factors known to impact alcohol-related crashes.

16.4.7.5 State-Level Studies of the Effect of Interlock Laws

State crash records have not been conducive to the study of the impact of alcohol-related crashes because of the limited number of fatal crashes for which BAC data are generally available and the limited availability of BAC data for less serious crashes. Further, as noted, with the pressure to install the units created by the passage of all DWI laws, the comparison of users with non-installers is challenged by the difficulty in creating a control group that adequately accounts for the biasing effect of the installation decision. This suggests that within-group, before-after, time series designs are likely to produce more credible evaluations of interlock programs. Two state studies using implementation of interlock laws have measured alcohol-related crashes. Vanlaar et al. (2015) reported on a study of the 2008 interlock law in Nova Scotia, Canada, in which DWI conviction rates were significantly lower following the implementation of the law, and there was a reduction in serious and fatal crashes that approached significance ($p = .10$) but was not statistically significant (Vanlaar et al. 2015). Another study (McCartt et al. 2012) found that the implementation of an interlock law in the state of Washington was associated with an 8.3% reduction in single-vehicle late-night crashes (a proxy measure for an alcohol-related crash).

16.4.7.6 National-Level Studies of Alcohol-Related Fatal Crashes

FARS provides a census of all fatal crashes in the United States together with a measured or imputed BAC for each driver involved in the crash. Three studies have made use of FARS to determine whether fatal alcohol-related crashes are reduced in states following the introduction of an interlock law. Kaufman and Weibe (2016) found a 15% reduction in alcohol-involved (BAC ≥ 0.00%) crashes in the 18 states that enacted all DWI laws between 2004 and 2013. McGinty et al. (2017) in a study covering a longer period (1982–2013) reported a 9% reduction in alcohol-related (BAC ≥ 0.08%) fatal crashes. Finally, a yet-to-be-published national study (Teoh et al. 2018), which covered the 22 states that enacted all DWI laws between 2001 and 2014, examined the impact of three types of interlock laws on alcohol-involved crashes (BAC > 0.01%). The study reported 16% reductions for the states with all DWI laws and 8% reductions for states with laws applying only to multiple offenders and high-BAC drivers. They found no significant alcohol-related crash reductions for states with laws applying only to multiple offenders. All three of these investigations used a panel-study procedure in which the states are treated as fixed effects with the implementation of an interlock law as the variable to be evaluated based on the change in the prevalence of alcohol-related fatal crashes. A key challenge to this method is to account for trends in the enactment of other potentially confounding traffic laws and secular trends in alcohol-related fatal crashes. All three of the studies appear to have gone to some length to meet this challenge.

16.4.7.7 National Studies Suggest That Interlock Laws Produce a General Deterrent Effect

An important feature of this methodology is that it measures the impact of interlock laws over an extended period of time beyond when the units are installed on offenders' vehicles. Since these analyses were not limited to offenders with prior DWI offenses, they encompassed all drivers using the roads, suggesting that all DWI laws may have a general deterrent effect. This interpretation is supported by the evidence reported above that DWI offenders find the interlock to be a more severe penalty than license suspension. If this is the case, then the interlock would appear to be having its impact through increased deterrence on all drivers produced by a more severe penalty rather than as a result of the incapacitation period experienced by offenders on the interlock. While the mechanism by which all DWI laws are having their effect may be unclear, together these studies comprise the strongest evidence for the safety benefit of interlock legislation.

16.4.8 Interlock Summary: A Limited Application of an Apparently Beneficial Program

The interlock appeared to be an important opportunity for DWI offenders to continue driving while serving the sanction for their offense. However, offenders rejected this opportunity and license suspension proved to be too weak a penalty to motivate more than a small percentage of DWI offenders to install interlocks. Other stronger sanctions such as home confinement proved to be more effective for motivating installation, but courts have not moved to impose such requirements. All DWI laws, which encouraged courts to impose stronger sanctions and state motor vehicle departments to make interlock installation a requirement for reinstatement of the driver's license, have substantially increased installations. Despite the impact of all DWI laws, states vary substantially in the proportion of their DWI offenders covered by interlock laws, as shown in Figure 16.12, and installation rates remain below 50% in most states (Figure 16.14).

16.4.8.1 Structural Features of Current Interlock Laws and Programs

The structural features of current interlock laws and programs are listed below:

- Of the two methods or proposed concepts of alcohol sensing and driver performance, only alcohol sensing has been implemented.
- Of the two implementation opportunities—placing interlocks on all vehicles or only on offender vehicles—units were only placed on offender vehicles.
- The requirement to install an interlock on a car empowers offenders to avoid installation by claiming not to have a car.

- DWI offenders resist installing the interlock: Avoiding license suspension is too weak a sanction to motivate installation; only 1/3 of offenders arrested for DWI install interlocks.
- Tampering with the interlock sensing system is prevented or detected but circumvention through use of a non-interlock-equipped car is not well controlled.
- New technology provides for remote, real-time reporting.
- New technology speeds and simplifies maintenance checks.
- The data-logger system provides an offender-performance measurement system.
- Social media provide for real-time education programs.
- In states in which time on the interlock is a prerequisite for license reinstatement, installers are substantially different from non-installers. Comparisons between installers and non-installers should be viewed caution.

16.4.8.2 Interlock Effectiveness

Despite the limitations listed above, interlocks have been demonstrated to reduce recidivism and alcohol-related crashes. This, despite that in comparison with non-interlock users they may drive more and be more exposed to non–alcohol-related crashes. Key features related to current interlock effectiveness can be described as follows:

- Interlocks while on the offender's vehicle reduce recidivism by approximately two-thirds.
- Following removal, recidivism returns to the normal level.
- Non–alcohol-related crashes are not affected while on the interlock.
- Alcohol-related crashes are presumably reduced while on the interlock, but their frequency is low—typically, the time on the interlock is too short for reliable measurement.
- Lockouts decrease during the period on the interlock, while total vehicle starts remain constant, suggesting a learning process.
- Lockouts predict recidivism following interlock removal.
- Lockouts provide a screening method for detecting offenders in need of an intervention program.
- The effectiveness of compliance-based removal (extending the time on the interlock based on excessive lockouts) in reducing postremoval recidivism remains to be demonstrated.
- Treatment of offenders identified by poor interlock performance reduces recidivism.
- Panel studies of the relationship of interlock laws to a reduction in alcohol-related crashes appear to be the best evidence for the effectiveness of the interlock.
- The reductions of 9% to 15% in alcohol-related crashes in state panel study results may indicate that the interlock produces a general deterrent effect.

16.4.9 Opportunities to Extend the Alcohol Interlock to All Vehicles

The current impact of the alcohol-detecting ignition interlock is extremely limited by its application only to DWI offenders when compared to an application of the interlock to all drivers by requiring it as a feature of all vehicles on the road. An update of the analysis by Lund et al. (2012) of the potential benefit of requiring interlocks on all cars has been published by Carter et al. (2015). They employed data from FARS and the National Automotive

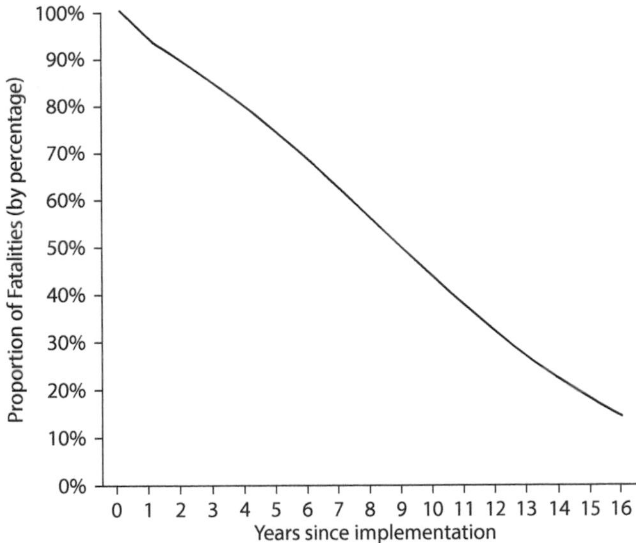

Figure 16.17 Remaining proportion of fatalities resulting from drinking drivers, by years since implementation of universal alcohol interlocks and by fatalities. (Reproduced (with modification) from Carter, P.M. et al., *Am. J. Public Health*, 105, 1028, 2015.)

Sampling System's General Estimates System (2006–2010) to estimate the impact of a universal interlock installation policy. They calculated the proportion of alcohol-related crashes that would be preventable in vehicles < 1 year old and then applied that fraction to the subsequent 15-year period required for the interlock to spread though the full vehicle population. They estimate that over that period interlocks would save 59,000 lives and reduce fatal alcohol-related crashes by 85% (Figure 16.17).

NHTSA has the power to make a rule requiring alcohol-detecting ignition interlocks on all cars using US roads, but would that actually be feasible? The NHTSA experience with safety belt interlocks in the 1970s (mentioned earlier in this review) suggests that there could be substantial opposition once drivers begin to experience delays associated with having to provide a breath sample every time they start their cars. Approximately 20% of the American public do not consume alcohol but they would potentially be required to provide a breath sample multiple times on every day they drive. Thus, immediate enforcement of an all-vehicle interlock rule might be counterproductive. Still, safety belt use in the United States was increased to its current 80% level over a 30-year period through safety campaigns, safety belt laws levying fines for non-use, and particularly by annoying warning systems. A similar approach might be successful for current interlocks. However, several issues arise in pursuing such a policy:

- **Cost to Vehicle Owners.** The $400 estimate of the cost of installing and maintaining the equipment and monitoring the driver in the first year and subsequent monitoring and maintenance costs would be borne by the vehicle owner. The $400 cost estimate is based on experience with relatively short periods on the interlock. The vast majority of first and second offenders have spent only 1 or 2 years on the interlock. Actual costs over a lifetime period remain to be determined.
- **Owner Time Requirement.** Most current interlocks require the owner to bring the vehicle to the service agency on a monthly or bimonthly basis. New technology

may reduce that requirement, but whether such checks can be reduced to the once-a-year frequency of emission tests is doubtful.

- **Rolling Retests.** Currently all interlocks require random retests while driving to prevent drinking in the car following ignition. That safeguard will probably need to be abandoned.
- **Circumvention.** Frustration with the demands of the system may increase over time, increasing efforts to disable or circumvent the interlock and reducing its effectiveness.

Thus, it is not clear (despite limited polling data, which indicate some public support) that interlocks on all cars would follow the path of safety belts and become accepted by 80% to 90% of Americans.

16.4.10 Driver Alcohol Detection System for Safety (DADSS)

The principal problem in obtaining public support for equipping all vehicles with interlocks is the requirement for action by the driver (providing a breath sample) every time the vehicle is started, not just at times such as weekends when the driver has been drinking. Even among DWI offenders, positive BACs on the interlock only occur in about 1 in 20 start attempts. A passive system that detected a high-BAC driver without requiring a breath test would be expected to be more attractive to vehicle owners. Alcohol-sensing technology has progressed to the point where passive alcohol sensing in the vehicle appears capable of detecting a drinking driver without requiring a special test or, if not, it at least signals when a breath test should be required.

A national effort to develop such a passive driver BAC test, labeled the Driver Alcohol Detection System for Safety (DADSS) (Ferguson et al. 2009), is sponsored by the Automotive Coalition for Traffic Safety (ACTS), which represents the world's leading automakers, NHTSA, and MADD. Two systems for detecting alcohol-impaired drivers have been developed. One collects air from in front of the driver, relying on the ratio of carbon dioxide to alcohol to distinguish between the driver and other passengers who may have been drinking. The other makes use of infrared spectroscopy to measure BAC through the skin when the driver pushes the start button. As of 2019, both systems are being demonstrated in vehicle tests. Both systems involve highly sensitive technology (US National Highway Traffic Safety Administration 2019).

As with the 1970 Borg Warner version of the interlock, the reliability of and ability to resist tampering with the DADSS remains to be demonstrated in 2019. Consider the effort that went into developing tamperproof systems for current interlock devices described above.

Arguably, the need to prevent tampering and the requirement for external monitoring may be less critical given that the vast majority of users will not be DWI offenders, who presumably will continue to be controlled by current criminal interlock programs. Nor will users be as likely to circumvent the test by driving a substitute vehicle since most possible substitute vehicles available will have the DADSS system installed. Nevertheless, it will certainly be an important consideration since many non-DWI heavy drinkers will be tempted to circumvent the device and external monitoring of its function will be considerably more intrusive and frequent than the monitoring programs applied by the states in emission control and safety check programs of current vehicles. The balance between false negatives that lead to crashes and false positives that will provoke user opposition, which results in program cancellation (as with seat belt interlocks), will be critical to the DADSS.

16.5 Simplifying Driving to Reduce Challenges to Impaired Drivers

NHTSA's vehicle driver assistance technologies program includes five "eras" of vehicle safety technology (Figure 16.18). Not included are the evolutions in the first half of the twentieth century, which accompanied the development of the basic design and production of the automobile. While these developments undoubtedly improved vehicle safety per mile, that safety impact was overwhelmed by the explosive growth of the industry and the increase in the number of cars on the road so that their impact on reducing crash involvements was difficult to assess. The current and projected safety-technology systems are directed at simplifying the driving task by removing challenges that lead to driver errors and crashes. None of these features are specifically motivated by the impaired driving problem, although some technologies (e.g., safety belts, automatic emergency braking) do appear to have special relevance to drinking drivers, who are at greater risk of being involved in a crash. As the driving task becomes less challenging, the impact of alcohol on driver performance is expected to diminish.

16.5.1 Driver Performance Interlocks and Remote Driver Monitoring

Examination of the technological safety programs (Figure 16.18), such as forward crash warning and control of lane-keeping, indicates that current vehicles are closely monitoring driver behavior related to safe driving. Further, a number have crash-avoidance systems for taking over if unsafe behavior is detected (e.g., "Frontal Emergency Braking"). These capabilities suggest that an opportunity exists to create an impaired-driver detection system. Early efforts to develop performance interlock were frustrated by the substantial differences between drivers in their respective performances, which would require the development of a baseline level for every user of the vehicle. The improvements in vehicle computer systems required for development of automated functions have resulted in expanded recording of vehicle maneuvers, which characterize driver performance. In the course of normal driving, vehicles accumulate the driver's "signature" performance against which unsafe departures can be calibrated. Evidence for such a possibility was developed by a study funded in 2010 by NHTSA (DOT HS 811 358), at the National Advanced Driving Simulator in Iowa, of 108 individuals driving on different types of roadways at 0.00%, 0.05%, and 0.10% BAC

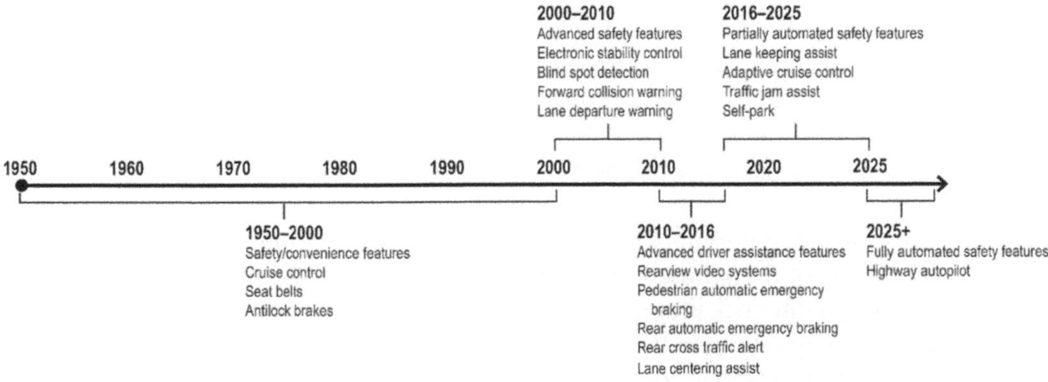

Figure 16.18 US National Highway Traffic Safety Administration's five eras of vehicle driver assistance technologies programs; https://www.nhtsa.gov/technology-innovation/automated-vehicles-safety (Accessed December 12, 2019).

levels to develop algorithms that could detect driver impairment. They found that with 8 minutes of driving data, the algorithms they developed could identify at or above 0.08% BAC with an accuracy of 73% to 86%, when compared to the standardized field sobriety tests used by police to generate probable cause to make an arrest. The report notes, however, that differences between drivers and driving situations suggested that the algorithms needed to be tailored to the individual driver.

16.5.1.1 Vehicle Performance Interlocks

The potential application of this performance-sensing system would seem to depend upon the intervention applied. It appears unlikely that the detection can be made sufficiently accurate and reliable to support its use as a basis for barring a driver from use of the vehicle, given the experience with safety belt interlocks. However, given the driving behaviors measured (speed and lane keeping are related to crash involvement for all drivers), it might be possible to implement limits on speed or increased automatic lane-keeping on all cars. Future safety vehicles might be equipped with a "safety mode" that could be actuated by tired or sleepy as well as alcohol- or drug-impaired drivers; the safety mode would limit vehicle operations known to increase crash risk (speed, short following distances), by increasing the sensitivity of the safety warnings and facilitating automated driving.

16.5.1.2 Remotely Monitoring Drivers for Impairment by Alcohol and Other Substances

The driving safety data being gathered and processed in vehicles with partial as well as full automation provides a method for external monitoring of driver performance that can be employed for law enforcement purposes—if the public will accept its use for that purpose and buy vehicles with that capability and appropriate state legislation is enacted. Driving data collected on a 24/7 basis can be analyzed, and compared with preset standards (e.g., the normal behavior of the driver, or the highway safety requirements of the roadway on which the vehicle is traveling). That type of information is currently displayed to the driver. Such information can be transmitted by internet systems to monitoring authorities. Aside from the accuracy and reliability of the data, two major factors should be expected to influence community and official acceptance of vehicle-managed monitoring programs:

- The population on which it is applied: criminals, drivers of limited capacity (children, elderly drivers, and handicapped drivers), or all drivers.
- The audience that has access to the data: the police, court or motor vehicle department monitors, parents, health professionals, or the general driving public.

Currently there are several examples of monitoring offenders through vehicle data. Global position monitoring of the vehicle is being used by the courts to provide no-drive zones in harassment cases. In interlock programs, vehicle starts without a prior breath test and failure to respond to a rolling retest are transmitted by some providers to monitoring agencies on a 24/7 basis. Failure to respond to a rolling retest is also broadcast to the public by a loud horn and flashing headlights. Whether such limited examples of external vehicle-monitoring systems proliferate as vehicle onboard technology provides greater and more detailed data remains to be seen.

Table 16.3 The Society of Automotive Engineers Visions of Five Steps in the Progress to Fully Automated Vehicles on the Nation's Roads

Level of Automation		Description
0	No automation	The driver performs all driving tasks
1	Drive assistance	Vehicle is controlled by the driver, but some driving assist features may be included in the vehicle design
2	Partial automation	Vehicle has combined automated functions, like acceleration and steering, but the driver must remain engaged with the driving task and monitor the environment at all times
3	Conditional automation	Driver is a necessary, but is not required to monitor the environment. The driver must be ready to take control of the vehicle at all times with notice
4	High automation	The vehicle is capable of performing all driving functions under certain conditions The driver may have the option to control the vehicle
5	Full automation	The vehicle is capable of performing all driving functions under all conditions The driver may have the option to control the vehicle

Source: https://www.nhtsa.gov/technology-innovation/automated-vehicles-safety#issue-road-self-driving (Accessed December 12, 2019).

16.5.2 Development of Autonomous Vehicles

Using the twentieth-century motor vehicle, where the driver is in control of all maneuvers, as the zero point, Table 16.3 displays the five steps (beyond the zero condition where the driver is in charge of all maneuvers) identified by the Society of Automotive Engineers as required to reach an environment given over almost entirely to autonomous vehicles. The first four phases involve different levels of self-driving cars, which retain a requirement for driver participation but in a gradually diminishing role as more and more elements of the driving task become automated (US Department of Transportation, National Highway Traffic and Safety Administration 2013). Reducing the driver's role should be particularly beneficial to the safety of the high-risk impaired driver. Paralleling this development of automated systems will be the application of intervehicle communications systems, which will allow initiating maneuvers based on unseen traffic events occurring ahead of the car. This communication system will also lend itself to interaction with a central traffic-management facility. This may provide the basis for the construction by the end of this century of a radically changed urban transportation system in which traditional twentieth century family cars are replaced by autonomous vehicles.

16.5.2.1 The Vision of an Autonomous Vehicle Environment

The fifth phase provides a vision of a future world urban environment, which, with minor exceptions, will contain only autonomous vehicles that communicate with each other and with a local control center. In that world, traditional vehicles would, for the most part, be banned from urban areas and highways, and individuals (with the possible exception of hobbyists) would not own cars but depend on an "Uber style" system for calling public-use autonomous vehicles. If this vision of dramatic change in the travel environment materializes, passenger vehicles will not need operators whose driving can be impaired by psychoactive substances, and alcohol- or drug-related vehicle crashes will be rare and no longer a major societal problem. This is the situation where all, or essentially all, motorized transportation (aside perhaps from police and fire department vehicles, motorcycles, electric pedicycles, and scooters) involves commercial or official vehicles.

However, building the infrastructure to support the transformed system is challenging and not expected to be in operation before the end of the century. If this situation materializes, the individual driver with little training and no supervision will no longer be driving a high-power, high-speed vehicle, and the source of alcohol-related crashes will be greatly diminished or eliminated.

16.5.3 Determining the Effect of Automation on Impaired Driving Enforcement

In the United States the proportion of fatally injured drivers with BACs greater than or equal to 0.08% has remained at 31%–32% for the past 10 years. This is stimulating an effort to strengthen enforcement of impaired driving laws by lowering the BAC limit to 0.05%. Thus, it appears that alcohol-related safety laws will be actively enforced for the foreseeable future—a future during which the slow but steady progress in vehicle safety engineering will gradually reduce the difficulty of the driving task—presumably producing greater ability for impaired drivers to avoid crashes. This will continue until the driver's task is eliminated in stage 5 of the development of the autonomous vehicle. Then toward the end of the twenty-first century, cars may simply become one additional method of public transportation.

This vision of a self-driving vehicle world may or may not materialize, but in moving toward it, the extent of vehicle automation will steadily increase, challenging our current policy of imposing heavy sanctions for the DWI offense in order to deter impaired drivers. Stage 4 automatic vehicles such as the Google car are already being tested. Uber is testing the use of self-driving vehicles (albeit with a backup driver). If the Google car or similar experiments succeed in demonstrating that autonomous vehicles can function safely in the current driving environment, states will probably allow the sale and provide for the registration of such vehicles to individual owners. This will set up a confrontation with current punitive impaired driving laws. Physically challenged drivers and the elderly will be seen as key beneficiaries of these new vehicles, and it will be logical to encourage drivers who are heavy drinkers, patients on medication, and other drug users to purchase and use fully automatic vehicles. This would be expected to bring pressure on the states to decriminalize impaired driving in an automated vehicle.

Easing restrictions on impaired drivers operating fully automatic vehicles with no controls available to them may be a relatively easy legal issue to resolve. More challenging will be the autonomous vehicle, which retains full or partial capability for normal driver control. This is likely to be the most popular version of the autonomous vehicle stages, prior to establishing the vision of the automated vehicle environment described above. It is probable that most owners will opt for the ability to influence the operation of the vehicle in order to travel on favorite routes and be able to take over in cases of traffic delays and emergencies. As suggested above, such vehicles might have an easy-to-actuate "safety mode" that would put the vehicle under automatic control, as in current cruise-control systems. Presumably an impaired driver riding in safety mode would not be stopped because police officers must have probable cause to make a stop. However, in states with primary safety belt laws, unbelted drivers can be stopped and ticketed, and, in the course of that action, impairment can be detected leading to an arrest.

During that interim period, the current relatively severe sanctions for the DWI offense will come under considerable pressure for modification to recognize the reduced risk of crashing and to establish provisions that encourage impaired drivers to make use of vehicles with automatic functions. It will be important for policymakers to have information

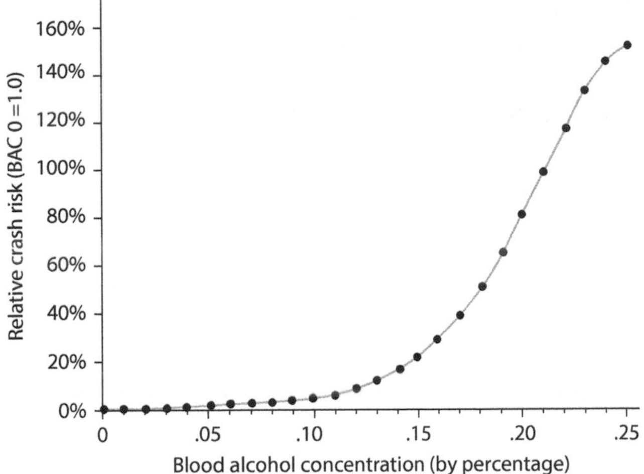

Figure 16.19 Relative risk curve of involvement in a road traffic crash in relation to the driver's BAC determined by breath analysis. (Reproduced (with modification) from Blomberg, R.D. et al., *Crash Risk of Alcohol Involved Driving*, National Highway Traffic Safety Administration, Washington, DC, 2004. A publication of the US government.)

on the extent to which vehicle automation is producing safety benefits. Periodic national roadside breath test surveys (Voas et al. 1998b) when combined with data from Fatality Analysis Record System (Zador et al. 2000b) have established a basis for measuring changes in risk as they occur from the implementation of new technology. Risk curves such as the one shown in Figure 16.19 (Blomberg et al. 2009) should flatten out and move to the right if an impaired driver no longer has control of the vehicle.

16.6 Summary—Five Stages of the Vehicle Safety Program

This review has focused on the role of the automobile and auto safety programs in the growth and decline of alcohol-related crashes in the United States. The presentation has covered five eras:

- **1900–1950 Growth of the Problem.** During this period, road-traffic safety became a major social problem because of the invention and mass production of the passenger vehicle, which places a high-powered and dangerous device in the hands of individuals without training and supervision.
- **1950–1990 Crashworthiness.** While public attention was focused on speed and power during the early years of the growth in the vehicle population, by mid-century the exploding highway fatality rate called attention to the dangers of automobile use and resulted in a change in public attitudes toward vehicle safety, resulting in an industry effort to increase vehicle crashworthiness and the founding of the National Highway Traffic Safety Administration to monitor vehicle safety. Although various crashworthiness measures were implemented with the intention of reducing injuries to all drivers, since impaired drivers have substantially higher crash rates, it is probable that they particularly benefitted from such vehicle improvements.

- **1990–2010 Alcohol-Detecting Ignition Interlock Devices.** Interlocks offered the potential, if mandated for use with every vehicle, to overcome the drinking-and-driving problem. However, they were only employed as an alternative to the license-suspension sanction for a DWI offense. In this application they played a substantial role in reducing recidivism and reducing alcohol-related fatal crashes by as much as 15%. However, DWI offenders strongly resist installing interlocks and currently only about one third of drivers arrested for DWI install these units.
- **2010–2025 Development of Driver Assistance and Crash Prevention Systems.** Growth in automobile technology is providing safety systems for assisting the driver with lane-keeping, backing up the vehicle, and, most importantly, emergency braking and crash avoidance. Because drinking drivers are at particularly high risk of crashing, these aids are of special benefit to them. Moreover, with the growing ability of vehicles to detect and ameliorate risky driving maneuvers, there is a possibility that a vehicle safety system can be developed specifically to detect an impaired driver and take over the control of the vehicle.
- **2025–2099 Development of the Automated Vehicle Environment.** Self-driving vehicles are currently being demonstrated under controlled protocols. They suggest the possibility that by the end of this century an environment can be created that would see only autonomous vehicles on US roads, at least in populated areas. In such a transportation environment, it is proposed that no one would own a car; rather, there would be a movement to a system of on-call autonomous vehicles to pick up passengers and deliver them to their destinations. In that environment, the drivers, as we know them, would be eliminated. Each vehicle would communicate with other cars on the road and a central guidance system. The absence of a driver will mean that we have stopped placing powerful, high-speed vehicles in the hands of relatively untrained and unsupervised individuals. Subsequently, alcohol-related crashes should disappear as a major societal problem, not because we have learned to cure problem drinking or prevent intoxicated people from driving but because the individually owned automobile of the twentieth century, an element of the problem, will no longer exist.

Acknowledgments

Work on this review was partially funded by the National Institute on Alcohol Abuse and Alcoholism (NIAAA), grant number 5R01AA022312. Important support was provided by Jill Dougherty in preparing the manuscript and Eileen Taylor in helping assemble the information for the text, and by Dr. Paul Marques and Dr. Eduardo Romano in reviewing and editing the manuscript. Also, this manuscript would not have been possible without the editorial assistance of Dr. Wayne Jones and Dr. Ray Liu. Finally, the author would like to express special appreciation to Dr. Robert Borkenstein, who mentored his entry into the field, and to 50-year associates Jim Fell, John Lacey, and Dr. Jim Nichols, who helped shape the author's career.

References

Blais É, Sergerie D, Maurice P: The effect of ignition interlock programs on drinking-and-driving: A systematic review; *Proceedings—23rd Canadian Multidisciplinary Road Safety Conference*; Montréal, Canada; May 26–29; 2013.

Blomberg RD, Peck RC, Moskowitz H, Burns M, Fiorentino D: *Crash Risk of Alcohol Involved Driving*; National Highway Traffic Safety Administration: Washington, DC; 2004.

Blomberg RD, Peck RC, Moskowitz H, Burns M, Fiorentino D: The Long Beach/Fort Lauderdale relative risk study; *J Safety Res* 40:285; 2009.

Carter PM, Flannagan CA, Bingham CR, Cunningham RM, Rupp JD: Modeling the injury prevention impact of mandatory alcohol ignition interlock installation in all new US vehicles; *Am J Public Health* 105:1028; 2015.

Collier DW: Second generation interlocks lead to improved program efficiencies (TRB ID Number: CF076); Presentation—73rd Annual Transportation Research Board; 1994.

Collier DW, Comeau FJE, Marples IR: *Experience in Alberta with Highly Sophisticated Anti-Circumvention Features in a Fuel Cell Based Ignition Interlock*; NHMRC Road Accident Research Unit: Adelaide, Australia; 1995.

Corbin JH, Larkin GL: Effectiveness of ignition interlock devices in reducing drunk driving recidivism; *Am J Prev Med* 16:81; 1999.

Crosby IB: Portland's asset forfeiture program: The effectiveness of vehicle seizure in reducing rearrest among problem drunk drivers; *Reed College Public Policy Workshop*; Portland, OR; 1995.

DeYoung DJ: An evaluation of the general deterrent effect of vehicle impoundment on suspended and revoked drivers in California; *J Safety Res* 31:51; 2000.

DeYoung DJ: An evaluation of the implementation of ignition interlock in California; *J Safety Res* 33:473; 2002.

DeYoung DJ: An evaluation of the specific deterrent effects of vehicle impoundment on suspended, revoked, and unlicensed drivers in California; *Accid Anal Prev* 31:45; 1999.

DeYoung DJ, Tashima HN, Masten SV: *An Evaluation of the Effectiveness of Ignition Interlock in California: Report to the Legislature of the State of California* (CAL-DMV-RSS-04-210/AL0357); California Department of Motor Vehicles: Sacramento, CA; 2004.

Elder RW, Voas R, Beirness D, Shults RA, Sleet DA, Nichols JL, Compton R, Task Force on Community Preventive Services: Effectiveness of ignition interlocks for preventing alcohol-related crashes: A community guide systematic review; *Am J Prev Med* 40:362; 2011.

Fell JC, Tippetts AS, Voas RB: Fatal traffic crashes involving drinking drivers: What have we learned? *Ann Adv Automot Med* 53:63; 2009.

Ferguson SA, Zaouk A, Dalal N, Strohl C, Traube E, Strassburger R: *Driver Alcohol Detection System for Safety (DADSS)—Phase I prototype testing and findings* (Paper No. 11-0230); *Proceedings—21st International Technical Conference on the Enhanced Safety of Vehicles*; Stuttgart, Germany; June 15–18; 2009.

Kaufman EJ, Wiebe DJ: Impact of state ignition interlock laws on alcohol-involved crash deaths in the United States; *Am J Public Health* 106:865; 2016.

Klein RH, Jex HR: Effects of alcohol on a critical tracking task; *J Stud Alcohol* 36:11; 1975.

Li R, Pickrell TM: *Seat Belt Use in 2017—Overall Results* (Traffic Safety Facts Research Note. Report No. DOT HS 812 465); National Highway Traffic Safety Administration: Washington, DC; 2018.

Lund AK, McCartt AT, Farmer CM: *Contribution of Alcohol-Impaired Driving to Motor Vehicle Crash Deaths in 2010*; Insurance Institute for Highway Safety: Arlington, VA; 2012.

MADD: Ignition interlock laws in the United States of America; 2018; https://madd.org/wp-content/uploads/2018/06/State-IID-overview.6-18-18.pdf (Accessed December 12, 2019).

MADD: Ignition interlocks: Every state, for every convicted drunk driver; 2016; https://www.madd.org/wp-content/uploads/2018/11/MADDmodelinterlocklawcomponents.pdf (Accessed August 4, 2019).

Marques P, Bjerre B, Dussault C, Voas RB, Beirness DJ, Marples IR, Rauch WR, Guthrie D, Bailey J, Ahlin EM, et al.: *Alcohol Ignition Interlock Devices—I: Position Paper*; International Council on Alcohol, Drugs and Traffic Safety; 2001; www.icadts.org/reports/Alcoholinterlockreport.pdf (Accessed August 4, 2019).

Marques P, Tippetts S, Allen J, Javors M, Alling C, Yegles M, Pragst F, Wurst F: Estimating driver risk using alcohol biomarkers, interlock blood alcohol concentration tests and psychometric assessments: Initial descriptives; *Addiction* 105:226; 2010a.

Marques PR, Tippetts AS, Voas RB: Comparative and joint prediction of DUI recidivism from alcohol ignition interlock and driver records; *J Stud Alcohol* 64:83; 2003a.

Marques PR, Tippetts AS, Voas RB, Beirness DJ: Predicting repeat DUI offenses with the alcohol interlock recorder; *Accid Anal Prev* 33:609; 2001.

Marques PR, Tippetts AS, Yegles M: Ethylglucuronide in hair is a top predictor of impaired driving recidivism, alcohol dependence, and a key marker of the highest BAC interlock tests; *Traffic Inj Prev* 15:361; 2014.

Marques P, Voas R: Are we near a limit or can we get more safety from vehicle alcohol interlocks? *Addiction* 108:657; 2013.

Marques PR, Voas RB, Roth R, Tippetts AS: *Evaluation of the New Mexico Ignition Interlock Program* (DOT HS 811 410); National Highway Traffic Safety Administration: Washington, DC; 2010b.

Marques PR, Voas RB, Timken DS, Field CT: Motivational enhancement of ignition interlock offenders to reduce DUI; *Alcohol Clin Exp Res* 28:154A; 2004.

Marques PR, Voas RB, Tippetts AS: Behavioral measures of drinking: Patterns in the interlock record; *Addiction* 98(S2):13; 2003b.

Marques PR, Voas RB, Tippetts AS, Beirness DJ: Behavioral monitoring of DUI offenders with the alcohol ignition interlock recorder; *Addiction* 94:1861; 1999.

Mayer R: *Ignition Interlocks—A Toolkit for Program Administrators, Policymakers, and Stakeholders*, 2nd ed (Report No. DOT HS 811 883); National Highway Traffic Safety Administration: Washington, DC; 2014.

McCartt AT, Geary LL, Nissen WJ: *Observational Study of the Extent of Driving While Suspended for Alcohol-Impaired Driving* (DOT HS 809 491); National Highway Traffic Safety Administration: Washington, DC; 2002.

McCartt AT, Leaf WA, Farmer CM, Eichelberger AH: *Washington State's Alcohol Ignition Interlock Law: Effects on Recidivism Among First-Time DUI Offenders*; Insurance Institute for Highway Safety: Arlington, VA; 2012.

McGinty EE, Tung G, Shulman-Laniel J, Hardy R, Rutkow L, Frattaroli S, Vernick JS: Ignition interlock laws: Effects on fatal motor vehicle crashes, 1982–2013; *Am J Prev Med* 52:417; 2017.

Nader R: *Unsafe at Any Speed*; Grossman Publishers: New York; 1965.

Peck R, Voas R: *Forfeiture Programs in California: Why So Few?* National Highway Traffic Safety Administration: Washington, DC; 2000.

Peck R, Voas R: Forfeiture programs in California: Why so few? *J Safety Res* 33:245; 2002.

Robertson RD, Vanlaar WGM, Hing MM: Annual Ignition IID Survey 2016 & 2017: United States; Traffic Injury Research Foundation USA, Inc.: Washington, DC; 2018.

Rodgers A: Effect of Minnesota's license plate impoundment law on recidivism or multiple DWI violators; *Alcohol Drugs Driving* 10:127; 1994.

Ross HL, Gonzales P: Effects of license revocation on drunk-driving offenders; *Accid Anal Prev* 20:379; 1988.

Roth R: How do offenders get arrested? *Presentation—8th International Interlock Conference*; Seattle, WA; August 26–27, 2007.

Safir H, Grasso G, Messner R: The New York City Police Department DWI Forfeiture Initiative; In Laurell H, Schlyter F (Eds): *Alcohol, Drugs and Traffic Safety T 2000: Proceedings of the 15th International Conference on Alcohol, Drugs and Traffic Safety* Vol. 3; Stockholm, Sweden; 2000.

Sussman ED, Abernethy CN: *Laboratory Evaluation of Alcohol Safety Interlock Systems*, Volume 1: Summary Report (Report No. DOT HS 800-925); National Highway Traffic Safety Administration: Washington, DC; 1973.

Tashima HN, Helander CJ: *1999 Annual Report of the California DUI Management Information System* (CAL-DMV-RSS-99-179); California Department of Motor Vehicles, Research and Development Section: Sacramento, CA; 1999.

Teoh ER, Fell JC, Scherer M, Wolfe DE: *State Alcohol Ignition Interlock Laws and Fatal Crashes*; Insurance Institute for Highway Safety: Arlington, VA; 2018.

Timken DS, Nandi A, Marques P: *Interlock Enhancement Counseling: Enhancing Motivation for Responsible Driving—A Participant's Workbook*; Center for Impaired Driving Research and Evaluation: Boulder, CO; 2012.

Tippetts AS, Voas RB: The effectiveness of the West Virginia interlock program; *J Traffic Med* 26:19; 1998.

US Department of Transportation, National Highway Traffic and Safety Administration: *Preliminary Statement of Policy Concerning Automated Vehicles*; 2013; https://www.nhtsa.gov/staticfiles/rulemaking/pdf/Automated_Vehicles_Policy.pdf. (Accessed September 9, 2019).

US Federal Bureau of Investigation. https://www.fbi.gov/services/cjis/ucr, 2018.

US National Center for Statistics and Analysis: *Fatality Analysis Reporting System* (FARS); 2003; https://www.nhtsa.gov/research-data/fatality-analysis-reporting-system-fars (Accessed August 4, 2019).

US National Highway Traffic Safety Administration: *Driver Alcohol Detection System for Safety*; 2019; https://one.nhtsa.gov/Vehicle-Safety/DADSS (Accessed August 4, 2019).

US National Highway Traffic Safety Administration: *Model Guideline for State Ignition Interlock Programs* (Report No. DOT HS 811 859); National Highway Traffic Safety Administration Washington, DC; 2013.

US National Highway Traffic Safety Administration: Model specifications for breath alcohol ignition interlock devices (BAIIDs); *Fed Regist* 80:16720; 2015; https://www.govinfo.gov/content/pkg/FR-2015-03-30/pdf/2015-07161.pdf (Accessed August 4, 2019).

Vanlaar W, Mainegra Hing M, Robertson R: *Nova Scotia Alcohol Ignition Interlock Program: Outcome Evaluation Executive Report*; Traffic Injury Research Foundation: Ottawa, Canada; 2015.

Vanlaar W, Robertson R, Schaap D, Vissers J: *Understanding Behavioral Patterns of Interlocked Offenders to Inform the Efficient and Effective Implementation of Interlock Programs: How Offenders on an Interlock Learn to Comply*; Traffic Injury Research Foundation: Ontario, Canada; 2010.

Vezina L: The Quebec Alcohol Ignition Interlock Program: Impact on recidivism and crashes; In Mayhew D, Dussault C (Eds): *Proceedings—16th International Conference on Alcohol, Drugs and Traffic Safety*; Montreal, Canada; August 4–9; 2002.

Voas RB: Cars that drunks can't drive; *Presentation—Annual Meeting of the Human Factors Society*; San Francisco, CA; 1970.

Voas RB: Enhancing the use of vehicle alcohol interlocks with emerging technology; *Alcohol Res* 36:81; 2014.

Voas RB: *Final Report on Assessment Impoundment and Forfeiture Laws for Drivers Convicted of DWI* (NHTSA Contract No. DTNH22-89-4-07026); National Highway Traffic Safety Administration: Washington, DC; 1992.

Voas RB: Have the courts and the motor vehicle departments adequate power to control the hard-core drunk driver? *Addiction* 96:1701; 2001.

Voas RB, Blackman KO, Tippetts AS, Marques PR: Evaluation of a program to motivate impaired driving offenders to install ignition interlocks; *Accid Anal Prev* 34:449; 2002.

Voas RB, DeYoung DJ: Vehicle action: Effective policy for controlling drunk and other high-risk drivers? *Accid Anal Prev* 34:263; 2002.

Voas RB, Marques PR: *Alcohol Ignition Interlock Service Support* (Final Report DOT HS 807 923 to National Highway Traffic Safety Administration); National Technical Information Service: Springfield, VA; 1992.

Voas RB, Marques PR: Barriers to interlock implementation; *Traffic Inj Prev* 4:183; 2003.

Voas RB, Marques PR, Roth R: Incapacitating the DUI offender: Dealing with the No-Car Problem. In Logan BK, Isenschmid DS, Walsh JM, Beirness D, Mørland J (Eds): *T2007, Abstracts of the Joint International Meeting of TIAFT/ICADTS/IIS*; Seattle, WA; August 26–30; 2007.

Voas RB, Marques PR, Tippetts AS, Beirness DJ: The Alberta Interlock Program: The evaluation of a province-wide program on DUI recidivism; *Addiction* 94:1849; 1999.

Voas RB, Tippetts AS: A note on compliance-based removal; Unpublished working paper; 2013.

Voas RB, Tippetts AS: Impact on recidivism of requiring time on the interlock as a pre-requisite for license reinstatement; Unpublished working paper; 2014.

Voas RB, Tippetts AS, Bergen G, Grosz M, Marques P: Mandating treatment based on interlock performance: Evidence for effectiveness; *Alcohol Clin Exp Res* 40:1953; 2016.

Voas RB, Tippetts AS, Lange JE: Evaluation of a method for reducing unlicensed driving: The Washington and Oregon license plate sticker laws; *Accid Anal Prev* 29:627; 1997a.

Voas RB, Tippetts AS, McKnight AS: DUI offenders delay license reinstatement: A problem? *Alcohol Clin Exp Res* 34:1282; 2010.

Voas RB, Tippetts AS, Taylor EP: Temporary vehicle immobilization: Evaluation of a program in Ohio; *Accid Anal Prev* 29:635; 1997b.

Voas RB, Tippetts AS, Taylor EP: Temporary vehicle impoundment in Ohio: A replication and confirmation; *Accid Anal Prev* 30:651; 1998a.

Voas RB, Wells J, Lestina D, Williams A, Greene M: Drinking and driving in the United States: The 1996 National Roadside Survey; *Accid Anal Prev* 30:267; 1998b.

Willis C, Lybrand S, Bellamy N: Alcohol ignition interlock programmes for reducing drink driving recidivism; *Cochrane Database Syst Rev* 18:CD004168; 2004.

Zador PL, Ahlin EM, Rauch WJ, Howard JM, Duncan GD: The effects of closer monitoring on driver compliance with interlock restrictions; *Accid Anal Prev* 43:1960; 2011.

Zador PL, Krawchuk SA, Moore B: *Drinking and Driving Trips, Stops by the Police, and Arrests: Analyses of the 1995 National Survey of Drinking and Driving Attitudes and Behavior* (Report No. DOT HS 809 184); National Highway Traffic Safety Administration: Washington, DC; 2000a.

Zador PL, Krawchuk SA, Voas RB: Alcohol-related relative risk of driver fatalities and driver involvement in fatal crashes in relation to driver age and gender: An update using 1996 data; *J Stud Alcohol Drugs* 61:387; 2000b.

Approaches for Reducing Alcohol-Impaired Driving

17

Evidence-Based Legislation, Law Enforcement Strategies, Sanctions, and Alcohol-Control Policies*

JAMES C. FELL

Contents

* This chapter is an updated version (format only) of a review article previously published in *Forensic Science Review*: Fell JC: Approaches for reducing alcohol-impaired driving: Evidence-based legislation, law enforcement strategies, sanctions, and alcohol-control policies; *Forensic Sci Rev* 31:161; 2019.

17.1 Introduction

This chapter presents an overview of evidence-based policies and programs designed to reduce highway crashes involving alcohol-impaired drivers. Scholars, researchers, or practitioners with an interest in this area should also consult a recent article (Voas 2020), and a report published by the US National Highway Traffic Safety Administration (NHTSA) (Goodwin et al. 2015) on "Countermeasures That Work," which lists over 100 specific traffic-safety countermeasures with evidence of effectiveness, covering all areas of traffic-safety behavioral programs. The latest in the series of NHTSA Alcohol and Highway Safety reviews also presents evidence up through 2006 (Voas and Lacey 2011). Other articles relevant to this chapter include "Effectiveness of Behavioral Highway Safety Countermeasures" (Preusser et al. 2008), "Preventing Impaired Driving: Opportunities and Problems" (Voas and Fell 2011), and "Programs and Policies Designed to Reduce Impaired Driving" (Voas and Fell 2014).

A popular public health approach is used in this chapter (Voas and Fell 2014) that provides a good logical structure for understanding the characteristics and impacts of alternative approaches. Alcohol-impaired driving countermeasures that are proven effective or that have great potential are classified here under three headings: Primary Prevention,

Secondary Prevention, and Tertiary Prevention. Primary Prevention countermeasures reduce high-risk drinking and high-risk driving directly, by limiting alcohol availability and reducing high-risk nighttime driving. Secondary Prevention countermeasures are intended to deter alcohol-impaired driving by adopting and enforcing effective impaired-driving laws. Tertiary Prevention focuses on countermeasures directed at preventing recidivism by convicted impaired-driving offenders, and include license and vehicle actions, treatment and rehabilitation programs, and alcohol-monitoring programs. The research described in this chapter primarily concerns the United States, although a few international approaches are considered.

17.1.1 Impaired Driving: A Worldwide Problem

Alcohol-impaired driving has been recognized as a problem almost as long as automobiles have existed (*Quart Inebriety* 1904). Worldwide, it is estimated that alcohol-impaired driving crashes account for anywhere from 5% (e.g., Turkey, Nicaragua) to 35% (e.g., the United States, Australia) of the 1.35 million traffic deaths each year. Chapter 13 covers "International Trends in Alcohol and Drug Use Among Motor Vehicle Drivers," presenting detailed evidence on the prevalence of alcohol-impaired driving in several different countries (Christophersen et al. 2016).

The World Health Organization (WHO) recommended four policies to reduce impaired driving in their 2018 report on the global status of road safety (WHO 2018):

- Adoption of a national drink-driving law;
- Setting blood alcohol concentration (BAC) limits for adult drivers at 0.05 g/dL or lower;
- Setting zero-alcohol limits for young novice drivers; and
- Conducting random breath testing (RBT) programs similar to those developed in Australia as a key enforcement strategy.

This chapter covers all four of these evidence-based recommendations and goes beyond these basic strategies to consider additional approaches. A brief overview of the alcohol-impaired driving problem in the United States is presented in the remainder of this introduction below, with detailed evidence on potential countermeasures provided in the following sections of the chapter.

Numerous laboratory and simulator studies have shown that impairment in driving performance begins with the first drink (a BAC = 0.02 g/dL) and increases substantially with each subsequent one. The risk of a crash is significant beginning at 0.04–0.05 g/dL BAC, and increases exponentially as BAC rises. Lowering the BAC limit to 0.05 g/dL has been shown to be an effective strategy that has reduced alcohol-impaired traffic fatalities in several countries. Impaired-driving laws, including administratively suspending the licenses of driving under the influence (DUI) offenders and requiring alcohol ignition interlock devices be installed on the vehicles of all convicted DUI offenders, have been effective in deterring impaired driving. The most important and the most immediately effective strategy, however, is DUI enforcement, especially sobriety checkpoints and RBT.

A continuing problem with few solutions is alcohol involvement in pedestrian and bicyclist crash fatalities. In the United States, about 34% of pedestrians killed in crashes have BACs ≥ 0.08 g/dL while in the UK, 48% of pedestrian deaths involve alcohol. That proportion is even higher in South Africa, where 61% of pedestrian deaths involve alcohol (Stewart 2004).

A system being developed called the Driver Alcohol Detection System for Safety (DADSS) in the United States and future fully autonomous vehicles worldwide promise to be the ultimate solution to eliminating alcohol-impaired driving.

17.1.2 Alcohol Impairment and Blood-Alcohol Concentration

Laboratory and test-track research has shown that a vast majority of drivers, even experienced drinkers who typically reach BACs of 0.15 g/dL or greater, are impaired in performing critical driving tasks at 0.05 g/dL BAC and higher. There are significant decrements in performance in areas such as braking, steering, lane changing, judgment, and divided attention at 0.05 g/dL BAC. Some studies report that performance decrements in some of these tasks are as high as 30%–50% at 0.05 g/dL BAC (Ferrara et al. 1994; Gjerde et al. 2015, 2019; Howat et al. 1991; Jones 1996; Moskowitz et al. 2000; Moskowitz and Fiorentino 2000).

17.1.3 Relative Risk of Being Involved in a Crash by Blood-Alcohol Concentration

The risk of being involved in a crash increases with increasing BAC level in general, but rises very rapidly after a driver reaches or exceeds 0.05 g/dL BAC (Blomberg et al. 2005, 2009; Compton and Berning 2015). Other studies indicate that the relative risk of being killed in a single-vehicle crash for drivers with BACs of 0.05 g/dL to 0.079 g/dL is at least 7 times that of drivers at 0.00 g/dL BAC (no alcohol), and could be as much as 21 times that of non-drinking drivers depending on the age of the driver (Voas et al. 2012; Zador et al. 2000b). These risks are significant (see Figure 17.1 [Blomberg et al. 2005]).

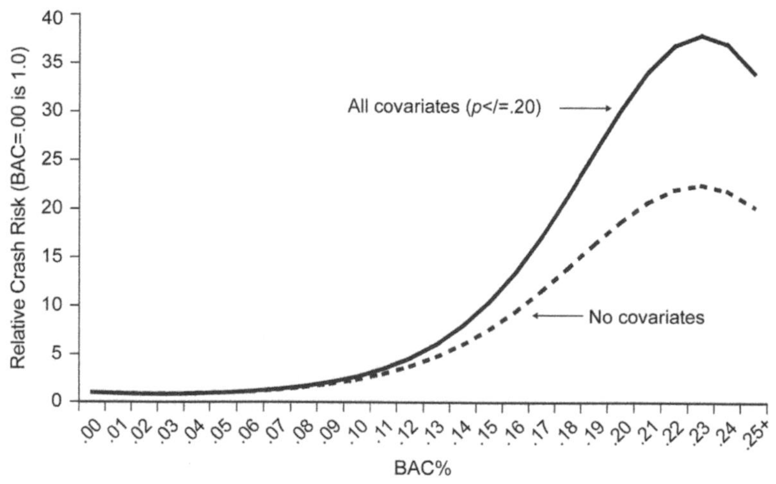

Figure 17.1 Relative risk of a crash by BAC with covariates and without covariates. (Reproduced from Blomberg, R.D. et al., *Crash Risk of Alcohol Involved Driving: A Case-Control Study* (Final Report), Dunlap & Associates: Stamford, CT, 2005. With permission.)

17.1.4 Impaired Drivers on the Roads in the United States

Since 1973, five national surveys of US drivers have estimated the prevalence of drinking and driving, showing how this prevalence has changed over time (1973, 1986, 1996, 2007, 2013–2014). In the first three National Roadside Surveys (NRS) (1973, 1986, 1996), breath alcohol tests were given to drivers on the roads on weekend nights. In 2007 and in 2013–2014, the fourth and fifth NRS studies changed their methodology to become a national field study to estimate the prevalence of alcohol-, drug-, and alcohol-plus-drug-involved driving among daytime drivers on Friday as well as nighttime weekend drivers (Berning et al. 2015; Lacey et al. 2009; Ramirez et al. 2016). These two NRSs involved randomly stopping drivers at 300 locations across the continental United States. The locations were selected through a stratified random-sampling procedure. Researchers collected the data during a 2-hour Friday daytime session (either 9:30 am to 11:30 am or 1:30 pm to 3:30 pm) at 60 locations and during four 2-hour nighttime periods (10 pm to midnight and 1 am to 3 am on Friday and Saturday nights) at 240 locations, for the total of 300 locations.

The data collected in these surveys included both self-reported use of alcohol and other drugs and biological measures such as BAC levels. The goal was to obtain at least 7,500 oral fluid samples for analysis. Oral fluid and blood samples were subjected to laboratory screening and liquid or gas chromatography-mass spectrometry confirmation respectively for alcohol and six classes of drugs, allowing researchers to estimate a national prevalence of alcohol and other drugs used by drivers. All drivers' responses were completely voluntary and anonymous. Figure 17.2 shows the percentages of drivers who had been drinking alcohol as estimated in these surveys (see [Christophersen et al. 2016] for the international perspective).

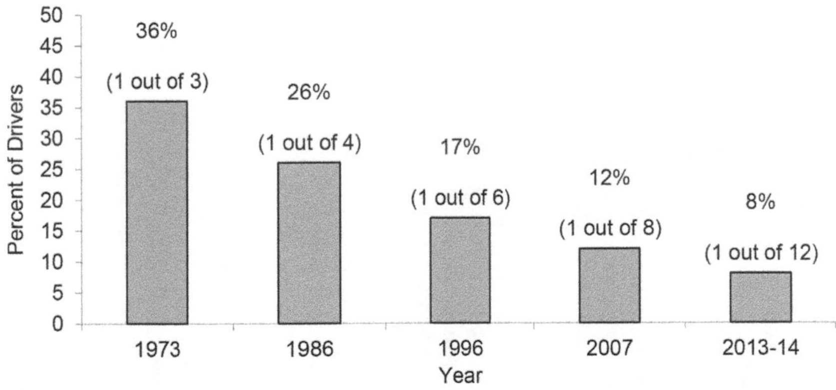

Figure 17.2 Percent of drivers on US roads with positive BAC levels (BAC ≥ 0.01) (weekend evenings). (Figure is constructed based on data appearing in Berning, A. et al., *Results of the 2013–2014 National Roadside Survey of Alcohol and Drug Use by Drivers* (DOT HS 812 118), US National Highway Traffic Safety Administration, Washington, DC, 2015; Lacey, J.H. et al., *National Roadside Survey of Alcohol and Drug Use by Drivers: Alcohol Results* (Report No. DOT HS 811 248), US National Highway Traffic Safety Administration, Washington, DC, 2009; Ramirez, A., *2013–2014 National Roadside Study of Alcohol and Drug Use by Drivers: Alcohol Results* (Report No. DOT HS 812 362), US National Highway Traffic Safety Administration, Washington, DC, 2016.)

17.1.5 Impaired Drivers in Fatal Crashes in the United States

Since 1982, the United States has been tracking the BACs of drivers fatally injured in traffic crashes. Trends in BACs in fatally injured drivers were examined and reported under the US Fatality Analysis Reporting System (FARS) from 1982 to 2016 (US National Highway Traffic Safety Administration 2019). In 2016, BAC levels could be determined for 61% of driver fatalities. When BAC data were unavailable, the estimated BAC was statistically imputed using crash, driver, and other characteristics to obtain more complete and accurate alcohol data (Subramanian 2002). In 2016, 30% of fatally injured drivers had impairing BACs (≥0.05 g/dL); 28% were at or above the illegal BAC limit in the United States (BAC ≥ 0.08 g/dL); and 12% had very high BACs (≥0.20 g/dL). These percentages are a vast improvement over 1982 when the percentages were, respectively, 52% (≥0.05 g/dL), 49% (≥0.08 g/dL), and 22% (≥0.20 g/dL). However, most of the reductions occurred before 1997, and the percentages of fatally injured drivers with BACs in the above ranges have changed little since then. While the number of drivers killed in crashes decreased 4% between 1997 and 2016, the proportion with impairing BAC levels (≥0.05 g/dL) has ranged from 36% in 2008 and 2009 to 30% in 2016 (see Figure 17.3). (Drugs other than alcohol are not consistently tested for in FARS so they are not included in the analyses presented below.)

17.1.6 Arrests for Driving Under the Influence in the United States

In 1989 there were an estimated 1,940,000 arrests for DUI in the United States (US Federal Bureau of Investigation 2019). Figure 17.4 shows that arrests had declined by 49%, to an estimated 990,000, by 2017 (US Federal Bureau of Investigation 2019). As demonstrated in Figure 17.3, this decline was not due to a decrease in the prevalence of impaired driving in fatal crashes. So, a research dilemma is to determine why the percent of impaired drivers in roadside surveys decreased significantly, and DUI arrests decreased significantly, yet the percent of drivers in fatal crashes who are alcohol-impaired has not decreased since 1997.

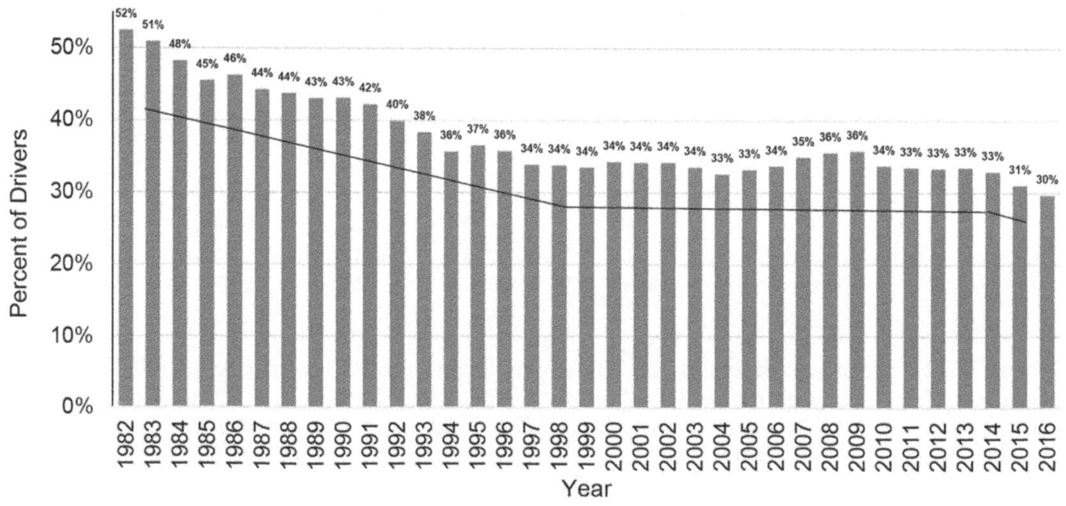

Figure 17.3 Proportion of all fatally injured drivers estimated to have been impaired (BAC ≥ 0.05), 1982–2016 (−42%). (Figure is constructed based on data appearing in US National Highway Traffic Safety Administration 1982–2016.)

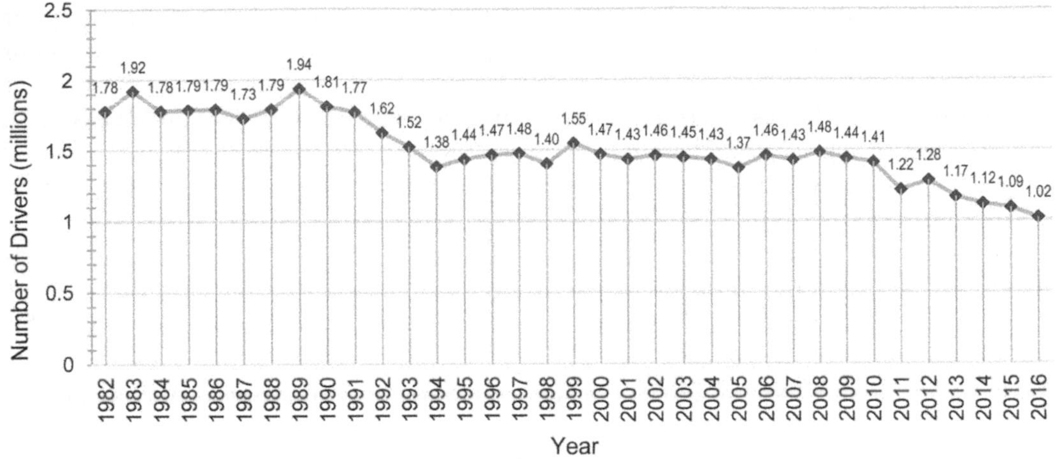

Figure 17.4 DUI arrests in the United States: 1982–2016. (Figure is constructed based on data appearing in US Federal Bureau of Investigation 1982–2016.)

While DUI arrest rates in a community have been shown to correlate with impaired driving on the roads and with crashes in that community (Fell et al. 2015), the actual risk of arrest for DUI in the United States is quite small. Estimates have varied from 1 in 2,000 impaired drivers, based on an analysis of average annual officer arrest rates (2 per year per officer) (Borkenstein 1975), to about 1 in 88 impaired drivers, based on responses to a national telephone survey and FBI crime statistics (Zador et al. 2000a). The most carefully developed risk estimates were those reported in (Beitel et al. 2000; Hause et al. 1982), based on studies in which field researchers rode with police. They found a probability of arrest for 6 in 1,000 drivers with BACs of 0.10 or higher. A more recent study estimated that only about 1 in 1,000 drivers on the roads with illegal BACs (>0.08 g/dL) is ever arrested for DUI (Zaloshnja et al. 2013). The US public is generally not aware of these low probabilities (Royal 2000).

The next sections of this chapter present evidence-based countermeasures that have been associated with valid measures of reductions in alcohol-impaired driving. These countermeasures have proven to be effective or to have strong potential to reduce impaired driving in the future.

17.2 Primary Prevention: Reducing High-Risk Drinking and High-Risk Driving

17.2.1 Alcohol-Control Policies: Limiting Alcohol Availability

17.2.1.1 Minimum Legal Drinking Age Laws

Minimum legal drinking age (MLDA) laws were established in the United States after the repeal of Prohibition in 1933. Many states set the MLDA at 21 during that time. When the voting age was lowered from 21 to 18 in 1971, many states lowered their legal drinking age to 18 or 19. Studies in the 1970s and 1980s showed significant increases in alcohol-related crashes involving youth aged 18 to 20 in states that lowered their drinking age (Brown and Maghsoodloo 1981; Cook and Tauchen 1984; Ferreira and Sickerman 1976; Wagenaar et al. 1995; Williams et al. 1975). Later, several studies showed that raising the drinking age lowered traffic crashes and crash fatalities (Hingson et al. 1983; Wagenaar 1981; Williams et al. 1983). Consequently, the US Congress adopted the National Uniform Drinking Age 21 Act, which provided a substantial financial incentive for states to adopt an MLDA of 21, and President Reagan signed the bill into law in 1984. Since 1988, the MLDA has applied to age 21 for both the purchase and possession of alcohol in all 50 states and the District of Columbia (DC).

Between 1982 and 1998, the population-adjusted fatal crash rate involving drinking drivers aged 20 and younger in the United States decreased 59% (Hedlund et al. 2001). MLDA-21 laws have been shown to be independently associated with part of this decline (O'Malley and Wagenaar 1991; Shults et al. 2001; Toomey et al. 1996; Voas et al. 2003; Wagenaar and Toomey 2002). The National Highway Traffic Safety Administration (NHTSA) has estimated that MLDA laws save approximately 900 lives a year in traffic fatalities alone (Arnold 1985; Kindelberger 2005; US National Center for Statistics and Analysis 2005; Womble 1989). Other studies have shown that homicides (Jones et al. 1992; Parker and Rebhun 1995), suicides (Birckmayer and Hemenway 1999), and unintentional injuries (Jones et al. 1992) by 18- to 20-year-olds have also fallen as the MLDA has risen to 21.

Numerous studies (Klepp et al. 1996; O'Malley and Wagenaar 1991; Voas et al. 2000b; Wagenaar 1983; Wagenaar and Toomey 2002), including a comprehensive review of literature from 1960 to 1999 (Wagenaar and Toomey 2002), have uniformly shown that increasing the minimum drinking age has significantly decreased self-reported drinking by young people, the number of fatal traffic crashes, and the number of arrests for DUI involving youths aged 20 and younger. Meta-analysis of 33 studies of the MLDA reported a change of 10% to 16% in fatal crashes: increasing fatal crashes if the MLDA was lowered, and decreasing fatal crashes if it was raised (Shults et al. 2001). Another study found that when New Zealand lowered its drinking age from 20 to 18, crash injuries among 15- to 19-year-olds increased (Kypri et al. 2006). While many youth under age 21 still drink alcohol, raising the legal drinking age makes it more difficult to obtain alcohol and to drink and drive. The MLDA-21 law has been considered one of the most important public health policies adopted in the United States (Shults et al. 2001).

17.2.1.2 Law Components Associated with MLDA

Legal research involving the use of the Alcohol Policy Information System (APIS) (US National Institute on Alcohol Abuse and Alcoholism 2019) has indicated that there are at least 20 MLDA-21 laws that have been adopted at the state level in the United States (Fell et al. 2016b). Table 17.1 contains a brief summary of those 20 laws; in parentheses is the number of states (including DC) that have currently adopted each law.

In a study assessing all 20 MLDA laws, nine were found to be associated with significant decreases in fatal crash ratios of underage drinking drivers (Fell et al. 2016b): penalties for possession of alcohol (–7.7%), penalties for purchase of alcohol (–4.2%), license loss with alcohol use (–7.9%), 0.02 BAC limit for underage drivers (–2.9%), bartenders required to be over 21 (–4.1%), institution of a state responsible-beverage-service program (–3.8%), fake-identification-detection support provisions for retailers (–11.9%), dram-shop liability for underage-drinking-related crashes (–2.5%), and social-host civil liability for underage-drinking–related crashes (–1.7%). The nine effective MLDA-21 laws were estimated to save approximately 1,135 lives annually, yet only five states have enacted all nine. If all states adopted these nine laws, an additional 210 lives could be saved in the United States every year.

Table 17.1 US Minimum Legal Drinking Age 21 (MLDA-21) Law Components and Descriptions

MLDA-21 Law Components	Description
	Core Laws That Apply to Youths
1. Possession	Illegal for youths under age 21 to possess alcohol (50 states + DC)
2. Purchase	Illegal for youths under age 21 to purchase or attempt to purchase alcohol (47 states + DC)
	Expanded Laws That Apply to Youths
3. Consumption	Illegal for youths under age 21 to consume alcohol (34 states + DC)
4. Internal possession	Evidence of possession and consumption via a BAC test (9 states)
5. Use and lose	Alcohol citation for a youth under age 21 results in driver's license suspension (39 states + DC)
6. Use of fake identification	Fake ID minor—Illegal for a youth under age 21 to use a fake identification to purchase alcohol (50 states + DC)
	Apply to Youth Driving
7. Zero tolerance	ZT—Illegal for drivers under age 21 to have any alcohol in their system when driving (50 states + DC)
8. Graduated driver licensing with night restrictions	GDL—Youths with intermediate or provisional license prohibited from driving without an adult in the vehicle past a certain hour at night (50 states + DC)
	Apply to Providers
9. Furnishing or selling	Illegal to furnish or sell alcohol to youths under age 21 (50 states + DC)
10. Age of on-premise servers	Minimum age 21 set for selling/serving alcohol (13 states)
11. Age of on-premise bartenders	Minimum age 21 for bartenders (23 states + DC)
12. Age of off-premise sellers	Minimum age 21 set for selling/serving alcohol (23 states)
13. Keg registration	Identification number for beer keg and purchaser required (30 states + DC)
14. Responsible beverage service training	RBS—Responsible beverage training mandatory or voluntary (37 states + DC)
15. Retailer support provisions for fake	Fake ID retailer—Provisions to assist retailers in avoiding sales to youths identification under age 21 (45 states)
16. Social host prohibition	SHP—Prohibits social hosting of underage drinking parties (28 states)
17. Dram shop liability	Action against commercial provider of alcohol (44 states + DC)
18. Social host civil liability	Action against non-commercial (private) provider of alcohol (33 states)
	Apply to Manufacturers or Suppliers of Fake Identification
19. Transfer/production of fake identification	Fake ID supplier—Prohibits manufacturing and/or supplying fake identification to youths for the purposes of buying alcohol (24 states)
	Apply to States Concerning Control of Alcohol Distribution
20. State control of alcohol sales	State control—A state-run retail distribution system of alcoholic beverages, i.e., beer, wine spirits (11 states)

17.2.1.3 Responsible-Beverage-Service Training and Enforcement

In a systematic review of interventions designed to reduce alcohol use and related harms in drinking environments, a study included seven studies that evaluated server-training interventions to increase responsible-beverage-service (RBS) practices (Jones et al. 2011). Three of the seven studies specifically examined the impact of server training on

RBS-intervention practices by servers. One found no impact, and the other two found some increases in server intervention. Both studies, however, indicated a low frequency of intervention among the trained servers. Evidence on the effects of server-intervention programs on patrons' alcohol consumption has also been mixed. One study of statewide-mandated server training (Holder and Wagenaar 1994) showed that it had a statistically significant effect on single-vehicle nighttime crashes. Another study (Graham et al. 2004) found that an intervention designed to reduce aggression among bar patrons (better lighting, visible presence of bouncers) had a modest impact on severe and moderate patron aggression (reduction in verbal arguments and physical fights).

Other research on RBS programs has shown that RBS practices can be a valuable tool in lowering rates of high-risk alcohol consumption and impaired driving. For example, server-training programs were found to help reduce the level of intoxication of bar patrons (Johnsson and Berglund 2003). In their study, the average BACs of patrons of bars given a server-training program were reduced more than the BACs of patrons at the control bars at a one-month follow-up. In a study (Toomey et al. 2001), the owners and managers of five bars in Minnesota received information on risk level, policies to prevent illegal sales, legal issues, and communication on alcohol-serving issues. The result of underage and pseudo-intoxicated (actors pretending to be drunk) purchase attempts conducted before and after the intervention showed that underage sales decreased by 11.5% and pseudo-intoxicated sales fell by 46% compared to the control bars.

Two communities in the United States—Rochester, NY and Cleveland, OH—participated in a demonstration and evaluation of a set of bar-related interventions (Fell et al. 2017). The intervention programs applied RBS training, targeted enforcement, and corrective actions by law enforcement to a random sample of 10 identified problem bars in each community, and results were compared to those for 10 matched problem bars without interventions. In Rochester, the percentage of intervention-bar patrons who were intoxicated decreased from 44% before the intervention to 27% after the intervention, which was statistically significant relative to the comparison bars. The average BAC of patrons in the intervention bars decreased from 0.097 g/dL (over the 0.08 g/dL limit for driving) to 0.059 g/dL pre- to post-intervention relative to the comparison bar patrons. In Cleveland, the percentage of pseudo-intoxicated patrons (actors pretending to be intoxicated) who were denied service in the intervention bars increased from 6% to 29%. This was significant relative to the comparison bars. It appears that when bar managers and owners are aware of the program and its enforcement and when servers are properly trained in RBS, fewer patrons may become intoxicated and greater efforts may be made to deny service to obviously intoxicated patrons. Given that about a third to half of all arrested impaired drivers had their last drink at a licensed establishment (bar, tavern, or restaurant) (Anglin et al. 1997; Eby 1995; O'Donnell 1985), widespread implementation of this strategy has the potential to help reduce impaired driving.

17.2.2 Citizen-Activist Organizations (e.g., Mothers Against Drunk Driving)

In the early 1980s, the public's attitude toward drinking and driving in the United States was substantially transformed by the victim-activist movement, marked by the founding and growth of Mothers Against Drunk Driving (MADD). Media coverage of drinking and driving increased (Clark and Hilton 1991; Moulden and Russell 1994). Most observers credit victim-activist groups, particularly MADD, for this sudden increase in press coverage (McCarthy et al. 1987). The sanctions for impaired driving also increased. A study (Merki and Lingg 1987) concluded that MADD has been a major force behind the adoption by states and communities of eight effective impaired-driving strategies. Another study (McCarthy and Ziliak 1990) found that the presence of a MADD chapter significantly reduced the number of DUI crashes resulting in injuries.

It has been estimated that 300,000 lives were saved between 1982 and 2004 due to the reduction in traffic fatalities involving impaired driving (Fell and Voas 2006a). The reduction in alcohol-related fatalities following the emergence of MADD supports the hypothesis that the group had an important effect on impaired driving in the 1980s. The continuation of substantial reductions into the early 1990s, when MADD emerged as the primary victim-activist organization, suggests that it had the primary influence on the observed reduction. Marshall and Oleson described the beneficial effects of MADD's victim services (Marshall and Oleson 1996), and McCarthy and Wolfson (1996) concluded that an affiliation with MADD appeared to energize local leaders in countering drunk driving. Compton found an effect of the adjudication of DUI offenders due to MADD's court-monitoring program (Compton 1987).

MADD is still an active organization working to reduce impaired driving in the United States. But progress has stagnated due to many competing issues that decrease attention to alcohol-impaired driving—by the public and by law enforcement (e.g., distracted, drowsy, and drugged driving).

17.2.3 Reducing High-Risk Driving by the Young

17.2.3.1 Graduated Driver-Licensing Laws

Research has shown that the first few months of licensure for young novice drivers entail the highest crash risk (Mayhew et al. 2003; McCartt et al. 2003; Sagberg 1998; Williams 1985). To address this issue, all US states and numerous other countries (e.g., Australia, New Zealand, the UK, South Africa, Canada) have adopted graduated driver licensing (GDL) laws that require a staged progression to full license privileges.

GDL laws generally require three-staged licensing for novice drivers: (a) a learner's permit period—practice driving with a licensed driver aged 21 or older; (b) an intermediate or provisional stage—drive solo only under certain conditions (e.g., restricts late-night driving and limits teen passengers); and (c) a full license with no restrictions (minimum age of 18 in some states and most other countries). The young driver must meet certain requirements to "graduate" to each stage. Evaluations of state programs in Florida (Ulmer et al. 2000), North Carolina (Foss and Goodwin 2003; Foss et al. 2001), and Michigan (Shope and Molnar 2004; Shope et al. 2001) showed reductions in crashes involving 16- and 17-year-olds that ranged up to 26%. A study (Chen et al. 2006) found that GDL programs appeared to be associated with an 11% reduction in fatal crashes involving 16-year-olds in the states that had implemented them. Several national studies of GDL systems in the United States have indicated they help reduce the crash rates of young novice drivers aged 15 to 17 (Dee et al. 2005; McCartt et al. 2009; Vanlaar et al. 2009).

17.2.3.2 Nighttime Driving and Passenger Restrictions for Young Drivers

A study explored the influence of nighttime curfew policies by comparing crash rates for young teenagers (aged 15, 16, or 17, depending on the state) in states with and without curfew laws (Preusser et al. 1984). These researchers estimated reductions in the crash involvement of 16-year-old drivers during curfew hours ranging from 25% to 69% and concluded that the laws were beneficial relative to their costs. Consequently, nighttime and passenger restrictions were incorporated into all GDL laws.

The nighttime and passenger restrictions under the GDL laws have been evaluated for their effectiveness (Fell et al. 2011b). Nighttime restrictions reduced 16- and 17-year-old driver involvements in nighttime fatal crashes by an estimated 10% and 16- and 17-year-old drinking drivers in nighttime fatal crashes by 13%. Passenger restrictions were found to reduce 16- and 17-year-old driver involvements in fatal crashes with teen passengers by an estimated 9%. These results confirm the effectiveness of these provisions in GDL systems.

In a study of GDL laws (Masten et al. 2011), substantial reductions (down 26%) in fatal crashes for 16-year-old drivers were found to be associated with the adoption of strong GDL laws, but for 18-year-olds fatal crashes increased in those same states (up 12%). The authors suggested that strong GDL laws might have delayed licensure of many youth until they were aged 18 to avoid all the GDL provisions and requirements. An analysis (Fell et al. 2013) indicated similar results. Estimates based on the statistically significant ($p < 0.05$) findings for each age group found that for 16-year-olds, 1,945 lives were saved by GDL-related reductions in fatal crashes, but these were offset by increases in fatal crashes for older teens. For the strong GDL laws, there was a net increase in fatalities of 377 due to the increase in fatal crashes by drivers aged 18, with an additional increase of 855 fatalities if the 19-year-old increase is included. Strong GDL laws resulted in 2,347 lives saved due to the reduction of drivers aged 16 in fatal crashes but were associated with an increase of 2,724 fatalities from fatal crash involvements of drivers aged 18.

The outcome of these two studies indicate once more that GDL laws save the lives of the population they target: novice drivers aged 15 to 17 and especially drinking novice drivers. This favorable impact is even larger for the better GDL programs (i.e., the enacted GDL is "good"). These results also indicate that the lives of some drivers aged 15 to 17 saved by GDL laws are offset by the associated increases in fatal crashes by drivers aged 18 and 19. The reasons for the conflict in GDL benefits are still unclear. Factors include: (a) drivers aged 18 and 19 skipping the GDL phases and beginning to drive at a later age, reducing their driving experience; (b) drivers aged 18 and 19 exhibiting more risk-taking behaviors (e.g., impaired driving, lack of safety belt use, distracted driving) than younger drivers; (c) drivers aged 18 and 19 having increased exposure to risk for a fatal crash (e.g., more late-night driving; more driving on high-speed roads); and/or (d) drivers aged 18 and 19 who have gone through the two phases of GDL lacking driving experience under risky conditions because of all the restrictions in the GDL laws. Whatever the reasons, this finding suggests that perhaps GDL laws should be applied to protect novice drivers older than ages 16 and 17, for example up to age 21 (although this might just postpone the increase in crashes to drivers over age 21). Further research to clarify this dilemma is needed.

17.3 Secondary Prevention: Reducing Drinking and Driving

17.3.1 Evidence-Based Legislation

17.3.1.1 Illegal BAC Limits for Driving

The BAC levels that are used by states to define impaired driving for enforcement purposes are based on case-controlled relative-risk studies (Borkenstein et al. 1975; Blomberg et al.

2005, 2009; Voas et al. 2012; Zador et al. 2000b). Initially set at 0.15 g/dL BAC in the 1950s, state BAC limits in the United States were generally lowered to 0.10 g/dL BAC by the 1980s. The strong evidence that BACs as low as 0.05 g/dL increased crash risk motivated several states to lower their limit to 0.08 g/dL in the 1990s. By 2000, the US Congress passed legislation encouraging all states to adopt 0.08 g/dL BAC laws by threatening to withhold a portion of a state's federal highway funds for noncompliance. This movement stimulated many research studies of the effectiveness of lowering the BAC limit from 0.10 to 0.08 g/dL. Most of these studies found sizable decreases in alcohol-related crashes associated with the 0.08 g/dL BAC limit. Between 1991 and 2000, nine evaluations of 0.08 g/dL laws involving 11 states were conducted in the United States (Apsler et al. 1999; Foss et al. 1998; Hingson et al. 1996, 2000; Johnson and Fell 1995; Research and Evaluation Associates 1991; Rogers 1995; Voas et al. 2000a, 2000b). A meta-analysis (Shults et al. 2001) of 25 studies on the enactment of the 0.08 law found that the median crash reduction among the studies they reviewed was 7%. A more recent panel study of the overall effects of the 0.08 BAC law in all 50 states and DC in the United States found a 10.4% reduction in the drinking-driver fatal crash rate associated with the lowered BAC (Scherer and Fell 2019).

A general review (Fell and Voas 2014) of studies of the effect of lowering the BAC limit in foreign countries and the United States, and concluded that further lowering the BAC limit to 0.05 g/dL would be likely to reduce alcohol-related crashes. In 1988, the illegal BAC limit was lowered from 0.08 to 0.05 g/dL in Austria. A study of the law found that there was an overall 9.4% decrease in alcohol-related crashes relative to the total number of crashes (Bartl and Esberger 2000). However, they noted that intense media and enforcement campaigns also occurred around the time that the limit was lowered, making it nearly impossible to attribute the reductions to any one of these factors, at least in the short term. A study (Bartl and Esberger 2000) concluded that "lowering the legal BAC limit from. 08 to 0.05 g/dL in combination with intensive police enforcement and reporting in the media leads to a positive short-term effect." This provided support for the view that a limit of 0.05 g/dL BAC or less, as part of a comprehensive approach to fighting impaired driving, can have beneficial effects.

It was found that lowering the BAC limit from 0.08 to 0.05 g/dL, in New South Wales, Australia, significantly reduced fatal crashes on Saturdays by 13% (Homel 1994). A rigorous time-series analysis of RBT and 0.05 g/dL BAC laws, in Australia, included many controlling factors such as seasonal effects, weather, economic trends, road use, alcohol consumption, and day of the week (Henstridge et al. 1997). Although the primary focus of the Australian study was the impact of RBT, the findings on the effect of 0.05 g/dL BAC laws were also significant. The study statistically accounted for the effect of other alcohol countermeasures to determine the specific values of the declines that were attributable directly to either RBT or the lower 0.05 g/dL BAC limit. The study analyzed traffic data for periods ranging from 13 to 17 years and found Australian states that lowered their BAC limits from 0.08 to 0.05 g/dL experienced meaningful declines in alcohol-related crash measures. For example, after Queensland, Australia, reduced its *per se* (i.e., no other evidence needed; just exceeding the BAC limit is illegal) BAC limit to 0.05 g/dL in 1982, it experienced an 18% reduction in fatal collisions and a 14% reduction in serious collisions. These results were not confounded by the effects of RBT, as it was not introduced until 8 years later. Similarly, the 0.05 g/dL BAC limit in New South Wales was estimated to have reduced serious collisions by 7%, fatal collisions by 8%, and single-vehicle nighttime collisions by 11%.

The effects of lowering the BAC limit in Queensland from 0.08 to 0.05 g/dL BAC was specifically evaluated (Smith 1988). A proxy measure of changes in nighttime crashes as compared to daytime crashes was used. There was a significant 8.2% reduction in nighttime serious injury crashes (requiring hospitalization) and a 5.5% reduction in nighttime property-damage crashes associated with the 0.05 g/dL BAC limit in the first year. Smith partially attributes the crash reductions in the second and third years after the adoption of 0.05 g/dL BAC to increased enforcement. Smith concludes that when lowering the BAC limit stimulates increased enforcement, it should be considered a benefit rather than a drawback of the law.

The evidence for lowering the BAC limit for driving, especially to 0.05 g/dL, is very strong. It apparently sends a message to would-be drinking drivers that the government is getting tougher on impaired driving and serves as a general deterrent to drinking and driving.

17.3.1.2 Zero-Tolerance Laws for Novice Drivers

By 1988, all states in the United States had enacted MLDA laws making it illegal for those younger than 21 to purchase or possess alcohol. This provided a basis for implementing a zero-BAC limit for drivers aged 20 and younger. In 1995, the US Congress passed a law creating a financial penalty (a reduction in their highway construction funds) for states that did not adopt zero-tolerance laws for drivers younger than 21. By 1998, all states and DC had passed laws making it illegal for any driver younger than 21 to have a positive BAC (generally defined as a BAC of 0.02 g/dL or greater). These zero-tolerance laws for youth have proven effective in reducing fatal crashes involving underage drinking drivers (Blomberg 1992; Fell et al. 2008b; Hingson et al. 1992, 1994; Voas et al. 2003; Zwerling and Jones 1999). A meta-analysis of the studies of zero-tolerance laws found reductions of 9% to 24% in fatal crashes (Shults et al. 2001). Zero-tolerance laws for young drivers are now being adopted in several countries.

17.3.1.3 Administrative License Revocation

Administrative license revocation (ALR) or suspension (ALS) is the administrative revocation or suspension of the driver's license of a driving while intoxicated (DWI) or DUI offender at the time of arrest (Lacey et al. 1991). ALS differs from traditional judicial license actions in several ways. First, anyone arrested for DUI in the United States in a state with an ALS law is immediately subject to ALS. Usually, the arresting officer confiscates the license and issues a notice of ALS. Often, the notice of ALS may serve as a temporary license for a period (e.g., 10–30 days) during which the driver may request an administrative hearing for license reinstatement. Regardless of the outcome of such a hearing, the arrestee is still subject to a separate criminal charge that may lead to additional penalties, including judicial license actions (Williams et al. 1991).

At the end of the suspension period, some states reissue the license back to the driver, often charging a license-reinstatement fee and requiring verification of insurance. Other states require a complete driver's license reexamination, including a reinstatement fee, before driving privileges are restored. Some states suspend the license but issue a hardship license while the suspension remains in effect (US National Highway Traffic Safety Administration 1992).

ALR or ALS laws have been shown in a nationwide study to reduce fatal crashes involving drinking drivers by 13% to 19% (Voas et al. 2000b). ALR laws were found (Wagenaar and Maldonado-Molina 2007) to have statistically significant and substantially important effects in reducing impaired-driving fatal crashes pooled across states; the 5% reduction in crashes represented at least 800 lives saved per year. Other earlier studies (Klein

1989; Ross and Gonzales 1988; Shults et al. 2001; Voas et al. 2000; Wagenaar et al. 1995; Williams 1992; Zador et al. 1988) have shown similar effects for ALR/ALS laws. An econometric analysis (Kenkel 1993) evaluated ALR laws along with mandatory jail sentencing, preliminary breath testing, sobriety checkpoints, and prohibition of plea bargaining, and concluded that stricter laws could decrease drunk-driving crashes by 20%.

License suspension generally has been shown to reduce DUI offender recidivism when suspended offenders are compared with offenders that avoid suspension (Hagen 1977; Lacey et al. 1990; McKnight and Voas 1991). There is also strong evidence that ALR laws have had a general deterrent effect on impaired-driving fatal crashes (Jones and Lacey 2001). Studies in other countries have confirmed the effectiveness of ALR (Beirness et al. 1997; Mann et al. 2002; Stoduto et al. 2000). NHTSA has sponsored studies on the effects of publicizing ALR laws (Lacey et al. 1986), on the cost benefit of ALR (Lacey et al. 1991), on the effects of ALR on employment (Knoebel and Ross 1996), and on the effectiveness of allowing telephonic testimony at ALR hearings (Wiliszowski et al. 2003).

ALR laws have been challenged but ruled constitutional by the US Supreme Court (US Supreme Court 1979). The Supreme Court found that the right to due process is not violated if a driver's license is suspended prior to an administrative hearing as long as it is a swift post-suspension hearing. All other legal cases in which state appellate courts have ruled on ALR/ALS issues have held that a separate criminal trial following an ALR action does not constitute double jeopardy under federal or state laws.

A study (Fell and Scherer 2017a) found that ALR laws are effective and that the ALR suspension length does matter. The implementation of any ALR law (with any suspension length) was associated with a 13.1% decrease in the drinking/nondrinking driver Fatality Analysis Reporting System (FARS) ratio, but only a 1.8% decrease in the intoxicated/non-intoxicated fatal crash ratio. So, the ALR law affects drinking drivers (BAC > 0.01 g/dL) substantially, but not intoxicated drivers (BAC > 0.08 g/dL). The risk of a fatal crash increases at each increase in the BAC level (Voas et al. 2012), so it appears that ALR laws send a message to not drink and drive (BAC = 0.01–0.07 g/dL) or you will lose your license, but apparently does not reach drivers who get intoxicated and then drive (BAC ≥ 0.08 g/dL). According to the fatal-crash data, more than half of intoxicated drivers (BAC ≥ 0.08 g/dL) in fatal crashes have very high BACs (BAC ≥ 0.15 g/dL). These are binge drinkers and/or abusive drinkers. Perhaps moderate drinkers (BAC = 0.01–0.07 g/dL), the majority of drinking drivers on US roads (Berning et al. 2015), fear the loss of their license more than binge drinkers (BAC ≥ 0.08 g/dL) do, or have more ability to moderate their alcohol-related behaviors in response to perceived risks.

Regarding ALR suspension length, even a short suspension period of 1–30 days has a significant effect on the drinking-driver ratio ($p < 0.001$) compared to having no ALR law. However, suspension periods of 31–90 days are no better than periods of 1–30 days. States with ALR suspension periods of 91–180 days had significantly larger ($p < 0.001$) reductions in drinking drivers than states with suspension periods of 1–90 days, as did the three states with suspension periods greater than 180 days compared to states with suspension lengths of 1–180 days ($p = 0.013$) (Fell and Scherer 2017b).

17.3.1.4 Primary Enforcement Safety-Belt Laws

NHTSA estimates that safety belts, when worn in a passenger car involved in a serious crash, are 45% effective in preventing fatalities (Klein and Walz 1998). A study (Klein and Walz 1998) also tracked vehicle safety belt use in the FARS from 1982 through 1995 and found non-use to be positively correlated with BAC levels for every year. In 1995, 75% of drivers at 0.10 g/dL BAC did not use safety belts compared to 34% of the drivers at zero BACs. There are two types of state laws regarding safety belt use: secondary laws, which allow officers to cite unbelted drivers only if they are stopped for some other traffic offense, and primary laws, which permit stopping the vehicle of an unbelted user.

It was found that when California moved from a secondary to a primary law, belt wearing increased from 70% to 90% among nondrinking drivers (Lange and Voas 1998). In contrast, the usage rate among drivers with BACs of 0.10 or higher increased from 50% to 90%. Aside from their direct effect in reducing the severity of injuries, primary safety-belt laws may be particularly effective in deterring impaired drivers because they allow the officer to stop the car, leading to the detection of drinking. Further evidence for the potential effectiveness of primary safety-belt laws in reducing impaired-driving crashes was provided (Voas et al. 2007). In a study of five states that passed primary safety-belt laws, four experienced significant declines in alcohol-related fatal crashes relative to non-alcohol-related fatal crashes.

17.3.2 Law Enforcement Strategies

17.3.2.1 Sobriety Checkpoints and Random Breath Testing

The highly successful random breath testing (RBT) enforcement procedure used in Australia, Sweden, and other countries allows officers to stop any vehicle on the road at random and to require the driver to take a breath test. Operators with BACs higher than the legal limit are transported to the police station for an evidential test. A study in 1997 found that RBT was twice as effective as "selective" checkpoints similar to those conducted in the United States (Henstridge et al. 1997). An earlier study in 1990 found that in Queensland, Australia, RBT resulted in a 35% reduction in fatal crashes, compared with 15% for checkpoints (Sherman 1990). The researchers estimated that every increase of 1,000 in the daily RBT testing rate corresponded to a decline of 6% in all serious crashes and 19% in single-vehicle nighttime crashes. Moreover, analyses revealed a measurable continuing deterrent effect of RBT on the motorist population after the program had been in place for 10 years. A study in 1988 showed that the deterrent influence of RBT also provided heavy drinkers with a legitimate excuse to drink less when drinking with friends (Homel 1988). A review of the effectiveness of sobriety checkpoints in Thailand was conducted in 2011 and concluded that barriers to successful enforcement needed to be overcome for the strategy to be effective (Ditsuwan et al. 2015). In a follow-up study of the cost-effectiveness of sobriety checkpoints in Thailand (Ditsuwan et al. 2013), the authors concluded that checkpoints need to be conducted with greater intensity to complement the investment in publicity campaigns.

In contrast, vehicles in the United States can only be stopped at random at specially designated "checkpoints" and drivers cannot be required to take a breath test. Rather, the officer must conduct an interview to determine whether the driver is impaired, and if there is evidence of impairment, the officer must require the driver to perform a set of field sobriety tests to establish impairment before transporting the offender to the police station. Studies of the US sobriety-checkpoint procedure found that checkpoints are associated with significant decreases in alcohol-related crashes (Epperlein 1987; Lacey et al. 1986; Levy et al. 1988, 1990; Voas 2008; Voas et al. 1985; Wells et al. 1992). Two related meta-analyses of 15 US checkpoint programs occurring between 1985 and 1999 found that the median reduction in crashes associated with checkpoints was 20% (Elder et al. 2002; Shults et al. 2001). A cost-benefit study of sobriety checkpoints indicated that, for every $1 invested in the checkpoint strategy, the community conducting the checkpoint saved $6 (Miller et al. 1998).

17.3.3 Impaired-Driving Enforcement Technology

17.3.3.1 Passive Alcohol Sensors

In the United States, police departments have resisted implementing checkpoints, partly because few DUI arrests are made in checkpoint operations (Fell et al. 2004). An important factor limiting arrests is the fact that officers cannot test every driver stopped, as they do in Australia, but must first determine that the individual has been drinking and may be impaired. A device designed to aid the officer in detecting drinking is the passive alcohol sensor, a standard police flashlight with a built-in passive alcohol sensor (see Figure 17.5). It draws in a mix of expired and environmental air from in front of a person's face and is not considered a search prohibited by the Fourth Amendment. These sensors can provide a good estimate of the driver's BAC (Farmer et al. 1999; Voas et al. 2006). The PAS is particularly effective when observation time is short, as it is at checkpoints.

However, efforts to persuade officers to make greater use of passive sensors have generally failed (Fell et al. 2008a) (e.g., PAS devices are too expensive; officers can detect alcohol as well as the PAS, etc.). A series of studies has demonstrated that when officers use passive sensors at a checkpoint, more drinking drivers are detected and the arrest rate increases by approximately 50% (Ferguson et al. 1995; Lestina and Lund 1989; Lund and Jones 1987; Lund et al. 1991). Aside from its effectiveness in increasing the detection of drinking drivers, the most important effect of the PAS on impaired driving may be its potential to increase the perceived risk of being apprehended for DUI if driving after drinking. If police use of the PAS is well publicized, it should increase general deterrence to impaired driving. Heavy drinkers who count on their increased tolerance to alcohol to avoid detection (Ross 1973; Ross and Gonzales 1988) might be deterred by the police's ability to detect drinking in an otherwise sober-appearing driver. Further, making underage drivers aware that even very small amounts of alcohol in the blood can be detected should increase their concern about being cited under the zero-tolerance law. Although the PAS has been used in many enforcement programs, relatively few (Voas et al. 1997; Wells et al. 1992) have actively publicized its use. More comprehensive research on the effects of publicizing PAS use in DUI enforcement is needed.

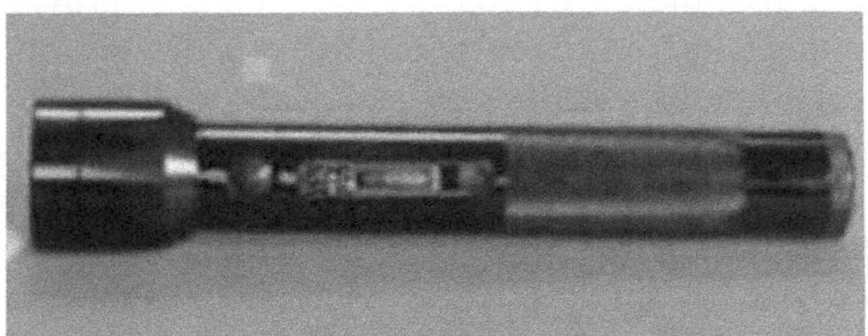

Figure 17.5 A police flashlight with a built-in passive alcohol sensors (PAS V Flashlight Passive Alcohol Tester by ALCOPRO Drug & Alcohol Testing Products: Knoxville, TN). Figure is for open access; https://www.alcopro.com/product/p-a-s-v-flashlight/ (Accessed May 21, 2019).

17.3.4 Publicizing Enforcement Programs

17.3.4.1 Paid Media Campaigns

Because deterrence depends on the perceived rather than the actual probability of being arrested, it is generally accepted that enforcement programs must be well publicized to be effective. General safety publicity without a related enforcement program is usually ineffective in reducing crashes. Publicizing general safety messages such as *If You Drink Don't Drive*, without an associated law or enforcement effort, has generally failed to demonstrate an effect on highway safety (Williams 1992). However, studies have also documented crash reductions produced by publicity in advance of the application of a change such as a new law (Ross 1973) or enforcement effort (Voas and Hause 1987). Sometimes, an enforcement program by itself produces enough public visibility and media attention to make the public aware of the program without a special media program, e.g., (Holder and Treno 1997; Voas 2008; Voas and Hause 1987).

Aside from free publicity provided by the press because of an ongoing enforcement effort, three types of information campaigns help educate the public on impaired-driving laws and enforcement: (a) public service announcements (PSAs); (b) paid media campaigns; and (c) media advocacy programs. Each program has its strengths and limitations. Few media campaigns of any type have been adequately evaluated.

In relation to impaired driving, paid media campaigns have been used most frequently in national *Click It or Ticket* campaigns to increase the use of safety belts or campaigns directed at impaired driving during holidays, such as Labor Day and Christmas, when many local police departments receive funding to implement special enforcement efforts (Tison et al. 2008). Mass media efforts alone are insufficient, however. Results from a comprehensive review (Friend and Levy 2002) of mass media campaigns on tobacco suggested that well-funded and implemented mass media campaigns targeted at smokers, with a comprehensive tobacco-control program, were associated with reduced smoking rates among both adults and youths. Similar strong effects of paid media on impaired driving remain to be demonstrated.

17.4 Tertiary Prevention: Preventing Repeated Infractions by Offenders

17.4.1 Sanctions for Impaired-Driving Offenders

17.4.1.1 Driving While Intoxicated (DWI)/DUI Drug Courts

Based on the effectiveness of drug court models, DUI courts are gradually increasing. Modeled after drug courts, these DUI courts are designed to provide constant supervision to offenders by judges and other court officials, who closely administer and monitor compliance with court-ordered sanctions coupled with treatment. DUI courts generally involve frequent interaction of the offender with the DUI court judge, intensive supervision by probation officers, intensive treatment, random alcohol and other drug testing, community service, lifestyle changes, positive reinforcement for successful performance in the program, and jail time for noncompliance. In jurisdictions that have DUI courts, nonviolent offenders who have had two or more prior DUI convictions typically are assigned to DUI court.

DUI courts are intended to hold offenders accountable for their actions, change offenders' behavior to end recidivism, stop alcohol abuse, treat the victims of DUI offenders in a fair and just way, and protect the public (Freeman-Wilson and Wilkosz 2002; Tauber and Huddleston 1999). It was reported (Breckenridge et al. 2000) that these programs significantly reduce recidivism among alcoholic DUI offenders. At the end of 2003, there were approximately 70 DUI courts and 1,200 Drug courts operating in the United States. By the end of 2007, there were an estimated 400 DUI courts and 2,000 Drug courts overall (Huddleston et al. 2008). A survey by NHTSA (Block 2016) found that there were 473 DUI courts by the end of May 2015. One report on a DUI court in New Mexico indicated that recidivism was reduced by more than 50% for offenders completing the program compared to similar offenders not assigned to the DUI court (Guerin and Pitts 2002). Those results, however, were preliminary and did not include statistical tests.

Three DUI courts in Georgia (Chatham, Clarke, Hall) were evaluated (Fell et al. 2011a). Levels of recidivism for DUI court participants (designated as the Intent to Treat Group) were compared to the recidivism rates for similar DUI offenders during the same time period but in other Georgia jurisdictions (Contemporary Group) and DUI offenders in the same three jurisdictions but before the DUI court was established (Retrospective Group). After four years of exposure, the DUI court participants (combined for all three courts) displayed a recidivism rate of 15%. This was compared to a recidivism rate of 24% for the Contemporary Group and 35% for the Retrospective Group.

The DUI court participants' rates were lower by statistically significant amounts: 38% lower ($p < 0.001$) than rates for the Contemporary Group and 65% lower ($p < 0.001$) than rates for the Retrospective Group. In addition, the DUI graduates had a significantly lower recidivism rate (63.5% lower) ($p < 0.001$) than the matched contemporary offenders from other counties who completed traditional programs and 79.3% lower ($p < 0.001$) than the retrospective offenders from the same counties who would have been eligible for the DUI court had it been operating at the time. Recidivism was also lower than the rate for the group of offenders whose licenses were terminated by DUI court, who had an overall rate of 26%. The 9% recidivism rate for the DUI court graduates was 65.1% lower ($p < 0.001$) than the rate for offenders who were terminated. Results were similar across DUI courts: the Chatham graduates had a recidivism rate of 10%, the Clarke graduates had an 11% rate, and the Hall graduates had a 7% rate. It is estimated that the DUI courts prevented between 47 and 112 repeat DUI arrests.

DUI courts are effective in reducing DUI recidivism and in helping offenders stop excessive drinking and return to a normal life. However, they are labor-intensive and expensive. Cost-benefit studies are needed.

17.4.1.2 Screening and Brief Interventions

When all three levels of prevention—primary, secondary, and tertiary—fail, many drivers become involved in crashes and wind up in hospital emergency rooms or regional trauma centers. This provides an opportunity outside the criminal justice system for the health care system to intervene with high-risk drivers. The trauma of being involved in a crash is viewed as providing a "teachable moment," when individuals may be open to undertaking a behavioral change that will reduce their risk of future crashes and injuries.

Research suggests that 30% to 50% of injured, crash-involved drivers admitted to emergency departments or trauma centers have BAC levels higher than the legal limit for driving (Cornwell et al. 1998; Maio et al. 1997; US National Highway Traffic Safety Administration 2002; Soderstrom et al. 2001). Some of these offenders may receive a court-based treatment intervention because of a DUI arrest; however, many are not charged because they are taken to the hospital before police officers have an opportunity to examine them for impairment, and hospital staff rarely notify the police when they receive a high-BAC driver. When screened for alcohol-use disorders, an estimated 27% of injured patients (including those with non-crash-related injuries) admitted to emergency departments or trauma centers test positive for alcohol abuse or dependence, indicating a large number of people entering emergency rooms who are potential DUI offenders (Gentilello et al. 2005). Thus, emergency rooms and trauma centers have an important opportunity to intervene with high-risk individuals who need treatment for alcohol problems—problems that may well lead to impaired-driving and alcohol-related crashes.

Evaluations indicate that brief interventions can decrease alcohol use (Fleming et al. 2002; Gentilello et al. 1999), including excessive and binge-drinking occasions. Other alcohol-related problems and negative consequences also decreased following such interventions (Mello et al. 2005; Monti et al. 1999). Most importantly, brief interventions effectively reduce driving-related infractions and other consequences, such as moving traffic violations (Gentilello et al. 1999; Monti et al. 1999), drunk-driving violations (Gentilello et al. 1999; Monti et al. 1999; Schermer et al. 2006), motor-vehicle-crash involvement (Runge et al. 2002), crash-sustained injuries (Fleming et al. 2002), and motor-vehicle fatalities (Fleming et al. 2002). A study (Schermer et al. 2006) demonstrated that one re-arrest for DUI could be prevented for every ten cases needing treatment who are treated. Other studies have also found that brief interventions reduce alcohol-related arrests (Fleming et al. 2002; Gentilello et al. 1999), as well as other types of arrests (Fleming et al. 2002) and general legal involvement (Fleming et al. 2002).

Screening and brief interventions (SBI) in medical and public health settings have great potential to reduce excessive drinking and impaired driving. But they have yet to be implemented on a widespread basis, and further evaluation of the effectiveness and cost/benefit ratios of specific types of intervention are needed.

17.4.2 Controlling Impaired Driving by DUI Offenders

17.4.2.1 Alcohol Monitoring

An alternative to controlling the driving of DUI offenders is to control their drinking (Voas 2010). Judges frequently admonish offenders to remain abstinent while on probation, but unless a program exists that monitors the BAC, this action has little force other than allowing the judge to impose more severe penalties if the offender returns to court during the probation period. In the past, offender abstinence has been monitored in several ways. Some courts have implemented closely supervised and intensive-supervision programs in which probation officers make surprise visits to the homes of offenders and conduct breath tests. As noted, DUI/drug courts generally provide for intensive monitoring of abstinence. Such systems are labor-intensive and expensive for the courts. In the last couple of decades, innovative technological methods for collecting BAC data have received considerable attention.

The South Dakota 24/7 Sobriety Program is a sobriety-monitoring program aimed at repeat DUI offenders, first DUI offenders with very high BACs, and similar offenders who have had repeated convictions related to alcohol abuse. Offenders report to the Sheriff's Office twice a day (at about 7 am and 7 pm) for alcohol breath testing. If the offenders have any positive BACs or they miss a scheduled test, they go to jail for 12 to 36 hours. South Dakota adopted legislation in 2007 that established the 24/7 program statewide. Depending on the circumstances, judges may also require these offenders to undergo treatment, attend victim-impact panels and/or perform a certain number of hours of community service. Some offenders (because of their working hours, the distance they must travel in rural counties, and other legitimate reasons) agree to wear a transdermal alcohol-monitoring (TAM) ankle bracelet instead of the twice-per-day breath testing. The TAM system records any alcohol use via sweat vapor every 30 minutes.

According to the Mountain Plains Evaluation report (Loudenburg et al. 2010), the DUI recidivism rates after three years for 24/7 first offenders (with BACs > 0.17 upon arrest) was 14.3% compared to 14.8% for similar offenders not on 24/7 (no difference). However, there was a statistically significant 74% reduction in recidivism after three years for DUI second offenders (13.7% for comparison offenders vs. 3.6% for the 24/7 offenders); a 44% reduction in recidivism for DUI third offenders (15.3% vs. 8.6%); and a 31% reduction in recidivism for DUI fourth offenders (15.5% vs. 10.7%).

The Rand Corporation conducted an independent evaluation of the South Dakota 24/7 program. According to a study (Kilmer et al. 2013), there was a 12% reduction in repeat DUI arrests and a 9% reduction in domestic violence arrests associated with the adoption of the 24/7 program.

More direct transdermal monitoring systems that are worn on the body and monitor the BAC level 24 hours a day/7 days a week are just beginning to be used by the judicial system (Swift 2003). Two devices have been studied—the Secure Continuous Remote Alcohol Monitoring (SCRAM™) ankle bracelet and the WrisTAS™, which is about the size of a large wristwatch. Introduced about 10 years ago, the SCRAM device is currently being used in 48 states and DC (excluding Hawaii and Massachusetts) in the United States. The company that produces the SCRAM bracelet reports that it works with more than 200 service providers in more than 1,800 courts and agencies around the United States and that close to 250,000 offenders have been monitored to date. Thirty-four states have had more than 1,000 offenders on SCRAM and eight states have had more than 10,000 offenders using SCRAM over the years. The SCRAM incorporates a system for detecting circumvention attempts such as inserting an object between the ankle skin and the SCRAM sensor to block the sweat vapor (Marques and McKnight 2007).

A method for monitoring drinking that is just emerging in the United States but is more widely used in Europe is to analyze the biomarkers in blood, urine, or hair that result from consumption of alcohol. Although alcohol is cleared relatively rapidly from the body, usually even after heavy drinking within 8 to 12 hours, alcohol biomarkers persist in hair and in urine long after the BAC level has fallen to zero. These biomarkers provide a way to measure total consumption over an extended time span. Longer-lasting markers reflecting alcohol use, such as urinary ethylglucuronide (EtG), offer a window of detection of 36 h or more following drinking (Borucki et al. 2005; Helander and Beck 2005; Wurst et al. 2003). These biomarkers are currently being used in Europe to manage the drinking of offenders. Tests for such biomarkers can be required on a regular schedule with the probability that they will detect illicit drinking because they are present in the blood for an extended period following drinking. Hair EtG is being used in Germany as a relicensing criterion for participants in the driver's license restitution processes following conviction for impaired-driving. To be eligible for reinstatement, a person's hair EtG level must be below 3 pg/mg, which is known to reflect abstinence.

Monitoring alcohol consumption by DUI offenders is a key component of DUI courts and is becoming more popular in US courts. The evidence indicates that when offenders are monitored, they tend to remain abstinent or at least refrain from excessive drinking.

17.5 Future Directions

17.5.1 Future Opportunities in Primary Prevention

17.5.1.1 Strengthen Enforcement of MLDA Laws

There is clear evidence that MLDA laws reduce alcohol-related crashes involving underage drivers. Although there are effective measures for enforcing MLDA laws, they are not widely and consistently used. Increased enforcement is needed. Countries around the world should consider establishing age 21 as the MLDA.

17.5.1.2 Strengthen Enforcement of Prohibitions on Serving Drinks to Obviously Intoxicated Patrons

Bars, restaurants, and other on-the-premises alcohol outlets are a major source of impaired drivers. Laws making it illegal to serve obviously intoxicated patrons are poorly enforced. Research suggests that refusal of service can be greatly increased through increased enforcement. This opportunity to reduce the number of impaired drivers on the road should be exploited.

17.5.1.3 Promote Ridesharing (e.g., Uber, Lyft) and Other Alternative Transportation Options

Ride-sharing applications on smart phones have substantially changed the landscape on alternative transportation. Uber and Lyft are the two largest ride-sharing programs in the United States. These programs enable passengers to hail nearby private drivers using geolocation technology. Uber and Lyft have introduced flexible pricing, automated payments, and shorter wait times than traditional taxi services. Both Uber and Lyft are in most major cities and counties in the United States and are growing rapidly in other countries. While there are potential safety risks to unregulated ride-sharing services, there also appear to be several benefits: convenience, affordability, and an alternative to drinking and driving. Three studies have been conducted on the effects of Uber on alcohol-impaired driving. The first study, sponsored by Uber and MADD, found that Uber's entry in Seattle, WA, was associated with a 10% decrease in DUI arrests (Uber, Mother Against Drunk Driving 2015). In Chicago, 45.8% of Uber rides requested within 50 m of a bar, restaurant, or other alcohol outlet came during peak drinking hours (10 pm to 3 am) compared to only 28.9% at off-peak hours. In California, monthly alcohol-related crashes declined 6.5% among drivers under age 30 following the launch of Uber. Providence College (Providence, RI) also studied the relationship between Uber, fatal crashes, and criminal arrests (Dills and Mulholland 2016). They examined over 150 cities and counties that introduced Uber between 2010 and 2013, and found that Uber was associated with decreases in fatal vehicular crashes and in arrests for DUI, assaults, and disorderly conduct. A third recent study (Brazil and Kirk 2016) conversely found that Uber had no association with the number of traffic fatalities, drunk-driving fatalities, and weekend and holiday fatalities after Uber entered the county. A study (Brazil and Kirk 2016) analyzed the FARS for several Uber counties, but it is unclear how drunk-driving fatalities were defined. It also appears that the alcohol-imputation FARS file was not used in that study, which is a standard procedure for researchers using FARS data. While alternative transportation programs have had some effect on impaired driving, ride-sharing programs such as Uber and Lyft hold promise to have substantial effects as the market penetration increases. However, very few of the alternative transportation studies are truly scientific, e.g., (Wilde et al. 1971). A properly designed, scientifically rigorous, controlled study that would be both approved by experts and understood by the public is therefore required.

17.5.2 Future Opportunities in Secondary Prevention

17.5.2.1 Increase Use of Low-Staff Checkpoints and RBT

Sobriety checkpoints and RBT, when well publicized, are highly effective in reducing alcohol-related crashes but are underused because of staffing requirements. Research has shown that checkpoints with a smaller number of officers can be equally successful, particularly if the officers use passive sensors to detect drinking. Low-staff checkpoints equipped with passive sensors conducted on a weekly basis in numerous communities in the United States and countries around the world would have a substantial effect on impaired-driving fatal crashes.

Canada's federal government recently introduced an RBT program that allows drivers to be breath-tested at any time and in any place on their roads. If RBT is successful and effective in Canada, this could affect similar legislation in the United States.

17.5.2.2 Reduce the BAC Limit for Driving to 0.05 g/dL

Virtually all drivers are impaired with regard to driving performance at 0.05 g/dL BAC. Laboratory and test track research shows that the vast majority of drivers, even experienced drinkers who typically reach BACs of 0.15 g/dL or greater, are impaired at 0.05 g/dL BAC and higher with regard to critical driving tasks. Further, the risk of being involved in a crash rises very rapidly after a driver reaches or exceeds 0.05 g/dL BAC, compared to drivers with no alcohol in their blood systems. Recent studies indicate that the relative risk of being killed in a single-vehicle crash for drivers with BACs of 0.05 to 0.079 g/dL is at least 7 times that of drivers at 0.00 g/dL BAC (no alcohol) and could be as much as 21 times that of drivers at 0.00 g/dL BAC depending on the age of the driver (Voas et al. 2012; Zador et al. 2000b).

Lowering the limit for legal driving to 0.05 g/dL BAC is a proven-effective countermeasure that has reduced alcohol-related traffic fatalities in several countries, most notably Australia. While studies in Europe and Australia use different methodologies to evaluate these effects, the evidence is consistent and persuasive that fatal and injury crashes involving drinking drivers decrease on the order of at least 5%–8% and up to 18% after a country lowers their BAC limit from 0.08 to 0.05 g/dL BAC (Brooks and Zaal 1993; Homel 1994; Nagata et al. 2008). A meta-analysis of international studies on lowering the BAC limit in general found a 5.0% decline in nonfatal alcohol-related crashes, a 9.2% decline in fatal alcohol-related crashes from lowering the BAC from 0.10 to 0.08 g/dL, and an 11.1% decline in fatal alcohol-related crashes from lowering the BAC to 0.05 g/dL or lower. The study estimated that 1,790 lives would be saved each year if all states in the United States adopted a 0.05 g/dL BAC limit (Fell and Scherer 2017b).

A 0.05 g/dL BAC is a reasonable standard to set. A 0.05 g/dL BAC is not typically reached with a couple of beers after work or with a glass of wine or two with dinner. It takes at least four US standard drinks (i.e., 12 oz. of beer at 5% alcohol; 5 oz. of wine at 12% alcohol; 1.5 oz. of distilled spirits at 40% alcohol; all equal 0.60 oz. of alcohol per drink) for the average 170-lb male to exceed 0.05 g/dL BAC in 2 hours on an empty stomach (three drinks for the 137-lb female) (US National Highway Traffic Safety Administration 1994). The BAC level reached depends on a person's age, gender, weight, whether there is food in their stomach, and their metabolism rate (US National Highway Traffic Safety Administration 1994). No matter how many drinks it takes to reach 0.05 g/dL BAC, people at this level are too impaired to drive safely (McKnight et al. 2002).

The US public generally supports levels below 0.08 g/dL BAC. NHTSA surveys show that most people would not drive after consuming two or three drinks in an hour and believe the limit should be no higher than the BAC level associated with that (Royal 2000). That would be 0.05 g/dL BAC or lower for most drivers. A recent survey indicated that 63% of drivers in the United States support lowering the illegal BAC from 0.08 to 0.05 g/dL (Arnold and Teftt 2016).

Most industrialized nations around the world have set BAC limits at 0.05 g/dL BAC or lower. All states in Australia now have a 0.05 g/dL BAC limit. France, Austria, Italy, Spain, and Germany lowered their limit to 0.05 g/dL BAC, whereas Sweden, Norway, Japan, and Russia have set their limit at 0.02 g/dL BAC (WHO 2018).

Further progress is needed in reducing alcohol-impaired driving in the United States and in many countries around the world. Progress in reducing impaired driving has stalled over the past 20 years in several countries (Dang 2008; Fell et al. 2016a). Lowering the BAC limit from 0.08 to 0.05 g/dL will serve as a general deterrent to all those who drink and drive by indicating that the government is getting tougher on impaired driving and society will not tolerate impaired drivers (Fell and Voas 2006b; 2014). Such legislation typically reduces the number of drinking drivers involved in fatal crashes at all BAC levels (BACs $\geq$ 0.01 g/dL; BACs $\geq$ 0.05 g/dL; BACs $\geq$ 0.08 g/dL; BACs $\geq$ 0.15 g/dL) (Hingson et al. 1996; Voas et al. 2000b; Wagenaar et al. 2007).

At the time of publication, Utah was the only state in the United States that had lowered its BAC limit from 0.08 to 0.05 g/dL. However, several states had introduced legislation to lower the limit to 0.05 g/dL, including California and New York. Utah did not change their DUI enforcement strategy for 0.05 g/dL BAC; it is the same as it was for 0.08 g/dL BAC. A new standardized field sobriety test (SFST) will need to be developed and validated at 0.05 g/dL BAC.

17.5.3 Future Opportunities in Tertiary Prevention

17.5.3.1 Interlock Alternative Programs: Secure Continuous Remote Alcohol Monitoring (SCRAM) and NO-DRIV Ankle Bracelet That Detects Driving

Ignition interlocks are highly effective in reducing offender recidivism (Voas 2020), but only a small portion of the eligible DUI offenders can be motivated to install them. An alternative to the interlock program is needed for those offenders without cars or who are willing to take the risk of driving illicitly rather than installing the interlock, because experience shows that offenders do continue to drive and become involved in crashes. Monitoring offenders' BACs appears to be an effective alternative to the interlock.

On the horizon is a developing technology that detects driving via an ankle bracelet with accelerometers that measure the foot movements required to operate a vehicle. When perfected, this will allow the court to monitor offenders to ensure they are not driving. This could be offered as an alternative to the interlock. Programs need to be created that require electronically monitored abstinence or electronically monitored driving as alternatives to the interlock. More offenders will then decide to choose the interlock instead of the other more stringent alternatives.

17.5.4 Silver Bullet: Cars That Drunks Can't Drive

17.5.4.1 Driver Alcohol Detection System for Safety Program

A long-term development program has been inaugurated by the NHTSA, automobile manufacturers, and MADD to develop a system for all cars that can passively sense the BAC of the driver and prevent ignition of the vehicle's motor if the driver is over the BAC legal limit. The program is called Driver Alcohol Detection System for Safety (DADSS) and is currently being funded by the NHTSA and most of the motor vehicle manufacturers. If such a vehicle can be produced, it would finally fulfill the objective enunciated 50 years ago—to build "Cars that Drunks Can't Drive" (Voas 1969). One of these monitors passively detects alcohol in the breath of the driver, making it unnecessary for the driver to blow into an interlock breath tube. Another developing technology measures BAC passively through the skin, providing a substitute for blowing into the interlock (Ennis 2006).

These systems may have value as a method for activating a driver interlock system only when there is evidence of a drinking driver in the vehicle. Thus, the not-too-distant future offers the possibility of equipping all new vehicles with a system that would make impaired driving less likely.

17.5.4.2 Autonomous Vehicles

New automated in-vehicle technologies are being developed and deployed to counteract driver errors and prevent crashes. Automated driver systems (ADSs) are a class of vehicle technologies that provide drivers timely warnings and/or actions. Some ADSs actively and automatically intervene to avoid hazardous situations.

Many manufacturers offer these technologies as options on some or all of their vehicles, and may offer these systems as standard in the future. ADS technologies are the precursor to autonomous vehicles and, depending on the combination of ADS equipment installed in a vehicle, can allow autonomous driving at the present time (Abraham et al. 2017; SAE International 2014). Currently, the effectiveness of each crash-avoidance technology relies on both the presence of the technology and the appropriate responses from drivers (Blower 2014; Jermakian 2011). In many cases, drivers may be unaware of the presence of the system within their car or may not fully understand its performance limits in terms of objects detected, speed of operation, or conditions where degraded performance is expected (Aziz et al. 2013). Since near-collisions are rare events, owners may rarely experience audible, visual, or haptic feedback and may not appropriately respond. Nomenclature and branding for each system also pose serious challenges since each carmaker may choose a name for marketing purposes that differs from other brands or even other vehicles in their fleet, making it harder for drivers to learn about the capabilities of the systems in their vehicles.

To achieve optimal safety, it is important for drivers to understand their vehicles and appropriately rely on ADSs for safe navigation. Today, drivers are educated about their vehicles in a number of ways including: (a) mainstream media; (b) original equipment manufacturers (OEM) websites and educational material; and (c) dealership experiences (Abraham et al. 2017). Several OEMs have implemented programs to educate new vehicle drivers. For example, Toyota currently integrates an overview of safety systems including Toyota Safety Sense in their vehicle overview. Toyota also equips all dealerships with handheld and large-format touchpads to allow existing and future customers to explore the content and performance of systems offered in each new car.

Studies are needed to determine if automated features will help impaired drivers avoid crashes and to monitor the performance of autonomous vehicles as they become available.

17.6 Conclusion: Where Do We Go from Here?

In January 2018, the US National Academies of Sciences, Engineering, and Medicine in the United States released a comprehensive report on accelerating progress to reduce alcohol-impaired driving fatalities in the United States (US National Academies of Sciences, Engineering, and Medicine 2018; Teutsch and Naimi 2018). The report (written by a highly qualified committee assembled to review the impaired-driving problem) provides a blueprint to solving the problem by identifying evidence-based and promising policies, programs, strategies, and system changes to increase progress in reducing alcohol-impaired drivers' traffic fatalities.

Among many other recommendations, those pertinent to this article include the following:

- Jurisdictions should adopt and/or strengthen laws and dedicate enforcement resources to stop illegal alcohol sales (i.e., sales to already intoxicated adults and sales to underage persons).
- Law enforcement agencies should conduct sobriety checkpoints in conjunction with widespread publicity to promote awareness of these enforcement initiatives.
- Municipalities should support policies and programs that increase the availability, convenience, affordability, and safety of transportation alternatives for drinkers who might drive otherwise. This includes permitting transportation network company ride-sharing, enhancing public transportation options (especially during nighttime and weekend hours), and boosting or incentivizing transportation alternatives in rural areas.
- Implement DUI courts that include available consultation or referral for evaluation by an addiction-trained clinician.
- All-offender, alcohol-detecting, ignition-interlock laws should be enacted. To increase effectiveness, jurisdictions should consider increased monitoring periods based on the offender's BAC at the time of arrest and past recidivism.
- Laws against alcohol-impaired driving should be enacted defining impairment at 0.05 BAC, and enactment should be accompanied by media campaigns and robust and visible enforcement efforts.

For developing countries with high traffic-fatality rates, the cost of those deaths and injuries is draining their economies. It will be cost-effective for them to use limited resources to reduce drunk-driving crashes. Drunk driving should be illegal in every country of the world and it should be based on the driver's BAC. Setting a BAC limit for the general population of 0.05 g/dL or lower will be a good start (WHO 2013).

Conducting RBT and/or sobriety checkpoints is an enforcement strategy that is effective in every country if it is done frequently and if it is visible and it is publicized.

For high-income countries, doubling down on what works and taking advantage of new technologies should be the norm. Technologies that passively detect BACs of motor vehicle operators have great potential to reduce impaired driving in the future.

While numerous countries have made progress in reducing drunk driving, much more work must be accomplished. Drunk-driving laws and their serious enforcement have been effective in most countries and have an immediate effect. A general deterrent effect (i.e., deter all drivers from drunk driving) gives the "biggest bang for the buck" in countermeasures and is cost-effective. A general approach to deterrence affecting all drivers involves laws, enforcement, reasonable sanctions, and publicity. Specific deterrence (i.e., affecting only drivers arrested for drunk driving and providing sanctions against repeating the behavior) works to some extent but does not have the magnitude of impact that a general deterrent strategy has.

It will most likely take a combination of strategies for drunk driving to be reduced in countries around the world. But for that to happen, some priority to deterring drunk driving must be established by key country officials. Data, analysis, and evaluations of specific strategies will be key needs. If countries can obtain measures of the BACs of drivers involved in fatal crashes and of drivers on the roads, those data will be extremely informative. Information on arrests and convictions for drunk driving will also provide important information. Countries must collect vital information that can be used to assess and bolster progress in reducing drunk driving.

References

Abraham H, McAnulty H, Mehler B, Reimer B: Case study of today's automotive dealerships: Introduction and delivery of advanced driver assistance systems; *Transport Res Rec* (Journal of the Transportation Research Board) 2660:7; 2017; doi:10.3141/2660-02 (Accessed May 22, 2019).

Anglin L, Caverson R, Fennel R, Giesbrecht N, Mann RE: *A Study of Impaired Drivers Stopped by Police in Sudbury*; Addiction Research Foundation: Ontario, Canada; 1997.

Apsler R, Char AR, Harding WM, Klein TM: *The Effects of 0.08 BAC Laws*; US National Highway Traffic Safety Administration: Washington, DC; 1999.

Arnold LS, Tefft BC: *Driving Under the Influence of Alcohol and Marijuana: Beliefs and Behaviors, United States, 2013–2015*; AAA Foundation for Traffic Safety: Washington, DC; 2016.

Arnold R: *Effect of Raising the Legal Drinking Age on Driver Involvement in Fatal Crashes: The Experience of Thirteen States* (DOT HS 806 902); US National Highway Traffic Safety Administration: Washington, DC; 1985.

Aziz T, Horiguchi Y, Sawaragi T: An empirical investigation of the development of driver's mental model of a lane departure warning system while driving; *Proceedings—12th Symposium on Analysis, Design, and Evaluation of Human-Machine Systems*; Las Vegas, VA; August 11–15; 2013.

Bartl G, Esberger R: Effects of lowering the legal BAC limit in Austria; In Laurell H, Schlyter F (Eds): *Proceedings—15th International Conference on Alcohol, Drugs and Traffic Safety* (T'2000); Stockholm, Sweden; May 22–26, 2000.

Beirness D, Simpson H, Mayhew D, Jonah B: The impact of administrative license suspension and vehicle impoundment for driving under the influence in Manitoba; In Mercier-Guyon C (Ed): *Proceedings—14th International Conference on Alcohol, Drugs and Traffic Safety*; Annecy, France; September 21–26, 1997.

Beitel GA, Sharp MC, Glauz WD: Probability of arrest while driving under the influence of alcohol; *Inj Prev* 6:158; 2000.

Berning A, Compton R, Wochinger K: *Results of the 2013–2014 National Roadside Survey of Alcohol and Drug Use by Drivers* (DOT HS 812 118); US National Highway Traffic Safety Administration: Washington, DC; 2015.

Birckmayer J, Hemenway D: Minimum-age drinking laws and youth suicide, 1970–1990; *Am J Public Health* 89:1365; 1999.

Block A: *Survey of DWI Courts* (DOT HS 812 283); US National Highway Traffic Safety Administration: Washington, DC; 2016.

Blomberg RD: *Lower BAC Limits for Youth: Evaluation of the Maryl and 0.02 Law* (DOT HS 806 807); US National Highway Traffic Safety Administration: Washington, DC; 1992.

Blomberg RD, Peck RC, Moskowitz H, Burns M, Fiorentino D: *Crash Risk of Alcohol Involved Driving: A Case-Control Study* (Final Report); Dunlap & Associates: Stamford, CT; 2005.

Blomberg RD, Peck RC, Moskowitz H, Burns M, Fiorentino D: The Long Beach/Fort Lauderdale relative risk study; *J Safety Res* 40:285; 2009.

Blower D: *Assessment of the Effectiveness of Advanced Collision Avoidance Technologies* (UMTRI-2014-3); University of Michigan Transportation Research Institute: Ann Arbor, MI; 2014.

Borkenstein RF: Problems of enforcement, adjudication and sanctioning; In Israelstam S, Lambert S (Eds): *Proceedings—6th International Conference on Alcohol, Drugs and Traffic Safety Alcohol, Drugs and Traffic Safety*; Toronto, Ontario; September 8–13, 1975.

Borucki K, Schreiner R, Dierkes J, Jachau K, Krause D, Westphal S, Wurst FM, Luley C, Schmidt-Gayk H: Detection of recent ethanol intake with new markers: Comparison of fatty acid ethyl esters in serum and of ethyl glucuronide and the ration if 5-hydroxytryptophol to 5-hydroxyindole acetic acid in urine; *Alcohol Clin Exp Res* 29:781; 2005.

Brazil N, Kirk DS: Uber and metropolitan traffic fatalities in the United States; *Am J Epidemiol* 183:192; 2016.

Breckenridge JF, Winfree LT, Maupin JR, Clason DL: Drunk drivers, DWI "Drug Court" treatment, and recidivism: Who fails? *JRP* 2:87; 2000.

Brooks C, Zaal D: Effects of a reduced alcohol limit in driving; In Utzelmann HD, Berghous G, Kroj G (Eds): *Alcohol, Drugs and Traffic Safety*; Verlag TÜV Rheinland: Cologne, Germany; p 860; 1993.

Brown DB, Maghsoodloo SA: A study of alcohol involvements in young driver accidents with the lowering of the legal age of drinking in Alabama; *Accid Anal Prev* 13:319; 1981.

Chen LH, Baker SP, Li G: Graduated driver licensing pro-grams and fatal crashes of 16-year-old drivers: A national evaluation; *Pediatrics* 118:56; 2006.

Christophersen AS, Mørland JG, Stewart K: International trends in alcohol and drug use among motor vehicle drivers; *Forensic Sci Rev* 28:37; 2016.

Clark WB, Hilton ME: *Alcohol in America: Drinking Practices and Problems*; State University of New York Press: Albany, NY; 1991.

Compton RP: Preliminary analysis of the effect of selected citizen group court monitoring programs; *J Traffic Safety Educ* 35(1):8; 1987.

Compton RP, Berning A: *Drug and Alcohol Crash Risk* (DOT HS 812 117); US National Highway Traffic Safety Administration: Washington, DC; 2015.

Cook PJ, Tauchen G: The effect of minimum drinking age legislation on youthful auto fatalities, 1970–1977; *J Leg Stud* 13:169; 1984.

Cornwell EE, Belzberg H, Velmahos G, Chan LS, Deme-triades D, Stewart BM, Oder DB, Kahaku D, Asensio JA, Berne TV: The prevalence and effect of alcohol and drug abuse on cohort-matched critically injured patients; *Am Surg* 64:461; 1998.

Dang JN: *Statistical Analysis of Alcohol-Related Driving Trends, 1982–2005* (DOT HS 810 942); US National Highway Traffic Safety Administration: Washington, DC; 2008.

Dee TS, Grabowski DC, Morrisey MA: Graduated driver licensing and teen traffic fatalities; *J Health Econ* 24:571; 2005.

Dills AK, Mulholland S: Ride-sharing, fatal crashes, and crime; *South Econ J* 84:965; 2016.

Ditsuwan V, Veerman JL, Bertram M, Vos T: Cost-effectiveness of interventions for reducing road traffic injuries related to driving under the influence of alcohol; *Value Health* 16(1):23; 2013.

Ditsuwan V, Veerman JL, Bertram M, Vos T: Sobriety checkpoints in Thailand: A review of effectiveness and developments over time; *Asia Pac J Public Health* 27(2):NP2177; 2015.

Eby DW: The convicted drunk driver in Michigan: A profile of offenders; *UMTRI Research Review* 25(5):1; 1995.

Elder RW, Shults RA, Sleet DA, Nichols JL, Zaza S, Thompson RS: Effectiveness of sobriety checkpoints for reducing alcohol-involved crashes; *Traffic Inj Prev* 3:266; 2002.

Ennis M: Impairment detection of Lumidigm's biometric platform; *Mothers Against Drunk Driving Technology Symposium*: Albuquerque, NM; 2006.

Epperlein T: Initial deterrent effects of the crackdown on drunken drivers in the state of Arizona; *Accid Anal Prev* 19:271; 1987.

Farmer CM, Wells JK, Ferguson SA, Voas RB: Field evaluation of the PAS III passive alcohol sensor; *Traffic Inj Prev* 1:55; 1999.

Fell JC, Beirness, J, Voas RB, Smith GS, Jonah B, Maxwell JC, Price J, Hedlund J: Can progress in reducing alcohol-impaired driving fatalities be resumed? Results of a workshop sponsored by the Transportation Research Board, Alcohol, Other Drugs, and Transportation Committee (ANB50); *Traffic Inj Preven* 17:771; 2016a.

Fell JC, Compton C, Voas RB: A note on the use of passive alcohol sensors during routine traffic stops; *Traffic Inj Prev* 9:534; 2008a.

Fell JC, Fisher DA, Voas RB, Blackman K, Tippetts AS: The relationship of underage drinking laws to reductions in drinking drivers in fatal crashes in the United States; *Accid Anal Prev* 40:1430; 2008b.

Fell JC, Fisher D, Yao J, McKnight S: Evaluation of a responsible beverage service and enforcement program: Effects on bar patron intoxication and potential impaired driving by young adults; *Traffic Inj Prev* 16:557; 2017.

Fell JC, Lacey JH, Voas RB: Sobriety checkpoints: Evidence of effectiveness is strong, but use is limited; *Traffic Inj Prev* 5:220; 2004.

Fell JC, Romano E, Voas RB: A national evaluation of graduated driver licensing laws in the United States; *Proceedings—20th International Conference on Alcohol, Drugs and Traffic Safety*; Brisbane, Australia; August 25–28, 2013.

Fell JC, Scherer M: Administrative license suspension: Does length of suspension matter? *Traffic Inj Prev* 18:577; 2017a.

Fell JC, Scherer M: Estimation of the potential effectiveness of lowering the blood alcohol concentration (BAC) limit for driving from 0.08 to 0.05 grams per deciliter in the United States; *Alcohol Clin Exp Res* 41:2128; 2017b.

Fell JC, Scherer M, Thomas S, Voas RB: Assessing the impact of twenty underage drinking laws; *J Stud Alcohol Drugs* 77:249; 2016b.

Fell JC, Tippetts AS, Ciccel JD: An evaluation of three driving-under-the-influence courts in Georgia; *Ann Adv Automot Med* 55:301; 2011a.

Fell JC, Todd M, Voas, RB: A national evaluation of the nighttime and passenger restricted components of graduated driver licensing; *J Safety Res* 42:283; 2011b.

Fell JC, Voas RB: Mothers Against Drunk Driving (MADD): The first 25 years; *Traffic Inj Prev* 7:195; 2006a.

Fell JC, Voas RB: The effectiveness of a 0.05 blood alcohol concentration (BAC) limit for driving in the United States; *Addiction* 109:869; 2014.

Fell JC, Voas RB: The effectiveness of reducing illegal blood alcohol concentration limits for driving: Evidence for lowering the limit to 0.05 BAC; *J Safety Res* 37:233; 2006b.

Fell JC, Waehrer G, Voas RB, Auld-Owens A, Carr K, Pell K: Relationship of impaired-driving enforcement intensity to drinking and driving on the roads; *Alcohol Clin Exp Res* 39:84; 2015.

Ferguson SA, Wells JK, Lund AK: The role of passive alcohol sensors in detecting alcohol-impaired drivers at sobriety checkpoints; *Alcohol Drugs Driving* 11:23; 1995.

Ferrara SD, Zancaner S, Georgetti R: Low blood alcohol levels and driving impairment. A review of experimental studies and international legislation; *Inter J Legal Med* 106:169; 1994.

Ferreira J, Sickerman A: The impact of Massachusetts' reduced drinking age on auto accidents; *Accid Anal Prev* 8:229; 1976.

Fleming MF, Mundt MP, French MT, Manwell LB, Stauffacher EA, Barry KL: Brief physician advice for problem drinkers: Long-term efficacy and benefit-cost analysis; *Alcohol Clin Exp Res* 26:36; 2002.

Foss R, Goodwin A: Enhancing the effectiveness of graduate driver licensing legislation; *J Safety Res* 34:79; 2003.

Foss RD, Feaganes JR, Roggman LA: Initial effects of graduated driver licensing on 16-year-old driver crashes in North Carolina; *JAMA* 286:1631; 2001.

Foss RD, Stewart JR, Reinfurt DW: *Evaluation of the Effects of North Carolina's 0.08% BAC Law*; US National Highway Traffic Safety Administration: Washington, DC; 1998.

Freeman-Wilson K, Wilkosz MP: *Drug Court Publications Resource Guide*, 4th ed; US National Drug Court Institute: Alexandria, VA; 2002.

Friend K, Levy DT: Reductions in smoking prevalence and cigarette consumption associated with mass-media campaigns; *Health Educ Res* 17:85; 2002.

Gentilello LM, Ebel BE, Wickizer TM, Salkever DS, Rivara FP: Alcohol interventions for trauma patients treated in emergency departments and hospitals: A cost benefit analysis; *Ann Surg* 241:541; 2005.

Gentilello LM, Rivara FP, Donovan DM, Jurkovich GJ, Daranciang ED, Christopher W, Villaveces A, Copass M, Ries RR: Alcohol interventions in a trauma center as a means of reducing the risk of injury recurrence; *Ann Surg* 230:473; 1999.

Gjerde H, Ramaekers JG, Mørland JG: Methodologies for establishing the relationship between alcohol/drug use and driving impairment—Differences between epidemiological, experimental, and real-case studies; *Forensic Sci Rev* 31:141; 2019.

Gjerde H, Strand MC, Mørland JG: Driving under the influence of non-alcohol drugs—An update Part I: Epidemiological studies; *Forensic Sci Rev* 27:89, 2015.

Goodwin A, Thomas L, Kirley B, Hall W, O'Brien N, Hill K: *Countermeasures That Work: A Highway Safety Countermeasure Guide for State Highway Safety Offices*, 8th ed (DOT HS 812 202); US National Highway Traffic Safety Administration: Washington, DC; 2015.

Graham K, Osgood DW, Zibrowski E, Purcell J, Gilksman L, Leonard K, Pemanen K, Saltz RF, Toomey TL: The effect of the safer bars programme on physical aggression in bars: Results of a randomized controlled trial; *Drug Alcohol Rev* 23:31; 2004.

Guerin P, Pitts WJ: *Evaluation of the Bernalillo County Metropolitan DWI/Drug Court: Final Report;* University of New Mexico Center for Applied Research and Analysis: Albuquerque, NM; 2002.

Hagen R: *The Effectiveness of License Suspension or Revocation for Drivers Convicted of Multiple Driving Under the Influence Offenses* (Report #59); California Department of Motor Vehicles: Sacramento, CA; 1977.

Hause JM, Voas RB, Chavez E: Conducting voluntary roadside surveys: The Stockton experience; In Valverius MR (Ed): *Proceedings—8th International Conference on Alcohol, Drugs and Traffic Safety*; Umea, Sweden; June 23–25. 1982.

Hedlund JH, Ulmer RG, Preusser DF: *Determine Why There Are Fewer Young Alcohol-Impaired Drivers* (DOT HS 809 348); US Department of Transportation: Washington, DC; 2001.

Helander A, Beck O: Ethyl sulfate: A metabolite of ethanol in humans and a potential biomarker of acute alcohol intake; *J Anal Toxicol* 29:270; 2005.

Henstridge J, Homel R, Mackay P: *The Long-Term Effects of Random Breath Testing in Four Australian States: A Time Series Analysis*; Federal Office of Road Safety: Canberra, Australia; 1997.

Hingson R, Heeren T, Winter M: Effects of recent 0.08% legal blood alcohol limits on fatal crash involvement; *Inj Prev* 6:109; 2000.

Hingson R, Heeren T, Winter M: Lower legal blood alcohol limits for young drivers; *Public Health Rep* 109:739; 1994.

Hingson R, Heeren T, Winter M: Lowering state legal blood alcohol limits to 0.08 percent: The effect on fatal motor vehicle crashes; *Am J Public Health* 86:1297; 1996.

Hingson R, Howland J, Heeren T, Winter M: Reduced BAC limits for young people (impact on night fatal) crashes; *Alcohol Drugs Driving* 7:117; 1992.

Hingson R, Scotch N, Mangione T, Meyers A, Glantz L, Heeren T, Lin N, Mucatel M, Pierce G: Impact of legislation raising the legal drinking age in Massachusetts from 18 to 20; *Am J Public Health* 73:63; 1983.

Holder H, Treno AJ: Media advocacy in community prevention: News as a means to advance policy change; *Addiction* 92:S189; 1997.

Holder HD, Wagenaar AC: Mandated server training and reduced alcohol-involved traffic crashes: A time series analysis of the Oregon experience; *AcciD Anal Prev* 26: 89; 1994.

Homel R: Drink-driving law enforcement and the legal blood alcohol limit in New South Wales; *Accid Anal Prev* 26:147; 1994.

Homel R: *Policing and Punishing the Drinking Driver—A Study of General and Specific Deterrence.* Springer-Verlag, New York, NY; 1988.

Howat P, Sleet D, Smith I: Alcohol and driving: Is the 0.05% blood alcohol concentration limit justified? *Drug Alcohol Rev* 10:151; 1991.

Huddleston CW, Marlowe DB, Casebolt R: *Painting the Current Picture: A National Report Card on Drug Courts and Other Problem-Solving Court Programs in the United States;* National Drug Court Institute, Bureau of Justice Assistance: Washington, DC; 2008.

Jermakian JS: Crash avoidance potential of four passenger vehicle technologies; *Accid Anal Prev* 43:732; 2011.

Johnson D, Fell JC: The impact of lowering the illegal BAC limit to 0.08 in five states in the U.S.; *Ann Adv Automot Med* 39:45; 1995.

Johnsson KO, Berglund M: Education of key personnel in student pubs leads to a decrease in alcohol consumption among the patrons: A randomized controlled trial; *Addiction* 98:627; 2003.

Jones AW: The analysis of ethanol in blood and breath for legal purposes—A historical review; *Forensic Sci Rev* 8:13; 1996.

Jones L, Hughes K, Atkinson AM, Bellis MA: Reducing harm in drinking environments: A systematic review of effective approaches; *Health Place* 17:508; 2011.

Jones NE, Pieper CF, Robertson LS: The effect of legal drinking age on fatal injuries of adolescents and young adults; *Am J Public Health* 82:112; 1992.

Jones R, Lacey J: *Alcohol and Highway Safety 2001: A Review of the State of Knowledge* (DOT HS 809 383); US National Highway Traffic Safety Administration: Washington, DC; 2001.

Kenkel DS: Drinking, driving and deterrence: The effectiveness and social costs of alternative policies; *JL & Econ* 36:877; 1993.

Kilmer B, Nicosia N, Heaton P, Midgette, G: Efficacy of frequent monitoring with swift, certain, and modest sanctions for violations: Insights from South Dakota's 24/7 sobriety project; *Am J Public Health* 103:37; 2013.

Kindelberger J: *Calculating Lives Saved Due to Minimum Drinking Age Laws* (Traffic Safety Facts Research Note); US National Center for Statistics and Analysis: Washington, DC; 2005.

Klein TM: *Changes in Alcohol-Involved Fatal Crashes Associated with Tougher State Alcohol Legislation* (DOT HS 807 511); US National Highway Traffic Safety Administration: Washington, DC; 1989.

Klein TM, Walz MC: *Estimating Alcohol Involvement in Fatal Crashes in Light of Increases in Restraint Use*; US National Center for Statistics and Analysis: Washington, DC; 1998.

Klepp KI, Schmid LA, Murray DM: Effects of the increased minimum drinking age law on drinking and driving behavior among adolescents; *Addict Res* 4:237; 1996.

Knoebel K, Ross HL: *Effects of Administrative License Revocation on Employment* (DOT HS 808 462); US National Highway Traffic Safety Administration: Washington, DC; 1996.

Kypri K, Voas RB, Langley JD, Stephenson SCR, Begg DJ, Tippetts AS, Davie GS: Minimum purchasing age for alcohol and traffic crash injuries among 15- to 19-year-olds in New Zealand; *Am J Public Health* 96:126; 2006.

Lacey J, Jones R, Stewart J: *Cost-Benefit Analysis of Administrative License Suspension* (DOT HS 807 689); US National Highway Traffic Safety Administration: Washington, DC; 1991.

Lacey JH, Kelley-Baker T, Furr-Holden D, Voas RB, Romano E, Torres, P, Tippetts AS, Ramirez A, Brainard K, Berning A: *2007 National Roadside Survey of Alcohol and Drug Use by Drivers: Alcohol Results* (Report No. DOT HS 811 248); US National Highway Traffic Safety Administration: Washington, DC; 2009.

Lacey JH, Rudisill LC, Popkin CL, Stewart JR: Education for drunk drivers: How well has it worked in North Carolina? *Pop Gov* 51:44; 1986.

Lacey J, Stewart J, Marchetti L, Jones R: *Assessment of the Effects of Implementing and Publicizing Administrative License Revocation for DWI in Nevada*; US National Highway Traffic Safety Administration: Washington, DC; 1990.

Lange JE, Voas, RB: Patterns of border crossings associated with Tijuana binge drinking by U.S. young people; *1998 Scientific Meeting of the Research Society on Alcoholism*: Hilton Head Island, SC; June 20–25, 1998.

Lestina DC, Lund AK: *Laboratory Evaluation of Two Passive Alcohol Sensors*; Insurance Institute for Highway Safety: Arlington, VA;1989.

Levy D, Asch P, Shea D: An assessment of county programs to reduce driving while intoxicated; *Health Educ Res*; 5:247; 1990.

Levy D, Shea D, Asch P: Traffic safety effects of sobriety checkpoints and other local DWI programs in New Jersey; *Am J Public Health* 79:291;1988.

Loudenburg R, Drube G, Leonardson G: *South Dakota 24-7 Sobriety Program Evaluation Findings Report*; Mountain Plains Evaluation: Salem, SD; 2010.

Lund AF, Jones IS: Detection of impaired drivers with a passive alcohol sensor; In Noordzij PC, Roszbach R (Eds): *Alcohol, Drugs and Traffic Safety'T86*; Excerpta Medica: New York, NY; P 379; 1987.

Lund AK, Kiger S, Lestina D, Blackwell T: Using passive alcohol sensors during police traffic stops; *70th Annual Meeting of Transportation Research Board*; Transportation Research Board: Washington, DC; 1991.

Maio RF, Waller PF, Blow FC, Hill FM, Singer KM: Alcohol abuse/dependence in motor vehicle crash victims presenting to the emergency department; *Acad Emerg Med* 4:256; 1997.

Mann R, Smart R, Stoduto G, Beirness D, Lamble R, Vingilis E: The early effects of Ontario's Administrative Driver's License Suspension Law on driver fatalities with BAC >80 mg%; *Can J Public Health* 93:176; 2002.

Marques PR, McKnight AS: *Evaluating Transdermal Alcohol Measuring Devices*; US National Highway Traffic Safety Administration: Washington, DC; 2007.

Marshall M, Oleson A: MADDer than hell; *Qual Health Res* 6:6; 1996.

Masten SV, Foss RD, Marshall SW: Graduated driver licensing and fatal crashes involving 16- to 19-year-old drivers; *JAMA* 306:1098; 2011.

Mayhew DR, Simpson HM, Pak A: Changes in collision rates among novice drivers during the first months of driving; *Accid Anal Prev* 35:683; 2003.

McCarthy JD, Wolfson M: Resources mobilization by social movement organizations: Agency, strategy, and organization in the movement against drinking and driving; *Am Sociol Rev* 61:1070; 1996.

McCarthy JD, Wolfson M, Harvey DS: *Chapter Survey Report of the Project on the Citizens' Movement Against Drunk Driving*; The Catholic University of America Center for the Study of Youth Development: Washington, DC; 1987.

McCarthy PS, Ziliak J: Effect of MADD on drinking-driving activities: An empirical study; *Appl Econ* 22:1215; 1990.

McCartt AT, Shabanova VI, Leaf WA: Driving experience, crashes and traffic citations of teenage beginning drivers; *Accid Anal Prev* 35:311; 2003.

McCartt AT, Teoh ER, Fields M, Braitman KA, Hellinga LA: *Graduated Licensing Laws and Fatal Crashes of Teenage Drivers: A National Study*; Insurance Institute for Highway Safety: Arlington, VA; 2009.

McKnight AJ, Langston E, McKnight AS, Lange J: Sobriety tests for low blood alcohol concentrations; *Accid Anal Prev* 34:305; 2002.

McKnight AJ, Voas R: The effect of license suspension on DUI recidivism; *Alcohol Drugs Driving* 7:43; 1991.

Mello MJ, Nirenberg TD, Longabaugh R, Woolard R, Minugh AP, Becker B, Baird J, Stein L: Emergency department brief motivational interventions for alcohol with motor vehicle crash patients; *Ann Emerg Med* 45:620; 2005.

Merki D, Lingg M: Combating the drunk driving problem through community action: A proposal; J Alcohol Drug Educ 32(3):42; 1987.

Miller TR, Galbraith M, Lawrence BA: Costs and benefits of a community sobriety checkpoint program; *J Stud Alcohol* 59:465; 1998.

Monti PM, Colby SM, Barnett NP, Spirito A, Rhsenow DJ, Myers M, Woolard R, Lewander W: Brief intervention for harm reduction with alcohol-positive older adolescents in a hospital emergency department; *J Consult Clin Psychol* 67:989; 1999.

Moskowitz H, Burns M, Fiorentino D, Smiley A, Zador P: *Driver Characteristics and Impairment at Various BACs* (DOT HS 809 075); US National Highway Traffic Safety Administration: Washington, DC; 2000.

Moskowitz H, Fiorentino D: *A Review of the Literature on the Effects of Low Doses of Alcohol on Driving-Related Skills* (DOT HS 809 028); US National Highway Traffic Safety Administration: Washington, DC; 2000.

Moulden JV, Russell A: Is it MADD trying to rate the states? A citizen activist approach to DWI prevention; *Alcohol Drugs Driving* 10:317; 1994.

Nagata T, Setoguchi S, Hemenway D, Perry MJ: Effectiveness of a law to reduce alcohol-impaired driving in Japan; *Inj Prev* 14:19; 2008.

O'Donnell MA: Research on drinking locations of alcohol-impaired drivers: Implications for prevention policies; *J Public Health Policy* 6:510; 1985.

O'Malley PM, Wagenaar AC: Effects of minimum drinking age laws on alcohol use, related behaviors and traffic crash involvement among American youth: 1976–1987; *J Stud Alcohol* 52:478; 1991.

Parker RN, Rebhun L: *Alcohol and Homicide: A Deadly Combination of Two American Traditions*; State University of New York Press: Albany, NY; 1995.

Preusser DF, Williams A, Nichols J, Tison J, Chaudhary N: *National Cooperative Highway Research Program: Effectiveness of Behavioral Highway Safety Counter-measures*; Transportation Research Board: Washington, DC; 2008.

Preusser DF, Williams AF, Zador PL, Blomberg RD: The effect of curfew laws on motor vehicle crashes; *Law Policy* 6:115; 1984.

Quart Inebriety: Editorial; *Quart Inebriety* 26:308; 1904.

Ramirez A, Berning A, Kelley-Baker T, Lacey JH, Yao J, Tippetts AS, Scherer M, Carr K, Pell K, Compton R: *2013–2014 National Roadside Study of Alcohol and Drug Use by Drivers: Alcohol Results* (Report No. DOT HS 812 362); US National Highway Traffic Safety Administration: Washington, DC; 2016.

Research and Evaluation Associates (REA): *The Effects Following the Implementation of an 0.08 BAC Limit and an Administrative per se Law in California*; US National Highway Traffic Safety Administration: Washington, DC; 1991.

Rogers P: *The General Deterrent Impact of California's 0.08% Blood Alcohol Concentration Limit and Administrative per se License Suspension Laws*; California Department of Motor Vehicles: Sacramento, CA; 1995.

Ross HL: Law, Science and Accidents: The British Road Safety Act of 1967; *J Legal Stud* 2:1; 1973.

Ross HL, Gonzales P: The effect of license revocation on drunk-driving offenders; *Accid Anal Prev* 20:379; 1988.

Royal D: *National Survey of Drinking and Driving: Attitudes and Behavior: 1999* (DOT HS 809 190—Vol I: Findings); US National Highway Traffic Safety Administration: Washington, DC; 2000.

Runge J, Garrison H, Hall W, Waller A, Shen G: *Identification and Referral of Impaired Drivers Through Emergency Department Protocols*; US National Highway Traffic Safety Administration: Washington, DC; 2002; http://www.nhtsa.dot.gov/people/injury/research/Idemergency/index.htm (Accessed May 15, 2019).

SAE International: *Standard J3016 Titled Taxonomy and Definitions for Terms Related to On-Road Motor Vehicle Automated Driving Systems*; Society of Automotive Engineers: Warrendale, PA; 2014.

Sagberg F: Month-by-month changes in accident risk among novice drivers; *Proceedings—14th International Congress of Applied Psychology*; Washington, DC; 1998.

Scherer M, Fell JC: Effectiveness of lowering the blood alcohol concentration (BAC) limit for driving from 0.10 to 0.08 grams per deciliter in the United States; *Traffic Inj Prev* 20:1; 2019.

Schermer CR, Moyers TB, Miller WR, Bloomfield LA: Trauma center brief interventions for alcohol disorders decrease subsequent driving under the influence arrests; *J Trauma* 60:29; 2006.

Sherman LW: Police Crackdowns: Initial and Residual Deterrence; *Crime and Justice—A Review of Research* (The University of Chicago Press Journal) 12:1; 1990.

Shope JT, Molnar LJ: Michigan's graduated driver licensing program: Evaluation of the first four years; *J Safety Res* 35:337; 2004.

Shope JT, Molnar LJ, Elliott MR, Waller PF: Graduated driver licensing in Michigan: Early impact on motor vehicle crashes among 16 year-old drivers; *JAMA* 286:1593; 2001.

Shults RA, Elder RW, Sleet DA, Nichols JL, Alao MO, Carande-Kulis VG, Zaza S, Sosin DM, Thompson RS: Task Force on Community Preventive Services: Reviews of evidence regarding interventions to reduce alcohol-impaired driving; *Am J Prev Med* 21(4 Suppl):66; 2001.

Smith DI: Effect on traffic safety of introducing a 0.05% blood alcohol level in Queensland, Australia; *Med Sci Law* 28:165; 1988.

Soderstrom CA, Dishinger PC, Kerns TJ, Kufera JA, Motchell KA, Scalea TM: Epidemic increases in cocaine and opiate use by trauma center patients. Documentation with a large clinical toxicology database; *J Trauma* 51:557; 2001.

Stewart K: *Alcohol Involvement in Fatal Crashes: Comparisons Among Countries*; US National Highway Traffic Safety Administration: Washington, DC; 2004.

Stoduto G, Mann R, Smart R, Adlaf E, Vingilis E, Beirness D, Lamble R: The impact of the administrative driver's License Suspension Law in Ontario; *15th International Conference on Alcohol, Drugs and Traffic Safety*; Stockholm, Sweden; May 22–26, 2000.

Subramanian R: *Transitioning to Multiple Imputation—A New Method to Estimate Missing Blood Alcohol Concentration (BAC) Values in FARS* (DOT HS 809 403); US National Highway Traffic Safety Administration: Washington, DC; 2002.

Swift RM: Direct measurement of alcohol and its metabolites; *Addiction* 98(Suppl 2):73; 2003.

Tauber J, Huddleston CW: *DUI/Drug Courts: Defining a National Strategy*; National Drug Court Institute: Alexandria, VA; 1999.

Teutsch SM, Naimi TS: Eliminating alcohol-impaired driving fatalities: What can be done? *Ann Intern Med* 168:587; 2018.

Tison J, Solomon MG, Nichols J, Gilbert SH, Siegler JN, Cosgrove LA: *May 2006 Click It or Ticket Seat Belt Mobilization Evaluation*; US National Highway Traffic Safety Administration: Washington, DC; 2008.

Toomey TL, Rosenfeld C, Wagenaar AC: The minimum legal drinking age: History, effectiveness, and ongoing debate; *Alcohol Health Res World* 20:213; 1996.

Toomey TL, Wagenaar AC, Gehan JP, Kilian G, Murray DB, Perry CL: Project Arm: Alcohol risk management to prevent sales to underage and intoxicated patrons; *Health Educ Behav* 28:186; 2001.

Uber, Mother Against Drunk Driving: *More Options, Shifting Mindsets, Driving Better Choices*; 2015; https://newsroom.uber.com/wp-content/uploads/2015/01/UberMADD-Report.pdf (Accessed May 15, 2019).

Ulmer RG, Preusser DF, Williams AF, Ferguson SA, Farmer CM: Graduated licensing program on the crash rate of teenage drivers; *Accid Anal Preven* 32:527; 2000.

US Federal Bureau of Investigation: *Uniform Crime Reporting Handbook*; US Department of Justice: Washington, DC; 2019; https://ucr.fbi.gov/about-us/cjis/ucr/crime-in-the-u.s/ (Accessed May 22, 2019).

US National Academies of Sciences, Engineering and Medicine: *Getting to Zero Alcohol-Impaired Driving Fatalities: A Comprehensive Approach to a Persistent Problem*; The National Academies Press: Washington, DC; 2018.

US National Center for Statistics and Analysis: *Traffic Safety Facts: 2005 Data—Young Drivers* (DOT HS 810 630); US National Highway Traffic Safety Administration: Washington, DC; 2005.

US National Highway Traffic Safety Administration: *Administrative License Revocation: Resource Manual* (DOT HS 807 873); US National Highway Traffic Safety Administration: Washington, DC; 1992.

US National Highway Traffic Safety Administration: *Computing a BAC Estimate*; US Department of Transportation: Washington, DC; 1994.

US National Highway Traffic Safety Administration: *Fatality Analysis Reporting System (FARS)*; US National Highway Traffic Safety Administration; *ftp://ftp.nhtsa.dot.gov/fars/* (Accessed May 15, 2019).

US National Highway Traffic Safety Administration, American College of Emergency Physicians: *Alcohol Screening and Brief Intervention in the Medical Setting*; US Department of Transportation: Washington, DC: 2002; http://www.nhtsa.dot.gov/people/injury/ems/alcohol_screening/Overview.html (Accessed May 15, 2019).

US National Institute on Alcohol Abuse and Alcoholism: *Alcohol Policy Information System (APIS)*; National Institute on Alcohol Abuse and Alcoholism: Bethesda, MD; 2019; http://alcoholpolicy.niaaa.nih.gov (Accessed May 15, 2019).

US Supreme Court: *Mackeay v. Montrym* 443 U.S. 1; 1979.

Vanlaar W, Mayhew D, Marcoux K, Wets G, Brijs Tom, Shope J: *An Evaluation of Graduated Driver Licensing Programs in North America*; Traffic Injury Research Foundation: Ottawa, Canada; 2009.

Voas RB: A new look at NHTSA's evaluation of the 1984 Charlottesville sobriety checkpoint program: Implications for current checkpoint issues; *Traffic Inj Prev* 9:22; 2008.

Voas RB: *Cars That Drunks Can't Drive*; US National Highway Safety Research Center: Washington, DC; 1969.

Voas RB: Monitoring drinking: Alternative to suspending license to control impaired drivers? *Transportation Research Record* (Journal of the Transportation Research Board) 2182:1; 2010.

Voas RB: Vehicle safety features aimed at preventing alcohol-related crashes; *Forensic Sci Rev* 32:81; 2020.

Voas RB, Fell JC: Preventing impaired driving: Opportunities and problems; *Alcohol Res Health* 34:225; 2011.

Voas RB, Fell JC: Programs and policies designed to reduce impaired driving; In Sher KJ (Ed): *The Oxford Handbook on Substance Use Disorders*, Vol 2; Oxford University Press: Oxford, UK; 2014.

Voas RB, Fell JC, Tippetts AS, Blackman K, Nichols J: Impact of primary safety belt laws on alcohol-related front-seat occupant fatalities: Five case studies; *Traffic Inj Prev* 8:232; 2007.

Voas RB, Hause JM: Deterring the drinking driver: The Stockton experience; *Accid Anal Prev* 19:81; 1987.

Voas RB, Holder HD, Gruenewald PJ: The effect of drinking and driving interventions on alcohol-involved traffic crashes within a comprehensive community trial; *Addiction* 92(Suppl 2):S221; 1997.

Voas RB, Lacey JC: *Alcohol and Highway Safety 2006: A Review of the State of Knowledge* (DOT HS 811-374); US National Highway Traffic Safety Administration: Washington, DC; 2011; https://www.nhtsa.gov/sites/nhtsa.dot.gov/files/811374.pdf (Accessed May 15, 2019).

Voas RB, Rhodenizer AE, Lynn C: *Evaluation of Charlottesville Checkpoint Operations*; US National Highway Traffic Safety Administration: Washington, DC; 1985.

Voas RB, Romano E, Peck R: Validity of the passive sensor for identifying high BAC drivers at the crash scene; *J Stud Alcohol* 67:714; 2006.

Voas RB, Taylor EP, Kelley-Baker T, Tippetts AS: *Effectiveness of the Illinois 0.08 Law*; US National Highway Traffic Safety Administration: Washington, DC; 2000a.

Voas RB, Tippetts AS, Fell J: Assessing the effectiveness of minimum legal drinking age and zero tolerance laws in the United States; *Accid Anal Prev* 35:579; 2003.

Voas RB, Tippetts AS, Fell JC: The relationship of alcohol safety laws to drinking drivers in fatal crashes; *Accid Anal Prev* 32:483; 2000b.

Voas RB, Torres P, Romano E, Lacey JH: Alcohol-related risk of driver fatalities: An update using 2007 data; *J Stud Alcohol Drugs* 73:341; 2012.

Wagenaar AC: Raising the legal drinking age in Maine: Impact on traffic accidents among young drivers; *Inter J Addict* 18:365; 1983.

Wagenaar AC: The minimum legal drinking age: A time-series impact evaluation; *Dissertation Abstracts International* 41(8B):2984; 1981.

Wagenaar AC, Maldonado-Molina MM: Effects of drivers' license suspension policies on alcohol-related crash involvement: Long-term follow-up in forty-six States; *Alcohol Clin Exp Res* 31:1399; 2007.

Wagenaar AC, Maldonado-Molina MM, Ma L, Tobler A, Komro K: Effects of legal BAC limits on fatal crash involvement: Analyses of 28 states from 1976 through 2002; *J Safety Res* 38:493; 2007.

Wagenaar AC, Toomey TL: Effects of minimum drinking age laws: Review and analyses of the literature from 1960 to 2000; *J Stud Alcohol Suppl* 14:206; 2002.

Wagenaar AC, Zobeck TS, Hingson R, Williams GD: Studies of control efforts: A meta-analysis from 1960 through 1991; *Accid Anal Prev* 27:1; 1995.

Wells JK, Preusser DF, Williams AF: Enforcing alcohol-impaired driving and seat belt use laws, Binghamton, New York; *J Safety Res* 23:63; 1992.

Wilde CJS, Hoste JL, Sheppard D, Wind G: *Road Safety Campaigns: Design and Evaluation*; Organization for Economic Co-Operation and Development: Paris, France; 75 pp; 1971.

Williams A: 1980's decline in alcohol impaired driving and crashes and why it happened; *Alcohol Drugs Driving* 8:71; 1992.

Williams AF: Young driver accidents: In search of solutions; In Mayhew DR, Simpson HM, Donalsen AC (Eds): *Laws and Regulations Applicable to Teenagers or New Drivers: Their Potential for Reducing Motor Vehicle Injuries*; The Traffic Injury Research Foundation: Ottawa, Canada; p 43; 1985.

Williams AF, Rich RF, Zador PI: The legal minimum drinking age and fatal motor vehicle crashes; *J Legal Stud* 12:169: 1975.

Williams AF, Zador PL, Harris SS, Karpf RS: The effect of raising the legal minimum drinking age on involvement in fatal crashes; *J Legal Stud* 12:169; 1983.

Williams AK, Weinberg K, Fields M: Effectiveness of administrative license suspension laws; *Alcohol Drugs Driving* 7:55; 1991.

Wiliszowski C, Jones R, Lacey J: *Examining the Effectiveness of Utah's Law Allowing Telephonic Testimony at ALR Hearings* (DOT HS 809 602); US National Highway Traffic Safety Administration: Washington, DC; 2003.

Womble K: Impact of minimum drinking age laws on fatal crash involvements: An update of the NHTSA analysis; *J Traffic Safety Educ* 37:4; 1989.

World Health Organization (WHO): *Global Status Report on Road Safety*; WHO: Geneva, Switzerland; 2018.

World Health Organization (WHO): *List of Countries' BAC Limits for Driving; World Health Organization*; Geneva, Switzerland; 2013; http://apps.who.int/gho/athena/data/GHO/SA_0000001520.html?profile=ztable&filter=COUNTRY:*;BACGROUP:* (Accessed May 15, 2019).

Wurst FM, Vogel R, Jachau K, Varga A, Alling C, Alt A, Skipper GE: Ethyl glucuronide discloses recent covert alcohol use not detected by standard testing in forensic psychiatric inpatients; *Alcohol Clin Exp Res* 27:471; 2003.

Zador P, Krawchuck S, Moore B: *Drinking and Driving Trips, Stops by Police, and Arrests: Analyses of the 1995 National Survey of Drinking and Driving Attitudes and Behavior* (DOT HS 809 184); US National Highway Traffic Safety Administration: Washington, DC; 2000a.

Zador PL, Krawchuk SA, Voas RB: Alcohol-related relative risk of driver fatalities and driver involvement in fatal crashes in relation to driver age and gender: An update using 1996 data; *J Stud Alcohol* 61:387; 2000b.

Zador PL, Lund AK, Field M, Weinberg K: *Alcohol-Impaired Driving Laws and Fatal Crash Involvement*; Insurance Institute for Highway Safety: Washington, DC; 1988.

Zaloshnja E, Miller T, Blincoe L: Costs of alcohol-involved crashes, United States, 2010; *Ann Adv Automot Med* 57:3; 2013.

Zwerling C, Jones MP: Evaluation of the effectiveness of low blood alcohol concentration laws for younger drivers; *Am J Prev Med* 16(1 Suppl):76; 1999.

Index

Note: Page numbers in italic and bold refer to figures and tables, respectively.

C

D

Milton Keynes UK
Ingram Content Group UK Ltd.
UKHW050447071024
449327UK00007B/188